Brief Contents

NURSING *for* Wellness in Older Adults

NURSING *for* Wellness in Older Adults

Fifth Edition

Carol A. Miller, MSN, RN-BC, AHN-BC
Gerontological Clinical Nurse Specialist and Nurse Case Manager
Care & Counseling, Miller/Wetzler Associates
Cleveland, Ohio

Clinical Faculty
Frances Payne Bolton School of Nursing
Case Western Reserve University
Cleveland, Ohio

Wolters Kluwer Health | Lippincott Williams & Wilkins
Philadelphia • Baltimore • New York • London
Buenos Aires • Hong Kong • Sydney • Tokyo

Senior Acquisitions Editor: Elizabeth Nieginski
Development Editor: Betsy Gentzler
Editorial Assistant: Laura Scott
Senior Production Editor: Debra Schiff
Director of Nursing Production: Helen Ewan
Senior Managing Editor/Production: Erika Kors
Art Director, Design: Joan Wendt
Manufacturing Manager: Karin Duffield
Indexer: Hassman Indexing Services
Compositor: Spearhead

5th Edition

9 8 7 6 5 4 3 2 1

Printed in China

Library of Congress Cataloging-in-Publication Data

Miller, Carol A.
Nursing for wellness in older adults / Carol A. Miller. — 5th ed.
p. ; cm.
Includes bibliographical references and index.
ISBN 978-0-7817-7175-7
1. Geriatric nursing. I. Title.
[DNLM: 1. Geriatric Nursing. 2. Aged—psychology. 3. Health Promotion. 4. Nursing Theory.
WY 152 M647n 2009]
RC954.M55 2009
618.97′0231—dc22

2007036449

Care has been taken to confirm the accuracy of the information presented and to describe generally accepted practices. However, the author, editors, and publisher are not responsible for errors or omissions or for any consequences from application of the information in this book and make no warranty, expressed or implied, with respect to the currency, completeness, or accuracy of the contents of the publication. Application of this information in a particular situation remains the professional responsibility of the practitioner; the clinical treatments described and recommended may not be considered absolute and universal recommendations.

The author, editors, and publisher have exerted every effort to ensure that drug selection and dosage set forth in this text are in accordance with the current recommendations and practice at the time of publication. However, in view of ongoing research, changes in government regulations, and the constant flow of information relating to drug therapy and drug reactions, the reader is urged to check the package insert for each drug for any change in indications and dosage and for added warnings and precautions. This is particularly important when the recommended agent is a new or infrequently employed drug.

Some drugs and medical devices presented in this publication have Food and Drug Administration (FDA) clearance for limited use in restricted research settings. It is the responsibility of the health care provider to ascertain the FDA status of each drug or device planned for use in his or her clinical practice.

LWW.COM

I lovingly dedicate this book to my parents, Margaret 'n' Bob Miller, who have always given me boundless support, encouragement, and inspiration—they have been shining examples of living long and full lives.

This book also is dedicated to the many older adults and their families who teach invaluable lessons about successfully navigating the challenges of older adulthood.

Contributors

Georgia Anetzberger, PhD, ACSW
Assistant Professor of Health Care Administration
Cleveland State University
Cleveland, Ohio

Cynthia Capers, PhD, RN
Professor of Nursing
University of Akron College of Nursing
Akron, Ohio

Mary Alice Momeyer, MSN, RN, ANP, GNP
Clinical Faculty
The Ohio State University College of Nursing
Columbus, Ohio

Mary Ann Osborne Schwenka, FNP
Integrative Family Nurse Practitioner, Private Practice
Clinical Faculty
University of Washington
Seattle, Washington

Casey R. Shillam, MSN, RN
Instructor
University of Portland School of Nursing
Portland, Oregon

A Student's Perspective Contributors

These features were contributed by students from the following programs:

Brigham Young University
Provo, Utah

Western Michigan University
Kalamazoo, Michigan

Angelo State University
San Angelo, Texas

Reviewers

Myra Aud, PhD, RN
Assistant Professor
University of Missouri-Columbia
Columbia, Missouri

Christine Bradway, PhD, CRNP
Assistant Professor
University of Pennsylvania
Philadelphia, Pennsylvania

Janet Brown, PhD, RN
Assistant Professor
University of Tennessee, Knoxville
Knoxville, Tennessee

Virginia Burgraff, DNS, RN, FAAN
Endowed Professor
Radford University
Radford, Virginia

Darlene Clark, MS, RN
Senior Lecturer
Pennsylvania State University
University Park, Pennsylvania

Darlene Copley, MS, APRN, BC
Assistant Professor
St. Cloud State University
St. Cloud, Minnesota

Gretchen Cornell, PhD, RN, CNE
Professor
Utah Valley State College
Orem, Utah

Sherri Cozzens, MS, RN
Nursing Instructor
De Anza College
Cupertino, California

Barbara Daniel, MS, APRN, BC, CRNP
Nurse Educator
Veterans Affairs, Maryland Health Care System
Baltimore, Maryland

Evelyn Duffy, NP, APRN, BC
Assistant Professor, Director—Adult and Gerontological NP Programs
Case Western Reserve University
Nurse Practitioner
University Hospitals of Cleveland
Cleveland, Ohio

Renee Dugger, MSN, APRN, BC
Assistant Professor
University of Southern Indiana
Evansville, Indiana

Julie Eggert, PhD, APRN, BC, AOCN
Associate Professor
Clemson University
Clemson, South Carolina

Dorothy Fraser, MSN, FNP
Faculty, ATI Coordinator/Lecturer
California State University
Fresno, California

Patricia Fuehr, MSN, RN, FNP-C
Faculty Specialist
Western Michigan University
Kalamazoo, Michigan

Susan Gardner, MS, RN
Assistant Professor
Southern Utah University
Cedar City, Utah

Earl Goldberg, EdD, APRN, BC
Associate Professor
La Salle University
Philadelphia, Pennsylvania

Darlene Hanson, MS, RN
Clinical Associate Professor
University of North Dakota
Grand Forks, North Dakota

Barbara Heise, PhD, APRN, BC
Assistant Professor
Brigham Young University
Provo, Utah

Susan Hinck, PhD, RN
Associate Professor
Missouri State University
Springfield, Missouri

Rosemary Macy, PhD, RN
Associate Professor
Boise State University
Boise, Idaho

Sharon Mailey, PhD, RN
Professor
Shenandoah University
Winchester, Virginia

Joyce S. Maynor, MSN, BA, RN, BC
Assistant Professor
Southeastern Louisiana University
Hammond, Louisiana

Sianne McDermid, BN, Med, RN
Coordinator, Gerontology Program
Mount Royal College
Calgary, Alberta, Canada

Dorothea McDowell, PhD, RN
Associate Professor
Salisbury University
Salisbury, Maryland

Krista Meinersmann, PhD, RN
Associate Director—Undergraduate Program
Georgia State University
Atlanta, Georgia

Mary Alice Momeyer, MSN, RN, ANP, GNP
Clinical Instructor, Adjunct Faculty
Ohio State University
Columbus, Ohio

Gaile Nellett, PhD, MSN, RN
Associate Professor
University of St. Francis Joliet
Joliet, Illinois

Shirley Newberry, PhD, RN
Associate Professor
Winona State University
Winona, Minnesota

Pat O'Leary, DSN, RN, COI
Associate Professor
Middle Tennessee State University
Murfreesboro, Tennessee

Lisa Onega, PhD, RN, FNP, GNP, CNF
Professor
Radford University
Radford, Virginia

Teresa O'Neill, PhD, MN, APRN
Associate Professor
Our Lady of Holy Cross
New Orleans, Louisiana

Lillian Parker, MS, APRN, ABD
Assistant Professor
Clayton State College
Morrow, Georgia

Regina Phillips, PhD, RN
Associate Professor
Villa Julie College
Stevenson, Maryland

Jean Raymond, ANCC, APRN, BC
Clinical Specialist, Gerontological Nursing
French Hospital Medical Center
San Luis Obispo, California

Denise Rohr, MSN, RN
Instructor
Cincinnati State Technical and Community College
Cincinnati, Ohio

Karen Moor Schaefer, PhD, RN
Assistant Professor; Director, Undergraduate Program
Temple University, College of Health Professionals
Philadelphia, Pennsylvania

Nuananong Seal, PhD, RN
Assistant Professor
University of North Dakota
Grand Forks, North Dakota

Barbara Servatka, MSN, RN
Associate Professor
Palomar College
San Marcos, California

Casey Shillam, MSN, RN
Instructor
University of Portland
Portland, Oregon

Janice Stephenson, MSc(A), BScN, RN
Clinical Nurse Specialist, Geriatrics and Transition Care
McGill University Health Centre
Montreal, Quebec, Canada

Ardith Sudduth, APRN-BC, FNP-BC
Assistant Professor
University of Louisiana
Lafayette, Louisiana

Tracey Szirony, PhD, RNC, CHPN
Associate Professor
University of Toledo
Toledo, Ohio

Marilyn Terrado, PhD, RNC, CHPN
Associate Professor
Loyola University, Marcella Niehoff School of Nursing
Chicago, Illinois

Karen Tetz
Professor
Walla Walla College
Walla Walla, Washington

Jeanine Tweedie, MSN, RN, CNE
Assistant Professor
Hawaii Pacific University
Honolulu, Hawaii

Linda Wagner, MA, RN, CNE
Assistant Professor
College of St. Scholastica
Duluth, Minnesota

Molly Walker, PhD, RN, CNS
Assistant Professor
Angelo State University
San Angelo, Texas

Dawn Weiler, MS, RN, ANP
Assistant Professor
Boise State University
Boise, Idaho

Mary Alice Welhaven, PhD, RN
Professor
Winona State University-Rochester
Rochester, Minnesota

Brenda Wheeler, MSN, BSN, RN
Assistant Professor
Truman State University
Kirksville, Missouri

Nancy Whestzel, MSN, CNS
Visiting Professor
Colorado State University-Pueblo
Pueblo, Colorado

Anita White, MSN, RN, CCRN
Critical Care Nurse Educator
Elyria, Ohio

Sarah Wilson, PhD, RN
Associate Professor, Director—Institute for End-of-Life Care Education
Marquette University
Milwaukee, Wisconsin

Charlotte Wood, PhD
Professor
Mississippi College
Clinton, Mississippi

Mary Ellen Yonushonis, RN, MS
Instructor
Pennsylvania State University
University Park, Pennsylvania

Tamara Zurakowski, PhD, CRNP
Practice Assistant Professor
University of Pennsylvania
Philadelphia, Pennsylvania

Preface

During the 2 decades since I wrote the first edition of this text, "wellness" has been emerging as a major focus of health care. The concept is usually associated with physical fitness and "preventing aging"; however, a major premise of this text is that there is no age limit to achieving wellness when it is holistically conceptualized in the context of one's body, mind, and spirit. Another major premise is that nurses have essential roles in promoting wellness for older adults because we holistically address the needs of our patients, which for older adults involves supporting their optimal level of functioning and quality of life. Thus, the intent of this text is to serve as a foundation for providing wellness-oriented nursing care for older adults in any health care setting.

This fifth edition of *Nursing for Wellness in Older Adults* has been extensively updated to incorporate wellness concepts and evidence-based information related to nursing care of older adults. In addition, it is updated to incorporate recent research findings pertinent to aging, older adults, health promotion, and gerontological nursing. As in previous editions, this text focuses on the aspects of physiologic and psychosocial function that are most relevant to nursing care of older adults. The Functional Consequences Theory provides a framework for identifying the many interacting factors that affect the level of functioning and quality of life of older adults within the context of the nursing process. For each aspect of functioning, nurses can use the assessment and intervention guidelines to identify and address factors that affect the functioning and quality of life for older adults. Nursing interventions focus on health promotion and many of the intervention guides can be used as health education tools to teach older adults, their families, and their caregivers about actions they can take to promote wellness. Chapters also include information about applicable wellness nursing diagnoses and wellness outcomes. Theory illustrations at the beginning of many chapters show how the Functional Consequences Theory is integrated with the nursing process with regard to specific aspects of functioning.

ORGANIZATION

Nursing for Wellness in Older Adults has 29 chapters, organized into five parts. Chapters in Parts 1 and 2 introduce topics relevant to aging, wellness, older adults, and the role of nurses in promoting wellness in older adults. Chapters in Parts 3 and 4 are organized around the functional consequences theory of gerontological nursing, so each facet of physiologic or psychosocial function is presented according to age-related changes, risk factors, functional consequences, nursing assessment, nursing diagnosis, outcomes, nursing interventions, and evaluation of nursing care. The three **new** chapters in Part 5 have been added to help nurses promote wellness during all stages of health and illness.

The intent of Part 1 (Chapters 1 through 4), *Older Adults and Wellness,* is to help nurses apply a wellness philosophy to their care of older adults. It begins with a discussion of how nurses can view older adults from a wellness perspective. In addition, it explicates the Functional Consequences Theory and provides an overview of theories that are pertinent to aging well. Chapter 4 provides information about culture and diversity in the older adult population.

Part 2 (Chapters 5 through 10), *Nursing Considerations for Older Adults,* introduces gerontological nursing as a subspecialty within nursing and addresses the unique challenges of caring for older adults, with an extensive discussion of health promotion in relation to older adults. Roles for gerontological nurses are described in relation to diverse settings that comprise the continuum of care for older adults. This section also covers the complex topics of assessment, medications, and legal and ethical concerns because nurses address these aspects of care with the majority of the older adults for whom they provide care. Elder abuse and neglect also is addressed in this section because nurses need be aware of this concern when caring for older adults.

Part 3 (Chapters 11 through 15), *Promoting Wellness in Psychosocial Function,* extensively reviews cognitive and psychosocial function and provides guidelines for a comprehensive nursing assessment of psychosocial function, with emphasis on healthy older adults. In addition, this part covers delirium, dementia, and depression, which are three of the most commonly occurring pathologic conditions that have serious psychosocial consequences for older adults.

Part 4 (Chapters 16 through 26), *Promoting Wellness in Physical Function,* includes chapters that address each of the following specific aspects of functioning in older adults: hearing, vision, digestion and nutrition, urinary function, cardiovascular function, respiratory function, mobility and safety, integument, sleep and rest, thermoregulation, and sexual function. Although the emphasis of this book is on wellness, coverage of selected common pathologic conditions is included when these conditions affect a particular aspect of functioning in older adults.

Part 5 (Chapters 27 through 29), *Promoting Wellness in All Stages of Health and Illness,* has been added to address topics of caring for older adults during illness and when they are experiencing pain or are at the end of life.

NEW AND SPECIAL FEATURES

Special features from past editions have been retained in this edition, and several new features have been added.

Pedagogical Features

- **Learning Objectives** help the reader identify important chapter content and focus his or her reading.
- ***NEW!* Key Terms** listed at the beginning of the chapter and bolded in the text highlight important vocabulary.
- ***NEW!* Theory Illustrations** at the beginning of each chapter on specific aspects of functioning present an overview of the Functional Consequences Theory in the context of the nursing process.
- **Icons** identify the five major components of the Functional Consequences Theory:

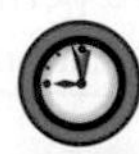 Age-related changes

 Risk factors

 Functional consequences

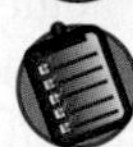 Nursing assessment

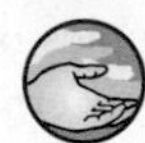 Nursing interventions

- **Progressive Case Studies** provide real-life examples of the effects of age-related changes and risk factors, beginning in young-old adulthood and continuing through all the stages of later adulthood. **Thinking Points** after each segment of the case assist the student in applying the content of the chapter to the case example. Many chapters include a concluding Case Study with a sample **Nursing Care Plan**.
- ***NEW!* Chapter Highlights** in an easy-to-read bulleted format facilitate review of the material.
- **Critical Thinking Exercises,** at the end of each chapter, help readers to gain insight and develop problem-solving skills through purposeful, goal-directed thinking.
- **References** give readers additional information about the most up-to-date research that supports evidence-based practice.

Practice-Oriented Features

- ***NEW!* Wellness Opportunities** are sprinkled throughout the clinically oriented chapters to draw attention to ways in which nurses can promote wellness during the usual course of their care activities.
- ***NEW!* A Student's Perspective** provides reality-based stories written by nursing students that illustrate the application of wellness concepts in clinical practice.
- **Cultural Considerations** boxes help the reader to appreciate cultural differences that may influence his or her approach to a patient, resident, or client.
- **Diversity Notes** give brief information about differences among specific groups (e.g., men and women, whites and African Americans).
- **Assessment Boxes** provide the reader with specific approaches for nursing assessment. Commonly used assessment tools are described (and, in many cases, illustrated).
- **Interventions Boxes** provide succinct guides for nursing interventions, with a strong focus on health promotion. Guides for "best practices" in nursing interventions are given. Many of the interventions boxes can be used as tools for teaching older adults and their caregivers about how to improve functional abilities. Interventions boxes that double as teaching tools can be downloaded from thePoint at http://thepoint.lww.com/miller5e.
- ***NEW!* Clinical Tool Resources** direct the reader to sources for clinical tools such as the assessment tools recommended by the Hartford Institute for Geriatric Nursing.
- **Educational Resources** direct the reader to sources of additional information and patient education materials. Internet addresses are provided. Key resources for Canadian readers are noted as well.

TEACHING AND LEARNING PACKAGE

The following tools and resources are available upon textbook adoption to instructors on thePoint http://thePoint.lww.com/miller5e:

- The **Test Generator** lets you generate new tests from a bank of NCLEX-style questions to help you assess your students' understanding of the course material.
- **PowerPoint Presentations** provide an easy way for you to integrate the textbook with your students' classroom experience, either via slide shows or handouts. Multiple-choice and True/False questions are integrated into the presentations to promote class participation and allow you to use i-clicker technology.
- A sample **Syllabus** provides guidance for structuring your course.
- An **Image Bank** contains illustrations from the book in formats suitable for printing and incorporating into PowerPoint presentations and Internet sites.
- **Journal Articles**, corresponding to book chapters, offer access to current research available in Lippincott Williams & Wilkins journals.

Students can also visit thePoint at http://www.thePoint.lww.com/miller5e and access student resources using the codes printed in the front of their textbooks. Resources include access to journal articles, an NCLEX alternate-item format tutorial, a Spanish–English audio glossary, and Learning Objectives and Interventions Boxes from the textbook.

SUMMARY

Providing holistic nursing care for older adults is an opportunity to care for people who are striving to meet the challenges of remaining healthy and functional as they cope with age-related changes and risk factors that affect their functioning and quality of life. The goal of *Nursing for Wellness in Older Adults* is to provide nurses and nursing students with a practical approach to assisting older adults in meeting the many challenges of older adulthood in positive and creative ways.

Carol A. Miller, ***MSN, RN-BC, AHN-BC***

Acknowledgments

I am deeply grateful to my family, friends, and colleagues who have supported me on my journey as this book has grown from a dream to a reality and now into its fifth edition. Pat Rehm, in particular, has constantly supported and encouraged me to pursue my goals as a nurse and author. My work with older adults and their families provides valuable lessons that have become part of this text. These experiences, which cannot be learned in books, have taught me to care deeply about, and to care sensitively for, older adults. I thank these older adults and their families and I appreciate their contributions to my life and my writings.

I appreciate and acknowledge the many people who have helped bring this text to fruition. I want to extend my deepest appreciation to the staff at Lippincott Williams & Wilkins who assisted with all phases of development and production. I am grateful for the enthusiasm and encouragement of Elizabeth Nieginski, Senior Acquisitions Editor. Betsy Gentzler and Melanie Cann, the Development Editors, deserve a special word of appreciation for their unending support, guidance, attention to detail, and thought-provoking discussions that helped me fine-tune and articulate important concepts. I also thank and acknowledge Sara Moses and Season Evans, Ancillary Editors; Debra Schiff, Senior Production Editor; Sara Krause, Art Coordinator; and Joan Wendt, Designer. I thank all these people, and many unnamed people, for the advice, guidance, support, assistance, and encouragement on my journey through all five editions of *Nursing for Wellness in Older Adults.*

I extend a very special appreciation to Patricia F. Brown, Artist, for creating a painting that was used in the cover design for this text.

Contents

PART 1
Older Adults and Wellness 1

PART 2
Nursing Considerations for Older Adults 61

CHAPTER 26
Sexual Function 541

PART 5
Promoting Wellness in All Stages of Health and Illness 565

CHAPTER 27
Caring for Older Adults During Illness 565

CHAPTER 28
Caring for Older Adults Experiencing Pain 577

CHAPTER 29
Caring for Older Adults at the End of Life 592

Appendix: Age-Related Variations in Laboratory Values 605

Index 607

Assessment and Interventions Boxes

ASSESSMENT BOXES

Safety and Functioning

Medications

Psychosocial Assessment

Impaired Cognitive Function

Impaired Affective Function

Hearing

Vision

Digestion and Nutrition

Urinary Function

Cardiovascular Function

Respiratory Function

Mobility and Safety

Integument

Sleep and Rest

Thermoregulation

Sexual Function

Illness

Pain

INTERVENTIONS BOXES

Health Promotion

Medications

Cognitive Function

Psychosocial Function

Impaired Cognitive Function

Impaired Affective Function

Hearing

Vision

Digestion and Nutrition

Urinary Function

Cardiovascular Function

Respiratory Function

Mobility and Safety

Integument

Sleep and Rest

Thermoregulation

Sexual Function

Illness

End of Life

Older Adults and Wellness

PART 1

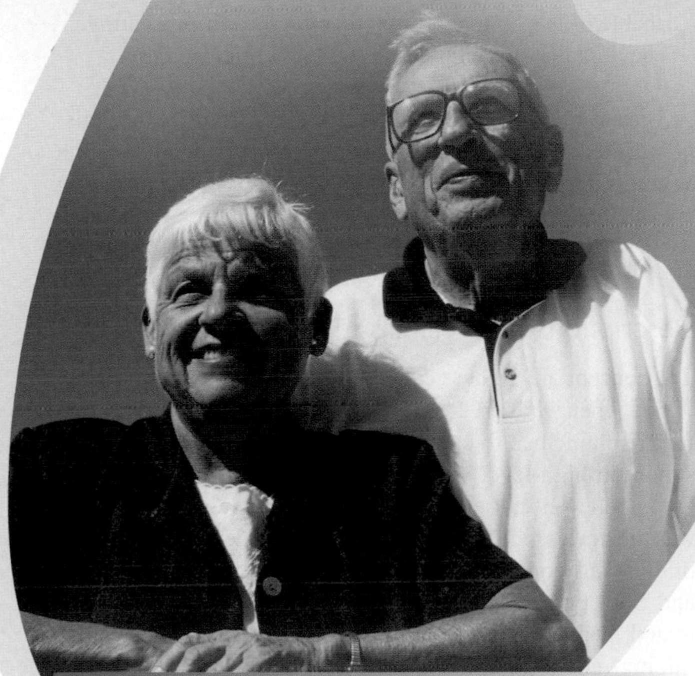

Learning Objectives

After reading this chapter, you will be able to:

1. Describe the relationship between aging and wellness.
2. Identify barriers to and opportunities for nurses to promote wellness in older adults.
3. Define aging from several perspectives.
4. Recognize the effects of ageism and attitudes about aging.
5. Identify myths that affect nursing care of older adults.
6. Describe demographic, health, and socioeconomic characteristics of older adults in the United States.
7. Discuss how population trends affect relationships of older adults and their families.
8. Describe living arrangements of older adults.

Key Terms

age identity
ageism
aging
aging anxiety
baby boomers
chronologic age
downward extension of households
functional age
gerontocratic
gerontophobia
high-level wellness
implicit ageism
multiple jeopardy
parent support ratio
sandwich generation
skipped-generation households
upward extension of households

CHAPTER 1

Seeing Older Adults Through the Eyes of Wellness

IMAGES OF AGING

In most modern societies, describing someone or something as "old" connotes images of decline, disease, disability, decrepitude, and death. These images, however, do not accurately describe the realities of aging, but rather reflect myths and stereotypes arising from a lack of knowledge about aging. Many of these images of aging arise from long-term patterns of incorrectly attributing pathologic conditions and undesirable characteristics to "normal" aging. Unfortunately, these misperceptions have been reinforced by terms such as "senility" that equate aging with impaired functioning. In fact, most older adults function well with little or no assistance and report being satisfied with their health and quality of life, despite a high prevalence of chronic conditions (Depp & Jeste, 2006; Montross et al., 2006). Moreover, at any age, most adults aspire to grow old, but also to enjoy good health and functioning into old age.

Most older adults recognize that they have less time in which to continue achieving their goals, so they face their challenges with resilience and determination. Gerontologists are increasingly recognizing that older adults who are aging successfully possess wisdom, which includes (among other characteristics) factual knowledge, problem-solving strategies, and the ability to manage uncertainty (Blazer, 2006; Brugman, 2006). Because many of the challenges of older adulthood involve health and functioning, older adults need accurate information, not only about normal aging, but also about interventions to promote wellness. Nurses are ideally positioned to teach older adults about health and aging and empower them to implement problem-solving strategies directed toward wellness, improved functioning, and quality of life.

The intent of this gerontological nursing book is to provide comprehensive and research-based information so nurses can distinguish between the changes in health and quality of life that result from normal aging and those that result from risk factors. Moreover, it provides tools for nursing assessment, interventions, and health education in relation to all aspects of physical and psychosocial functioning. This chapter provides an overview of concepts related to wellness and aging and reviews some myths about aging and older adults. To combat myths about aging, this chapter also presents information about older adults in the United States in terms of demographic, health, and socioeconomic characteristics; family relationships; and living arrangements.

THE RELATIONSHIP BETWEEN WELLNESS AND AGING

If asked to define "wellness" and "aging," most people associate wellness with peak achievement in younger adulthood, and aging with declining health that eventually leads to death. Although somewhat accurate with regard to physical performance, this description of wellness does not include well-being of the body, mind, and spirit. Similarly, many definitions of aging narrowly focus on physical health and functioning, rather than viewing humans as more complex bio-psycho-social-spiritual beings. Thus, the apparent disconnect between definitions of wellness and aging results not only from misunderstandings about aging but from a narrow focus on physical health and functioning.

Promoting wellness in older adults is an ideal; however, nurses may not believe it is achievable in practice because of barriers such the following:

- Older adults may be pessimistic about being able to improve their health and functioning.
- Survival needs and a multitude of health problems may take precedence over the "luxury" of being able to focus on wellness and quality of life.
- Despite the purported emphasis on wellness and health promotion, health care environments focus more on treatment of disease than on preventing illness and addressing whole-person needs.
- Older adults and health care providers often mistakenly attribute symptoms to aging rather than identifying and addressing reversible and treatable contributing factors.
- Health care providers may not believe that older adults are capable of learning and implementing health-promoting behaviors that are inherent in wellness-oriented care.

Because many of these barriers arise from myths, misperceptions, and lack of knowledge, accurate information about older adults and the relationship between aging and wellness is an indispensable tool for addressing these barriers.

Descriptions of Wellness

The concept of wellness came to public attention in the early 1960s when Halbert L. Dunn, MD, PhD, retired from his formal public health career and became a "lecturer and consultant in high-level wellness work" (Dunn, 1961, p. 244). Dunn believed that education at all points in a person's life was the key to high-level wellness, and he developed a series of radio talks on the theme of "High-Level Wellness for Man and Society." He defined **high-level wellness** as an "integrated method of functioning that is oriented toward maximizing each person's potential, while maintaining a continuum of balance and purposeful direction within the person's environment" (Dunn, 1961, pp. 4–5). In one radio program, Dunn addressed stereotypes about aging and emphasized that "healthy maturity" is characterized not only by physical decline but by wisdom. Moreover, he discussed the relationship between mind, body, and spirit and stressed the importance of older adults having a purpose in life, communicating with others, maintaining personal dignity, and contributing to society (Dunn, 1961).

Even before addressing aging in his public education series, Dunn had published an article in *Geriatrics* while he was chief of the National Office of Vital Statistics. In the article, he advised all health care workers to foster a sense of value and dignity for older adults by directing interventions toward improved health and functioning (Dunn, 1958). Dunn described the role of health care professionals with regard to older adults as follows (1958, p. 51):

> *The later years of life will come to be more widely regarded as years of opportunity for older people and for society if, in addition to prevention, care, and various health-related activities, direct attention is devoted to the promotion of high-level wellness. This will require a major reorientation.*

Nurses have opportunities to promote wellness for older adults through actions such as:

- Addressing the body–mind–spirit interrelatedness of each older adult
- Identifying and challenging ageist attitudes (including their own), especially those that interfere with optimal health care
- Assessing each older adult from a whole-person perspective
- Incorporating wellness nursing diagnoses as a routine part of care
- Planning for wellness outcomes, which are directed toward improved health, functioning, and quality of life
- Using nursing interventions to address the factors that interfere with optimal functioning (including lack of accurate information about aging)
- Recognizing each older adult's potential for psychological and spiritual growth during all phases of physical health and functioning
- Teaching about self-care behaviors to improve health and functioning (or teaching caregivers of dependent older adults)
- Promoting wellness for caregivers and other people who provide care for older adults (including self-care for nurses)

Definitions of Aging

Gerontologists and lay people define aging from many perspectives. Objectively, **aging** is a universal process that begins at birth; in this context, it applies equally to young and old people. Subjectively, however, aging is typically associated with being "old" or reaching "older adulthood," and people define aging in terms of personal meaning and experience. Children usually do not view themselves as aging, but they delight in announcing how old they are. They view birthdays as positive experiences that will permit them to enjoy additional opportunities and responsibilities. Adolescents, likewise, perceive aging as the mechanism that allows them to participate legally in coveted activities, such as driving. In adulthood, however, aging is negatively associated with being "old," and "old age" is often arbitrarily defined as an age that is several years or a decade beyond a person's current age. For example, many people whose chronologic age is 70 years, 75 years, or older refer to "old people" as if they were a group older than and distinct from themselves.

Gerontologists define **age identity** from various perspectives, and all of the following terms have been applied to this concept: feel-age, subjective age, cognitive age, stereotype age, comparative age, and perceived or self-perceived age. Since the 1980s, gerontologists have viewed age identity on a continuum based on the assumption that old age is accompanied by a decline in health. Consequently, people who feel good will feel younger, and people who feel poorly will feel older (Bowling et al., 2005). In addition, lower socioeconomic status is associated with having an older age identity.

Because cultural views significantly influence age identity, people in societies that place a high value on youth are likely to adopt age identifications that are younger than their chronologic age. That is, beginning around the fourth decade, people are likely to report their age identity as younger than their chronologic age; however, this may be changing. Two almost identical surveys of public and personal perceptions of aging found that Americans in 2000 dated the beginning of older adulthood to later chronologic ages than they did in 1974. Moreover, they do not necessarily use chronologic age as a factor that defines people as "old" (Bradley & Longino, 2001).

Objectively, people define **chronologic age** as the length of time that has passed since birth. North American culture is particularly fascinated by numbers, quantities, and relative values that can be measured. Among the questions frequently asked and answered are *How much? How far? How often?* and *How old?* Our fascination with age is particularly evident in newspaper articles, which invariably state the age of the subjects, regardless of the relevance of age to the topic. In addition to being easily measured, another advantage of chronologic age is that it serves as an objective basis for social organization. For example, societies establish chronologic age criteria for certain activities, such as education, driving, marriage, employment, alcohol consumption, military service, and the collection of retirement benefits. To participate legally in these activities, people must provide documentation of a certain chronologic age.

With the passage of the 1935 Social Security Act and the 1965 amendment that created Medicare, the age of 65 years was established as the standard age criterion for eligibility for retirement and health care benefits in the United States. This age-based determination for retirement was based in part on the socioeconomic condition of the United States after the Depression. Retirement of older workers was seen as a solution to providing much-needed jobs for younger workers, and the establishment of Social Security was seen as a solution to the social burden caused by increasing numbers of older people (Hirshbein, 2001). Thus, in America, 65 years of age has been accepted as the designated age for becoming a "senior citizen" and enjoying the benefits of the so-called Golden Age. Even this government-established chronologic age criterion, however, is subject to cross-cultural variation when it is applied to some government-sponsored programs, such as the Older Americans Act (OAA). For example, the qualifying age for Native Americans' participation in OAA-funded programs is 45 years in Montana, but it is 55 years in all other states.

In the early decades of gerontology, gerontologists also viewed 65 years of age as an acceptable chronologic criterion for aging processes. In recent decades, however, gerontologists agree that aging is too complex to be defined only by one's birth date. Consequently, older adulthood is commonly divided into subgroups, such as young-old, middle-old, old-old, and oldest-old. As one of the first gerontologists to challenge the original criterion stated:

We have used sixty-five as the economic marker, then as the social and psychological marker, of old age. A set of stereotypes has grown up that older persons are sick, poor, enfeebled, isolated, and desolated. While these stereotypes have been greatly overdrawn even for the old-old, they have become uncritically attached to the whole group over sixty-five (Neugarten, 1978, pp. 47–48).

The trend in gerontology to divide old age into chronologic subcategories is an improvement over the categorization of all people older than 65 years of age as one homogeneous group, but it has the disadvantage of creating additional stereotypes and age biases. For example, if a chronologically old-old person needs a complicated or expensive medical treatment to maintain or potentially improve his or her health status, such treatment may be ignored, denied, or withheld based on advanced age.

Although chronologic age has the advantages of being easily measured, widely accepted, and readily understood, it has many disadvantages, especially in gerontology. From both scientific and humanistic perspectives, a person's age is relatively insignificant. From the perspective of biogerontology, chronologic age has little or no value because no biologic measurement applies to everyone at a specific age; from this perspective, therefore, there is no way of measuring age objectively (International Longevity Center—USA, 2001).

For gerontological practitioners, as well as for most older adults, the important indicators of age are physiologic health, psychological well-being, socioeconomic factors, and the ability to function and participate in desirable activities. Based on this understanding of aging, gerontologists have used the term **functional age** for several decades. This concept is associated with a shift in emphasis from chronologic factors to factors such as whether individuals can contribute to society and benefit others and themselves. Functional age is a concept that is used worldwide, but its definition varies according to different cultural contexts. For example, industrialized societies may associate functional age with self-sufficiency and physiologic function, whereas other cultures might associate it more closely with social or psychological function than with physiologic function.

One advantage of functional definitions of age over chronologic definitions is that the former are associated with higher levels of well-being and with more positive attitudes about aging. From a holistic perspective, the concept of functional age provides a more rational basis for care than the measurement of how many years have passed since the person was born. Thus, the question *How functional?* is more relevant than *How old?* Even more relevant for promoting wellness in older adults are questions such as:

- How well do you feel?
- What goals do you have for improving your level of wellness?
- Is there anything that you would like to do that you cannot do?
- What goals do you have for improving your quality of life?

In this text, the term "older adult" applies to individuals experiencing the cumulative effects of age-related changes and risk factors that affect their health and functioning (discussed in Chapter 2). From a holistic perspective, this conceptualization addresses all aspects of bio-psycho-social-spiritual health and functioning, as discussed in the next section in relation to successful aging.

Descriptions of Successful Aging

In recent decades, gerontologists have focused much attention on identifying components of successful aging, addressing all aspects of health and functioning. A large-scale longitudinal study identified three components of successful aging as an active engagement with life, high cognitive and physical function, and low probability of disease and disability (Rowe & Kahn, 1997). Other studies have confirmed the importance of active engagement with life as a component of successful and healthy aging (Depp & Jeste, 2006). One study found that psychosocial factors exert an influence on functioning, particularly in older adults with chronic conditions such as diabetes and high blood pressure (Seeman & Chen, 2002). Gerontologists agree that successful aging is multifaceted and includes lifestyle and social factors (George, 2006; Hendricks & Hatch, 2006). Moreover, each older adult defines successful aging based on personal values and experiences. For example, one study found that older women viewed successful aging in the context of their relationships with home, family, body images, and religious beliefs (Covan, 2005). Additional aspects of successful aging are discussed in Chapter 3 in the context of biologic, sociologic, and psychological theories.

ATTITUDES TOWARD AGING

Historical Attitudes

Although old age has not always been viewed as something to look forward to, historically it was at least viewed as something to be respected. Fischer (1977) has analyzed trends in attitudes toward old people in the United States from the early 1600s through the 1970s. Data from this analysis indicate that the early 1600s were characterized by **gerontocratic** attitudes (i.e., veneration of old people) (Fischer, 1977). The median age during that time was barely 16 years, so respect for age was at least partly attributable to its relative rarity. A revolution in attitudes that began in the late 1700s sparked a long period of **gerontophobia** characterized by a fear of aging and an idealization of youth.

According to Fischer, the "cult of youth...became most extreme in the 1960s, when mature men and women followed fashions in books, music, and clothing which were set by their adolescent children....But always, old was out and youth was in" (pp. 132–133). As youth was being idealized, old age was being labeled as a medical and social problem. Although Fischer did not use the term *ageism* in his book, he discussed the importance of efforts "to oppose the age prejudice which has grown so strong in America" (p. 195).

Another analysis of views of old age in America between 1900 and 1950 concluded that a shift in perception of aging began in the 1930s when "national enthusiasm about extending life and avoiding old age was waning" (Hirshbein, 2001, p. 1558). During the mid-1940s, the trend toward significant increases in life expectancy brought attention to aging-related issues as a social concern and a problem to be solved. During this time, American society began to see older adults as a group of people with economic needs. Professional organizations became interested in aging and old age, and by the 1950s, "old age was seen as an economic, social, and medical problem that demanded management by a variety of professional groups" (Hirshbein, 2001, p. 1558). During the 1950s, gerontologists initiated longitudinal studies to identify normal aging, and by the 1980s the paradigm had shifted to focusing on successful aging (Blazer, 2006). Despite the progress in research, however, long-held misperceptions continue to influence attitudes toward aging today (Hess, 2006).

Ageism

The term *ageism* was coined by Robert Butler in 1968 and was first used in a publication, *The Gerontologist*, the next year (Butler, 1969). With the publication of Butler's Pulitzer Prize–winning book *Why Survive? Being Old in America* (1975), *ageism* became an accepted new word in the English language. Butler defines **ageism** as "the prejudices and stereotypes that are applied to older people sheerly on the basis of their age....Ageism, like racism and sexism, is a way of pigeonholing people and not allowing them to be individuals with unique ways of living their lives" (Butler et al., 1991, p. 243). Devaluing the contributions of older adults and viewing the pathologic processes of later life as normal aging processes are common forms of ageism today (Cummings et al., 2000). Myths that are perpetuated today promote stereotypes of social isolation, asexual behavior, lack of creativity, physical and mental decline, and economic and familial burden (Angus & Reeve, 2006). A study of ageism in the United States and six other countries found common stereotypes of older adults as warm, incompetent, noncompetitive, and low status (Cuddy et al., 2005).

Ageism can be considered an outcome of urbanization and industrialization because the emphasis on the negative and debilitative aspects of old age correlates with perceptions of older people as unproductive (Covey, 1988). Another perspective is that ageism affects only those old people who are disabled, and this group is similar to other groups who have fought against prejudices (Cohen, 1988). Cohen further suggests that discrimination against older disabled people arises from the societal perception of them as "biologically inferior and hence incapable of levels of self-fulfillment and self-realization comparable to those of the dominant reference group" (Cohen, 1988, p. 25). **Multiple jeopardy** is a similar concept that describes older adults who are likely to experience added discrimination because of their race or gender. Older women of color, for example, encounter "triple jeopardy," or discrimination based on ageism, sexism, and racism (Cummings et al., 2000).

Ageism continues to be a frequent topic in current gerontological literature, with some emphasis on identifying and addressing its causes (Hess, 2006). Some gerontologists advocate for addressing ageist myths with the same kind of attention that is given to racism and sexism (Thornton, 2002). Gerontologists have developed a 20-item survey to answer questions about types and prevalence of ageism and which subgroups of older people report more ageism (Fig. 1-1). Results of studies using this survey indicate that the experience of ageism continues to be widespread and frequent in the United States (Palmore, 2001).

Gerontologists also are recognizing and raising questions about the serious and detrimental effects of **implicit ageism**. This is defined as "the thoughts, feelings, and behaviors toward elderly people that exist and operate without conscious awareness or control, with the assumption that it forms the basis of most interactions with older individuals" (Levy, 2001, p. 578). Implicit ageism is detrimental in several ways. First, because individuals are not aware that a person's older age has automatically triggered their negative stereotypes of aging, they may attribute their own response to other factors. For example, an employer will attribute the preferential hiring of a younger person to training or experience rather than to age discrimination. Second, Levy points out that older people themselves may accept false explanations for ageist behavior because they do not want to admit that they are members of a stigmatized group (Levy, 2001). Implicit ageism and other forms of ageism can have serious implications for gerontological nurses, as discussed later in this chapter. Although the concept of ageism is most often used in reference to discrimination against older people, ageism can also apply to other stages of life. For example, older people may hold prejudices against young people, and old people may feel anger and ambivalence toward middle-aged people.

Cultural Influences and Ageism

Although ageism is not unique to the United States, it does not exist in all cultures. In the United States, ageism has developed and grown as a result of dominant cultural beliefs and trends, such as the glorification of youth, the ideal of socioeconomic competition, the perception of the individual as autonomous, and the equating of human worth with eco-

The Ageism Survey

Please put a number in the blank that shows how often you have experienced that event: Never = 0; Once = 1; More than once = 2.
("Age" means older age.)

____ 1. I was told a joke that pokes fun at old people.
____ 2. I was sent a birthday card that pokes fun at old people.
____ 3. I was ignored or not taken seriously because of my age.
____ 4. I was called an insulting name related to my age.
____ 5. I was partronized or "talked down to" because of my age.
____ 6. I was refused rental housing because of my age.
____ 7. I had difficulty getting a loan because of my age.
____ 8. I was denied a position of leadership because of my age.
____ 9. I was rejected as unattractive because of my age.
____10. I was treated with less dignity and respect because of my age.
____11. A waiter or waitress ignored me because of my age.
____12. A doctor or nurse assumed my ailments were caused by my age.
____13. I was denied medical treatment because of my age.
____14. I was denied employment because of my age.
____15. I was denied promotion because of my age.
____16. Someone assumed I could not hear well because of my age.
____17. Someone assumed I could not understand because of my age.
____18. Someone told me,"You're too old for that."
____19. My house was vandalized because of my age.
____20. I was victimized by a criminal because of my age.

Please write in your age: ____

Please check: Male ___ Female ___

What is the highest grade in school that you completed? ________

FIGURE 1-1 The Ageism Survey is being used to measure the prevalence and identify types of ageism. (From Palmore, E. [2000]. *The ageism survey*. Durham, NC: Duke Center for the Study of Aging. Used with permission.)

nomic worth. These values create a cultural environment in which the drawbacks of aging are emphasized, the benefits of aging are ignored, and individual elders are blamed for problems they have not created (McGowan, 1996). A potentially positive outcome of the increasing cultural diversity in the United States is that the dominant cultural values that foster ageism may be challenged by cultural values of other groups. For example, a study of the self-perceptions of older Anglo Americans, Chinese Americans, and Chinese in Taiwan found that all three groups held positive views of aging, and that the group that represented the highest degree of industrialization and modernization held the most positive view of aging (Tien-Hyatt, 1986–1987).

As the so-called baby boom generation, one of the most diverse generations in American history, reaches older adulthood, some of the long-held American values that have promoted ageism may be challenged and perhaps even replaced with different values that do not foster ageism. The questions that follow are among those that need to be addressed by gerontologists and others in the United States as planning for the aging baby boom cohort proceeds.

> *Should society automatically marginalize one fifth of its population because of a chronological age?...What roles and responsibilities ought older people to have as individuals to families and to society?...Should society care about the quality of life of older persons?...Ought society to be concerned if significant numbers of older people are economically poor and/or experience significant health problems?...How might we best support the efforts of family members to provide care to persons with significant functional disabilities? (Cornman & Kingston, 1996, p. 24)*

Effects of Ageism

The effects of negative stereotypes are hard to measure, but gerontologists have attempted to identify specific effects of negative stereotypes on older adults. For example, Ryan and colleagues (2002) explored the potential effects of "age excuses," which is the tendency to attribute problems such as forgetfulness to old age rather than to pathologic and potentially treatable conditions. These researchers concluded that age excuses could undermine the self-perceptions of older people and threaten self-esteem if the older person believes the excuse. A recent review of literature on the effects of subliminal messages conveying either positive or negative age stereotypes drew the following conclusions (Hess, 2006):

- Negative attitudes about aging are pervasive and are reflected in affective, cognitive, and behavioral responses of individuals and groups.
- Implicit attitudes may be even more strongly negative than explicit ones.
- Most stereotypes are negative, but even the positive ones usually have a subtle negative component.
- Stereotype-influenced responses of others have a negative impact on older adults.

- Stereotypes held by others can cause negative self-referent beliefs in older adults.
- Performance of older adults is negatively influenced by stereotypes.

Age stereotypes may also influence health-related behaviors. For example, a negative age stereotype may influence an older adult to perceive health problems as normal aging. Sarkisian and colleagues (2001) found that 13.5% of older women falsely attributed a new disability to old age. These researchers concluded that "despite great advances in geriatric medicine, old age is still perceived as a causal agent in functional decline, especially among our oldest patients" (p. 134). When older adults or health care professionals falsely attribute symptoms of pathologic conditions to normal aging, they are likely to overlook treatable conditions, and significant harm can result from this negligence. An important responsibility of gerontological nurses is to be knowledgeable about the differences between age-related changes and pathologic conditions, so appropriate nursing interventions can be initiated. An essential first step in planning interventions, especially health promotion interventions, is to identify those factors that are not inherent consequences of aging. Throughout this text, emphasis is placed on differentiating between age-related changes, which cannot be modified, and those factors that can be addressed through interventions.

Negative attitudes about aging that are held by health care workers can negatively affect the care older adults receive. Health care workers are likely to be influenced not only by ageism in society but by their own experiences in health care, which often are with those older adults who are the most impaired and in need of interventions. It is important, therefore, that all health care workers who care for older adults understand that most older adults are healthy and functional and strive toward improved levels of wellness and functioning.

Attitudes are changed through education, but changing attitudes requires first recognizing their existence. Because ageism is subtle but pervasive in American society, nurses first need to become aware of the attitudes they hold toward older adults. The first Critical Thinking Exercise at the end of this chapter suggests ways of becoming aware of one's own attitudes about older adults.

Aging Anxiety and Anti-Aging

Gerontophobia, a narrower concept than ageism, refers to an "unreasonable fear and/or irrational hatred of older people" (Palmore, 1972). Although gerontophobia has received less attention than ageism, gerontologists have focused some attention on the similar concept of aging anxiety. **Aging anxiety** is defined as "the combination of people's concerns or fears about getting older" (Lynch, 2000, p. 533). Indicators of aging anxiety include worries about social losses, cognitive ability, financial well-being, changes in physical appearance, and declines in health and physical functioning (Lynch, 2000). Aging anxiety is related to negative stereotypes of older adults and the perceptions of younger adults that these problems are likely to occur in their own later life. People with greater knowledge about the aging process are less likely to experience anxiety and worries about later life (Cummings et al., 2000). Gerontologists have found that aging anxiety is lower in people with better health, and higher in women and nonwhites (Cummings et al., 2000; Lynch, 2000). The study by Cummings and colleagues suggests that exposure to serious consequences of aging and the experience of caring for older family members are two factors that may increase a younger adult's insecurity and fears about growing older.

In the 1990s, anti-aging interventions emerged as popular approaches to staving off the negative consequences of aging. One example of the anti-aging movement is the American Academy of Anti-Aging Medicine, founded in 1993 and publicized as a "healthcare model promoting innovative science and research to prolong the healthy lifespan in humans" (Klatz, 2001–2002, p. 59). This movement has largely been discredited as pseudoscientific by many prominent geriatricians and gerontologists (Butler et al., 2002; Olshansky et al., 2002; Whitehouse & Juengst, 2005). A commentary on the movement suggests that the term *anti-aging* attempts to separate us from our bodies and presumes "that we can choose whether we are 'for' or 'against' our very existence as biologic and temporal beings" (Cole & Thompson, 2001–2002, p. 7). Cole and Thompson see anti-aging as a "broad cultural impulse" that has come about because aging has gone out of style and is currently associated with negative images of decay and decline. Butler (2001–2002) proposes that the term *longevity medicine* be used to convey a more positive approach to extending healthy life.

Addressing Attitudes of Nurses

One way of addressing attitudes of nurses and other health care workers toward older adults is through experiential educational activities. For example, *Into Aging* is a simulation game developed by nurses in the late 1980s to challenge the myths of aging (see the Educational Resources section of this chapter). This game has been used successfully to improve attitudes and staff behaviors toward care of older adults in a variety of settings (e.g., Pacala et al., 2006). A simpler method of addressing attitudes is to listen carefully to older adults as they talk about beliefs, values, hopes, and experiences that are integral to their self-identities. Nurses have daily opportunities to learn about aging and older adulthood simply by listening to the older adults for whom they provide care.

In addition, nurses should equip themselves with accurate information about the older adult population. Accurate information may be the most effective antidote to negative attitudes that result from misunderstandings or myths. Thus, the next two sections address myths about aging by providing an accurate snapshot of older adults in the United States.

DEBUNKING MYTHS: UNDERSTANDING REALITIES ABOUT OLDER ADULTS IN THE UNITED STATES

As a consequence of ageism and negative attitudes about aging, many myths and negative stereotypes about older adults have been perpetuated, especially with regard to aspects of health and functioning. These myths and stereotypes can be particularly detrimental when health care providers base their decisions or actions on lack of accurate information about aging because these misconceptions lead to suboptimal goals for care. At best, older adults do not experience the benefits of wellness-focused care; at worst, they experience unnecessary decline.

Providing accurate information about aging has been found to be an effective intervention for reducing negative stereotypes and improving attitudes about aging (Harris & Dollinger, 2001; Lynch, 2000). Chapters in Part 3 of this book address aspects of functioning that can be significantly affected by myths and misunderstandings about aging. Table 1-1 lists some of the myths and misperceptions about aging that are commonly held by older adults and health care professionals. The related realities about each aspect of health and functioning also are identified, along with a reference to the chapter that provides accurate information to dispel the myths. The information in this section is intended to provide a realistic picture of older adults in the United States in terms of their population characteristics, family relationships, and living arrangements.

Characteristics of the Older Adult Population

The characteristics of the older adult population in the United States that are reviewed in this section are based on census data and other reliable sources; however, this information can only reflect trends and compilations. The intent

TABLE 1-1 Myths and Realities of Aging

Myth	Reality
Older adulthood is something to anticipate with dread; it is essentially the end of life.	Demographics show that the older adult population is growing and life expectancy is increasing. In addition, emphasis is being placed on living long and living well. *(Chapter 1)*
People consider themselves to be old at the age of 65 years.	People usually feel old based on their health and function, rather than on their chronologic age. *(Chapter 1)*
Gerontologists have discovered that, by the age of 75 years, people are quite homogeneous as a group.	The more gerontologists learn about aging, the more they realize that, with increased age, people become more diverse, and individuals become less like their age peers. *(Chapters 3 and 4)*
Ageism is endemic in all societies.	Ageism is much more common in industrialized societies and is highly influenced by stereotypes and cultural values. *(Chapter 1)*
Gerontologists have recently discovered a theory that explains biologic aging.	Theories about biologic aging continue to evolve, and there is little agreement on any one theory. *(Chapter 3)*
In today's society, families no longer care for older people.	In the United States, 80% of the care of older adults is provided by their families. *(Chapter 1)*
In the United States, there is an increasing trend toward fewer multigenerational families in which people age 65 years and older live in households with younger generations.	There is an increasing trend toward "downward extension of households," in which older generations live with and provide care for grandchildren. *(Chapter 1)*
As people grow older, it is natural for them to want to withdraw from society.	Because older people are unique individuals, each of them responds differently to society. *(Chapter 3)*
By the age of 70 years, an individual's psychological growth is complete.	People never lose their capacity for psychological growth. *(Chapters 3 and 12)*
Increased disability in older people is attributable to age-related changes alone.	Although age-related changes increase one's vulnerability to functional impairments, the disabilities are attributable to risk factors, such as diseases and adverse medication effects. *(Chapter 2)*
Health promotion efforts are not beneficial to older adults who have two or more chronic conditions.	Research has debunked the myths that prevention is not effective after onset of chronic illness. *(Chapter 5)*
About 20% of people age 65 years and older live in nursing homes as long-term residents.	Between 4% and 5% of older adults live in a nursing home at any time. *(Chapter 6)*
Widowhood and other specific life events have been found to have a consistently negative impact on older people.	No one life event affects all older people negatively. The most important consideration governing the impact of an event is its unique meaning for the individual. *(Chapter 12)*
In old age, there is an inevitable decline in all intellectual abilities.	A few areas of cognitive ability decline in older adulthood, but other areas show improvement. *(Chapter 11)*
Older adults cannot learn complex new skills.	Older adults are capable of learning new things, but the speed with which they process information slows with age. *(Chapter 11)*

continued on following page

TABLE 1-1 Myths and Realities of Aging (continued)

Myth	Reality
Constipation develops primarily because of age-related changes.	Constipation is attributable primarily to risk factors, such as restricted activity and poor dietary habits. *(Chapter 18)*
Urinary incontinence is a normal consequence of aging that is best managed by using incontinence products.	In most cases, underlying causes of urinary incontinence can be addressed and a variety of self-care methods can be initiated. *(Chapter 19)*
Skin wrinkles can be prevented by using oils and lotions.	The best way to prevent skin wrinkles is to avoid exposure to ultraviolet light. *(Chapter 23)*
Older people decrease the level of their sexual activity because they are less able to perform sexually.	If sexual activity in older people declines, it is because of social reasons (e.g., loss of partner) or risk factors, such as diseases and adverse medication effects. *(Chapter 26)*
Health care professionals readily recognize adverse medication effects in older adults.	Adverse medication effects are often overlooked in older adults because they are mistakenly attributed to aging or pathologic conditions. *(Chapter 8)*
Some degree of "senility" is normal in very old people.	"Senility" is an inaccurate term used to refer to dementing conditions, which are always caused by pathologic changes. *(Chapter 14)*
Most old people are depressed and should be allowed to withdraw from society.	About one third of older people exhibit depressive symptoms; however, depression is a very treatable condition at any age. *(Chapter 15)*

is to provide an overview of health and socioeconomic characteristics of older adults that are most pertinent to holistically caring for older adults. Nurses need to keep in mind that older adults are a highly diverse group and this general information will not apply to every individual older adult.

Demographics of Aging

Discussions of current demographic trends in the United States inevitably focus on the so-called **baby boomers** (i.e., the large group of people born between 1946 and 1964). This group, which comprised about 30% of the population in 1994, will begin turning 65 years old in 2011, and will bring about major demographic changes. The influence of this and other population trends (e.g., increasing life expectancy, greater cultural diversity) is reflected in statistics such as the following from the 2000 census and later (He et al., 2005):

- In July 2003, 35.9 million people were 65 years of age or older and accounted for 12% of the population; projections for 2030 are that 72 million older adults will comprise nearly 20% of the population (Fig. 1-2).
- The median age of 35.3 years is the highest it has ever been; it is expected to peak at 39.1 years in 2035, after which it will decrease slightly (Fig. 1-3).
- The proportion of older adults who are non-Hispanic white (83%) has been decreasing in the past several decades and will continue to decline to 72% by 2030.
- Life expectancy at birth has increased from 47.3 years in 1900 to 76.9 years in 2000; projections for men and women in 2050 are 81 and 87 years, respectively.
- Remaining life expectancy for people who reach the age of 65 is 12 years, for those who reach 85 it is 6.3 years, and for centenarians it is 2.6 years.
- The older adult population can be divided by age groups as follows: 53% aged 65 to 74 years, 35% aged 74 to 84 years, and 12.1% aged 85 years and older.
- Increases by age groups are highest for those aged 85 years and older and lowest for those aged 65 to 74 years; this trend is expected to reverse starting in 2011, when the largest increase will be in the group of people aged 65 to 74 years.
- The number of centenarians increased by 35%, from 37,306 to 50,454, between 1990 and 2000; 80% of centenarians are women.

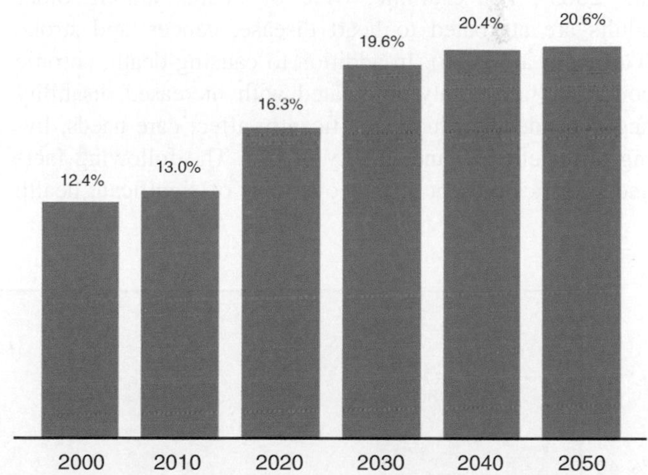

FIGURE 1-2 Projected percentage of the total population aged 65 years and older: 2000 to 2050. (From He, W., Sengupta, M., Velkoff, V. A., & DeBarros, K. A. [2005]. *65+ in the United States: 2005.* U.S. Census Bureau, Current Population Reports, P23-209. Washington, DC: U. S. Government Printing Office.)

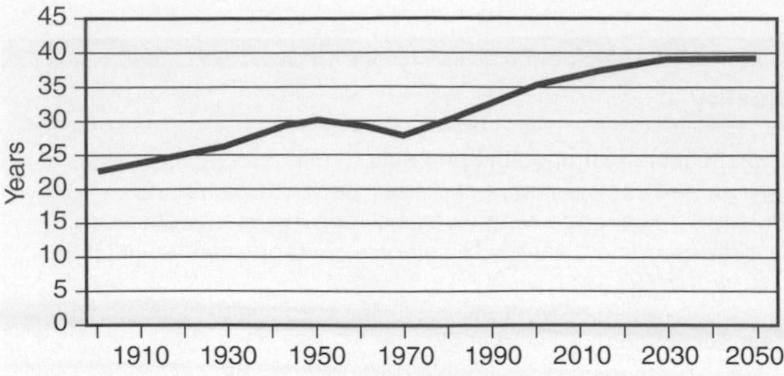

FIGURE 1-3 Projected median age: 1900 to 2050. (From He, W., Sengupta, M., Velkoff, V. A., & DeBarros, K. A. [2005]. *65+ in the United States: 2005.* U.S. Census Bureau, Current Population Reports, P23-209. Washington, DC: U. S. Government Printing Office.)

In summary, the older adult population in the United States is increasing, living longer, and reflecting greater diversity.

Health Characteristics

Because much of the focus of health care for older adults is on preventing disabilities and maintaining and improving function, gerontologists and health care providers are particularly interested in statistics about chronic conditions and impaired function in daily life. Economists, politicians, and health care planners also are interested in health characteristics of older adults because of the significant implications related to cost and types of health care services. Much attention is directed toward chronic conditions, which have been the predominant causes of death among older adults during the past 50 years (He et al., 2005). For example, 61% of deaths among older adults are attributed to heart disease, cancer, and stroke (Gorina et al., 2006). In addition to causing death, chronic conditions are highly associated with increased disability and dependency, which significantly affect care needs, living arrangements, and quality of life. The following facts and statistics present a brief overview of significant health characteristics of older adults in the United States (He et al., 2005):

- 80% of older adults have at least one chronic condition, and 50% have at least two.
- 43% of older women and 40% of older men experience disability (see also Fig. 1-4).
- The most prevalent chronic conditions that affect the daily functioning of older adults are arthritis, hypertension, heart disease, diabetes, stroke, cataracts, hearing impairments, sinusitis, and orthopedic impairments.
- The percentage of older adults who rated their health as fair or poor in 1996 was 26% of whites, 35.1% of Hispanics, and 41.6% of African Americans.

Because of the dramatic increases in life expectancy during the 20th century, gerontologists are focusing on concerns about extending quality of life by avoiding or delaying the onset of disability due to chronic conditions. Research indicates that health and functioning of older adults have been improving during the past decade, and these improvements are attributed to factors such as healthier lifestyles, improved environments, higher educational levels, advances in medical care, and greater use of assistive devices (Fries, 2002; He et al., 2005; Lan et al., 2002).

Socioeconomic Characteristics

Socioeconomic characteristics such as income, education, and marital status vary significantly among various groups (e.g., gender, cultural background, young-old versus old-old). Overall, there are many indications of socioeconomic trends that contribute to improved health and functioning for many older adults. For example, present and projected census data indicate gradual and continuing increases in level of education, which will be accompanied by better health and higher incomes (He et al., 2005). Despite the optimistic outlook, however, data point toward economic insecurity for older adults in the next decades and persistent disparities in economic well-being for disadvantaged groups (Holden & Hatcher, 2006). For example, women are more likely than men to be poor and living alone, and members of minority

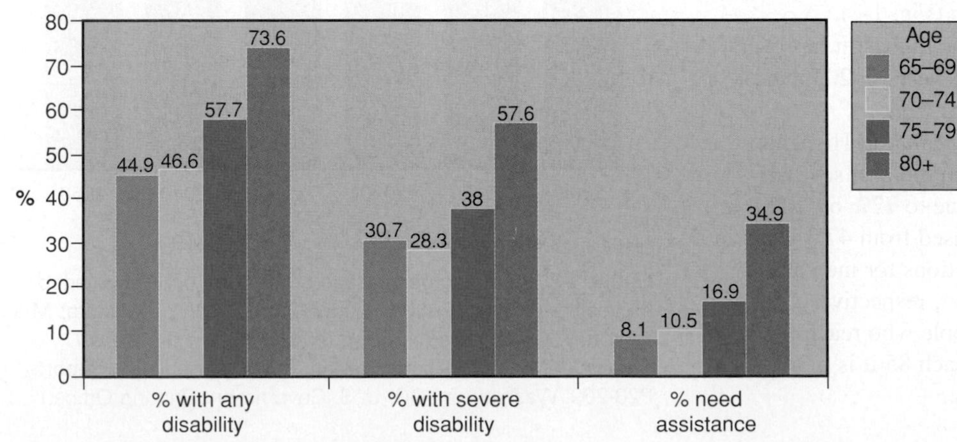

FIGURE 1-4 Percentage of older adults with disabilities, by age group. (Data from Federal Interagency Forum on Aging-Related Statistics. [2000]. *Older Americans 2000: Key indicators of well-being.* Washington, DC: U.S. Government Printing Office.)

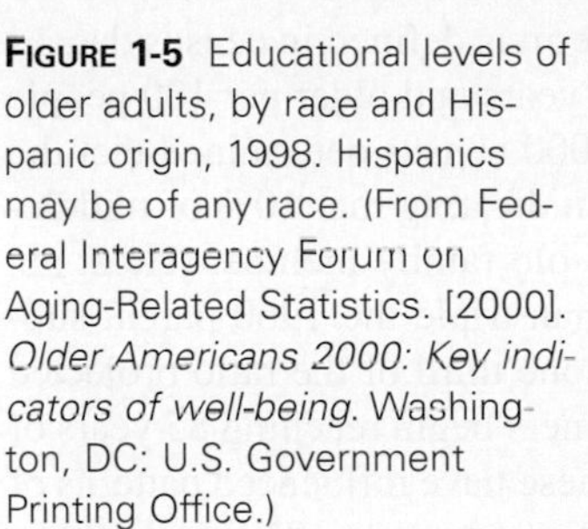

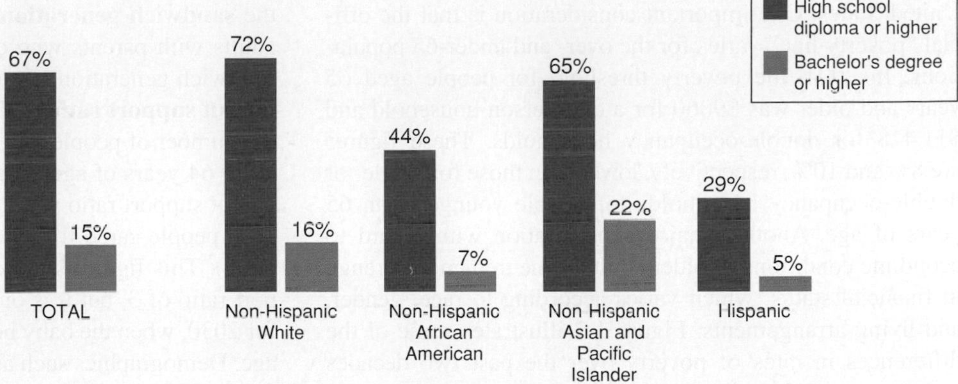

FIGURE 1-5 Educational levels of older adults, by race and Hispanic origin, 1998. Hispanics may be of any race. (From Federal Interagency Forum on Aging-Related Statistics. [2000]. *Older Americans 2000: Key indicators of well-being.* Washington, DC: U.S. Government Printing Office.)

groups are more likely to be poor and less educated, but more likely to be living with other relatives.

The following statistics reflect current trends with respect to some socioeconomic conditions of older adults (He et al., 2005):

- *Income*: The number of older people living below the poverty line has diminished from almost 30% in 1967 to 10.2% in 2003.
- *Education levels*: The percentage of people age 65 years and older who have completed high school has increased from 18% in 1950, to 28% in 1970, and to 70% in 2000; however, education levels vary by race (Fig. 1-5).
- *Gender*: The ratio of women to men increases with older age, as indicated by the following number of men for every 100 women: 86 between 65 and 69 years, and 41 at age 85 years and older.
- *Widowhood/widowerhood*: Women are more likely than men to survive their spouse and live alone because of their longer life expectancy and tendency to marry older men.
- *Marriage*: The percentages of men and women from 65 to 74 years of age who are married are 79% and 55%, respectively; and at 85 years and older, 50% and 13%, respectively (Fig. 1-6).

Although the overall poverty rate for older adults has been declining, this does not mean that all older people are economically better off today than they were 40 years ago. Gerontologists and sociologists emphasize that statistics about poverty should be interpreted in relation to a broader

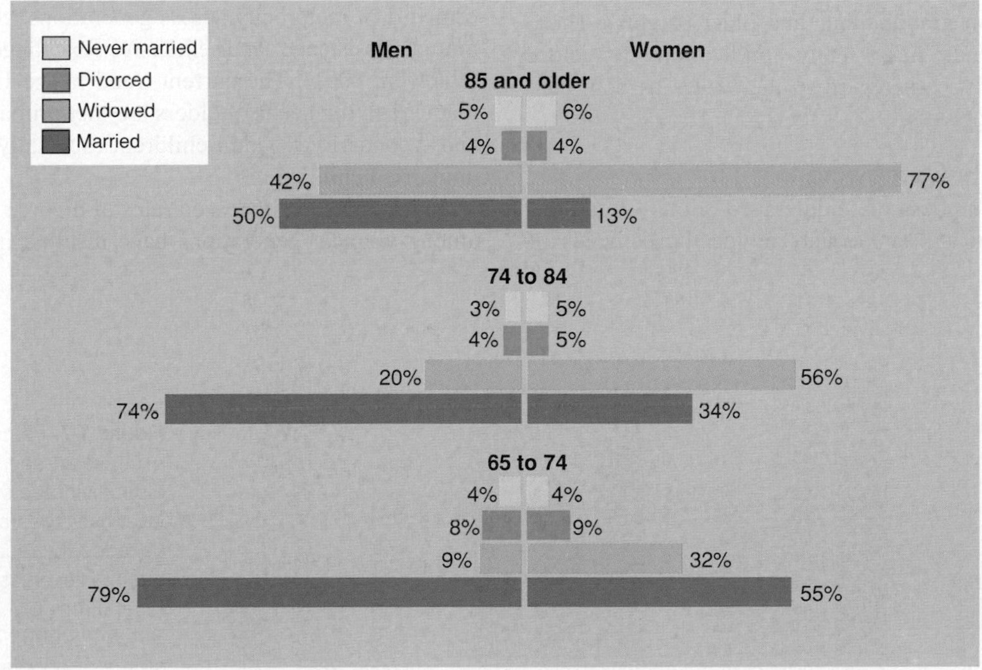

FIGURE 1-6 Marital status of older adults, by sex and age groups, 1998. These data refer to the civilian noninstitutional population. (From Federal Interagency Forum on Aging-Related Statistics. [2000]. *Older Americans 2000: Key indicators of well-being.* Washington, DC: U.S. Government Printing Office.)

perspective on the economic conditions of older adults in the United States. One important consideration is that the official "poverty line" varies for the over- and under-65 populations. In 2004, the poverty threshold for people aged 65 years and older was $9060 for a one-person household and $11,418 for double-occupancy households. These figures are 8% and 10%, respectively, lower than those for single- or double-occupancy households for people younger than 65 years of age. Another major consideration with regard to economic conditions of older adults is the tremendous range in financial status, which varies according to race, gender, and living arrangements. Figure 1-7 illustrates some of the differences in rates of poverty over the past two decades among groups of older adults classified by race and Hispanic origin. Other factors that increase the likelihood of an older adult living in poverty are female sex, living alone, advanced old age, having poor health, and not completing high school.

Family Relationships of Older Adults

Increased life expectancy and other demographic trends in the United States have brought about major changes in, and increasing diversity of, family relationships in recent decades. For example, multigenerational families are now the norm; 25% of people aged 58 to 59 years have at least one living parent, and 10% of older people have at least one child who is also older than 65 years of age. Gerontologists describe relationships among several generations of family members in terms of **upward extension of households** (i.e., older adults reside with adult children or grandchildren to receive care) and **downward extension of households** (i.e., grandchildren or adult children live with and are in some way dependent on grandparents and older parents). These demographic trends have many implications for older adults, particularly with regard to their roles as both care receivers and caregivers.

Trends in Family Caregiving

The increasing numbers of middle-aged adults—traditionally women—who simultaneously juggle the demands of caring for older and younger generations are referred to as the **sandwich generation**. Responsibilities of middle-aged adults with parents who depend on them for care (i.e., the sandwich generation) are described demographically by the **parent support ratio**. This term is defined in census data as the number of people age 85 years and older per 100 people 50 to 64 years of age. The 2000 census determined that the parent support ratio was 10, indicating that 10% of middle-aged people cared for an old-old family member (He et al., 2005). This figure is more than triple the 1960 parent support ratio of 3, but it is only one third of the ratio projected for 2030, when the baby boomers begin reaching 85 years of age. Demographics such as these have influenced patterns of family caregiving, particularly for women. The mid-1980s, for example, marked the beginning of an era in which the average woman in the United States spent more time caring for her parents than for her children.

Since the preindustrial period, nuclear family living arrangements have been predominant in Western Europe and the United States. Typically, younger family members establish separate households after marriage, and older family members attempt to maintain independent households for as long as possible. For much of American history, the "ideal" relationship between older and younger generations in families has been to be far enough away to preserve independent lifestyles but close enough for social support and emotional connectedness. Moreover, this kind of family relationship provides for meeting occasional caregiving needs of family members while allowing for the maintenance of differing lifestyles for both younger and older generations. Family relationships have been based on the principle of reciprocity across generations, characterized by mutual assistance and extensive exchanges among kin (Hareven, 2001). The current trend in the United States is that caregiving needs of elders are met primarily by spouses and secondarily by adult children, especially daughters and unmarried children.

In recent years, increased rates of divorce and remarriage among younger generations have resulted in the prolifera-

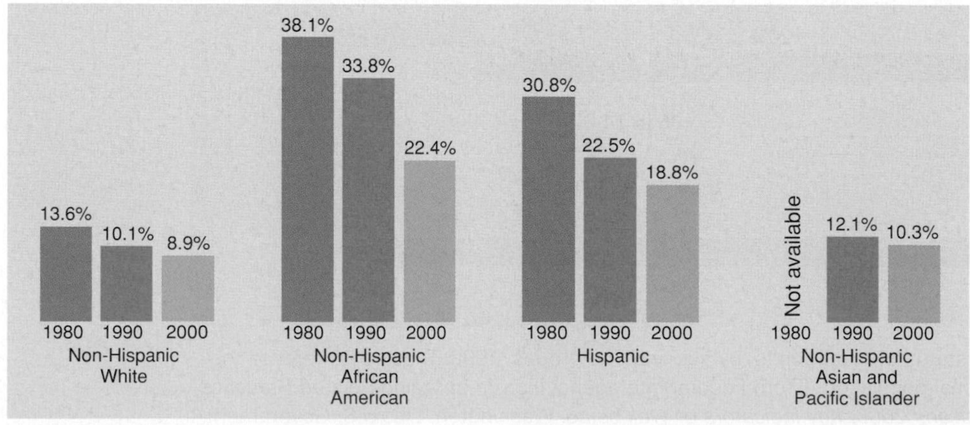

FIGURE 1-7 Percentages of Americans, age 65 years and older, living below the poverty level over the past two decades, by race and Hispanic origin. Hispanics may be of any race. (From U.S. Census Bureau. [2000]. Table 3: Poverty status of people by age, race, and Hispanic origin, 1959–2000. In *Current population survey*. Washington, DC: Author.)

tion of varieties of blended families across several generations. In addition, increased rates of remarriage among older adults who are widowed or divorced have led to increasing numbers of later-life blended families. One consequence of these trends is that family dynamics can become quite complex, particularly when adult stepchildren assume new roles as caregivers or decision makers for dependent older adults. For example, adult children may share caregiving and decision-making responsibilities regarding their impaired parent with a parent's spouse who they hardly know. Similarly, adult children may assist their parent with caregiving or decision making about a stepparent who they are just getting to know. Relationships among blended families usually are complicated by concerns regarding financial resources and questions about inheritance.

Another trend that affects relationships between older adults and their families is differing expectations and attitudes about caregiving practices. In the early 1900s, for example, the tradition of deep involvement in generational assistance, reinforced by strong family and ethnic values, was dominant in American culture. After World War II, however, a tradition of individualistic values and lifestyles emerged with an acceptance of reliance on institutions and public agencies to provide care for dependent elderly (Hareven, 2001). Also, in current families, middle-aged daughters have been influenced by the trend toward having careers independent of their roles in families. These trends can lead to conflict between the younger generation of adult children, especially daughters, and older family members who need care.

Even with complex and evolving social and demographic trends in the United States, some aspects of the relationship between older adults and their families have remained unchanged for many decades. For example, studies consistently show that older adults are satisfied with their family relationships and maintain close emotional ties and frequent contact with children and grandchildren (Field & Gueldner, 2001). Another consistent relationship between older adults and their families is that about 80% of care for dependent older adults is provided by family members and other "informal" sources. Spousal and filial responsibilities are traditions that have directed family caregiving in the United States for centuries, and this continues even though the specific dynamics of the care are changing.

Cultural Considerations 1-1 presents cultural perspectives related to older adults and family caregiving.

Diversity Note

Studies indicate that, in comparison with white families, some ethnic minority families use fewer formal services but provide more informal support from a broader range of family members (Dilworth-Anderson et al., 2002).

Cultural Considerations 1-1

Cultural Perspectives on Elders and Family Caregiving Relationships

African Americans

- Elders are a source of wisdom and deserve respect.
- Grandparents are often involved with caring for grandchildren and may live in the same household.

American Indians/Alaskan Natives

- Elder status is characterized by health status and roles as counselors, teachers, or grandparents.
- Grandparents often care for grandchildren, who then are expected to care for the elders; grandmother may be called "Mother."

Chinese

- Traditional Chinese values place family and society above the individual.
- Elders are highly respected and honored.
- Multigenerational households are common.

Filipinos

- Respect for elders is a cornerstone of Filipino values, demonstrated by deference in verbal and nonverbal communication.
- Children (especially the oldest daughter) are expected to care for parents to repay their debt of gratitude (*utang na loob*).

Germans

- Close intergenerational relationships are maintained by first- and second-generation German Americans, but family mobility may affect this.
- Children are expected to help their parents stay in their own homes as long as possible.
- Because Amish and German Baptists view family relationships as reciprocal throughout life, grandparents usually live with their children or move from child to child.

Greeks

- Elderly women have higher status and more power within the family than younger women do and are expected to live with or near adult children, especially daughters.

Haitians

- Elders assume roles as family advisers, babysitters, historians, and consultants.
- Children are expected to care for elders at home.

Japanese

- Elders are highly respected and those who are able help in caring for children and grandchildren.
- Elders commonly maintain separate households; when they need help, the eldest son's family is expected to care for them at home.

continued on following page

Continued

Koreans

- Caring for elderly kin is a family duty that is associated with respect for elders and family bonds inherent in Confucianism.
- Grandparents frequently provide care for grandchildren; elders are welcome to live with family during times of need.

Mexican Americans

- Elders are revered, but acculturation reduces the sense of obligation toward providing care.
- Obligation to care for an elder parent or relative does not preclude placement in long-term-care facility.

Puerto Ricans

- *La abuela(o)* (elder or grandparent) is a figure of respect, wisdom, and admiration.
- Both men and women care for elderly and share caregiving responsibilities with family members and a close family network.

Russians

- Elders are highly respected and remain close to their children.
- Even if elders do not live with their children, they are expected to help raise grandchildren and participate in decision making.

Vietnamese

- They believe that the more one respects the elderly, the greater one's chance is of reaching old age.
- Young adults are expected to assume full responsibility for caring for elders at home.

From Lipson, J. G., & Dibble, L. (2005). *Culture & clinical care.* San Francisco: UCSF Nursing Press.

Grandparents Raising Grandchildren

Another phenomenon that is increasingly being addressed by gerontologists, organizations such as the AARP, and the federal government is the dramatic increase in the number of children younger than 18 years of age living in households maintained by a grandparent, which are referred to as **skipped-generation households**. Questions about grandparental caregiving were included in the 2000 census because the practice is becoming more common, particularly among culturally diverse groups. The following conclusions about this trend are based on census data, studies, and a review of research (Fuller-Thomson & Minkler, 2005; Hayslip & Kaminski, 2005; Kataoka-Yahiro et al., 2004; Simmons & Dye, 2003):

- Approximately 6 million grandparents live with grandchildren who are 18 years of age or younger; 2.4 million were raising these grandchildren.
- Between 1970 and 1997, the number of grandchildren being raised by grandparents increased by 76%.
- Grandparental coresidence with grandchildren was highest among the following groups: 10% for Pacific Islanders; 8% for Hispanics, African Americans, and American Indians/Alaskan Natives, and 6% for Asians.
- Overall, 42% of grandparents who live with grandchildren assume primary responsibility for their care; Asians and Hispanics were less likely than African Americans or American Indians/Alaskan Natives to be responsible for these grandchildren.
- Common reasons for grandparent custody include adult parent drug abuse; child abuse; teen pregnancy; and death, disability, or incarceration of adult parents.
- African Americans are more likely to raise their grandchildren because of parent-absent circumstances.
- Negative consequences associated with being a custodial grandparent include significant stresses, role overload, social isolation, detrimental effects on health and functioning, and increased likelihood of being poor.
- Rewards of grandparent caregiving include role enhancement, sense of purpose in life, close relationships with younger generations, and satisfaction with maintaining family well-being.

Living Arrangements of Older Adults

Living arrangements for older adults are significantly influenced by such factors as health, marital status, family relationships, and socioeconomic conditions. Health is a significant variable, particularly in relation to functional level and ability to meet one's daily needs. Older people who are able to meet their basic needs with little or no help are likely to live alone or with a spouse. For people who are dependent on others for their daily needs, the willingness and availability of a caregiver is the factor that most strongly determines whether they remain at home or move to a nursing facility. About 90% of the older adult population in the United States lives in houses or apartments, with the remaining 10% about equally divided between nursing facilities and facilities that provide some assistance with daily needs. These living arrangements vary by gender, however, as shown in Figure 1-8. Data from the 2000 census indicate a decline in the percentage of people 65 years and older living in nursing homes (from 5.1% in 1990 to 4.5% in 2000) for the first time in history. This decline occurred in all age subgroups but was most marked for the group 85 years of age and older, in which the percentage of people in nursing homes declined from 24.5% in 1990 to 18.2% in 2000. Similarly, the percentage of women age 75 years and older who live alone increased during the past several decades from 37% in 1970 to 53% in 1998; for men age 75 years and older during this same period, the percentage increased from 19% to 22%.

These trends toward more independent living arrangements are due to a combination of factors, including improved health and functioning, especially for people 75 years of age and older, as well as a broader range of community-

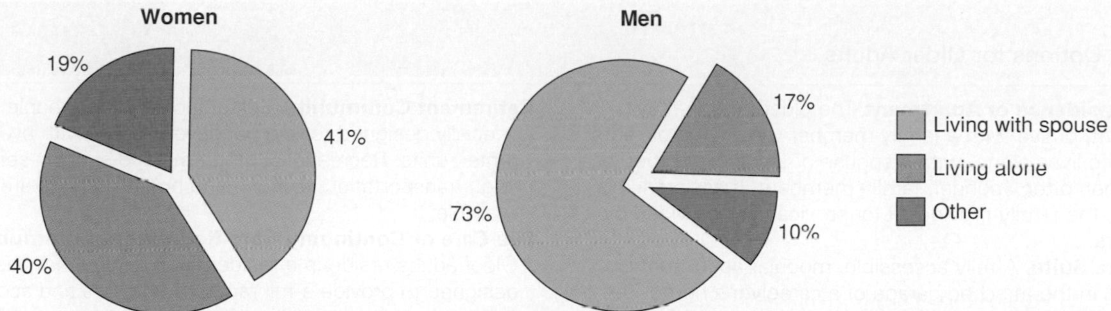

FIGURE 1-8 Living arrangements of people age 65 years and older, 2000. (Data from the U.S. Census Bureau. [2001]. *America's families and living arrangements; population characteristics: June, 2001.* Current Population Reports, P20-537; and *The 65 years and over population: 2000, Census 2000 Brief, October, 2001.* Washington, DC: Author.)

based services to provide assistance to people who need help with daily activities but wish to remain in their own homes (discussed in Chapter 6). In addition to the growth of community-based services for people who live in their own homes, a wide range of housing options has evolved in recent decades to address the needs of the growing number of older adults who require daily assistance but do not need full-time care. For example, life-care and continuing-care retirement communities provide a wide range of integrated and comprehensive services addressing health and social needs. Older adults typically enter this type of residential setting when they are relatively healthy and independent, but the arrangement guarantees that their health needs will be met at the most appropriate level until their death. Residents initially reside in an apartment or single home and move to assisted-living, skilled nursing, or other areas within the large complex as their needs change. Cost of care is covered primarily through a combination of the entrance fee, a monthly service fee, and long-term care insurance. Some aspects of care may require fee-for-service payment, and some nursing care services may be covered by Medicare and Medicaid. The continuing-care retirement community model provides the most comprehensive type of care, but there are significant financial and other barriers to its use.

Assisted-living facilities have become very popular in recent years and are available in most areas of the country. Although the services provided by these facilities vary widely, basic services generally include a single residential unit, at least one daily meal, and 24-hour availability of assistance. People who live in assisted-living facilities usually need help with three or more daily activities and some facilities are designed specifically for people who have cognitive impairments. Residence in an assisted-living facility generally costs less than nursing home care or extensive home care services, but it is usually not covered by Medicaid. Recently, assisted-living facilities have come to be seen as cost-effective ways of providing care to people who otherwise would need care in nursing facilities. Because there is no consistent licensure or regulation of these facilities, however, states have been reluctant to provide Medicaid funds for assisted-living care. Consequently, most people who live in these facilities pay out of-pocket and move to a nursing facility when their funds are exhausted. This is likely to change in the near future because there is growing recognition of the need for public financial support of this type of facility. Most states are currently considering implementing regulations and licensing for assisted-living facilities, and the Joint Commission for the Accreditation of Healthcare Organizations (JCAHO) began accreditation for assisted-living facilities in 2001.

Because the range of housing options as well as community-based services is rapidly increasing, decisions about staying in one's own home or moving to another type of living facility are becoming more complex. Although nurses may not be familiar with all the housing options in their communities, at a minimum, they need to know about the various types of facilities that are commonly available. Moreover, nurses are responsible for suggesting referrals to social service agencies and offices on aging so older adults and their families can find additional information. Box 1-1 describes various housing options for older adults that are available in most parts of the United States.

CHAPTER HIGHLIGHTS

The Relationship Between Wellness and Aging

- Since the late 1950s, health care professionals have recognized the importance of incorporating wellness goals in their care of older adults; however, there are many conceptual and practical barriers.
- Barriers to promoting wellness in older adults include older adults' negative attitudes about being able to improve, the existence of more serious or pressing health concerns, the focus of health care environments on disease treatment rather than prevention or health promotion, the false attribution of symptoms of pathologic conditions to normal aging processes, and the belief that older adults are not capable of learning and implementing health-promoting behaviors inherent in wellness-oriented care.

Box 1-1
Housing Options for Older Adults

Family Residence or Apartment. The older person may own, rent, or live with a family member who owns or rents. He or she lives alone, with a spouse or significant other, or with other, often younger, family members. If assistance is needed, the family provides it, or services are provided by outsiders.

Homecare Suite. A fully accessible, modular apartment is installed in the attached garage of a caregiver's home. The unit is fully insulated and contains its own water, heating, and air conditioning systems. It can be purchased, rented, or leased for whatever length of time it is needed.

Foster Care or Board-and-Care Home. The older person lives with unrelated people in a private home. Each resident has a private or shared bedroom and shared use of common space, such as a living room and dining room. The foster family or board-and-care operator usually provides meals, housekeeping, and supervision of, or assistance with, basic and instrumental activities of daily living.

Shared Housing. The older person shares a house or apartment with one or more unrelated people. Each occupant has a private or semiprivate bedroom and shares the rest of the dwelling, expenses, and chores. Offices on aging may coordinate these programs and provide some services.

Congregate Housing. Older people occupy individual apartments within a specially designed, multiunit dwelling. Supportive services, such as meals, housekeeping, transportation, and social and recreational activities, are provided.

Retirement Community. Self-sufficient older people live in a specially designed residential development with owned or rented units. Recreational programs and support services (e.g., transportation, laundry, and housekeeping) are usually available.

Life-Care or Continuing-Care Retirement Community. Older adults reside in a residential complex that has been designed to provide a full range of services and accommodations to meet each resident's needs as they change. The development includes independent housing, congregate housing, assisted living, and nursing home care. Each resident usually pays a significant fee and enters into a contract with the organization. This legal agreement guarantees lodging, nursing services, and other health-related services for a specified term or for the remainder of the resident's life. Strict admission criteria may apply.

Assisted-Living Facility. Older adults live in their own apartment (usually one or two rooms and a bathroom), and they share common areas for meals and social activities. One to three meals a day are provided. Assistance with laundry, housekeeping, transportation, personal care, and medication administration usually is available, as is some degree of protective supervision and 24-hour emergency services. Fees vary depending on the number of services used, and service agreements may be adjusted as the needs of the resident change.

- Rather than having a narrow focus on physical health and functioning, wellness-focused nursing considers the older adult's physical, mental, social, and spiritual well-being.
- Definitions of aging can be understood in terms of chronologic age, age identity, or functional age. Addressing functional age is most appropriate in wellness-oriented nursing care.

Attitudes Toward Aging

- Negative images of aging and ageism are pervasive in modern societies and can have a negative impact on care provided to older adults, especially when health care providers—including nurses—base their care on myths and inaccurate information (Fig. 1-1).
- Nurses need to identify myths about older adults, examine attitudes toward aging (including their own), and use accurate information as an antidote so they can provide wellness-oriented care for older adults (Table 1-1).
- Cultural perspectives have a significant influence on attitudes about aging, older adults, and family caregiving relationships (Cultural Considerations 1-1).

Debunking Myths: Understanding Realities About Older Adults in the United States

- The older adult population in the United States is increasing, living longer, and reflecting greater diversity.
- Multigenerational families and households are increasingly common.
- The current trend in the United States is that caregiving needs of elders are met primarily by spouses and secondarily by adult children, especially daughters and unmarried children.
- Older adults may be responsible for raising grandchildren in skipped-generation households.
- Living arrangements for older adults are significantly influenced by such factors as health, marital status, family relationships, and socioeconomic conditions (Fig. 1-1 and Box 1-1).

Critical Thinking Exercises

1. Increase your awareness of attitudes toward aging and older adults through the following exercises:
   - During the next 2 weeks, as you go about your usual activities, keep a small notebook handy and jot down examples of images of older adults that you see or hear in the following media: newspapers, magazines, Internet, television, greeting cards, and social conversations. Note whether the images convey a neutral, positive, or negative image.
   - During the next 2 weeks, pay attention to your thoughts and conversations about older adults and identify the perceptions you hold, the terms you use, and the images you convey.
   - Rephrase each of the 20 questions in the Ageism Survey (Fig. 1-1) and ask yourself how often you have done any of those activities in the past few months (e.g., "How often did I tell a joke that pokes fun at old people?").

- Ask an older relative, friend, or acquaintance to fill out the Ageism Survey and discuss his or her experiences.

2. Define old age and aging from each of the following perspectives: chronologic age, age identity, and functional age.

EDUCATIONAL RESOURCES

Into Aging: Understanding Issues Affecting the Later Stages of Life

(Boxed simulation game)
www.slackbooks.com

REFERENCES

Angus, J., & Reeve, P. (2006). Ageism: A threat to "aging well" in the 21st century. *Journal of Applied Gerontology, 25*(2), 137–152.

Blazer, D. G. (2006). Successful aging. *American Geriatric Psychiatry, 13*(1), 2–5.

Bowling, A., See-Tai, S., Ebrahim, S., Gabriel, Z., & Solanki, P. (2005). Attributes of age-identity. *Ageing and Society, 25*, 479–500.

Bradley, D. E., & Longino, C. F. (2001). How older people think about images of aging in advertising and the media. *Generations, 25*(3), 17–21.

Brugman, G. M. (2006). Wisdom and aging. In J. E. Birren & K. W. Schaie (Eds.), *Handbook of the psychology of aging* (6th ed., pp. 445–476). San Diego: Academic Press.

Butler, R. N. (1969). Ageism: Another form of bigotry. *The Gerontologist, 9*, 243–246.

Butler, R. N. (1975). *Why survive? Being old in America*. New York: Harper & Row.

Butler, R. N. (2001–2002). Is there an "anti-aging" medicine? *Generations, 25*(4), 63–64.

Butler, R. N., Fossel, M., Harman, S., Heward, C. B., Olshansky, S. J., Perls, T. T., et al. (2002). Is there an antiaging medicine? *Journals of Gerontology: Series A, Biological Sciences and Medical Sciences, 57*, B333–B338.

Butler, R. N., Lewis, M. I., & Sunderland, T. (1991). *Aging and mental health* (4th ed.) New York: Merrill/Macmillan.

Cohen, E. S. (1988). The elderly mystique: Constraints on the autonomy of the elderly with disabilities. *The Gerontologist, 28*(Suppl.), 24–31.

Cole, T. R., & Thompson, B. (2001–2002). Introduction: Anti-aging: Are you for it or against it? *Generations, 25*(4), 6–8.

Cornman, J. M., & Kingston, E. R. (1996). Trends, issues, perspectives, and values for the aging of the baby boom cohorts. *The Gerontologist, 36*, 15–26.

Covan, E. K. (2005). Meaning of aging in women's lives. *Journal of Women & Aging, 17*(3), 3–22.

Covey, H. C. (1988). Historical terminology used to represent older people. *The Gerontologist, 28*, 291–297.

Cuddy, A. J. C., Norton, M. I., & Fiske, S. T. (2005). This old stereotype: The pervasiveness and persistence of the elderly stereotype. *Journal of Social Issues, 61*, 267–285.

Cummings, S. M., Kropf, N. P., & DeWeaver, K. L. (2000). Knowledge of and attitudes toward aging among non-elders: Gender and race differences. *Journal of Women & Aging, 12*(1/2), 77–91.

Depp, C. A., & Jeste, D. V. (2006). Definitions and predictors of successful aging: A comprehensive review of larger quantitative studies. *American Journal of Geriatric Psychiatry, 14*(1), 6–20.

Dilworth-Anderson, P., Williams, I. C., & Gibson, B. E. (2002). Issues of race, ethnicity, and culture in caregiving research: A 20-year review (1980–2000). *The Gerontologist, 42*, 237–272.

Dunn, H. L. (1958). Significance of levels of wellness in aging. *Geriatrics, 13*(1), 51–57.

Dunn, H. L. (1961). *High-level wellness*. Arlington, VA: R. W. Beatty.

Field, D., & Gueldner, S. H. (2001). The oldest old: How do they differ from the old-old? *Journal of Gerontological Nursing, 27*(8), 20–27.

Fischer, D. H. (1977). *Growing old in America*. New York: Oxford University Press.

Fries, J. F. (2002). Successful aging: An emerging paradigm of gerontology. *Clinics in Geriatric Medicine, 18*, 371–382.

Fuller-Thomson, E., & Minkler, M. (2005). American Indian/Alaskan Native grandparents raising grandchildren: Findings from the Census 2000 Supplementary Survey. *Social Work, 50*, 131–139.

George, L. K. (2006). Perceived quality of life. In R. H. Binstock & L. K. George (Eds.), *Handbook of aging and the social sciences* (6th ed., pp. 320–336). San Diego: Elsevier Academic Press.

Gorina, Y., Hoyert, D., Lentzner, H., & Goulding, M. (2006). *Trends in causes of death among older persons in the United States*. Aging Trends, No. 6. Hyattsville, MD: National Center for Health Statistics.

Hareven, T. K. (2001). Historical perspectives on aging and family relations. In R. H. Binstock & L. K. George (Eds.), *Handbook of aging and the social sciences* (5th ed., pp. 141–159). San Diego: Academic Press.

Harris, L. A., & Dollinger, S. (2001). Participation in a course on aging: Knowledge, attitudes and anxiety about aging in oneself and others. *Educational Gerontology, 27*, 657–667.

Hayslip, B., Jr., & Kaminski, P. L. (2005). Grandparents raising their grandchildren: A review of the literature and suggestions for practice. *The Gerontologist, 45*, 262–269.

He, W., Sengupta, M., Velkoff, V. A., & DeBarros, K. A. (2005). *65+ in the United States: 2005*. U.S. Census Bureau, Current Population Reports, P23-209. Washington, DC: U. S. Government Printing Office.

Hendricks J., & Hatch, L. R. (2006). Lifestyle and aging. In R. H. Binstock & L. K. George (Eds.), *Handbook of aging and the social sciences* (6th ed., pp. 301–319). San Diego: Academic Press.

Hess, T. M. (2006). Attitudes toward aging and their effects on behavior. In J. E. Birren & K. W. Schaie (Eds.), *Handbook of the psychology of aging* (6th ed., pp. 379–406). San Diego: Academic Press.

Hirshbein, L. D. (2001). Popular views of old age in America, 1900–1950. *Journal of the American Geriatrics Society, 49*, 1555–1560.

Holden, K., & Hatcher, C. (2006). Economic status of the aged. In R. H. Binstock & L. K. George (Eds.), *Handbook of aging and the social sciences* (6th ed., pp. 219–237). San Diego: Elsevier Academic Press.

International Longevity Center—USA. (2001). *Biomarkers of aging: From primitive organisms to man*. New York: Author.

Kataoka-Yahiro, M., Ceria, C., & Caulfield, R. (2004). Grandparent caregiving role in ethnically diverse families. *Journal of Pediatric Nursing, 19*, 315–328.

Klatz, R. (2001–2002). Anti-aging medicine: Resounding, independent support for expansion of an innovative medical specialty. *Generations, 25*(4), 59–62.

Lan, T.-Y., Melzer, D., Tom, B. D. M., & Guralnik, J. M. (2002). Performance tests and disability: Developing an objective index of mobility-related limitation in older populations. *Journals of Gerontology: Series A, Biological Sciences and Medical Sciences, 57*, M294–M301.

Levy, B. R. (2001). Eradication of ageism requires addressing the enemy within. *The Gerontologist, 41*, 578–579.

Lipson, J. G., & Dibble, S. L. (2005). *Culture & clinical care*. San Francisco: UCSF Nursing Press.

Lynch, S. M. (2000). Measurement and prediction of aging anxiety. *Research on Aging, 22*, 533–558.

McGowan, T. G. (1996). Ageism and discrimination: In J. E. Birren (Ed.), *Encyclopedia of gerontology: Age, aging, and the aged*. Vol. 1. (pp. 71–80). San Diego: Academic Press.

Montross, L. P., Depp, C., Daly, J., Reichstadt, J., Golshan, S., Moore, D., et al. (2006). Correlates of self-rated successful aging among community-dwelling older adults. *American Journal of Geriatric Psychiatry, 14*(1), 43–51.

Neugarten, B. L. (1978). The rise of the young-old. In R. Gross, B. Gross, & S. Seidman (Eds.), *The new old: Struggling for decent aging* (pp. 47–49). Garden City, NY: Anchor Press/Doubleday.

Olshansky, S. J., Hayflick, L., & Carnes, B. A. (2002). Position statement on human aging. *Journals of Gerontology: Series A, Biological Sciences and Medical Sciences, 57*, B292–B297.

Pacala, J. T., Boult, C., & Hepburn, K. (2006). Ten years' experience conducting the aging game workshop: Was it worth it? *Journal of the American Geriatrics Society, 54*, 144–149.

Palmore, E. (1972). Gerontophobia versus ageism. *The Gerontologist, 12*, 213.

Palmore, E. (2001). The ageism survey: First findings. *The Gerontologist, 41*, 572–575.

Rowe, J. W., & Kahn, R. L. (1997). Successful aging. *The Gerontologist, 37*, 433–440.

Ryan, E. B., Bieman-Copland, S., See, S. T. K., Ellis, C. H., & Anas, A. P. (2002). Age excuses: Conversational management of memory failures in older adults. *Journals of Gerontology: Series B, Psychological Sciences and Social Sciences, 57*, P256–P267.

Sarkisian, C. A., Liu, H., Ensrud, K, E., Stone, K. L., & Mangione, C. M. (2001). Correlates of attributing new disability to old age. *Journal of the American Geriatrics Society, 49*, 134–141.

Seeman, T., & Chen, X. (2002). Risk and protective factors for physical functioning in older adults with and without chronic conditions: MacArthur Studies of Successful Aging. *Journals of Gerontology: Series B, Psychological Sciences and Social Sciences, 57*, S135–S144.

Simmons, T., & Dye, J. L. (2003). Grandparents living with grandchildren: 2000. U.S. Census Bureau, Census 2000 Brief. Available at: www.census.gov/prod/2003pubs/c2kbr-31.pdf.

Thornton, J. E. (2002). Myths of aging or ageist stereotypes. *Educational Gerontology, 28*, 301–312.

Tien-Hyatt, J. L. (1986–1987). Self-perceptions of aging across cultures: Myth or reality? *International Journal of Aging and Human Development, 24*, 129–148.

Whitehouse, P. J., & Juengst, E. T. (2005). Antiaging medicine and mild cognitive impairment: Practice and policy issues for geriatrics. *Journal of the American Geriatrics Society, 53*, 1417–1422.

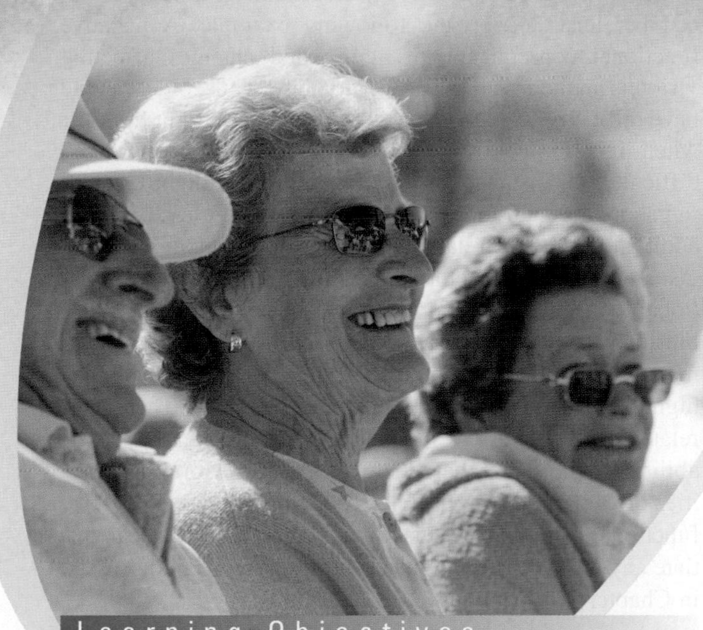

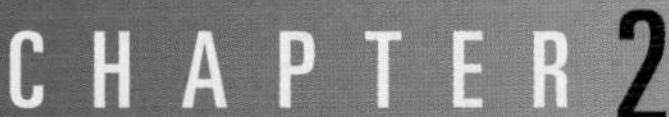

CHAPTER 2

Applying a Nursing Model for Promoting Wellness in Older Adults

Learning Objectives

After reading this chapter, you will be able to:

1. Discuss the basic premises that underpin the Functional Consequences Theory in older adults.
2. Define concepts of age-related changes, risk factors, and functional consequences as they relate to nursing care of older adults.
3. Describe the domains of nursing (i.e., person, nursing, health, environment) in the context of the Functional Consequences Theory.
4. Apply the Functional Consequences Theory to the practice of nursing to promote wellness in older adults.

Key Terms

age-related changes
competence-press model
environment
functional consequences
Functional Consequences Theory for Promoting Wellness in Older Adults
health
negative functional consequences
nursing
older adult
person
positive functional consequences
risk factors
wellness outcomes

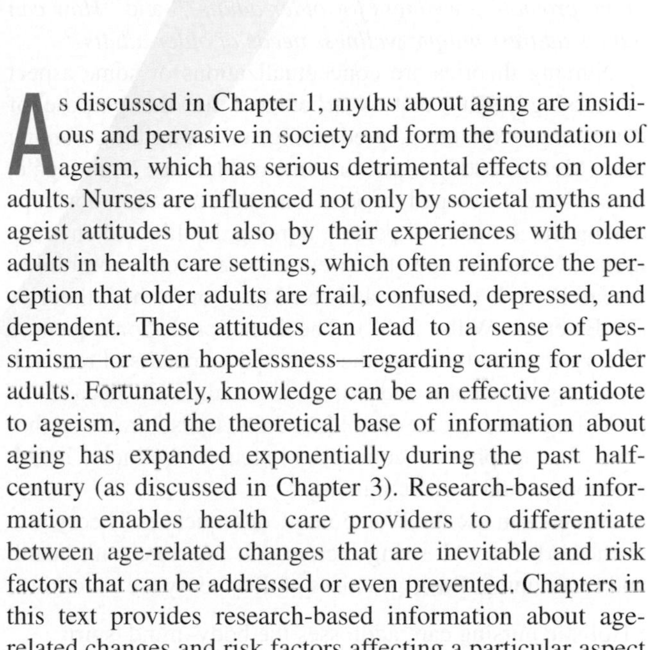

As discussed in Chapter 1, myths about aging are insidious and pervasive in society and form the foundation of ageism, which has serious detrimental effects on older adults. Nurses are influenced not only by societal myths and ageist attitudes but also by their experiences with older adults in health care settings, which often reinforce the perception that older adults are frail, confused, depressed, and dependent. These attitudes can lead to a sense of pessimism—or even hopelessness—regarding caring for older adults. Fortunately, knowledge can be an effective antidote to ageism, and the theoretical base of information about aging has expanded exponentially during the past half-century (as discussed in Chapter 3). Research-based information enables health care providers to differentiate between age-related changes that are inevitable and risk factors that can be addressed or even prevented. Chapters in this text provides research-based information about age-related changes and risk factors affecting a particular aspect of functioning, with emphasis on the changes and factors that nurses can address. Nurses can apply this information to help older adults identify ways of improving functioning and quality of life.

Theories and studies about aging and older adults attempt to answer questions about why and how people age, and they provide a base for identifying the risk factors that health care providers can address. However, they do not address *nursing* care of older adults, as does a nursing theory that explains relationships among the core concepts of person, nursing, health, and environment. The Functional Consequences Theory for Promoting Wellness in Older Adults, which is the focus of this chapter, is a framework for applying the nursing process to holistically caring for older adults.

A NURSING THEORY FOR WELLNESS-FOCUSED CARE OF OLDER ADULTS

During the 1980s, this author proposed a model for gerontological nursing, which was the organizational framework for the first edition of this book (Miller, 1990). Since its inception, this model has emphasized the significant role of nurses in using health education interventions to promote optimal health, functioning, and quality of life for older adults. For the fifth edition, some terminology has been revised to reflect current emphasis on adding life to years in conjunction with adding years to life. Thus, the model is now called the **Functional Consequences Theory for Promoting Wellness in Older Adults**. In addition, the revised model reflects and incorporates the increased understanding of wellness that is evolving as an integral aspect of health care. Nurses can apply this model in any situation where a goal of nursing care is to promote wellness for older adults. The theory was developed to explain questions such as *"What is unique about promoting wellness for older adults?"* and *"How can nurses address unique wellness needs of older adults?"*

Nursing theories are conceptualizations of some aspect of nursing reality that is articulated for the purpose of describing, explaining, predicating, or prescribing nursing care (Meleis, 2007). Since the time of Florence Nightingale, nurses have developed theories that address the relationships among the domains of person, nursing, health, and environment. Middle-range theories evolve from combining research and practice and building on other theories (McEwen & Wills, 2007). The Functional Consequences Theory is a middle-range theory based on results of research on aging and health and this author's almost 4 decades of providing nursing care for older adults. It also draws on theories that emphasize concepts related to wellness, health promotion, and holistic nursing.

Nurses can use the Functional Consequences Theory as a framework for addressing factors that interfere with health and functioning. Basic premises of this theory are as follows:

- Holistic nursing care addresses the body–mind–spirit interconnectedness of each older adult and recognizes that wellness encompasses more than physiologic functioning.
- Although age-related changes are inevitable, most problems affecting older adults are caused by risk factors.
- Older adults experience positive or negative functional consequences because of a combination of age-related changes and additional risk factors.
- Most functional consequences are negative, but they can be addressed through interventions directed toward alleviating or modifying the effects of risk factors.
- Nurses can promote wellness in older adults through health promotion interventions and other nursing actions that address the negative functional consequences.
- Nursing interventions result in positive functional consequences (also called **wellness outcomes**), which enable older people to function at their highest level despite the presence of age-related changes and risk factors.

This theoretical framework, diagrammed in Figure 2-1, can be illustrated by the following example. A negative functional consequence of age-related changes affecting vision is an increased sensitivity to glare. Thus, older people have difficulty seeing clearly when they face bright lights or when lights reflect off shiny surfaces. They have increased difficulty, for instance, driving toward the sunlight or reading shopping mall maps that are enclosed in glass cases. In addition to this age-related change, older adults might have disease-related risk factors that cause similar negative functional consequences. For example, cataracts may cause blurred vision and increased sensitivity to glare. Environmental conditions that intensify glare include bright lights, highly polished floors, and white or glossy paint. These age-related changes and risk factors can interfere with the visual abilities to the extent that older adults stop performing activities or perform them unsafely. To counteract these negative functional consequences, the older person or a nurse can initiate any of the following interventions, which are discussed in Chapter 17:

- Wearing sunglasses and using glare-reducing glasses (self-care)
- Addressing environmental conditions by using adequate nonglare lighting (self-care)
- Obtaining periodic evaluations from an ophthalmologist (self-care)
- Teaching about the use of sunglasses and glare-reducing glasses (nursing action)
- Teaching about environmental modifications (nursing action)
- Taking actions to avoid glare (e.g., not standing in front of a bright window when talking with an older adult) (nursing action)
- Teaching older adults about the importance of having their eyes evaluated at least annually for treatable conditions (nursing action)

Wellness outcomes resulting from these interventions include improved safety, function, and quality of life.

CONCEPTS UNDERLYING THE FUNCTIONAL CONSEQUENCES THEORY

The Functional Consequences Theory draws from theories that are pertinent to aging, older adults, and holistic nursing. The nursing domain concepts of person, environment, health, and nursing are linked together specifically in relation to older adults. Before discussing these domain concepts, however, the concepts of functional consequences, age-related changes, and risk factors are explained. Box 2-1 summarizes the key concepts in the Functional Consequences Theory for promoting wellness in older adults.

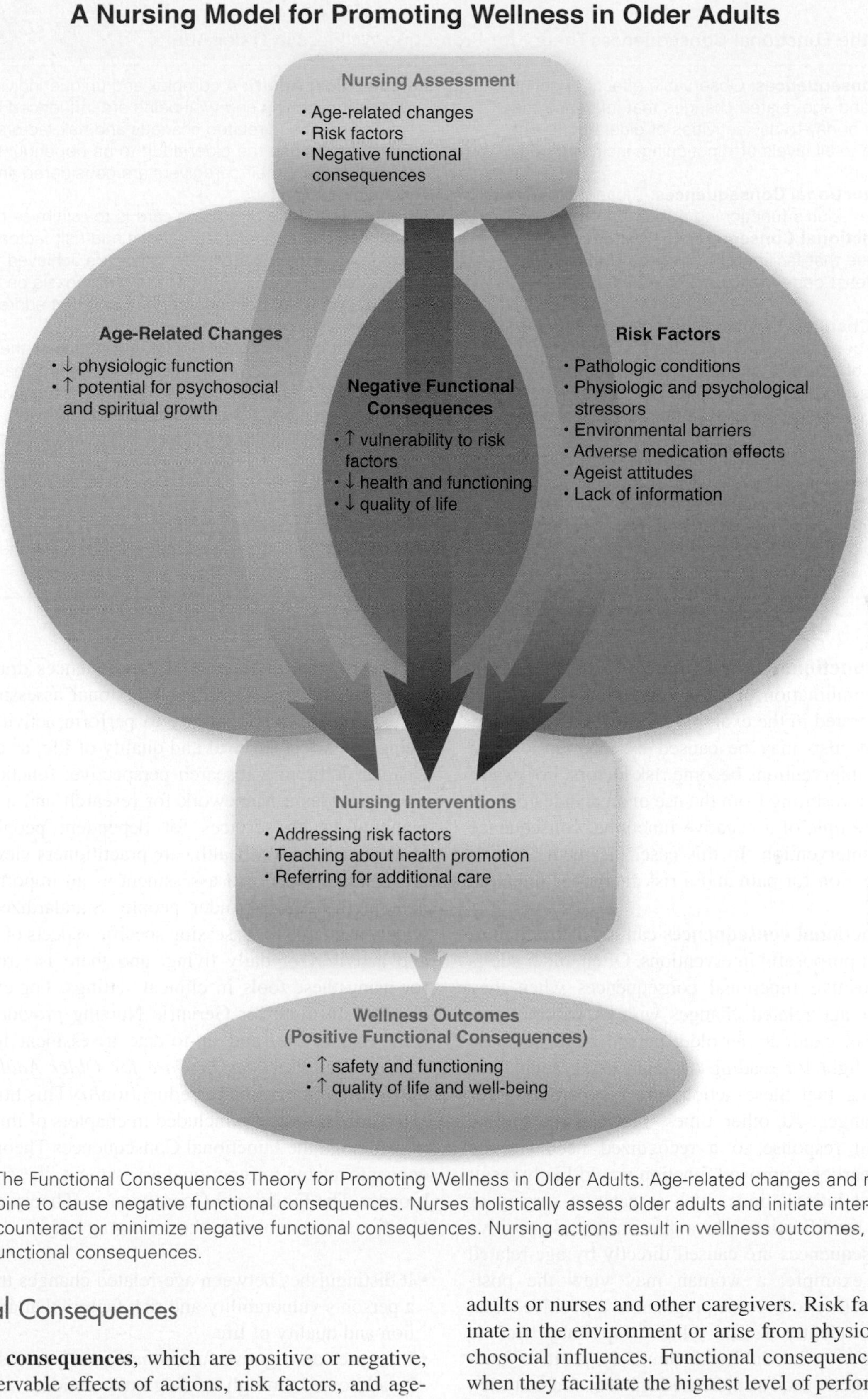

A Nursing Model for Promoting Wellness in Older Adults

Nursing Assessment
- Age-related changes
- Risk factors
- Negative functional consequences

Age-Related Changes
- ↓ physiologic function
- ↑ potential for psychosocial and spiritual growth

Negative Functional Consequences
- ↑ vulnerability to risk factors
- ↓ health and functioning
- ↓ quality of life

Risk Factors
- Pathologic conditions
- Physiologic and psychological stressors
- Environmental barriers
- Adverse medication effects
- Ageist attitudes
- Lack of information

Nursing Interventions
- Addressing risk factors
- Teaching about health promotion
- Referring for additional care

Wellness Outcomes (Positive Functional Consequences)
- ↑ safety and functioning
- ↑ quality of life and well-being

FIGURE 2-1 The Functional Consequences Theory for Promoting Wellness in Older Adults. Age-related changes and risk factors combine to cause negative functional consequences. Nurses holistically assess older adults and initiate interventions to counteract or minimize negative functional consequences. Nursing actions result in wellness outcomes, or positive functional consequences.

Functional Consequences

Functional consequences, which are positive or negative, are the observable effects of actions, risk factors, and age-related changes that influence the quality of life or day-to-day activities of older adults. Actions include, but are not limited to, purposeful interventions initiated by either older adults or nurses and other caregivers. Risk factors can originate in the environment or arise from physiologic and psychosocial influences. Functional consequences are positive when they facilitate the highest level of performance and the least amount of dependency. Conversely, they are negative when they interfere with a person's level of function or quality of life or increase a person's dependency.

Box 2-1
Concepts in the Functional Consequences Theory for Promoting Wellness in Older Adults

Functional Consequences: Observable effects of actions, risk factors, and age-related changes that influence the quality of life or day-to-day activities of older adults. The effects relate to all levels of functioning, including body, mind, and spirit.

- **Negative Functional Consequences:** Those that interfere with the older adult's functioning or quality of life.
- **Positive Functional Consequences (Wellness Outcomes):** Those that facilitate the highest level of functioning, the least dependency, and the best quality of life.

Age-Related Changes: Inevitable, progressive, and irreversible changes that occur during later adulthood and are independent of extrinsic or pathologic conditions. On the physiologic level, these changes are typically degenerative; however, on psychological and spiritual levels they include potential for growth.

Risk Factors: Conditions that increase the vulnerability of older adults to negative functional consequences. Common sources of risk factors include diseases, environment, lifestyle, support systems, psychosocial circumstances, adverse medication effects, and attitudes based on lack of knowledge.

Person (Older Adult): A complex and unique individual whose functioning and well-being are influenced by the acquisition of age-related changes and risk factors. When risk factors cause the older adult to be dependent on others for daily needs, their caregivers are considered an integral focus of nursing care.

Nursing: The focus of nursing care is to minimize the negative effects of age-related changes and risk factors and to promote wellness outcomes. Goals are achieved through the nursing process, with particular emphasis on health promotion and other nursing interventions that address the negative functional consequences.

Health: The ability of older adults to function at their highest capacity, despite the presence of age-related changes and risk factors. It is not limited to physiologic function and encompasses psychosocial and spiritual function. Thus, it addresses well-being and quality of life as defined by each older adult.

Environment: External conditions, including caregivers, that influence the body, mind, spirit, and functioning of older adults. Environmental conditions are risk factors when they interfere with function, and they are interventions when they enhance function.

Negative functional consequences typically occur because of a combination of age-related changes and risk factors, as illustrated in the example of impaired visual performance. They also may be caused by interventions, in which case the interventions become risk factors. For example, constipation resulting from the use of an analgesic medication is an example of a negative functional consequence caused by an intervention. In this case, the medication is both an intervention for pain and a risk factor for impaired bowel function.

Positive functional consequences can result from automatic actions or purposeful interventions. Often, older adults bring about positive functional consequences when they compensate for age-related changes with or without conscious intent. For example, an older person might increase the amount of light for reading or begin using sunglasses without realizing that these actions are compensating for age-related changes. At other times, older adults initiate interventions in response to a recognized need. In the example cited earlier, improved function would likely result from purposeful interventions, such as cataract surgery or environmental modifications. In a few instances, positive functional consequences are caused directly by age-related changes. For example, a woman may view the postmenopausal inability to become pregnant as a positive effect of aging. Consequently, sexual relationships may become more satisfying in later adulthood. Similarly, positive functional consequences, such as increased wisdom and maturity, can result from psychological growth in older adulthood. In the context of the nursing process, positive functional consequences are equivalent to wellness outcomes.

The concept of functional consequences draws on concepts and research regarding functional assessment, which focuses on a person's ability to perform activities of daily living that affect survival and quality of life, as discussed in Chapter 7. From a research perspective, functional assessment provides a framework for research and a method for planning health services for dependent people. From a clinical perspective, health care practitioners view the multidimensional functional assessment as an important component in the care of older people. Standardized tools are widely available for assessing specific aspects of functioning and activities of daily living, and there is strong support for using these tools in clinical settings. For example, the Hartford Institute for Geriatric Nursing provides standardized, easy-to-use, and up-to-date assessment tools identified as *Best Practices in Care for Older Adults* at www.hartfordign.org/resources/education/tryThis.html. Many standardized tools are included in chapters of this book.

Although the Functional Consequences Theory draws on concepts related to functional assessment, its scope is much broader. The Functional Consequences Theory differs from functional assessment in the following ways:

- It distinguishes between age-related changes that increase a person's vulnerability and risk factors that affect function and quality of life.
- It focuses on negative functional consequences that can be addressed through nursing interventions.
- It focuses on assessment of conditions that affect functioning, rather than simply identifying a person's functional level.

- It leads to interventions that address negative functional consequences.
- It leads to wellness outcomes, such as improved functioning and quality of life.

Age-Related Changes and Risk Factors

A unique challenge of caring for older adults is the need to differentiate between age-related changes and risk factors, because the interventions for age-related changes differ from those for risk factors. Age-related changes cannot be reversed or altered, but it is possible to compensate for their effects so that wellness outcomes are achieved. By contrast, risk factors can be modified or eliminated to diminish or prevent negative functional consequences.

In the Functional Consequences Theory, **age-related changes** are the inherent physiologic processes that increase the vulnerability of older people to the negative impact of risk factors. From a body–mind–spirit perspective, however, age-related changes are not limited to physiologic aspects, but include potential for increased cognitive, emotional, and spiritual development. Thus, nurses holistically focus on the whole person by identifying age-related changes that can be strengthened to improve the older adult's ability to adapt to physiologic decline. For example, nurses can work with older adults to strengthen their coping skills, as discussed in Chapter 12. In addition, nurses have many opportunities to build on the wisdom of older adults, especially their "everyday problem-solving" skills (as discussed in Chapter 11) by teaching about interventions to address risk factors.

The definition of age-related changes in the context of the Functional Consequences Theory draws primarily on research on aging. Biologic theories can help differentiate between age-related and disease-related processes; however, there usually is some overlap among these processes, as discussed in Chapter 3. In addition to biologic theories of aging, other theories about aging and older adulthood can shed light on age-related changes that contribute to the ability of older adults to respond to the challenges of aging.

A Student's Perspective

Most older adults live outside nursing homes and are actively involved in maintaining their independence and functional abilities as much as possible. Having worked in an acute care setting for many years, it is very easy for me to assume that all older adults have many underlying chronic diseases and do very little to comply with their medical therapies. It does help to separate what is a part of the aging process from what is part of a chronic condition, since problems resulting from chronic conditions may be receptive to medical and nursing interventions.

Darris C.

Chapters in Parts 3 and 4 of this book discuss research on age-related changes pertinent to specific aspects of functioning.

Risk factors are the conditions that are likely to occur in older adults and have a significant detrimental effect on their health and functioning. Risk factors commonly arise from environments, acute and chronic conditions, psychosocial conditions, or adverse medication effects. Although many risk factors also occur in younger adults, they are more likely to have serious functional consequences in older adults because of the following characteristics:

- They are cumulative and progressive (e.g., long-term effects of smoking, obesity, inadequate exercise, or poor dietary habits).
- The effects are exacerbated by age-related changes (e.g., effects of arthritis are exacerbated by diminished muscle strength).
- The effects may be mistakenly viewed as age-related changes rather than reversible and treatable conditions (e.g., mental changes from adverse medication effects may be attributed to normal aging or dementia).
- They would not have negative functional consequences in a younger person (e.g., glare or background noise would not affect the vision or hearing of someone who is not experiencing age-related sensory changes).

Researchers and health care providers commonly address risk factors in relation to prevention and treatment of medical conditions. For example, evidence-based practice emphasizes weighing the probable risks versus benefits for pharmacologic or surgical treatments. Similarly, studies are focusing on identifying factors that increase the chance of developing conditions, such as heart disease, so these risks can be addressed through health promotion interventions.

Nurses incorporate the concept of risk factors in many aspects of the nursing process. For example, many nursing diagnoses, interventions, and outcomes address Risk Control, Risk Identification, or Risk Detection. In particular, nurses identify risk factors that they can address through health promotion interventions. For example, from a holistic perspective, nurses routinely assess for risks associated with stress, smoking, obesity, poor nutrition, and inadequate physical activity. A unique aspect of caring for older adults is the need to assess for risk factors associated with myths or ageist attitudes that can affect interventions. For example, if urinary incontinence is mistakenly attributed to "normal" aging, then the older adult will not receive appropriate evaluation and interventions. Environmental risks are also particularly pertinent to older adults because additional risk factors, such as sensory, mobility, or cognitive impairments, can compromise their safety and functioning. Risk factors are a major focus of the Functional Consequences Theory because nurses have numerous opportunities for promoting wellness by identifying and addressing the many modifiable factors that affect functioning and quality of life for older adults.

Person

In the Functional Consequences Theory, the concept of **person** applies specifically to older adults. Because the holistic approach of the theory views each **older adult** as a complex and unique individual whose functioning and well-being is influenced by many internal and external factors, older adults are not defined simply according to chronologic criteria. From this perspective, an older adult is characterized by the acquisition of physiologic and psychosocial characteristics that are associated with increasing maturity. These characteristics include slowing down of physiologic processes, increased vulnerability to pathologic conditions and other risk factors, and compromised ability to respond to physiologic stress. In addition, older adults are characterized by an increased potential for wisdom, creativity, and other psychosocial strengths, and the potential for advanced levels of personal and spiritual growth.

Because aging is a complex and gradual process involving all aspects of body, mind, and spirit, a person does not suddenly become an older adult at a particular chronologic age. Rather, people who live long enough recognize at some point that they have reached a stage of life that society categorizes as older adulthood. When they reach this point, they may or may not identify with social labels, such as elder, senior, or older adults. Although this concept has the distinct disadvantage of being difficult to measure, it has the advantage of accurately reflecting the realities of older adulthood as a continuum within the life-course continuum. Because people become more heterogeneous rather than homogeneous as they age, any definition of the older adult must, by its nature, be broad. In the context of the Functional Consequences Theory, an individual is an older adult when he or she manifests several or many functional consequences attributable to age-related changes alone, or to age-related changes in combination with risk factors. Stated simply, the accumulation of age-related functional consequences defines someone as an older adult. Moreover, because aging involves many gradual, interacting, and cumulative processes, each older adult experiences his or her own unique continuum. This concept is applied in the progressive case examples in chapters of Parts 3 and 4 of this book, which illustrate the progression of one person from young–old to old–old as he or she is affected by functional consequences pertinent to a particular aspect of functioning.

The older adult is further conceptualized in the context of his or her relationships with others because a person is not an isolated entity, but a dynamic being who continually influences and is influenced by the environment and other people. This context is particularly important for older adults because the more functionally impaired a person is, the more important are support resources and environmental factors. When negative functional consequences accumulate to the extent that the older adult is very dependent on others for daily needs, nurses shift their primary focus to working with caregivers to identify and implement interventions. Even for older adults who do not rely on others for assistance, this context is important because older people have a long history of interpersonal relationships that influence their health behaviors and well-being. Thus, nurses assess and address the needs of older adults in the context of their relationships.

Madeleine Leininger's Theory of Culture Care Diversity and Universality is particularly relevant to this conceptualization of older adults because it emphasizes the importance of honoring individuality and respecting each person's values (Leininger & McFarland, 2002). Although no characteristics apply universally to all older adults, the cumulative effects of aging affect them all and they are all vulnerable to the effects of risk factors. Nurses need to be knowledgeable about both the facts and myths about normal aging so that they can implement interventions to address negative functional consequences. Moreover, nurses need to assess each older adult's unique response to the effects of aging and risk factors in order to implement appropriate interventions to improve function and quality of life. For example, Leininger's theory reminds nurses that an important part of every assessment is to identify cultural factors that are likely to influence the person. Similarly, the Functional Consequences Theory emphasizes the importance of identifying and respecting the unique characteristics of each older adult that affect his or her functioning and well-being.

Nursing

The conceptualization of **nursing** in the Functional Consequences Theory draws on many nursing theorists, including the following examples (McEwen & Wills, 2007; Meleis, 2007):

- Florence Nightingale: Nurses foster an environment conducive to healing and health promotion.
- Virginia Henderson: Nurses provide assistance with daily activities to help gain independence as rapidly as possible.
- Modeling and Role-Modeling Theory: Nursing is an interactive, interpersonal process that nurtures strengths to achieve a state of perceived holistic health.
- Imogene King: Nurse and client interact to achieve a specific health-related goal.
- Jean Watson: Nursing consists of knowledge, thought, values, philosophy, commitment, and action with passion in human care transactions.
- Martha Rogers: Nurses promote person–environment interactions for unitary human beings.
- Margaret Newman: Nursing is the act of assisting people to use their power to evolve toward higher levels of consciousness.

In addition to drawing on many nursing theories, the concept of nursing in the Functional Consequences Theory is consistent with the American Nurses Association statement on the scope of gerontological nursing, as discussed in Chapter 5.

Health

The Functional Consequences Theory defines **health** as the ability of older adults to function at their highest capacity, despite the presence of age-related changes and risk factors. It encompasses psychosocial as well as physiologic function, including well-being and quality of life as defined by each older adult. According to this theory, health is individually determined, based on the functional capacities that are perceived as important by that person. For example, one person might define the desired level of function as a capacity for intimate relationships, whereas another might define it as being able to perform aerobic exercise for half an hour daily. Wellness is a closely related concept (defined in Chapter 1) that is used throughout this book in reference to outcomes that address the person's highest potential for well-being.

Some nursing definitions that expand on and support the conceptualization of health in the Functional Consequences Theory include the following (Leininger & McFarland, 2002; McEwen & Wills, 2007):

- Florence Nightingale: to be well, but to be able to use well every power we have
- Imogene King: a dynamic life experience involving continuous adjustment to stressors through optimum use of one's resources to achieve maximum potential for daily living
- Calista Roy: a state and process of being and becoming integrated and whole
- Jean Watson: unity and harmony within the mind, body, and soul; congruence between the self as perceived and the self as experienced
- Margaret Newman: expanding consciousness; evolving pattern of the whole of life
- Rosemarie Parse: a way of being in the world; the living of day-to-day ways of being
- Madeleine Leininger: a state of well-being that is culturally constituted, defined, valued, and practiced by individuals or groups that enables them to function in their daily lives

Many non-nursing definitions view health of older adults in relation to fitness, functioning, and quality of life.

Older adults themselves associate successful aging with good health and high-level functioning; however, they view optimal aging as the ability to "maximize whatever health one has by having the good judgment to avoid agents that accelerate the aging process and promoting those that retard it. Nonetheless, a certain level of detachment and wisdom may be necessary to learn to accept whatever level of illness and disability one has, thereby preserving mental health and as much social functioning as possible within the confines of disability" (Aldwin et al., 2006, pp. 98–99). A nursing study found that perceptions of health for people aged 65 to 79 years was associated with self-esteem and a sense of coherence; for people aged 80 and older a sense of mastery was strongly associated with perceived health (Forbes, 2001). Other studies also indicate that older adults view health in relation to optimal functioning in physical as well as psychosocial dimensions (Damron-Rodriguez et al., 2005; Radcliffe-Branch & Tannenbaum, 2006; Young & Cochrane, 2004).

Environment

In the Functional Consequences Theory, **environment** is a broad concept that includes all aspects of the setting in which the care is provided; for dependent older adults, the environment also includes their caregivers. Some aspects of the conceptualization may seem to be contradictory because the environment can be both a risk factor for negative functional consequences and a source of interventions for positive functional consequences. For example, the environment is a risk factor when it interferes with functioning (e.g., glare or poor lighting), but it is an intervention when it is used to improve functioning (e.g., grab bars, or bright and nonglare lighting).

The following are some definitions of environment from nursing theories that are pertinent to the Functional Consequences Theory (McEwen & Wills, 2007):

- Florence Nightingale: a healthy environment is essential for healing and includes specific aspects such as noise level, cleanliness, and nutritious food
- Madeleine Leininger: the totality of an event, situation, or particular experience that gives meaning to human expressions, interpretations, and social interactions in particular physical, ecologic, sociopolitical, and cultural settings
- Imogene King: the background for human interactions, which is both internal and external to the individual
- Margaret Newman: all internal and external factors of influences that surround the client or system
- Calista Roy: all conditions, circumstances, and influences that surround and affect the development and behavior of humans

Since the 1970s, gerontologists have studied the influence of the environment on functioning of older adults. For example, the **competence-press model** suggests that the relationship between personal competence and environmental demands determines behavioral outcomes (Scheidt & Windley, 2006). According to this model, the more impaired a person is, the more the environment influences the person's health and functioning. The following questions, which are based on this model, are pertinent to the Functional Consequences Theory (Windley & Scheidt, 1980):

- Is the environment comfortable?
- How does the spatial organization influence orientation and direction finding?
- Can the type and amount of visual and auditory stimuli be controlled?
- How does the environment compensate for sensory deficits?

- Does the environment allow for choices in the degree of privacy and personal use of space?
- How does the environment affect activities of daily living?

The Functional Consequences Theory provides a framework for addressing questions such as these as an integral part of the nursing assessment and interventions.

APPLYING THE THEORY TO PROMOTE WELLNESS IN OLDER ADULTS

In the context of the Functional Consequences Theory, nurses direct their care toward minimizing the effects of negative functional consequences and promoting wellness outcomes for older adults. The focus and goals of this type of care vary in different settings. For acute care, the focus is on treatment of pathologic conditions that create serious risks; goals include helping vulnerable older adults recover from illness and maintain or improve their level of functioning. For long-term care, the focus is on addressing multiple risk factors that interfere with functional abilities; goals include improved functioning and quality of life. For home and community settings, the focus is on short- and long-term interventions aimed at age-related changes and risk factors; goals include improving or preventing declines in functioning and addressing quality-of-life concerns. In all settings, nurses can incorporate wellness outcomes to address each older adult's personal aspirations toward well-being of body, mind, and spirit.

Nurses apply the nursing process to assess age-related changes and risk factors, identify nursing diagnoses, plan wellness outcomes, implement nursing interventions to address negative functional consequences, and evaluate the effectiveness of their interventions. A major focus of nursing care is on educating older adults and the caregivers of dependent older adults about interventions that will eliminate risk factors or minimize their effects. The educational aspects are particularly important when myths and misunderstandings contribute to negative functional consequences. For example, nurses can provide information about age-related changes and risk factors to an older person who believes that functional impairments are a necessary consequence of old age and identify ways of minimizing the effects of risk factors and compensating for the effects of age-related changes.

Nurses have recently developed a middle-range theory for fostering generative quality of life for the elderly that is pertinent to the concepts in the Functional Consequences Theory. According to this model, nurses direct their care toward establishing "patient-centered connections that would result in generative elders who would seek to establish or sustain a variety of connections in response to the forces and processes they encounter on a daily basis" (Register & Herman, 2006, p. 347). Register and Herman suggest the following examples of generative nursing interventions, which are based on this model, to address specific aspects of quality of life for older adults:

- Metaphysical connectedness: teaching about guided imagery, journaling activities, and activities that increase self-esteem and a sense of optimism
- Spiritual connectedness: arranging transportation to local church services or making referrals to faith-based groups
- Biologic connectedness: facilitating participation in congregate meals, doing group exercises to big band music
- Connectedness to others: providing comfort touch, encouraging participation in social and educational activities
- Environmental connectedness: encouraging and facilitating activities out in nature, referring for transportation resources
- Connectedness to society: providing information about support resources, helping older adults develop contingency plans for emergencies

Providing nursing care for older adults is both challenging and rewarding, despite the common perception that it is futile and discouraging. Unfortunately, negative attitudes about aging carry over to attitudes about gerontological nursing, so nursing care of older adults is often associated with limited goals and little chance of helping patients achieve a higher level of functioning (Gething et al., 2004; Lovell, 2006; Wells et al., 2004). This perception may be applicable in situations in which the older adult is experiencing terminal or progressive conditions; however, even in those situations, it applies only to the physical aspects of care. There is still potential for achieving higher levels of psychological or spiritual functioning. Even older adults who have dementia and other progressive conditions that can profoundly affect psychological function may have potential for spiritual growth in ways that are not always observable or measurable.

The Functional Consequences Theory helps nurses see older adults as more than an accumulation of age-related physiologic changes and pathologic conditions leading to diminished functioning. Thus, it provides a framework for promoting wellness because it addresses the whole-person needs of the older adult and his or her relationships with self, others, and the environment. It reminds nurses to identify strengths and potentials in relation not only to physical aspects of functioning but to psychological and spiritual well-being. Moreover, it leads to nursing interventions directed toward achieving wellness outcomes, such as improved quality of life for older adults.

CHAPTER HIGHLIGHTS

A Nursing Theory for Wellness-Focused Care of Older Adults

- The Functional Consequences Theory explains the unique relationships among the concepts of person, health, nursing, and environment in the context of promoting wellness for older adults.

Concepts Underlying the Functional Consequences Theory

- Combinations of age-related changes and risk factors increase the vulnerability of older people to negative functional consequences, which interfere with the person's level of functioning or quality of life.
- Nurses assess the age-related changes, risk factors, and negative functional consequences, with particular emphasis on identifying the risk factors that can be addressed through nursing interventions.
- Wellness outcomes are achieved by enabling older adults to function at their highest level despite the presence of age-related changes and risk factors.

Applying the Theory to Promote Wellness in Older Adults

- Nurses can incorporate wellness outcomes to address each older adult's personal aspirations for well-being of body, mind, and spirit.
- Nurses educate older adults and caregivers about interventions to minimize risk factors or their effects.
- Providing nursing care for older adults is rewarding when approached from a holistic perspective that sees opportunities for wellness in physical, psychological, and spiritual aspects of function.

Critical Thinking Exercises

Bring to your mind a vivid image of an older friend, relative, or patient who is at least 80 years old, and apply the following questions to one obvious negative functional consequence (e.g., impaired mobility). Develop an opportunity to talk with that person about what you have learned about the Functional Consequences Theory for Promoting Wellness in Older Adults, and use Figure 2-1 as a basis for discussion.

1. What age-related changes and risk factors interact to contribute to this negative functional consequence?
2. What environmental conditions either improve or interfere with the affected aspect of functioning?
3. How can you use your nursing knowledge to improve health and quality of life in relation to that aspect of functioning?

Educational Resources

Hartford Institute for Geriatric Nursing
www.hartfordign.org

National Gerontological Nursing Association (NGNA)
www ngna.org

National Institute of Nursing Research
www.nih.gov/ninr

References

Aldwin, C. M., Spiro III, A., & Park, C. L. (2006). Health, behavior, and optimal aging: A life span developmental perspective. In J. E. Birren & K. W. Schaie (Eds.), *Handbook of the psychology of aging* (6th ed., pp. 85–104). San Diego: Elsevier Academic Press.

Damron-Rodriguez, J., Frank, J. C., Enriquez-Haass, V. L., & Reuben, D. B. (2005). Definitions of health among diverse groups of elders: Implications for health promotion. *Generations, 29*(2), 11–16.

Forbes, D. A. (2001). Enhancing mastery and sense of coherence: Important determinants of health in older adults. *Geriatric Nursing, 22*, 29–32.

Gething, L., Fethney, J., McKee, K., Persson, L. O., Goff, M., Churchward, M., et al. (2004). Validation of the Reactions to Ageing Questionnaire: Assessing similarities across several countries. *Journal of Gerontological Nursing, 30*(9), 47–54.

Leininger, M., & McFarland, M. R. (2002). *Transcultural nursing: Concepts, theories, research and practice* (3rd ed.). New York: McGraw-Hill.

Lovell, M. (2006). Caring for the elderly: Changing perceptions and attitudes. *Journal of Vascular Nursing, 24*(1), 22–26.

McEwen, M., & Wills, E. M. (2007). *Theoretical basis for nursing* (2nd ed.). Philadelphia: Lippincott Williams & Wilkins.

Meleis, A. I. (2007). *Theoretical nursing: Development and progress* (4th ed.). Philadelphia: Lippincott Williams & Wilkins.

Miller, C. A. (1990). *Nursing care of older adults: Theory and practice.* Glenview, IL: Scott, Forsman/Little, Brown Higher Education.

Radcliffe-Branch, D., & Tannenbaum, C. (2006). A review of older women's health priorities. *Geriatrics and Ageing, 9*, 124–128.

Register, M. E., & Herman, J. (2006). A middle range theory for generative quality of life for the elderly. *Advances in Nursing Science, 29*, 340–350.

Scheidt, R. J., & Windley, P. G. (2006). Environmental gerontology: Progress in the post-Lawton era. In J. E. Birren & K. W. Schaie (Eds.), *Handbook of the psychology of aging* (6th ed., pp. 105–125). San Diego: Elsevier Academic Press.

Wells, Y., Foreman, P., Gething, L., & Petralia, W. (2004). Nurses' attitudes toward aging and older adults. *Journal of Gerontological Nursing, 30*(9), 5–13.

Windley, P. G., & Scheidt, R. J. (1980). Person-environment dialectics: Implications for competent functioning in old age. In L. W. Poon (Ed.), *Aging in the 1980s* (pp. 407–423). Washington, DC: American Psychological Association.

Young, H. M., & Cochrane, B. B. (2004). Healthy aging for older women. *Nursing Clinics of North America, 39*, 131–143.

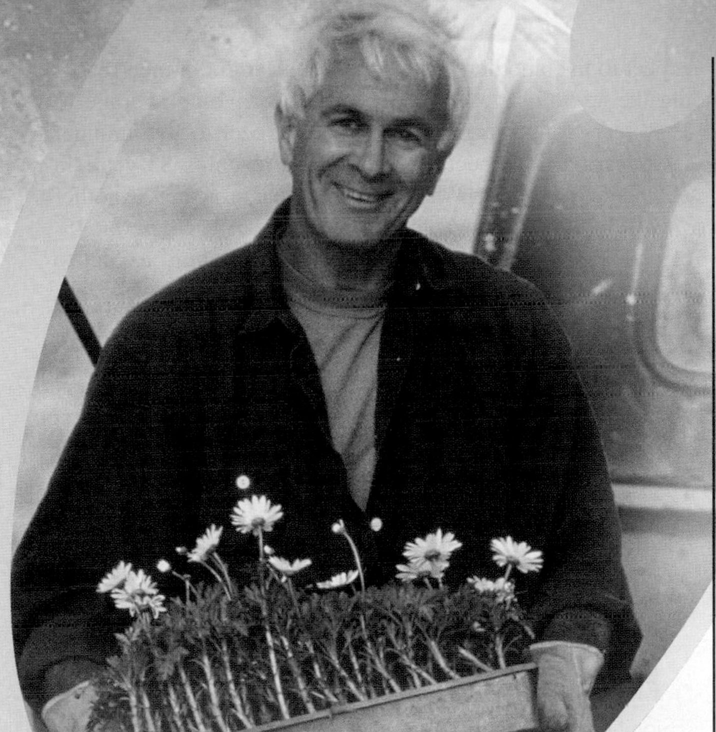

CHAPTER 3

Theoretical Perspectives on Aging Well

Learning Objectives

After reading this chapter, you will be able to:

1. Describe perspectives on the relationships among aging, disease, health, and quality of life.
2. Discuss pertinent concepts from biologic theories of aging and their relevance to nursing care of older adults.
3. Discuss pertinent concepts from sociologic theories of aging and their relevance to nursing care of older adults.
4. Discuss pertinent concepts from psychological theories of aging and their relevance to nursing care of older adults.

Key Terms

active life expectancy
activity theory
age stratification theory
apoptosis
compression of morbidity
continuity theory
cross-linkage theory
disengagement theory
free radicals theory
genetic theories
gerotranscendence
human needs theory
immunity theories
immunosenescence
life-course theories
life expectancy
life span
neuroendocrine theories
person–environment fit theory
primary aging
rectangularization of the curve
secondary aging
senescence
subculture theory
wear-and-tear theory

People have always looked for answers to universal questions such as *How long can we live? Why do we age?* and *How can we prevent the unwanted effects of aging?* Since early times, scientists and philosophers have tried to answer these questions, beginning with early theories that addressed biologic aging. For example, Aristotle, Hippocrates, Galen, and other early philosopher-scientists associated aging with a decrease in body heat and fluid. As scientists learned more about aging, it became clear that aging is, in fact, an extremely complex and variable process. During the 20th century, theorists explained aging from the following three perspectives: (1) biologic age, encompassing measures of functional capacities of vital or life-limiting organ systems; (2) sociologic age, involving the roles and age-graded behaviors of people in response to the society of which they are a part; and (3) psychological age, referring to the behavioral capacities of people to adapt to changing environmental demands.

Today, the foremost question about aging is *How can we live both long and well?* There is no simple answer to this question; however, there are many theoretical perspectives on aging that lead toward answers. Increasingly, all health care practitioners are recognizing that adults of all ages view health as a resource for doing the things they want to do and see their goal as longevity with good function (Breslow, 2006). By drawing on knowledge from biologic, sociologic, and psychological theories of aging, gerontologists and health care professionals identify the factors that contribute to a long and healthy life. This chapter addresses questions about aging from various theoretical perspectives and focuses on perspectives about how we can live both long and well. A major emphasis of this chapter is on concepts that are most relevant to the role of nurses in supporting "successful aging" through nursing interventions that promote wellness in older adults.

HOW CAN WE LIVE LONG AND WELL?

One way of addressing the question *How long can we live?* is by measuring life span, life expectancy, morbidity, and mortality rates. Another way to address this question—and an approach that is particularly relevant to health care practitioners—is through exploring the relationship among aging, health, and disease. Early theories focused on problems of aging and diseases associated with aging, but more recent theories address the relationships among aging, health, and health-related behaviors. The ultimate goal of gerontology research is to apply the discoveries about health and aging to enhance quality of life and reduce the likelihood of premature morbidity, disability, and death (Ferraro, 2006).

Life Span and Life Expectancy

Two measures that gerontologists use to address questions about how long we can live are life span and life expectancy. **Life span**, defined as the maximum survival potential for a member of a species, is about 116 years for humans. **Life expectancy** is the predictable length of time that one is expected to live from a specific point in time, such as birth. Life span is relatively fixed, as evident by the barely perceptible extensions that occur over the evolutionary time scale; however, life expectancy has been increasing rapidly. For example, in developed countries, life expectancy increased as much between 1900 and 2000 as it had increased over the previous 2000 years (Hayflick, 2001-02) (Fig. 3-1). Similarly, in 1900, people reaching the age of 65 years could expect to live another 12 years; in the year 2000, men reaching the age of 65 years could expect to live an average of 16.3 years longer and women could expect to live another 19.2 years. Life expectancy for people reaching 85 years in 2000 is 6.7 years for women and 5.6 years for men. Another way of looking at this is to consider that, in 1940, about 7% of people who reached the age of 65 years could expect to survive to 90 years of age. In 2000, that percentage was 26%, and by 2050, that percentage is expected to increase to 42%. Projections for 2050 estimate that life expectancy will be 82 years, and that people aged 65 years and older will represent about 20% of the population. Projections for the mid-21st century are that average life expectancy will level off at the age of 85 years, barring unforeseen breakthroughs in biotechnology (Hazzard, 2001). This is because the inherent teleology of human beings indicates that we are genetically programmed to live for about 100 years, even under the best of circumstances.

Diversity Note

Significant racial variation exists in life expectancy rates. In 2003, life expectancy for whites and African Americans, respectively, was 78 and 72.8 years at birth. The life expectancy of Asians and Pacific Islanders is higher than that of any other group in the United States.

Mortality Rates and the Rectangularization of the Curve

Mortality rates are graphically represented in a survivorship curve, which illustrates the changes occurring in death rates over different periods of time (Fig. 3-2). The vertical axis designates the percentage of survivors, whereas the horizon-

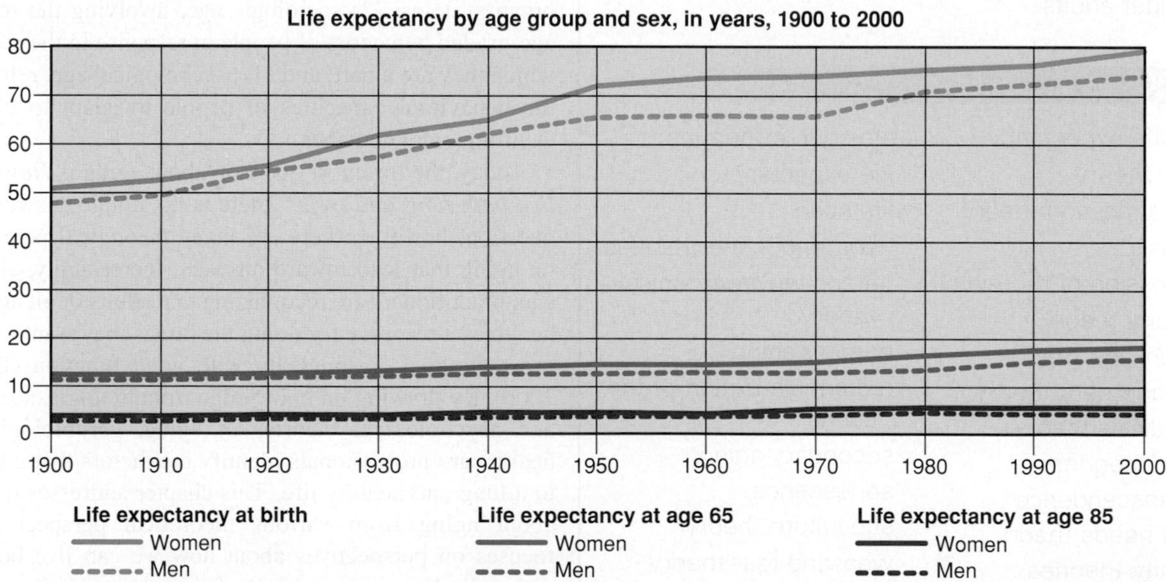

FIGURE 3-1 Changes in life expectancy from 1900 to 2000 for men and women, at birth, age 65 years, and age 85 years. (From National Vital Statistics System.)

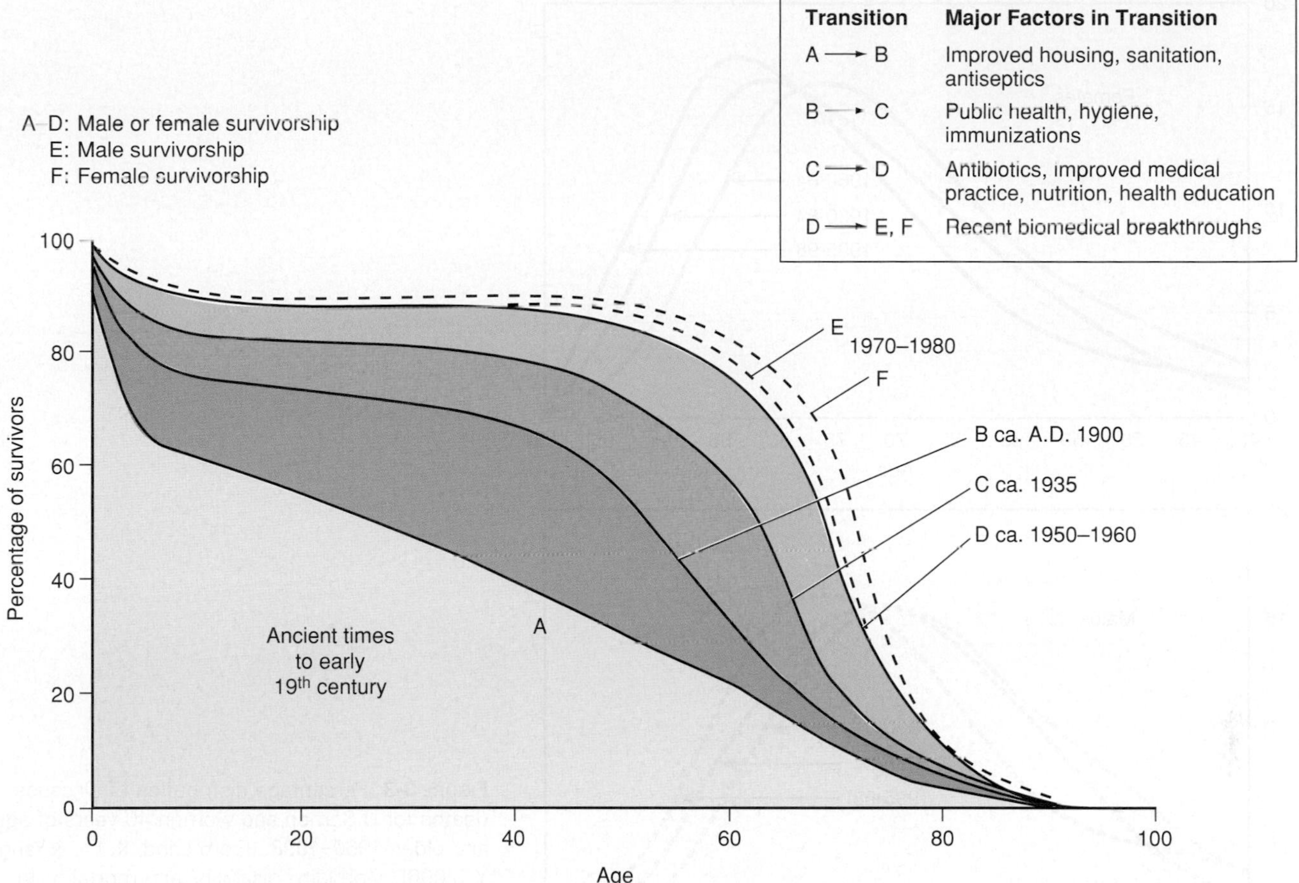

FIGURE 3-2 Human survivorship curve. (Adapted from Strehler, B. L. [1975]. Implications of aging research for society. *Proceedings of the Federation of American Societies for Experimental Biology, 34*, 6. Used with permission.)

tal axis represents the age of survivorship. Since the 1980s, the rate of increase in average longevity has continued to rise, but the pace of increase has slowed. This change in pace has resulted in the squaring of the human survival curve, meaning that life expectancy is not significantly prolonged at the age of 75 or 80 years. This **rectangularization of the curve** is attributed to changes caused by various significant factors occurring at different points in time. The first major change in survival resulted from improved housing and sanitation practices, and the second major change was brought about by the advent of immunization programs and other advances in public health practices. The third major change, occurring between 1960 and 1980, is attributable to biomedical breakthroughs, such as organ transplants, heart–lung machines, and increasingly effective cancer treatments. As one public health physician noted, we have progressed beyond the two eras of communicable and chronic disease and entered the third era of health, in which "people in their 70s and 80s are increasingly free of disease burdens" (Breslow, 2006, p. 17).

For many years, gerontologists identified the three stages of the epidemiologic shifts in causes of mortality as the ages of (1) pestilence and famine, (2) receding pandemics, and (3) degenerative and man-made diseases. More recently, gerontologists identified a fourth stage—the age of delayed degenerative diseases—characterized by the later onset of death from diseases that cause disability and chronic illness (Land & Yang, 2006). Figure 3-3 illustrates differences in the survival curve that occurred between 1960 and 1998 for men and women, indicating that the peak ages at death are older for women during all periods. There is much agreement that continued extension of life expectancy depends on integration of health behaviors related to weight, nutrition, exercise, blood pressure, and smoking cessation.

Active Life Expectancy

Although it is clear that increased life expectancy involves a longer time in chronic illness, it is less clear whether this is necessarily associated with a longer time in a state of disability. Thus, the focus of geriatric research and practice shifted from an emphasis on disease processes per se to an emphasis on the functional losses that are of key importance to older people. James Fries, a physician, first brought attention to this concern in an article on the **compression of morbidity**, in which he argued that the onset of significant illness could be postponed, but that one's life expectancy

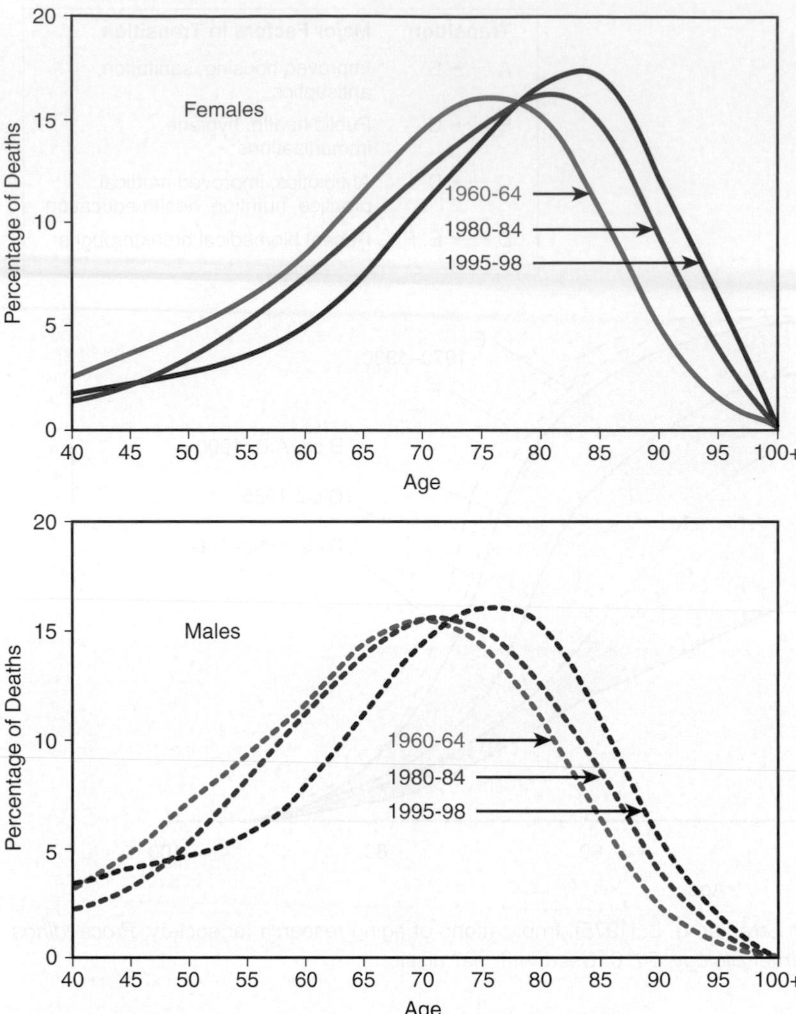

FIGURE 3-3 Percentage distribution of all-cause deaths for U.S. men and women 40 years of age and older, 1960–1998. (From Land, K. C., & Yang, Y. [2006]. Morbidity, disability, and mortality. In R. H. Binstock & L. K. George [Eds.], *Handbook of aging and the social sciences* [6th ed., pp. 41–58]. San Diego: Elsevier Academic Press. Used with permission.)

could not be extended to the same extent. Consequently, disease, disability, and functional decline are "compressed" into a period averaging 3 to 5 years before death. Fries and a colleague emphasized that preventive approaches must be directed toward preserving health by postponing the onset of chronic illnesses (Fries & Crapo, 1981).

In response to Fries' hypothesis, gerontologists developed the concept of **active life expectancy** as an indicator of quality of life during later adulthood. Active life expectancy is measured on a continuum of four states, ranging from inability to perform activities of daily living to full independent functioning (Crimmins et al., 1996). Since the 1990s, many studies of older adults in developed countries concluded that there has been a significant reduction in the rate of functional decline over the last three decades (Mor, 2005). There is now much agreement that the period of coping with functional decline is being pushed further into later adulthood (Ferraro, 2006). Improvements in level of functioning are attributed to factors such as a more educated population of older adults and environments and medical interventions that improve function and accessibility. Increasingly, gerontologists as well as health care consumers and professionals are recognizing that continuation of this trend toward improved functioning depends on the degree to which individuals engage in healthy behaviors.

Spurred partly by the compression of morbidity theory, gerontologists have been trying to predict the probable active life expectancy for older people. This issue is of particular interest because gerontologists and older adults identify physical and functional health as a critical determinant of successful aging (Phelan et al., 2004). Using life-table methods and the activities of daily living index as a measure of health, Katz and coworkers (1983) analyzed data for community-living older people in an attempt to predict active (healthy) life expectancy. The results showed that people entering the age category of 65 to 69 years had 10 years of functional well-being remaining, whereas those in older groups had progressively fewer years. For people 85 years of age or older, the active life expectancy was 2.5 years. More recently, the U.S. Department of Health and Human Services calculated and published life expectancy and active life expectancy data for white women in the United States (Fig. 3-4).

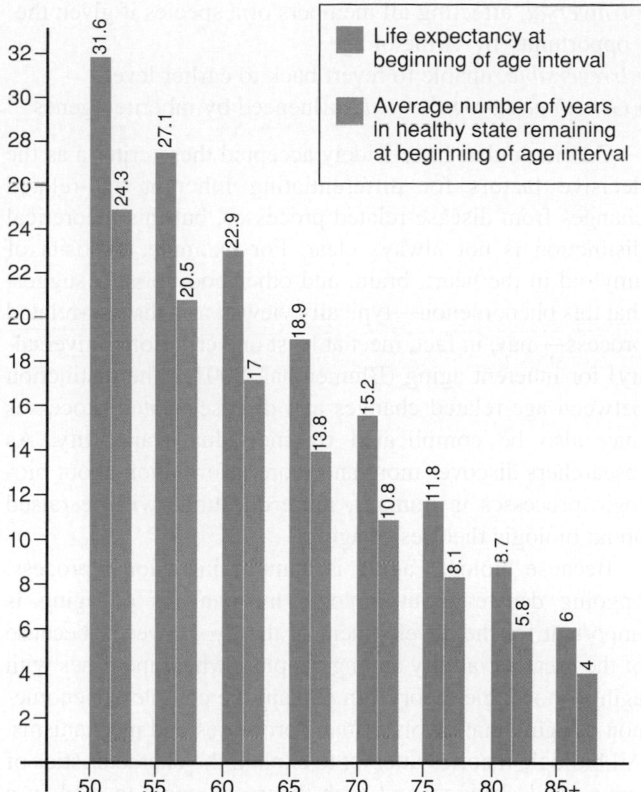

FIGURE 3-4 Graphic illustration of life expectancy and active (healthy) life expectancy for white women in the United States, 1995. (Data from Molla, M. T., Wagener, D. K., & Madans, J. H. [2001]. *Summary measures of population health: Methods for calculating healthy life expectancy.* Washington, DC: U.S. Department of Health and Human Services.)

Relationships Among Aging, Disease, and Disability

Studies of long-lived people who are healthy and functional explore the most important question of all: *How can we live a life that is not only long, but functional, productive, and satisfying?* This question is particularly relevant to the growing attention to adding quality, not just quantity, to life. Gerontologists emphasize that the ability to survive to extreme old age is the result of a complex blend of genetics, environment, lifestyle, and luck; the goal is to develop preventive and therapeutic approaches that will allow more people to age in good health (Perls, 2005).

The New England Centenarian Study is an example of longitudinal research that challenges the common perception that advanced age is always associated with increased illness and disability. Conclusions such as the following suggest advanced age may be accompanied by high levels of functioning (Evert et al., 2003; Perls, 2005):

- 90% of centenarians were functionally independent at the average age of 92 years.
- The older an individual gets, the healthier he or she has been.
- 43% and 24% of women and men, respectively, attained their 100th year as "Survivors" of an age-associated illness with onset before the age of 80 years.
- 42% and 44% of women and men, respectively, were in the "Delayers" group, in which the onset of age-associated illness occurred after the age of 80 years.
- 15% and 32% of women and men, respectively, reached their 100th birthday in the "Escapers" group, without having any age-associated condition.

Although many studies of centenarians have found that people who live to age 100 and older are relatively healthy and functional, other studies have found a high prevalence of chronic illness among centenarians (Andersen-Ranberg et al., 2001). An autopsy study of 40 nonhospitalized centenarians who experienced sudden unexpected death found that all subjects had died from a medically identifiable cause involving acute organ failure, despite the fact that 60% of the subjects were evaluated by their families and physicians as healthy before their death. Cardiovascular disease was the cause of death for 68% of the subjects, and respiratory disease accounted for 25% of the deaths. A major conclusion of this study is that centenarians are not necessarily free of disease during their later life, but they possess the ability to live longer with chronic conditions. Moreover, chronic conditions do not necessarily interfere with functioning because 29 of the 40 centenarians lived unaccompanied in their own homes, and 14 of these received no assistance with care (Berzlanovich et al., 2005).

Attempts to answer questions about the relationships between aging and death have resulted in theories about senescence. **Senescence** is defined as the progressive deterioration during adulthood that underlies an increasing vulnerability to challenges and a decreasing ability to survive (Masoro, 2006). Kohn (1982) proposed a senescence theory based on postmortem studies of 200 people who died at the age of 85 years or older. Death certificates of at least 26% of that group listed no disease process that experienced pathologists would accept as a cause of death. Kohn determined this by comparing findings from extensive postmortem examinations with the listed cause of death. When decisions about the accuracy of the cause of death were questionable, the evaluations were weighted in favor of the listed cause. Based on the results of these autopsies, Kohn concluded that, had the same degree of disease occurred in middle-aged people, the condition would not have been fatal. Thus, aging itself was thought to be the actual cause of death in a large fraction of the aged population (Kohn, 1982). Kohn further suggested that, when death in older people cannot be ascribed to a disease process that would cause death in middle-aged people, the cause of death should be listed on the death certificate as senescence. According to Kohn (1982), the relationship between aging and disease is very clear: "The aging syndrome should be viewed as a universal, progressive, and ultimately fatal disease" (p. 2797).

A variation of the senescence theory has been proposed to explain the relationships among aging, health beliefs, and health behaviors (Newquist, 1987). According to Newquist, there are three models for viewing these relationships. In the siege model, illness is viewed as a necessary concomitant of being old. The attitude of people with this perspective is "Get ready to be sick, you're old." In the senescence model, illness and aging represent the same entity. Illnesses are viewed as age-induced changes ("just old age") and are not seen as pathologic conditions. In the vanquished model, sickness is viewed as pathologic, but it is seen as something to be accepted if one is old. According to this model, not only does sickness invariably accompany old age, it is untreatable because of old age (Newquist, 1987). Newquist's perspective illustrates an approach that is in stark contrast to that taken currently by gerontological health care practitioners and it has important implications with regard to attitudes about aging.

Whether age-associated diseases are an integral part of aging is an important question related to living both long and well. Biogerontology is a subspecialty of gerontology that addresses this question. Growing evidence supports the view that at least some age-associated diseases are, in fact, an integral part of aging (Masoro, 2006). One discussion about biologic theories of aging concluded that aging and disease are not synonymous and that aging proceeds even in the absence of disease, but that "aging clearly includes increased *vulnerability* to disease" (Austad, 2001). The noted gerontologist Leonard Hayflick described the complex relationship between aging and disease as analogous to the "weak links" in automobiles. According to his analogy, both humans and particular makes and models of cars are characterized by weak links that increase the probability of component failure. For cheap cars, the "mean time to failure" is 4 or 5 years; for Americans born today, it is about 76 years. The weakest links for people in developed countries are the vascular system and the cells in which cancer commonly occurs. As Hayflick (2001-02) stated, "The aging process increases vulnerability to the pathologies that become the leading causes of death" (p. 21).

HOW DO WE EXPLAIN BIOLOGIC AGING?

Biologic theories of aging address questions about the basic aging processes that affect all living organisms. These theories answer questions such as *How do cells age?* and *What triggers the process of aging?* Gerontologists have emphasized that a biologic theory of aging must explain age-related changes that meet the following criteria (Blumenthal, 1999; Hayflick, 1988):

- *Deleterious*, resulting in reduced function
- *Progressive*, occurring gradually
- *Intrinsic*, not attributable to modifiable environmental agents
- *Universal*, affecting all members of a species if given the opportunity by virtue of age
- *Irreversible*, unable to revert back to earlier level
- *Genetically programmed*, influenced by inherited genes

Gerontologists have widely accepted these criteria as the decisive factors for differentiating inherent age-related changes from disease-related processes, but this theoretical distinction is not always clear. For example, deposits of amyloid in the heart, brain, and other body organs suggest that this phenomenon—typically viewed as a disease-related process—may, in fact, meet at least one criterion (universality) for inherent aging (Blumenthal, 2001). The distinction between age-related changes and disease-related processes may also be complicated by individual variability. As researchers discover more and more information about biologic processes in humans, more questions will be raised about biologic theories of aging.

Because biologic aging is a multidimensional process, ongoing debate about biologic mechanisms of aging is important for the development of theory. However, because of the great variability among people—which increases with aging—no single theory can explain the complex phenomenon of aging that involves many processes and mechanisms. All biologic theories attempt to explain the characteristics of age-related changes, and each theory attempts to explain a particular aspect of aging from a particular perspective. Major biologic theories are considered in this chapter, but these are only a sampling of the various perspectives that have been proposed and that continue to evolve.

Genetic Theories

Genetic theories, which emphasize the role of genes in the development of age-related changes, are one of the most complex types of biologic theories. They are also among the most intensely studied and rapidly evolving types of theories in the 21st century. One of the earliest of the genetic theories is the program theory of aging, proposed by Hayflick in the 1960s. This theory states that the life span of animals is predetermined by a genetic program, or a so-called biologic clock (Hayflick, 1965). In humans, for instance, the program allows for a maximum of about 110 years. Hayflick (1974) estimates that normal human cells divide 50 times in this number of years, and argues that cells are genetically programmed to stop dividing after achieving 50 cell divisions, at which time they begin to deteriorate. The number of times cell division takes place is different for each species of animal, and the longer a species' life expectancy, the more cell divisions that animal has in its genetic program. Abnormal cells, however, are not subject to this predictable program, and can proliferate an indefinite number of times. Some genetic theories, called *mutation theories*, suggest that aging is the result of mutations of somatic cells or alterations in DNA repair mechanisms.

Genetic theories of aging are supported by studies that indicate that life expectancy is genetically preprogrammed within a species-specific range. Many studies of life expectancies of twins, siblings, and several generations of family members have confirmed a genetic component to aging and to extreme longevity. Willcox and colleagues (2006) found that 1142 siblings of centenarians experienced approximately half the mortality as that of 1890 of their birth-cohort counterparts. Researchers are focusing on the relative effects of genetic and environmental influences and on how the influence of genetic factors changes with increased age. Results of one study found that the genetic advantage did not diminish with age, in contrast to the influence of environmentally based variables such as income and education (Willcox et al., 2006). A different perspective is that the influence of genetic factors diminishes over time because environmental insults and physiologic breakdown accumulate and have a stronger effect (Vogler, 2006).

The year 2000 saw many advances in genetic research as scientists involved with the Human Genome Project successfully identified the location of each human gene, facilitating the identification of specific genes that influence both biologic aging and age-related diseases. Ongoing developments of the Human Genome Project are likely to contribute significantly to emerging biologic theories of aging, particularly with regard to the complex interactions between aging and disease processes. For example, researchers have identified specific chromosomes that are linked to both familial and nonfamilial types of Alzheimer's disease (Vogler, 2006). A current focus of genetic research is on methods of mutating a single gene to extend longevity in humans (Binstock et al., 2006).

Wear-and-Tear Theories

The first **wear-and-tear theory** was based on a 19th-century attempt to explain the difference between immortal "germ plasm" cells—those that are capable of reproducing—and mortal "somatic" cells—those that die. In the late 1880s, August Weismann theorized that normal somatic cells were limited in their ability to replicate and function. He further postulated that death occurred because worn-out tissues could not forever renew themselves and living organisms surrendered to the "wear and tear" of life. According to the wear-and-tear theory, the body can be likened to a machine that is expected to function well during the period of its warranty, but that will wear out at a fairly predictable time. Parts can be fixed or replaced, but eventually, the machine no longer functions because of the extensive accumulation of wear and tear. Like the machine, the longevity of the human body will be affected by the care it receives, as well as by its genetic components. Unlike the machine, however, the human body can repair many of its own parts well into old age.

Harmful stress factors, such as smoking, poor diet, alcohol abuse, or muscular strain can exacerbate the wearing-out process. Microscopic signs of wear and tear in all nerve and striated muscle cells support the wear-and-tear theory of aging. Osteoarthritis, a degenerative joint condition, is an age-related process that can be explained by this theory.

Immunity Theories

Immunity theories are based on the knowledge that immune system components—particularly the thymus and immunocompetent cells in the bone marrow—are affected by the aging process. Because of this age-related diminished function of the immune system, called **immunosenescence** or immunodeficiency, the older person has fewer defenses against foreign organisms. Consequently, older people are more susceptible to cancer, infections, and autoimmune diseases, such as lupus or rheumatoid arthritis. Immunosenescence may also explain the significant increase in incidence and severity of diarrhea and other gastrointestinal infectious diseases because the gastrointestinal tract represents more than half of the human immune system (Effros, 2001).

Immunity theories also attempt to explain a relationship between diminished immune functioning and an increase in the body's autoimmune responses. When autoimmunity occurs, the body reacts against itself and produces antibodies in response to its own constituents. Age-related autoimmunity could explain the fact that older adults often manifest allergies to food and environmental conditions that they previously never experienced. Research on immunity theories is focusing on links between immune function and age-associated diseases such as Alzheimer's disease and cardiovascular disease (Effros, 2001).

Cross-Linkage Theory

The **cross-linkage theory** proposes that molecular structures that normally are separated may be bound together through chemical reactions. According to this theory, a cross-linking agent attaches itself to a single strand of a DNA molecule and damages that strand. Natural defense mechanisms usually repair the damage, but increasing age weakens these defense mechanisms, allowing the cross-linkage process to continue until irreparable damage occurs. The end result is an accumulation of cross-linking compounds that causes mutations in the cell and renders the cell unable to eliminate wastes and transport ions. This irreversible damage to the cells that form collagen-type substances eventually leads to tissue and organ failure because the protein system becomes inelastic and ineffective. This theory would explain arteriosclerosis and age-related skin changes.

Free Radicals Theory

The **free radicals theory**, first proposed in the mid-1950s (Harman, 1956), continues to provide the basis for much of the current research on aging. One discussion of biologic theories of aging suggested that "the free radicals theory of aging is the only aging theory to have stood the test of time" (Grune & Davies, 2001, p. 41). Free radicals are highly unstable and reactive molecules (particularly oxygen molecules) that form when an electron pair is separated. Free radicals can be produced by normal metabolism, reactions to irradiation, chain reactions with other free radicals, and oxidation of certain environmental pollutants, such as ozone, pesticides, and air pollutants.

Free radicals and their conjugated compounds are capable of attacking other molecules because they possess an extra electric charge, or free electron. Because they are so highly reactive, free radicals rapidly interact with and damage cellular components such as lipids, proteins, and nucleic acids. Fortunately, the human body has protective mechanisms that can interfere with oxidation activity and remove and repair damaged cells. Antioxidants, including beta-carotene and vitamins C and E, are one of the major defense mechanisms against oxidative damage from free radicals. Despite these natural mechanisms that guard against free radicals, however, a low level of oxidation occurs continuously.

The free radicals theory postulates that protective mechanisms decrease, or free radical formation increases, with advancing age. When free radicals attack molecules, they damage the cell membranes; aging is thought to occur because of cumulative cell damage that eventually interferes with function. Early support for the free radicals theory came from the discovery of lipofuscin, a pigmented waste material that is rich in lipids and proteins. This discovery led to research on lipid peroxidation, with many studies showing an age-related increase in oxidation of lipids after stress (Grune & Davies, 2001).

Research currently is focusing on developing interventions to modify or prevent the age-related accumulation of free radicals. One approach is through supplementation with natural or synthetic antioxidants, such as melatonin, L-carnitine, and vitamins C and E. Of the substances studied to date, vitamin E is one agent that has been shown to have beneficial antioxidant actions in humans (Grune & Davies, 2001). Studies also are addressing interventions that diminish the formation of free radicals through restricted intake of calories, proteins, or certain types of fats (Sinclair & Howitz, 2006).

Neuroendocrine Theories

Neuroendocrine theories (also known as *neurochemical theories*) are the focus of intense interest, but they are still in the early stage of development. These theories postulate that changes in the brain and endocrine glands cause aging. One such theory—the neurotransmitter theory—proposes that an imbalance of nerve impulse–transmitting chemicals in the brain interferes with cell division throughout the body. Neuroendocrine theories are based on the understanding that the neuroendocrine system integrates body functions and facilitates adaptation to changes in both internal and external environments. These theories suggest that the numerous alterations of the endocrine system may actually represent the mechanisms of age-related changes in organ function (Bartke & Lane, 2001).

Apoptosis Theory

In recent years, gerontologists have expressed much interest in exploring the relationship between apoptosis and aging, and new biologic theories of aging are emerging based on this concept. **Apoptosis** is a mechanism of cell death, first described in the 1970s, that is distinct from necrosis (Kerr et al., 1972). Whereas necrosis is an inflammatory response to trauma, apoptosis is a noninflammatory, gene-driven process. Necrosis is characterized by cell swelling and loss of membrane integrity, whereas apoptosis is characterized by cell shrinkage and maintenance of membrane integrity (Kerr et al., 1972). Apoptosis is considered a normal developmental process that occurs continuously throughout life. When apoptosis is properly regulated, it is beneficial to the organ because a balance is maintained between cells that should be retained and those that should be eliminated. Apoptosis can be described as a gene-directed biologic program that has evolved to remove extra cells during development in order to optimize the pattern and shape of each organ (Wang et al., 2001). This process is analogous to the process involved in writing a research paper. Researchers collect large amounts of data, then select the information that actually will be incorporated into the text and discard the information that is not germane.

Recent research suggests that this process is regulated by interplay between two opposing families of genes. Members of one gene family promote elimination of cells, and members of the opposing gene family promote survival of cells. Gerontologists are currently trying to answer questions about "why, during aging, the apoptotic program is dysregulated and how this dysregulation precipitates the disability and degeneration associated with the aging process" (Wang et al., 2001, p. 260). Some studies suggest that one cause of this dysregulation is age-related changes in the levels of proteins and other factors that control apoptosis (Joaquin & Gollapudi, 2001). The apoptosis theory might explain the increased incidence of cancer, autoimmune disease, and cardiovascular and neurodegenerative disorders in older adults.

Conclusions About Biologic Theories

Biologic theories attempt to explain how biologic changes associated with the aging process affect the physiologic function of the human body. These theories address questions about the relationships between aging and disease processes and unique aspects of providing medical care to older people. Some conclusions that can be drawn from biologic theories of aging include the following:

- Biologic aging affects all living organisms.
- Biologic aging is natural, inevitable, irreversible, and progressive with time.
- The course of aging varies from individual to individual.
- The rate of aging for different organs and tissues varies within individuals.

- Biologic aging is influenced by nonbiologic factors.
- Biologic aging processes are different from pathologic processes.
- Biologic aging increases one's vulnerability to disease.

In this book, theoretical explanations of specific functional aspects of aging are discussed in the sections on age-related changes; however, conclusions are not always clearly delineated because much research is ongoing. Whenever possible, theories and conclusions that have generated the greatest concordance are summarized. In all cases, an attempt is made to reflect accurately the current theoretical base. It is important to keep in mind, however, that all theories of aging are in a state of flux and growth. As knowledge of the older adult population continues to expand, new theories may challenge or supplant current theories.

Relevance of Biologic Perspectives on Aging to Nurses

The relevant question for nurses that is addressed in biologic theories of aging is *How does aging affect physiologic function?* The answers to this question provide a basis for identifying ways to use the nursing process to improve the health and functioning of older adults, which is the focus of this text. Many theories support the increasing attention to the significant effects of lifestyle, environment, and other factors on aging and health. This focus is reflected in *Healthy People 2010*, which emphasizes that the increased life expectancy in the United States has led to a shift in focus from longevity to improving functioning and preventing disability (Molla et al., 2001). This trend is likely to continue as gerontologists and older adults themselves increasingly view quality-of-life issues as equal to or even more important than the simple extension of life.

Closely related to this trend, gerontologists have attempted to distinguish between "primary" and "secondary" aging. **Primary aging** is defined as the universal changes occurring with age that are independent of disease or environmental factors (Masoro, 2006). This process occurs late in life and involves a gradual decline in physiologic efficiency in all systems that eventually leads to "natural death" at the age genetically programmed for the individual (Hazzard, 2001). In contrast, **secondary aging** is defined as changes involving interactions of primary aging processes with disease processes and environmental influences (Masoro, 2006). Differentiating between aging and disease is important because people often mistakenly ascribe changes in their own abilities, or those of a family member or patient, to age ("What do you expect? I'm/he's/she's old!"). Unfortunately, many older people still have not been hearing (or do not agree with) the message "that *old age itself is not a disease* and as such should not cause health problems such as disability" (Sarkisian et al., 2001, p. 139).

Distinguishing between aging and disease is essential for identifying interventions aimed at delaying the onset of secondary aging processes. Ideally, health promotion practices would be implemented throughout life, beginning at conception, and these practices would lead to a long and healthy life. Although these health promotion interventions are most effective when they are initiated early in life, people of any age can move toward better health. For example, contrary to common assumptions, older adults respond as well as younger adults to smoking cessation interventions (Aldwin et al., 2006). A primary role of nurses is to help older adults identify the modifiable factors that are associated with secondary aging and to plan interventions to address these factors. With this knowledge of the primary and secondary aging processes, nurses can better understand the differences between age-related changes and the risk factors that affect the functional status of older adults. Nurses then can use this knowledge to implement interventions that promote wellness and a higher level of functioning.

Nurses and primary care providers alike are asking questions that address the uniqueness of caring for older people, as well as questions pertaining to how the functional abilities of older adults can be improved. Unlike nurses, however, primary care providers focus primarily on disease processes. When function is compromised in an older person, the goal of medical care is to identify a pathologic cause so appropriate medical interventions can be initiated. Theories about disease and aging therefore provide a basis for addressing the disease-related factors that influence functional abilities. As is emphasized throughout this text, nurses consider not only the pathologic factors involved, but the many additional risk factors that may significantly influence the health, functioning, and well-being of older adults.

Attitudes about aging exert a strong influence on health care for older adults. If, for example, a primary care provider practices from the perspective of "what do you expect, you're old," reversible disease conditions may go untreated. Similarly, if primary care providers subscribe to the theory that aging is an ultimately fatal disease, their attitude may reflect a hopelessness that pervades their care for older patients. Regardless of the medical approach, however, nurses can base their care on a holistic perspective. Nurses often are in positions to serve as teachers and advocates for older adults whose care might be based on outdated or narrow approaches that incorrectly equate aging and disease. The Functional Consequences Theory for Promoting Wellness in older adults (discussed in Chapter 2) provides a framework for a holistic approach that identifies the risk factors and addresses those that are modifiable in older adults. This book addresses each aspect of functioning from this perspective, with emphasis on those factors that nurses can address through health promotion interventions.

Biologic theories highlight the need for health promotion interventions to prevent disease conditions and minimize the negative effects of aging. However, these theories do not address the significant influence of nursing, medical, and psychosocial interventions that can improve a person's functioning and life expectancy. From a broader perspective, aging is more than an unrelenting progression of cellular deterioration. Survival to old age is an accomplishment that denotes strong will and the ability to adapt. As emphasized throughout this text, older adulthood is a dynamic part of the life span continuum and has the potential to be a most rewarding part of the life cycle, during which one experiences personal growth and self-understanding, fulfillment of potential, and the ability to establish clear priorities. These aspects of aging are addressed in the following sections, which describe sociologic and psychological theories of aging.

Imagine that you are 72 years old and your parents are still living. Your mother is 96 and your father is 95 and they live in an assisted-living apartment. You have a brother who died last year at the age of 70 and you have a sister who is 69 years old. You have two children, three grandchildren, and two great-grandchildren. Your mother is moderately obese, and has osteoarthritis, hypertension, glaucoma, and type 2 diabetes. Functionally, she uses a walker, needs help with getting in and out of the bathtub, and has some trouble reading but can still see well enough to watch television and get around familiar environments. Your father has hypertension, osteoarthritis, and a recent diagnosis of prostate cancer. Functionally, he is independent in his basic activities of daily living but is quite hearing impaired. Both of your parents have some memory impairment, but the support services at the facility where they live address their needs for meals, medication administration, and reminders about getting to activities.

THINKING POINTS

- Using the concepts of rectangularization of the curve and compression of morbidity, what would you expect the health, functioning, and life expectancy to be for each of the five generations in your family?
- Pick the biologic theory of aging that you think is most applicable for your family and use it to explain to your great-grandchildren why their great-great grandparents are still living.
- Pick a theory about the relationships among age, disease, and death or a theory about active life expectancy and functional health and use it to respond to your mother's statement, "I'm 96 years old—what does it matter if I follow a diabetic diet? If the sugar hasn't killed me so far, then eating two donuts this morning isn't going to kill me. It's old age that will take me, not my diet."
- Pick a theory about the relationships among age, disease, and death or a theory about active life expectancy and functional health and use it to respond to your father's declaration that "Of course, I have prostate cancer! I'm 95 years old!"
- What perspectives on aging would you want your father's primary care provider to use in addressing your father's prostate cancer?

SOCIOLOGIC PERSPECTIVES ON AGING

Sociologic theories of aging attempt to explain how a society influences its older adults and how older adults influence their society. Early sociologic theories of aging, developed during the 1960s, focused on adjustments of older people to losses within the context of roles and reference groups. For example, disengagement, activity, and subculture theories viewed older adults from a narrow perspective. Beginning in the 1970s, social gerontologists broadened their perspective to focus on larger societal influences, but theirs were similar to earlier theories in viewing older adults in the context of societal problems. More recent theories explore the complex interrelationship between older people and their physical, political, and socioeconomic environments. Currently, sociologic theories of aging address issues related to the tremendous diversity of older adults in industrialized as well as developing societies. Similarly, emerging sociologic theories are addressing inequality in aging societies by attempting to explain how and why group differences emerge. The following sections present a sampling of the more well-developed sociologic theories of aging.

Disengagement Theory

In 1961, Cumming and Henry published the first sociologic theory of aging in their book, *Growing Old: The Process of Disengagement* (Cumming & Henry, 1961). According to **disengagement theory**, a society and older people engage in a mutually beneficial process of reciprocal withdrawal to maintain social equilibrium. This process occurs systematically and inevitably and is governed by society's needs, which override individual needs. Moreover, older people desire this withdrawal and are happy when it occurs. As the number, nature, and diversity of the older person's social contacts diminish, disengagement becomes a circular process that further limits opportunities for interaction. Disengagement theory was later amended to reflect better the complexity and diversity of older people.

The usefulness of this theory lies in the controversies it has inspired by challenging traditional beliefs about the relationship between a person and society. For instance, there is considerable controversy regarding whether the disengagement process is, in fact, universal, inevitable, and beneficial to the person. Questions have also been raised about how this theory ignores the unique responses of individuals to aging and society. Gerontologists no longer widely accept disengagement theory, but it still influences thought on some aspects of aging. For example, the disengagement theory has been used to explain the widespread withdrawal of older adults from productive activities such as work and volunteering (Uhlenberg, 2000).

Activity Theory

Aging successfully was first associated with keeping active in the early days of social gerontology, when Havighurst and Albrecht (1953) published the first explicit statement about the importance of social role participation in positive adjustment to old age. During the next two decades, social gerontologists formalized this perspective as the **activity theory**. The activity theory is based on the supposition that older people remain socially and psychologically fit if they remain actively engaged in life. For example, one's self-concept is affirmed through activities associated with various roles and the loss of roles in old age negatively affects life satisfaction. Lemon and colleagues (1972) tested this theory and found a significant relationship between informal activity and life satisfaction. They concluded that the quality or type of interaction was more important than the quantity of activity. Studies continue to validate the positive relationship between successful aging and having a range of meaningful activities, including social, physical, and solitary (George, 2006).

Subculture Theory

The **subculture theory**, first proposed by Rose in the early 1960s, states that old people, as a group, have their own norms, expectations, beliefs, and habits; therefore, they have their own subculture (Rose, 1965). The theory also maintains that older people are less well integrated into the larger society and interact more among themselves, compared with people from other age groups. Moreover, the theory holds that the formation of an aged subculture is primarily a response to the loss of status resulting from old age, which is so negatively defined in the United States that people do not want to be viewed as old. In the aged subculture, individual status is based on health and mobility, rather than on the occupational, educational, or economic achievements that were previously important. Rose (1965) envisioned that one outcome of the aged subculture would be the development of an aging group consciousness that would serve to improve the self-image of older people and change the negative cultural definition of aging.

Because the aged subculture has millions of members in this country, it constitutes a minority group that can organize and make public demands. The growth of groups, such as the American Association of Retired Persons (AARP), whose membership exceeds 34 million people, is evidence of the social importance of the aged subgroup. When considered along with the activity theory, the subculture theory supports the social gerontological view that there is a strong relationship between peer group participation and the adjustment process of aging.

A Student's Perspective

My comfort level at the nursing home increases each and every week, and I find myself enjoying my time there more and more. Today there was a children's program in the dining room for all the residents. It was very cute. The kids were great, and most of the residents expressed true appreciation and enjoyment while the kids visited. For instance, my patient Mr. B. was chatting with a young boy and his mother. As the boy got more and more involved in the conversation, Mr. B.'s attitude changed completely; he became so happy and engaged with the young boy. I had seen Mr. B. smile a couple of times before, but not to the extent of how he smiled and laughed with the little one. After the boy left, Mr. B. told me that the boy reminded him of his own grandson, whom he doesn't get to see very much. I think it brought Mr. B. joy and a sense of comfort because he felt like he was with his family. Personally, I was quite touched. Sometimes everyone gets so caught up in current tasks or problems, when really at the end of the day it comes down to making people smile and helping them to enjoy life to the best of one's abilities.

Caitlin B.

Age Stratification and Age Integration Theories

The **age stratification theory**, first proposed by Riley and colleagues (1972), addresses the interdependencies between age as an element of the social structure and the aging of people and cohorts as a social process. This theory emphasizes the following concepts:

- People pass through society in cohorts that are aging socially, biologically, and psychologically.
- New cohorts are continually being born and each experiences a unique sense of history.
- A society can be divided into various strata according to age and roles.
- Society itself is continually changing, as are the people and their roles in each age stratum.
- A dynamic interplay exists between individual aging and social change.

Thus, aging people and the larger society are constantly influencing each other and changing both the cohorts and the society. In a societal context, the related concept of cohort-centrism is illustrated by the perception that people in the so-called Baby Boomer generation behave and act as one cohesive group (Walker, 2006).

Social gerontologists in recent years have studied age segregation, particularly in relation to residential settings for older adults (Hagestad & Dannefer, 2001). There is increasing recognition of the importance of age integration, defined as a community in which chronologic age is not a criterion for entrance, exit, or participation. Two additional components of age integration are the absence of age barriers and the presence of cross-age interactions (Uhlenberg, 2000). Age integration is on a continuum, with the following variations (Uhlenberg, 2000):

- Some societies and social structures are more age integrated than others.
- The degree of age integration in any society changes over time.
- Some people may experience more age integration than others.

Age integration is seen as an important factor in combating ageism and improving quality of life, not only for older adults, but for younger generations.

Person–Environment Fit Theory

The **person–environment fit theory** considers the interrelationships between personal competence and the environment (Lawton, 1982). According to this theory, personal competence involves the following factors, which collectively contribute to a person's functional ability: ego strength, motor skills, biologic health, cognitive capacity, and sensory-perceptual capacity. The environment is viewed in terms of its potential for eliciting a behavioral response from the person. Lawton asserts that for each person's level of competence, there is a level of environmental demand, or environmental press, that is most advantageous to that person's function. People who function at relatively lower levels of competence can tolerate only low levels of environmental press, whereas people who function at higher levels of competence can tolerate increased environmental demands. An often-quoted correlate is that the more impaired the person, the greater the impact of the environment. This theory is often used in planning appropriate environments for older adults with disabilities.

The person–environment fit theory has stimulated further research and theory development in the field of environmental gerontology, which is the interdisciplinary study of behavioral and psychological implications of the relationship between older adults and their environments (Scheidt & Windley, 2006). Information gleaned from these theories is particularly relevant to designing environments that are most supportive of optimal functioning for older adults.

Relevance of Sociologic Theories of Aging to Nurses

Sociologic theories of aging help nurses view older adults in relation to society and environments. Thus, these perspectives contribute to a better understanding of influences such as culture, family, education, community, ascribed roles, cohort effects, home and living setting, and personal and political economics. These theories remind health care practitioners that there are patterns of similar responses among cohorts, but within those larger patterns, each person is unique. Some older people achieve their identity in a subculture, others may define successful aging in relation to their activities, and still others may find new roles in society. Sociologic theories of aging can shed light on the unique ways that older people cope with stress, respond to illness, and achieve healthy aging.

Emerging theories about age integration and person–environment interactions are stimulating interest in broadening the environments of institutional settings to include pets and intergenerational activities. Theories addressing questions of diversity encourage nurses to consider the cultural needs of individual older adults. Similarly, theories addressing power hierarchies and inequalities encourage nurses to be more aware of opportunities to empower older adults. For example, many of the health promotion interventions discussed throughout this text emphasize the importance of educating older adults about choices they can make that influence their health and functioning. Another implication of theories addressing inequalities is the increased recognition of residents' rights in the institutional setting, as well as increased recognition of the importance of respecting autonomy for all older adults.

Concepts from the person–environment fit theory help nurses appreciate the importance of environmental adaptations as interventions to improve functional status, especially when working with dependent older adults. In addition, these theories emphasize the importance of assessing both environmental and psychosocial factors that influence the functioning of an older person. Lawton's theory also suggests that when an older person has difficulty, coping interventions can be directed toward improving personal competency or decreasing environmental demands, or both. Some of the risk factors discussed throughout this text identify environmental factors that interfere with the health and functioning of older adults. Similarly, many of the nursing interventions discussed in this text identify ways of modifying the environment to improve the functioning of older adults.

Imagine that you are 87 years old and have been retired for 10 years. Create an image of yourself at that age, making sure that you incorporate some changes that are likely to occur as you grow older. Describe the people who are an active part of your relationships during a typical month. Describe the activities you would engage in during a typical week for each of the following aspects of your life: leisure activity, physical activity, intellectual stimulation, emotional growth, social interaction, and spiritual nurturing. Are you active in any volunteer organizations? What would your health and functioning be and where would you be living? Based on the

(case study continues on page 41)

image of yourself at 87 years old that you just created, answer the following questions:

THINKING POINTS

- How could you apply either the activity theory or the disengagement theory to your life as it compares with your life at your present age?
- Would any of the concepts in the subculture, age stratification, or age integration theories explain your activities and relationships?
- How would the person–environment fit theory explain the relationship between you and your environment?

PSYCHOLOGICAL PERSPECTIVES ON AGING

Psychological theories of aging address questions about the behavioral and developmental aspects of later adulthood, such as the following:

- How does aging affect behavior?
- How do factors such as perceptions, relationships, personality, and behaviors affect aging?
- How is longevity and quality of life influenced by factors such as values and perceived control?
- Does personality change or remain the same with aging?
- Do patterns of behavior change over time in any identifiable way?
- How does gender influence aging?

These theories are especially relevant to psychosocial aspects of functioning because they address variables such as learning, memory, feelings, intelligence, and motivation. The following sections review some of the major psychological theories of aging. In addition, relevant psychological theories about wisdom, creativity, cognitive function, spiritual outlook, stress and coping, and depression are discussed in Chapters 11, 12, and 15.

Human Needs Theory

Maslow's hierarchy of needs framework forms the basis of the **human needs theory**, one of the psychological theories that gerontologists use to address the concepts of motivation and human needs. According to Maslow's (1954) theory, the five categories of basic human needs, ordered from lowest to highest, are physiologic needs, safety and security needs, love and belongingness, self-esteem, and self-actualization. The attainment of lower-level needs takes priority over higher-level needs; self-actualization can occur only when lower-level needs are met to some degree. People continually move between the levels, but always strive toward higher levels. This theory is particularly applicable to older adults because Maslow describes self-actualized people as fully mature humans who possess such desirable traits as autonomy, creativity, independence, and positive interpersonal relationships.

Life-Course and Personality Development Theories

Some psychological theories of aging, referred to as personality development theories, identify personality types as predictive forces for successful or unsuccessful aging. Other theories, referred to as **life-course theories** (also called life span theories), attempt to address old age within the context of the person's life span or life cycle. Life-course theories address the series of role transitions and trajectories that people experience as they move through their lives, entering and exiting roles over time (Moen & Spencer, 2006).

According to these theories, one's life course is divided into stages, and one moves through these stages in certain patterns. Like Maslow's human needs theory, life-course theories describe some progression through various stages and suggest that successful progression is related in some way to successful accomplishments in prior stages. A central theme of life span models is that successful aging is accomplished when older adults can engage in life tasks that they consider important despite a reduction in their energy (Birren & Schroots, 2001). There is a great deal of overlap between some of the concepts in personality development theories and those in life-course theories; indeed, these terms are often used interchangeably by different authors to refer to the same theories.

Neugarten and colleagues (1968) proposed the **continuity theory** because they believed that a theory of aging needed to address the relationship of personality to successful aging. Thus, they proposed a personality-continuity, or developmental, theory of aging (Neugarten et al., 1968). According to this theory, a person's characteristic coping strategies are in place long before old age, even though personality features are dynamic and continually evolving. Continuity theory proposes that the best way to predict how a person will adjust to being old is to examine how that person has adjusted to changes throughout life. A review of studies concluded that personality shows considerable stability over time, but changes occur during middle and later years (Hendricks & Hatch, 2006). Another recent conclusion is that the question of whether personality changes or remains the same is complex and the most accurate answer is that some people's personalities are stable and others are not (Mroczek et al., 2006).

Personality development theories, like the theory of continuity, address the question of whether the personality changes or remains the same throughout the life course. Neugarten and colleagues (1968) conducted a study of personality types and identified four basic personality patterns in older adults: integrated, armored-defended, passive-dependent, and unintegrated. Most of their older subjects had made positive adjustments to aging and were assigned to the mature, or integrated, personality group. They further divided this group of high-functioning older subjects into three categories based on their level of role activity: (1) reorganizers, who were engaged in a wide variety of activities; (2) focused people, who had become selective in their activities; and (3) disengaged people, who had voluntarily moved away from role commitments. People in the armored-defended group either held on to patterns of middle age as long as possible, or closed themselves off from the world. Those with passive-dependent personalities had strong dependency needs or were described as apathetic "rocking-chair" people. Those in the unintegrated personality group formed the smallest group and were the least well adjusted. This group included those with psychological problems, those who exhibited irrational behavior, and those who failed to cope with activities of daily living (Neugarten et al., 1968).

Most theories of adult personality development are based on the theories of Carl Jung or Erik Erikson. Jung's (1960) theory categorizes personalities as either extroverted and oriented toward the external world, or introverted and oriented toward subjective experiences. A balance between the two orientations, both of which are present to some degree in all people, is essential for mental health. Jung further theorized that people tend to be more extroverted in their younger years because of the nature of the demands and responsibilities associated with family and social roles. As these demands change and diminish, beginning around the age of 40 years, people become more introverted. Jung (1954) describes later adulthood as a period of taking stock, a time during which a person looks backward rather than forward and is responsible for devoting serious attention to self. Successful aging, according to Jung's theory, depends on accepting one's diminishing capacity and increasing number of losses.

Jung's theory set the stage for later revisions in the disengagement theory of Cumming and Henry (1961) and for Neugarten's (1968) theory of interiority. Based on studies of middle-aged and older adults, Neugarten (1968) suggested replacing the term "disengagement" with the phrase "increased interiority of the personality." Neugarten's definition of interiority was similar to Jung's definition of introversion, but she identified the middle years as beginning at 50, rather than 40 years of age. Neugarten described the middle years of life as the time when "introspection seems to increase noticeably, and contemplation and reflection and self-evaluation become characteristic forms of mental life" (Neugarten, 1968, p. 140). Like Jung, she proposed that, with increasing age, ego functions are increasingly turned toward the self and away from the outer world.

Erik Erikson's (1963) original theory about the eight stages of life has been used widely in relation to older adulthood. Erikson defines the stages of life as trust versus mistrust, autonomy versus shame and doubt, initiative versus guilt, industry versus inferiority, identity versus identity diffusion, intimacy versus self-absorption, generativity versus stagnation, and ego integrity versus despair. Each of these stages presents the person with certain conflicting tendencies that must be balanced before he or she can move successfully from that stage. As in other life-course theories, how one stage is mastered lays the groundwork for successful or unsuccessful mastery of the next stage. In works published between 1950 and 1966, Erikson emphasized the life course from childhood to young adulthood; in later publications, however, he reconsidered the meaning of these stages. In 1982, when he was 80 years old, Erikson described the task of old age as balancing the search for integrity and wholeness with a sense of despair. He believed that the successful accomplishment of this task, achieved primarily through life review activities, would result in wisdom. A current focus on relationships between religion and aging suggests that Erikson's theory links religion with meaning in life, as evidenced by the report that when he was 80 years old, he had replaced the word "integrity" with "faith" (Krause, 2006).

Peck (1968) expanded Erikson's original theory and divided the eighth stage—ego integrity versus despair—into additional stages occurring during middle age and old age. The stages described by Peck as specific to old age are ego differentiation versus work-role preoccupation, body transcendence versus body preoccupation, and ego transcendence versus ego preoccupation. Recent psychological theories on aging continue to use Erikson's construct of generativity in addressing questions about how generativity is linked to other aspects of personality and about how the life-course shifts into and out of midlife generativity (Ryff et al., 2001).

Departing from theories that begin with infancy or childhood, life-course theories concentrate on middle or later adulthood. Some tasks of late life that these theories address include the following (Havighurst, 1972; Newman & Newman, 1984):

- Adjusting to decreasing physical strength and health
- Coping with physical changes of aging
- Adjusting to retirement and reduced income
- Adjusting to the death of a spouse
- Redirecting energy to new roles and activities, such as retirement, widowhood, and grandparenting
- Establishing an explicit association with one's age group
- Adapting to social roles in a flexible way
- Establishing satisfactory physical living arrangements
- Accepting one's own life
- Developing a point of view about death

Theory of Gerotranscendence

The theory of **gerotranscendence** was proposed in the early 1990s by Lars Tornstam (1994) and has become widely recognized in Sweden and other Scandinavian countries. This theory proposes that human aging is a process of shifting from a rational and materialistic metaperspective to a more cosmic and transcendent vision. This shift includes the following aspects (Tornstam, 1996):

- Decreased self-centeredness
- Less concern with body and material things
- Decreased fear of death
- Discovery of hidden aspects of self
- Increased altruism
- Increased time spent in meditation and solitude
- Decreased interest in superfluous social interaction
- Urge to abandon roles
- Increased understanding of moral ambiguity
- Increased feelings of cosmic union with the universe
- Increased feelings of affinity with past and coming generations
- A redefinition of one's perception of time, space, and objects

Gerotranscendence is sometimes viewed as an extension of the disengagement theory because it attempts to "reenchant aging" by replacing performance-oriented characteristics of people in midlife with "spiritual" qualities such as play, rest, wisdom, creativity, and relaxation (Dalby, 2006; Jonson & Magnusson, 2001). Thus, gerotranscendence is associated with a deepening wisdom and spirituality, a greater sense of intergenerational continuity, and a greater ability to counterbalance losses and focus on what is important in life (Aldwin et al., 2006).

Theories About Gender and Aging

Over the past decade, a number of psychological theories of aging, particularly those with life span perspectives, have focused on relationships between gender and aging. Some of these studies have addressed diverse populations, such as lesbians, gay men, and transgendered persons. Three purposes of gender-related psychological theories of aging studies have been (1) to compare and contrast male and female performance data, (2) to examine the nature of change in gender roles, and (3) to study the relationship between gender role differences and social roles and social power (Sinnott & Shifren, 2001). Some of the gender-specific aspects of psychology and aging that gerontologists are addressing include intelligence, personality, caregiving, self-efficacy, body attitudes, verbal ability, social ties, self-reported health, sense of control, and medical decision-making processes (Sinnott & Shifren, 2001).

A recent longitudinal study found gender differences in socioeconomic and psychosocial predictors of mortality (Fry & Debats, 2006). For men, the greatest predictors were lower levels of education, perceived control, personal commitment, and physical functioning. For women, the greatest predictors were lower levels of perceived social support and social engagement. The factors that were most influential for men were inconsequential for women, and vice versa.

Psychological theories of aging also address gender role development across the life span. They address questions such as *Why is there a gender difference as we age?* (Sinnott & Shifren, 2001). Many researchers believe that gender roles evolve from being narrowly defined in adolescence and younger adulthood to becoming more amorphous in later adulthood. An analysis of research on this subject concluded that gender role development in older adulthood involves transcending roles as they were conceptualized in earlier life and continuing to develop a sense of individual identity, meaning, and community (Sinnott & Shifren, 2001). A more recent analysis suggested that older men and women have more choices about roles and relationships, but they are strongly influenced by age- and gender-graded norms based on outmoded scripts (Moen & Spencer, 2006). Gender differences relevant to health and aging are discussed throughout this text, and pertinent information about gender differences is designated in the Diversity Notes.

Relevance of Psychological Theories of Aging to Nurses

In caring for older adults, nurses can use psychological theories of aging as a framework for addressing certain issues, such as response to losses and continued emotional development. Maslow's hierarchy of needs framework is useful for conceptualizing the nature of interventions in institutional or home settings. For instance, if older adults are unable to purchase food, they are unlikely to feel secure. Likewise, if older adults feel insecure about being able to meet their shelter needs, they are unlikely to have a sense of trust. Older adults who have already met their lower-level needs, however, can be encouraged to focus on higher-level achievements such as self-actualization.

In addition, psychological theories imply that older adults should devote some time and energy to life review and self-understanding. Nurses can facilitate this process by asking sensitive questions and by listening attentively to older adults as they share information about their past. Reminiscence is a positive experience that is essential for continued psychological development, and it can be promoted by nurses either on an individual or group basis.

Life-course models can help nurses identify those areas of personality that are likely to change and those that are more likely to remain stable. Nurses have used life span theories to develop a multidisciplinary Theory of Thriving (Haight et al., 2002). This model proposes that thriving is achieved when there is concordance between the person and the human and nonhuman environment; that is, when these three elements are mutually engaged, supportive, and harmonious. In contrast, failure to thrive is the result of discordance among these three elements, causing a failure of engagement and mutual support, and disharmony (Haight et al., 2002). In addition to these implications, nurses consider implications regarding specific aspects, such as cognitive function and coping responses (see Chapters 11 and 12), in the context of psychological theories of aging.

Imagine, again, that you are 87 years old and add the following information to the description of yourself that you created for the discussion of sociologic theories. Describe your personality, including, but not limited to, the following characteristics: emotional stability, adjustments to losses, contentedness with life, optimism versus pessimism, engagement in activities versus withdrawal from activities, and feelings of self-efficacy versus feelings of powerlessness. Describe your beliefs about your gender-specific roles (i.e., those aspects of roles that are defined by you being a woman, or a man). Based on this image of yourself at 87 years old, answer the following questions:

THINKING POINTS

- Where do you think you would be in Maslow's or Erikson's stages and how would you have moved between the levels in the past decades?
- What aspects of your lifestyle at 87 years old could be explained by the continuity theory?
- How would any concepts in the personality development theories apply to you?
- Based on your own experiences, how has your perception of your role as a woman or man changed over time?

A HOLISTIC PERSPECTIVE ON AGING AND WELLNESS

From a holistic perspective—the perspective that is most pertinent to promoting wellness—it is necessary to consider the body–mind–spirit interconnectedness of each older adult for whom nurses provide care. Thus, questions about how we can live long and well must be answered in the context of the interplay among the many factors that influence health and aging. This requires an integrated perspective on aging, an avoidance of stereotypes, and a commitment to identifying the factors that most directly affect—both negatively and positively—health and quality of life for each unique older adult. At present, gerontologists are trying to develop a paradigm that both explains aging and accounts for individual differences in biologic aging and psychosocial factors (Aldwin et al., 2006). Current theories point to the following determinants of living long and well:

- Inherit good genes.
- Avoid oxidative damage (e.g., from tobacco, environmental conditions).
- Protect from oxidative damage with antioxidants from natural sources (e.g., fruits and vegetables).
- Maintain optimal weight.
- Engage in physical exercise.
- Engage in meaningful social interactions.
- Develop close personal relationships.
- Maintain a sense of spiritual connectedness.
- Reject ageist stereotypes.

The Functional Consequences Theory for Promoting Wellness that was presented in Chapter 2 provides a nursing framework for addressing the factors that affect the health and functioning of older adults. Although it is beyond the scope of any nursing text to address all aspects of body–mind–spirit interconnectedness, nurses can use the functional consequences perspective, in conjunction with information from theories discussed in this chapter, to help older adults answer their own questions about aging. When older adults express resignation in the "What-do-you-expect-you're-old?" outlook, nurses can rephrase that viewpoint and ask "So, what *do* you expect because you are older?" or "What *will* you expect when you are older?" Nurses can challenge ageist stereotypes and approach the question from a holistic perspective that acknowledges the interconnectedness among one's body, one's mind, and one's spirit. From this point of view, nurses can emphasize that even though some degenerative changes affect one's body with increasing age, one's mind and spirit can continue to thrive and even improve.

Because self-responsibility is an essential component of wellness, nurses can ask older adults to identify for themselves those factors that most significantly influence their health and functioning and can focus care on those aspects that are within the scope of nursing. Nurses also need to avoid communicating ageist stereotypes, which requires that we examine our own attitudes about aging and make sure that our nursing care of older adults is based on accurate, theory-based information. Nurses can check their attitudes about their own aging and periodically ask, *What do I expect (or wish) for my own wellness when I am older tomorrow? ...a week from now? ...a month from now? ...a year? ...ten years? ...twenty years?* Even more important, ask, *What am I doing today that will affect how well I am aging tomorrow? ...ten years from now?* If we acknowledge that no matter what else is happening, we are aging biologically, we are likely to pay careful attention to health-related behaviors that affect how well we age. Likewise, if we approach our care of older adults holistically, we will be able to identify interventions that promote wellness of body, mind, and spirit.

CHAPTER HIGHLIGHTS

How Can We Live Long and Well?

- Gerontologists develop theories to answer questions about how and why we age. From a holistic perspective, the most important question is *How can we live a life that is both long and healthy?* Nurses address this question by promoting wellness and facilitating optimal level of functioning for older adults.
- One way of addressing the question *How long can we live?* is by measuring life span, life expectancy, and morbidity and mortality rates.

- Another way to address this question is through exploring the relationship between aging, health, and disease.

How Do We Explain Biologic Aging?

- Biologic theories of aging address questions about basic age-related changes, which are characterized as deleterious, progressive, intrinsic, universal, irreversible, and genetically programmed.
- Biologic theories include genetic, wear-and-tear, immunity, cross-linkage, free radicals, neuroendocrine, and apoptosis theories.

Sociologic Perspectives on Aging

- Sociologic theories of aging attempt to explain how a society influences its old people and how old people influence their society.
- Sociologic theories include disengagement, activity, subculture, age stratification and age integration, and person–environment fit theories.

Psychological Perspectives on Aging

- Psychological theories of aging provide a framework for addressing certain psychosocial issues that are common among older adults (e.g., responses to losses and continued emotional development).
- Psychological theories include human needs, life-course and personality development, gerotranscendence, and gender theories.

A Holistic Perspective on Aging and Wellness

- Nurses can use theories of aging developed by other disciplines in conjunction with the Functional Consequences Theory (see Chapter 2) to develop and implement a holistic approach to promoting wellness in older adults.

Critical Thinking Exercises

You are assessing an 87-year-old woman who is being admitted to the hospital with congestive heart failure for the third time in the past 2 years. She does not have any cognitive impairment and she lives alone in her own home. When you ask her why she came to the hospital, she states, "I'm 87 years old, you know, isn't that a good enough reason to be sick? Don't you think you'll be in the hospital when you're my age?"

1. How do you respond to her?
2. What additional assessment information would you want?
3. What health teaching would you think about incorporating into your care plan?

Educational Resources

American Federation for Aging Research
www.afar.org *and* www.infoaging.org

International Longevity Center—USA
www.ilcusa.org

National Institute on Aging Information Center
www.nih.gov/nia

References

Aldwin, C. M., Spiro III, A., & Park, C. L. (2006). Health, behavior, and optimal aging: A life span developmental perspective. In J. E. Birren & K. W. Schaie (Eds.), *Handbook of the psychology of aging* (6th ed., pp. 85–125). San Diego: Elsevier Academic Press.

Andersen-Ranberg, K., & Schroll, M., & Jeune, B. (2001). Healthy centenarians do not exist, but autonomous centenarians do: A population-based study of morbidity among Danish centenarians. *Journal of the American Geriatrics Society, 49*, 900–908.

Austad, S. N. (2001). Concepts and theories of aging. In E. J. Masoro & S. N. Austad (Eds.), *Handbook of the biology of aging* (5th ed., pp. 3–22). San Diego: Academic Press.

Bartke, A., & Lane, M. (2001). Endocrine and neuroendocrine regulatory functions. In E. J. Masoro & S. N. Austad (Eds.), *Handbook of the biology of aging* (5th ed., pp. 297–323). San Diego: Academic Press.

Berzlanovich, A. M., Keil, W., Waldhoer, T., Sim, E., Fasching, P., & Fazeny-Dorner, B. (2005). Do centenarians die healthy? An autopsy study. *Journals of Gerontology: Series A, Biological Sciences and Medical Sciences, 60*, 862–865.

Binstock, R. H., Fishman, J. R., & Johnson, T. E. (2006). Anti-aging medicine and science: Social implications. In R. H. Binstock & L. K. George (Eds.), *Handbook of aging and the social sciences* (6th ed., pp. 436–455). San Diego: Elsevier Academic Press.

Birren, J. E., & Schroots, J. J. F. (2001). The history of geropsychology. In J. E. Birren & K. W. Schaie (Eds.), *Handbook of the psychology of aging* (5th ed., pp. 3–28). San Diego: Academic Press.

Blumenthal, H. T. (1999). A view of the aging–disease relationship from age 85. *Journals of Gerontology: Series A, Biological Sciences and Medical Sciences, 54*, B255–B259.

Blumenthal, H. T. (2001). Milestone or genomania? The relevance of the human genome project to biological aging and the age-related diseases. *Journals of Gerontology: Series A, Biological Sciences and Medical Sciences, 56*, M529–M537.

Breslow, L. (2006). Health measurements in the third era of health. *American Journal of Public Health, 96*, 17–19.

Crimmins, E. M., Hayward, M. D., & Saito, Y. (1996). Differentials in active life expectancy in the older population of the United States. *Journals of Gerontology: Series B, Psychological Sciences and Social Sciences, 51*, S111– S120.

Cumming, E., & Henry, W. (1961). *Growing old: The process of disengagement.* New York: Basic Books.

Dalby, P. (2006). Is there a process of spiritual change or development associated with aging? A critical review of research. *Aging & Mental Health, 10*(1), 4–12.

Effros, R. B. (2001). Immune system activity. In E. J. Masoro & S. N. Austad (Eds.), *Handbook of the biology of aging* (5th ed., pp. 324–350). San Diego: Academic Press.

Erikson, E. H. (1963). *Childhood and society* (2nd ed.). New York: W. W. Norton.

Evert, J., Lawler, E., Bogan, H., & Perls, T. (2003). Morbidity profiles of centenarians: Survivors, delayers, and escapers. *Journals of Gerontology: Series A, Biological Sciences and Medical Sciences, 58*, 232–237.

Ferraro, K. F. (2006). Health and aging. In R. H. Binstock & L. K. George (Eds.), *Handbook of aging and the social sciences* (6th ed., pp. 238–256). San Diego: Elsevier Academic Press.

Fries, J. F., & Crapo, L. M. (1981). *Vitality and aging: Implications of the rectangularization of the curve.* San Francisco: W. H. Freeman.

Fry, P. S., & Debats, D. L. (2006). Sources of life strengths as predictors of late-life mortality and survivorship. *International Journal of Aging and Human Development, 62*, 303–334.

George, L. K. (2006). Perceived quality of life. In R. H. Binstock & L. K. George (Eds.), *Handbook of aging and the social sciences* (6th ed., pp. 320–336). San Diego: Elsevier Academic Press.

Grune, T., & Davies, K. J. A. (2001). Oxidative processes in aging. In E. J. Masoro & S. N. Austad (Eds.), *Handbook of the biology of aging* (5th ed., pp. 25–58). San Diego: Academic Press.

Hagestad, G. O., & Dannefer, D. (2001). Concepts and theories of aging: Beyond microfication in social sciences approaches. In R. H. Binstock & L. K. George (Eds.), *Handbook of aging and the social sciences* (5th ed., pp. 3–21). San Diego: Academic Press.

Haight, B. K., Barba B. E., Tesh, A. S., & Courts, N. F. (2002). Thriving: A life span theory. *Journal of Gerontological Nursing, 28*(3), 14–22.

Harman, D. (1956). Aging: A theory based on the free radical and radiation chemistry. *Journal of Gerontology, 11*, 298–300.

Havighurst, R. J. (1972). *Developmental tasks and education* (3rd ed.). New York: David McKay.

Havighurst, R. J., & Albrecht, R. (1953). *Older people*. New York: Longmans, Green.

Hayflick, L. (1965). The limited in vitro lifetime of human diploid cell strains. *Experimental Cell Research, 37*, 614–636.

Hayflick, L. (1974). The longevity of cultured human cells. *Journal of the American Geriatrics Society, 22*, 1–12.

Hayflick, L. (1988). Aging in cultured human cells. In B. Kent & R. N. Butler (Eds.), *Human aging research: Concepts and techniques*. New York: Raven Press.

Hayflick, L. (2001-02). Anti-aging medicine hype, hope, and reality. *Generations, 20*, 20–26.

Hazzard, W. R. (2001). Aging, health, longevity, and the promise of medical research: The perspective of a gerontologist and geriatrician. In E. J. Masoro & S. N. Austad (Eds.), *Handbook of the biology of aging* (5th ed., pp. 445–456). San Diego: Academic Press.

Hendricks, J., & Hatch, L. R. (2006). Lifestyle and aging. In R. H. Binstock & L. K. George (Eds.), *Handbook of aging and the social sciences* (6th ed., pp. 301–319). San Diego: Elsevier Academic Press.

Joaquin, A. M., & Gollapudi, S. (2001). Functional decline in aging and disease: A role for apoptosis. *Journal of the American Geriatrics Society, 49*, 1234–1240.

Jonson, H., & Magnusson, J. A. (2001). A new age of old age? Gerotranscendence and re-enchantment of aging. *Journal of Aging Studies, 15*, 317–331.

Jung, C. G. (1954). Marriage as a psychological relationship. In W. McGuire, H. Reed, M. Fordham, & G. Adler (Eds.) (R. F. C. Hull, trans.), *Collected works: Vol. 17: The development of personality*. New York: Pantheon Books.

Jung, C. G. (1960). The stages of life. In W. McGuire, H. Reed, M. Fordham, & G. Adler (Eds.) (R. F. C. Hull, trans.), *Collected works: Vol. 8: The structure and dynamics of the psyche* (pp. 387–403). New York: Pantheon Books.

Katz, S., Branch, L. G., Branson, M. H., Papsidero, J. A., Beck, J. C., & Greer, D. S. (1983). Active life expectancy. *New England Journal of Medicine, 309*, 1218–1224.

Kerr, J. F., Wyllie, A. H., & Currie, A. R. (1972). Apoptosis: A basic biologic phenomenon with wide-ranging implications in tissue kinetics. *British Journal of Cancer, 26*, 239–257.

Kohn, R. R. (1982). Cause of death in very old people. *Journal of the American Medical Association, 247*, 2793–2797.

Krause, N. (2006). Religion and health in late life. In J. E. Birren & K. W. Schaie (Eds.), *Handbook of the psychology of aging* (6th ed., pp. 499–518). San Diego: Elsevier Academic Press.

Land, K. C., & Yang, Y. (2006). Morbidity, disability, and mortality. In R. H. Binstock & L. K. George (Eds.), *Handbook of aging and the social sciences* (6th ed., pp. 41–58). San Diego: Elsevier Academic Press.

Lawton, M. P. (1982). Competence, environmental press, and the adaptation of older people. In M. P. Lawton, P. G. Windley, & T. O. Byerts (Eds.), *Aging and the environment: Theoretical approaches* (pp. 33–59). New York: Springer.

Lemon, B., Bengston, V. L., & Peterson, J. A. (1972). An exploration of the activity theory of aging: Activity types and life satisfaction among in-movers to retirement community. *Journal of Gerontology 27*, 511–523.

Maslow, A. H. (1954). *Motivation and personality*. New York: Harper & Row.

Masoro, E. J. (2006). Are age-associated diseases an integral part of aging? In E. J. Masoro & S. N. Austad (Eds.), *Handbook of the biology of aging* (6th ed., pp. 43–62). San Diego: Elsevier Academic Press.

Moen, P., & Spencer, D. (2006). Converging divergences in age, gender, health, and well-being: Strategic selection in the third age. In R. H. Binstock & L. K. George (Eds.), *Handbook of aging and the social sciences* (6th ed., pp. 129–144). San Diego: Elsevier Academic Press.

Molla, M. T., Wagener, D. K., & Madans, J. H. (2001). *Summary measures of population health: Methods for calculating healthy life expectancy*. Washington, DC: U.S. Department of Health and Human Services.

Mor, V. (2005). The comprehension of morbidity hypothesis: A review of research and prospects for the future. *Journal of the American Geriatrics Society, 53*, S308–S309.

Mroczek, D. K., Spiro III, A., & Griffin, P. W. (2006). Personality and aging. In J. E. Birren & K. W. Schaie (Eds.), *Handbook of the psychology of aging* (6th ed., pp. 363–378). San Diego: Elsevier Academic Press.

Neugarten, B. L. (1968). Adult personality: Toward a psychology of the life cycle. In B. L. Neugarten (Ed.), *Middle age and aging* (pp. 137–1477). Chicago: University of Chicago Press.

Neugarten, B. L., Havighurst, R. J., & Tobin, S. S. (1968). Personality and patterns of aging. In B. L. Neugarten (Ed.), *Middle age and aging* (pp. 173–177). Chicago: University of Chicago Press.

Newman, B. M., & Newman, P. R. (1984). *Development through life: A psychosocial approach* (3rd ed.) Homewood, IL: Dorsey Press.

Newquist, D. D. (1987). Voodoo death in the American aged. In J. E. Birren & J. Livingston (Eds.), *Cognition, stress, and aging* (pp. 111–133). Englewood Cliffs, NJ: Prentice-Hall.

Peck, R. C. (1968). Psychological developments in the second half of life. In B. L. Neugarten (Ed.), *Middle age and aging* (pp. 88–92). Chicago: University of Chicago Press.

Perls, T. T. (2005). The different paths to age one hundred. *Annals of the New York Academy of Sciences, 1055*, 13–25.

Phelan, E. A., Anderson, L. A., LaCroix, A. A., & Larson, E. B. (2004). Older adults' views of "successful aging": How do they compare with researchers' definitions? *Journal of the American Geriatrics Society, 52*, 211–216.

Riley, M. W., Johnson, M., & Foner, A. (1972). *Aging and society. Vol. 3: A sociology of age stratification*. New York: Russell Sage Foundation.

Rose, A. M. (1965). The subculture of the aging: A framework for research in social gerontology. In A. M. Rose & W. Peterson (Eds.), *Older people and their social worlds*. Philadelphia: F. A. Davis.

Ryff, C. D., Kwan, C. M. L., & Singer, B. H. (2001). Personality and aging: Flourishing agendas and future challenges. In J. E. Birren & K. W. Schaie (Eds.), *Handbook of the psychology of aging* (5th ed., pp. 477–499). San Diego: Academic Press.

Sarkisian, C. A., Liu, H., Ensrud, K. E., Stone, K. L., & Mangione, C. M. (2001). Correlates of attributing new disability to old age. *Journal of the American Geriatrics Society, 49*, 134–141.

Scheidt, R. J., & Windley, P. G. (2006). Environmental gerontology: Progress in post-Lawton era. In J. E. Birren & K. W. Schaie (Eds.), *Handbook of the psychology of aging* (6th ed., pp. 105–125). San Diego: Elsevier Academic Press.

Sinclair, D. A., & Howitz, K. T. (2006). Dietary restriction, hormesis, and small molecule mimetics. In E. J. Masoro & S. N. Austad (Eds.), *Handbook of the biology of aging* (6th ed., pp. 63–104). San Diego: Elsevier Academic Press.

Sinnott, J. D., & Shifren, K. (2001). Gender and aging: Gender differences and gender roles. In J. E. Birren & K. W. Schaie (Eds.), *Handbook of the psychology of aging* (5th ed., pp. 454–476). San Diego: Elsevier Academic Press.

Tornstam, L. (1994). Gerotranscendence: A theoretical and empirical exploration. In L. E. Thomas & S. A. Eisenhandler (Eds.), *Aging and the religious dimension*. Westport, CT: Greenwood.

Tornstam, L. (1996). Gerotranscendence: A theory about maturing into old age. *Journal of Aging & Identity, 1*, 37–50.

Uhlenberg, P. (2000). Why study age integration? *The Gerontologist, 40*, 261–266.

Vogler, G. P. (2006). Behavior genetics and aging. In J. E. Birren & K. W. Schaie (Eds.), *Handbook of the psychology of aging* (6th ed., pp. 41–56). San Diego: Elsevier Academic Press.

Walker, A. (2006). Aging and politics: An international perspective. In R. H. Binstock & L. K. George (Eds.), *Handbook of aging and the social sciences* (6th ed., pp. 339–359). San Diego: Elsevier Academic Press.

Wang, E., Autexier, C., & Chen, E. (2001). Apoptosis and aging. In E. J. Masoro & S. N. Austad (Eds.), *Handbook of the biology of aging* (5th ed., pp. 246–266). San Diego: Academic Press.

Willcox, B. J., Willcox, D. C., He, Q., Curb, D. J., & Suzuki, M. (2006). Siblings of Okinawan centenarians share lifelong mortality. *Journals of Gerontology: Series A, Biological Sciences and Medical Sciences, 61*, 345–354.

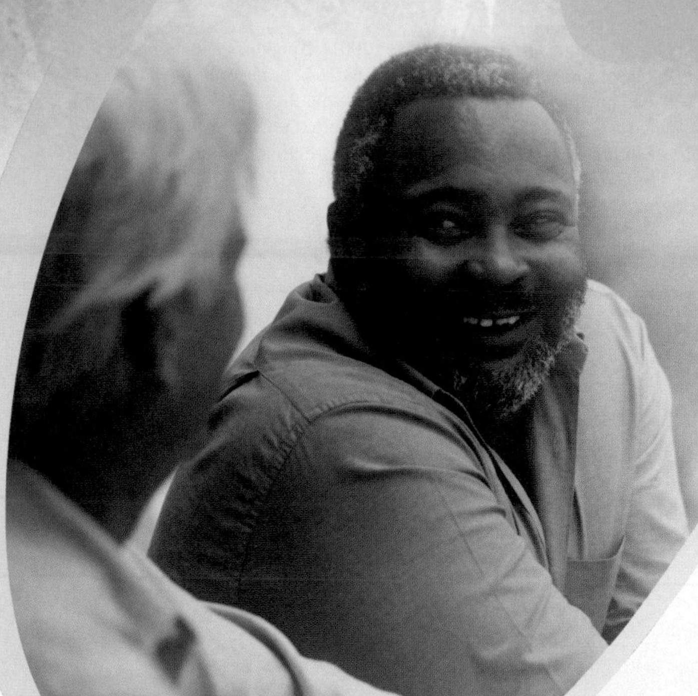

CHAPTER 4

Perspectives on Culture and Diversity of Older Adults

Learning Objectives

After reading this chapter, you will be able to:

1. Identify steps nurses can take to achieve cultural competence.
2. Discuss the importance of providing linguistically and culturally competent care for older adults.
3. Identify sources of information that nurses can use to improve their cultural competence.
4. Describe characteristics of the following four groups of older adults in the United States: African American, Hispanics, Asians, and American Indians.
5. Describe characteristics of rural and homeless older adults.

Key Terms

cultural competence
cultural rooting
linguistic competence
rural
transcultural nursing

Increasing diversity is a hallmark of the older adult population in the United States. This increasing diversity affects almost every facet of nursing care for older adults because cultural background significantly affects communication, values, health beliefs and health-related behaviors, and many other aspects of functioning. This is especially true for older adults from racially and ethnically diverse backgrounds because seven or more decades of cultural influences affect their health beliefs and behaviors. Moreover, these factors can significantly affect their relationships with health care providers and their receptivity to interventions. This chapter discusses the importance of cultural competence and transcultural nursing for the older adult population and describes diverse groups of older adults in the United States.

CULTURAL DIVERSITY OF OLDER ADULTS IN THE UNITED STATES

Much of the focus on cultural diversity in gerontological research centers on population trends in the United States that significantly affect the health care of older adults. Most commonly cited is the trend toward increasing diversity among older adults and the continuation of this trend through the next decades, as illustrated in Figure 4-1. Conclusions drawn from the 2000 census data that are pertinent to health care for older adults are as follows (Angel & Angel, 2006; Fuller-Thomson & Minkler, 2005; Murdock et al., 2005):

- Life expectancies at birth and at 65 years of age are increasing for all racial and ethnic groups; however, the highest life expectancy (as well as projected increases in

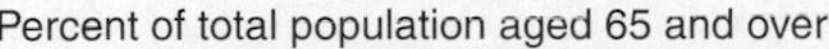

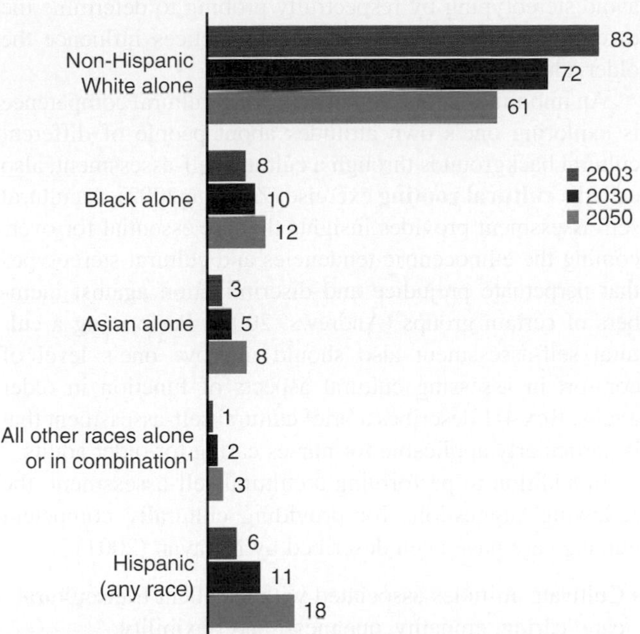

[1]The race group "All other races alone or in combination" includes American Indian and Alaska Native alone, Native Hawaiian and Other Pacific Islander alone, and all people who reported two or more races.

Note. The reference population for these data is the resident population.

FIGURE 4-1 Actual and projected population aged 65 years and older by race and Hispanic origin: 2003, 2030, and 2050. (From He, W., Sengupta, M., Velkoff, V. A., & DeBarros, K. A. [2005]. *65+ in the United States: 2005.* U.S. Census Bureau, Current Population Reports, P23-209. Washington, DC: U.S. Government Printing Office.)

life expectancy) is for Hispanic women, and the lowest is for African Americans.

- Dependency in activities of daily living is twice as high among older African Americans and Hispanics than among whites.
- American Indians and Alaskan Natives report disproportionately high levels of functional limitations (28% of those aged 45 years and older), with the higher rate being associated with increased age, lower income, less education, and unmarried and unemployment status.
- Minority populations will account for nearly 54% of the net increase in older adult population between 2000 and 2050.
- For every category of disease/disorder, the proportion of minority elderly who need treatment will increase between 2000 and 2050.
- Between 2000 and 2020, the percentage of total patient care hours spent caring for minority patients will increase from 31% to 40%.

These trends underscore the need for nurses to consider the older adult's cultural background when assessing health and wellness and planning care.

CULTURAL COMPETENCE AND TRANSCULTURAL NURSING FOR OLDER ADULTS

For several decades, nurses have recognized the importance of **transcultural nursing** (i.e., the provision of nursing care across cultural boundaries), and more recently, the importance of providing culturally competent care has been widely addressed by nurses and nursing organizations. For example, in the early 1990s both the American Academy of Nurses (1992, 1993) and the American Nurses Association (1994) published statements about culturally competent care. Holistic nursing literature, in particular, addresses cultural care as an essential component of caring (e.g., Barnes et al., 2000; Engebretson & Headley, 2005). In addition, many other regulatory, accrediting, and professional organizations (e.g., Joint Commission for Accreditation of Healthcare Organizations, American Nurses Credentialing Center Magnet Recognition Program) are calling attention to the need to ensure that people of diverse cultural, racial, ethnic, and linguistic groups receive care that is culturally congruent and linguistically appropriate (Narayan, 2001). The U.S. Department of Health and Human Services (USDHSS) Office of Minority Health is addressing issues related to cultural competence in health care (Fortier & Bishop, 2003). Also, elimination of health disparities is an aspect of cultural competence that is addressed by *Healthy People 2010* and other federal initiatives (USDHHS, 2000), by the Institute of Medicine's (2002) report on unequal treatment, and increasingly in medical journals (Appel et al., 2006; Rosa, 2006). Organizations such as the Gerontological Society of America and AARP (American Association of Retired Persons) also are emphasizing the need to address cultural diversity in the aging population. Clearly, there is a challenge, and support, for nurses to address cultural factors and seek cultural competence in caring for older adults.

Cultural competence in nursing is defined as "a process, as opposed to an end point, in which the nurse continuously strives to work effectively within the cultural context of an individual, family, or community from a diverse cultural background" (Andrews, 2003, p. 15). Similarly, cultural care in nursing is defined as "the subjectively and objectively learned and transmitted values, beliefs, and patterned lifeways that assist, support, facilitate, or enable another individual or group to maintain their health and well-being, to improve their human condition and lifeway, or to deal with illness, handicaps, or death" (Leininger & McFarland, 2002, p. 83).

Several nursing models conceptualize cultural competence as a continuum that reflects a progression from negative practices to positive approaches within an individual or organization (Engebretson & Headley, 2005). Stages of this continuum, from negative to positive, are cultural destructiveness, cultural incapacity, cultural blindness, cultural precompetence, cultural competence, and cultural proficiency (Luna, 2002). Purnell and Paulanka (2003) also view cultural competence as a continuum that begins with *unconscious incompetence* as a state of not being aware that one is lacking knowledge about another culture. When the person becomes aware of this knowledge gap, he or she progresses to a state of *conscious incompetence* and takes actions to learn about the cultural group. The person progresses to a stage of *conscious competence* by verifying generalizations and incorporating culture-specific interventions in care. The final stage is *unconscious competence* when knowledge of the cultural group is fully integrated into one's thinking and approach.

Health care professionals rarely achieve high levels of cultural competency (i.e., cultural proficiency or unconscious competence) in relation to a broad spectrum of different ethnic/cultural groups. However, health care professionals are expected to achieve cultural competency (or conscious competence) in relation to the specific cultural groups for whom they provide care. Moreover, they are expected to avoid stereotyping by respectfully probing to determine the extent to which cultural views and practices influence the older adults receiving care.

> **A Student's Perspective**
>
> *I found myself in a situation today in which I quickly recognized the importance of the lesson on cultural sensitivity in nursing. My aging client unfortunately had a significant change over the weekend, and her husband requested for her to be transported to the hospice inpatient unit. As she and I sat on her bed, she verbalized her acceptance that her disease is terminal. She wept as she voiced her heartache in telling her family of her "disappointment." Even though she is Catholic, because of her Chinese heritage and her family's Buddhist belief in "saving face," she worries that she has let her family down. While she expressed her thoughts, I listened and provided emotional support, which seemed to ease some of her grief. We transported her to the hospice unit, and I assisted in making her comfortable with the new environment. When I went out to the nurses' station to give my report, the receiving nurse's first comment to me was, "I see she is Asian and you have her religious preference documented as Catholic. Are you sure that is correct?" Because of our recent discussions and reading on cultural sensitivity, I quickly realized how we as nurses can make incorrect assumptions in categorizing individuals based on their ethnicity. I reported about my client's childhood history, her parents' belief in Buddhism, the Catholicism she was taught in school, and her long and strong Catholic faith. I found myself really understanding the importance of educating ourselves as nurses about different cultures and the effect of cultural belief systems on individualized health care. As difficult as it was for me to leave my client in a strange environment, I felt that the information I had learned and shared would enable the staff to be respectful of her beliefs, which in turn would be a positive experience for my client during her stay.*
>
> *Deborah L.*

An important initial step in achieving cultural competence is exploring one's own attitudes about people of different cultural backgrounds through a cultural self-assessment, also called a **cultural rooting** exercise (Zoucha, 2002). A cultural self-assessment provides insights that are essential for overcoming the ethnocentric tendencies and cultural stereotypes that perpetuate prejudice and discrimination against members of certain groups (Andrews, 2003). Performing a cultural self-assessment also should improve one's level of comfort in assessing cultural aspects of function in older adults. Box 4-1 describes a brief cultural self-assessment that is particularly applicable for nurses caring for older adults.

In addition to performing a cultural self-assessment, the following suggestions for providing culturally competent nursing care have been described by Narayan (2001):

- Cultivate attitudes associated with excellent transcultural care: caring, empathy, openness, and flexibility.
- Develop an awareness of the impact culture has on the beliefs, values, and practices of the patient and clinician and identify and avoid potential areas of cultural conflict (e.g., social values, communication patterns, and health beliefs and values).
- Become informed about cultural norms of the populations commonly served.
- Perform a cultural assessment and include questions that address cultural influences on nutrition, medication management, pain assessment, and psychosocial assessment.
- Individualize care plans that are culturally congruent.
- When unfamiliar with different cultural norms, avoid mistakes by taking cues from the other person and mirroring their behaviors; observe for cues that your actions or words are not culturally sensitive (e.g., discomfort, withdrawal).

A Nursing Model for Providing Culturally Sensitive Care

Nurses use many theoretical approaches to guide practice, spur research, and frame nursing curricula. For example, the Neuman Systems Model is a holistic nursing conceptual model that addresses a wide range of nursing concerns (Neuman & Fawcett, 2002). The explicit attention to sociocultural and spiritual variables is particularly applicable to providing culturally appropriate care to older adults under conditions of illness and wellness. According to this nursing model, the recipient of care can be individuals, families, groups, and communities with innate variables that relate to physiologic, psychological, sociocultural, developmental, and spiritual aspects. Nurses ask questions of the client, answer parallel questions from their own perspectives (Table 4-1), and then compare the answers to identify similarities and discrepancies, and mediate when there are differences (Neuman & Fawcett, 2002). Nursing interventions focus on primary, secondary, and tertiary prevention. When nurses mediate differ-

Box 4-1
Cultural Self-Assessment for Nurses Working With Older Adults

What self-identity influences my world view?

- With what sociocultural and religious groups do I most closely identify?
- What does it mean to belong to these groups?
- Is there any stigma associated with any of these groups?
- What do I like and dislike about these groups and my sociocultural identity?

How has my cultural background influenced me?

- How has (does) the society in which I grew up (currently live in) influenced the dominant values that I now hold?
- What is my perception of concepts such as time, work, leisure, health, family, relationships?
- How do my perceptions differ from those of people who come from different cultural backgrounds?

What is my attitude toward people, especially older adults, ...

- Who are immigrants?
- Who have difficulty with the English language?
- Who have difficulty communicating?
- Who have a cultural background different from my own?

What are my attitudes about and experiences with health practices that differ from my own?

- Do (did) my parents, grandparents, great-grandparents have health care practices that differed from conventional Western medicine practices (e.g., herbs, poultices, folk remedies)?
- Do (did) they consult with folk, indigenous, religious, or spiritual healers?
- How do I feel about alternative or complementary health care practices for myself and for older adults?

What do I do and how do I feel when I have difficulty understanding people whose accents and primary language are different from my own?

What have I learned about myself because of this self-assessment?

ences, they consider the use of cultural interventions, including folk and traditional care, as complementary to modalities such as medications, diagnostic tests, monitoring devices, special diets, and behavioral therapeutics.

Nurses can also use transcultural nursing theories to guide their care. The first of these theories is attributed to Madeleine Leininger, a nurse-anthropologist who established transcultural nursing as a formal and legitimate area of study in the mid-1950s (Leininger & McFarland, 2002). In recent decades, the influence of transcultural nursing has spread worldwide and has significantly influenced all areas of nursing practice (Andrews & Boyle, 2008). Thus, gerontological nurses have rich resources for gaining a deeper understanding of the complexities of cultural influence on the health of older adults.

Sources of Information for Developing Cultural Competence

Besides using nursing models and theoretical frameworks, nurses can increase their cultural competency by using research-based sources of information pertinent to health

TABLE 4-1 Questions Derived From the Neuman Systems Model for Guiding Culturally Sensitive Care

Questions to Ask the Client	Questions for the Nurse to Reflect On
"What are your major health care concerns?" (Or use other words that the client will understand.)	What do you consider to be the major health concerns for the older adult?
"How do your present circumstances differ from your usual pattern of living?" (e.g., ask about changes in schedules and responsibilities).	How do the present circumstances differ from the client's usual pattern of living? (Add observations about apparent importance of this change.)
"Have you ever experienced a similar problem? If so, what was the problem and how did you handle it? Were you successful?" (e.g., ask about folk and traditional health care practices).	Has the client ever experienced a similar situation? If so, how would you evaluate what the client did? How successful do you think it was? (Look for use of cultural care interventions as self care and the impact of these interventions.)
"What do you anticipate for yourself in the future as a consequence of your present situation?"	What do you anticipate for the future as a consequence of the client's present situation?
"What are you doing and what can you do to help yourself?" (e.g., ask the client to share information about folk and traditional health care practices).	What can the client do to help himself or herself? (Examine congruence between cultural and professional health care practices.)
"What do you expect caregivers, family, friends or others to do for you?"	What do you think the client expects from caregivers, family, friends, or other resources? (Use information to develop a synergistic and culturally sensitive plan of support that incorporates family, community, and professional resources.)

From Neuman, B., & Fawcett, J. (Eds.). (2002). Appendix C. In *The Neuman Systems Model* (4th ed., p. 351). Upper Saddle River, NJ: Prentice Hall.

care for older adults. Types of published works that are particularly useful in this regard are (1) studies that examine the effectiveness of a treatment in a specific patient population; (2) studies that compare similar actions or outcomes of two or more culturally diverse groups; and (3) randomized clinical trials, which are recommended by the federal government to determine the extent to which specific treatments ameliorate health disparities among ethically diverse populations.

In addition, nursing texts on transcultural nursing (e.g., Andrews & Boyle, 2008; Leininger & McFarland, 2002) are helpful sources of comprehensive information about cultural competence that is both theoretical and clinically relevant. Some nursing texts address specific cultural groups in relation to health care. For example, *Culture & Clinical Care* (Lipson & Dibble, 2005) is an excellent clinical reference describing characteristics of 35 culturally diverse groups in the United States. Another text, *Transcultural Health Care: A Culturally Competent Approach* (Purnell & Paulanka, 2003) applies a model for transcultural nursing to 20 diverse groups in the United States. Another excellent resource, *A Core Curriculum in Ethnogeriatrics* (2nd ed.), which was funded by the Bureau of Health Professions Health Resources and Services Administration, is available from the Stanford Geriatric Education Center (www.Stanford.edu/group/ethnoger/). This curriculum contains modules related to providing culturally competent geriatric care and includes information about 12 specific ethnic groups of older adults in the United States.

In this text, culturally specific information that is pertinent to nursing assessment of, and interventions for, older adults is highlighted in Cultural Considerations and Diversity Note features. Nurses are encouraged to supplement this information by reading journals and other references, and by obtaining information from the Internet and other sources listed in the Educational Resources section of this chapter. In addition, many of the organizations listed in the Educational Resources sections at the end of other chapters provide culturally appropriate educational materials. These materials can be important resources for health promotion interventions and are usually available at little or no cost; many can be downloaded from the Internet. In addition, all health care professionals are encouraged to obtain culturally specific information about groups that reside in their locale; such information is often available from local organizations.

Linguistic Competence in Care of Older Adults

Linguistic competence, which refers to health care services that are respectful of and responsive to a person's linguistic needs, is a form of cultural competence. This concept is important for gerontological nurses because they frequently work with older adults whose primary language differs from their own. Older adults who immigrated as adults may be particularly disadvantaged as regards English proficiency because they had few opportunities to learn English (Enslein et al., 2002). The challenge of communicating with people who do not speak the same language or dialect is magnified when the person also has dementia or sensory impairments, as is often the case in long-term care settings. Gerontological literature describes interventions to address cultural differences and communication needs of residents of long-term care facilities (e.g., Burgio et al., 2000; Gorek et al., 2002).

Because the Civil Rights Act of 1964 upholds the rights of individuals with limited English proficiency to have equal access to health and social services programs, health care providers must ensure effective use of interpretation services. At key decision-making points in health care encounters, circumstances that require the use of an interpreter include the following (Enslein et al., 2002):

- When client and practitioner speak different languages
- When the client has limited understanding of the practitioner's language
- When the practitioner has only a rudimentary understanding of the client's primary language
- When cultural tradition prohibits the client from speaking directly to the practitioner

Gerontological nurses have developed an excellent evidence-based protocol, called Interpreter Facilitation for Individuals with Limited English Proficiency, that provides comprehensive guidelines to facilitate the effective use of language interpretation services with older adults who have limited English proficiency (Enslein et al., 2002). Some nurses have found the AT&T Language Line Service to be a useful resource when interpreters are unavailable (see Educational Resources at the end of this chapter). Box 4-2 summarizes guidelines for using interpreters in health care settings with older adults.

OVERVIEW OF CULTURAL GROUPS OF OLDER ADULTS IN THE UNITED STATES

To provide culturally competent care, nurses need to educate themselves about the cultural groups in their patient populations. The study of the aging population in the United States has primarily been a study of white Americans, but gerontologists are increasingly recognizing the growing diversity and heterogeneity of older adults in the United States and the importance of identifying the interrelationships among race, ethnicity, aging, and health. Research regarding cultural aspects of aging began with a focus on African Americans during the 1960s and then extended to Hispanic Americans in the 1970s and to other groups in the 1980s. Little or no census data or other information about various subgroups was available until the early 2000s. Even today, terminology used in reference to subgroups is inconsistent and there is tremendous variation in definitions of specific groups. To add to the confusion, even the United States government defines groups differently. For example, Native Hawaiians are categorized as Asian American or Pacific Islanders in the United States Census, but as Native Americans in the Older

Box 4-2
Guidelines for Using Interpreters

Before the Interaction

- Whenever possible, use the services of a professional interpreter. Avoid using visitors or staff from auxiliary services unless permission to do so has been obtained from both the older adult and the interpreter.
- Given that there are more than 140 languages spoken in North America, be certain that the correct language and dialect have been identified before arranging for an interpreter. For example, does the person speak Cantonese or Mandarin Chinese?
- If an interpreter for the primary language is unavailable, determine whether the older adult speaks other languages. For example, many older adults from Vietnam and some African nations are also fluent in French.
- Be aware of age, gender, and socioeconomic class considerations in selecting an interpreter. In general, it is best to use an interpreter who is the same gender and of the same approximate age and socioeconomic class as the older adult.
- Organize your thoughts and plan ahead to ensure that the most important topics are covered.
- Allow sufficient time for the interaction and expect that it will take longer than an interaction with an older adult for whom English is the primary language.

During the Interaction

- Review the importance of confidentiality.
- Talk to the older adult, not the interpreter.
- Talk about only one topic at a time.
- Use short sentences and simple vocabulary.
- Use the active voice. Avoid vague modifiers.
- Avoid professional jargon, idioms, and slang.
- Be aware that many words do not translate into another language. For instance, the English word *depression* has no equivalent in many Asian and other languages.

Americans Act and in other contexts. Some of the commonly used cultural groupings and subgroupings are:

- Black or African American: African, West Indian, and Caribbean Islander
- Hispanic or Latino: Cuban, Spaniard, Mexican, Puerto Rican, and Central or South American
- Asian: Chinese, Japanese, Korean, Filipino, Asian Indians, and Vietnamese
- Native Hawaiian and Other Pacific Islander: Native Hawaiian, Samoan, Fijian, and Guamanian
- Native American and Native Alaskan (also known as American Indian, First Nation, and Alaska Native): Aleut, Eskimo, and more than 500 tribes of American Indian

Thus, although much progress has been made in research related to diverse groups of older adults, many subgroups continue to be lumped together. For example, cultural groups generally share a common language, but the category of Asian typically includes people who speak Hindi, Japanese, Vietnamese, Cambodian, and numerous Chinese dialects.

Information about some specific cultural groups of older adults is presented in the following sections. Nurses can use this information to learn about the cultural traditions of their patient populations but, as stated earlier, must be careful not to generalize or stereotype on the basis of a person's race or ethnicity.

African Americans

Africans were brought to America and bound into slavery beginning in 1619; by the end of the 19th century, more than 10 million Africans had been sold as slaves. Slavery, therefore, became the way of life that formed the roots of African American (black) culture in a European American (white) society. Inherent effects of slavery included poverty, discrimination, and social and psychological obstacles.

Racism continues in our society today and has a particularly negative impact on African Americans. However, consequences of racism affect all of society and have been a significant factor in the prevalence of health care disparities. Considerable evidence indicates that systemic discrimination is the most likely explanation for racial disparities in the provision of health care services for older African Americans (Williams & Wilson, 2001). For example, great disparity exists between the health status of African Americans and whites in the United States as well as in their access to health care. Stroke, cancer, arthritis, diabetes, glaucoma, hypertension, alcoholism, heart disease, and cerebrovascular disease are some of the conditions that have an excess prevalence in African Americans. African American older adults are more likely than whites to be impaired in daily activities, and functional declines occur at earlier ages for African Americans than they do for whites. African Americans also have worse self-perceptions of health than do whites. Studies suggest that racial differences significantly affect the kind and quality of medical care received, even under the Medicare system. Overall, the life expectancy for African Americans born in 1999 was 6 years lower than that for white Americans. A health difference that favors African Americans is the lower rate of osteoporosis compared with whites.

Older adults who identify themselves as black or African American are an extremely heterogeneous group, as indicated by the following (Yeo, 2000):

- Many are low income, but increasing numbers are in the middle and upper income categories
- Some are retired professionals, and many have children with professional careers
- Religious affiliations include Protestant, Catholic, Muslim, and none
- Educational levels vary from very little education to having doctorates
- Although many are dependent on children, grandchildren, and "fictive kin" for care, others are raising grandchildren or great-grandchildren

Female-headed households are a common family structure, and African American older adults are likely to have a broad base of extended family and social support. African American men are more likely to live alone (24%) and less likely to live with a spouse (54%) than men from any of the four other major older racial/ethnic populations (Yeo, 2000).

Geographically, African Americans live in all states, but their largest populations are in the South, in large metropolitan areas, and in the states of New York, California, Texas, Florida, Georgia, and Illinois. African Americans generally speak Standard English, but many also speak Black English (Ebonics) or another dialect. Black English is more common in urban areas, whereas Creole dialect is more common in the rural South. Compared with white older adults, African Americans are more likely to live with their children, grandchildren, or extended family and are less likely to live alone or in a nursing home. However, with an increase in single-parent families and dual working young adults as children of older parents, nursing homes are becoming more acceptable. African Americans may associate good health with harmony in life and may view illness as a punishment for sin.

Mrs. A. is an 81-year-old African American who lives with her daughter, Mildred, and teenage great-grandson in a two-bedroom apartment in a large metropolitan area of Ohio. Mildred works as a nursing assistant in a nearby nursing home and often works double shifts. Mrs. A. was born in Alabama and lived there until 20 years ago, when her husband died and she moved in with her daughter (who lived alone at the time). Seven years later, Mildred took on responsibility for raising her infant grandson, who is now 13 years old. Mrs. A. has glaucoma, arthritis, and hypertension, and she had a stroke several years ago. She admits to having "a little problem with my memory" but Mildred says "she remembers what she wants to remember." She takes an over-the-counter analgesic as needed for her arthritis and has two prescription medications for hypertension. She also uses prescription eye drops twice daily. Mrs. A. has her blood pressure checked by the parish nurse about once monthly; she sees a doctor and nurse practitioner at a neighborhood clinic for check-ups about twice yearly. The parish nurse often tells her that her blood pressure is "a little on the high side" and encourages her to see her doctor, but Mrs. A. has difficulty getting to appointments because she depends on Mildred to take her there. Mrs. A. is about 30 pounds overweight and she walks very slowly. When she is out of the house, Mildred provides a supportive hand to assist her with steadiness and mobility. Mildred shops for groceries, but Mrs. A. prepares most meals for the family.

THINKING POINTS

- How might Mrs. A's living arrangements influence her health and functioning, both positively and negatively?
- What factors are likely to influence the kind of health care Mrs. A. receives?
- If you were the parish nurse, what actions would you take to decrease health risks and promote quality of life for Mrs. A?
- What additional resources could be used to improve Mrs. A's situation?

Hispanics or Latinos

Because the federal government counts race and Hispanic origin as two separate categories, the 2000 census categorizes people by race and by whether or not they are Hispanic or Latino. People are considered Hispanic or Latino if their origin is Cuba, Mexico, Puerto Rico, South or Central America, or Spain, regardless of race. Thus, the category of Hispanic includes many heterogeneous groups that immigrated from these countries. Although they have some characteristics in common, they actually represent culturally diverse groups that are categorized together for reasons such as census and research. According to the 2000 census data, 12.5% of the total U.S. population, but only 5.6% of older Americans, is Hispanic or Latino. This group is expected to increase by 3.9% every year after 1990, so they will comprise 16.4% of the older adult population in the United States by 2050 (Yeo, 2000).

Hispanic older adults are divided as follows: 48% Mexican Americans, 15% Cuban, 12% Puerto Rican, and 25% mainly from Central and South American countries (Yeo, 2000). In the general U.S. population, Mexican Americans represent the largest proportion of Hispanics (61%), and there are almost three times as many Puerto Ricans (13%) as Cubans (5%). The differences in proportions of younger and older groups of Hispanics can be explained by the immigration patterns of each group.

The initial wave of Mexicans immigrating to America came to what was then the southwest territory during colonial times to build railroads. During the *bracero* period (1940s to 1960s), Mexicans came as agricultural laborers. (*Braceros* were experienced farm laborers who worked in cotton, sugar beet, and other agricultural fields.) The people who came during the *bracero* period currently comprise the population of older Mexican Americans. Recent Mexican immigrants are younger people, including many who are undocumented immigrants. This group will contribute to the significant increase in older Hispanics that is expected to occur over the next decades.

Cubans initially immigrated to the United States in the late 1800s to work in the tobacco industry, and a second influx occurred between 1940 and 1950 when Cubans came to help with the war industry. The largest number of Cuban immigrants came to the United States between 1959 and 1979 when many middle- and upper-class citizens fled Cuba for political reasons. This accounts for the higher number of older Cubans in relation to younger Cubans.

Puerto Ricans first came to the United States in the 1830s and began settling in New York City, but they did not come in great numbers until after World War II. By the 1970s, over

1 million Puerto Ricans had immigrated to more than 20 cities, motivated primarily by economics, employment, social mobility, and family relationships. Puerto Ricans were granted citizenship status in 1917.

Most Hispanics in the United States are concentrated in major cities in Arizona, California, Florida, New Jersey, New Mexico, New York, and Texas. Despite the significant diversity among these groups, information about them is generally lumped together under the classification of "Hispanics." Health conditions that disproportionately affect Hispanics include diabetes, obesity, malnutrition, and tuberculosis. The rate of heart disease in Mexican Americans is lower than it is in non-Hispanic whites. Like African Americans, Hispanics have lower rates of osteoporosis but higher rates of functional impairments compared with whites. Hispanics have high regard (*respecto*) for people by virtue of their age, service, or experience, and this carries over to a strong respect for older people. Hispanic groups have a strong sense of family and they tend to place the needs of the group or family over those of the individual. Hispanics, like African Americans, are more likely than whites to be living with family or extended family and less likely to be living in a nursing home. Hispanic older Americans, especially those who are Puerto Rican, have higher poverty rates than whites. The educational level of older Hispanics is lower than that of whites or African Americans. Most Hispanics in the United States speak both Spanish and English.

Both Mr. and Mrs. H. are 64-year-old Mexican Americans who came to an urban area of Texas to live with their son, Jose, and daughter-in-law, Maria, about 10 years ago. Mr. and Mrs. H. provide child care for their four grandchildren, Jose works as a farm laborer, and Maria does domestic work. Mr. and Mrs. H. prefer to speak and read in Spanish, and all family members speak Spanish in the home, but they can speak English well enough to communicate when necessary. Jose and Mr. H. each smoke a couple packs of cigarettes a day. None of the family members has health insurance, but this is not of concern to Mr. and Mrs. H. because they have relied on folk healers for many years and this has been effective for them. In their *curandismo* (traditional healing) system, Mrs. H. is the first person consulted and she applies the remedies that have been passed on to her from her mother and grandmother. Her remedies are directed toward restoring balance between hot and cold, and she also encourages prayers and lighting of candles at church. In the rare instances when a family member has not gotten better within a couple days, Mrs. H. takes him or her to a *yerbero* (herbalist) for herbs and other remedies. Once, when Maria had a more serious "female" problem, Mrs. H. took her to a *curandero* (folk healer), who was able to cure the problem.

You are a community health nurse in the county where Mr. and Mrs. H. reside and you are told to develop a planning committee for a health fair, which is being held at and cosponsored by the Catholic church attended by many of the community's Mexican Americans. The county health department received a grant from the National Institutes of Health to identify people most at risk for cancer, diabetes, and hypertension as part of the *Healthy People 2010* initiative. At least part of the motivation for receiving this grant was to cut the cost of providing care for people who are not diagnosed until these diseases are advanced. Statistics verify that Hispanics in your county have unusually high rates of diabetes, hypertension, and lung and breast cancer. Statistics also confirm that the cost of treating these conditions is disproportionately high because of complications from untreated and undiagnosed cases. The goal of this health fair, which is part of a larger initiative, is to screen for diabetes and to motivate people to return to future fairs for additional preventive measures. Your target population for this health fair is Hispanic people 45 years of age and older.

THINKING POINTS

- Who would you want to be on your committee?
- What factors will significantly influence participation in this health fair, both positively and negatively? What plans would you suggest for overcoming barriers to participation?
- What health topics would you be sure to address for health promotion?
- How might you incorporate a family perspective in the plans for the health fair?
- What could be done to incorporate folk healers in the planning and implementation of the health fair? What are the benefits and risks in doing this?
- What additional information would you want to have so you could proceed with planning a successful health fair? How would you go about finding this information?

Asians and Pacific Islanders

The category of "Asian and Pacific Islanders," like the category of "Hispanics," refers to numerous diverse subgroups of people in the United States who are clustered together for purposes of simplifying data. The 2000 census data distinguish between the Asian population and the Native Hawaiian and Other Pacific Islander population, but previous census data, and much of the available information about subgroups in the United States, lump together at least 30 subgroups in the one category of "Asian/Pacific Islanders." In the 2000 census, "Asian" refers to people having origins in any of the original peoples of the Far East, Southeast Asia, or the Indian subcontinent (including China, India,

Japan, Korea, Thailand, Vietnam, Pakistan, Cambodia, Malaysia, and the Philippine Islands). The largest Asian subgroup in the United States is the Chinese, who account for 30% of the Asian elderly. The next largest groups are the Japanese and Filipinos, each accounting for 24% of the Asian elderly (Williams & Wilson, 2001). Older Chinese and Japanese Americans are the two groups that are represented by both recent immigrants and American-born generations of earlier immigrants. Older Koreans, Vietnamese, Cambodians, and Asian Indians are likely to be recent immigrants to the United States.

The Chinese first migrated as laborers between 1840 and 1882, after which immigration of Chinese people to America was suspended until 1924, when annual quotas were established. Many of these immigrants came for political or socioeconomic reasons and had little or no education. In 1965 the Quota Act was abolished and many professional and highly educated Chinese came to the United States. Many Chinese live in metropolitan areas; the states with the largest Chinese populations are California, Hawaii, New York, Illinois, and Texas.

Japanese people began immigrating to America in 1885, and immigration peaked in the early 1900s. In 1924, they were barred from entering the United States, and in 1942, all Japanese people living in the United States were relocated to internment camps. Immigration resumed in the 1950s and increased after 1965 when immigration restrictions were eased. Japanese Americans are the only immigrant group whose members identify themselves according to their generation of birth in the United States. Generation groupings are *issei*, first-generation immigrants; *nisei*, first American-born generation; *sansei*, third generation; and *yonsei, gosei*, and *rokusei* for fourth, fifth, and sixth generations.

Filipinos came to the United States in three waves, beginning in the early 1700s when the "pioneer" group came to New Orleans. This first wave continued through the early 1900s and included agricultural workers in Hawaii and the western states. Beginning in 1934, Filipino immigrants were limited to an annual quota of 50. The second wave of Filipino immigrants took place between 1946 and 1965 when the annual quota was raised to 100. During this period many became United States citizens by joining the armed services or coming as students, professionals, or war brides. The third wave began after quotas were expanded and includes a large proportion of families and young professionals.

Koreans began immigrating to the United States in the 1900s, particularly to Hawaii, where they sought plantation work. Between 1950 and 1965, a second major wave of Koreans came, including many war brides of American servicemen. After 1965, many middle-class and college-educated Koreans, including many health care professionals, came to the United States.

The Vietnamese, who comprise the most recent Asian immigrant group, began arriving in the mid-1970s seeking political refuge because of the Vietnam War. Second and third waves of Vietnamese, Cambodians, and Laotians have come to the United States as refugees, including many older adults and other extended family members.

Despite the great diversity among Asian and Pacific Islander groups, some general characteristics may be summarized. Asian and Pacific Islander cultures are very family oriented and place a strong value on care of older family members. Asian older adults are less likely to live alone than the older population in general in the United States. Most American-born Asians speak English, but some immigrants speak only their native language or are bilingual. In Asian cultures, health is viewed as a state of spiritual and physical harmony, and illness occurs when the yin and yang are out of balance. "Yin" refers to female energy and is associated with wet, cold, and dark; "yang" refers to male energy and is associated with dry, hot, and light. Asians and Pacific Islanders have an excess prevalence of diabetes, hypertension, certain cancers, thalassemias (anemia), hepatitis B and other liver diseases, and tuberculosis (including multiple-drug–resistant strains). They have a lower rate of osteoporosis than whites.

Mrs. C. is a 76-year-old Chinese American widow who lives in an apartment in the Chinatown section of San Francisco. She has lived within the same 1-mile radius since her parents brought her to the United States from mainland China when she was 9 years old. All three of her children are married; two live about an hour away, and the other one lives on the East Coast. Although she can speak and read English, she prefers to use her native Chinese dialect, and all of her reading materials are in Chinese. She completed a high school education in Chinatown and married a Chinese immigrant when she was 19 years old. She served as her husband's primary caregiver after he developed lung cancer several years ago until his death last year.

Mrs. C. is enrolled in the On Lok Senior Health Program, a health maintenance organization that provides a wide range of health and social services. She attends a daily meal program and sees the nurse at the center for blood pressure checks every month. She has hypertension, arthritis, and coronary artery disease. Mrs. C. sees a local herbalist every few weeks to obtain the herbal medicines that will keep her yin and yang energies in balance, and she chooses foods according to their yin and yang characteristics. She periodically has acupuncture treatments when her arthritis bothers her. Although Mrs. C. believes she can control her heart problem and high blood pressure with herbs and diet, she takes her two medications as prescribed because the nurse at the On Lok clinic has emphasized that these pills are essential for keeping her energy in balance.

Mrs. C. recently had a stroke and received medical treatment and rehabilitation services. She is being discharged to her apartment with a referral to the On

Lok home care services for skilled nursing and speech, physical, and occupational therapies. Discharge orders also include the need to instruct Mrs. C. in a low-sodium diet. In addition to having some aphasia and left-sided paralysis, Mrs. C. has some residual memory impairment from the stroke. Before discharge from the rehabilitation program she said she would not need any home health aide assistance because she expected that her daughter and daughter-in-law would take turns coming over every day and that they would take care of her. You are the nurse assigned to do the initial assessment and your visit is scheduled for the day after discharge, when the daughter-in-law will be there. Although you have been a visiting nurse for several years, you have recently moved to San Francisco and you began working for On Lok 2 weeks ago.

THINKING POINTS

- How would you use the Neuman Systems Model (Table 4-1) to assess Mrs. C.'s situation, particularly with regard to expectations for family caregiving?
- What cultural factors might influence Mrs. C.'s acceptance of you, as the skilled care nurse, and of home care services in general?
- What would you do to gain cultural competence to work more effectively with Mrs. C. and other patients in the On Lok health care program?
- What are your specific health care concerns for Mrs. C., and what strategies would you use to develop an effective and acceptable care plan?

American Indians and Alaska Natives

In the 2000 United States census, the phrase "American Indian and Alaska Native" was used in reference to people having origins in any of the original peoples of North and South America (including Central America), and who maintain a tribal affiliation or community attachment. Native Hawaiians are sometimes categorized as Native Americans, but this is not done consistently, and the 2000 census designates Native Hawaiians and Other Pacific Islanders as a distinct group. In the United States, there are more than 500 federally recognized American Indian and Native Alaskan tribes, and an additional 100 to 200 native societies (unrecognized tribes). American Indians are the only minority group indigenous to the United States. Census 2000 reports that of all the American Indian respondents, 43% lived in the West, 31% in the South, 17% in the Midwest, and 9% in the Northeast. Twenty-five percent of the American Indian population lives in California and Oklahoma, and another 37% lives in Arizona, Texas, New Mexico, New York, Washington, North Carolina, Michigan, Alaska, and Florida.

The typical older American Indian is poor, has less than a high school education, and lives in a rural area with family or alone. Younger American Indians are likely to speak English, but older American Indians may speak little or no English and are likely instead to speak one of the more than 150 indigenous languages that continue to be spoken. American Indians have the highest prevalence of diabetes and the lowest cancer survival rate of any group. Diabetes is a significant health problem among American Indians as manifested by high rates of complications such as blindness, lower extremity amputations, and end-stage renal disease. In some American Indian communities, as many as half of all adults have diabetes, and the overall rate of diabetes in American Indians 65 years of age and older is almost 21%. Other diseases that are more prevalent among American Indians include cancer, obesity, arthritis, cataracts, alcoholism, tuberculosis, kidney disease, rheumatoid arthritis, and liver and gallbladder disease. American Indians also have a higher-than-average risk of dying from accidents such as falls, fires, and motor vehicle accidents. Compared with whites, they are more likely to have functional impairments and require assistance with daily activities.

Mrs. I. is a 72-year-old Navajo who lives with her daughter and son-in-law. In accordance with Navajo traditions, Mrs. I. believes that health is closely linked with being in harmony with the environment, family members, and supernatural forces. She regularly attends native healing ceremonies, and protects her family and herself from sickness through songs, stories, rituals, prayers, and sand paintings. Mrs. I.'s mother kept a medicine bundle, called a *jish*, containing stones, feathers, arrowheads, and corn pollen and used this for healing and blessings. Mrs. I.'s older sister now uses the jish that was passed on from their mother. Mrs. I. has had diabetes and hypertension for several years, and is about 30 pounds over her ideal weight. She receives medical care at the Indian Health Service, where you are the nurse. During a recent visit, you find that Mrs. I.'s blood pressure was 164/98 mm Hg and her random blood sugar as measured on the glucometer was 196 mg/dL. You know from previous visits that Mrs. I. does not want to take any prescription medications because she thinks they are not in harmony with spiritual forces. When you explain that both her blood sugar and blood pressure are high, she promises you that she will ask her older sister to use the jish for healing. You know from your experience with the Indian Health Service that nurses have been successful in persuading Navajos to perform physical exercise if it is viewed in a larger cultural context. For example, when the nurse consulted a tribal leader in developing an exercise program, the American Indians at a community health center were receptive to incorporating mild aerobic exercise into their daily routines in the form of traditional dance movements.

(case study continues on page 58)

THINKING POINTS

- What cultural factors are likely to influence Mrs. I.'s understanding of diabetes and hypertension?
- How would you use metaphors and cultural knowledge to help Mrs. I. understand her diabetes and hypertension?
- What questions would you ask Mrs. I. in order to identify teaching strategies and other interventions that might be successful with regard to her diabetes and hypertension?
- What strategies are likely to be successful in implementing dietary and lifestyle interventions for Mrs. I.?
- What steps would you take to improve your cultural competence in working with Mrs. I.?

OLDER ADULTS IN OTHER DIVERSE COMMUNITIES

In addition to exploring the unique needs of older adults of various cultural backgrounds, recent gerontological literature also examines the needs of other diverse groups, such as older adults living in rural areas and homeless older adults. Although most gerontological nurses do not provide care for rural or homeless older adults, they should recognize the numerous, highly diverse subculture groups of older adults who have unique health care needs.

Older Adults in Rural Areas

Rural is generally used in reference to people who live outside areas designated as "urban" or "metropolitan" and is determined by population density. Estimates of the percentage of older adults living in rural areas range from one fourth to one third, with only a small minority of these living in farming regions. In many rural areas, older adults comprise more than 20% of the population, in contrast to their comprising 12.4% of the population in the entire United States. Although significant local differences exist among rural areas and generalizing about rural older adults is difficult, some common characteristics and needs have been identified. Rural older adults are usually socioeconomically disadvantaged and have poor housing, higher poverty rates, and less formal education. Moreover, health care services are fewer and less accessible. Thus, older adults experience concomitant problems such as underdiagnosis, more disability, poorer health outcomes, and lower rates of monitoring chronic conditions. Of particular concern are the disproportionately higher rates of cardiovascular disease among rural older adults and of diabetes and hypertension among rural African Americans (Caldwell et al., 2005; Mainous et al., 2004).

Rural older adults are self-reliant and politically conservative; they are likely to have strong bonds with family, church, and community (Rosswurm, 2001). A 10-year series of ethnographic studies of a rural subculture of older adults, their families, and their health care providers in Colorado identified major cultural themes applicable to health care services for rural older adults. These themes included (1) availability of significant circles of formal and informal care; (2) a strong integration of faith, spirituality, and family with health status; (3) crisis-oriented decision making during health care transitions; and (4) use of nursing homes as a housing option because of few alternatives (Congdon & Magilvy, 2001).

Appalachia is a specific, federally defined rural nonfarming region of the United States that was established by an Act of Congress in 1965. The region spans more than 1000 miles across 13 states, including Ohio, Georgia, Virginia, Alabama, Mississippi, Pennsylvania, New York, and South Carolina. Much of the designated area lies in mountainous territory, causing geographic isolation and lack of access to health care. Appalachian people have been characterized as white, of British or Scotch-Irish descent, and predominantly fundamentalist Protestant in religion. Appalachia has a higher poverty rate and lower levels of formal education than the general population. Appalachian families maintain strong bonds, and older family members are honored for their role in transmitting their culture to younger generations. Older family members are likely to live with or very close to their children.

Appalachian people may be reluctant to seek medical care, particularly in a hospital, because they view the hospital as a place to go to die. Similarly, they may be reluctant to use rehabilitative services because they tend to view illness as the will of God and disability as an inevitable consequence of aging. These beliefs can present challenges for health care professionals who are attempting to address preventive, rehabilitative, or health promotion needs. An important aspect of providing culturally sensitive care to older adults in Appalachia is recognizing that women assume strong roles in maintaining health and preventing health risks within their families (Denham et al., 2004). In addition, studies have found that nurses can build on the cultural value of self-reliance by teaching about good health practices that can be incorporated into daily lives (Lohri-Posey, 2006).

Homeless Older Adults

The category of "older homeless" typically extends downward to the age of 50 years because some researchers have observed that homeless people look and behave as if they were 10 to 20 years older than their actual ages and have significant health problems (Brush, 2001). Increased homelessness among older adults is associated with increased poverty rates among certain segments and declining availability of affordable housing. Homeless people age 65 years and older are entitled to Medicare and Social Security benefits, but homeless people between the ages of 50 and 64 years usually do not qualify for these benefits unless they have been disabled for 2 years. Health characteristics of homeless older adults include significantly higher mortality rates, higher levels of disability, and higher overall rates of chronic illnesses and mental illness than younger homeless adults or older adults who are not homeless (Brush, 2001). Since the mid-1980s, social service and health care providers have recognized the need to provide rehabilitative services to address health, social, and behavioral problems of homeless older adults, in addition to addressing their basic needs for food and shelter. Services that have been developed in recent years specifically for the older homeless include resettlement and rehabilitation programs, drop-in and day care centers, and a variety of long-term housing options (Warnes & Crane, 2000).

Chapter Highlights

Cultural Diversity of Older Adults in the United States

- The population of the United States, including older adults, is increasing in diversity.
- Projections for 2050 estimate that 61.3% of older adults will be white, 12% black, 17.5% Hispanic, 7.8% Asian, and 1.4% other (Fig. 4-1).

Cultural Competence and Transcultural Nursing for Older Adults

- Numerous nursing, gerontological, and health care organizations recognize the importance of transcultural nursing (i.e., providing nursing care across cultural boundaries).
- All nurses are expected to develop cultural competence by assessing their own attitudes (Box 4-1) and learning about culturally diverse groups.
- Nurses can use the Neuman Systems Model as a guide for providing culturally sensitive care (Table 4-1).
- All health care providers need to be linguistically competent and to use resources to address needs of patients who are not proficient in English (Box 4-2).

Overview of Cultural Groups of Older Adults in the United States

- Some predominant cultural groups of older adults include African Americans, Hispanics or Latinos, Asian and Pacific Islanders, and American Indians and Alaska Natives.
- Nurses can develop cultural competence by educating themselves about the cultural traditions of the older adults in their geographic areas.

Older Adults in Other Diverse Communities

- Nurses must also take into consideration the subcultures of rural and homeless older adults when providing care to these populations.

Critical Thinking Exercises

1. Complete the cultural self-assessment in Box 4-1.
2. Identify one culturally diverse group that you are likely to work with if you practice nursing in your current geographic area. Contact the agencies and organizations that serve these groups and find out what services they offer; ask about unique health care issues affecting these particular groups.
3. Go to the Internet site of one of the culturally specific organizations and find information that you might use if you were presenting a health education program to a group of older adults who are of a particular cultural background (e.g., Chinese, African American).
4. Think of the various settings in which you work with older adults and describe what you would do or who you would call if you needed to communicate with a patient who did not speak English.

Educational Resources

Association of Asian Pacific Community Health Organizations
www.aapcho.org

AT&T Language Line
www.languageline.com

National Alliance for Hispanic Health
www.hispanichealth.org

National Asian Pacific Center on Aging
www.napca.org

National Caucus and Center on Black Aged, Inc.
www.ncba-aged.org

National Hispanic Council on Aging
www.nhcoa.org

National Indian Council on Aging
www.nicoa.org

National Resource Center on Native American Aging
www.und.edu/dept/nrcnaa/

National Rural Health Association
www.nrharural.org

Native Elder Health Care Resource Center University of Colorado Health Sciences Center
www.uchsc.edu/ai/nehcrc/

Office of Minority Health Resource Center
www.omhrc.gov

Organization of Chinese Americans
www.ocanatl.org

References

American Academy of Nursing. (1992). AAN expert panel report: Culturally competent health care. *Nursing Outlook, 40*, 277–283.

American Academy of Nursing, Subpanel on Nursing Education. (1993). *Promoting cultural competence in and through nursing education.* New York: Author.

American Nurses Association. (1994). *Position statement on cultural diversity in nursing practice.* Washington, DC: American Nurses Association Board of Directors.

Andrews, M. M. (2003). Cultural competence in the health history and physical examination. In M. M. Andrews & J. S. Boyle (Eds.), *Transcultural concepts in nursing care* (4th ed., pp. 15–35). Philadelphia: Lippincott Williams & Wilkins.

Andrews, M. M., & Boyle, J. S. (2008). *Transcultural concepts in nursing care* (5th ed. Philadelphia: Lippincott Williams & Wilkins.

Angel, R. J., & Angel, J. L. (2006). Diversity and aging in the United States. In R. H. Binstock & L. K. George (Eds.), *Handbook of aging and the social sciences* (6th ed., pp. 94–110). San Diego: Academic Press.

Appel, A., Everhart, R., Mehler, P. S., & MacKenzie, T. D. (2006). Lack of ethnic disparities in adult immunization rates among underserved older patients in an urban public health system. *Medical Care, 44*, 1054–1058.

Barnes, D. M., Craig, K. K., & Chambers, K. B. (2000). A review of the concept of culture in holistic nursing literature. *Journal of Holistic Nursing, 18*, 207–221.

Brush, B. (2001). Homelessness. In M. D. Mezey (Ed.), *The encyclopedia of elder care* (pp. 354–355). New York: Springer.

Burgio, L. D., Allen-Burge, R., Roth, D. L., Bourgeois, M. S., Dijkstra, K., Gerstle, J., et al. (2000). Come talk with me: Improving communication between nursing assistants and nursing home residents during care routines. *The Gerontologist, 41*, 449–460.

Caldwell, M. A., Peters, K. J., & Dracup, K. A. (2005). A simplified education program improves knowledge, self-care behavior, and disease severity in heart failure patients in rural settings. *American Heart Journal, 150*, 983.e7–983.e12.

Congdon, J. G., & Magilvy, J. K. (2001). Themes of rural health and aging from a program of research. *Geriatric Nursing, 22*, 234–238.

Denham, S. A., Meyer, M. G., Toborg, M. A., & Mande, M. J. (2004). Providing health education to Appalachia populations. *Holistic Nursing Practice, 18*, 293–301.

Engebretson, J. C., & Headley, J. A. (2005). Cultural diversity and care. In B. M. Dossey, L. Keegan, & C. E. Guzetta (Eds.), *Holistic nursing: A handbook for practice* (4th ed., pp. 307–336). Boston: Jones and Bartlett.

Enslein, J., Tripp-Reimer, T., Kelley, L. S., Choi, E., & McCarty, L. (2002). Interpreter facilitation for individuals with limited English proficiency. *Journal of Gerontological Nursing, 28*(7), 5–11.

Fortier, J. P., & Bishop, D. (2003). *Setting the agenda for research on cultural competence in health care: Final report.* Rockville, MD: U.S. Department of Health and Human Services Office of Minority Health, and Agency for Healthcare Research and Quality.

Fuller-Thomson, E., & Minkler, M. (2005). Functional limitations among older American Indians and Alaska Natives: Findings from the Census 2000 supplementary survey. *American Journal of Public Health, 95*, 1945–1948.

Gorek, B., Martin, J., White, N., Peters, D., & Hummel, F. (2002). Culturally competent care for Latino elders in long-term care settings. *Geriatric Nursing, 23*, 272–275.

Institute of Medicine. (2002). *Unequal treatment: Confronting racial and ethnic disparities in health care*. Washington, DC: National Academies Press.

Leininger, M., & McFarland, M. R. (2002). *Transcultural nursing: Concepts, theories, research and practice*. New York: McGraw-Hill.

Lipson, J. G., & Dibble, S. L. (2005). *Culture & clinical care*. San Francisco: University of California Nursing Press.

Lohri-Posey, B. (2006). Middle-aged Appalachians living with diabetes mellitus: A family affair. *Family and Community Health, 29*, 214–220.

Luna, I. (2002). Diversity issues in the delivery of healthcare. *Lippincott's Case Management, 7*(4), 138–146.

Mainous, A. G., King, D. E., Garr, D. R., & Pearson, W. S. (2004). Race, rural residence, and control of diabetes and hypertension. *Annals of Family Medicine, 2*, 563–568.

Murdock, S. H., Hoque, N., & McGehee, M. (2005). Population change in the United States. *Annual Review of Gerontology and Geriatrics, 25*, 19–63.

Narayan, M. C. (2001). Six steps toward cultural competence: A clinician's guide. *Home Health Care Management & Practice, 14*, 40–48.

Neuman, B., & Fawcett, J. (Eds.). (2002). *The Neuman Systems Model* (4th ed.). Upper Saddle River, NJ: Prentice Hall.

Purnell, L. D., & Paulanka, B. J. (2003). *Transcultural health care: A culturally competent approach*. Philadelphia: F. A. Davis.

Rosa, U. W. (2006). Impact of cultural competence on medical care: Where are we today? *Clinics in Chest Medicine, 27*, 395–399.

Rosswurm, M. A. (2001). Rural elders. In M. D. Mezey (Ed.), *The encyclopedia of elder care* (pp. 580–582). New York: Springer.

U.S. Department of Health and Human Services (USDHSS). (2000). *Healthy people 2010* (2nd ed.). Washington, DC: U.S. Government Printing Office.

Warnes, A. M., & Crane, M. A. (2000). The achievements of a multiservice project for older homeless people. *The Gerontologist, 40*, 618–626.

Williams, D. R., & Wilson, C. M. (2001). Race, ethnicity, and aging. In R. H. Binstock & L. K. George (Eds.), *Handbook of aging and the social sciences* (5th ed., pp. 160–178). San Diego: Academic Press.

Yeo, G. (Ed.). (2000). *Core curriculum in ethnogeriatrics* (2nd ed.). Stanford, CA: Stanford Geriatric Education Center. (Developed by the members of the Collaborative on Ethnogeriatric Education, supported by the Bureau of Health Professions, Health Resources and Services Administration, U.S. Department of Health and Human Services.)

Zoucha, R. (2002). Understanding the cultural self in promoting culturally competent care in the community. *Home Health Care Management & Practice, 14*, 452–456.

Nursing Considerations for Older Adults

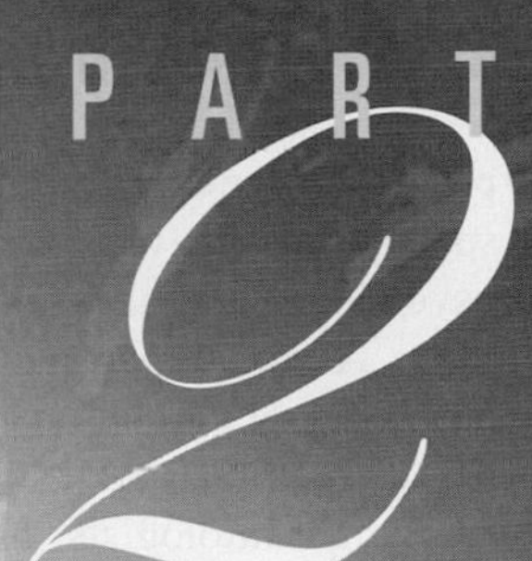

CHAPTER 5

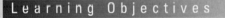

Gerontological Nursing and Health Promotion

Learning Objectives

After reading this chapter, you should be able to:

1. Describe the scope of gerontology and geriatrics.
2. Discuss the practice of gerontological nursing as a specialty.
3. Identify and use resources for improving competence in care of older adults.
4. Describe health promotion programs and interventions that are pertinent to older adults.
5. Identify and use resources for health promotion programs for older adults.

Key Terms

geriatrics
gerontology
gerontological nursing
health promotion
health-related quality of life
Transtheoretical Model

What emerges from the information in Part 1 is an image of older adults as a diverse group of individuals with various sociocultural backgrounds who are more heterogeneous than homogeneous. What is becoming clear is that, even among the same-age cohorts, as people age, they become less and less like others of the same age. Indeed, the most universal characteristic of increasing age is increasing uniqueness and diversity. Because the provision of health care and other services to this complex and heterogeneous population is so complicated, several branches of science have evolved to address the unique issues related to aging and older adults. This chapter introduces these branches of science and discusses health promotion for the older adult population.

GERONTOLOGY AND GERIATRICS

Gerontology is the study of aging and older adults. Gerontology was first recognized as a specialty in the mid-1940s with the establishment of the Gerontological Society of America and the publication of the first issue of the *Journal of Gerontology*. Since its inception, gerontology has addressed problems that "transcend the knowledge and methods of any one discipline or profession" (Frank, 1946,

p. 1). Gerontology continues to be multidisciplinary and is a specialized area within various disciplines, such as nursing, psychology, social work, and certain allied health professions. Although gerontologists initially focused on various problems of aging and older adults, they recently have begun to emphasize healthy and successful aging.

As gerontologists have become more aware of the increasing diversity among older people, health care providers also have become more aware of the increasing complexity of caring for older people. Consequently, the health care specialties of geriatric medicine and gerontological nursing have emerged. **Geriatrics** is associated with the diseases and disabilities of old people, and geriatric medicine is a subspecialty of internal medicine or family practice that focuses on the medical problems of older people. In 1942, the American Geriatrics Society was established and the editorial of its first publication, *Geriatrics*, called for physicians to "alleviate the inevitable deficiencies and limitations inherent in growing old" (Touhy, 1946, p. 17). In 1953, the society changed the name of their journal to the *Journal of the American Geriatrics Society* and broadened its focus to address a variety of issues that affect the health and functioning of older adults. These changes reflected the shift in geriatrics from medically oriented care to care that is more preventive—a shift from curing to caring. Consistent with this shift in orientation, the current foci of geriatrics include quality-of-life issues, interventions to maintain optimal functioning, and the importance of health promotion as a means of delaying the onset of disability.

GERONTOLOGICAL NURSING

History of Gerontological Nursing

In the early 1900s, nurses first recognized the need for a specialization to address the unique nursing needs of older adults, but it was not until the 1960s that geriatric nursing evolved as a nursing subspecialty (Fig. 5-1). In 1962, the American Nurses Association (ANA) convened a focus group on gerontological nursing practice. Four years later they formally recognized this specialty area by establishing a Division of Geriatric Nursing Practice and publishing a monograph titled *Exploring Progress in Geriatric Nursing Practice*. In 1969, the ANA published its first nursing practice standards, *Standards of Practice for Geriatric Nursing*. By the mid-1970s, the ANA was advocating the use of the

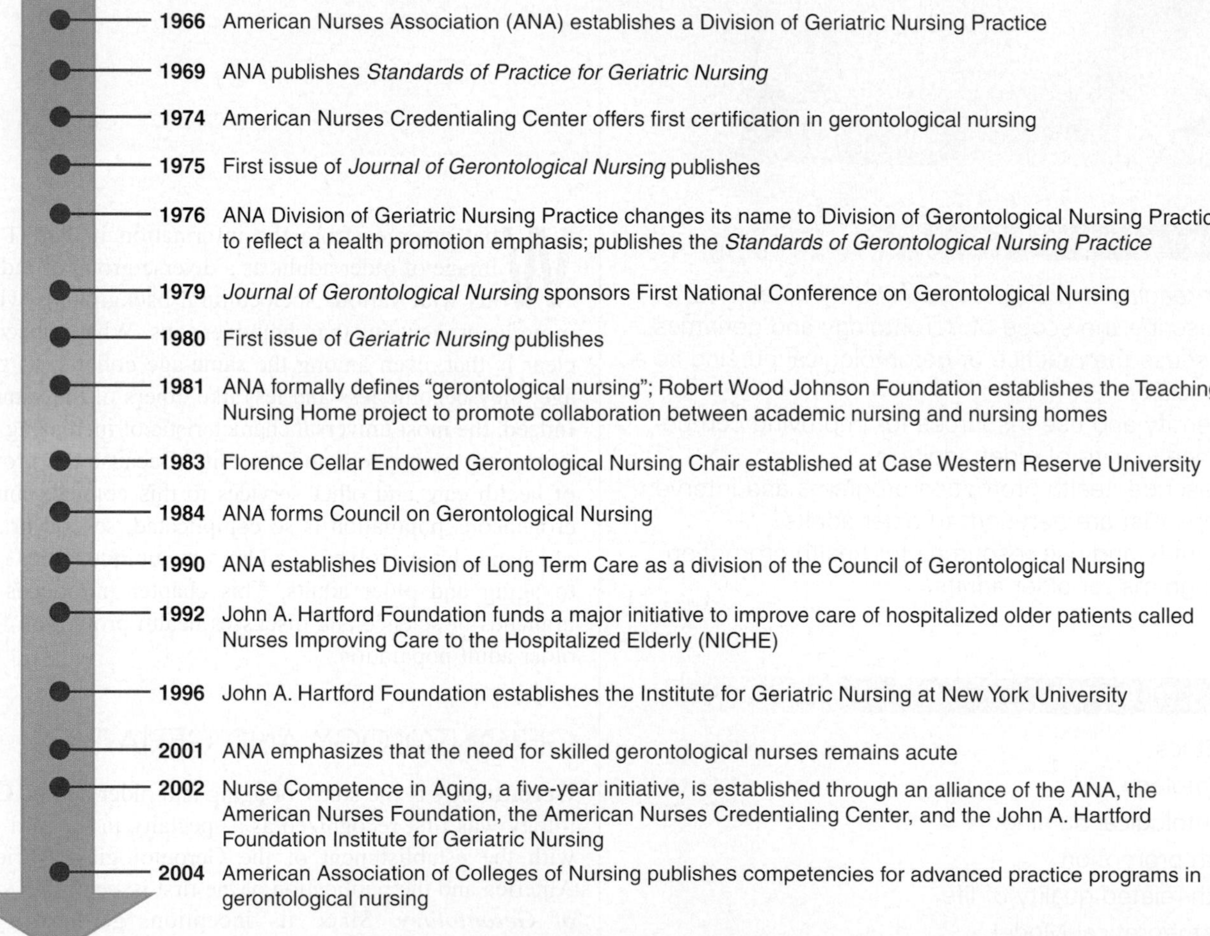
1966 American Nurses Association (ANA) establishes a Division of Geriatric Nursing Practice
1969 ANA publishes *Standards of Practice for Geriatric Nursing*
1974 American Nurses Credentialing Center offers first certification in gerontological nursing
1975 First issue of *Journal of Gerontological Nursing* publishes
1976 ANA Division of Geriatric Nursing Practice changes its name to Division of Gerontological Nursing Practice to reflect a health promotion emphasis; publishes the *Standards of Gerontological Nursing Practice*
1979 *Journal of Gerontological Nursing* sponsors First National Conference on Gerontological Nursing
1980 First issue of *Geriatric Nursing* publishes
1981 ANA formally defines "gerontological nursing"; Robert Wood Johnson Foundation establishes the Teaching Nursing Home project to promote collaboration between academic nursing and nursing homes
1983 Florence Cellar Endowed Gerontological Nursing Chair established at Case Western Reserve University
1984 ANA forms Council on Gerontological Nursing
1990 ANA establishes Division of Long Term Care as a division of the Council of Gerontological Nursing
1992 John A. Hartford Foundation funds a major initiative to improve care of hospitalized older patients called Nurses Improving Care to the Hospitalized Elderly (NICHE)
1996 John A. Hartford Foundation establishes the Institute for Geriatric Nursing at New York University
2001 ANA emphasizes that the need for skilled gerontological nurses remains acute
2002 Nurse Competence in Aging, a five-year initiative, is established through an alliance of the ANA, the American Nurses Foundation, the American Nurses Credentialing Center, and the John A. Hartford Foundation Institute for Geriatric Nursing
2004 American Association of Colleges of Nursing publishes competencies for advanced practice programs in gerontological nursing

FIGURE 5-1 Development of gerontological nursing as a specialty.

term **gerontological nursing**, rather than *geriatric nursing*, because the former more accurately reflects the scope of nursing and the latter term implies a focus of care primarily on the disease conditions of older people, which, for the most part, are much the same as those that affect all adults. In recognition of this, the ANA Division of Geriatric Nursing Practice changed its name to the Division on Gerontological Nursing Practice in 1976 and published the *Standards of Gerontological Nursing Practice*. These standards emphasize the role of gerontological nurses in maximizing independence in daily activities and promoting, maintaining, and restoring health (ANA, 1976).

In 1981, the ANA formally defined gerontological nursing in *A Statement on the Scope of Gerontological Nursing Practice*. In 1987, the ANA issued a combined *Standards and Scope of Gerontological Nursing Practice*, which was revised in 1995 and 2001. The 2001 revision identified gerontological nursing as "one of the profession's most challenging practice areas" and called for gerontological nurses to "meet the special needs of the increasing numbers of older adults, particularly those over 85 years of age, minorities, and those with decreased financial and social resources" (ANA, 2001, p. 7). The ANA published the 2001 edition jointly with the National Gerontological Nursing Association, the National Conference of Gerontological Nurse Practitioners, and the National Association of Directors of Nursing Administration in Long Term Care. The document summarizes the scope of practice for gerontological nursing and emphasizes that older adults in home, hospital, or various community and long-term care agencies require "comprehensive care that focuses on individualized health promotion and disease prevention, ongoing assessment of functional and cognitive status, rapid identification of acute problems, rehabilitation and restorative care, ongoing education, and appropriate referrals" (ANA, 2001, pp. 7–8). The document also delineates standards of clinical gerontological nursing care and professional gerontological nursing performance (Box 5-1).

Box 5-1
Standards of Professional Gerontological Nursing Performance

- I. **Quality of Care.** The gerontological nurse systematically evaluates the quality of care and effectiveness of nursing practice.
- II. **Performance Appraisal.** The gerontological nurse evaluates his or her own nursing practice in relation to professional practice standards and relevant statutes and regulations.
- III. **Education.** The gerontological nurse acquires and maintains current knowledge applicable to nursing practice.
- IV. **Collegiality.** The gerontological nurse contributes to the professional development of peers, colleagues, and others.
- V. **Ethics.** The gerontological nurse's decisions and actions on behalf of older adults are determined in an ethical manner.
- VI. **Collaboration.** The gerontological nurse collaborates with the older adult, the older adult's caregivers, and all members of the multidisciplinary team to provide comprehensive care.
- VII. **Research.** The gerontological nurse interprets, applies, and evaluates research findings to inform and improve gerontological nursing practice.
- VIII. **Resource Utilization.** The gerontological nurse considers factors related to safety, effectiveness, and cost in planning and delivering patient care.

The development of professional journals and the establishment of certification provide additional evidence of the growth of gerontological nursing as a specialty. The *Journal of Gerontological Nursing* was first published in 1975, followed by *Geriatric Nursing* in 1980; both journals continue to be published today. The American Nurses Credentialing Center offered the first certification in gerontological nursing in 1974. Today, certification is offered in the following gerontological nursing areas: Gerontological Nurse, Clinical Specialist in Gerontological Nursing, and Gerontological Nurse Practitioner. Home Health Nurse and Nursing Case Manager are additional certification areas that are particularly relevant to gerontological nurses.

Education of Gerontological Nurses

Care of older adults is compromised when the health care practitioner lacks knowledge about the unique manifestations of aging and disease and the relationships between diseases and age-related changes. Although this knowledge deficit is diminishing, nurses and other health care practitioners still lack the necessary skills to assess and treat common geriatric conditions accurately and effectively (Mezey & Fulmer, 2002).

In the 1980s, nursing organizations, schools of nursing, and institutions of higher learning began developing undergraduate, graduate, and continuing educational programs to prepare nurses and nursing students for gerontological nursing. Despite these efforts, however, the Bureau of Health Professions of the Health Resources and Service Administration reported a serious shortage of registered nurses that most seriously affected the following groups of older adults: rural elders, older women, minority elders, people in long-term care settings, and older adults with mental health problems (Klein, 1997). The current nursing shortage has important implications for the delivery of health care to all people, but its impact on older adults is likely to be even more serious.

Nationally recognized leaders in gerontology published a document titled *A National Agenda for Geriatric Education* (Klein, 1997), which summarized recommendations to address the identified needs. Two recommendations in this document were mandatory continuing education in gerontological nursing and the incorporation of model gerontological nursing curricula at both undergraduate and graduate levels. Some progress has been made in implementing these recommendations, but articles in a variety of nursing and health care journals continue to emphasize the need for educational programs to prepare nurses for gerontological nursing practice. One emphasized "the responsibility of the nursing profession as a whole" to address negative attitudes about and misperceptions of gerontological nursing and to "produce a more accurate and positive representation of gerontology" (Happell & Brooker, 2001).

Advanced practice gerontological nurses are registered nurses who hold a master's, nursing doctorate, or higher degree, and demonstrate advanced knowledge and clinical expertise in the care of older adults (ANA, 2001). Categories include gerontological nurse practitioners (GNPs) and gerontological clinical nurse specialists (GCNSs). Because state boards of nursing define and regulate the practice of advanced practice nurses, their scope varies to some extent. In general, however, all have some degree of prescriptive authority and are viewed as expert practitioners in their specialty area. Roles of advanced practice nurses include teacher, researcher, consultant, administrator, expert clinician, independent practitioner, care/case manager, individual/group counselor, and multidisciplinary team member/leader. Advanced practice nurses often manage acute and chronic conditions of older adults in their roles as primary care practitioners. Gerontological advanced practice nurses are knowledgeable about normal aging changes as well as common pathologic conditions of older adults, and their skills include comprehensive assessments of older adults and provision of in-depth prevention and health promotion services. There is increasing recognition of the important role of advanced practice nurses in long-term care facilities in improving quality of care through direct care and staff education (Futrell & Melillo, 2005).

Gerontological Nursing Resources

Since the late 1990s, the nursing profession has recognized that it is imperative to "prepare all practicing nurses with basic geriatric competencies as a way to ensure that older adults experience appropriate nursing care" (Mezey & Fulmer, 2002, p. M439). To accomplish this, the John A. Hartford Foundation established and funded the Hartford Institute for Geriatric Nursing to promote excellence in nursing care and increase all nurses' understanding of geriatric practice. This mission is accomplished through major initiatives in practice, research, policy, and professional and consumer education. A widely used and actively developing resource provided by the Hartford Foundation is a series of assessment tools to provide knowledge of best practices in care of older adults. These two-page tools are easy to access and use, and the Hartford Foundation encourages nurses to download them for use with older adults (available at www.hartfordign.org/resources/education/tryThis.html).

Current efforts of gerontological nursing leaders are directed toward improving competencies of all nurses, especially those in specialty practice, to address unique care needs of older adults. In 2002, the Hartford Institute formed an alliance with the ANA, the American Nurses Foundation, and the American Nurses Credentialing Center to fund a 5-year initiative called Nurse Competence in Aging. Major goals of the initiative are to (1) enhance geriatric activities of national specialty nursing organizations, (2) promote gerontological nursing certification nationally, and (3) provide an Internet resource center for specialty nurses (Stierle et al., 2006). A very practical outgrowth of this initiative is the availability of a free web-based resource center with information about nursing care issues specific to older adults. Nurses can access this wealth of information at http://www.consultgerirn.org.

Research Imperatives for Gerontological Nurses

Standard VII of the *Standards of Professional Gerontological Nursing Performance* states that gerontological nurses "are responsible for improving current nursing practice and the future healthcare for older adults by participating in the generation, testing, utilization, and evaluation of research findings" (ANA, 2001, p. 25). This standard mandates that nurses at the basic level of practice ask questions about the care of older adults, participate in studies to address these questions, and apply research findings to improve clinical care of older adults. At the Advanced Practice Nursing level, the gerontological nurse can fully participate in the generation, testing, utilization, critical evaluation, and dissemination of knowledge related to gerontological health care research (ANA, 2001). For example, in long-term care facilities, a geriatric clinical nurse specialist can improve quality of care by identifying resident care problems and developing solutions that are relevant, clinically correct, and up to date (Popejoy et al., 2000). Major accomplishments of gerontological nursing research in the last two decades include changing the paradigm for the use of physical restraints, improving the assessment and management of pressure ulcers and urinary incontinence, and developing strategies to improve bathing, feeding, and managing difficult and disruptive behaviors (Mezey & Fulmer, 2002).

In 1993, the 7-year-old National Center for Nursing Research was elevated to the status of a national institute within the National Institutes of Health (NIH). The National Institute of Nursing Research (NINR) supports multidisciplinary studies on innovative approaches to promoting health and preventing disease, minimizing the effects of acute and chronic illness and disability, and speeding recovery from disease. In the late 1990s, NINR-funded studies addressed such issues as prevention of pressure sores, decisions about hormonal therapy, the use of hip pads to prevent fractures, and quality of life for Alzheimer's patients and their caregivers. NINR-funded studies during the early 2000s that contribute to improved care for older adults address topics such as hydration, urinary incontinence, arthritis self-efficacy, continuity of care, cancer in older adults, care of people with Alzheimer's disease, and racial differences among caregivers. Nurses are encouraged to contact the NINR or visit its Internet site (www.nih.gov/ninr) for information about results of studies or funding for nursing research with regard to topics such as aging, self-management, and long-term care.

A working paper on the state of the art in gerontological nursing identified research priorities of the Hartford Foundation Centers for Geriatric Nursing Excellence in addressing needs of frail elders. Priorities included addressing specific care issues; preventing, delaying, or shortening institutionalization; improving outcomes and decreasing costs of care; facilitating transitions for older adults across the continuum of care; testing effective ways to promote health and improve quality of life; and demonstrating the unique contributions of professional nurses in the care of at-risk and vulnerable older adults and their caregivers (Strumpf, 2000). Another working paper, described as a "think piece" for The John A. Hartford Foundation, proposed the following goal for nursing's research–practice agenda in the third millennium: "May we prevent disease where possible, may we minimize morbidity and maximize quality of life where we cannot prevent disease, and may we have the wisdom to reconcile the two" (McBride, 2000, p. 26).

One of the nation's most recognized gerontological nursing leaders, May L. Wykle, PhD, RN, FAAN, also proposed an agenda for gerontological nursing research addressing the following priorities (Wykle, 2001):

- Developing interdisciplinary research activities
- Addressing diversity issues related to race, gender, and culture
- Promoting health and preventing disease for individuals, families, and communities
- Providing elder care resources that are community focused and home care based
- Testing of various gerontological nursing practice models for providing evidence-based practice
- Addressing long-term care issues such as physical care activities, interventions for behavior problems, end-of-life care, and staffing patterns and nursing staff mix
- Attracting students to gerontology and nurses to employment in long-term care

HEALTH, WELLNESS, AND HEALTH PROMOTION

Nurses often use the terms *health* and *wellness* interchangeably because of the shifting paradigm from the traditional health–illness continuum to a whole-person model. This paradigm shift is evident in holistic nursing definitions of health and wellness. For example, holistic nurses define health as "the state or process in which the individual (nurse, client, family, group, or community) experiences a sense of well-being, harmony, and unity where subjective experiences about health, health beliefs, and values are honored" (Dossey & Guzzetta, 2005, p. 6). Similarly, a holistic nursing definition of wellness is "integrated, congruent functioning aimed toward reaching one's highest potential" (Gaydos, 2005, p. 58). In this book, *health* is defined as the ability of older adults to function at their highest capacity despite the presence of age-related changes and risk factors, whereas *wellness* is an outcome for older adults whose quality of life is improved through nursing interventions.

The growing emphasis on health and wellness has resulted in increasing recognition of the importance of health promotion. **Health promotion** refers to programs or interventions that focus on behavior changes directed toward improved health and well-being of individuals, groups, communities, and nations in relation to their environments. Traditionally, health promotion programs have focused primarily on physical health and functioning and screening programs to detect disease. In recent years, the focus and scope of health promotion has broadened to emphasize wellness behaviors in addition to disease prevention actions. For example, some health promotion activities that promote wellness include

- Regularly engaging in various types of physical exercise
- Assuring optimal nutritional intake and avoiding foods associated with risk for disease
- Using stress reduction methods, such as yoga, meditation, relaxation, and imagery
- Fostering healthy relationships with others
- Engaging in self-wellness actions (e.g., getting adequate rest and sleep, taking time for enjoyable activities alone or with others)
- Attending to spiritual growth

This broader perspective on wellness in older adults emphasizes not only body–mind–spirit interconnectedness but the need for health promotion programs to address the relationship between individual behaviors and the social environment (Gordon, 2006). Gordon provides the following example of such a health promotion program:

> *A health promotion program that seeks to change social norms such as the belief that it is unsafe for older adults to do strength training could intervene at the interpersonal ("between people") level by inviting families to participate in strength training at a physical-activity health fair. The same program might also intervene at the community and public policy levels by starting a walking club and encouraging the participants to become involved in a local effort to create a walk/bike path (p. 2).*

Health Promotion Initiatives for Older Adults

Health promotion is evolving as a major focus of health care services in the United States, as evidenced by the development of several major national health initiatives since 1979. These initiatives, which apply the concept of healthy aging to adults of all ages, emphasize that everyone can benefit from preventive health care (Infeld & Whitelaw, 2002).

Healthy People 2010, launched in January 2000 as an extension of the *Healthy People 2000* campaign of the 1990s, is a well-known national health initiative with many aspects particularly applicable to older adults. The program—designed as a road map for improving the health of all people in the United States—outlines a comprehensive, nationwide agenda for promoting health and preventing illness, disability, and premature death. The two major goals are increasing quality and years of healthy life and eliminating health disparities. For older adults, the first goal is associated with preventing chronic illness as well as exacerbations of illnesses that already exist. The second goal addresses some of the health disparities that disproportionately affect specific older populations. Common health disparities include hypertension in African Americans, diabetes in Hispanic and Native American groups, obesity in Hispanic and African American women, and smoking in American Indians and Alaska Natives (Burggraf & Barry, 2000).

Beginning in the early 2000s, the Centers for Disease Control and Prevention (CDC) has focused on health promotion research and program implementation addressing specific health concerns of older adults. For example, in 2001 researchers began examining factors that influenced the low rate of immunization among older African Americans. In 2002, they established a healthy aging research network to identify ways of improving health and functioning of older Americans with regard to healthy lifestyles, early detection of diseases, immunizations, injury prevention, and self-management techniques. The CDC also maintains a website devoted to providing reliable, science-based, high-quality information on health of older adults (www.cdc.gov/aging), with emphasis on dispelling myths about health promotion and aging. Core projects for 2004 to 2009 include a community outreach and demonstration project through the Center for Healthy Aging and a health promotion program called Physical Activity for Lifetime Success (PALS). Other current focus areas for healthy aging sponsored by the Prevention Research Centers of the CDC include nutrition, immunizations, depression, diabetes, oral health, and physical activity. Nurses are encouraged to use the websites listed in the Educational Resources section of this chapter to find more information and to keep up to date on health promotion programs specific for older adults.

The *Live Well, Live Long: Health Promotion and Disease Prevention for Older Adults* program is another source of useful information about topics such as cultural competence and health literacy as well as specific aspects of health promotion. This program, which is a joint effort of the CDC and the American Society on Aging, provides teaching modules that nurses can use for health promotion on topics such as diabetes, nutrition, medications, mental wellness, cognitive vitality, and driving wellness. They also publish issue briefs and a monthly newsletter called *Healthword: Putting Health Promotion Back in Motion* (available at www.asaging.org/cdc/HealthWord.cfm). Box 5-2 summarizes some national health initiatives that are applicable to health promotion for older adults. Resources for health promotion materials that are especially useful for gerontological nurses (including

Box 5-2
National Health Initiatives and Resources Important to Older Adults

Medicare. Medicare covers the following preventive services: glaucoma screening, breast examinations, screening mammograms, bone density measurements, influenza and pneumonia immunizations, Pap smears and pelvic examinations, colorectal cancer screening procedures, prostate-specific antigen tests and digital rectal examinations, and diabetes education and self-management benefits.

Healthy People 2010. *Healthy People 2010* focuses on leading health indicators for which measurable baseline and target levels have been established (e.g., mental health, physical activity, and access to quality health services).

Eliminating Racial and Ethnic Disparities in Health. This initiative addresses disparities in health status that are applicable to racial and ethnic older adults (e.g., diabetes, immunizations, cardiovascular disease, and cancer screening and management).

Healthy Aging Project. Part of the Centers for Medicare and Medicaid Service, the Healthy Aging Project reviews available literature on health promotion and disease prevention interventions for older people and publishes evidence-based recommendations (e.g., *Smoking Cessation and Medicare*).

Program of All-Inclusive Care for the Elderly (PACE). PACE provides an integrated, community-based multidisciplinary care model with a strong emphasis on health promotion.

National Institute on Aging. The Institute's goals for 2001 to 2005 include understanding healthy aging processes, reducing health disparities among older people and groups, improving health and quality of life for older people, and enhancing resources to support high-quality research.

Put Prevention in Practice: Staying Healthy at 50+. This educational booklet offers recommendations about living habits, screening tests, and immunizations.

Exercise: A Guide From the National Institute on Aging. This video and booklet focus on a safe and effective exercise program for older adults.

Healthfinder. From the U.S. Department of Health and Human Services, Healthfinder provides reliable information on the Internet about health topics (e.g., prevention, self-care).

National Resource Center on Aging and Injury. The Center provides information about preventing unintentional injuries to older adults. It is a division of the National Center for Injury Prevention of the Centers for Disease Control and Prevention.

National Center for Chronic Disease Prevention and Health Promotion. The Center provides educational materials on healthy aging.

From Infeld, D. L., & Whitelaw, N. (2002). Policy initiatives to promote healthy aging. *Clinics in Geriatric Medicine, 18*, 627–642.

Internet sites for many of the national health initiatives) are listed in the Educational Resources section at the end of this chapter.

Focus of Health Promotion Programs

The emergence and expansion of interest in health promotion can be attributed in part to the national initiatives and in large part to the current emphasis on both cost-effectiveness of health care services and quality of life for health care consumers of all ages. Health care planners are increasingly recognizing that health promotion activities can be cost-effective when they prevent or delay the onset of disease or disability. Although Medicare and many managed care systems have traditionally focused on acute and episodic care, the focus is now shifting, and health care systems are addressing and managing risk factors and helping people maintain independence as ways of controlling health care costs (Given & Given, 2001). A discussion of health promotion and disease prevention specifically with regard to older adults concluded that "concepts such as function preservation, disability prevention and postponement, chronic-disease management, and independence enhancement must become central concerns of our health care system" (Given & Given, 2001, p. 220). Another article concluded that "the net effect of primary prevention will be to reduce and compress disability into a shorter period toward the end of life, to decrease overall lifetime disability, and consequently, to reduce the associated health care burden" (Hubert et al., 2002, p. M347).

A dominant theme of current gerontological health promotion efforts is to *add life to years, not just more years to life* (Drewnowski & Evans, 2001a; Mehr & Tatum, 2002; Rejeski & Mihalko, 2001). The concept of **health-related quality of life**—a phrase that is becoming commonplace in gerontological literature—is being promoted as an alternative to morbidity and mortality data as an indicator of health status. Definitions of health-related quality of life include characteristics such as social functioning, emotional well-being, a personal sense of physical and mental health, and overall life satisfaction and happiness (Drewnowski & Evans, 2001a). Health promotion activities, such as exercise, nutrition, and other lifestyle modifications, improve health-related quality of life by improving the ability of older adults to live independently and care for themselves (Chernoff, 2002). Gerontologists emphasize that "there is no single segment of our society that can benefit more from regular exercise and improved diet than older adults. Maintenance of function permits older adults to care for themselves, maintain their independence, and enjoy improved quality of life" (Drewnowski & Evans, 2001b, p. 5). One recent review of preventive interventions concluded that "perhaps the best antiaging medicine is exercise" (Fisher & Morley, 2002, p. M637). Because older adults are likely to view nurses as important providers of health education and other health promotion interventions, nurses have numerous opportunities for improving the quality of life for older adults through health promotion interventions (Dubbert et al., 2002; Hawranik & Pangman, 2002).

The focus of health promotion activities varies for different age groups. For older adults, health promotion activities focus on (1) prevention and postponement of disease and disability, and (2) early identification and effective management of disease conditions. Specific goals for health promotion and disease prevention for older adults include reduced premature mortality, enhanced quality of life, expanded active life expectancy, and maintenance of functional independence for as long as possible (Bloom, 2001). Major emphasis is placed on modifiable lifestyle factors because lifestyle choices account for as much as 10 years of life expectancy and strongly influence health, functioning, quality of life, and the onset of disability (Fraser & Shavlik, 2001; Hubert et al., 2002; Mehr & Tatum, 2002).

Despite the proliferation of evidence that health promotion interventions are cost-effective ways of preventing disease and disability and improving functioning and quality of life for older adults, evidence indicates that older adults as a group receive fewer prevention and screening health care services than other populations. Misconceptions that have interfered with the development of health promotion programs for older adults include (1) normal aging processes diminish the benefits of prevention, (2) prevention is not effective after the onset of chronic illness, and (3) older adults are less responsive to health education and promotion interventions. Researchers have recently debunked all three of these myths (Bhalotra & Mutschler, 2001), providing even more impetus for the development of health promotion programs for older adults.

Many organizations disseminate guidelines for health promotion interventions, and they are not always in agreement, especially with regard to recommendations for older adults. The American Cancer Society, the United States Preventive Services Task Force, and the Agency for Healthcare Research and Quality are some of the organizations that play a prominent role in developing and promulgating guidelines for preventive care. Box 5-3 summarizes some of the more widely agreed-on guidelines for older adults, which gerontological nurses can follow when educating older adults about health promotion interventions.

Types of Health Promotion Interventions for Older Adults

Interventions to promote physical and psychosocial well-being include screening programs, risk reduction interventions, environmental modifications, and health education to promote good health practices. In addition to addressing all aspects of physical function, health promotion activities for older adults address psychosocial aspects of function such as dementia, depression, mental health, substance abuse, and elder abuse and neglect. Another focus of health promotion that nurses address is self-care, especially for

Box 5-3
Guidelines for Prevention and Health Promotion Interventions for Older Adults

Immunizations

For All Older Adults

- **Tetanus-diphtheria** pertussis boaster shot every 10 years
- **Influenza** annually at beginning of influenza season
- **Pneumovax** once after age 65 years; booster after 5 years if initial vaccination was before age 65 years or if other risk factors are present
- **Herpes zoster**

For At-Risk Older Adults

- **Hepatitis A and B**
- **Measles, mumps, rubella** if evidence of lack of immunity and significant risk for exposure
- **Varicella** if evidence of lack of immunity and significant risk for exposure

Screening

For All Older Adults

- **Blood pressure** checks at least annually, more frequently if range is 130–139 mm Hg systolic or 85–90 mm Hg diastolic or if other risk factors are present (e.g., diabetes, African American race)
- **Serum cholesterol** every 5 years, more frequently in people with risk such as personal or family history of cardiovascular disease
- **Fecal occult blood and rectal exam** annually
- **Sigmoidoscopy** every (3 to) 5 years after age 50 years
- **Visual acuity and glaucoma screening** annually
- **Breast exam:** self-exam monthly, annually by primary care practitioner

For Women

- **Pap smear and pelvic exam** annually until three consecutive negative exams, then every 2 to 3 years; discontinue after 65 years of age if three consecutive negative exams
- **Mammogram** annually or biannually between 50 and 69 years, every 1 to 3 years between 70 and 85 years

For Men

- **Digital rectal exam** annually

For At-Risk Older Adults

- **Blood glucose level**
- **Thyroid function**
- **Heart function (electrocardiograph)**
- **Bone density**
- **Mental status assessment**
- **Screening for dementia, depression, substance abuse**
- **Urinary incontinence assessment**
- **Functional assessment**
- **Screening for adverse medication effects and drug interactions**
- **Skin cancer assessment**
- **Fall risk assessment**
- **Pressure ulcer assessment**
- **Elder abuse or neglect assessment**

For Men

- **Prostate-specific antigen (PSA) blood test**

Health Promotion Counseling

For All Older Adults (Unless Contraindicated)

- **Exercise:** at least 30 minutes of moderate-intensity physical activity daily
- **Nutrition:** adequate intake of all vitamins and minerals, especially calcium and antioxidants
- **Dental care and prophylaxis:** every 6 months
- **Protective measures:** seatbelts, sunscreens, smoke detectors, fall risk prevention

For Older Adults if Applicable

- **Smoking cessation**
- **Substance abuse cessation**
- **Weight loss**

community-living older adults (Leenerts et al., 2002). For example, nurses have developed and tested a model for Self-Care for Health Promotion in Aging that was effective for older adults who were caregivers (Teel & Leenerts, 2005). Nurses used this model to teach older adults skills related to communicating effectively, practicing healthy habits, building self-esteem, focusing on the positive, avoiding role overload, and building meaning.

Additional types of health promotion interventions that are relevant for some older adults include addressing their pain and comfort concerns and issues related to the use of multiple medications. Active management of pain (discussed in Chapter 28) is an essential aspect of disability prevention because chronic pain leads to depression and diminished physical activity (Morley & Flaherty, 2002). Interventions for polypharmacy are health promotion activities when they are directed toward identifying and preventing medication interactions and other adverse effects of medications. As discussed in Chapter 8, nurses have important responsibilities for monitoring therapeutic as well as adverse medication effects and for educating older adults and their caregivers about medication effects.

Social supports and social interaction on a regular basis have positive effects on many aspects of mental health and some aspects of physiologic function, such as cardiovascular health. Religion and spiritual practices are increasingly being recognized as a focus of health promotion directed toward successful aging (Parker et al., 2002).

Screening Programs

Screening programs are particularly important for the early detection of serious and progressive conditions that can readily be detected and treated, such as glaucoma, diabetes, hypertension, hyperlipidemia, osteoporosis, hypothyroidism, and skin cancer. The following criteria have been identified for effectiveness of screening tests: (1) the test must be able to detect the condition or risk factor earlier than without screening and without excessive false-positive or false-negative results, and (2) early intervention must be superior to waiting until signs or symptoms of disease are present (Mehr & Tatum, 2002).

Although the incidence of many types of cancer increases with age, and cancer screening programs have been widely recommended for skin, breast, colon, prostate, and other cancers, cancer screening for older adults, particularly for those older than 75 years of age, has always been somewhat controversial. Recently, controversy about mammography for older women and prostate-specific antigen (PSA) testing for older men has increased because of conflicting study findings, concerns about cost-effectiveness, and questions about the risks and benefits of treatment options. Because geriatric practitioners are focusing more on increasing years of healthy living and less on extending the quantity of life, decisions about screening tests can be based on the person's active life expectancy and health-related quality of life. These decisions also are based on individual values, which are shaped in large part by culture and religion (Mehr & Tatum, 2002). For example, if these principles were applied to the use of the PSA screening test, this test would not be recommended for a man with a life expectancy of less than 10 years, nor would it be offered to a man with dementia because the interventions would not contribute to short-term well-being. However, it would be given to a man older than 70 years if he still requested it after a discussion of its advantages and disadvantages (Mehr & Tatum, 2002).

Risk Reduction Interventions

Risk reduction interventions include any activity that is directed toward reducing the chance that a disease condition will develop; these interventions are based on an assessment of the degree of risk for development of a particular condition. Some risk reduction interventions (e.g., vaccinations) are applicable to all older adults, and other interventions vary according to the specific risk factors and the level of health or frailty of an older person. Risk assessment tools have been developed for a variety of conditions, including falls, incontinence, heart disease, pressure ulcers, and elder abuse and neglect. These tools often include a rating scale to identify people who are most likely to develop a particular condition so that health care professionals can plan and implement preventive interventions for people at higher risk. These tools also serve as a way of identifying the risk factors that can be addressed through preventive interventions.

Even without assessment tools, health care professionals can usually identify risk factors that can be addressed to prevent disease or disability. Priority usually is given to reducing the risk factors that are most dominant or are likely to have the most serious negative consequences. For example, health promotion interventions for a relatively healthy older adult with a history of hypertension, hypercholesterolemia, and family history of heart attacks would address risk factors for heart disease for that person. Health promotion interventions for a frail older adult who is in a skilled care unit recovering from a fractured hip would focus on fall prevention and safe mobility. For any older adult, risk reduction interventions include lifestyle factors such as exercise, optimal nutrition, physical activity, stress-relieving techniques, and smoking cessation (if applicable). Health promotion activities to reduce risk may also include the use of over-the-counter medications (e.g., low-dose aspirin), nutritional supplements (e.g., vitamins), and complementary and alternative medicine (e.g., yoga). The Health Enhancement Program is one example of a risk reduction program for community-dwelling older adults at risk for functional decline in which a nurse works with each participant to develop a "health action plan" that addresses at least one disability risk factor identified in an initial assessment (Phelan et al., 2002). Positive outcomes of this program after 1 year's participation include improved health status, decreased burden of disability, and no decline in functional status.

Environmental Modifications

Environmental modifications are within the realm of health promotion activities when they are implemented to reduce risks or improve a person's level of functioning. For example, reduction of fall risks involves numerous environmental modifications (discussed in Chapter 22). Environmental modifications also are effective in improving hearing and vision, and in preventing urinary incontinence, as discussed in Chapters 16, 17, and 19. The National Resource Center on Supportive Housing and Home Modifications (listed in the Educational Resources section) is an example of an initiative to promote healthy aging through environments designed to facilitate optimal functioning. This center disseminates information, conducts research, and provides training and education for older adults, caregivers, providers, and policymakers (Infeld & Whitelaw, 2002).

Health Education to Promote Good Health Practices

Health education is a key component of most health promotion interventions, with a focus on teaching people to engage in self-care activities that are preventive in their scope. Health education addresses health practices such as nutrition, dental care, exercise and physical activity, and avoidance of smoking and environmental tobacco smoke. Because health education about nutrition, dental care, and smoking cessation is addressed in Chapters 18 and 21, this chapter focuses on health education related to exercise and physical activity.

Articles about the need for increased physical activity are ubiquitous in lay and professional literature, and physical activity is probably the most widely promulgated health promotion intervention today. Gerontologists emphasize that physical inactivity is an independent risk factor for a wide range of chronic conditions, and older adults are at particular risk for leading sedentary lifestyles (King, 2001). A summary of research concluded that older adults should be screened for sedentariness at all major encounters with health care professionals, "given its role as a potent risk factor for all-cause and cardiovascular mortality, obesity, hypertension, insulin resistance, cardiovascular disease, diabetes, stroke, colon cancer, depression, osteoporosis, recurrent falls, and disability, among other conditions" (Singh, 2002, p. M276). Numerous well-designed studies support the recommendation that exercise should be the standard of care for all older adults because "there is no group of individuals who can benefit more from increased levels of physical activity than elderly people" (Evans, 2002, p. M260). Even moderate levels of physical activity—defined as 30 minutes of participation in activities of moderate intensity such as walking or gardening on most days of the week—can have substantial health benefits (DiPietro, 2001).

Despite the wealth of undisputed evidence about the beneficial effects of physical activity for older adults, less than one third of older people in the United States engage in it regularly. Factors associated with lower levels of physical activity are female sex, being a smoker, having poor health or medical concerns, having lower income and less education, and lacking experience with physical activity. Barriers that have been identified in older adults include impaired health, fear of injury, unpleasant sensations associated with exercise, lack of access to appropriate facilities, and lack of knowledge about the benefits of exercise (Resnick, 2002). Motivational factors that are associated with higher levels of physical activity include a desire to improve physical fitness and appearance, fewer perceived barriers to being physically active, positive beliefs about the value of physical activity, and a higher level of confidence about being able successfully to undertake physical activity (King, 2001).

Nurses take many roles in promoting physical activity for older adults. Because many older adults do not perceive the benefits of physical activity and, in fact, may falsely believe that physical activity should be avoided, nurses need to assess the person's beliefs about and understanding of both the beneficial and detrimental effects of physical activity. Nurses also assess for and address other factors that positively or negatively influence an older adult to participate in regular physical activity. Nurse researchers found an association between self-efficacy and motivation to participate in exercise and physical activity (e.g., Allison & Keller, 2000). Health-related barriers that interfere with physical activity in older adults include pain, fatigue, and sensory and mobility impairments (Cooper et al., 2001). Cooper and colleagues proposed a variety of nursing interventions to help overcome these barriers. For example, pacing the exercise program and taking prescribed anti-inflammatory medications before physical activity are interventions that address pain. The WALC model—**W**alk, **A**ddress pain, fear, fatigue, **L**earn about exercise, **C**ue by self-modeling—is one example of a nursing intervention that has been used effectively to increase participation of older adults in exercise and can be implemented in a variety of settings (Resnick, 2002). The University of Iowa Gerontological Nursing Interventions Research Center has developed an evidence-based protocol that provides nursing guidelines for teaching older adults about exercise promotion (Titler, 2002). Singh (2002) summarizes current research on exercise and aging and makes comprehensive recommendations for an exercise and physical activity program for health promotion and disease prevention in older adults. Other examples of nursing interventions to promote exercise interventions for older adults are found in nursing journals (e.g., Melillo et al., 2001; Resnick & Spellbring, 2000; Schlicht, 2000). Nurses can use Box 5-4 as a guide to teaching older adults about recommended exercises.

THE TRANSTHEORETICAL MODEL OF HEALTH PROMOTION

Many disease prevention and health promotion interventions require a change from detrimental health-related behaviors to those that prevent disease and promote wellness. Once behavior change has been initiated, the new healthier behaviors must be maintained. Initiation and maintenance of these changes involve both motivation and action steps. The more ingrained and rewarding or pleasurable the behaviors that must be changed, the more difficult it is to refrain from these activities. Some unhealthy behaviors, such as cigarette smoking, have a strong addictive component that increases the difficulty of behavior change. Similarly, the more comfortable a person is with the absence of healthy behaviors, such as physical activity, the more difficult it will be to develop healthier behaviors. The role of gerontological health care professionals in health promotion interventions is to lead and support the older person through the stages of change involved in replacing unhealthy behaviors with health-promoting behaviors.

The **Transtheoretical Model** (TTM), developed two decades ago (Prochaska & DiClemente, 1982), has been widely used by health care professionals to explain stages of behavior change. Stress management, sun exposure, smoking cessation, medication compliance, alcohol and drug cessation, diet and weight control, and screening for breast and cervical cancer are health promotion areas in which the TTM has been used successfully (Burkholder & Evers, 2002). One gerontological nursing article described the TTM as "an integrative model of behavior change that is applicable to older adults and can be used easily by nurses in any health care setting.... Further, the recommendations from the TTM are well suited to nurses working with older people and can be used both in individual interactions or group sessions" (Burbank et al., 2000, p. 32). Application of this model specifically in gerontological health care settings is described in detail in *Promoting Exercise and Behavior Change in Older Adults* (Burbank & Riebe, 2002).

The TTM is called the *stages-of-change model* because it describes five specific stages through which a person progresses in accomplishing behavior changes. In the first stage, *Precontemplation*, the person is unaware of the problem, is in denial of the need for change, or is resistant to

Box 5-4
Health Education About Types of Exercise

Physical activity is any skeletal muscle activity that causes energy expenditure.
Exercise refers to structured and repetitive body movements performed with the goal of attaining physical fitness.

	Definition	Benefits	Intensity	Frequency	Examples
Aerobic (dynamic or endurance) activity	Activity that requires the body to use oxygen to produce the energy necessary for the activity	Lowers blood pressure, strengthens heart muscle, decreases triglycerides, increases high-density lipoproteins, diminishes blood glucose, decreases intra-abdominal fat, decreases risk for cardiovascular disease, improves self-esteem, relieves symptoms of anxiety and depression	Identify your target heart rate by subtracting your age in years from 220 (this is the maximum heart rate) and multiplying by 0.65	30 minutes, 5 times weekly	Brisk walking, jogging, walking up stairs
Strength training (resistance training, weight-training, muscle-building) activity	Performance of muscle contractions against a resistance that is greater than usual for that muscle; slow and controlled movements of major muscled groups such as arms, back, hips, chest, and shoulders, with exhalation during exertion and inhalation during return to the starting position	Improves balance and diminishes risk for falls, strengthens musculoskeletal system, improves function and independence, decreases risk for osteoporosis, favorably modifies risk factors for cardiovascular disease and type 2 diabetes	You should be able to repeat the movement 8 consecutive times, but not more than 12 times, before experiencing significant muscle fatigue	8 to 10 different sets of exercises working all major muscle groups, each repeated 8 to 12 times, several days a week	Resistance bands, weight training, strap-on sandbags, bicep curls for the arms, bench presses for the chest, bent-over rows for the upper back
Stretching	Activity that improves body flexibility	Increases flexibility, reduces muscle soreness, improves performance of daily activities	Stretch muscle groups, but not to the point of pain, and hold for 10 to 30 seconds	Repeat each stretch at least 4 times, a minimum of 2 to 4 times weekly	Yoga, stretching of all joints and muscle groups, range-of-motion exercises

change. At this stage, the person has no intention of changing his or her behaviors within the next 6 months. Appropriate health promotion interventions for a person in this stage include providing information about the problem behavior and providing unconditional encouragement for thinking about behavior change. When working with an older adult in this stage, gerontological nurses can offer information, discuss their own beliefs, and help the person identify the personal benefits of the health-promoting behaviors. The nurse also can acknowledge the person's perspective and point out the negative consequences of current behaviors.

The second stage, *Contemplation*, is characterized by an intention to change in the foreseeable future, based on some acknowledgment of the negative consequences of current behaviors and positive consequences of different behaviors. The person is likely to ask questions and to seek information about the short- and long-term risks and benefits of various behaviors. He or she is likely to be ambivalent about giving up a rewarding activity or taking on an activity that is viewed as difficult or less enjoyable. During this stage, the gerontological nurse can help the person see that the benefits outweigh the disadvantages, even though the person may not experience the benefits immediately. Appropriate health promotion interventions for this stage include providing additional information about the risks and benefits and exploring with the person how he or she can begin establishing personal goals for a healthier lifestyle. Interventions also include increasing the person's sense of self-efficacy by helping the person to see himself or herself practicing these new behaviors. When working with an older adult in this stage, it is helpful to express confidence in the person's ability to develop health-promoting behaviors.

Stage three, the *Preparation* stage, is characterized by some ambivalence about the unhealthy behavior, but a stronger inclination to change to healthier behaviors. The person acknowledges the need for change, expresses serious intent to adopt the healthier behaviors within the next month, and begins to identify strategies for implementing them. During this stage, people usually benefit from support from family and friends, and they are likely to state their intentions and seek help from others in accomplishing their goals. Gerontological nurses can support and provide positive reinforcement for the person's intent to change; they also can point out the progress that the person already has made in developing an action plan. An important role for nurses is to assist with developing a plan and identifying the person's goals and small-step strategies to achieve them. Although discussing the barriers to changing behaviors might be necessary, it is important to focus on the benefits of the new behavior. Planning strategies for dealing with anticipated difficulties in implementing the plan is also helpful.

Action, the fourth stage, occurs when the person has already made the behavior change, but the changes have been in place for less than 6 months. At this stage, people usually do not fully experience the benefits of the new behavior and are vulnerable to resuming prior unhealthy behaviors or giving up the new healthy behaviors. At the same time, they are likely to have high levels of self-efficacy and to feel good about the progress they have made. Health promotion interventions during this stage are directed toward reinforcing the progress that has been made as well as toward identifying any barriers to continuing the healthy behaviors. Gerontological nurses can help the older adult identify motivators, establish a reward system, and plan strategies for overcoming the identified obstacles. They also can ask about support from friends and family and help the person identify ways of extending their support system if necessary.

Stage five, *Maintenance*, occurs when the person has continued the healthy behaviors for 6 months or longer. By this time, the person is experiencing positive effects of the healthier behavior and the risk of relapse is less. During this stage, levels of self-efficacy are usually high and the person is motivated to maintain the healthier lifestyle. Because the person has less need for external support, the role of the gerontological nurse diminishes. Health promotion interventions during this stage include reinforcement of progress and positive feedback about the healthier behaviors. In addition, the nurse can ask about any difficulties in maintaining the progress and help the person identify strategies to overcome any difficulties.

Mrs. H. is 72 years old and visits the local senior center three times weekly for meals and social activities. Once a month she comes to see you to have her blood pressure checked. You have recently studied the Transtheoretical Model and are interested in applying it to your clinical work in the Senior Wellness Program. Mrs. H. takes medication for high blood pressure and has expressed concern about heart disease. When you discuss risk factors for heart disease with Mrs. H., she says that she would like to incorporate more physical activity into her daily life, as long as it doesn't worsen her arthritis. She agrees to begin meeting with you regularly to develop a plan. Table 5-1 shows how you might apply the Transtheoretical Model to your work with Mrs. H.

THINKING POINTS

Precontemplation Stage

- From a health promotion perspective, how would you assess Mrs. H.'s understanding of the role of exercise in prevention of heart disease? What misconceptions would you want to address?
- What are the goals of your teaching interventions at this stage?

Contemplation Stage

- How would you assess Mrs. H.'s perception of the advantages and disadvantages of increased levels of exercise?
- What are the goals of your teaching interventions at this stage?
- What additional teaching points would you incorporate in your health promotion interventions at this time?

(case study continues on page 73)

Preparation Stage

- What additional assessment questions would you ask Mrs. H.?
- What are the goals of your teaching interventions at this stage?
- What additional teaching points would you incorporate, particularly with regard to Mrs. H.'s concerns about her arthritis?

Action Stage

- What concerns would you have about Mrs. H. during this stage, and what additional questions would you ask?
- What additional teaching points would you make?

Maintenance Stage

- What additional assessment questions would you ask Mrs. H.?
- What additional teaching points would you make?

TABLE 5-1 Applying the Transtheoretical Model to Mrs. H.

Stage	Nurse	Mrs. H.
I: Precontemplation		
Assessment	"I know you're concerned about preventing heart disease because you've talked with me about your high blood pressure and you pay attention to avoiding high-fat foods. How do you think you rate on a scale of 1 to 10, with 1 being the lowest level and 10 being the best, in level of physical activity for preventing heart disease?"	"I would rate myself about 10. I take the dog out for a 5-minute walk every morning. My friend says we don't need more than 10 minutes of walking a day after we're 70 years old."
Intervention	"Did you know that there is extremely good evidence that 30 minutes of physical activity every day—even if it's not done all at once—is a good measure for protecting against heart disease? Would you be willing to read this pamphlet from the American Heart Association and let me know what you think when I see you again next week?"	"I've seen that before, but I'll try to read it this week if I have a chance."
II: Contemplation		
Assessment	"Now that you've had a chance to read that brochure, what's your understanding of the role of physical activity in preventing heart problems?"	"I think the Heart Association is on an exercise kick—they must think we all want to participate in marathons! Maybe they have a point about walking more than 15 minutes a day, but don't they realize that those of us who are in our 70s have a lot of problems walking? Most of us have arthritis. I think that brochure was written for people in their 20s, but on the other hand, maybe they do know what they're talking about."
Intervention	"From what I know, the Heart Association focuses on helping people prevent heart disease through healthy habits. They strongly urge everyone to do physical exercise for 30 minutes every day to keep the heart healthy. Many studies of people of all ages support this recommendation. You already walk 5 minutes with your dog every day, so you've gotten a good start on daily exercise. I bet your dog would love to go just a little farther each day and you would be quite capable of increasing your walk by just a little bit."	"Well, the dog is getting pretty fat, and it would probably do her good to get out for another walk in the evening. But it's hard enough for me to get out once a day with the weather as cold as it is right now. With my arthritis, I think I should wait a couple of months until the weather is warmer."
III: Preparation		
Assessment	"Since we met a couple of months ago, what are your current thoughts about increasing your walking?"	"I've been doing a lot of thinking about what we discussed, and now that spring is finally here, I think it's time to increase my walking time by a little bit each day. I just hope my arthritis doesn't get worse if I walk more."

continued on following page

TABLE 5-1 Applying the Transtheoretical Model to Mrs. H. (continued)

Stage	Nurse	Mrs. H.
Intervention	"So, have you thought of a plan that might work for you? Can you identify people who might be helpful in supporting your efforts?"	"Well, to begin with, I thought I could walk for 10 minutes every morning instead of 5—my dog sure would like that. I could increase that by 5 minutes every few weeks until I get up to 30 minutes a day. I've told my daughter that I'm trying to do more walking, and she said she might come over and walk with me and the dog on Saturdays. I do worry about my arthritis, though."
IV: Action		
Assessment	"It's so good to hear that you've been increasing your walking time for 3 months now. Congratulations on getting up to 30 minutes a day. How are you feeling about that?"	"My dog sure likes it, but I'm not sure that it's doing any good for me. I guess it feels good to pay attention to my health, but I haven't noticed that I'm feeling any better physically—at least not yet. My daughter came with me for the first few weeks and that was a good chance to see her, but she hasn't been coming for the last 3 weeks."
Intervention	"You deserve a lot of credit for accomplishing your goal—do you give yourself any rewards? It sounds as though you're disappointed that your daughter stopped walking with you—is there anyone else who might walk with you?"	"I guess I do deserve some credit—I did buy myself a new pair of walking shoes last week. A neighbor lady has talked to me about my walking and she said she'd like to get out there and join me, but I didn't encourage that because I thought my daughter would be coming with me. Maybe I'll invite her along—she could use the exercise, too."
V: Maintenance		
Assessment	"Congratulations on walking for 30 minutes every day for 7 months—that's quite an accomplishment and a nice gift for yourself and your health. You also deserve credit for getting your neighbor to join you at least a couple of days a week. Are you concerned about any temptations to cut down on your walking routine?"	"Thanks for the encouragement—my neighbor says she appreciates me inviting her along, and I enjoy the chance to keep up on neighborhood happenings by chatting with her when we walk. I am a little concerned about keeping up with the walking during the winter. I don't even take the dog out when it snows."
Intervention	"Have you thought about walking in the mall when the weather is bad? I'm not sure if you can take the dog along, but the mall opens every day an hour before the stores open so that walkers can come. I understand there's quite a group that walks there in the mornings."	"That sounds like a good idea—my neighbor mentioned that we might go there in bad weather. I think I'll try that out—maybe if I went to the mall, I could get my daughter to meet me there on Saturdays."

Chapter Highlights

Gerontology and Geriatrics

- Geriatrics and gerontology are areas of professional specialization that have evolved since the mid-1940s to address the unique needs of older adults.
- These specialties initially focused on problems associated with aging, but the current focus is on quality-of-life issues and promoting optimal health and functioning.

Gerontological Nursing

- Gerontological nursing was first recognized as a nursing specialty during the 1960s, and major initiatives continue to encourage the development of this much-needed area of expertise.
- Major initiatives promote geriatric competencies for all nurses and nursing research that focuses on nursing interventions to meet the unique needs of older adults.

Health, Wellness, and Health Promotion

- Major national initiatives such as *Healthy People 2010* highlight the focus on health promotion in U.S. health care and on improved health and functioning in older adults.
- Health promotion interventions are essential if older adults are to achieve and maintain high levels of health and functioning.
- Goals of health promotion for older adults focus on (1) prevention and postponement of disease and disability, and (2) early identification and effective management of disease conditions.
- Types of health promotion interventions applicable to older adults include screening programs, risk reduction interventions, environmental modifications, and health education to promote good health practices.

The Transtheoretical Model of Health Promotion

- Gerontological nurses can apply the Transtheoretical Model (TTM) of Health Promotion to address the many disease prevention and health promotion interventions that require a change in health-related behaviors.
- The TTM describes five specific stages in accomplishing behavior changes: precontemplation, contemplation, preparation, action, and maintenance.

CRITICAL THINKING EXERCISES

1. Describe the development of gerontological nursing from the 1960s to the present.
2. You are asked to give a presentation to beginning nursing students to recruit them for an elective class called "Nursing for Wellness in Older Adults." What topics would you expect to be covered in this course and what points would you make to encourage them to enlist in this course?
3. You are discussing with your fellow students the choices you will be making about a practice area after graduation. You tell them that you are planning to specialize in gerontological nursing, and they challenge your decision with statements such as, "You'll be bored to death taking care of old fogies. Why don't you specialize in something exciting like trauma care? Besides, there's not much to do about the conditions of older folks, and what's the challenge in taking care of people who aren't going to get better?" How do you respond to these statements?
4. Identify one health-related behavior that you would like to change in your life (e.g., smoking cessation, increased level of exercise, decreased dietary fat intake) and develop a care plan for your behavior change using the Transtheoretical Model of Health Promotion (as in the case study).

EDUCATIONAL RESOURCES

AARP (formerly American Association of Retired Persons)
www.aarp.org

American Nurses Association (ANA)
www.nursingworld.org

Centers for Medicare & Medicaid Services
www.cms.hhs.gov

Fifty Plus Fitness Association
www.50plus.org

National Center for Chronic Disease Prevention and Health Promotion
www.cdc.gov/nccdphp

National Gerontological Nursing Association (NGNA)
www.ngna.org

National Institute on Aging
www.nia.nih.gov

National Institute of Nursing Research
www.nih.gov/ninr

Office of Disease Prevention and Health Promotion
U.S. Department of Health and Human Services
www.cdc.gov

Office of Minority Health Resource Center
www.cdc.gov/omhd

Partnership for Prevention
www.prevent.org

REFERENCES

Allison, M. J., & Keller, C. (2000). Physical activity maintenance in elders with cardiac problems. *Geriatric Nursing, 21*, 200–203.

American Nurses Association. (1976). *Standards of gerontological nursing practice*. Kansas City, MO: Author.

American Nurses Association. (2001). *Scope and standards of gerontological nursing practice* (22nd ed.). Washington, DC: Author.

Bhalotra, S. M., & Mutschler, P. H. (2001). Primary prevention for older adults: No longer a paradox. *Journal of Aging and Social Policy, 12*(2), 5–22.

Bloom, H. G. (2001). Preventive medicine: When to screen for disease in older patients. *Geriatrics, 56*(4), 41–45.

Burbank, P. M., Padula, C. A., & Nigg, C. R. (2000). Changing health behaviors of older adults. *Journal of Gerontological Nursing, 26*(3), 26–33.

Burbank, P. M., & Riebe, D. (Eds.). (2002). *Promoting exercise and behavior change in older adults*. New York: Springer.

Burggraf, V., & Barry, R. J. (2000). Healthy People 2010: Protecting the health of older individuals. *Journal of Gerontological Nursing, 26*(12), 16–22.

Burkholder, G. J., & Evers, K. A. (2002). Application of the transtheoretical model to several problem behaviors. In P. M. Burbank & D. Riebe (Eds.), *Promoting exercise and behavior change in older adults* (pp. 85–145). New York: Springer.

Chernoff, R. (2002). Health promotion for older women: Benefits of nutrition and exercise programs. *Topics in Geriatric Rehabilitation, 18*, 59–67.

Cooper, K. M., Bilbrew, D., Dubbert, P. M., Kerr, K., & Kirchner, K. (2001). Health barriers to walking for exercise in elderly primary care. *Geriatric Nursing, 22*, 258–262.

DiPietro, L. (2001). Physical activity in aging: Changes in patterns and their relationship to health and function. *Journals of Gerontology: Series A, Biological Sciences and Medical Sciences, 56*(Special Issue II), 13–22.

Dossey, B. M., & Guzzetta, C. E. (2005). Holistic nursing practice. In B. M. Dossey, L. Keegan & C. E. Guzzetta (Eds.), *Holistic nursing: A handbook for practice* (4th ed., pp. 5–30). Boston: Jones and Bartlett.

Drewnowski, A., & Evans, W. J. (2001a). Nutrition, physical activity, and quality of life in older adults: Summary. *Journals of Gerontology: Series A, Biological Sciences and Medical Sciences, 56*(Special Issue II), 89–94.

Drewnowski, A., & Evans, W. J. (2001b). Introduction. *Journals of Gerontology: Series A, Biological Sciences and Medical Sciences, 56*(Special Issue II), 5.

Dubbert, P. M., Cooper, K. M., Kirchner, K. A., Meydrech, E. F., & Bilbrew, D. (2002). Effects of nurse counseling on walking for exercise in elderly primary care patients. *Journals of Gerontology: Series A, Biological Sciences and Medical Sciences, 57*, M733–M740.

Evans, W. J. (2002). Guest editorial: Exercise as the standard of care for elderly people. *Journals of Gerontology: Series A, Biological Sciences and Medical Sciences, 57*, M260–M261.

Fisher, A., & Morley J. E. (2002). Antiaging medicine: The good, the bad and the ugly. *Journals of Gerontology: Series A, Biological Sciences and Medical Sciences, 57*, M636–M639.

Frank, L. K. (1946). Gerontology. *Journal of Gerontology, 1*(1), 1–11.

Fraser, G. E., & Shavlik, D. J. (2001). Ten years of life: Is it a matter of choice? *Archives of Internal Medicine, 161*, 1645–1652.

Futrell, M., & Melillo, K. D. (2005). Gerontological nurse practitioners: Implications for the future. *Journal of Gerontological Nursing, 31*(4), 19–24.

Gaydos, H. L. B. (2005). The art of holistic nursing and the human health experience. In B. M. Dossey, L. Keegan, & C. E. Guzzetta (Eds.), *Holistic nursing: A handbook for practice* (4th ed., pp. 57–76). Boston: Jones and Bartlett.

Given, B. A., & Given, C. W. (2001). Health promotion for older adults in a managed care environment. In E. A. Swanson, T. Tripp-Reimer, &

K. Buckwalter (Eds.), *Health promotion and disease prevention in the older adult* (pp. 219–241). New York: Springer.

Gordon, C. (2006). Health promotion for older adults: Meeting the challenges of the future. American Society on Aging's Live Well, Live Long Issue Brief Series. San Francisco: American Society on Aging. Available at www.asaging.org/cdc.

Happell, B., & Brooker, J. (2001). Who will look after my grandmother? Attitudes of student nurses toward the care of older adults. *Journal of Gerontological Nursing, 27*(12), 12–17.

Hawranik, P., & Pangman, V. (2002). Perceptions of a senior citizens' wellness center: The community's voice. *Journal of Gerontological Nursing, 28*(11), 38–44.

Hubert, H. B., Bloch, D. A., Oehlert, J. W., & Fries, J. F. (2002). Lifestyle habits and compression of morbidity. *Journals of Gerontology: Series A, Biological Sciences and Medical Sciences, 57*, M347–M351.

Infeld, D. L., & Whitelaw, N. (2002). Policy initiatives to promote healthy aging. *Clinics in Geriatric Medicine, 18*, 627–642.

King, A. C. (2001). Interventions to promote physical activity by older adults. *Journals of Gerontology: Series A, Biological Sciences and Medical Sciences, 56*(Special Issue II), 36–46.

Klein, S. M. (1997). *A national agenda for geriatric education*. New York: Springer.

Leenerts, M. H., Teel, C. S., & Pendleton, M. (2002). Building a model of self-care for health promotion in aging. *Journal of Nursing Scholarship, 34*, 355–361.

McBride, A. B. (2000). Nursing and gerontology. *Journal of Gerontological Nursing, 26*(7), 18–27.

Mehr, D. R., & Tatum, P. E. (2002). Primary prevention of disease in old age. *Clinics in Geriatric Medicine, 18*, 407–430.

Melillo, K. D., Williamson, E., Houde, S. C., Futrell, M., Read, C. Y., & Campasano, M. (2001). Perceptions of older Latino adults regarding physical fitness, physical activity, and exercise. *Journal of Gerontological Nursing, 27*(9), 38–46.

Mezey, M., & Fulmer, T. (2002). The future history of gerontological nursing. *Journals of Gerontology: Series A, Biological Sciences and Medical Sciences, 57*, M438–M441.

Morley, J. E., & Flaherty, J. H. (2002). It's never too late: Health promotion and illness prevention in older persons. *Journals of Gerontology: Series A, Biological Sciences and Medical Sciences, 57*, M338–M342.

Parker, M. W., Bellis, J. M., Bishop, P., Harper, M., Allman, R. M., Moore, C., et al. (2002). A multidisciplinary model of health promotion incorporating spirituality into a successful aging intervention with African American and white elderly groups. *The Gerontologist, 42*, 406–415.

Phelan, E. A., Williams, B., Leveille, S., Snyder, S., Wagner, E. H., & LoGerfo, J. P. (2002). Outcomes of a community-based dissemination of the Health Enhancement Project. *Journal of the American Geriatrics Society, 50*, 1519–1524.

Popejoy, L. L., Rantz, M. J., Conn, V., Wipke-Tevis, D., Grando, V. T., & Porter, R. (2000). Improving quality of care in nursing facilities: Gerontological clinical nurse specialist as research nurse consultant. *Journal of Gerontological Nursing, 26*(4), 6–13.

Prochaska, J. O., & DiClemente, C. C. (1982). Transtheoretical therapy: Toward a more integrative model of change. *Psychotherapy: Theory, Research, and Practice, 19*, 276–288.

Rejeski, W. J., & Mihalko, S. L. (2001). Physical activity and quality of life in older adults. *Journals of Gerontology: Series A, Biological Sciences and Medical Sciences, 56*(Special Issue II), 23–35.

Resnick, B. (2002). Testing the effect of the WALC intervention on exercise adherence in older adults. *Journal of Gerontological Nursing, 28*(6), 40–49.

Resnick, B., & Spellbring, M. (2000). Understanding what motivates older adults to exercise. *Journal of Gerontological Nursing, 26*(3), 34–42.

Schlicht, J. (2000). Strength training for older adults: Prescription guidelines for nurses in advanced practice. *Journal of Gerontological Nursing, 26*(8), 25–32.

Singh, M. A. F. (2002). Exercise comes of age: Rationale and recommendations for a geriatric exercise prescription. *Journals of Gerontology: Series A, Biological Sciences and Medical Sciences, 57*, M262–M282.

Stierle, L. J., Mezey, M., Schumann, M. J., Esterson, J., Smolenski, M. C., Horsley, K. D., et al. (2006). The Nurse Competence in Aging initiative: Encouraging expertise in the care of older adults. *American Journal of Nursing, 106*(9), 93–96.

Strumpf, N. E. (2000). Improving care for the frail elderly: The challenge for nursing. *Journal of Gerontological Nursing, 26*(7), 36–44.

Teel, C. S., & Leenerts, M. H. (2005). Developing and testing a self-care intervention for older adults in caregiving roles. *Nursing Research, 54*, 193–200.

Titler, M. (2002). *Evidence-based protocol. Exercise promotion: Walking in elders*. Iowa City, IA: University of Iowa Gerontological Nursing Interventions Research Center.

Touhy, E. L. (1946). Geriatrics: The general setting. *Geriatrics: Official Journal of the American Geriatrics Society, 1*(1), 17–20.

Wykle, M. L. (2001). Gerontological nursing research: Challenges for the new millennium. *Journal of Gerontological Nursing, 27*(4), 7–9.

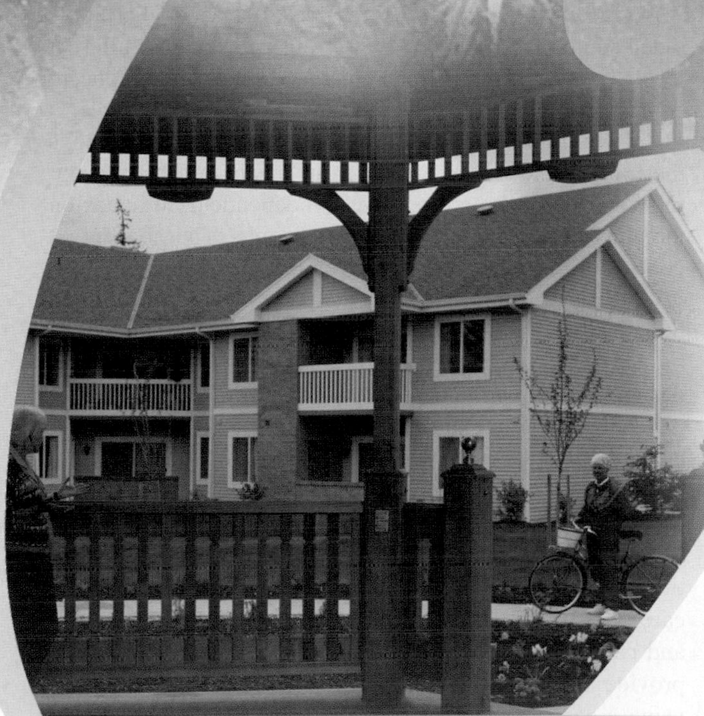

CHAPTER 6

Diverse Health Care Settings for Older Adults

Learning Objectives

After reading this chapter, you will be able to:

1. Describe the services that are included in a continuum of care for older adults.
2. Describe characteristics of several models of acute care programs for older adults.
3. Describe models of and trends in long-term care settings.
4. Describe the types of home care services, including sources of payment and scope of services.
5. Describe each of the following types of community-based services: adult day centers, respite services, parish nursing, health promotion programs, and care management programs.
6. Discuss the roles of nurses caring for older adults in acute care, long-term care, and home and community settings.
7. Discuss the role of public and private insurance programs in paying for health care services for older adults.

Key Terms

acute care for elders (ACE)
aging in place
assisted-living facilities
continuum of care
geriatric care manager
intermediate nursing home care
long-term care
nursing facility
nursing home
parish nursing
resident-centered care
respite
skilled home care
skilled nursing home care
special care units (SCUs)
subacute care
telehealth
transitional care

Although nurses have always cared for older adults, it has been only since the late 1960s that health care organizations have recognized and addressed the unique health care needs of older adults by developing new programs. Because of these programs, a continuum of care for older adults has gradually evolved over the past several decades, and health care services are increasingly addressing specific needs of older adults during different phases of health and illness. Another outcome of these programs is the emergence of new roles for nurses, particularly for those who specialize in care of older adults. This chapter presents an overview of the continuum of health care services for older adults that began in the late 1960s and continues to evolve today; it also discusses roles of nurses working with older adults in these programs.

DEVELOPMENT OF A CONTINUUM OF CARE FOR OLDER ADULTS

The establishment of Medicare in 1965 (discussed later in this chapter) stimulated major changes in the delivery of health care services to older adults, and nurses have taken prominent roles in developing gerontological health care programs. For example, during the early 1970s, home care and community health nurses recognized the central role they played in coordinating services for older adults, and they spearheaded the development of multidisciplinary models of health care in home and community settings. Around this same time, nurses in long-term care settings recognized the vital leadership roles they played in developing models for skilled, rehabilitative, restorative, and chronic care of older adults. By the 1980s, health care providers acknowledged that most existing acute care models did not comprehensively address the health and functioning of older adults, and they began developing innovative and cost-effective models for inpatient care. During the 1990s, health care programs began emphasizing health promotion, prevention of disease, improvement in functioning, and enhancement of quality of life. In 1992, an amendment to the Older Americans Act enabled the federal Administration on Aging to expand its support of health promotion and wellness programs nationwide. By the early 2000s, a continuum of innovative health care services had emerged, and programs continue to be developed to meet the complex needs of diverse groups of older adults in numerous settings. Although some of these programs have arisen from an increased concern about health expenditures, many are the result of an increased awareness of the importance of meeting chronic care needs of older adults in a way that addresses both financial concerns and quality-of-life issues.

Long-term care refers to a variety of services and supports provided by formal and informal (i.e., paid and unpaid) providers that help people function as well as possible and maintain their lifestyles despite the presence of long-term disability or chronic illness (Stone, 2006). Traditionally, this term was associated with care provided in nursing homes because they were the primary resource, and usually the only formal resource, for people who needed more care on a long-term basis than could be provided by family members in home settings. However, in recent years this narrow perception of long-term care has become outdated because many types of services address the long-term care needs of people of all ages. Many long-term care services are provided in nursing homes, assisted-living facilities, and other institutional settings, but these services are also provided in apartments, private homes, and other community settings. Current descriptions of long-term care services include assistance not only with activities of daily living (ADLs), but with activities such as transportation, household chores, money management, and medication management. In addition, it may include services such as provision of assistive devices (e.g., walkers), technology (e.g., emergency alert systems), and home modifications (e.g., ramps, grab bars) (Stone, 2006).

Aging in place refers to a range of services that allow older adults to remain in one setting and receive different levels of care as their needs change. Although the concept of aging in place initially referred to supporting people in their own homes, it also is applied to institutional settings that provide services ranging from meals and housekeeping for people who are relatively independent, to hands-on nursing care for more dependent people. The concept of **continuum of care** (sometimes called *seamless continuum of care*) is a similar concept that refers to programs that holistically address the comprehensive needs of older adults in a variety of settings and include all those services designed to provide care for people at different stages of dependence for an extended period. Life care or continuing care retirement communities (described in Chapter 1) are examples of continuum-of-care programs. Continuum-of-care models usually include all or most of the following services: primary and preventive care, acute care, transitional care, rehabilitation services, extended care, respite care, social services, home health care, adult day centers, and care management services. By nature, these programs provide multidisciplinary and coordinated services, often using a care manager. Some models use a continuing care pathway to assess a person's readiness for transition from one part of the program to another. For example, the Pathway Project uses a care management model to assess, plan, implement, coordinate, monitor, and evaluate services effectively to meet the acute and long-term care needs of frail older adults (Tichawa, 2002).

Programs providing a continuum of care covered by health care insurance are not widely available in the United States, but two well-known and relatively long-standing programs are the On Lok Program and the Program of All-inclusive Care for the Elderly (PACE), which are discussed later in this chapter. Even without formal continuum-of-care models, however, numerous long-term care services are provided in many settings ranging from traditional nursing homes to innovative community-based settings. People with complex needs usually require a combination of services. For example, a person with early dementia who lives with her daughter may attend an adult day center three days a week, receive home-delivered meals twice weekly, and have a companion service on weekends. Combinations of services also are needed when two or more people with long-term care needs live together (e.g., siblings, couples, or parents and adult children). When combinations of long-term care services are needed, family members or care managers must coordinate care.

ACUTE CARE SETTINGS

Models for Acute Care of Older Adults

Inpatient hospital stays are one part of a continuum of care that necessitates careful preadmission and postdischarge planning and coordination of services. As with other aspects of health care, hospital care of older adults is rapidly changing, with many of these changes being determined in large part by health insurance coverage. For example, because the current Medicare reimbursement policy provides financial incentives for earlier discharge from acute care settings, hospitals have developed **subacute care** units (also called **transitional care** units). These units provide skilled nursing care under Medicare and other insurance programs, so reimbursement is lower than that for acute care. In general, subacute care patients are medically complex or need skilled rehabilitation after acute episodes such as a stroke or orthopedic surgery. Examples of typical subacute care services include chemotherapy; intravenous therapy; complex wound care; enteral and parenteral nutrition; speech, physical, and occupational therapies; and management of complex respiratory care (e.g., ventilator, tracheostomy). In recent years, some nursing homes also have developed subacute care units.

Many hospitals are addressing acute care needs of older adults by establishing separate geriatric units—often referred to as **acute care for elders (ACE)** units—staffed by a specially trained multidisciplinary team. The rationale for these units is that older adults have unique needs that can be anticipated and addressed to prevent functional decline during hospitalization (Miller, 2002). Compared with patients who receive usual hospital care, patients who receive care in ACE units have improved functional status, fewer discharges to nursing homes, and a better 1-year survival rate (Thomas, 2002), and there is increasing evidence of the effectiveness of these units (Morley, 2003). The focus of ACE programs is to assist older adults who have complex problems to remain at their highest level of function. Key elements of ACE units are (Benedict et al., 2006):

- A specially adapted environment (e.g., homelike rooms, carpeted floors)
- Functional assessment
- Assessment and interventions for common geriatric syndromes (e.g., mobility, fall risk, self-care, skin integrity, continence, confusion, depression, anxiety)
- Interdisciplinary team care, with a strong role for the clinical nurse specialist
- Patient-centered care, including care plans that address needs of the patient and family within the community
- Intensive review of care to identify and address risks for iatrogenic complications (e.g., adverse effects of medications and procedures)
- Discharge planning with the goal of returning the patient to his or her home

In addition to gerontological nurses, the health care teams in ACE units typically include a geriatrician, pharmacist, social worker, various rehabilitation therapists (e.g., speech, physical, or occupational therapists), and mental health professionals (e.g., psychologists or psychiatrists). Some teams also include a geriatric care manager and music, activity, or horticultural therapists.

Other acute care programs focus on specific target conditions, such as delirium, with an emphasis on comprehensive improvement of one aspect of geriatric care in hospital settings (Fulmer et al., 2002). For example, the Hospital Elder Life Program (HELP) is a hospital-wide program that screens patients on admission for the risk factors of immobility, dehydration, sleep deprivation, vision impairment, hearing impairment, and cognitive impairment (Inouye, 2000). This program uses a multidisciplinary team to implement interventions to prevent cognitive and functional decline in older patients. Another model, called Together We Improve Care of the Elderly (TWICE), has achieved significant improvements in care of hospitalized older adults using nursing protocols, staff development, and geriatric resource staff (Swauger & Tomlin, 2002). The Older Adult Services Inpatient Strategies (OASIS) program is another example of an inpatient model that has a strong role for a full-time clinical nurse specialist and is cost-effective (Tucker et al., 2006). Positive outcomes for patients include reduced costs, shorter length of stay, decreased readmission rate, no decline in function, and no incidence of iatrogenic complications (e.g., delirium, pneumonia, thrombus, pressure ulcer, or urinary tract infection) during the initial 6-month period (Tucker et al., 2006).

Emergency departments of acute care settings also have developed innovative programs to address the complex needs of frail elders. The Systematic Intervention for Geriatric Network of Evaluation and Treatment (SIGNET) model was developed to improve case finding of at-risk older patients, improve care planning and referral of at-risk older people, and create a coordinated network of existing medical, nursing, and social services (Mion et al., 2001). This program demonstrated the feasibility of implementing an assessment and linkage model to address the needs of frail older adults in emergency departments.

Roles for Gerontological Nurses in Acute Care Settings

As acute care settings have developed programs to address the unique needs of hospitalized older patients, new roles have emerged for gerontological nurses, particularly for advanced practice nurses. Gerontological nurses are likely to serve as consultants and role models for staff nurses and often take leadership roles in developing and implementing specialized care programs and protocols for hospitalized older adults. The Geriatric Resource Nurse Model has been successful in developing bedside experts in geriatric care through mentoring by advanced practice nurses (Turner et al., 2001). The following positive outcomes have been associated with the use of advanced practice nurses in acute care settings (Mezey, 2001):

- Shorter lengths of stay
- Reduced morbidity after discharge
- Fewer readmissions and less use of emergency department after discharge
- Significant reductions in morbidity, including preventing or reducing the incidence of delirium and other syndromes that commonly occur in hospitalized older patients

Since the early 1990s, the Yale Geriatric Care Program has been using a unit-based and nursing-centered model of care to prevent functional decline in hospitalized older adults (Fulmer, 1991; Inouye et al., 1993a, 1993b). Primary nurses, designated as Geriatric Resource Nurses, identify risks for conditions associated with functional decline in older adults and implement preventive measures. Older patients who receive care in a unit staffed with Geriatric Resource Nurses have less functional decline in ADLs than patients on similar units without the specialized care (Turner et al., 2001). This model has been supported by the Nurses Improving Care for Healthsystem Elders (NICHE) program of the John A. Hartford Foundation and is now widely used (Fulmer et al., 2002; Guthrie et al., 2002; Lee and Fletcher, 2002; Pfaff, 2002; Salinas et al., 2002).

LONG-TERM CARE SETTINGS

Nursing Home Models for Long-Term Care

The term **nursing home**, or **nursing facility**, refers to a residential institutional setting for people who need assistance with several ADLs. Nursing homes are licensed by a state or federal agency and must be certified as a Medicare or Medicaid facility if they receive funds from those programs. Nursing homes are required to have continuous on-site supervision by a registered nurse or licensed practical nurse. Sixty-five percent of all nursing homes are for-profit, whereas 29% percent are not-for-profit and 6% are government owned (Stone, 2006). In addition to medical care and nursing services, nursing homes must provide dental, podiatry, medical specialty consultation services, and rehabilitation therapies (e.g., physical and occupational therapies).

Gerontologists have identified the reasons older people are admitted for nursing home care. Factors that increase the likelihood of being admitted to a nursing home include poverty, white race, female sex, living alone, advanced age, hospital admission, functional dependence, impaired mental status, lack of informal supports, and loss of self-care ability (Bharucha et al., 2004; Mitty, 2001). The most common diagnoses leading to nursing home admission are dementia, heart disease, and hypertension (Mitty, 2001). People with a combination of cognitive impairment and ADL limitations are significantly more at risk of being admitted to a nursing home, and this risk increases with the severity of the cognitive impairment (Borrayo et al., 2002).

Although the basic criterion for admission to a nursing home is that the person be sick enough to require continuous nursing care but not sick enough to require hospital care, not everyone meeting this criterion goes to a nursing home. Many people needing continuous nursing care—as well as less intense levels of nursing care—are cared for in their own homes or in other settings. Since the 1970s, gerontologists have recognized that admission to a nursing home for long-term care is determined not only by the person's dependence in performing ADLs but by the availability of capable and willing caregivers. Thus, many older people move to a nursing home not because their condition has changed, but because there has been a change in the availability or abilities of the caregiver. Researchers found that the most commonly cited reasons for admitting a family member to a nursing facility were caregivers' perceptions that skilled care was needed, that their own health was in jeopardy, and that dementia-related behaviors were too difficult to manage (Buhr et al., 2006).

Nursing home care is generally categorized as skilled nursing or skilled rehabilitation (usually short-term) or intermediate care (usually long-term). **Skilled nursing home care**, usually provided for 6 months or less, is associated with post-hospital care. Medicare and other health insurance programs cover the cost of skilled nursing or skilled rehabilitation services for up to 100 days if the care is medically necessary and the person is progressing; however, people generally meet these criteria for only 32 days (Mitty, 2001). Long-term or **intermediate nursing home care** refers to nursing services provided for chronically ill people who need assistance with daily activities. The average length of stay for long-term residents is 2.5 years (Mitty, 2001). Medicare does not cover costs of long-term nursing care, but some long-term care insurance policies provide limited coverage. Sources of payment for long-term nursing home care are as follows: Medicaid (approximately 50%); private pay, which is also called *out-of-pocket* (approximately 33%); and other insurance (Yeaworth, 2002). Seventy-five to 85% of all public long-term care dollars (primarily from Medicaid and Medicare) is spent for care in institutions such as nursing homes rather than for community-based care (Borrayo et al., 2002).

Newer Models for Long-Term Care

Recent changes in health care services for older adults have significantly influenced both long-term and short-term nursing home care. On any given day, between 4% and 5% of people older than 65 years of age in the United States live in a nursing home. This percentage has declined slightly since the 1970s (Hays et al., 2003). However, about 40% of people older than 65 years are likely to spend some time in a nursing home, and this is likely to increase to 46% by the year 2020 (Spillman & Lubitz, 2002). These statistics reflect the following major trends in health care for older adults in the United States (Hays et al., 2003; Stone, 2006):

- Shorter lengths of hospital stays and increased use of short-term postacute care in nursing homes
- Higher percentages of nursing home residents returning to community settings (e.g., an increase from 18% to 30% between 1985 and 1997)
- Increased use of skilled home care services
- Rapid growth of assisted-living facilities and community-based long-term care services that substitute for nursing home care

Because of these trends, most nursing homes provide a combination of skilled care services for short-term residents and intermediate care services for long-term residents. Increasingly, the boundaries between long-term care and acute care settings are becoming blurred (Stone, 2006). Because the skilled care provided in nursing homes today is similar to the care that used to be provided to patients in hospitals, residents often are able to stay in the nursing facility during acute illnesses rather than being admitted to a hospital. Another result of these trends is that the percentage of long-term residents who are more dependent in ADLs has gradually increased in recent years because people who are less dependent now receive care in other settings.

Assisted-living facilities provide some of the basic nursing home services (e.g., meals and laundry) at a lower cost, and additional services (e.g., dementia care and medication management) can often be purchased as the need arises (Hujer et al., 2000). Because these facilities are considered "nonmedical," they are not eligible for Medicare reimbursement. Regulations for assisted-living facilities vary, with some states requiring the presence of a licensed nurse (RN or LPN). Nurses in these settings focus on wellness, and their responsibilities include conducting assessments, teaching and counseling residents, managing medications, and even chaperoning field trips (Wallace, 2003). The following are key characteristics of assisted-living facilities (Stone, 2006):

- Provision of lifestyle and service choices similar to what one could have in his or her own home
- Explicit focus on privacy, autonomy, and independence
- Emphasis on apartment settings in which residents can choose to share their living space
- Opportunity for resident to assume responsibility for possible untoward consequences of individual actions and decisions

Additional types of housing options that address needs of older adults are discussed in Chapter 1.

A recent development in long-term care settings is the establishment of **special care units (SCUs)**, which are separate units designed to address the needs of specific groups of residents who meet explicit admission criteria. Dementia care units, or Alzheimer's units, are a common type of SCU; other types are AIDS, subacute care, oncology, ventilator-dependent, pressure ulcers, and traumatic brain injury units. SCU staff receive specialized training, and care plans address unique needs of the residents. Support and educational programs often are provided for residents and families. Dementia care units or programs are increasingly available in both nursing homes and assisted-living facilities. Another type of specialized care in nursing homes is the development of "niche" services, such as hospice, wound care, subacute care, bariatric care, or short-term rehabilitation (Jarchin, 2006).

In recent years, health care providers have emphasized quality of care and quality of life in nursing homes. This focus stems in part from consumer pressure that began during the 1970s, and in part from legislation passed during the late 1980s (see Chapter 9). Terms such as **resident-centered care** refer to the shift from the traditional medical model of efficiently providing physical care to frail and impaired individuals to a focus on quality of life for residents. Goals for resident-centered care include supporting opportunities for continued growth, encouraging meaningful connections with family and the community, respecting the individualized needs and desires of each resident, and honoring the life patterns and accomplishments of each person in the setting (Calkins, 2002).

Concerns about quality of care and quality of life have prompted a limited but growing effort to bring about a "culture change" focusing on putting the concept of "home" back in the provision of nursing home care (Stone, 2006). For example, the Pioneer Network in Long-Term Care is a group of providers who strive to implement care in nursing homes that exemplifies values such as putting people before tasks and responding to the needs of the spirit, mind, and body. To this end, nursing homes are making efforts to permit spontaneity, foster neighborhood groupings, include residents in decision making, break down the rigidities of routines, empower both residents and certified nursing assistants, and foster more normal and meaningful relationships between residents and staff (McGilton, 2002; Stone, 2006). Other examples of this movement include the Greenhouse Project, Regenerative Change, and Deep Culture Change (Stone, 2006).

The Eden Alternative is a model developed in the mid-1990s by William Thomas, MD, with the intent of creating a "human habitat" to combat boredom, loneliness, and lack of meaning in nursing homes (Thomas, 1994). The Eden Alternative is a comprehensive program of transforming the organizational culture as well as the physical, spiritual, psychosocial, and interpersonal environments of a facility. An essential component is the systematic introduction of pets, plants, and children to create a homelike setting and improve the quality of life of residents. The program incorporates strategies to engage and empower staff in bringing about the environmental change (Thomas, 1994). Many nursing homes are adopting this comprehensive model or implementing some components of it.

Nurses in particular have expressed much interest in incorporating aspects of the Eden Alternative in nursing homes. Nursing research "supports the conclusion that the Eden Alternative or other environmental transformation may be feasibly undertaken by facilities of any sort, large or small, private or public, rural or urban" (Tesh et al., 2002, p. 33). Barba and colleagues (2002) describe the implementation of this model in one nursing home and discuss some of its risks, benefits, and challenges from a nursing perspective. A nursing study found that interventions based on the Eden Alternative could improve quality of life for residents by reducing feelings of boredom, loneliness, and helplessness (Bergman-Evans, 2004). The Eden Alternative website (www.edenalt.org) provides further information about this program.

Roles for Gerontological Nurses in Long-Term Care Settings

Nurses have always assumed strong leadership roles in nursing homes and other long-term care settings, and opportunities for role expansion are skyrocketing because of some of the trends and newer models of care just discussed. The focus on improved quality of care and quality of life led nursing homes and other long-term care facilities to use nurses to implement innovative changes in delivery of care. Currently, gerontological nurses have almost unlimited opportunities to develop and implement cost-effective programs directed at improving care in nursing homes and other long-term care settings. Some of the most common roles for gerontological nurses in long-term care settings include team leader, restorative nurse, wellness nurse, and director of nursing.

In the late 1990s, numerous opportunities opened up for gerontological nurses in long-term care settings when Medicare and Medicaid began to reimburse for advanced practice nurses. For example, advanced practice nurses in assisted-living facilities may provide staff education, assist with program development, develop plans for clients with dementia, provide for acute and chronic care needs, establish support groups for clients and families, and act as advocates for clients and their families (Bonnel, 2002). The following positive outcomes of the use of advanced practice nurses in nursing homes have been identified (Allen et al., 2000; Mezey, 2001; Ryden et al., 2000):

- Fewer hospitalizations
- Better resident assessments
- Decreased use of emergency departments
- Better illness prevention and case finding
- Lower use of physical restraints and psychotropic medications
- Improved nursing outcomes for health problems such as pressure ulcers, urinary incontinence, and aggressive behaviors
- Successful and cost-effective management of medical conditions

Other roles for advanced practice nurses in long-term care include consultation regarding conditions such as dementia and depression. Eisch and colleagues (2000) found that positive behavioral changes occurred in 62% of the residents who had been referred by the nursing home staff for agitation, disruptive behaviors, depressive symptoms, or a decline in ADLs when recommendations of a geriatric nurse practitioner consultant were implemented.

HOME CARE SERVICES

Older people and other dependent populations have always received much of their health care at home, and visiting nurse services have existed in the United States since the late 1880s. But the delivery of home care services dramatically changed after 1965 when Medicare funds became available for these services. In 1975, the Older Americans Act and Title XX Social Services Act allocated federal funds for home-based services, and the federal Health Services Program funded grants for the establishment, operation, or expansion of programs providing home health services. By the late 1970s, thousands of home care agencies had been established, and their number escalated exponentially over the course of the next two decades.

Although the federal government had envisioned Medicare home health care services as a short-term supplement to acute care services for people who needed skilled care, consumers came to view these services as an extension of long-term care for people with chronic illnesses. By the 1990s, home care had become the fastest-growing component of the Medicare program, and costs had increased so drastically that Congress included cost-containment measures in the Balanced Budget Act of 1997. A major goal of the Act was to substantially reduce Medicare payments for home health care services. In practical terms, however, home care agencies reduced their spending through screening, fewer visits, earlier discharges, and reduction or elimination of specialized staffing (Smith et al., 2000). In the 2 years after this legislation went into effect, Medicare spending on home health care decreased 45%, the number of beneficiaries dropped from 3.6 to 3.0 million, and approximately 3000 home health agencies closed for financial reasons (Leff & Burton, 2001; Martin, 2001). The new payment system established by the Act "wrought the biggest changes to the home care industry since the inception of the Medicare program 30 years ago" (Marrelli, 2001, p. 217). The impact was larger on people in rural areas where home care was already in short supply (Anetzberger, 2002).

While the federal government was cutting funding for home care, state governments were recognizing the need for increased funding for home- and community-based services. Motivated both by cost containment and by consumer preference, state long-term care policy shifted from a focus on institutional care to a focus on noninstitutional services. As a result, more state funds became available for home care and other community-based long-term care services. Although many state-funded programs are limited to people who would be eligible for Medicaid if they were in a nursing home, many affordable services have become widely available through public, private, and nonprofit agencies. Skilled home care services and long-term home care services are the main types of home care services for older adults in the United States that evolved because of these trends.

Skilled Home Care

Home care services provided under Medicare and some other health insurance programs have always been limited to **skilled home care** and restricted to people who meet all of the following criteria:

- The person must be homebound (i.e., leaving the home requires considerable and taxing effort).

- The services must be ordered by a primary care provider.
- There must be a need for skilled nursing or rehabilitative services.
- The person must require intermittent, but not full-time, care.

People often qualify for skilled home care after a hospitalization or a stay in a skilled nursing or rehabilitation setting for an acute illness. Studies of outcomes of home-based interventions for people with chronic conditions, such as stroke and congestive heart failure, have identified the following benefits (with the exception of services for chronic obstructive pulmonary disease) (Pearson et al., 2006):

- Improved disease control
- Reduced mortality
- Reduced rate of recurrent hospitalizations
- Overall decrease in cost of care

Medicare covers the following types of home care services for people who meet the criteria: skilled nursing, physical therapy, occupational therapy, nutrition counseling, speech–language therapy, medical social work, the assistance of a home health aide, and medical supplies and equipment. A licensed professional nurse or therapist provides or directs the services. Types of skilled nursing services covered by Medicare home care benefits include case management, medication management, infusion therapy, intravenous antibiotics, and psychiatric nursing services. Home health aides can provide some of the care (e.g., assistance with bathing, linen changes, range-of-motion exercises, and assistance with transfers and ambulation), and their services are provided under the directions of a licensed nurse or therapist. Because skilled home care services are meant to be short-term, a major focus is on teaching the older person and caregivers about self-care activities.

Typical skilled care recipients are (1) people who are homebound but able to manage most of their daily care at some level of independence; and (2) people who, although homebound and dependent in many functional areas, receive help from families, friends, or paid caregivers to supplement the skilled care services. If people reach a level of independence such that they are no longer homebound, they cannot continue receiving skilled care services. Likewise, people no longer qualify for skilled care after they achieve self-care goals. Many people receiving skilled care, however, still need some level of home care services after the skilled services are discontinued.

Long-Term Home Care

A wide spectrum of long-term home care services are available for the large majority of older adults who need home care but do not meet the criteria for skilled care. At one end of the spectrum is nonskilled care provided by companions, homemakers, and home health aides. The most common services are meal preparation, light housekeeping, assistance with personal care, accompaniment to medical appointments, and grocery shopping and other errands. These services are often supplemented by community-based services such as transportation and home-delivered meals. Frequency of service ranges from periodic to 24 hours daily, and some agencies and independent caregivers require a minimum number of hours weekly. A licensed nurse may assess the client and supervise the services, and a registered nurse usually assists with medication management, if needed. At the other end of the spectrum is skilled care for people who need this type of care but do not meet Medicare criteria. Virtually any skilled service available under Medicare is available as a self-pay service, but these services are usually quite expensive.

Payment for Home Care Services

Sources of payment for home care services are self-pay, public funds for people who qualify, and some long-term care insurance for the small minority of older adults who have these policies. Self-pay has been the primary source of payment for long-term home care, but public funds through Medicaid waiver programs have been increasing gradually since the early 1990s. In addition, sliding-scale fees for home care and other community-based services are increasingly becoming available through public and nonprofit agencies. For example, in recent years, third-party payment for private duty home care is increasingly covered by armed services programs, workers' compensation policies, and long-term care insurance (McMackin, 2006).

Home care services are available through formal sources (e.g., agencies) or informal sources (e.g., independent caregivers). Agencies usually provide initial assessments, arrange for services, assign workers, provide ongoing supervision, and collect payment for services. They are responsible for hiring, training, directing, scheduling, and firing workers. Some agencies provide a wide range of services, including care management. Other agencies provide only a limited type of service, such as the provision of home health aides. Some so-called agencies, however, are little more than a registry or referral service. When services are obtained from informal sources rather than from agencies, the care recipient or a surrogate decision maker is responsible for performing the organizational tasks that agencies normally perform (e.g., hiring, firing, and supervising the caregiver). In this case, sometimes the aid of a geriatric care management service (discussed later in this chapter) is enlisted to arrange for services and oversee the care. A common way of finding independent caregivers and other home care resources is through a word-of-mouth network, in which names are obtained from friends, families, churches, or local offices on aging.

People who self-pay for home care obtain services from agencies or from informal sources. Traditionally, when home care services are covered by insurance or public funds, they have been provided by agencies under contractual arrangements. This is changing, however, as an increasing number of states are allowing care recipients to choose and direct independent providers (Wiener, 2001). In some situations, Medicaid waiver programs compensate family members for providing home care services.

Roles for Gerontological Nurses in Home Care Settings

Nursing services have always been the foundation of skilled home care services, but the roles of nurses have been limited and determined largely by Medicare policies. Two recent trends in health care—a change in the Medicare reimbursement system and the development of telehealth technology—are creating opportunities for expanded roles for home care nurses. Because of the October 2000 change in the Medicare reimbursement system, home health agencies have more incentives and fewer barriers to using advanced practice nurses (Pierson, 2001). Several models have demonstrated the effectiveness of advanced practice nurses in home care settings for consultation, home visits, comprehensive assessments, and staff education and mentoring (Milone-Nuzzo & Pike, 2001). The transitional care model, which uses advanced practice nurses to promote continuity of care from hospital to home for older hospitalized patients at high risk for readmission, has consistently demonstrated reduced costs, fewer hospital readmissions, and reduced lengths of stay when readmissions were necessary (Bourbonniere & Evans, 2002). Home care roles for gerontological nurses are likely to continue expanding as Medicare and other health insurance programs address cost-effectiveness and quality-of-care issues.

Developments in telecommunication technology also are creating new roles for nurses, particularly in home care settings. **Telehealth**, also called *telecare*, refers to the use of a wide range of information and communication technologies (e.g., audio, video, Internet-based devices) to transmit information that is essential for patient assessment and monitoring (Coughlin et al., 2006). Subsets of telehealth include telemedicine (remote health care facilities interact with facilities that provide specialized services), telenursing (nurses deliver services through telecommunication devices), telehomecare (home health care services are delivered through telecommunication devices), and telemonitoring (health data are transmitted from site to site over a telecommunications network (Tran et al., 2002). Nurses are advocating for the use of telehealth technology to improve access to and availability of health care services for older adults, particularly those who are homebound or live in rural, remote, or underserved areas (Wakefield et al., 2001). For example, nurses have found that telehealth technology could be used in hospice programs to accomplish desired outcomes, increase patient and family satisfaction, and decrease cost and utilization (Williams & Bassett, 2006). Telehealth technology typically is used to collect information through physiologic monitors connected to a computer in the home. Assessment data are then sent through a telephone connection to a nurse or other health care professional who verbally communicates with the patient to obtain additional information. Some systems use videophones to allow for visual as well as audio communication.

Since the late 1990s, Medicare and a few other health insurance programs have reimbursed providers for telehealth services, and insurance coverage is likely to increase as studies demonstrate the effectiveness and cost benefits of particular telehealth programs. For example, Jenkins and McSweeney (2001) found that telehealth assessments provided information that was comparable with in-home nursing assessments of older adults with congestive heart failure. Assessment parameters included weight, edema, blood pressure, respiratory effort, heart rate and rhythm, lung and heart sounds, and color of the patient's lips, face, and nails. Nurses and older clients expressed satisfaction with the telehealth assessment. Additional benefits of telehealth technology include quicker access of home health nurses to their patients, decreased patient anxiety and stress, and substantial cost and time savings without any loss of quality of care (Jenkins & McSweeney, 2001). Telehealth technology in home care settings also can reduce hospital readmissions for people who have congestive heart failure and patients who are recovering from cardiac surgery (Frantz et al., 2002). Tran and colleagues (2002) describe the effective use of telehealth technology in home care settings to support and educate caregivers of patients with stroke.

COMMUNITY-BASED SERVICES

Public and private agencies have provided many types of community support resources for older adults for decades, and the range of these services is continually broadening. For example, home-delivered meals programs have been available in most metropolitan areas for decades, and in recent years a variety of home-delivered groceries and prepared meals have become available for delivery within 24 hours through Internet sites or toll-free phone numbers. For older adults who need assistance with daily activities these services are essential components of the continuum of care. Although community-based services are widely available, only about one fifth of older adults take advantage of these programs (Anetzberger, 2002). Older adults and their caregivers often are not aware of the great variety of services available to meet the health needs of older adults in their own homes. Even when they are aware of the availability of such services, they may not know the eligibility criteria for publicly funded services to which they are entitled. Also, if community-based services are not culturally relevant, older adults or their families may not use them, even when they are aware of their existence. Because the use of these resources may improve the health, functioning, and quality of life of the older adult, nurses need to address any lack of information about these services. Also, nurses need to assess barriers to the use of community services, as discussed in Chapter 13. Nurses in all settings have many opportunities to suggest the use of the community-based services that are described in Box 6-1.

Box 6-1
Community Resources for Older Adults

National Eldercare Locator (800-677-1116). This program provides free information about state or local resources in any part of the United States according to the zip code of the location where services are desired. This is a collaborative project of the U.S. Administration on Aging, the National Association of Area Agencies on Aging, and the National Association of State Units on Aging.

Senior Information and Referral Service. This service is often listed in the front of telephone directories under the heading "Community Services" and is sometimes referred to as "Infoline." Callers are given the names of agencies that might address their needs.

Area Agency on Aging. Funded through state, county, and local resources, these agencies provide a range of services. Some area agencies on aging employ social workers and registered nurses to make assessments and provide supportive services (e.g., referrals, case management, assistance with daily living needs). Eligibility for these services is based on economic need and the ability to address the safety and quality-of-life needs of older people living in their home environment.

Senior Centers. Sometimes the sites for hot meals, these community centers provide social, educational, and recreational programs for older adults.

Home-Delivered Meals. This program provides daily home delivery of hot meals to homebound people. Fees generally are based on a sliding scale. Special dietary needs can sometimes be addressed.

Companions and Friendly Visitors. Volunteers visit homebound older adults in their homes. Some also do errands or provide escort service to community activities.

Telephone Reassurance. Volunteers make scheduled, usually daily (sometimes more frequent) telephone calls to older people to provide support and reality orientation.

Personal Emergency Response Systems. This type of program is a home emergency response system that initiates a phone call to designated people when it is activated by a remote-control device. Public funding is available in some areas to assist low-income older adults in acquiring such a system.

Energy Assistance Programs. State and local programs offer financial assistance for utility bills for qualifying people. Older adults should check with local utility companies or the local office on aging.

Home Weatherization and Home Repair Service. Home repairs and maintenance (e.g., insulation, window caulking, and installation) are provided for low-income people by contractors paid by government agencies.

Adult Day Centers

Adult day centers, first developed in the 1970s, have become a major community-based resource for care of dependent older adults. They offer structured, comprehensive programming to functionally impaired older people in a congregate setting for less than 24 hours per day (Anetzberger, 2002). Adult day centers provide meals and structured social and recreational activities in a group setting and they may also provide transportation services. Some adult day centers provide medication management, assistance with personal care, and other health-related services and therapies. Adult day centers generally provide supervised care on weekdays for 8 hours a day, with approximately 5 hours of formal programming during that time and 3 hours of social interaction and other unstructured activities. Less commonly, services are available for longer hours and on weekends and holidays. The number of adult day centers in the United States doubled from 2000 in 1985 to 3500 in 2003 (Stone, 2006).

Participants in adult day centers usually are impaired to the point that they need supervision or assistance in several functional areas. The majority of participants are cognitively impaired, but depression and physical disabilities also are common conditions among adult day center participants. Participants typically live with a family member, but some live independently or in group settings. Because participants in adult day centers typically have multiple health-related needs, nurses have essential roles in assessment, health education, and implementation of interventions (Jennings-Sanders, 2004).

The goals of these programs are to maintain or improve the functional abilities of impaired older people; to delay or prevent the need for institutional care; to provide relief for caregivers of dependent older adults; and to improve the quality of life for impaired older adults and their caregivers. Researchers have evaluated the effects of adult day center care on both dependent older adults and their caregivers. For example, Zank and Schacke (2002) found a significant decline in health in the control group and an improvement or stabilization of subjective well-being and dementia symptoms in a group of adult day center participants.

Costs of adult day center programs vary widely, as does the source of payment. Although families have been the primary source of payment for most costs of adult day center care, public funds are increasingly becoming available because of the growing recognition of the benefits and cost-effectiveness of this kind of community-based service. Some programs are subsidized by nonprofit organizations and some have a sliding fee scale. Only a few health insurance policies cover adult day center programs. The PACE model (discussed later in this chapter) is a very successful, but atypical, model that uses adult day centers as a core component of long-term care services. It is projected that adult day centers will become more integral to the community. For example, they are likely to be located in places where caregivers work and may be regarded as an employment benefit in the future (Anetzberger, 2002).

Respite Services

Respite usually refers to any service whose primary goal is to relieve caregivers periodically from the stress of their usual caregiving responsibilities. The term first appeared in the gerontological literature in the late 1970s when gerontologists first recognized that caregivers had substantial risk of developing social isolation, clinical depression, psychological distress, and other problems directly related to the burden of caregiving. As such, respite services are provided for people who are living in a home setting and are being cared for by family members or other unpaid help. Goals of respite services include improved well-being for caregivers and delayed institutionalization of dependent older people. Types of respite services include adult day centers, overnight and short-term nursing home care, and provision of in-home companions or home health aides.

Parish Nursing Programs

Parish nursing, first established in the early 1970s, has been recognized by the American Nurses Association as a specialty practice since 1998. **Parish nursing** is a holistic approach to addressing the physical, emotional, and spiritual health care needs of members of church-based congregations, with a focus on health promotion activities such as screenings, education, and increased access to health care (Brudenell, 2003; Burkhart & Androwich, 2004). Although parish nurse programs serve people of all ages, a high percentage of care recipients are older adults or people with chronic illnesses. Roles for parish nurses specific to older adults include assessing and addressing health needs, providing spiritual counseling and health education, training volunteers to assist with visiting people, and acting as referral agent and liaison with other community services. Parish nurses promote wellness by empowering individuals to achieve their full potential, especially with regard to assuming responsibility for self-care (Weis et al., 2006).

Health Promotion Programs

Because of the growing emphasis on health promotion, many community-based programs address the needs of older adults who are relatively healthy and functional, as discussed in Chapter 5. Periodic health screenings and other health promotion activities are increasingly being offered in senior centers and other places where older adults gather. Among the health promotion activities offered by these programs are blood pressure checks; safe driving courses; smoking cessation classes; health screening (e.g., cancer, vision, hearing); flu shots and other immunizations; medication assessment, management, and education; and various types of exercise, such as walking, aerobics, aquatics, or t'ai chi. Health education topics include nutrition, stress management, general health care, and seasonal health issues such as hypothermia, heat-related illness, and colds and flu.

Organized group activities, such as senior wellness programs, frequently take place in or are sponsored by community-based senior centers that exist in almost every community. Hospitals and other health care institutions are becoming more involved in providing this kind of program, and are employing nurses to address the needs of older adults in the community. Programs are sometimes sponsored jointly by senior centers and health care agencies. For example, senior health fairs, which address the specific health needs of a specific population, provide the opportunity for follow-up and referral of identified medical issues. Thus, they can provide a valuable health promotion service for older adults while they increase the potential patient base for health care providers. Recommended health promotion activities for a senior health fair include the provision of information about interventions for maintaining good health and screenings for diabetes, glaucoma, cholesterol, and blood pressure (Hatchett & Duran, 2001).

Geriatric Care Management Services

Services provided to older adults in their own homes constitute one of the most rapidly growing components of health care services. Although family and other unpaid workers provide 85% of all in-home care, informal and formal paid caregivers provide the remaining 15%. Family caregiving has become more complex and difficult as more and more family members have moved away from their hometowns. In addition, the entry of more women into the paid workforce has significantly diminished the availability of traditional family caregivers. These trends, along with the significant increase in the number of people aged 85 years and older, have led to the need for professional geriatric care management services.

As the range of services for older adults has expanded, identification of appropriate services and coordination of care has become more necessary and more challenging. Although family members sometimes take on these tasks, many family members are not prepared to assume this challenge, and many older adults do not have any family members available. In these situations, the older adult may receive care (or case) management services. A **geriatric care manager** serves as the primary coordinator who is responsible for implementing a long-term care plan in the absence of family members who have the ability to do so.

Care management involves comprehensive assessment, care planning, implementation, monitoring, and reassessment. Professional geriatric care management services are provided by individual professionals and by nonprofit and for-profit groups and organizations. These services are often provided by a nurse who assesses the needs for a variety of long-term care services and then plans, coordinates, and oversees the services. Care management has created many opportunities for gerontological nurses in agencies or in private practice settings. Outcomes of nurse care management services in a pilot project called the Frail Elderly Community-Based Case Management Project included decreases in hospital admission (13%), emergency department visits (38%), length of stay (22%), and total hospital costs (73%) (Duke, 2005).

Roles for Gerontological Nurses in the Community

Gerontological nurses have leading roles in developing and implementing health services for older adults in community-based programs for older adults such as adult day care, senior centers, respite programs, and care management. Because wellness and health promotion are major foci of these programs, involvement of nursing is essential. For example, nurses have established wellness centers to provide screening, counseling, and skill enhancement programs for older adults. Services at wellness centers commonly include assessment of nutrition, blood glucose, blood pressure, mood states, and risks for falls (Belza & Baker, 2000).

Innovative roles are increasingly being developed for gerontological nurses involved in the care or counseling of older adults living in the community, dependent older adults in various institutional settings, and caregivers of dependent older adults. In addition to the health care needs of older adults, there is growing concern about the needs of the caregivers of dependent older adults; gerontological nurses have many opportunities for expanding their roles to address those needs. Geriatric care management services and caregiver counseling and education are rapidly becoming essential components of gerontological nursing, and gerontological nurses are frequently involved in formally assessing not only the needs of older adults, but the needs of their caregivers, who may or may not be older adults themselves. Interventions are directed as much toward the caregivers of dependent older people as toward the older people themselves. It has become increasingly common for gerontological nurses to work in collegial relationships with other members of a multidisciplinary team, including primary care providers, psychiatrists, social workers, physical therapists, and other health care providers to address the needs of older adults as well as their caregivers.

Attention in recent years also has focused on the health care needs of culturally diverse older adults and groups such as rural elders, as discussed in Chapter 4. There is a tremendous need for gerontological nurses who can develop and implement health care programs that are designed to meet specific needs of groups such as African Americans, Asian Americans, American Indians, and Hispanic Americans. Gerontological literature has also focused recently on the health care needs of two population groups that exhibit characteristics of old age beginning in their sixth decade: prisoners and homeless people (e.g., Dubler, 2001). Chow (2002) described the role of a gerontological nurse in organizing and implementing a long-term care nursing service for aging inmates. Clearly, there are no limits to the creativity that nurses can use in developing health care services for older adults.

PAYING FOR HEALTH CARE SERVICES FOR OLDER ADULTS

At a minimum, gerontological nurses must be knowledgeable enough about current health care policies relating to older people to understand some of the barriers to and challenges of implementing nursing care plans and discharge plans. For example, knowing the Medicare criteria for skilled home care services enables the nurse to make referrals for this type of nursing care when appropriate. In addition, nurses need to keep up to date on recent changes, not only so that they can guide older adults in the many choices of health care delivery systems that are now available, but so that they can identify opportunities for new roles for gerontological nurses. The roles of gerontological nurses are expanding rapidly, and much of this expansion directly relates to changes in health insurance and health care delivery systems. For example, after several decades of anticipation, Medicare reimbursement for advanced practice nurses finally became a reality in the late 1990s. Payment for health care services for older adults is commonly funded through Medicare, Medicaid, private insurance, out-of-pocket spending, or comprehensive models.

Medicare

Medicare is a health insurance program that was established by Congress in 1965 as an entitlement program for people who are eligible for Social Security benefits. Medicare covers primarily hospital and physician services, with very limited coverage for some skilled care services in homes and nursing homes. As of 2005, Medicare also offers some coverage for prescription drugs. It does not cover dental care, most vision care, most routine or preventive services, or nonskilled long-term care. The original Medicare plan is divided into Part A, funded through payroll taxes, and Part B, financed through monthly premiums paid by beneficiaries and by general revenues. Medicare, therefore, is part of the national budget and is subject to the same political processes that affect other budget items.

Hospital insurance (Part A) covers medical or psychiatric inpatient care in a hospital and in a skilled nursing facility after a hospital stay. It also covers some of the approved costs of durable medical equipment and skilled home care services and hospice care for those patients who qualify. Beneficiaries are responsible for a co-pay amount for hospital services that increases every year and is the equivalent of the average cost of 1 day of hospital care. Reimbursement for hospital and skilled nursing facility care is based on benefit periods. A benefit period begins on the first day of hospital admission and ends 60 days after the person no longer qualifies for care in a hospital or skilled nursing facility. Strict criteria must be met for coverage of services in a skilled nursing facility, and the number of days that are covered is limited. The Medicare home care benefit is intended to provide medically oriented, acute or restorative, skilled nursing care on an intermittent, short-term basis to homebound patients who are under the care of a physician.

Supplemental medical insurance (Part B) covers all or part of the cost of approved physician's services and other outpatient services, such as diagnostic imaging and laboratory services. Additional services covered under Part B include certain ambulance services, durable medical equipment used at home, and the services of certain specially qualified, nonphysician, health care practitioners (e.g., nurse practitioners).

A major limitation of traditional Medicare has been its lack of coverage for preventive services. This is changing, however, because of the increasing recognition of the importance of these services in delaying the onset of chronic illnesses and improving the health and function of older adults. In recent years, Medicare began paying for the following preventive services: diabetes education; glaucoma screening; bone density measurements; colorectal cancer screening; mammograms and breast examinations; Pap smears and pelvic examinations; influenza, pneumonia, and hepatitis B vaccinations; and prostate-specific antigen (PSA) tests and digital rectal examinations. Additional preventive and screening coverage that has been proposed for Medicare coverage includes hypertension screening, osteoporosis screening and counseling, and counseling for cessation of tobacco use (Infeld & Whitelaw, 2002).

In the past four decades, Medicare has always achieved its original goal of paying for basic medical services, but program implementation has undergone significant changes. When Medicare was first established, there was a limit on the types of services covered, but little regulation of the amount of reimbursement for these services. A fee-for-service system reimbursed providers directly for the cost of services. During the first 10 years of Medicare, health care costs increased an average of 141% per year, compared with 11.4% for the increase in gross national product. Causes of this unprecedented rise in health care costs included the availability of federal funds under Medicare, the high rate of inflation in the general economy, and the even higher rate of inflation in the health care industry. Other contributing factors were malpractice concerns, expensive technology, duplication of equipment and services, lack of less costly alternatives to institutional care, and the legal and ethical constraints that encourage the use of high technology to prolong life.

Because the federal government had not anticipated the dramatic rise in health care costs that began in the late 1960s, they grossly underestimated the projected spending for the 1970s and 1980s. In an attempt to control the rapidly growing costs of this federal program, Congress amended Medicare in 1972 and established Professional Standard Review Organizations to review use of services. Despite the need to control costs, these same amendments expanded Medicare coverage to include adults of any age who had end-stage renal disease or were disabled for 2 years or more as a result of any disease. Although these amendments provided some control over the use of services, the costs of the program continued to escalate far beyond the cost estimates.

In the early 1980s, the federal government took a serious look at health care expenditures and began to deal with the problem of cost containment. Other goals of the federal government during this period included increasing expenditures for defense and diminishing the role of the government in health and social programs. One way of accomplishing these goals was to target for reduction the large part of the federal budget that went toward Medicare, Medicaid, Social Security, and other programs for older people. The three-pronged approach that was adopted to cut health care costs included an increase in the amount paid by individual participants, restriction of the amount of Medicare payment for services, and promotion of voluntary reductions in costs of health care services.

In 1982, the federal government established a system of prospective payment as the basis of fee-for-service payments. This system reimbursed providers on a predetermined rate based on the expected cost of treating a patient with a specific diagnosis that was classified according to a diagnosis-related group (DRG). Initially this system was applied only to Medicare patients, but insurance companies now use it almost universally. Thus, hospitals are no longer guaranteed payment for actual services rendered. Rather, they are financially rewarded when the cost of patient care is less than that allowed for the relevant DRG and are penalized when the cost of patient care is more than that allowed for the relevant DRG. This system promotes the early discharge of hospitalized patients, who tend to be relatively sicker at the time of discharge, and shifts the burden of care from hospitals to families, nursing homes, and other community-based care providers. This approach has given rise to the phrase *quicker and sicker*, which became the theme of discharge planning in the 1980s. Other results are a dramatic increase in the number of outpatient procedures and the development of postacute and subacute care programs.

In addition to radically changing the Medicare reimbursement system, the 1982 federal legislation allowed Medicare beneficiaries to enroll in approved Medicare managed care organizations. This marked the first time that Medicare payments were based on criteria other than a fee-for-service basis. People in managed care programs pay little or nothing for premiums, deductibles, and coinsurance amounts. For each enrollee in their program, the managed care organization receives capitation payments of 95% of the average amount paid to fee-for-service providers in the same geographic area. The major advantage to participants is that these plans generally cover all or part of the costs of medications, vision care, and some other services not covered under traditional Medicare. In addition, preventive services are covered and many plans strongly encourage health promotion services. In contrast to the traditional Medicare plan, managed care plans do not require a 3-day hospital stay to qualify for skilled nursing services. The major disadvantage for some participants is that the choice of health care providers is limited, and permission is needed from a primary care provider before services can be obtained from specialists.

Medicare managed care organizations initially evolved very slowly, but the Balanced Budget Act of 1997 promoted the growth of managed care by creating Medicare Plus Choice (M+C) plans (also called Medicare Part C). This legislation provided Medicare funds for a variety of managed care organizations, including preferred provider organizations and provider-sponsored organizations. By the early 2000s, many types of managed care plans were available under Medicare as alternatives to the traditional fee-for-service Medicare plan. The main differences among managed care plans are the amount of choice allowed to participants, the amount of copayments and other out-of-pocket costs, and the optional services covered (e.g., dental care, eye care, and prescription drugs).

In 2005, the Medicare Modernization and Improvement Act created the Part D Drug Benefit, which provided limited coverage for prescription medications for the first time. All persons with Medicare Part A or B are eligible for this benefit, which involves the following conditions:

- A monthly premium and annual deductible, which increase every year
- Annual coverage of 75% of the cost of approved drugs up to $2510 in 2008
- A so-called donut hole, in which the next $1540 in costs are paid by the beneficiary
- After the beneficiary pays a total of $4050 out-of-pocket, Medicare pays for 95% of drug costs for the rest of the year
- Exclusions of some drugs (e.g., barbiturates, benzodiazepines, nonprescription drugs, drugs for anorexia, weight control, or relief of symptoms of coughs or colds)

Low-income people and those who also have Medicaid insurance are exempt from copayments and out-of-pocket expenses. Medicare beneficiaries have a choice of approved drug plans, and each plan varies in coverage for specific drugs. Beneficiaries are expected to compare available plans to determine which one best meets their needs. Major concerns about the drug plans include the complexity of decisions, restrictions on enrollment periods, penalties for not enrolling during certain periods, exclusion of some drugs, and the high out-of-pocket expenses. Medicare Part D is discussed further in Chapter 8.

Medicaid

Medicaid legislation was enacted at the same time as Medicare to provide health insurance for poor people. Although Medicare falls entirely under the jurisdiction of the federal government, Medicaid is a state-run program that receives partial funding from federal sources and is subject to certain federal guidelines. To qualify for Medicaid, people must meet medical and financial criteria. Financially, they must have a very low income and limited assets. States establish asset limits, with a typical upper limit between $2000 and $4000 for individuals and between $3000 and $6000 for couples (Moon, 2006). If income is more than the lower eligibility level and medical expenses account for a high proportion of income, people can qualify by spending down to the eligible income level. Each state determines the specific income and asset limits, and rules differ considerably among the states. State and federal regulations restrict the transfer of assets from one family member to another to qualify for Medicaid, but federal legislation enacted in 1988 protects the income and assets of a married person when his or her spouse is in a nursing facility for at least 30 days. Although a high proportion of nursing home residents qualify for Medicaid, less than 10% of noninstitutionalized older adults receive Medicaid (Crystal et al., 2000).

States have some discretion with regard to eligibility criteria for Medicaid, but the federal government mandates that they pay for certain medical services, including skilled and intermediate levels of nursing home care, for all eligible adults. Because the cost of nursing home care is so high—about $50,000 per year in the early 2000s—many older adults with modest incomes meet the eligibility criteria by having limited assets and medical expenses that account for a very high proportion of their income. Thus, Medicaid has become increasingly important as a source of payment for long-term care for older adults, covering about half of nursing home costs. It is less important for noninstitutionalized older adults, however, because it accounts for less than 2% of health care expenditures for this group (Crystal et al., 2000).

Traditionally, Medicaid has been biased toward paying for institutional care rather than community-based long-term care, but this is gradually changing. Since the 1980s, states have been able to apply for Medicaid waivers to provide community-based services to people who otherwise would need nursing home care. Between 1989 and 1999 the proportion of Medicaid funding for long-term care devoted to home-based care doubled from 13% to 26% (Feder et al., 2001). As with other components of Medicaid, the federal government mandates some long-term care services, whereas states have discretion over the provision of other services. Home care services are mandatory, but optional services include personal care, case management, and medically oriented day care (Wiener, 2001).

Private Insurance

Because of the many limitations of Medicare as a health insurance program, approximately three fourths of older adults purchase additional insurance coverage from private companies. Private health insurance policies include all of the following types: continuation of employer-provided policies, hospital indemnity, specific diseases, medigap, long-term care, and managed care. These supplemental policies attempt to fill the gap between the services covered by Medicare and the services paid for out-of-pocket. All supplemental policies cover the premiums and copayments for services covered by Medicare Parts A and B, but additional benefits vary according to each policy.

Employer-sponsored policies usually provide the best supplemental insurance—sometimes covering prescription drugs and limited long-term care services—but they are available only to retired people (or their spouses) who continue coverage under the health insurance policy offered by their employer. Retirees who held higher-paying jobs and attained higher educational levels are more likely to have these policies (Crystal et al., 2000). Because many retirees are required to pay all or part of the premium, it is estimated that 27% of people who are offered employer-sponsored health insurance do not accept the insurance (Crystal et al., 2000). As employers address current major economic concerns, employee-sponsored policies are likely to be less available and more costly for retirees.

Hospital indemnity policies pay cash amounts for each day of inpatient hospital care; they may also include benefits for surgical procedures or days spent in a skilled nursing facility. Specific disease policies are limited to paying for services related to a specific disease, and are likely to duplicate benefits covered under Medicare or other primary insurance policies.

Medigap policies are designed to supplement Medicare benefits, and are now regulated by federal and state laws. The National Association of Insurance Commissioners has developed 10 standard plans that insurance companies must follow in the provision of medigap policies. Plan A contains basic benefits, such as coverage for coinsurance payments and additional payments for hospital days. Other plans (B through J) cover Part A deductible and additional services, such as preventive medical care, skilled nursing coinsurance, and medical care in foreign countries. The most comprehensive policies cover the cost of medications. Limits are applied to the drug benefit and some of the other benefits. A relatively new type of supplemental policy is the Medicare Select policy, which provides the same coverage as medigap policies, but only when services are provided by a designated, preferred provider.

Long-term care insurance is a recent development in the health insurance industry. When these policies were introduced in the late 1980s they were unregulated, and many of the policies contained large loopholes and significant barriers to receiving benefits. During the 1990s, many states enacted laws mandating standards suggested by the National Association of Insurance Commissioners. Suggested requirements for long-term care insurance policies include inflation protection and caps on rates. A good long-term care policy will provide payment for a range of options, including home care services, assisted-living facilities, and nursing home care. In addition, policies should be open enough that they include services that may be developed in the future but are not available at the time the policy is initiated. For example, the first long-term care policies that were developed were limited to nursing home care because few other options were available at that time. A major drawback of this type of insurance for older people is that the premiums are based on the age of the person when he or she initially signs up for the policy. For most older adults, therefore, the cost of the policy will outweigh the benefits. These policies will likely become increasingly important, particularly for young-old and middle-aged people, because recent proposals promote private long-term care insurance rather than public programs (Wiener, 2001).

Out-of-Pocket Spending

Despite the major contribution of health insurance programs in paying for health care services, older adults currently spend a larger percentage of their income—about 20%—on their health care needs than ever before. Out-of-pocket health care expenses have been increasing steadily in the past four decades and that burden falls disproportionately on poor people. Crystal and colleagues (2000) found that increases in out-of-pocket expenses were consistent with increases in income, but that the out-of-pocket expenditures account for much larger proportions of income (31.5%) for people in the lowest income quintile than for those in the highest income group (8.5%).

In the early 2000s, this issue emerged as one of the most hotly debated aspects of Medicare reform legislation and stirred great conflict among groups concerned about the increasing costs of both providing and paying for health care services. In particular, many groups are concerned about the significant financial burden associated with prescription drugs and long-term care. Many of the proposals that Congress considered during the early 2000s attempted to limit the rate of Medicare growth. If this goal is accomplished, out-of-pocket expenses will inevitably increase, and the financial burden will fall most heavily on the people who already experience high out-of-pocket expenses—those with lower incomes and chronic illnesses (Crystal et al., 2000).

Comprehensive Models

Consumer demand for noninstitutional long-term care services and persistent increases in health care costs for Medicare and Medicaid programs have stimulated the development of new models of health insurance and health care delivery. Since the 1980s, the federal government has funded innovative models of long-term care for people with chronic conditions that are both comprehensive and cost-effective. These Medicare and Medicaid waiver programs—sometimes called Social Health Maintenance Organizations—provide a wide range of social and medical services on a capitated managed care basis. The prototype of this model is the On Lok Senior Services program, which was developed in the early 1970s in the Chinatown area of San Francisco and still exists today in a greatly expanded form. On Lok—Cantonese for "peaceful happy abode"—successfully addresses the health care system issues that most strongly affect older adults: expense, fragmentation, and lack of creativity in community-based care (Pierce, 2002).

The success of On Lok prompted the development of 10 similar programs, called Program of All-inclusive Care for the Elderly (PACE), in the late 1980s. Based on data from On Lok, it is estimated that the cost of care for participants in PACE programs is 15% less than the cost in traditional fee-for-service programs (Mui, 2002). The Balanced Budget Act of 1997 established PACE models as permanently recognized Medicare and Medicaid providers. By the end of 1998, 17 PACE programs were fully funded under dual Medicare and Medicaid capitation, and 14 programs were in development (Mui, 2002). In 2000, two private foundations—the Robert Wood Johnson Foundation and the John A. Hartford Foundation—supported the expansion of these models of care. By the end of 2002, 25 demonstration sites were eligible for permanent federal funding, and more than 70 organizations in 30 states were developing or implementing PACE models. Clearly, it is quite possible that this model will revolutionize how long-term care is provided in the future.

The target group for PACE is people who are eligible for both Medicare and Medicaid services, live in the community, and qualify for nursing home care. Distinguishing features of the model are (1) the provision of comprehensive and community-based long-term care services to nursing-home-eligible clients, (2) an emphasis on preventive services, (3) integrated service delivery through adult day health centers, (4) case management through multidisciplinary teams, and (5) full funding on a capitation basis (similar to health maintenance organizations). Core components of PACE programs are nutrition, transportation, home care, acute care, respite care, primary care, social services, restorative therapies, prescription drugs, long-term care, adult day care, medical specialty care, durable medical equipment, and multidisciplinary case management. The hallmarks of PACE programs are an emphasis on interdisciplinary teamwork, a reliance on day care centers as the base of services, and a commitment to keeping enrollees out of institutions (Kane et al., 2002).

Another federal initiative for integrating acute and long-term care is the EverCare model, in which teams of geriatric physicians and nurses provide intense primary care in nursing homes. In this model, all medical services are covered independent of the setting, so there is no financial incentive to provide services in a hospital setting if they can be provided in a nursing home (Stone, 2006).

Chapter Highlights

Development of a Continuum of Care for Older Adults

- The establishment of Medicare and Medicaid in 1965 provided a major financial stimulus for the development of health care programs for older adults.
- By the early 1970s, home care agencies and nursing home facilities had emerged as the primary avenue for addressing health care needs of older adults outside of acute care settings.
- During the 1980s, geriatricians, gerontologists, and health care providers became aware of the need to develop more cost-effective and innovative ways of providing health care services to older adults.
- By the early 2000s, a wide continuum of health care services was available to address the complex needs of older adults.
- Gerontological nurses assume many roles in the diverse settings that comprise the continuum of care for older adults.
- Changes in Medicare reimbursement policy have created opportunities for advanced practice nurses, particularly in acute care settings, nursing homes, and home care agencies.

Acute Care Settings

- Acute care settings, which are part of the continuum of care, have developed subacute care units and specialized geriatric units for addressing the complex needs of hospitalized older adults.

Long-Term Care Settings

- Older adults who have chronic conditions that affect their level of functioning and quality of life typically need long-term care services.
- Although long-term care has traditionally been associated with nursing home care, it is currently associated with continuum-of-care services that are provided in many institutional and community-based settings.
- Nursing homes provide short-term skilled nursing for people who are recovering from acute conditions and intermediate or long-term nursing care for chronically ill people who need assistance with daily activities.
- Because of federal legislation and consumer demand, long-term care facilities are currently addressing many issues about quality of care and quality of life for their residents.

Home Care Services

- Home care services are generally classified as skilled and long-term.
- Skilled home care services, which are covered under Medicare and other health insurance programs, provide short-term skilled nursing or rehabilitative services for homebound people who meet medical criteria.
- Long-term home care includes a wide spectrum of services ranging from unskilled care such as meal preparation and grocery shopping to full-time hands-on nursing care. Older adults or their families pay for the majority of these services out-of-pocket.

Community-Based Services

- Community-based services, which include adult day centers, respite services, parish nursing programs, health promotion programs, and care management services, play important roles in meeting the long-term needs of older adults.

Paying for Health Care Services for Older Adults

- Medicare is the health insurance program that covers hospital and medical care and some skilled care services. In the 1970s, Congress began making major changes to Medicare because costs were exceeding estimated expenditures, and these changes continue today. By the early 2000s, Medicare benefits to providers had been reduced significantly and many types of managed care plans were available as alternatives to the traditional fee-for-service Medicare plan.

- Medicaid is a health insurance program that was established to provide medical care for poor people, but it has evolved to being the primary source of payment for nonskilled long-term care for older adults. Medicaid has traditionally been slanted toward payment for nursing home care rather than community-based care, but this has been changing in recent years.
- Private insurance is available from many sources to supplement Medicare coverage, but older adults spend a larger percentage of their income—about 20%—on their health care than ever before.
- Program of All-inclusive Care for the Elderly (PACE), which are comprehensive models of health care first developed in the late 1980s, are becoming more widely available.

Critical Thinking Exercises

1. You are on a panel of nursing students who are presenting information about opportunities for nurses to work in various settings. Your topic is "Roles for Gerontological Nurses in Home, Institutional, and Community Settings." Describe the content of your 20-minute presentation.
2. Mrs. F. is a resident in the skilled care section of the nursing home where you work. She had been living alone in her own home before being admitted to the hospital with a fractured hip 4 weeks ago. She has regained much of her independence and walks with a walker and one-person assist. She expects to ambulate independently using a walker within 2 weeks, at which time she expects to return to her own home. She asks you what kind of services would be available in her home. What additional information would you want to know before you answered her questions? What information would you give to her? What suggestions would you make?
3. Your grandmother, who is 64 years old, asks your advice about health insurance choices that she needs to make when she is 65. How would you explain her choices and what suggestions would you make to her?

Educational Resources

AARP (American Association of Retired Persons)
www.aarp.org

Administration on Aging, Eldercare Locator
(800) 677-1116
www.aoa.gov

Centers for Medicare & Medicaid Services
www.cms.hhs.gov

National Association of Professional Geriatric Care Managers
www.caremanager.org

National Institute on Aging
www.nia.nih.gov

National PACE Association
www.npaonline.org

References

Allen, L. A., Mihalovic, S. J., & Narveson, G. G. (2000). Successful protocol-based practitioner management of warfarin anticoagulation in nursing home patients. *Annals of Long-Term Care, 8*, 60–71.

Anetzberger, G. J. (2002). Community resources to promote successful aging. *Clinics in Geriatric Medicine, 18*, 611–626.

Barba, B. A., Tesh, A. S., & Courts, A. F. (2002). Promoting thriving in nursing homes. *Journal of Gerontological Nursing, 28*(3), 7–13.

Belza, B., & Baker, M. W. (2000). Maintaining health in well older adults: Initiatives for schools of nursing and The John A. Hartford Foundation for the 21st Century. *Journal of Gerontological Nursing*, 26(7), 8–17.

Benedict, L., Robinson, K., & Holder, C. (2006). Clinical nurse specialist practice within the acute care for elders interdisciplinary team model. *Clinical Nurse Specialist, 20*, 248–252.

Bergman-Evans, B. (2004). Beyond the basics: Effects of the Eden alternative model on quality of life issues. *Journal of Gerontological Nursing, 30*(6), 27–34.

Bharucha, A. J., Pandav, R., Changyu, S., Dodge, H. H., & Ganguli, M. (2004). Predictors of nursing facility admission: A 12-year epidemiological study in the United States. *Journal of the American Geriatrics Society, 52*, 434–439.

Bonnel, W. B. (2002). Assisted living: Strategies for initiating an advanced practice nurse clinic. *Journal of Gerontological Nursing*, 28(1), 5–11.

Borrayo, E. A., Salmon, J. R., Polivka, L., & Dunlop, B. D. (2002). Utilization across the continuum of long-term services. *The Gerontologist, 42*, 603–612.

Bourbonniere, M., & Evans, L. K. (2002). Advanced practice nursing in the care of frail older adults. *Journal of the American Geriatrics Society, 50*, 2062–2076.

Brudenell, I. (2003). Parish nursing: Nurturing body, mind, spirit, and community. *Public Health Nursing, 20*(2), 85–94.

Buhr, G. T., Kuchibhatla, M., & Clipp, E. C. (2006). Caregivers' reasons for nursing home placement: Clues for improving discussions with families prior to the transition. *The Gerontologist, 46*, 52–61.

Burkhart, L., & Androwich, I. (2004). Measuring the domain completeness of the Nursing Interventions Classification in Parish Nurse documentation. *Computers, Informatics, Nursing, 22*, 72–82.

Calkins, M. C. (2002). The nursing home of the future: Are you ready? *Nursing Homes/Long Term Care Management, 51*(6), 42–47.

Chow, R. K. (2002). Initiating a long-term care nursing service for aging inmates. *Geriatric Nursing, 23*, 24–27.

Coughlin, J. F., Pope, J. E., & Leedle, B. R. (2006). Old age, new technology, and future innovations in disease management and home health care. *Home Health Care Management & Practice, 18*, 196–207.

Crystal, S., Johnson, R. W., Harman, J., Sambamoorthi, U., & Kumar, R. (2000). Out-of-pocket health care among older Americans. *Journals of Gerontology: Series B, Psychological Sciences and Social Sciences, 55*, S51–S62.

Dubler, N. N. (2001). Prison-residing elders. In M. D. Mezey (Ed.), *The encyclopedia of elder care* (pp. 528–531). New York: Springer.

Duke, C. (2005). The frail elderly community-based case management project. *Geriatric Nursing, 26*, 122–127.

Eisch, J. S., Brozovic, B., Colling, K., & Wold, K. (2000). Nurse practitioner geropsychiatric consultation services to nursing homes. *Geriatric Nursing, 21*, 150–155.

Feder, J., Komisar, H. L., & Niefeld, M. (2001). The financing and organization of health care. In R. H. Binstock & L. K. George (Eds.), *Handbook of aging and the social sciences* (5th ed., pp. 387–405). San Diego: Academic Press.

Frantz, A. K., Colgan, J., Palmer, K., & Ledgerwood, B. (2002). Lessons learned from telehealth pioneers. *Home Healthcare Nurse, 20*, 363–366.

Fulmer, T., Mezey, M., Bottrell, M., Abraham, I., Sazant, J., Grossman, S., et al. (2002). Nurses Improving Care for Healthsystem Elders (NICHE): Using outcomes and benchmarks for evidenced-based practice. *Geriatric Nursing, 23*, 121–123.

Fulmer, T. T. (1991). The geriatric nurse specialist role: A new model. *Nursing Management, 22*, 91–93.

Guthrie, P. F., Edinger, G., & Schumacher, S. (2002). A NICHE program at North Memorial Health Care. *Geriatric Nursing, 23*, 133–138.

Hatchett, B. F., & Duran, D. A. (2001). Older adults share opinions: Senior health fairs. *Activities, Adaptation & Aging, 25*(3/4), 59–71.

Hays, J. C., Pieper, C. F., & Purser, J. L. (2003). Competing risk of household expansion or institutionalization in late life. *Journals of Gerontology: Series B, Psychological Sciences and Social Sciences, 58*, S11–S20.

Hujer, M., Mann, A., & Mion, L. C. (2000). Assisted living facilities. In J. J. Fitzpatrick & T. Fulmer (Eds.), *Geriatric nursing research digest*. New York: Springer.

Infeld, D. L., & Whitelaw, N. (2002). Policy initiatives to promote healthy aging. *Clinics in Geriatric Medicine, 18*, 627–642.

Inouye, S. K. (2000). The hospital elder life program: a model of care to prevent cognitive and functional decline in older hospitalized patients: Hospital elder life program. *Journal of the American Geriatrics Society, 48*, 1697–1706.

Inouye, S. K., Acampora, D., Miller, R. L., Fulmer, T., Hurst, L. D., & Cooney, L. M. (1993a). The Yale Geriatric Care Program: A model of care to prevent functional decline in hospitalized elderly patients. *Journal of the American Geriatrics Society, 41*, 1345–1352.

Inouye, S. K., Wagner, D. R., Acampora, D., Horwitz, R. I., Cooney, L. M., & Tinetti, M. E. (1993b). A controlled trial of a nursing-centered intervention in hospitalized elderly medical patients: The Yale Geriatric Care Program. *Journal of the American Geriatrics Society, 41*, 1353–1360.

Jarchin, S. (2006). Finding your post-acute care niche. *Nursing Homes Magazine, March*, 32–36.

Jenkins, R., L., & McSweeney, M. (2001). Assessing elderly patients with congestive heart failure via in-home interactive telecommunication. *Journal of Gerontological Nursing, 27*(1), 21–27.

Jennings-Sanders, A. (2004). Nurses in adult day care centers. *Geriatric Nursing, 25*, 227–232.

Kane, R. L., Homyak, P., & Bershadsky, B. (2002). Consumer reactions to the Wisconsin Partnership Program and its parent, the Program for All-inclusive Care of the Elderly (PACE). *The Gerontologist, 42*, 314–320.

Lee, V. K., & Fletcher, K. R. (2002). Sustaining the geriatric resource nurse model at the University of Virginia. *Geriatric Nursing, 23*, 128–132.

Leff, B., & Burton, J. R. (2001). The future history of home care and physician house calls in the United States. *Journals of Gerontology: Series A, Biological Sciences and Medical Sciences, 56*, M603–M608.

Marrelli, T. M. (2001). Prospective payment in home care: An overview. *Geriatric Nursing, 22*, 217–218.

Martin, K. S. (2001). Home health care. In M. D. Mezey (Ed.), *The encyclopedia of elder care* (pp. 351–353). New York: Springer.

McGilton, K. S. (2002). Enhancing relationships between care providers and residents in long-term care: Designing a model of care. *Journal of Gerontological Nursing, 28*(12), 13–21.

McMackin, S. (2006). What is private-duty homecare? An industry overview. *Home Health Care Management & Practice, 18*(2), 92–97.

Mezey, M. M. (2001). Advanced practice nursing. In M. D. Mezey (Ed.), *The encyclopedia of elder care* (pp. 24–26). New York: Springer.

Miller, S. K. (2002). Acute care of the elderly units: a positive outcomes case study. *AACN Clinical Issues, 13*(1), 34–42.

Milone-Nuzzo, P., & Pike, A. (2001). Advanced practice nurses in home care: Is there a role? *Home Health Care Management & Practice, 13*, 349–355.

Mion, L. C., Palmer, R. M., Anetzberger, G. J., & Meldon, S. W. (2001). Establishing a case-finding and referral system for at-risk older individuals in the emergency department setting: The SIGNET model. *Journal of the American Geriatrics Society, 49*, 1379–1386.

Mitty, E. L. (2001). Nursing homes. In M. D. Mezey (Ed.), *The encyclopedia of elder care* (pp. 452–455). New York: Springer.

Moon, M. (2006). Organization and financing of health care. In R. H. Binstock & L. K. George (Eds.), *Handbook of aging and the social sciences* (6th ed., pp. 380–396). San Diego: Academic Press.

Morley, J. E. (2003). Editorial: Hot topics in geriatrics. *Journals of Gerontology: Series A, Biological Sciences and Medical Sciences, 53*, 30–36.

Mui, A. C. (2002). The Program of All-inclusive Care for the Elderly (PACE): An innovative long-term care model in the United States. *Journal of Aging and Social Policy, 13*(2/3), 53–67.

Pearson, S., Inglis, S. C., & McLennan, S. N. (2006). Prolonged effects of a home-based intervention in patients with chronic illness. *Archives of Internal Medicine, 166*, 645–650.

Pfaff, J. (2002). The geriatric resource nurse model: A culture change. *Geriatric Nursing, 23*, 140–144.

Pierce, C. A. (2002). Program of All-inclusive Care for the Elderly in 2002. *Geriatric Nursing, 23*, 173–174.

Pierson, C. (2001). APN elder home care: A successful model. *Home Health Care Management & Practice, 13*, 375–379.

Ryden, M. B., Snyder, M., Gross, C. R., Savik, K., Pearson, V., Kirchbaum, K., et al. (2000). Value-added outcomes: The use of advanced practice nurses in long-term care facilities. *The Gerontologist, 40*, 654–662.

Salinas, T. K., O'Connor, L. J., Weinstein, M., Lee, S. Y. V., & Fitzpatrick, J. J. (2002). A family assessment tool for hospitalized elders. *Geriatric Nursing, 23*, 316–319, 335.

Smith, B. M., Maloy, K. A., & Hawkins, D. J. (2000). An examination of Medicare home health services. *Care Management Journals, 2*, 238–247.

Spillman, B. C., & Lubitz, J. (2002). New estimates of lifetime nursing home use: Have patterns changed? *Medical Care, 40*, 965–975.

Stone, R. I. (2006). Emerging issues in long-term care. In R. H. Binstock & L. K. George (Eds.), *Handbook of aging and the social sciences* (6th ed., pp. 397–418). San Diego: Academic Press.

Swauger, K., & Tomlin, C. (2002). Best care for the elderly at Forsyth Medical Center. *Geriatric Nursing, 23*, 145–150.

Tesh, A. S., McNutt, K., Courts, N. F., & Barba, B. A. (2002). Characteristics of nursing homes: Adopting environmental transformations. *Journal of Gerontological Nursing, 28*(3), 28–34.

Thomas, D. R. (2002). Focus on functional decline in hospitalized older adults. *Journals of Gerontology: Series A, Biological Sciences and Medical Sciences, 57*, M567–M568.

Thomas, W. (1994). *The Eden Alternative: Nature, hope, and nursing homes*. New York: Eden Alternative Foundation.

Tichawa, U. (2002). Creating a continuum of care for elderly individuals. *Journal of Gerontological Nursing, 28*(1), 46–52.

Tran, B. Q., Buckley, K. M., & Prandoni, C. M. (2002). Selection and use of telehealth technology in support of homebound caregivers of stroke patients. *CARING Magazine, March*, 16–21.

Tucker, D., Bechtel, G., Quartana, C., Badger, N., Werner, D., Ford, I., et al. (2006). The OASIS program: Redesigning hospital care for older adults. *Geriatric Nursing, 27*, 112–117.

Turner, J. T., Lee, V., Fletcher, K., Hudson, K., & Barton, D. (2001). Measuring quality of care with an inpatient elderly population: The Geriatric Resource Nurse Model. *Journal of Gerontological Nursing, 27*(3), 8–18.

Wakefield, B., Flanagan, J., & Specht, J. K. P. (2001). Telehealth: An opportunity for gerontological nursing practice. *Journal of Gerontological Nursing, 27*(1), 10–14.

Wallace, M. (2003). Is there a nurse in the house? The role of nurses in assisted living: Past, present, and future. *Geriatric Nursing, 24*(4), 218–221.

Weis, D., Schank, M. J., & Matheus, R. (2006). The process of empowerment. *Journal of Holistic Nursing, 24*(1), 17–24.

Wiener, J. M. (2001). Long-term-care policy. In M. D. Mezey (Ed.), *The encyclopedia of elder care* (pp. 403–406). New York: Springer.

Williams, J., & Bassett, M. (2006). Telemanagement in hospice: A new frontier. *Caring, 25*(1), 22–24.

Yeaworth, R. C. (2002). Long-term care and insurance. *Journal of Gerontological Nursing, 28*(11), 45–51.

Zank, S., & Schacke, C. (2002). Evaluation of geriatric day care units: Effects on patients and caregivers. *Journals of Gerontology: Series B, Psychological Sciences and Social Sciences, 57*, P348–P357.

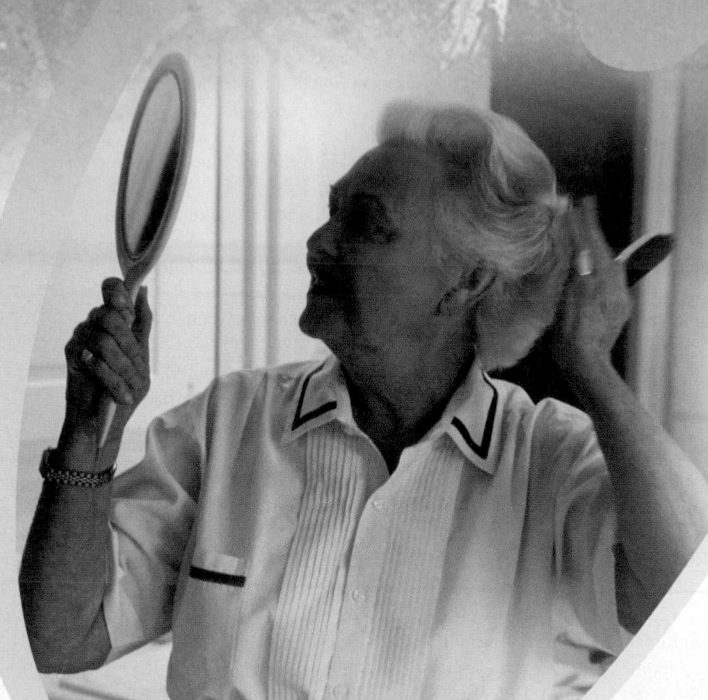

CHAPTER 7

Assessment of Health and Functioning

Learning Objectives

After reading this chapter, you will be able to:

1. Discuss factors that contribute to the complexity of assessing older adults.
2. Explain how to perform a functional assessment of an older adult.
3. Describe how the older adult's environment, use of adaptive and assistive devices, and cognitive abilities can affect functioning.
4. Explain how nurses can assess and address concerns about safe driving in older adults.

Key Terms

activities of daily living (ADLs)
everyday competence
functional assessment
instrumental activities of daily living (IADLs)

Assessment of older adults is complex. This chapter discusses the general approach to assessing the older adult's health and functioning and provides guidelines for functional assessment. This information supplements assessment information related to specific areas of function that is provided in other chapters. In addition, because health and functioning significantly affect the ability to drive a motor vehicle, this chapter discusses how nurses can assess and address risk factors that interfere with safe driving in older adults.

GENERAL APPROACH TO ASSESSING THE OLDER ADULT'S HEALTH AND FUNCTIONING

One of the major challenges of caring for older adults is the complexity of assessing their health, especially from a holistic perspective. As discussed in Chapter 3, there are more questions than clear answers about the complex relationship between aging and disease. Several factors contribute to the complexity of assessing health and functioning in older adults:

- Older adults commonly have one or more chronic conditions in addition to any acute health conditions for which they are being assessed. These conditions often interact, causing older adults' health to fluctuate unpredictably.
- Manifestations of illness, even acute illness, tend to be obscure and less predictable in older adults than in younger adults. For example, an older adult with an infection is likely to experience cognitive changes rather than an elevated body temperature. One of the most common manifestations of illness or an adverse medication

effect in older adults is a change in level of functioning or cognitive status.

- For any one manifestation of illness in an older adult, there are usually at least three possible explanations. For example, changes in function usually are related to a combination of several of the following conditions: (1) acute illness, (2) psychosocial factors, (3) environmental conditions, (4) age-related changes, (5) a new chronic illness, (6) an existing chronic illness, or (7) an adverse effect of medication(s) or other treatments.
- Because of the difficulty in identifying the underlying cause of a change in health or functioning, the source of a problem is likely to go undetected while treatment is initiated incorrectly for the symptoms. This treatment often creates additional problems, which, in turn, continue to mask the underlying problem. This is particularly common and problematic when adverse medication effects are not recognized as such and are treated with additional medications that further contribute to the problem (discussed in detail in Chapter 8).
- Impaired cognitive or psychosocial function can make it difficult for an older adult to accurately report or describe a physiologic problem. For example, cognitive impairment can diminish the ability to describe symptoms accurately, and depression can cause people either to ignore or exaggerate symptoms of physical illness. In many cases, by the time illness in an older adult is detected and addressed, the underlying physiologic disturbance is in an advanced stage, and additional complications have developed.
- Myths and misunderstandings can lead health care providers, family members, or older adults to falsely attribute treatable conditions to aging. This can cloud the assessment process, as discussed in Chapter 2.

Because of all of these factors, nurses must take a detective-like approach to assessing older adults. This approach requires nurses to assess all aspects of the person's body, mind, and spirit to look for clues to underlying causes of changes in health or functioning. The Functional Consequences Model for Promoting Wellness in Older Adults is described in Chapter 2 and applied to specific aspects of functioning throughout this text. This framework enables nurses to assess older adults holistically in order to plan and implement nursing interventions to improve functioning and well-being.

Health care practitioners are increasingly using screening tools and easy-to-use assessment guides for identifying specific problems that affect health and functioning in older adults. Since the early 1990s, the Nurses Improving Care for Healthsystem Elders (NICHE) project of the John A. Hartford Foundation for Geriatric Nursing has been in the forefront of developing brief assessment guides for nurses to use in acute care settings. The first assessment guide, called SPICES, addressed the following target conditions: Skin impairment, Poor nutrition, Incontinence, Confusion, Evidence of falls or functional decline, and Sleep disorders (Fulmer, 1991). Recently, the SPICES tool has been modified and expanded to include target conditions of pain, safety, restraints, bowel elimination, and elder mistreatment (Guthrie et al., 2002; Lee & Fletcher, 2002; Pfaff, 2002). NICHE also developed a family assessment guide called FAMILY for assessment of the following: Family involvement, Assistance needed, Members' needs, Integration into care plan, Links to community support, and Your intervention (Salinas et al., 2002). These types of tools do not replace a more focused or comprehensive assessment, but are commonly used, especially in acute care settings, to identify specific areas to address in the care plan. The Hartford Institute for Geriatric Nursing periodically updates their recommended assessment guides and encourages the use of these "Best Practice" tools, which are available at www.hartfordign.org/resources/education/tryThis.html.

Wellness Opportunity

When assessing older adults, nurses try to identify the conditions that affect not only health status and level of functioning, but quality of life.

FUNCTIONAL ASSESSMENT

A functional assessment is a necessary component of a holistic assessment because identifying areas where function can be improved is an integral part of promoting wellness for older adults. **Functional assessment** refers to the measurement of a person's ability to fulfill responsibilities and perform self-care tasks. It is associated with a rehabilitation approach, rather than a medical diagnosis approach, because it emphasizes improved functioning in daily life. For example, a functional assessment for a person with hemiparesis due to a stroke focuses on the limitations and abilities of the person in carrying out his or her usual activities so a care plan can be developed to meet goals for improved functioning.

Development of the Functional Assessment Approach

The concept of functional assessment was first used in relation to workers' compensation. In the 1920s, the primary purpose of such an assessment was to measure the loss of function in work activity so a cash value could be assigned to an impairment (Frey, 1984). Initially, no standards were used, and the determination was based solely on a physician's opinion. In the 1940s, primarily as a result of World War II, the number of people with functional impairments increased dramatically; with this increase came a new emphasis on rehabilitation. Concomitantly, there was a surge of interest in functional assessment for rehabilitation. In 1954, the term **activities of daily living (ADLs)** was coined to refer to the ability to meet one's basic needs independently (Frey, 1984).

Beginning in the late 1950s, a few forward thinking gerontologists published articles about the interrelationships between ADLs, chronic disease, and older people (e.g., Benjamin Rose Institute, 1959; Katz et al., 1963). During the 1960s, researchers developed functional assessment instruments that would be applicable to older people in a number of situations. For example, Lawton and Brody (1969) developed a point-system scale to measure six ADL items (toileting, feeding, dressing, grooming, bathing, and ambulation), as well as more complex tasks that they identified as **instrumental activities of daily living (IADLs),** such as shopping and housekeeping. Another development during the 1960s was the broadening of the concept of functional assessment to assess person–environment interactions. This approach identifies the impact of environmental modifications and other rehabilitation interventions on the person's level of function.

Although researchers and planners first used functional assessment measures during the 1970s, it was not until the 1980s that gerontological practitioners began recognizing the clinical value of these assessment tools. This appreciation of the functional assessment approach was closely related to a growing recognition of the inadequacy of diagnostic labels for describing the health needs of people with chronic illnesses. In 1983, an article in the *Journal of the American Medical Association* stated that "the most important and distinguishing aspect of good health care for the elderly is the switch in emphasis away from dealing strictly with pathology and organ-specific disease [and] toward restoring the patient's resultant loss of function" (Kennie, 1983, p. 770). The same year, the National Institute on Aging convened a special conference on functional assessment and encouraged physicians to use a functional assessment tool along with their traditional, disease-oriented, diagnostic evaluations. The following year, geriatricians proposed a conceptual framework for a functional approach to the care of the elderly and emphasized the complex relationships among social, biologic, and psychological variables that influence functioning and well-being (Becker & Cohen, 1984). Moreover, the functional assessment approach emphasized that age-related, as well as disease-related, changes can interfere with functional status. Accordingly, the goal of health care interventions is to restore, maximize, and maintain a person's functional status and independence for as long as possible. In the late 1980s, the American College of Physicians and the American Geriatrics Society cited the importance of incorporating a functional assessment into routine clinical geriatrics as a major component of quality of life and as a critical component of appropriate health care.

Application of Functional Assessment in Practice Settings

In 1987, the Omnibus Budget Reconciliation Act (OBRA) mandated that all Medicaid- and Medicare-funded nursing homes begin using a standardized assessment form, which was developed by the Health Care Financing Administration. This form, known as the Minimum Data Set (MDS) for Resident Assessment and Care Screening, included a Resident Assessment Instrument (RAI). The purpose of the RAI was "to improve assessment of residents by identifying strengths, preferences, and functional abilities, and improve the care planning process so resident needs would be addressed better by nursing home staff" (Rantz et al., 1999, p. 36). The value of the MDS/RAI has been internationally recognized; it has been translated and validated in more than 15 countries (Yamada & Ikegami, 2001). In 1995, a second version of the MDS replaced the initial assessment tool; subsequent nursing research has supported the reliability and clinical utility of this version as well (Morris et al., 1997). Currently, the MDS is viewed as an essential source of data related to quality indicators such as falls, dehydration, weight loss, and restraint use (Rantz et al., 1999).

Because the use of the MDS/RAI as an assessment instrument has been successful in improving care in nursing homes, the federal government and accrediting organizations (e.g., the Joint Commission) have promoted the use of standardized functional assessment tools in all gerontological health care settings. For example, a home version of the MDS (MDS-HC) is currently used in Medicaid- and Medicare-funded home care agencies. Positive outcomes of programs that use the MDS-HC include fewer hospital readmissions and shorter lengths of stay (Landi et al., 2001). Currently, functional assessments are viewed as a core component of comprehensive health care for older adults.

Wellness Opportunity

Keep in mind that formal assessment tools fulfill requirements for documentation, but their primary purpose is to improve care and quality of life for older adults.

Tools for Functional Assessment

Functional assessment tools generally include a scale for measuring a person's level of independence in performing specific ADLs and IADLs. ADLs include activities that are essential to personal care, whereas IADLs comprise the more complex activities that are essential in community-living situations. The assessment of ADL performance is important in determining the level of assistance needed on a daily basis and is particularly helpful in planning long-term care for older adults. Likewise, an evaluation of IADLs is important in determining the level of assistance needed by people in independent or semi-independent settings. Functional assessment instruments measure changes that occur over time, identify factors that influence functional abilities, and provide a base for planning care. The functional assessment tool illustrated in Figure 7-1 was developed by nurses in a geriatric rehabilitation setting and can be used to measure a person's functional status at different times. An initial functional assessment can be done at the time of admission to provide information on which to base goals for care. The form also includes a column for information about the person's reported level of function before admission, which is helpful in determining the person's potential level of function. At the time of discharge, the reassessment information enables the staff to determine whether the goals were met. In settings in which postdischarge follow-up is possible, or in settings in which the person is readmitted at different times, the same assessment form is used to measure changes over time. Each category of activity is assigned a numeric value based on the criteria listed in Boxes 7-1 and 7-2. The numeric values are then used as a guide to measure progress toward goals as the person's level of function changes.

The functional assessment form in Figure 7-1 differs from many others in two ways. First, allowance is made for measurement of changes over time. The three time designations indicated on the form signify the period prior to admission (PTA), the time of admission (ADM), and the day of discharge (DISCH). The unmarked columns may be used at any time after discharge, or upon readmission. In a rehabilitative or long-term care setting, these measurements over time are particularly helpful in evaluating progress and reevaluating goals. Second, for each activity category, the number 1 rating is used to indicate that the person does not depend on others, but depends on some adaptive device or equipment for independent function in that area. The adaptive device might be as small as a shoehorn or as complex as an electric wheelchair. The importance of this designation is that the staff is then aware that the person has compensated for a deficit, but that the compensatory mechanism must be available for the person's use.

Nurses obtain information for the functional assessment from several sources. When older adults are able to provide reliable information about their level of function before admission, the nurse obtains data for the column marked "PTA" by interviewing the patient/resident within 24 hours of the admission to the care facility. When, as is often the case, older adults are not able to provide this information, the nurse interviews a family member or other person who is knowledgeable about the person's level of function before admission. Nurses directly observe the person's current level of function in performing ADLs to complete the columns marked "ADM" and "DISCH." In institutional settings, nurses must obtain much of the information on IADLs by questioning the older adult or his or her caregivers because many of these activities pertain only to community-based settings. The source of information is noted on the chart, and any discrepancies between objective and subjective information also are noted.

In interviewing the older adult or caregiver, it is important to ask for specific details about how tasks are accomplished, rather than ask open-ended questions such as "Do you have any difficulty with ...?" Also, it is important to find out whether the task is meaningful to the person, rather than assuming that the person wants or needs to do the task. For example, in the IADL categories, a person who lives with other people might never have to participate in grocery shopping or money management. Therefore, assessment information, particularly regarding IADLs, must be considered in relation to the person's support system and living arrangements.

Wellness Opportunity

Nurses identify factors that affect the older adult's quality of life by asking a question such as "Are there enjoyable activities that you used to do but are no longer able to do because of health problems?"

Assessment of Activities of Daily Living (ADLs)

The following areas of function are those generally considered in an assessment of ADLs: grooming, bathing, dressing, eating, elimination, and mobility. The assessment format illustrated in Figure 7-1 further specifies these activities as follows: bathing, dressing, mouth care, hair care, dietary intake, transfer mobility, ambulation, bed mobility, and bladder and bowel elimination. In addition, a brief mental status assessment is included on the ADL form. Including mental status in the functional assessment rather than using a separate mental status assessment tool reinforces the fact that cognitive function is an integral component of ADLs. In addition, it helps to determine whether ADL impairments are attributable, at least in part, to cognitive impairments, rather than primarily to physical limitations. See Box 7-1 for the functional assessment criteria for each of the ADLs, as well as for mental status.

Assessment of Instrumental Activities of Daily Living (IADLs)

IADLs are less important in institutional settings than they are in community settings. In institutional settings, however, an assessment of IADLs is an important consideration in discharge planning. When older adults cannot perform IADLs independently, caregivers often provide the assistance that enables the person to remain in a community setting. When older adults cannot perform IADLs and have no caregiver to help with the task, community resources often are available to meet these needs. Home-delivered meals programs, for example, might be appropriate for older adults who have difficulty with shopping or meal preparation. Community resources often can be arranged with one or two phone calls, and they can be effective and efficient ways of improving an older adult's ability to perform IADLs. See Box 7-2 for assessment criteria for the IADLs that are included in Figure 7-1.

Assessing the Effect of the Older Adult's Environment on Functioning

In addition to assessing the older adult's health and functioning, nurses need to be aware of environmental factors that may influence the person's functional abilities. Researchers and practitioners increasingly are addressing the interrelationship between people and their environments, and this is particularly pertinent to care of older adults. For example, the concept of **everyday competence** was used in the

		Date	PTA	ADM	DISCH		
Personal Care	*Bathing* 5 completely dependent 4 dependent with some assist 3 heavy partial 2 light partial 1 independent with devices 0 independent						
	Dressing 5 complete assist 3 partial assist 1 compensated 0 independent						
	Mouth care 5 totally unable to do 3 some assist 1 independent with device 0 independent						
	Hair care 5 completely unable 3 some assist 1 independent with device 0 independent						
	Dietary intake 5 total assist 4 assist with feeding 3 supplements 2 set up/encouragement 1 independent with device 0 independent						
Mobility	*Transfer* 5 completely unable 4 3-person/portalift 3 2-person 2 1-person 1 independent with devices 0 independent						
	Ambulation 5 completely unable 4 3-person assist 3 2-person assist 2 1-person assist 1 independent with devices 0 independent						
	Bed 5 unable to move in bed 3 needs assist 1 independent with device 0 independent						
Mental Status	*Mental* 5 totally impaired 4 assist with simple tasks 3 assist with complex tasks 2 inconsistent 1 compensated 0 no impairment						

FIGURE 7-1 Functional assessment of older adults. This form allows for recording changes over time. The three time designations indicated on the form signify the period prior to admission (PTA), the time of admission (ADM), and the day of discharge (DISCH). The unmarked columns may be used at any time after discharge, or upon readmission. (From Fairview General Hospital, Cleveland, OH. Used with permission.)

	Date	PTA	ADM	DISCH		
Elimination	*Bladder* 5 completely incontinent 3 occasionally incontinent 1 continent with assist/device 0 continent/independent					
	Bowel 5 completely incontinent 3 occasionally incontinent 1 continent with assist/device 0 continent/independent					
	Assist/device codes A bedside commode B bathroom C urinal D bedpan E ostomy F incontinence pads G catheter, external H catheter, indwelling I catheter, intermittent J verbal cuing/supervision K other ______					
Instrumental Activities of Daily Living	*Meal preparation* 5 unable to do 3 assist/supervise 1 independent with resources 0 independent					
	Shopping 5 unable to do 3 assist/supervise 1 compensated 0 independent					
	Telephone 5 unable to do/doesn't have 3 assist 1 independent with device 0 independent					
	Transportation 5 completely homebound 3 assist 1 arranges own 0 independent					
	Medications 5 unable to take 3 assist 1 independent 0 doesn't use					
	Housekeeping 5 unable to do 3 assist 1 independent with resources 0 independent					
	Laundry 5 unable to do 3 assist 1 independent with resources 0 independent					
	Money management 5 unable to handle 3 assist 1 independent with resources 0 independent					
	Total Points					

FIGURE 7-1 (continued)

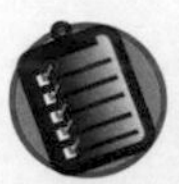

Box 7-1
Criteria for Assessing Activities of Daily Living (ADLs)

Bathing

5 Unable to assist in any way
4 Able to cooperate but cannot assist
3 Able to wash hands, face, and chest with supervision; needs help with completing the bath
2 Able to wash face, chest, arms, and upper legs; needs help with completing the bath
1 Bathes self but requires devices (e.g., long-handled sponge)
0 Bathes self independently

Dressing

5 Needs total assistance
4 Needs total supervision, but is able to dress self if clothing articles are given one at a time or set out in the order they are needed
3 Needs reminding and encouragement and some assistance with clothing selection, but can dress with little supervision
2 Dresses self, but needs help with activities requiring fine motor skills (e.g., zippers, shoelaces)
1 Dresses self using assistive devices (e.g., zipper pullers, long-handled shoehorn)
0 Dresses independently

Mouth Care

5 Cannot perform oral hygiene, but requires that it be done by others
4 Needs total supervision; needs toothpaste put on brush
3 Needs reminding and some supervision
2 Needs reminding but is otherwise independent
1 Performs oral hygiene using devices (e.g., toothbrush with built-up handle)
0 Performs oral hygiene independently

Hair Care

5 Cannot perform hair care, but requires that it be done by others
4 Needs total supervision
3 Needs some assistance with daily care
2 Performs daily care independently, but needs assistance with washing hair
1 Performs hair care using devices (e.g., hairbrush with built-up handle)
0 Performs all hair care (including washing) independently

Dietary Intake

5 Cannot prepare or obtain food; cannot feed self; nutritional requirements would not be met without total assistance
4 Needs assistance in obtaining and preparing food; needs total supervision with eating, but can feed self; nutritional requirements would not be met adequately without assistance
3 Needs assistance in tasks that involve complex skills (e.g., cutting meat, opening packages, preparing and obtaining food), but feeds self; nutritional needs would be met partially without assistance
2 Requires some assistance with obtaining and preparing food, but eats independently; would maintain adequate nutrition with encouragement or a little assistance
1 Needs assistive devices for food preparation and consumption (e.g., plate rings, rocker knife); adequately maintains nutritional requirements
0 Requires no assistance

Transfer Mobility

5 Cannot transfer, except with extreme difficulty
4 Needs assistance of three people for transfers, or needs two people and a lifting device
3 Needs the assistance of two people
2 Needs the assistance of one person
1 Transfers independently with a device (e.g., sliding board)
0 Transfers independently

Ambulation

5 Completely unable to walk
4 Walks with the assistance of three people
3 Walks with the assistance of two people
2 Walks with the assistance of one person
1 Walks independently with device (e.g., walker, quad cane)
0 Walks independently

Bed Mobility

5 Unable to move in bed
4 Needs the assistance of two people
3 Needs the assistance of one person
2 Needs to be encouraged and supervised
1 Moves indepedently with device (e.g., uses side rails or trapeze)
0 Moves independently in bed

Mental Status

5 Has extremely poor memory function; cannot follow directions; has minimal ability to identify and express needs; requires a totally structured environment
4 Has obvious memory impairment that interferes with daily life; has poor judgment and may undertake inappropriate actions; may be aware of the deficit and, consequently, may be anxious or depressed; can participate in daily routine but needs supervision; requires a strong orientation and reminder program
3 Fluctuates between levels two and four; unpredictable on a routine basis; requires monitoring and some supervision; may engage in risky behaviors at times
2 Minimal short-term memory loss; able to perform most daily tasks with only minimal reminding or supervision; has good to fair judgment and occasionally needs assistance, but does not engage in any risky behaviors
1 Is dependent on self-initiated reminders and cues for daily activities
0 No observable impairment in memory; no cognitive or psychosocial impairment that interferes with daily activities

Bladder and Bowel Elimination

5 Consistently soils self
4 Needs supervision and assistance on a regular basis
3 Needs reminding on a regular basis
2 Generally controls elimination; has accidents no more than once a week
1 Maintains control of elimination with devices (listed in Fig. 11-1)
0 Fully continent without any assistance

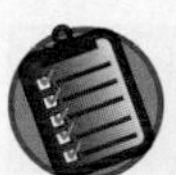

Box 7-2
Criteria for Assessing Instrumental Activities of Daily Living (IADLs)

Meal Preparation

5 Unable to prepare even simple meals
4 Can assist with meal preparation
3 Prepares meals, but cannot obtain groceries
2 Prepares meals with reminding or supervision
1 Prepares meals and obtains food using resources (e.g., specialized equipment, Meals on Wheels program, transportation to the grocery store)
0 Independent in obtaining and preparing food

Grocery Shopping

5 Cannot participate in shopping
4 Can accompany someone else and assist with food selection
3 Can shop and select appropriate food with some supervision
2 Can shop, but has difficulty obtaining transportation
1 Is able to arrange for necessary help with shopping
0 Shops independently

Telephone Use

5 Cannot dial or answer the phone, or carry on a routine phone conversation
4 Can talk on the phone, but cannot dial or answer it
3 Can use the phone with assistance (e.g., help in dialing)
2 Can use the phone with supervision
1 Depends on adaptive devices for telephone activities (e.g., automatic dialing system, speaker phone)
0 Independent in phone-related activities

Transportation

5 Does not leave home, even for medical care
4 Leaves home only for medical care or in rare circumstances
3 Needs assistance in arranging for transportation and needs special accommodations (e.g., wheelchair lift)
2 Needs assistance in arranging for transportation, but can get in and out of cars with little or no help
1 Arranges for own transportation, but depends on others for any transportation other than walking
0 Independent in traveling from one place to another (e.g., drives a car)

Medications

5 Unable to obtain or take medications without assistance or complete supervision
4 Cannot obtain medications, but can take them with assistance or supervision
3 Can obtain and take medications with reminders from others or with a system set up by others
2 Can obtain and take medications with a self-initiated reminder or set-up system
1 Safely takes and prepares all medications
0 Does not use medications

Housekeeping

5 Cannot perform any routine household tasks
4 Can assist with household tasks (e.g., bed making, dusting, vacuuming)
3 Can perform household tasks if supervised during the activity
2 Can perform household tasks if encouraged to do so
1 Arranges for housekeeping assistance
0 Is independent in all routine tasks

Laundry

5 Cannot perform any laundry tasks
4 Can assist with folding clothes; cannot wash or iron clothes
3 With assistance, can perform laundry tasks adequately
2 Can perform laundry tasks with supervision and reminding
1 Arranges for laundry to be done
0 Completes all laundry tasks independently

Money Management

5 Unable to manage any aspect of finances
4 Can handle simple cash transactions, but no other financial transactions (e.g., writing checks)
3 Can write checks with supervision or assistance; cannot handle any higher-level transactions (e.g., bank withdrawals)
2 Maintains checkbook, pays bills appropriately, and understands currency exchanges, but needs some assistance or supervision with these tasks
1 Arranges for someone else to handle financial matters
0 Handles all finances independently

late 1990s to describe the effects of cultural, physical, cognitive, emotional, social, and contextual factors on a person's daily functioning (Diehl, 1998). This is particularly important to consider when assessing older adults because these factors can appreciably hinder or improve functional abilities. For example, environmental factors that significantly affect hearing, vision, and mobility are discussed in Chapters 16, 17, and 22, respectively.

Wellness Opportunity

In addition to assessing conditions that affect functioning, nurses pay attention to environmental factors that affect quality of life.

Home assessments are essential not only for identifying fall risks (as discussed in Chapter 22), but also for addressing environmental factors that positively or negatively affect overall functioning. For example, proper lighting is essential for performing enjoyable activities such as reading, playing cards, and engaging in hobbies. Similarly, the ability to regulate the temperature is important not only as a safety consideration for preventing hypothermia and hyperthermia, but for comfort. Nurses can use Box 7-3 as a guide to assessing home environments for safety and optimal functioning.

During home visits it is especially important for nurses to respect autonomy and privacy and be nonjudgmental, and at the same time be able to identify all factors that affect the person's functioning and quality of life.

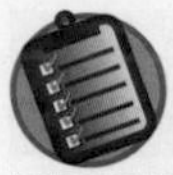

Box 7-3
Guidelines for Assessing the Safety of the Environment

Illumination and Color Contrast

- Is the lighting adequate but not glare producing?
- Are the light switches easy to reach and manipulate?
- Can lights be turned on before entering rooms?
- Are nightlights used in appropriate places?
- Is color contrast adequate between objects, such as a chair and the floor?

Hazards

- Are there highly polished floors, throw rugs, or other hazardous floor coverings?
- If area rugs are used, do they have a nonslip backing, and are the edges tacked to the floor?
- Are there cords, clutter, or other obstacles in pathways?
- Is there a pet that is likely to be running underfoot?

Furniture

- Are chairs the right height and depth for the person?
- Do the chairs have armrests? Are tables stable and of the appropriate height?
- Is small furniture placed well away from pathways?

Stairways

- Is lighting adequate?
- Are there light switches at the top and bottom of the stairs?
- Are there securely fastened handrails on both sides of the stairway?
- Are all the steps even?
- Are the treads nonskid?
- Should colored tape be used to mark the edges of the steps, particularly the top and bottom steps?

Bathroom

- Are grab bars placed appropriately for the tub and toilet?
- Does the tub have skid-proof strips or a rubber mat in the bottom?
- Has the person considered using a tub seat?
- Is the height of the toilet seat appropriate?
- Has the person considered using an elevated toilet seat?
- Does the color of the toilet seat contrast with surrounding colors?
- Is toilet paper within easy reach?

Bedroom

- Is the height of the bed appropriate?
- Is the mattress firm at the edges to provide enough support for sitting?
- If the bed has wheels, are they locked securely?
- Would full or partial side rails be a help or a hazard?
- When side rails are in the down position, are they completely out of the way?
- Is the pathway between the bedroom and bathroom clear of objects and adequately illuminated, particularly at night?
- Would a bedside commode be useful, especially at night?
- Is a light near the bed, and does the person have sufficient physical and cognitive ability to turn it on before getting out of bed?
- Is furniture positioned to allow safe use of assistive devices for ambulation?
- Is a telephone situated near the bed?

Kitchen

- Are storage areas used to the best advantage (e.g., are objects that are frequently used in the most accessible places)?
- Are appliance cords kept out of the way?
- Are nonslip mats used in front of the sink?
- Are the markings on stoves and other appliances clearly visible?
- Does the person know how to use the microwave safely?

Assistive Devices

- Is a call light available, and does the person know how to use it?
- What assistive devices are used?
- Would the person benefit from any assistive devices that are not being used?
- Are assistive devices being used safely and properly, or do they present additional hazards?

Temperature

- Is the temperature of the room(s) comfortable?
- Can the person read the markings on the thermostat and adjust it appropriately?
- During cold months, is the room temperature high enough to prevent hypothermia?
- During hot weather, is the room temperature cool enough to prevent hyperthermia?

Overall Safety

- How does the person obtain objects from hard-to-reach places?
- How does the person change overhead light bulbs?
- Are doorways wide enough to accommodate assistive devices?
- Do door thresholds create hazardous conditions?
- Are telephones accessible, especially for emergency calls? Would it be helpful to use a cordless portable phone?
- Would it be helpful to have some emergency call system available?
- Does the person wear sturdy shoes with nonskid soles?
- Does the person keep a list of emergency numbers by the phone?
- Does the person have an emergency exit plan in the event of fire?
- Are smoke alarms present and operational?
- Is there a carbon monoxide detector in an appropriate place (if the house has gas appliances, wood burning stoves, or another object that produces carbon monoxide)?

Assessing the Use or Potential Use of Adaptive and Assistive Devices

The actual or potential use of items such as mobility aids (e.g., canes, walkers, wheelchairs) and adaptive equipment (e.g., grab bars) also should be assessed as factors that can significantly affect everyday competence (Allen et al., 2001). Physical, occupational, and rehabilitation therapists are skilled in assessing for the use of these aids, but nurses need to be familiar with the array of adaptive and assistive devices so they can facilitate referrals for further evaluation. Nurses also can identify problems related to the use of assistive devices and request further evaluation by a qualified therapist. This is especially important with regard to wheelchairs because improper fit leads to specific problems such as those summarized in Table 7-1. In addition, improper wheelchair fit is likely to cause pain, fatigue, discomfort, agitation, and decreased tolerance for using a wheelchair (Rader et al., 2000).

Diversity Note

In a study of over 7000 older adults with impaired mobility, African Americans (21%) were more likely to use mobility devices than Hispanics (14%) and whites (13%) (Resnik & Allen, 2006).

Assessing the Effect of the Older Adult's Cognitive Abilities on Function

Another significant factor that can affect an older adult's function is his or her cognitive status. The influence of cognitive abilities on function is a specific aspect of assessment addressed in the gerontological literature (Njegovan et al., 2001; Tabbarah et al., 2002). For example, some functional assessment scales apply specifically to people with dementia in a variety of settings and at all levels of cognitive impairment and address the interplay between cognition and abilities to perform ADLs. One such scale that has been used since the early 1990s, the Cleveland Scale for Activities of Daily Living (CSADL), divides ADLs into smaller components that may be affected by the underlying cognitive impairment (Patterson et al., 1992). Because this scale is designed to evaluate the effect of dementia on the ability to perform ADLs, the items focus on potential effects of cognitive deficits (Patterson & Mack, 2001). Studies have found that this instrument, illustrated in Figure 7-2, is reliable and valid as a measurement of functional deficits in people with Alzheimer's disease (Patterson & Mack, 2001). The Alzheimer's Disease Activities of Daily Living International Scale (ADL-IS) was developed to fulfill the need for an ADL scale that is "useful for the earliest stages of AD, and which is simultaneously non-gender-biased and cross-nationally relevant" (Reisberg et al., 2001). The ADL-IS assesses 40 items divided into the following categories: conversation, recreation, self-care, household activities, general activities, medication, social functioning, telephone, reading, organization, food preparation, travel, and driving.

Wellness Opportunity

When assessing the impact of cognitive abilities on functioning, nurses can try to identify simple interventions, like putting labels on drawers, that can improve the person's self-esteem by promoting independence.

ASSESSING AND ADDRESSING DRIVING SAFETY

The ability to drive a vehicle safely is an aspect of daily living that merits special consideration when assessing the

TABLE 7-1 Negative Effects of Improper Wheelchair Fit

Seating Problem	Result on Body	Potential Effect
Wheelchair too high	Feet do not touch the floor Unable to self-propel Pelvis moves forward	Edema and decreased circulation in legs Decreased activity Poor sitting posture
Poor back support	Compression of trunk, chest, abdomen Sliding out of chair Increased pelvic tilt	Skin breakdown on back and sacrum Impaired gastrointestinal and respiratory function
Wheelchair too heavy	Difficulty moving chair	Decreased activity
Wheelchair too wide	Pelvic shifting laterally Forward leaning Difficulty using hand rims	Shear stress on skin Poor posture, circulation Decreased mobility
Seat not firm enough ("sling" effect)	Scoliosis Sliding out of chair	Poor posture, circulation Shear stress on skin
Footrest too high	Poor femoral support Unequal pressure distribution Increased ischial tuberosity	Poor posture Skin breakdown

From Rader, J., Jones, D., & Miller, L. (2000). The importance of individualized wheelchair seating for frail older adults. *Journal of Gerontological Nursing, 26*(11), 24–31.

CLEVELAND SCALE FOR ACTIVITIES OF DAILY LIVING (CSADL)

Name or ID of Subject ____________ Date __ __/__ __/__ __ (mm dd yy) Rater ________

Name of Informant ____________

Relation of Informant to Subject (*Circle one.*)		Contact with Subject	Interview Type
1 Spouse	4 Friend or other family	1 2 days/week	1 Visit
2 Child	5 Professional: ________	2 3-4 days/week	2 Telephone
3 Sibling	6 Other: ________	3 5 or more days/week	

To administer this scale, the rater must be thoroughly familiar with the Manual, which includes the full instructions. Place rating in blank after each item number. Several items have specific rating instructions. In particular, some require special questioning if the subject is rated as dependent (rating of 1, 2, or 3).

Rating	***Meaning of Rating***
0	**Never Dependent.** [S] does this effectively, quite independently, without any direction or help.
1	**Sometimes Dependent.** [S] usually does this independently, but sometimes or in some situations [S] needs direction or help.
2	**Usually Dependent.** [S] usually requires some direction or help, but sometimes or in some situations [S] does it independently.
3	**Always Dependent.** [S] always requires direction or help. [S] never does it independently.
9	Cannot rate because of insufficient information

Bathing

1. ____ Initiates bath or shower with appropriate frequency and at appropriate times
2. ____ Prepares bath/shower (draws water of proper temperature, ensures soap and towel are present, etc.)
3. ____ Gets in and out of tub or shower
4. ____ Cleans self

Toileting

5. ____ Able to physically control timing of urination
6. ____ Able to physically control timing of bowel movements
7. ____ Recognizes need to eliminate
8. ____ After toileting, cleans and re-clothes self appropriately

Personal Hygiene and Appearance

9. ____ Initiates personal grooming with appropriate frequency and at appropriate times
10. ____ Washes hands and face
11. ____ Brushes teeth
12. ____ Combs hair, shaves (as appropriate)

FIGURE 7-2 The Cleveland Scale for Activities of Daily Living (CSADL). This functional assessment form was specifically designed for use with people with Alzheimer's disease. (Used with permission from the University Memory and Aging Center, Case Western Reserve University, Cleveland, OH. Copyright 1994.)

Dressing

13. ____ Initiates dressing at appropriate time

14. ____ Selects clothes

15. ____ Puts on garments, footwear, etc.

16. ____ Fastens clothing (buttons, shoelaces, zippers, etc.)

Eating

17. ____ Initiates eating at appropriate times of day and with appropriate frequency

18. ____ Carries out physical acts of eating (including using utensils)

19. ____ Eats with acceptable manners, e.g. with appropriate speed, does not speak with food in mouth, etc.

20. ____ Prepares own meals (includes cooking on stove). *This item requires special questioning.*

Mobility

21. ____ Initiates actively moving about the environment, as opposed to sitting, not attempting to get about, etc.

22. ____ Actively moves about environment (with or without assisting device)

22a. Does subject have physical limitations of mobility? *(Circle one of following codes.)*

0 No physical limitations of mobility

1 Yes, there are physical limitations of mobility. *(Circle all that apply.)*

Needs assistance of other persons to walk	Trouble getting in or out of bed	Other Mobility Problems
Needs cane	Trouble getting in or out of chair	*(describe):*
Needs walker	Trouble getting on or off toilet	
Needs wheelchair	Trouble climbing or descending stairs	

Medications

23. ____ Takes medications as scheduled and in correct dosages. *If subject has taken no medications during prior year, rate item as 9. This item requires questioning.*

Shopping

24. ____ Does necessary grocery shopping, buying appropriate items and quantities. *This item requires special questioning.*

25. ____ Does necessary clothes shopping, buying appropriate items and quantities. *This item requires special questioning.*

Travel

26. ____ Finds way about in familiar surroundings

27. ____ Orients to unfamiliar surroundings without undue difficulty

28. ____ Travels beyond walking distance (i.e., driving own vehicle or using public transportation)

29. ____ Drives motor vehicle. *This item requires special questioning.*

FIGURE 7-2 (continued)

Hobbies, personal interests, employment

30. ____ Initiates activities of personal interest (e.g. card playing, woodworking, others). *This item requires special questioning.*

31. ____ Carries out such activities. *This item requires special questioning.*

32. ____ Does subject work for pay? *If subject does not work because of having reached an age appropriate to retirement from his or her occupation, rate 9. This item requires special questioning.*

Housework/home maintenance (as appropriate to individual situation)

33. ____ Initiates work around house as needed. *This item requires special questioning.*

34. ____ Carries out work effectively, e.g. cleanly, neatly, accurately, efficiently. *This item requires special questioning.*

Types of work done (*Don't score, just circle*)

Dish washing	Vacuuming	Mowing lawn
Sweeping	Scrubbing floors	Gardening
Personal laundry	Small home repairs	Minor car care

Other types of work (*Describe*):

Telephone

35. ____ Looks up numbers

36. ____ Dials numbers

37. ____ Answers phone

38. ____ Takes messages

Money Management

39. ____ Pays for purchases (selecting appropriate amount and determining correct change). *This item requires special questioning.*

40. ____ Manages financial responsibilities beyond paying for immediate purchases (e.g., paying monthly bills, managing checking or savings account, etc.). *This item requires special questioning.*

Communication Skills

41. ____ Spontaneously expresses thoughts and needs to others

42. ____ Responds accurately to spoken instructions and conversation

43. ____ Reads and understands single words and short phrases (signs, lists, etc.)

44. ____ Reads and understands complex material (books, newspapers, etc.)

45. ____ Writes short phrases (lists, brief messages)

46. ____ Writes complex material (letters, diary, etc.)

FIGURE 7-2 (continued)

Social Behavior

47. ____ Behaves in a socially appropriate manner. Socially inappropriate behaviors encompass a **wide** range of behavior, including but not limited to such things as making rude remarks, belching, touching private parts, showing little regard for personal privacy, etc. For this item, dependency refers to the extent to which other people must direct or manage the subject to ensure that he or she behaves in a socially appropriate fashion.

Other Problems — Are there any situations in which patient does not behave in an independent and responsible fashion that have not been covered by these questions? (*Circle one of following codes.*)

48. 0 No other dependent behaviors

1 Yes, there are other dependent behaviors. (*Please provide details below.*)

QUALITY OF INTERVIEW (Rater's Judgment)

Interview appeared valid	0
Some questions about interview, but it is probably acceptable	1
Information from interview is of doubtful validity	2

Rater should record the basis for judging the interview of questionable or doubtful validity.

Comments:

FIGURE 7-2 (continued)

older adult. Driving at an advanced age is a major focus of attention, not only for health care providers but for all members of society. Commentaries and news articles frequently address issues about people who continue to drive when they are in their 80s and 90s. Regardless of age, most driving-related problems arise from chronic conditions that affect cognitive abilities or neurologic or musculoskeletal function. However, even healthy older adults need to compensate for age-related changes in vision and other areas of function that affect driving, as discussed in Chapter 17.

Older drivers who recognize changes in their abilities commonly adjust their driving behaviors in the following ways (Klavora & Heslegrave, 2002; Messinger-Rapport, 2003; Ruechel & Mann, 2005):

- Driving shorter distances
- Driving more slowly
- Avoiding driving at night
- Not driving in rain or inclement conditions
- Not driving on freeways or interstate highways
- Avoiding driving in congested areas
- Not driving during rush hours
- Receiving navigation assistance from a passenger

When older drivers adjust their driving patterns, they often view these restrictions as the beginning of a process of driving cessation with subsequent loss of independence and quality of life (Ruechel & Mann, 2005). Decisions about driving are very complex because they are associated with many psychosocial implications, as discussed in Chapter 12.

Increasingly, nurses are among the health care professionals responsible for addressing concerns about driving, not only as a personal safety issue for older adults but as a moral obligation to protect society. As with other aspects of functioning, nurses are responsible for identifying potential risk factors for unsafe driving. Moreover, nurses need to be knowledgeable about resources for assessing and addressing this risk. Because decisions about driving are multidimensional, nurses work closely with other care providers, such as physicians and social workers, to address this important issue from a broad perspective. Thus, health care providers facilitate referrals not only for assessments of driving but for interventions that help people retain safe driving skills as long as possible.

Wellness Opportunity

Nurses can sensitively address issues about driving by expressing compassionate concern not only for the individual older adult but for the safety of others.

Identifying Risks

When motor vehicle accident rates are adjusted for miles driven, older drivers (age 65 years and older) represent a crash risk equivalent to that of younger drivers (age 25 years and younger), with these two groups accounting for the highest rate of fatalities. Increased age and number of miles driven are the two most consistently identified risk factors, but other factors associated with an increased risk for motor vehicle accidents among older adults include stroke, dementia, visual impairment, and use of certain medications (Margolis et al., 2002). Analyses have found that accidents involving older adults are associated with low speeds, involve multiple vehicles, and occur at intersections during the day and close to home (Messinger-Rapport, 2003; Ruechel & Mann, 2005). Conditions that contribute to the increased fatality rates for older adults in accidents include decreased bone density, an increased potential for sepsis and multiorgan failure, and increased morbidity and mortality from head injuries (Messinger-Rapport, 2003).

Health care providers are responsible for inquiring about changes that can affect driving skills, such as medical conditions, functional limitations, medication use, alcohol consumption, and changes in habits or personality. In addition, they are responsible for identifying risk factors for unsafe driving when they perform physical, functional, or mental status assessments. Age-related and disease-related changes in visual abilities, cognitive abilities, musculoskeletal function, and central nervous system function can affect the older adult's ability to drive safely. Even healthy older adults are likely to experience the following conditions that can affect driving safety (Mann et al., 2005; Messinger-Rapport, 2003, p. 18):

- Diminished field of vision
- Difficulty switching attention between tasks
- Limited range of motion affecting the trunk, neck, and extremities
- Slower motor response
- Delayed reaction time

As with all age groups, health care providers can inquire about any recent history of vehicular accidents, legal actions related to unsafe driving, or driving under the influence. Key behavioral indicators for unsafe driving that have been identified by experts include the following (Perkinson et al., 2005):

- Getting lost
- Driving at an inappropriate speed
- Reacting too slowly
- Failing to notice street signs
- Having more accidents
- Receiving indecent gestures from other drivers
- Miscalculating speed or distances
- Running into a building
- Knocking off side-view mirrors
- Showing poor judgment
- Being confused
- Having difficulty focusing attention

Health care professionals assess for risks by asking the older adult about these behavioral indicators as part of the usual assessment process. When appropriate, nurses also obtain information from family members who are likely to have observations and concerns.

Wellness Opportunity

Nurses promote personal responsibility by assessing the older adult's awareness of driving issues and their willingness to consider addressing these concerns.

Addressing Risk Factors

When risks are identified, nurses also try to identify contributing factors that can be addressed through appropriate interventions. For example, when vision impairments affect driving, older adults may benefit from a referral to ophthalmology, as discussed in Chapter 17. Similarly, because hearing impairments can affect safety while driving, nurses can discuss the importance of interventions to improve hearing, as discussed in Chapter 16.

Another approach to improving driving safety for some older adults is to address medication-related issues when these are likely to have a negative impact on driving. When adverse effects of medications affect safe driving, nurses can encourage older adults to discuss this with the prescribing practitioner to explore options. For example, it may be possible to adjust dosing of medications to minimize their effects on driving. Even over-the-counter products like diphenhydramine may have significant adverse effects on psychomotor skills needed for safe driving (Verster & Volkerts, 2004; Vuurman et al., 2004). Many states include diphenhydramine and other over-the-counter agents in laws pertaining to driving while impaired. Studies have found adverse effects of diphenhydramine on mood, speed, attention, vigilance, working memory, and level of activity. These effects may persist through the next day after an evening dose (Kay, 2000).

When pathologic conditions affect neuromuscular functioning, nurses may suggest a referral for physical or occupational therapy to improve particular aspects of functioning that affect driving. For example, an older person with arthritis or Parkinson's disease may benefit from working with a therapist who has additional training for driving rehabilitation. Even if the therapist does not have special training, the older adult can focus on the goal of improved safety and functioning for driving skills as part of the therapy program. Older adults may be more motivated to participate in exercises prescribed by physical or occupational therapists if they see a connection between the therapies and maintaining safe and independent functioning.

Wellness Opportunity

Nurses can promote quality of life for older adults by creatively identifying appropriate and acceptable ways of improving an older adult's ability to continue driving safety.

When nurses identify safety risks, they must assess the older adult's awareness and degree of cooperation for further assessment. If older adults self-restrict their driving to eliminate safety risks, health care professionals need to reassess the situation periodically. However, when any significant risks are identified, a referral to occupational therapy may be necessary for further evaluation and possible interventions. When medically warranted, these referrals are covered by Medicare and other health insurance plans. When suggesting this kind of referral, nurses can emphasize that the purpose is not to take away the person's driving privileges but rather to identify interventions to improve safety for the person and others. Recommendations fall within a wide range and may include having no or few driving restrictions, adding adaptive devices to the vehicle, participating in driving rehabilitation therapy, or refraining from driving.

Nurses need to be familiar with the range of programs for driving safety, education, and rehabilitation to facilitate referrals. Driving evaluation programs, which usually are administered by occupational therapy departments, provide appropriate follow-up when the person can benefit from education and rehabilitation. One function of driver rehabilitation programs is to assess the need for and provide education about adaptive driving equipment, such as the following (McCarthy, 2005):

- Pedal extenders
- Left foot accelerators
- Spinner knobs to assist with steering
- Adaptations to steering wheels
- Spot mirrors to compensate for visual and range-of-motion deficit
- In-vehicle controls to alert the driver about corrective actions that need to be initiated
- Units that take control of the vehicle
- Devices that detect the driver's level of alertness
- Intelligent cruise control that warns drivers or takes control of acceleration and braking
- Radar monitoring of other cars during lane changes
- Distance sensors for facilitating parking and backing up
- Touch pads to operate secondary controls (e.g., heating, headlights)

Adaptive equipment and driving rehabilitation can effectively improve safety for people who have the cognitive abilities to learn new driving behaviors. Unfortunately, these interventions are of little or no help in improving safe driving for people with impaired cognition.

Driving education programs are available through organizations such as AARP (Mature Driving Program) and the American Automobile Association (Safe Driving for Mature Operators). Numerous Internet resources provide excellent information about driving assessments and interventions to improve driving safety for older adults. Some of the resources that are most relevant to nurses are listed in the Educational Resources section of this chapter.

Chapter Highlights

General Approach to Assessing the Older Adult's Health and Functioning

- Assessment of older adults is a multidimensional process addressing the complex interactions among older adults, their health, and all contextual factors (e.g., culture, environments, medical conditions, adverse medication effects).
- Factors that contribute to the complexity of assessing older adults include unique manifestations of illness, multiple possible causes for changes in health, treatment for symptoms that may not be appropriate for the undetected underlying cause, potential for impaired cognitive or psychosocial function to interfere with the older adult's reporting of symptoms, and misunderstandings that may falsely attribute treatable conditions to aging.

Functional Assessment

- A functional assessment is a formal process of measuring a person's ability to fulfill responsibilities and perform self-care tasks.
- Functional assessment tools focus on the person's ability to perform ADLs and IADLs, as illustrated in Figure 7-1 and Boxes 7-1 and 7-2.
- Assessment of the home environment is important for identifying factors that affect safety, comfort, functioning, and quality of life (Box 7-3).

- Assessing the use of adaptive equipment and assistive devices is important for identifying factors that affect safety, comfort, and functioning (Table 7-1).
- Some assessment tools address the effect of cognitive impairment on ability to perform activities of daily living (Fig. 7-2).

Assessing and Addressing Driving Safety

- Nurses have an important role in identifying risk factors that compromise safe driving in older adults.
- Common risk factors include any chronic condition that affects cognition or functional abilities (e.g., dementia, Parkinson's disease, mobility limitations).
- Nurses address risk factors by facilitating referrals for further evaluation or for programs related to driving safety, education, and rehabilitation.

Critical Thinking Exercises

1. Identify an older adult who has some functional impairment but no cognitive impairment and perform a functional assessment on him or her, using Figure 7-1.
2. Identify another older adult (in a clinical setting or someone you know personally) who has some functional impairment as well as some cognitive impairment and perform a functional assessment on him or her, using Figure 7-2.
3. Identify an older adult in your personal life or a clinical setting who has risk factors that affect his or her driving safety; then explore one or more of the educational resources to find information applicable to addressing concerns about safe driving for this person.

Clinical Tool Resources

Hartford Institute for Geriatric Nursing
Try This: Best Practices in Nursing Care to Older Adults
Issue Number 1 (Revised 2007), SPICES: An Overall Assessment Tool of Older Adults
Issue Number 2 (Revised 2007), Katz Index of Independence in Activities of Daily Living (ADL)
Issue Number 23 (Revised 2007), The Lawton Instrumental Activities of Daily Living (IADL) Scale
www.hartfordign.org/resources/education/tryThis.html

Educational Resources

American Automobile Association (AAA)
Roadwise Review: A Tool to Help Seniors Drive Safely Longer (interactive CD-ROM for self-testing of skills that affect safe driving)
Car Fit brochure to assess how well a car "fits" a driver
Safe Driving for the Mature Operator (classes)
www.aaapublicaffairs.com

AARP (American Association of Retired Persons)
Information about when to stop driving, helping someone else stop or limit driving, links to other organizations
"55 Alive" (classes for older adults about driving)
www.aarp.org

American Medical Association
Patient resources on safe driving and helping older drivers
Physician's Guide to Assessing and Counseling Older Drivers (free resource with comprehensive information about assessing driver safety, resources for driver evaluation and rehabilitation, state laws regarding reporting requirements)
www.ama-assn.org

Driving Safely While Aging Gracefully
Information developed by the National Highway Traffic Safety Administration about aging and safe driving
www.nhtsa.dot.gov

Grand Driver
Advice about safe driving practices for older adults
Public service information and a speaker's bureau
www.granddriver.info

Hartford: Family Conversations With Older Drivers
Information provided by the Hartford Financial Services Group and the Massachusetts Institute of Technology (MIT) to help families talk with older adults about driving safety
Information about additional resources
www.thehartford.com/talkwitholderdrivers

Safe and Reliable Mobility Equipment
National Mobility Equipment Dealers Association (NMEDA)
Guidelines and regulations related to vehicle modifications
www.nmeda.org

Senior Drivers
Numerous reports and resources for consumers, providers, and researchers on aging and driving
Links to other organizations and resources
www.seniordrivers.org

References

Allen, S. M., Foster, A., & Berg, K. (2001). Receiving help at home: The interplay of human and technological assistance. *Journals of Gerontology: Series B, Psychological Sciences and Social Sciences, 56*, S374–S382.

Becker, P. M., & Cohen, H. J. (1984). The functional approach to the care of the elderly: A conceptual framework. *Journal of the American Geriatrics Society, 32*, 923–929.

Benjamin Rose Institute. (1959). Multidisciplinary studies of illness in aged persons: II. A new classification of functional status in activities of daily living. *Journal of Chronic Disease, 9*, 55–62.

Diehl, M. (1998). Everyday competence in later life: Current status and future directions. *The Gerontologist, 38*, 422–433.

Frey, W. D. (1984). Functional assessment in the '80s: A conceptual enigma, a technical challenge. In A. S. Halpern & J. J. Fuhrer (Eds.), *Functional assessment in rehabilitation* (pp. 11–43). Baltimore: Paul H. Brookes.

Fulmer, T. T. (1991). The geriatric nurse specialist role: A new model. *Nursing Management, 22*, 91–93.

Guthrie, P. F., Edinger, G., & Schumacher, S. (2002). A NICHE Program at North Memorial Health Care. *Geriatric Nursing, 23*, 133–138.

Katz, S., Ford, A. B., Moskowitz, R. W., Jackson, B. A., & Jaffee, M. W. (1963). Studies of illness in the aged: The index of ADL, a standardized measure of biological and psychosocial function. *Journal of the American Medical Association, 185*, 914–919.

Kay, G. G. (2000). The effects of antihistamines on cognition and performance. *Journal of Allergy and Clinical Immunology, 105*, 622–627.

Kennie, D. C. (1983). Good health care for the aged. *Journal of the American Medical Association, 249*, 770–773.

Klavora, P., & Heslegrave, R. J. (2002). Senior drivers: An overview of problems and intervention strategies. *Journal of Aging and Physical Activity, 10*, 322–335.

Landi, F., Onder, G., Tua, E., Carrara, B., Zuccala, Gambassi, G., et al. (2001). Impact of a new assessment system, the MDS-HC on function and hospitalization of homebound older people: A controlled clinical trial. *Journal of the American Geriatrics Society, 49*, 1288–1293.

Lawton, M. P., & Brody, E. M. (1969). Assessment of older people: Self-maintaining and instrumental activities of daily living. *The Gerontologist, 9*, 179–186.

Lee, V. K., & Fletcher, K. R. (2002). Sustaining the geriatric resource nurse model at the University of Virginia. *Geriatric Nursing, 23*, 128–132.

Mann, W. C., McCarthy, D. P., Wu, S. S., & Tomita, M. (2005). Relationship of health status, functional status, and psychosocial status to driving among elderly with disabilities. *Physical and Occupational Therapy in Geriatrics, 23*(2/3), 1–24.

Margolis, K. L., Kerani, R. P., McGovern, P., Songer, T., Cauley, J. A., & Ensrud, K. E. (2002). Risk factors for motor vehicle crashes in older women. *Journals of Gerontology: Series A, Biological Sciences and Medical Sciences, 57*, M186–M191.

McCarthy, D. P. (2005). Approaches to improving elders' safe driving abilities. *Physical and Occupational Therapy in Geriatrics, 23*(2/3), 25–42.

Messinger-Rapport, B. J. (2003). Assessment and counseling of older drivers: A guide for primary care physicians. *Geriatrics, 58*(12), 16–24.

Morris, J. N., Nonemaker, S., Murphy, K., Hawes, C., Fries, B. E., Mor, V., et al. (1997). A commitment to change: Revision of HCFA's RAI. *Journal of the American Geriatrics Society, 45*, 1011–1016.

Njegovan, V., Man-Son-Hing, M., Mitchell, S. L., & Molnar, F. J. (2001). The hierarchy of functional loss associated with cognitive decline in older persons. *Journals of Gerontology: Series A, Biological Sciences and Medical Sciences, 56*, M638–M643.

Patterson, M. B., & Mack, J. L. (2001). The Cleveland Scale for Activities of Daily Living (CSADL): Its reliability and validity. *Journal of Clinical Gerospychology, 7*(1), 15–28.

Patterson, M. B., Mack, J. L., Neundorfer, M., Martin, R. J., Smyth, K. A., & Whitehouse, P. J. (1992). Assessment of functional ability in Alzheimer's disease: A review and a preliminary report on the Cleveland Scale for Activities of Daily Living. *Alzheimer Disease and Associated Disorders, 6*, 145–163.

Perkinson, M. A., Berg-Weger, M. L., Carr, D. B., Meuser, T. M., & Palmer, J. L. (2005). Driving and dementia of the Alzheimer type: Beliefs and cessation strategies among stakeholders. *The Gerontologist, 45*, 676–685.

Pfaff, J. (2002). The geriatric resource nurse model: A culture change. *Geriatric Nursing, 23*, 140–144.

Rader, J., Jones, D., & Miller, L. (2000). The importance of individualized wheelchair seating for frail older adults. *Journal of Gerontological Nursing, 26*(11), 24–31.

Rantz, M., Popejoy, L., Zwygart-Stauffacher, M., Wipke-Tevis, D., & Grando, V. T. (1999). Minimum Data Set and Resident Assessment Instrument: Can using standardized assessment improve clinical practice and outcomes of care? *Journal of Gerontological Nursing, 25*(6), 35–43.

Reisberg, B., Finkel, S., Overall, J., Schmidt-Gollas, N., Kanowski, S., Lehfeld, H., et al. (2001). The Alzheimer's Disease Activities of Daily Living International Scale (ADL-IS). *International Psychogeriatrics, 13*, 163–181.

Resnik, L., & Allen, S. (2006). Racial and ethnic differences in use of assistive devices for mobility. *Journal of Aging and Health, 18*(1), 106–124.

Ruechel, S., & Mann, W. C. (2005). Self-regulation of driving by older persons. *Physical and Occupational Therapy in Geriatrics, 23*(2/3), 99–101.

Salinas, T. K., O'Connor, L. J., Weinstein, M., Lee, S. Y. V., & Fitzpatrick, J. J. (2002). A family assessment tool for hospitalized elders. *Geriatric Nursing, 23*, 316–319, 335.

Tabbarah, M., Crimmins, E. M., & Seeman, T. E. (2002). The relationship between cognitive and physical performance: MacArthur Studies of Successful Aging. *Journals of Gerontology: Series A, Biological Sciences and Medical Sciences, 57*, M228–M235.

Verster, J. C., & Volkerts, E. R. (2004). Antihistamines and driving ability: Evidence from on-the-road driving studies during normal traffic. *Annals of Allergy, 92*, 294–303.

Vuurman, E. F., Rikken G. H., Muntjewerff, N. D., de Halleux, F., & Ramaekers, J. G. (2004). Effects of desloratadine, diphenhydramine, and placebo on driving performance and psychomotor performance measurements. *European Journal of Clinical Pharmacology, 60*, 307–313.

Yamada, Y., & Ikegami, N. (2001). Multidimensional functional assessment: Instruments. In M. D. Mezey (Ed.), *The encyclopedia of elder care* (pp. 440–442). New York: Springer.

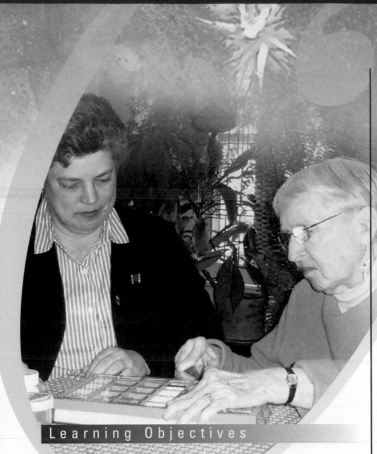

CHAPTER 8

Medications and Other Bioactive Substances

Learning Objectives

After reading this chapter, you will be able to:

1. Discuss considerations about herbs and homeopathic remedies that are pertinent to the care of older adults.
2. Examine age-related changes and risk factors that affect the action of bioactive substances in the body and the skills involved with taking them.
3. Describe interactions that can occur between medications and medications, herbs, or other bioactive substances.
4. Identify the adverse effects that are likely to occur in older adults because of age-related changes and risk factors.
5. Describe the purposes of a medication assessment and the relationship between the medication assessment and the overall assessment of older adults.
6. Describe observations and interview questions that nurses can use for a comprehensive medication assessment.
7. Identify interventions directed toward enhancing the therapeutic effectiveness of medications, reducing the risks for adverse effects, and minimizing the negative functional consequences of these effects.

Key Terms

adverse medication effects
Beers criteria
clearance rate
elimination half-time
herbs
inappropriate medications
Medicare Part D
medication nonadherence
nutrient
pharmacodynamics
pharmacokinetics
polypharmacy
prescribing cascade
prescription assistance programs
serum anticholinergic activity
tardive dyskinesia
total anticholinergic burden

INTRODUCTION TO BIOACTIVE SUBSTANCES

Although the topic of bioactive substances and the older adult is not a distinct category of function in the same sense as physiologic and psychosocial aspects (e.g., vision and cognition), it can be addressed from a similar perspective. Thus, this chapter presents information about age-related changes, risk factors, and functional consequences related to bioactive substances and the behaviors associated with taking them relative to older adults. As with other chapters, it

Promoting Safe and Effective Medication Use in Older Adults

Nursing Assessment
• Medication-taking patterns
• Use of all bioactive substances (herbs, vitamins, minerals)
• Barriers to adherence
• Cultural considerations
• Therapeutic and adverse medication effects
Age-Related Changes
• ↓ body water
• ↓ lean tissue
• ↑ body fat
• ↓ serum albumin
• ↓ liver and renal function
• Altered receptor sensitivity
Negative Functional Consequences
• Less predictable therapeutic effects
• ↑ risk for adverse effects
• ↑ risk for interactions
Risk Factors
• Pathologic processes
• Functional impairments
• Polypharmacy
• Inadequate monitoring
• Financial barriers
• Insufficient recognition of adverse effects
Nursing Interventions
• Teaching about safe and effective medications
• Teaching about herbs and other bioactive substances
• Decreasing the number of medications
Wellness Outcomes
• Improved safety and effectiveness of medications
• Prevention or alleviation of interactions and adverse effects
• Improved quality of life

addresses the role of nurses in assessing and managing bioactive substances in the context of the functional consequences theory for promoting wellness.

Considerations Regarding Medications

Effects of medications in the body are usually considered in relation to **pharmacokinetics** (i.e., how the drug is absorbed, distributed, metabolized, and excreted) and **pharmacodynamics** (i.e., how the body is affected by the drug at the cellular level and in relation to the target organ). *Absorption* refers to the passage of a medication from its site of introduction, usually the gastrointestinal tract, into the general circulation. Absorption of oral medications can be affected by diminished gastric acid, increased gastric pH, delayed gastric emptying, and the presence of other substances (e.g., food, nutrients, inert ingredients of medications). Because most oral medications are absorbed by passive diffusion across the small intestine—a process that is not pH dependent—they are not usually affected by any alterations in gastric acidity. The unique chemical properties of each medication determine the degree to which it is susceptible to any gastrointestinal changes, regardless of age. For example, pH-sensitive medications, such as penicillin and ferrous sulfate, are more likely to be affected by altered gastric acid levels or by prolonged exposure to these acids because of delayed emptying.

Two measures of the efficiency of metabolism and elimination of a drug are elimination half-time and clearance rate. **Elimination half-time** (also called *serum half-life*) is the time required to decrease the drug concentration by one half of its original value. It takes five half-times to reach steady-state concentrations after a drug is initiated or to completely eliminate a medication from the body after a drug is discontinued. The **clearance rate** measures the volume of blood from which the medication is eliminated per unit of time. An increase in serum half-time or a decrease in clearance rate may result in accumulation of the medication. The result is that the therapeutic effect is likely to be altered, and the risk of adverse effects is likely to be increased.

Considerations Regarding Herbs and Homeopathy

The use of complementary and alternative medicine is increasing dramatically in the United States, especially among older adults and people with chronic conditions. All health care practitioners need to know what products their patients are using so they can address concerns about safety, effectiveness, and potential interactions. This is particularly important with regard to bioactive substances, such as herbs and homeopathy, in relation to interactions with medications. In addition, health care practitioners need to be prepared to address questions that their patients may ask about alternative practices, as discussed in the Nursing Interventions section of this chapter.

Although herbs, homeopathy, and folk remedies are viewed as "nontraditional" or "alternative" approaches to preventing and treating illness, these remedies have been used for centuries in many non-Western cultures. Both herbal and homeopathic products have physiologic actions; however, herbal products are of particular concern because their actions can be similar to those of prescription and over-the-counter medications. Thus, they can have beneficial effects, adverse effects, and interactions. This section presents an overview of herbs and homeopathic remedies; additional aspects of herbs are discussed throughout this chapter with regard to physiologic considerations, adverse effects, and herb–medication interactions. Pertinent aspects also are addressed in the sections on Nursing Assessment and Nursing Interventions.

Diversity Note

The use of herbs and other dietary supplements is highest among people with chronic conditions and older, non-Hispanic white women with higher levels of income and education (Wold et al., 2005).

Herbs

Herbs were perhaps the original "over-the-counter" products, used by people who found these medicinal remedies in their natural environments. **Herbs** (also called *botanicals*) are plant-based products that have medicinal properties. Herbs and many other pharmaceutical preparations have common origins in nature. For example, warfarin, which currently is the most widely used oral anticoagulant worldwide, was discovered after it was observed that cattle that consumed sweet clover hay died from hemorrhage (Jacobs, 2006).

Information about the pharmacokinetics and pharmacodynamics that applies to medications (discussed later in the section on Changes That Affect the Action of Bioactive Substances in the Body) also applies to the action of herbs in the body. This is particularly pertinent with regard to herbs that are metabolized by the liver, because metabolism of substances in the liver is affected by many factors, including diet and genetic variations. Thus, it is important to keep in mind that even when taken alone, herbs can be affected by the same age-related changes and risk factors that affect medications in older adults.

Although herbs are commonly viewed as being safer than drugs, health care professionals are increasingly concerned about safety and interactions. Safety of herbs is particularly important for people who also take medications or more than one dietary supplement because, as with all bioactive substances, nothing is taken without risk and the risk increases in proportion to the number of substances consumed. Herbs that are similar in bioactivity to over-the-counter or prescription medications can potentiate the effects of the medication and increase the risk for adverse effects and drug interactions. Table 8-1 lists some herbs and medications that have similar bioactivity.

A factor that complicates safety issues is the limited amount of testing performed that meets the standards established by the U.S. Food and Drug Administration (FDA) for medications. Because herbs are considered dietary supplements, there is no requirement that they be tested for safety or efficacy, and there is little or no reliable information about additional ingredients, potential harmful effects, quantity of active ingredients, or suitability of form for human use. Manufacturers are required to ensure the accuracy of the ingredient list; however, there have been many cases of adulteration and contamination of supplements. In response to these problems, groups such as the United States Pharmacopoeia (USP) and National Sanitation Foundation (NSF) International have launched quality verification programs in an effort to assure the public that they are buying a quality product that has been held to rigorous standards.

TABLE 8-1 Medications and Herbs with Similar Bioactivity

Medication	Herb
Aspirin	Birch bark Willow bark Wintergreen Meadowsweet
Anticoagulants	Dong quai Feverfew Garlic Ginkgo biloba Wintergreen
Caffeine	Guarana Kola nut
Ephedrine	Ephedra
Estrogen	Black cohosh Fennel Red clover Stinging nettle
Lithium	Thyme Purslane
Monoamine oxidase inhibitors	Ginseng St. John's wort Yohimbe
Nicotine	Lobelia
Calcium channel blockers	Angelica

TABLE 8-2 Potential Adverse Effects of Some Herbs

Black cohosh	Bradycardia, hypotension, joint pains
Bloodroot	Bradycardia, arrhythmia, dizziness, impaired vision, intense thirst
Boneset	Liver toxicity, mental changes, respiratory problems
Coltsfoot	Fever, liver toxicity
Dandelion	Interactions with diuretics, increased concentration of lithium or potassium
Ephedra	Anxiety, dizziness, insomnia, tachycardia, hypertension
Feverfew	Interference with blood clotting mechanisms
Garlic	Hypotension, inhibition of blood clotting, potentiation of antidiabetic drugs
Ginseng	Anxiety, insomnia, hypertension, tachycardia, asthma attacks, postmenopausal bleeding
Ginkgo biloba	Increased anticoagulation
Goldenseal	Vasoconstriction
Guar gum	Hypoglycemia
Hawthorn	Hypotension
Hops, skullcap, valerian	Drowsiness, potentiation of antianxiety or sedative medications
Kava	Damage to the eyes, skin, liver, and spinal cord from long-term use
Licorice	Hypokalemia, hypernatremia
Lobelia	Hearing and vision problems
Motherwort	Increased anticoagulation
Nettle	Hypokalemia
Senna	Potentiation of digoxin
Yohimbe	Anxiety, tachycardia, hypertension, mental changes

These programs are voluntary, and the manufacturers who use theses labels are required to undergo strict auditing of their facilities, ensure good manufacturing practices (GMP), test product samples, review labeling, and periodically test off-the-shelf products. Nurses can educate themselves and their patients to buy products with these labels to ensure they are buying a quality product. Some websites that provide excellent assistance in finding high-quality manufacturing and other information are listed in the Educational Resources section.

Most herbs and dietary supplements are safe if they are obtained from reliable sources, but some of these products are potentially dangerous, even when taken alone. Moreover, the risk for adverse effects from some herbs is increased for people with certain conditions, such as a history of stroke, glaucoma, diabetes, hypertension, heart disease, thyroid disorder, and any disorder requiring anticoagulation therapy. There also is increasing concern about the effects of herbs during periods of physiologic stress. For example, herbs can have harmful effects before and after surgery because they can interfere with coagulation, prolong the effects of anesthesia, and cause electrolyte disturbances and cardiovascular disorders (Lee et al., 2006). Another example is the stimulation of the cytochrome P-450 system by St. John's wort, which changes the metabolism of immunosuppressants and cancer chemotherapy agents (Moss & Yuan, 2006). Some of the more serious effects of herbs (listed in Table 8-2) include altered liver function, electrolyte imbalance, elevated blood pressure, diminished blood clotting mechanisms, and alterations of the heart rate and rhythm. Less serious adverse effects include nausea, vomiting, and other gastrointestinal symptoms from oral preparations, especially if they are taken with medications that have similar adverse effects. Table 8-3 lists some of the herbs more commonly used by older adults and their uses, precautions, and doses.

Homeopathic Remedies

Three concepts are crucial to understanding homeopathy as a German physician, Samuel Hahnemann, initially proposed it 2 centuries ago. First, there is the law of similars, or "like cures like." According to this concept, homeopathy treats an illness by stimulating the body's self-healing abilities through the use of a small amount of a substance similar to that which caused the illness. For example, quinine can produce symptoms of malaria in a healthy person, and it can cure malaria when administered in minute doses. The second key concept is that the more a substance is diluted, the more potent it becomes. Based on this concept, homeopathic remedies are diluted repeatedly, and each dilution is vigorously

TABLE 8-3 Herbs Commonly Used by Older Adults

Herb	Uses	Actions and Precautions	Standardization and Dose
Bilberry	The German E Commission approves for acute nonspecific diarrhea and topical treatment of mild inflammation of the mouth, throat, and oral mucosa. Concentrated extracts are used for retinopathy (diabetic and hypertensive), venous insufficiency, and varicose veins.	High doses may inhibit platelet aggregation (in vitro study); monitor anticoagulants if patient is taking larger dosages. Avoid in patients with hemorrhagic disorders.	Concentrated extracts generally standardized to anthocyanosides (25%) Decoction: place 5–10 g dried fruit in 5 oz water and simmer for 10 minutes. This preparation is taken several times daily, principally for diarrhea.
Black cohosh	The German E Commission approves preparations of fresh or dried rhizome for menopausal symptoms (hot flashes, night sweats, sleep disturbances, irritability).	Cases of possible hepatotoxicity; monitoring liver function every 6 months is advised. Several NIH clinical trials are in progress that may answer the question of whether long-term use of black cohosh causes endometrial hyperplasia.	Standardized to triterpene glycosides as marker compound Decoction: Place 40–200 mg dried root/rhizome in 8 oz of water and simmer for 10 minutes. This is the total daily amount, usually taken in two to three divided doses. Tincture: 2–4 mL twice daily (1:10 [g/mL] in 40%–60% alcohol) Remifemin clinical trials have used 20- to 80-mg tablets twice daily.
Cat's claw	Osteoarthritis of the knee and rheumatoid arthritis There are no monographs from the German E Commission.	Avoid in patients with organ transplant or lymphocytosis (theoretically because of stimulation of immune system). Inhibits cytochrome P-450 CYP3A4 enzyme in vitro. Use with caution in patients with autoimmune disease (e.g., those taking cyclosporine or prednisone) and antiplatelet therapy. Caution with antihypertensive medication; may dilate peripheral blood vessels and increase heart rate.	Extracts in clinical trials standardized to either pentacyclic oxindole alkaloids (POA) or carboxyl alkyl esters (CAE). Decoction: Place 1 g root bark in 8 oz of water and simmer 10 minutes. This preparation is taken one to three times daily
Chamomile	The German E Commission approves for inflammation of GI tract and GI spasms. Topical preparation use includes inflammation of skin and mucous membranes and bacterial skin diseases.	Contraindicated with allergy to chamomile No herb–drug interactions reported in the literature	Standardization is not common, but may be standardized to contain 1.2% apigenin and 0.5% essential oil per dose. Infusion: Pour 5 oz boiling water over 1 heaping Tbsp (3 g) herb, steep 10 minutes. Take 1 to 4 cups per day. Tincture: 3–10 mL three times daily (1:5 g/mL in 45% alcohol)
Echinacea	The German E Commission approves for supportive therapy for colds and infections of the respiratory and urinary tract.	Caution should be used when coadministering with drugs dependent on CYP3A or CYP1A2 for elimination. Echinacea has a long history of adulteration, substitution, and products of poor quality. Contraindicated in progressive systemic diseases (e.g., HIV, AIDS, tuberculosis, multiple sclerosis, leukocytosis) Avoid in patients taking immunosuppressant drugs (e.g., transplant patients). German health authorities recommend limiting use to 8 weeks, but two studies have used for 10–12 weeks without any adverse effects.	Varies with preparation and part of the plant being used Decoction: Place 1 g root in 5 oz water, simmer for 10 minutes; repeat three times daily. Dried powdered herb capsules: 1 g three times daily Tincture dried root: 1.5–5 mL three times daily (1:5 g/mL 55% alcohol) Fresh pressed juice: 6–9 mL/day (expressed juice from fresh *E. purpurea* aerial parts 2.5:2, stabilized in 22% alcohol)
Evening primrose	There are no monographs from the German E Commission. Atopic dermatitis and eczema	Possible interaction with antipsychotic medications; however, it may be an "unmasking" of temporal lobe epilepsy.	Generally standardized to their content of linoleic (LA) and gamma-linoleic acid (GLA)

continued on following page

TABLE 8-3 Herbs Commonly Used by Older Adults (continued)

Herb	Uses	Actions and Precautions	Standardization and Dose
	May improve blood flow and nerve conduction deficits in diabetes	Anticonvulsants: theoretical risk of increased seizure activity	Dose: Typical dosage range in clinical trials is 1–6 g (2–12 capsules) per day, the higher dose being associated with more positive results, particularly in eczema.
Garlic	The German E Commission approves to lower cholesterol, prevent hardening of arteries, and to treat minor respiratory infections	Inhibits platelet aggregation (may increase risk of bleeding if taking warfarin, aspirin or NSAIDs); avoid with HIV patients taking saquinavir (decreased action). Discontinue garlic supplementation 7–14 days prior to surgery, except for garlic used in cooking.	Standardized to allicin Dried garlic powder: 0.5–1.0 g/d Fresh garlic: 4 g/d
Ginger	The German E Commission approves for prevention of motion sickness. Anti-inflammatory	Contraindicated in active gallbladder disease Antiplatelet aggregation is commonly listed as a contraindication; however, clinical trials have not substantiated when used in typical dose of 2–4 g/day. Discontinue supplementation 7–14 days before surgery, except for ginger used in cooking.	Root or rhizome used Dried ginger: 2–4 g/day; all three clinical trials for nausea and vomiting of pregnancy used 1 g/day. Fluid extract: 1:1 (g/mL) 0.25–1.0 mL three times daily, tincture 1.5 (g/mL) 1.25–5.0 mL three times daily
Ginkgo biloba	Standardized ginkgo extract has a positive German E Commission monograph for degenerative and vascular dementia, peripheral artery occlusive disease, vertigo, and tinnitus. Ginkgo leaf has a null German E Commission monograph.	American Herbal Products Association contraindicates use with MAO inhibitors. Potential for interaction with anticoagulant and antiplatelet medications (e.g., warfarin, aspirin) Rare case reports of spontaneous bleeding Potential to increase blood glucose in type 2 diabetes Discontinue 7–14 days before surgery.	Dry leaf extract standardized to 22%–27% flavone glycosides and 5%–7% terpene lactones Use as directed on product label.
Ginseng	The German E Commission and World Health Organization (WHO) recognize as a tonic, prophylaxis, or restorative agent for invigoration during times of fatigue, exhaustion, stress, and convalescence.	Hypoglycemic effects have been documented. One case report shows decreased INR; however, animal studies fail to show interaction. Avoid with MAO inhibitors. May increase blood pressure Contraindicated in acute asthma or acute infection	Generally standardized to 4% ginsenosides Clinical trials use 100–200 mg/day. Infusion: 5 oz boiling water is poured over 1–2 g powdered ginseng root and steeped for 10 minutes. This dose is repeated one to two times per day. Decoction: Place 3–9 g dried root in 24 oz water and simmer for 30–45 minutes. This preparation is divided into several doses taken throughout the day.
Hawthorn	The German E Commission approves leaf with flower for the treatment of congestive heart failure.	May potentiate action of digitalis and beta-blockers	Standardized to procyanidins Clinical trials have used 160–900 mg/day. Infusion: Pour 5 oz boiling water over 1.5 g herb (roughly 1 tsp) and steep for 10 minutes. This dose is repeated three to four times per day.
Horse chestnut	The German E Commission approves for treatment of chronic venous insufficiency, night cramps, and itching.	Monitor bleeding times in patients taking anticoagulants.	Dose is generally 100 mg aescin/day, achieved by taking 250–312.5 mg extract twice daily. Tablets (200 mg of 5:1 concentrated extract, standardized to 40 mg aescin): 2–3 tablets per day
Kava	Treatment option for anxiety The German E commission contradicts current use for anxiety or depression.	Serious concerns about liver toxicity have been raised because of multiple reports of hepatotoxicity (leading to 8 transplants and 3 deaths). Increased risk of decreased effectiveness of warfarin	Standardized to 30%–70% kava lactones Because of liability issues, many U.S. companies have discontinued product.

continued on following page

TABLE 8-3 Herbs Commonly Used by Older Adults (continued)

Herb	Uses	Actions and Precautions	Standardization and Dose
		May potentiate barbiturates Studies indicate that kava has a high potential for causing drug interactions.	Current ban on production of products in Germany
Licorice	The German E Commission approves the use of licorice root for inflammation of the upper respiratory tract and gastric/duodenal ulcers.	Contraindicated in liver disorders, congestive heart failure, or edema Avoid prolonged use of higher dosages. Licorice can increase blood pressure. Potential interactions with diuretics, corticosteroids, and antihypertensives	Dose 2–6 mL/day of 1:1 liquid extract; 0.4–1.6 g three times daily of deglycyrrhizinized licorice dry extract BP (British Pharmacopoeia)
Saw palmetto	The German E Commission and USP (U.S. Pharmacopoeia) recognize as treatment for benign prostatic hypertrophy.	No reported drug interactions Does not appear to affect prostate-specific antigen levels	Varies according to fruit, tea, tincture, or extract Fruit: 1–2 g berries or equivalent preparation Tea: Place 1/3 daily dose of saw palmetto berry in 8 oz water and simmer for 5 minutes. Repeat three times daily. Tincture: Fresh fruit 1:2, dried fruit 1:5, 80% alcohol; 1–2 mL three to four times daily Extract: Liquid (1:1) 0.6–1.5 mL/day
St. John's wort	The German E Commission recognizes use in mild to moderate depressive moods, anxiety, and nervousness.	Not indicated for use in severe depression Fewer adverse reactions than prescription antidepressants. Phototoxicity is extremely rare but can occur in light-skinned people. Potential for decreased cyclosporine levels; decreased effectiveness of warfarin; possible decreased digoxin levels; reduced levels of protease inhibitors (e.g., indinavir); decreased levels of simvastatin Avoid in patients taking multiple medications.	Extracts often standardized to hypericin or hyperforin (no consensus on which to standardize and at what level) Clinical trials used 500–1800 mg/day.
Valerian	Used for restlessness, mild sleep-promoting agent in nervous and anxiety-related sleep disturbances	In theory, there is potential additive effect when taken with central nervous system depressants.	Extracts standardized to contain 0.3–0.8% valerenic acid Infusion: Pour 5 oz over 3–5 g (1 tsp) valerian root and steep for 10–15 minutes. Drink before bed or two to three times per day as needed. Tincture: 1–3 mL one to three times per day (1:5, 70% alcohol)

GI, gastrointestinal; MAO, monoamine oxidase.

shaken to increase its potency. The third concept is that illnesses are highly individualized and, therefore, the treatment must be individualized. Based on this principle, homeopathic practitioners focus on treating the person, not the disease, and they spend a lot of time interviewing and assessing patients before prescribing a homeopathic remedy. Homeopathy is widely used in India, Russia, Mexico, and European countries, and it is gaining acceptance in the United States as a safe alternative to conventional medicine.

Although most homeopathic remedies are now available for self-treatment, a few are available only through health care practitioners. Unlike herbs, homeopathic remedies are regulated by the FDA as over-the-counter products. Remedies come in a variety of single-substance or combination forms, including powders, wafers, small tablets, and alcohol-based liquids. Over-the-counter homeopathic products are too weak to cause adverse effects, and there are very few precautions, interactions, or contraindications that apply to these products. People who are taking homeopathic remedies are advised to limit the amount taken and the length of time they are consumed. Other precautions include avoiding food, caffeine, beverages, toothpaste, and mouthwashes for 15 to 60 minutes before and after taking the substance. Also, oils of camphor, eucalyptus, and peppermint should be avoided during homeopathic treatments. Information about homeopathic remedies and homeopathic practitioners can be obtained from the National Center for Complementary and Alternative Medicine (see Educational Resources).

AGE-RELATED CHANGES THAT AFFECT BIOACTIVE SUBSTANCES IN OLDER ADULTS

Age-related changes that affect bioactive substances in older adults are discussed in relation to those that affect the actions of the agents in the body, and those that affect the skills involved with taking them. The factors that have the most significant impact on the effectiveness of bioactive substances in older adults are not age-related changes, but risk factors, and are considered in the section on Risk Factors.

Changes That Affect the Action of Bioactive Substances in the Body

An age-related decline in glomerular filtration rate, which begins in early adulthood and progresses at an annual rate of 1% to 2%, may affect the concentrations of bioactive substances in the body, particularly those that are cleared through the kidneys. For example, diminished renal function can decrease the clearance of water-soluble medications that depend on glomerular filtration (e.g., gentamicin) or tubular secretion (e.g., penicillin) for their removal. Likewise, the consequences of diminished renal function will be greater on substances that readily reach toxic levels because they have a narrow therapeutic index (e.g., digoxin). Box 8-1 lists some medications that are likely to be affected by age-related renal changes.

The gradual 30% to 50% decline in hepatic blood flow that begins around the age of 40 years can affect serum concentration and volume of distribution of substances that are metabolized more extensively by the liver (Blanda, 2006). For example, medications that normally are rapidly metabolized and, therefore, greatly influenced by the speed of delivery to the liver may be affected by diminished hepatic blood flow. In addition to age related changes, many other factors affect the liver metabolism of substances in people of all ages. The specific effects of these age-related liver changes on the metabolism of bioactive agents is unclear, however, because factors such as diet, caffeine, smoking, alcohol, genetic variations, and pathologic conditions are likely to simultaneously affect the metabolism of substances and exert a stronger influence than any age-related factors. Box 8-1 also lists some medications whose clearance is likely to be delayed because of age-related liver changes.

In recent years, there has been increasing attention paid to the role of the cytochrome P-450 system, which is composed of many specific enzymes responsible for the metabolism of medications and other bioactive substances, including herbs, nutrients, and nicotine. The cytochrome P-450 system is particularly important with regard to interactions between herbs, medications, and other substances because competition at the enzyme sites can affect clearance. Pathways most commonly involved with pharmaceutical agents are 1A2, 2C9, 2C19, 2D69, and 3A4. Because age-related changes slow the function of this system, clearance of substances that depend on the cytochrome P-450 system is likely to be delayed in older adults. Table 8-4 lists examples of some commonly used drugs and herbs according to their metabolic pathway.

An age-related decrease in total body water and an increase in the proportion of body fat to lean body mass can alter the action of bioactive substances in older adults. Between the ages of about 20 and 80 years, the following changes in body composition occur: body fat gradually increases by 15% to 20%, lean tissue decreases by about 20%, and total body water is reduced by 10% to 15%. Loss of lean body mass accelerates after the age of 80 years, even in healthy older adults (Kyle et al., 2001). Because these age-related changes in body composition will affect substances according to their degree of fat or water solubility, agents that are distributed primarily in body water or lean body mass may reach higher serum concentrations in older adults and their effects may be more intense. Similarly, the serum concentration of highly fat-soluble substances, which are distributed and stored in fat tissue, may be lowered, and these agents have an increased tendency to accumulate in adipose tissue. Consequently, fat-soluble substances may have a prolonged duration of action, be more erratic in their effects, and have less intense immediate effects. Box 8-2 lists some medications whose concentrations are likely to be increased or decreased because of age-related changes in body composition.

As bioactive substances are distributed and metabolized in the body, some molecules are bound to serum albumin and other proteins, so the bound portion becomes inactive

Box 8-1
Medications With Decreased Clearance Due to Age-Related Changes

Decreased Clearance Caused by Renal Changes	***Decreased Clearance Caused by Hepatic Changes***
amantadine	acetaminophen
amoxicillin	amitriptyline
ampicillin	barbiturates
atenolol	benzodiazepines
ceftriaxone	codeine
cephalexin	labetalol
chlorpropamide	lidocaine
cimetidine	meperidine
ciprofloxacin	morphine
colchicine	phenytoin
digoxin	propranolol
enalapril	quinidine
furosemide	salicylates
glyburide	theophylline
hydrochlorothiazide	warfarin
levofloxacin	
lisinopril	
metformin	
ranitidine	

TABLE 8-4 Metabolic Pathways of Some Commonly Used Bioactive Substances

CYP1A2	CYP2C9	2C19	2D6	3A4	2C8
*amitriptyline**	*carbamazepine*	ginkgo	bupropion	*alprazolam*	*gemfibrozil*
caffeine	cranberry	*carbamazepine*	celecoxib	*clarithromycin*	*phenobarbital*
charbroiled food	*diazepam*	*fluoxetine*	*codeine*	*erythromycin*	*rifampin*
clomipramine	ginkgo	*omeprazole*	*oxycodone*	*estrogens, oral*	quercetin
echinacea	*isoniazid*	*phenytoin*	*cimetidine*	*felodipine*	
estradiol	*phenobarbital*		*sertraline*	*fentanyl*	
imipramine	*phenytoin*			*sildenafil*	
nicotine	*St. John's wort*			*simvastatin*	
St. John's wort	warfarin			*tamoxifen*	
theophylline				*garlic*	
				St. John's wort	
				caffeine	
				progesterone/ progestins	
				grapefruit	
				pomegranate	

* *Italics* indicate that the drug or herb has been involved in a drug interaction of clinical relevance or associated with a strong drug interaction warning.

while the unbound molecules remain active. Because the unbound portion is the amount available for metabolism, tissue perfusion, and renal excretion, the protein-binding capacity of an agent is an important determinant of its potential for both therapeutic and adverse effects. The degree of protein binding of each substance varies, with some medications, such as warfarin, having a protein-binding capacity of 99%. The binding capacity of substances that are highly protein bound can be influenced by diminished serum albumin levels in older adults. Additional factors that affect the degree of protein binding for any agent include the strength of the binding and the number of chemicals competing for the binding sites.

Although gerontologists disagree about the extent and cause of decreased serum albumin levels in older adults, it is generally agreed that the level diminishes by as much as 20% in the later decades of life. Diminished serum albumin levels are associated with a combination of factors, including malnutrition, pathologic processes, decreased mobility, and age-related liver changes. Regardless of the cause, a decrease in the serum albumin level will lead to an increased amount of the active portion of protein-bound substances. Medications that are highly protein bound, which are commonly taken by older adults, are most strongly affected. This effect is intensified when more than one protein-bound substance is consumed because the agents compete for the same sites. Box 8-3 lists some medications that are most likely to have adverse effects when they are taken together or when serum albumin levels are low.

Independent of any changes that affect pharmacokinetics, age-related changes in receptor sensitivity can influence pharmacodynamics and cause older adults to be more or less sensitive to particular substances. For example, an increased sensitivity of the older brain to centrally acting psychotropic medications may potentiate both the therapeutic and adverse effects of these drugs. This is particularly true for benzodiazepines, which have stronger sedative effects in older adults. Box 8-4 lists examples of drugs that have increased or decreased sensitivity in older adults. Age-related change in homeostatic mechanisms, such as thermoregulation, fluid regulation, and baroreceptor control over blood pressure, also can affect pharmacodynamics. For example, inefficient fluid regulation may alter the action of medications, such as lithium, that are particularly sensitive to fluid and electrolyte balance.

Box 8-2
Medications Likely to Be Affected by Age-Related Changes in Body Composition

Medications With Increased Concentrations	***Medications With Decreased Concentrations***
cimetidine	phenobarbital
digoxin	prazosin
ethanol (alcohol)	thiopental
gentamicin	tolbutamide
morphine	
propanolol	
quinine	
warfarin	

Box 8-3
Some Medications Affected by Serum Albumin

aspirin	phenylbutazone
clofibrate	phenytoin
digoxin	sertraline
furosemide	sulfonamides
nonsteroidal anti-inflammatory drugs (NSAIDs)	theophylline
oral hypoglycemics	thyroid hormone
	warfarin

Box 8-4
Medications With Increased or Decreased Receptor Sensitivity in Older Adults

Increased Sensitivity (increased potency)	***Decreased Sensitivity (may have delayed signs of toxicity)***
Angiotensin-converting enzyme (ACE) inhibitors	Beta-blockers
Diazepam	Bemetamide
Digoxin	Dopamine
Diltiazem	Furosemide
Enalapril	Isoproterenol
Felodipine	Propranolol
Levodopa	Tolbutamide
Lithium	
Midazolam	
Morphine	
Temazepam	
Verapamil	
Warfarin	

Body size and sex are additional factors that can influence the action of bioactive substances in the body. Although these factors are not unique to older adults, they can add to the effects of age-related changes and need to be considered with regard to doses. Because body size can affect both the therapeutic and adverse effects of substances, doses need to be adjusted for older adults who are small or have lost or are losing weight. This consideration is particularly important for older adults who are losing muscle mass or have decreased renal function.

Changes That Affect Behaviors Related to Taking Bioactive Substances

For any adult, all the following factors affect the appropriate use of bioactive substances:

- Motivation
- Knowledge about the purpose of the substance
- Cultural and psychosocial influences
- Ability to obtain correct amounts (influenced by factors such as cost, accessibility)
- Ability to distinguish the correct container
- Ability to read and comprehend directions
- Ability to hear and remember verbal instructions
- Knowledge about correct timing for consumption
- Ability to follow the correct dosage regimen
- Physical ability to remove the substance from the container and administer it
- Ability to swallow oral preparations
- Additional skills related to coordination, manual dexterity, and visual acuity for substances that are administered nasally, transdermally, subcutaneously, or by other methods

Even for healthy older adults, age-related changes and functional impairments often interfere with these skills. For example, hearing or vision changes can interfere with the ability to understand instructions and read directions, especially labels on bottles. Any limitations in fine motor movement of the hands may interfere with the ability to remove lids from containers, especially when the lids are tamper resistant. Although the skills related to taking bioactive substances are sometimes influenced by age-related changes, more often they are influenced by risk factors that commonly occur in older adults.

RISK FACTORS THAT AFFECT BIOACTIVE SUBSTANCES

By approximately 75 years of age, even the healthiest of older adults have age-related changes that affect pharmacokinetics and pharmacodynamics in their bodies. Even more significant, however, are the numerous risk factors that have even greater effects on behaviors of older adults relative to taking bioactive substances. Risk factors can be the result of the patient's own attitudes, level of knowledge, and socioeconomic circumstances, or they can be attributed to outside sources (e.g., health care providers).

The consumption of more than one bioactive substance greatly increases the potential for adverse and altered therapeutic effects. Because older adults take a disproportionately greater number of medications than do younger people, they have an increased susceptibility to adverse or altered effects. Additional risks arise from myths and misunderstandings that affect the medication consumption patterns of older adults. Finally, certain factors unrelated to age, such as weight, sex, and smoking habits, combine with age-related changes and risk factors to increase further the risk of adverse and altered effects.

Wellness Opportunity

Nurses provide holistic care when they explore the wide range of factors that affect bioactive substances and substance-taking behaviors.

Pathologic Processes and Functional Impairments

Because the purpose of any medication is to relieve or control symptoms of pathologic conditions, it can be assumed that people who take medications have at least one disease-related symptom. The increased prevalence of chronic conditions in older adults adds to their vulnerability to medication–disease interactions (Petrone & Katz, 2005). Medication–disease interactions manifest themselves in any of the following ways:

- Pathologic processes can exacerbate age-related changes that would otherwise have little or no impact on the medication. (For example, malnutrition further decreases

serum albumin, thereby increasing both the therapeutic and adverse effects of highly protein-bound medications.)
- Pathologic processes can alter therapeutic and adverse effects of substances. (For instance, congestive heart failure decreases both the metabolism and the excretion of most medications.)
- Bioactive substances can cause serious adverse effects for people with pathologic conditions. (For example, anticholinergics may cause urinary retention in men with prostatic hyperplasia.)

Pathologic conditions not only influence the action of substances in the body, but can contribute to nonadherence, especially in combination with functional limitations. For example, dementia can significantly affect the older adult's ability to understand directions and remember instructions. This cognitive impairment interferes with the ability to self-manage medication regimens, especially in the absence of supervision or assistance (Ownby, 2006). Dysphagia or any condition that affects chewing and swallowing can interfere with the ability to take substances orally.

Behaviors Based on Myths and Misunderstandings

Myths and misunderstandings influence attitudes held by older adults, as well as their caregivers, about the consumption of bioactive substances. An attitude that can be potentially harmful for older adults is that medications, particularly over-the-counter products, provide a "quick fix" for any uncomfortable symptom. For example, messages promoting constipation remedies can reinforce false beliefs about bowel function and lead to laxative abuse. Although adults of any age can be influenced by these attitudes, older adults are more likely than their younger counterparts to experience negative consequences because they are more vulnerable to adverse effects and drug interactions when they take bioactive substances.

Another potentially harmful belief is that over-the-counter remedies are always safe, even in extra-strength doses. Although over-the-counter preparations may be relatively safe for healthy younger adults, they often create problems for older adults, particularly in the presence of pathologic conditions and in combination with other substances. For example, over-the-counter preparations for colds and insomnia typically contain antihistamines and anticholinergic ingredients that have serious adverse effects in older adults (e.g., cognitive impairment; decreased reflexes; and increased risk of falls, hip fractures, and motor vehicle accidents) (Blanda, 2006). In these situations, the addition of a seemingly harmless over-the-counter product to an already complex regimen of prescription medications can be the factor that tips the scale of safety and causes a serious adverse effect, such as delirium. Nonsteroidal anti-inflammatory drugs (NSAIDs) are another category of over-the-counter drugs that commonly have serious adverse effects in older adults, either alone or in combination with other substances (e.g., anticoagulants, prednisone, antihypertensive agents).

Attitudes and expectations about medications as quick-fix remedies also can influence the prescribing patterns of primary care practitioners. For example, when over-the-counter remedies are ineffective, people expect their health care practitioners to provide an otherwise unobtainable remedy—a prescription—for their discomfort. Sometimes a nonpharmacologic remedy is safer than, and just as effective as, a prescription medication, but these remedies usually demand more of the practitioner's time and some degree of patient motivation. For example, it is easier to prescribe an antihypertensive than to advise about diet and exercise interventions. Another factor contributing to the reluctance of practitioners to suggest nonpharmacologic remedies is that there are more controlled clinical trials supporting the use of medications. Sleep and anxiety complaints are examples of conditions that respond to nonpharmacologic treatments but that are often addressed by prescription medications because of the attitudes of the patient or primary care practitioner.

Wellness Opportunity

By taking time to identify an older adult's beliefs about illness and treatments (including pharmacologic and nonpharmacologic approaches), nurses pave the way for teaching about the safest and most effective interventions.

Communication Barriers

Another factor that may contribute to an increased use of prescriptions by older adults is their own reluctance to challenge or question the primary care practitioner because they perceive him or her as "all-knowing." Although the image of the infallible physician is subsiding, older adults are still inclined to accept advice from prescribing practitioners without question.

Communication barriers and lack of confidence in one's communication skills may further inhibit someone from discussing treatment options with a health care practitioner. Because medical knowledge has been expanding at a tremendous pace in recent years, treatment decisions have become increasingly more complex. Consequently, older adults may hesitate to ask questions about medical decisions out of fear of appearing ignorant. Hearing and other sensory impairments common in older adults also may interfere with patient-directed discussions of a treatment plan. Other communication barriers, such as an attitude of impatience on the part of the health care practitioner, also may thwart discussion. In addition, poor command of the English language, on the part of either the older adult or the health care practitioner, can interfere with a discussion of health issues and lead to misunderstandings. Language barriers and a low education level can present major impediments to many treatment decisions, including medication adherence.

Lack of Information

Despite the fact that older adults are the primary consumers of prescription and over-the-counter medications, our knowledge about medication effects in older adults is insufficient and still in an early phase. Before the 1980s, research on the influence of age on the action of specific medications was virtually nonexistent and pharmaceutical companies determined normal adult doses based on clinical trials of healthy younger men. In addition, the few studies of age-related influences on medications were cross-sectional rather than longitudinal and identified age differences rather than age-related changes. Moreover, older adults who are included in clinical trials tend to be healthier and young-old, rather than medically frail or old-old (Beyth & Shorr, 2002).

Information about medication–medication interactions also is lacking, especially for newly approved drugs. Because the FDA requires only limited testing of medication–medication interactions, these interactions are often identified only after the medication has been on the market for several years. Thus, any recently approved medication should be used cautiously in older adults who are taking more than one drug because of the increased risk of unpredictable interactions. Examples of medications that are likely to cause serious adverse effects when consumed with another medication include alcohol, analgesics, anticoagulants, anticholinergics, digoxin, phenytoin, theophylline, and warfarin.

In 1982, the USP, which sets the official standards for medications in the United States, established a geriatrics advisory panel to examine age-related influences on medication action. Since the late 1980s, three trends have emerged in the pharmaceutical industry that are beneficial for older adults: (1) pharmaceutical companies began testing medications on older adults; (2) they began focusing on adverse medication effects, including medication interactions; and (3) because of the emphasis on adverse reactions, new medications are now developed and promoted not only for their therapeutic effectiveness but for their lack of unwanted effects. Since 1997, pharmaceutical companies have been required to include a separate geriatric-use section in their labeling. However, because current legislation does not require the inclusion of older patients in clinical trials, there is a dearth of research-based evidence to support geriatric prescribing practices (Petrone & Katz, 2005).

Inappropriate Prescribing Practices

During the late 1980s, geriatricians began to address medication-related problems in older adults because of widespread concerns about the large numbers as well as the types of drugs prescribed for this population. The term **inappropriate medications** describes drugs that are not appropriate for use in older adults; in 1991, an international panel of experts used consensus criteria to identify drugs that should not be used by frail older adults (Beers et al., 1991). According to these explicit criteria, which are commonly called the **Beers criteria**, medications are deemed inappropriate if they are ineffective or have poor safety profiles, or if better drugs are available (Beers et al., 1991). The most recent update in 2003 identified 48 medications or classes of medications that are inappropriate for older adults, and it rated the risks associated with these medications as high or low (Fick et al., 2003). These criteria have been widely used in the United States and worldwide to guide research and clinical practice, and they are recommended as a Best Practice tool by the Hartford Institute for Geriatric Nursing (Molony, 2003). Some common themes in the Beers criteria include the following:

- Anticholinergic drugs and drugs with anticholinergic properties are inappropriate because of toxicity and serious side effects (e.g., seizures, delirium, agitation, hallucinations, cardiac arrhythmias, cognitive impairment, urinary retention).
- Tricyclic antidepressants are inappropriate not only because of anticholinergic effects, but because of their increased volume of distribution and slowed metabolism, which are particular concerns for older adults with cardiac conditions.
- Antipsychotic medications can produce extrapyramidal and anticholinergic effects, as well as tardive dyskinesia, even with low doses and short-term use.
- Barbiturates are inappropriate, except as anticonvulsants, because their high protein-binding capacity can lead to accumulation and toxicity.
- Benzodiazepines, especially those that have been on the market the longest (e.g., diazepam, chlordiazepoxide, flurazepam) have a high risk for accumulation and toxicity because of their prolonged half-life in older adults.

The use of psychotropic drugs in long-term care facilities has been a particular focus of concern since 1987, when the Nursing Home Reform Act mandated that the Health Care Financing Administration address this issue. Despite efforts to improve prescribing practices for older adults, however, recent studies indicate that little or no progress has been made in reducing inappropriate prescribing practices, either in general or with regard to psychotropic drugs in long-term care facilities (Blanda, 2006; Briesacher et al., 2005; Petrone & Katz, 2005; Simon et al., 2005). An analysis of data on 2.5 million Medicare beneficiaries who resided in long-term care facilities in 2000 and 2001 determined that the level of antipsychotic use was at the highest in over a decade (Briesacher et al., 2005). Moreover, this analysis found that only 42% of the antipsychotic therapy was in accordance with prescribing guidelines. Among the other findings of this survey were that 23.4% had no appropriate indication, 17.2% had a daily dose exceeding the recommended levels, and 17.6% had both inappropriate indications and high dosing (Briesacher et al., 2005).

In the last decade, numerous studies have used the Beers criteria to analyze prescribing patterns and health outcomes of inappropriate prescribing practices. Findings of some of the recent and larger-scale studies are as follows:

- An analysis of over 1 million outpatient visits at a Veterans Administration facility in 2000 found that 23% of the patients had at least one inappropriate medication; analgesics, benzodiazepines, antidepressants, and musculoskeletal agents were most common (Pugh et al., 2005).
- During a total of 24 months, the mean monthly prevalence of inappropriate medications for a study group of 546 older adults with and without dementia admitted to a long-term care facility was 20% and 23%, respectively, before admission and 19% and 28%, respectively, after admission (Zuckerman et al., 2005).
- In a group of 425 older adults admitted to seven Finnish nursing homes and two hospitals, 36.2% had at least one inappropriate medication; the most common were temazepam, oxybutynin, dipyridamole, and amitriptyline (Raivio et al., 2006).
- In a group of 1669 older adults admitted to 17 Japanese long-term care facilities, 21.1% had at least one inappropriate medication; the most common was ticlopidine (Niwata et al., 2006).
- A review of over 1000 records of residents of 15 long-term care facilities found that 46.5% received at least one inappropriate medication, and of those, 12.8% suffered an adverse health outcome. Propoxyphene was the medication most strongly associated with an adverse health outcome (Perri et al., 2005).
- A study of 3372 residents of long-term care facilities found that the use of any inappropriate medication was associated with a greater risk of being hospitalized or dying (Lau et al., 2005).
- A study of 800 community-residing rural older adults found that 26.6% used at least one inappropriate medication; factors associated with higher use included more medications, lower levels of social support, and higher levels of disability (Blalock et al., 2005).
- A longitudinal study of 9294 community-residing older adults in France found that nearly 40% of the participants used at least one inappropriate medication; cerebral vasodilators, long-acting benzodiazepines, and anticholinergics were most common (Lechevallier-Michel et al., 2005).

There is evidence that much of the inappropriate prescribing involves overuse and poor monitoring; however, there also is increasing concern about the underuse of medications that have proven efficacy. This concern is warranted, because studies indicate that underuse of beneficial medications by older adults is associated with increased morbidity and mortality and diminished quality of life (Terrell et al., 2006). Petrone and Katz (2005) cited studies that found underuse by older adults with regard to the following treatments, which have been substantiated by research to improve outcomes:

- Angiotensin-converting enzyme inhibitors for congestive heart failure
- Calcium supplements for osteoporosis
- Anticoagulants or antiplatelets for a history of cerebrovascular attack
- Aspirin or beta-blockers for coronary artery disease
- Osteoporosis treatments in the year after an osteoporotic fracture

Undertreatment of pain is of particular concern with regard to older adults, as discussed in detail in Chapter 28. Additional conditions that are undertreated in older adults include hypertension, depression, and hyperlipidemia (Terrell et al., 2006).

Wellness Opportunity

Nurses have many opportunities to prevent adverse medication effects by raising questions about the use of medications that are potentially inappropriate.

Polypharmacy and Inadequate Monitoring of Medications

Polypharmacy refers to the use of multiple medications, often from multiple sources. Studies have found that community-residing older adults in the United States take, on average, between 3 and 9 medications at a time, with 12% taking more than 10 (Blanda, 2006). Medication use is even higher among older adults in long-term care facilities. The high level of medication use is primarily associated with the increased prevalence of chronic illness among older adults, and it is usually appropriate and therapeutic; however, it can lead to drug interactions and adverse medication effects. One study found that the use of four or more medications was a significant independent risk factor for increased mortality, even when illness severity, level of functioning, and other factors were considered (Espino et al., 2006).

As the number and sources of medications increase, the need for monitoring becomes more important, from the time of the initial prescription until the termination of treatment. The following risk factors could potentially interfere with medication monitoring in older adults:

- Patient consultations with multiple health care providers, who usually do not communicate with each other about the patient's care
- Health care practitioners' lack of information about medications obtained from a variety of sources (i.e., prescription medications offered by friends and relatives, or nonprescription products, such as herbs, nutritional supplements, and over-the-counter products)
- Health care practitioners' lack of information about a patient's nonadherence to a treatment regimen
- A patient's fear of disclosing information about folk remedies or medications obtained from sources other than the prescribing health care practitioner
- A patient's reluctance to disclose information about self-directed changes in the medication regimen

- An assumption by the patient or health care practitioner that, once most medications are started, they should be continued indefinitely
- An assumption by the patient or health care practitioner that, once an appropriate medication dosage is established, it will not need to be changed
- An assumption by the patient or health care practitioner that a lack of adverse effects early in the course of treatment indicates that adverse effects will never occur
- Changes in the patient's weight, especially weight loss, which may affect pharmacokinetics
- Changes in the patient's daily habits, which may affect pharmacokinetics (e.g., smoking, activity level, or nutrient and fluid intake)
- Changes in the patient's mental–emotional status, which may affect medication consumption patterns
- Changes in the patient's health status, which may affect medication actions, increasing the potential for adverse effects

Medication Nonadherence: Financial Concerns and Other Contributing Factors

Medication nonadherence (also called *noncompliance*) refers to medication-taking patterns that differ from the prescribed pattern, including missed doses, failure to fill prescriptions, or medications taken too frequently or at inappropriate times. Although nonadherence is often viewed as a problem specific to older adults, studies indicate that 50% of adults of any age do not take drugs as prescribed (Schlenk et al., 2004). Factors that can contribute to nonadherence include depression, isolated living situation, financial considerations, disease category, adverse medication effects, complex medication regimen, inadequate understanding of the medication regimen, the use of two or more prescribing practitioners or pharmacies, and cognitive impairments, especially those affecting memory or executive function (Blanda, 2006; Insel et al., 2006; Schlenk et al., 2004).

Wellness Opportunity

Nurses can build on their trusting relationship with older adults to encourage open discussion of factors that interfere with adherence to medication regimens.

In recent years, there has been increasing attention paid to the rapidly increasing cost of medications and the lack of health insurance coverage for prescriptions. In 2002, community-residing older adults in the United States paid an average of $686 per year out of pocket for prescription drugs, and private insurance and public programs covered additional amounts of $634 and $419, respectively (Federal Interagency Forum, 2006). Of great concern is the even more dramatic increase in the cost of prescription drugs as a proportion of health care costs. For example, in 1992, prescription drugs accounted for 8% of health care expenditures for older adults, but in 2003, they accounted for 14% (Federal Interagency Forum, 2006). Another way of looking at the increasing cost is in terms of mean annual cost per older adult, which far exceeds inflation or the increase in price of other goods and services in the past decade. According to the Centers of Medicare & Medicaid Services price index, mean annual spending for prescriptions increased by 164% between 1992 and 2001; when adjusted for inflation, this increase is 88% (Goulding, 2005). Nonadherence is one consequence of this increase. A survey of almost 14,000 community-residing Medicare beneficiaries in the fall of 2004 (1 year before the implementation of the Medicare Prescription Drug program) found that 13% of older adults reported that the high cost of medications caused them to not fill prescriptions or to skip or otherwise reduce doses (Soumerai et al., 2006).

Increasing public pressure to address concerns about prescription drug costs led to the legislation creating the **Medicare Part D** prescription drug program, which became effective in January 2006. Unlike the basic Medicare program, which is a publicly funded insurance program operated by the Centers for Medicare & Medicaid Services, beneficiaries enroll in one of the many plans offered by private insurance companies.

A major intent of Medicare Part D was to substantially improve drug coverage for older adults and Medicare-eligible people with disabilities, with particular provisions for low-income Medicare beneficiaries. Preliminary analysis after the first 6 months of implementation indicated that Medicare beneficiaries with the lowest incomes (i.e., those who also qualified for Medicaid) were worse off with the new program. For example, more than half of the people eligible for both Medicare and Medicaid (referred to as "dually eligible") had higher copayments under the new system, and in the future, these higher copayments will affect all dually eligible beneficiaries unless additional legislation is passed (Families USA, 2006).

A larger concern about the Medicare prescription drug coverage is that the program fails to address the rapid and significant increase in the cost of drugs that has been occurring during the past decade. Despite the claim that Medicare Part D would achieve the best discounts on drugs, a comparative analysis of drug prices during 2006 did not support this assertion. In fact, the analysis indicates that the lowest negotiated price for each of the 20 drugs most commonly prescribed under the plan was an average of 58% higher than the lowest price negotiated by the Veterans Administration (Families USA, 2007). In 2007, Congress was considering a bill that would require the federal government to negotiate with the pharmaceutical companies for medication prices on behalf of the companies that provide prescription drug coverage for Medicare beneficiaries.

Concerns also have been raised about complexity of the plan and the need to compare different plans offered by private insurance companies, which vary widely with regard to premiums, specific drugs covered, and amount of coverage.

As an insurance program, Medicare Part D is unique in having three phases of coverage, with an initial phase beginning each year on January 1, and having limits for each phase established by the federal government annually. Beneficiaries pay monthly premiums during all phases, and during the initial phase they pay 25% of the drug costs until they have reached the limit of $2510 (in 2008) in out-of-pocket expenses. During the "doughnut hole" phase, they pay 100% of prescription costs until they reach the limit of $4050 (2008 amount), at which point the insurance coverage resumes and the beneficiary pays only 5% of the costs.

Insufficient Recognition of Adverse Medication Effects

Another problem specific to older adults is that adverse effects are likely to be misinterpreted or not recognized as such because of their similarity to age-related changes or commonly occurring pathologic conditions. Studies have found that nurses and physicians in acute care settings detect only 5% to 15% of ongoing adverse medication effects (Hohl et al., 2001). When an older adult experiences an adverse medication reaction, two or three potential causes other than the medication usually can be identified. The term **prescribing cascade** describes the following scenario that commonly occurs with older adults: an adverse drug reaction is misinterpreted as a new medical condition, a drug is prescribed for this condition, another adverse drug effect occurs, the patient is again treated for the perceived additional medical condition, and the sequence perpetuates new adverse events (Blanda, 2006). Examples of the prescribing cascade include the use of medications for parkinsonism induced by antipsychotics and for hypertension induced by NSAIDs (Petrone & Katz, 2005). Several studies found that the use of antipsychotics is strongly associated not only with the onset of parkinsonism but with the initiation of antiparkinson medications; furthermore, very few patients had their antipsychotic medication evaluated as a potential causative factor (Noyes et al., 2006). Although adverse effects are not unique to older adults, they occur more commonly with increasing age and are more likely to be attributed erroneously to pathologic conditions or age-related changes and circumstances. Table 8-5 summarizes adverse medication effects that are likely to remain unrecognized in older adults because of their similarity to age-related changes.

Wellness Opportunity

Nurses promote wellness when they challenge ageist attitudes and identify adverse effects falsely attributed to aging or pathologic conditions.

TABLE 8-5 Some Adverse Medication Effects That May Remain Unrecognized in Older Adults

Manifestation	Medication Type	Specific Examples
Cognitive impairment	Antidepressants; antipsychotics; antianxiety agents; anticholinergics; hypoglycemics; OTC cold, cough, and sleeping preparations	Perphenazine, amitriptyline, chlorpromazine, diazepam, chlordiazepoxide, benztropine, trihexyphenidyl, cimetidine, digoxin, barbiturates, tolazamide, tolbutamide, chlorpheniramine, diphenhydramine
Depression	Antihypertensives, antiarthritics, antianxiety agents, antipsychotics	Reserpine, clonidine, propranolol, indomethacin, haloperidol, barbiturates
Urinary incontinence	Diuretics, anticholinergics	Furosemide, doxepin, thioridazine, lorazepam
Constipation	Narcotics, antacids, antipsychotics, antidepressants	Codeine, chlorpromazine, calcium carbonate, aluminum hydroxide, amoxapine
Vision impairment	Digitalis, antiarthritics, phenothiazines	Digoxin, indomethacin, ibuprofen, chlorpromazine
Hearing impairment	Mycin antibiotics, salicylates, loop diuretics	Gentamicin, aspirin, furosemide, bumetanide
Postural hypotension	Antihypertensives, diuretics, antipsychotics, antidepressants	Guanethidine, furosemide, propranolol, chlorpromazine, imipramine, clonidine
Hypothermia	Antipsychotics, alcohol, salicylates	Haloperidol, aspirin, alcohol, fluphenazine
Sexual dysfunction	Antihypertensives, antipsychotics, antidepressants, alcohol, antihypertensives	Timolol, clonidine, thiazides, haloperidol, amitriptyline, alcohol, cimetidine, propranolol, methyldopa
Mobility problems	Sedatives, antianxiety agents, antipsychotics, ototoxic medications	Chloral hydrate, diazepam, furosemide, gentamicin
Dry mouth	Anticholinergics, corticosteroids, bronchodilators, antihypertensives	Chlorpromazine, haloperidol, prednisone, furosemide, sertraline, theophylline
Anorexia	Digitalis, bronchodilators, antihistamines	Digoxin, theophylline, diphenhydramine
Drowsiness	Antidepressants, antipsychotics, OTC cold preparations, alcohol, barbiturates	Amitriptyline, haloperidol, chlorpheniramine, secobarbital
Edema	Antiarthritics, corticosteroids, antihypertensives	Ibuprofen, indomethacin, prednisone, reserpine, methyldopa
Tremors	Antipsychotics	Haloperidol, chlorpromazine, thioridazine

OTC, over-the-counter.

MEDICATION INTERACTIONS

Medications can interact with almost any other substance, including other medications, herbs, nutrients, alcohol, caffeine, and nicotine. These interactions occur not only with prescription medications but with commonly used over-the-counter products, including antacids, analgesics, and remedies for coughs, colds, and sleep problems. Outcomes of medication interactions with other substances include altered or erratic therapeutic effect, increased potential for adverse effects, and in rare cases, a decreased potential for adverse effects.

Medication–Medication Interactions

The risk of adverse effects from interactions between two or more medications increases exponentially according to the number of medications being consumed. Because older adults are more likely than younger people to take two or more medications concurrently, they are at increased risk for medication–medication interactions. Medication–medication interactions are often caused by competitive action at binding sites, but they can be caused by any mechanism that influences the absorption, distribution, metabolism, or elimination of any of the medications. Effects of medication–medication interactions include increased or decreased serum levels of either one or both of the medications, with subsequent altered therapeutic effects and increased risk of adverse or toxic effects. Geriatricians and researchers are particularly concerned about interactions with warfarin because of the increasing use of this drug on a long-term basis for prevention of thrombosis by people who also take other medications, including over-the-counter analgesics. A review of almost 200 studies of warfarin found strong evidence of potentially serious interactions with the following medications, which are commonly used by older adults: omeprazole, amiodarone, lipid-lowering agents, selective serotonin reuptake inhibitors, antibiotics (including azoles, macrolides, and quinolones), and NSAIDs (including selective ones) (Holbrook et al., 2005). Table 8-6 summarizes specific mechanisms of medication–medication interactions and examples of each type that are most likely to occur in older adults.

Medications and Herbs

Many medication–herb interactions have been identified in recent years because of the increased use of herbs and increased attention to interactions. Although the more widely recognized medication–herb interactions are sometimes listed in pharmacology references, there is no requirement for identifying or publishing information about these interactions because these products are classified as dietary supplements. In general, herbs should be used very cautiously in combination with anticoagulants and medications for diabetes, and in people with compromised renal or hepatic function. Refer to Table 8-3 for common interactions and precautions regarding herbs.

Medications and Nutrients

Interactions between medications and nutrients can affect either the nutrient or the medication. Because the influence of medications on nutrients is addressed in Chapter 18, this chapter focuses on the effects of nutrients on medications. In the context of medication–nutrient interactions, the term

TABLE 8-6 Types and Examples of Medication–Medication Interactions

Type of Interaction	Example: Interaction	Example: Effect
Binding effect (e.g., an oral drug diminishes the absorption of another drug in the stomach)	Magnesium- or aluminum-containing antacids may bind with tetracycline in the stomach	Decreased effects of tetracycline
Metabolism interference effect (e.g., one drug interferes with liver metabolism of another drug)	Ciprofloxacin and anticonvulsants inhibit metabolism of warfarin	Increased effects of warfarin
Metabolism enhancing effect (e.g., one drug activates the drug-metabolizing enzymes in the liver)	Phenobarbital increases metabolism of warfarin	Decreased effects of warfarin
Elimination interference effect (e.g., one drug interferes with the renal elimination of another drug)	Furosemide can interfere with elimination of salicylates	Increased effects of salicylates
Elimination enhancement effect (e.g., renal reabsorption is blocked because of altered urinary pH)	Sodium bicarbonate can enhance excretion of lithium, tetracyclines, and salicylates	Decreased effects of lithium, tetracycline, or salicylate
Competitive or displacement effect (e.g., two drugs compete at receptor sites)	Diphenhydramine may interfere with effect of cholinergic agents (e.g., tacrine, donepezil)	Decreased effects of tacrine or donepezil
Potentiating effect (e.g., two drugs produce greater effects when taken together even though they have different actions)	Acetaminophen taken with codeine has a greater analgesic effect than either medication taken alone	Increased analgesic effect
Additive effect (e.g., two drugs produce greater effect because they have similar action)	Verapamil or diltiazem may have additive effect when taken with a beta-blocker	Increased effect on blood pressure

nutrient includes foods, beverages, enteral formulas, and dietary supplements. Commonly consumed foods that can affect medications include cocoa, coffee, fiber, alcohol, protein, cabbage, caffeinated tea, and brussels sprouts. In addition, food preparation methods, such as charcoal broiling, can affect certain medications. Medication–nutrient interactions affect people of all ages; however, they are likely to have more serious consequences in older adults because they occur in combination with age-related changes and other risk factors.

A common way that nutrients affect medications is by altering absorption in the stomach through any of the following mechanisms:

- Delayed transit time or slowed gastric emptying
- Competitive binding of molecules
- Diminished stomach secretions

In many situations, the effect of the nutrient is to diminish the absorption of the medication, causing the serum levels to be lower than expected. In other situations, however, the effect on the medication is delayed absorption, which increases the time required to reach peak serum levels, but does not necessarily affect the total amount absorbed. In some situations, delayed gastric emptying increases the amount of medication that is absorbed before it passes into the small intestine. Examples of some common medication–nutrient interactions, including those involving absorption, are listed in Table 8-7.

Medications and Alcohol

Alcohol interacts with medications in the same way as other central nervous system depressants, but because of societal attitudes about alcohol consumption, medication–alcohol interactions often are not addressed. Health care practitioners do not always inquire about a patient's use of alcohol, and even when people are asked, they might not accurately acknowledge the amount of alcohol used. Alcohol is consumed not only in beverages but in over-the-counter preparations, some of which are composed of up to 40% alcohol. Categories of over-the-counter preparations that are most likely to contain alcohol include mouthwashes, vitamin and mineral tonics, and liquid cough and cold preparations. When taken in combination with medications, alcohol can alter the therapeutic action of medications and increase the potential for adverse effects. Older adults may be more susceptible to medication–alcohol interactions because age-related changes in receptor sensitivity and body composition lead to higher serum levels of alcohol than those in a younger person who consumes an equivalent amount of alcohol. In addition, any condition that decreases the secretion of stomach enzymes that metabolize alcohol can increase the concentration of alcohol in the blood. As with other types of interactions, medication–alcohol interactions can alter the effect of either the alcohol or the medication. Table 8-8 lists some of the medication–alcohol interactions that can occur in older adults.

Diversity Note

Physiologically, women are more vulnerable to the toxic effects of alcohol compared with men of the same stature (Ludwick et al., 2000).

TABLE 8-7 Medication–Nutrient Interactions

Effect on Medication	Example of Interaction Effect
Delayed absorption rate, no effect on amount absorbed	Ingestion of food may delay absorption of cimetidine, digoxin, and ibuprofen.
Reduced rate and amount of absorption	Calcium decreases absorption of tetracycline. A high-protein or high-fiber meal decreases absorption of levodopa.
Reduced absorption because of non-nutrient components	Caffeinated tea and fiber intake interfere with iron absorption.
Increased absorption	High-fat foods increase serum levels of griseofulvin.
Decreased therapeutic effect	Vitamin K decreases the effectiveness of warfarin. Charcoal broiling of foods diminishes the effectiveness of aminophylline or theophylline.
Increased rate of metabolism	A high-protein diet increases the metabolism of theophylline.

TABLE 8-8 Medication–Alcohol Interactions

Type of Interaction	Example of Interaction Effect
Altered metabolism of benzodiazepines when combined with alcohol	Increased psychomotor impairment and adverse effects
Altered metabolism of barbiturates and meprobamate when combined with alcohol	Central nervous system depression
Competition between alcohol and chloral hydrate at metabolic sites	Increased serum levels of alcohol and chloral hydrate
Altered metabolism of alcohol when combined with chlorpromazine	Increased serum levels of alcohol and acetaldehyde; increased psychomotor impairment
Enhanced vasodilation as a result of a combination of alcohol and nitrates	Severe hypotension and headache, enhanced absorption of nitroglycerin
Altered hepatic gluconeogenesis, which influences the action of oral hypoglycemics, as a result of alcohol	Potentiation of oral hypoglycemics by alcohol

Medications and Caffeine

Medication–caffeine and medication–nicotine interactions have received little attention, despite the widespread use of caffeine and nicotine and the fact that interactions between these substances and medications can be as harmful as medication–medication interactions. Caffeine is found not only in food and beverages but in many over-the-counter analgesics and cold preparations. Most medication–caffeine interactions affect the action of the medication rather than that of the caffeine; however, a few medications alter caffeine metabolism and increase its serum half-time. Table 8-9 lists examples of medication–caffeine interactions.

Medications and Nicotine

Medication–nicotine interactions can be associated with the use of any nicotine product, including smoking and smokeless tobacco and nicotine substitutes used during smoking cessation. Nicotine can affect medications through any of the following actions: vasoconstriction, stimulation of the central nervous system, increased gastric acid secretions, and altered metabolism of liver enzymes. Most often, the medication–nicotine interaction interferes with the therapeutic action of the medication, and smokers may require higher doses of a medication than nonsmokers to achieve the same therapeutic effects. Studies indicate that smokers may require increased doses of fluvoxamine, imipramine, and clozapine to reach the same therapeutic level as that of nonsmokers (Metz et al., 2004). Prescribing practitioners may need to adjust medication doses not only for smokers, but in cases when the use of nicotine products is discontinued. Table 8-10 lists some common medication–nicotine interactions.

TABLE 8-9 Medication–Caffeine Interactions

Type of Interaction	Example of Interaction Effect
Caffeine-induced increase in gastric acid secretion	Decreased absorption of iron
Caffeine-induced gastrointestinal irritation	Decreased effectiveness of cimetidine; increased gastrointestinal irritation from corticosteroids, alcohol, and analgesics
Altered caffeine metabolism	Prolonged effect of caffeine when combined with ciprofloxacin, estrogen, or cimetidine
Caffeine-induced cardiac arrhythmic effect	Decreased effectiveness of antiarrhythmic medications
Caffeine-induced hypokalemia	Exacerbated hypokalemic effect of diuretics
Caffeine-induced stimulation of the central nervous system	Increased stimulation effects from amantadine, decongestants, fluoxetine, and theophylline
Caffeine-induced increase in excretion of lithium	Decreased effectiveness of lithium

TABLE 8-10 Medication–Nicotine Interactions

Type of Interaction	Example of Interaction Effect
Nicotine-induced alteration in metabolism	Decreased efficacy of analgesics, lorazepam, theophylline, aminophylline, beta-blockers, and calcium channel blockers
Nicotine-induced vasoconstriction	Increased peripheral ischemic effect of beta-blockers
Nicotine-induced central nervous system stimulation	Decreased drowsiness from benzodiazepines and phenothiazines
Nicotine-induced stimulation of antidiuretic hormone secretion	Fluid retention, decreased effectiveness of diuretics
Nicotine-induced increase in platelet activity	Decreased anticoagulant effectiveness (heparin, warfarin); increased risk of thrombosis with estrogen use
Nicotine-induced increase in gastric acid	Decreased or negated effects of H_2 antagonists (cimetidine, famotidine, nizatidine, ranitidine)

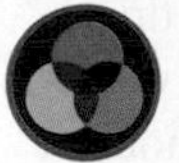

FUNCTIONAL CONSEQUENCES ASSOCIATED WITH BIOACTIVE SUBSTANCES IN OLDER ADULTS

The major functional consequence affecting bioactive agents in healthy older adults who take only one substance is an increased potential for both altered therapeutic action and adverse effects. Older adults who take more than one substance or have other risk factors are likely to have additional functional consequences, such as medication interactions with other substances. Age-related changes and risk factors also affect consumption patterns, increasing the possibility of nonadherence and the potential for adverse and altered therapeutic effects.

Altered Therapeutic Effects

Age-related changes alone can alter the therapeutic action of some substances; however, most of the altered therapeutic effects that occur in older adults are caused by risk factors, such as polypharmacy. Consequently, the therapeutic effectiveness of substances is less predictable, even in healthy older adults. The main implication is that bioactive agents need to be monitored more closely in older adults, especially initially and when there is any change in the person's medical status or treatment regimen. Thus, the commonly accepted principle for geriatric drug prescribing is "start low and go slow."

Increased Potential for Adverse Effects

Adverse medication effects are the unintended and undesired outcomes of a medication that occur in doses used in humans for prophylaxis, diagnosis, or therapy (Blanda, 2006). Consequences of adverse drug effects include a decline in function, an increased risk for falls and fractures, an increased number of visits for health care services, admission to a hospital or prolongation of a hospital stay, and death. There is much agreement that adverse medication effects occur commonly, have serious consequences, and frequently are avoidable. These conclusions are supported by research findings such as the following:

- Older adults are twice as likely as younger adults to experience adverse outcomes from medications (Beyth & Shorr, 2002).
- Thirty-five percent of community-residing older adults experience adverse medication effects on a yearly basis, and 29% require medical evaluation (Petrone & Katz, 2005).
- A study of more than 30,000 Medicare enrollees in an ambulatory clinical setting found that 28% of the adverse medication events were considered preventable, and 38% were categorized as serious, life-threatening, or fatal (Gurwitz et al., 2003).
- A 9-month record review of residents in two long-term care facilities found an overall rate of 9.8 adverse drug events per 100 residents per month; 42% of those were considered preventable and 28% were deemed serious or life-threatening (Gurwitz et al., 2005).
- Between 3% and 28% of hospital admissions are attributed to drug-related problems or toxic drug effects (Blanda, 2006).
- Between 7% and 11% of all emergency department visits by older adults are a result of adverse medication effects (Hohl et al., 2001).
- If ranked as a disease, adverse medication reactions would be the fifth leading cause of death in the United States (Petrone & Katz, 2005).

A study of long-term care residents identified the following most common types of adverse medication effects: hemorrhage, mental status changes (e.g., confusion, delirium, hallucinations, somnolence), gastrointestinal conditions (e.g., diarrhea, constipation, impaction, abdominal pain), electrolyte imbalances (e.g., azotemia, dehydration, hyperkalemia, hypokalemia), and metabolic or endocrine conditions (e.g., hypoglycemia, thyroid dysfunction) (Gurwitz et al., 2005).

Box 8-5 lists some of the characteristics of people who are at high risk for altered medication effects.

Several aspects of adverse medication effects are particularly important for the care of older adults. As discussed in the section on Risk Factors (and listed in Table 8-5), adverse effects may not be recognized as such because they are similar to the manifestations of pathologic conditions or they are mistakenly attributed to aging. Three concerns of particular importance are anticholinergic toxicity, changes in mental status, and tardive dyskinesia.

Box 8-5
Factors That Increase the Risk for Adverse Medication Effects

- Inclusion of several medications in the drug regimen
- Debilitated or frail state
- Malnourishment or dehydration
- Multiple illnesses
- An illness that interferes with cardiac, renal, or hepatic function
- Cognitive impairment
- Medication allergy
- History of adverse medication effects
- Exposure to certain environmental chemicals
- Fever, which can alter the action of certain medications
- Recent change in health or functional status (e.g., as a result of an accident, surgery, mental changes, or insertion of a nasogastric tube)

Anticholinergic Toxicity

In recent years, geriatricians have increasingly recognized that older adults are particularly susceptible to the anticholinergic action of many medications, including several that are not specifically designated as anticholinergic agents. Many over-the-counter agents commonly used for coughs, colds, and sleep problems contain anticholinergic ingredients. In fact, all nonprescription antihistamines have potent anticholinergic actions that can be even stronger than those of some prescription drugs (Fick et al., 2003). Anticholinergic toxicity also can occur from systemic absorption of commonly used ophthalmic agents such as mydriatics and cycloplegics (Marti et al., 2005). The types of medications with anticholinergic properties include antidepressants, antihistamines, antiparkinson agents, antipsychotics, cardiovascular agents, gastrointestinal agents, and urinary antispasmodics (see Box 8-6 for examples).

Older adults are likely to experience the usual adverse effects of anticholinergic agents (e.g., constipation, dry mouth, urinary retention, fecal impaction), even from drugs that have weak anticholinergic activity (Terrell et al., 2006). Additional adverse effects that are likely to occur in older adults include delirium, seizures, hallucinations, agitation, heart block, cardiac arrhythmias, and impaired thermoregulation (Blanda, 2006). Studies indicate that anticholinergic agents can impair cognition not only in older adults, but even in healthy young adults (Ancelin et al., 2006). Geriatricians and researchers are particularly concerned about the effects of anticholinergic agents in people with dementia because they have lower levels of acetylcholine in the brain. This concern is warranted because studies have found that the adverse effects of anticholinergic agents become worse as the dementia progresses (Chew et al., 2005). A related concern is that anticholinergics counteract the effects of cholinesterase inhibitors, which are used as a primary treatment for dementia. Despite the evidence that this combination is inappropriate, one study of 557 Medicaid beneficiaries found that 35%

Box 8-6
Examples of Medications With Anticholinergic Effects

Antidepressants
amitriptyline
doxepin
nefazodone
trazodone

Antihistamines
chlorpheniramine
diphenhydramine
fexofenadine
hydroxyzine
loratadine
meclizine
promethazine

Antiparkinson Agents
benztropine
trihexyphenidyl

Antipsychotics
chlorpromazine
clozapine
fluphenazine
haloperidol
prochlorperazine
promethazine
thioridazine
triflupromazine

Cardiovascular Agents
captopril
digoxin
dipyridamole
isosorbide dinitrate
nifedipine

Gastrointestinal Agents
belladonna
cimetidine
dicyclomine
hyoscyamine
ranitidine

Urinary Antispasmodics
oxybutynin

Miscellaneous Agents
furosemide
meclizine
prednisolone
theophylline
warfarin

of people had concurrent prescriptions for cholinesterase inhibitors and anticholinergics (Carnahan et al., 2004).

Because older adults are particularly vulnerable to anticholinergic effects and because many medications have anticholinergic properties, geriatricians are emphasizing the importance of assessing the **total anticholinergic burden**, which is the cumulative effect of medications that have anticholinergic effect. The **serum anticholinergic activity** is used in research and clinical practice to assess the cumulative effect of anticholinergic medications in the body (Carnahan et al., 2006).

Altered Mental Status

Although medications can cause mental changes in anyone, older adults are at increased risk for medication-induced altered mental status because of age-related changes and risk factors. In addition, when older adults experience changes in their mental status, these changes are likely to be attributed to dementia or another pathologic condition, rather than being recognized as adverse medication effects. Nurses need to be alert to the possibility that even a simple over-the-counter product such as diphenhydramine is a common cause of mental changes in older adults.

Delirium is an acute confusional state that can be precipitated by any medication or by medication interactions (refer to Chapter 14 for further discussion of delirium). Older adults are particularly susceptible to medication-induced delirium because of altered neurochemical activity in the brain. Moreover, some pathologic conditions (e.g., dementia, dehydration, malnutrition, head injury, or central nervous system infection) can increase the risk for medication-induced delirium. Even at nontoxic serum levels, or at doses considered normal, medications can cause mental changes in older adults. It is important to keep in mind that medication-induced mental changes do not always subside immediately after the offending medication is discontinued. In some cases, it may take several weeks or even months after the medication is decreased or discontinued for mental function to return to the premedication level. Some medications that are likely to cause mental changes in older adults, as well as the mechanisms underlying these adverse actions, are listed in Table 8-11.

Tardive Dyskinesia

Tardive dyskinesia refers to a constellation of rhythmic and involuntary movements of any of the following: the trunk and extremities; and the jaw, lips, mouth, and tongue (referred to as oro-buccal-lingual). The earliest signs are usually fine, wormlike movements of the tongue. Other early signs include chewing, grimacing, lip smacking, jaw clenching, eye blinking, and side-to-side jaw movements. Studies have concluded that tardive dyskinesia is caused by medications that block dopamine receptors in the brain, such as antipsychotics (Chou & Friedman, 2006). The strong association between tardive dyskinesia and the so-called "first-generation antipsychotics" (e.g., haloperidol and thioridazine) spurred more recent development of the so-called "atypical antipsychotics," which include clozapine, risperidone, olanzapine, quetiapine, amisulpride, and ziprasidone. Some

TABLE 8-11 Mechanisms of Action for Mental Changes Caused by Adverse Medication Effects

Mechanism of Action	Examples
Anticholinergic effects	Atropine, scopolamine, antihistamines, antipsychotics, antidepressants, antispasmodics, antiparkinsonian agents
Decreased cerebral blood flow	Antihypertensives, antipsychotics
Depression of respiratory center	Central nervous system depressants
Fluid and electrolyte alterations	Diuretics, alcohol, laxatives
Altered thermoregulation	Alcohol, psychotropics, narcotics
Acidosis	Diuretics, alcohol, nicotinic acid
Hypoglycemia	Hypoglycemics, alcohol, propranolol
Hormonal disturbances	Thyroid extract, corticosteroids
Depression-inducing action	Reserpine, methyldopa, indomethacin, barbiturates, fluphenazine, haloperidol, corticosteroids

studies suggest that the newer antipsychotics reduce the risk of tardive dyskinesia (Chou & Friedman, 2006). However, other studies have found that older adults with dementia are likely to experience tardive dyskinesia and other drug-induced movement disorders as a result of any type of antipsychotic (Lee et al., 2005).

Manifestations can begin as early as 3 to 6 months after initiation of antipsychotic medications, and they persist even after the causative agent is discontinued. Tardive dyskinesia deserves special attention with regard to older adults for the following reasons:

- For people taking antipsychotic medications, prevalence ranges from approximately 35% of community-residing older adults to more than 80% of institutionalized older adults (Chou & Friedman, 2006).
- Advanced age correlates with both an earlier onset and increased severity of tardive dyskinesia.
- The chance of reversing tardive dyskinesia decreases with increasing age.
- When combined with age-related changes and risk factors, tardive dyskinesia can seriously impair the older adult's ability to perform activities of daily living (ADLs).
- The risk of tardive dyskinesia can be eliminated by avoiding the use of antipsychotics when nonpharmaceutical therapies could be effective, as with behavioral and psychological symptoms of dementia.

Diversity Note

Female sex and African American race are possible risk factors for tardive dyskinesia (Chou & Friedman, 2006).

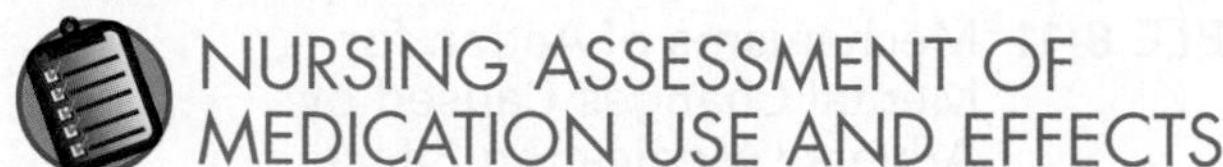

NURSING ASSESSMENT OF MEDICATION USE AND EFFECTS

Nurses assess medication regimens and medication-taking behaviors of older adults to accomplish the following:

- Determine the effectiveness of the medication regimen
- Identify any factors that interfere with the correct regimen
- Ascertain risks for adverse effects or altered therapeutic actions (with particular attention to older adults at increased risk)
- Detect adverse medication effects
- Identify teaching needs with regard to medications

During a medication assessment, nurses should clarify the prescribed medication regimen and identify actual medication-taking behaviors so that they can assess for adherence.

Communication Techniques for Obtaining Accurate Information

Some of the many barriers to obtaining accurate information about medications and medication-taking behaviors include time limitations, complex medication regimens, and lack of a trusting relationship. Because medication assessments often are very time-consuming, and because the older adult may not think of all the information during the first interview or may initially be reluctant to reveal accurate information, it may be necessary to conduct the medication assessment over the course of two or more visits. In addition, older adults may be reluctant to answer questions about their medications because they perceive this information, including information about the use of alcohol, as being very private. Many older adults have learned not to ask questions about their health care because they are unsure of what to ask or they falsely believe that they are not entitled to medical information. Although most older adults appreciate the opportunity to discuss medications with a nurse, they initially may hesitate to ask questions or share information. Some of this reluctance may be caused by fear of being judged, especially if the prescribed regimen is not being followed exactly, or if the person uses folk remedies, alternative therapies, or over-the-counter medications. When people do not follow the medication regimen exactly as prescribed, they are likely to recite the orders rather than describe their actual medication-taking behaviors. Another factor that contributes to this reluctance is anxiety about discussing the underlying reason for not following the regime. For example, older adults who cannot afford medications may be embarrassed to discuss their limited finances.

Nurses can address the barriers by asking open-ended questions in a matter-of-fact way and conveying a nonjudgmental attitude during the medication interview. They should also keep in mind that they need to elicit information about the use of herbs, folk remedies, over-the-counter preparations, and complementary and alternative care practices. For example, "What do you do to help you sleep?" is more open-ended than "Do you take any medications for sleep?" because the latter may be interpreted only in relation to prescription medications. Another interview technique is to use leading questions related to potential risk factors that interfere with the older person's ability to take medications accurately. For example, because the high cost of medications is a commonly acknowledged problem, nurses can ask a question such as "I know that some of these medications that are prescribed for you can be quite expensive; do you have any problems with getting them?" Similarly, asking a question such as "I know you don't drive—are you able to have your medications delivered, or do you have someone who helps you get them from the pharmacy?" may elicit information about transportation barriers.

Nurses should ask additional questions about the person's ability to take his or her medications as prescribed based on specific observations. For example, if a nurse observes that a pill is very large, a question such as "Do you have any trouble swallowing these capsules?" might be appropriate. Similarly, if the nurse knows that the older adult has limited hand strength, an appropriate assessment question would be "Do you have any difficulty getting the caps off your medication bottles?" Another technique for eliciting information is to ask about the person's method of organizing medications. For example, people taking medications often have a method of organizing their regimen by using divided medication boxes or written charts or schedules. They usually are willing to show this organizational system to the nurse and, in fact, may be proud to discuss their method with the nurse during the medication assessment.

Scope of a Medication Assessment

Medication assessments include information about all of the following:

- Prescription and over-the-counter medications, used orally and by all other routes (e.g., nasal, aural, topical, optical, injectable, dermal methods)
- Medications that are used only sporadically, or as needed
- Vitamins, minerals, and dietary supplements (including doses and frequency)
- Alcohol, caffeine, nicotine
- Folk remedies and complementary and alternative medicines, including all herbal products and homeopathic remedies

Information about doses of vitamins and minerals is important because megavitamins can be harmful, and even low doses can have adverse effects (e.g., iron or calcium carbonate can be constipating). Information about the brand names of over-the-counter medications can help identify additives that may be causing problems or increasing the risk of altered medication action (e.g., analgesics with caffeine, antacids with lactose, or bronchodilators with sulfites). Information about folk remedies and complementary and alternative health care practices can help identify health beliefs that affect adherence and other aspects of medication-taking behaviors.

Nurses also need to assess the person's understanding of the purpose of medications; doing so provides information about his or her understanding of health status and medical conditions. As with other parts of the medication assessment, it is essential to phrase questions in as open-ended and nonjudgmental a manner as possible. Asking "What do you take this pill for?" with a tone of curiosity will likely elicit more information than asking questions such as, "What do you take for your heart?" or "Why do you take digoxin?"

Obtaining information about allergies and adverse reactions is essential because anyone with a history of medication-related problems will need to be closely monitored, especially if the medications being administered are similar to those that caused the reaction. Sometimes people state that they are allergic to a medication, but when they are asked about the symptoms, they describe an adverse effect, rather than an allergic reaction. Therefore, rather than simply documenting that the person is allergic to a certain medication, nurses should document the specific reaction that occurred. Nurses can use Box 8-7 as a guide to assessing medications regimens and medication-taking behaviors.

Nurses should also obtain and document information about the person's perception of and preferences for various forms of medications because this information can influence prescribing decisions, especially when there are several options that may be equally effective. Similarly, nurses should identify any cultural factors that might influence

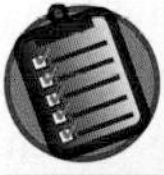

Box 8-7
Guidelines for Medication Assessment

Information About the Therapeutic Agents

- Prescription pills, liquids, injections, eye drops, ear drops, nasal sprays, transdermal methods, and topical preparations
- Over-the-counter preparations (identified by brand names) that are used regularly or occasionally
- Vitamins, minerals, and nutritional supplements
- Pattern of alcohol, caffeine, or tobacco use
- Herbs and herbal preparations
- Homeopathic remedies
- Home folk remedies
- Sources of health care

Interview Questions to Assess Medication-Taking Behaviors

- How would you describe your usual daily routine for taking medications and remedies, beginning when you get up in the morning?
- Is there anything else you do or use to treat illness or to maintain your health, such as using herbs, ointments, home remedies, or nutritional supplements?
- Are you taking anyone else's medications?
- What do you do when you miss a dose of medication?
- What do you take for constipation? What do you do to help you sleep (or to alleviate any other identified problem)?
- How do you get your prescriptions filled? (Where do you get your remedies?)
- Do you have any difficulty taking your pills?
- What method do you use to keep track of your medications and remedies?
- Is there anything you do to help you remember to take your medicines or remedies at the appropriate time?

Interview Questions to Assess the Person's Understanding of the Purpose of Medications and Other Remedies

- What is this medication (or herb, etc.) for?
- For medications (or remedies) that are used as needed (PRN): How do you decide when to take this pill (or remedy)?
- What did your health care practitioner tell you about this medication (or herb, etc.)?
- What problems were you having when the health care practitioner prescribed this medication (or suggested that you use this remedy)?

(continued on following page)

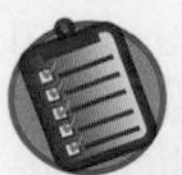

Box 8-7
Guidelines for Medication Assessment (continued)

Interview Questions to Elicit Additional Information

- Are there any medications or remedies you were taking at one time but are no longer taking?
- Have you ever had an allergic reaction, or any other bad reaction, to a medication or remedy? (If yes, describe what happened.)
- Where do you store your medications and remedies?

Questions and Observations Based on Reading of Prescription Labels

- Who is the prescribing health care practitioner?
- If there is more than one health care practitioner, does each practitioner know all the medications that are being used?
- Are any medications the same or similar and prescribed by different health care practitioners?
- If the dates on various prescriptions are different, were the later medications supposed to be added to the medication regimen, or were they intended to replace previously prescribed medications?
- Are the date of the last refill and the number of pills in the bottle consistent with the prescribed regimen?

medication-taking behaviors. For example, according to some Asian traditions, illness is perceived as an imbalance of hot and cold forces. If the illness makes the body hot, then the remedy should make it cooler. Cultural Considerations 8-1 lists some cultural factors that are pertinent to a medication assessment.

Another component of a comprehensive medication assessment is obtaining information about various sources of health care. This information is particularly important when someone receives care from more than one health care practitioner, as is often the case with older adults. Nurses can ask nonjudgmentally about whether the person receives care from non-Western health care practitioners, such as herbalists, spiritual healers, naturopathic practitioners, or Ayurvedic doctors. Cultural Considerations 8-2 summarizes some culturally specific sources of health care and treatment modalities that older adults might use.

Cultural Considerations 8-1

Cultural Considerations With Regard to Medication Assessment and Interventions

- Medications that are not readily available or that are available by prescription only in the United States may be available over the counter in other countries, such as Mexico, Canada, and Latin American countries.
- Older Hispanic people may view wine and other forms of alcohol as a food staple, not a social drug, because they may be used as a healthy alternative to potentially contaminated water in their home country.
- People of Vietnamese and other cultural groups may view injections as being more effective than pills, and pills as being more effective than drops.
- Some Chinese and other Asian people may have the following preferences:
  - Balms and ointments rather than pills for local pain
  - Teas and soups rather than antacids for indigestion
  - Herbs rather than prescription drugs
- Teaching about medications should be done in the context of culturally based beliefs about health, illness, and remedies.

Wellness Opportunity

Nurses promote personal responsibility for health by encouraging discussion of various sources of care.

Observing Patterns of Medication Use

In addition to using good communication techniques, nurses obtain essential assessment information by reviewing the person's array of medications. When nurses conduct the medication assessment in the home setting, they can ask to see all the medications that the older person uses. In settings other than the home, the nurse can ask the older adult ahead of time to bring in all of his or her medications. In community settings, nurses might sponsor a "brown bag" medication review session. Program participants are asked to bring all their medications to an educational session, during which the nurse provides group education and individual assessment and counseling regarding the medications. Because older people often are very comfortable discussing medications with their peers, this method is both nonthreatening and quite effective.

Direct observation of medication containers provides useful information about adherence, dates of original prescription and refills, duplication of similar medications, and pharmaceutical treatments for pathologic conditions. For example, if three types of antihypertensive medications have been prescribed at different times, the nurse can inquire whether the second or third medication was supposed to replace or supplement the original medication. Nurses can also assess whether the bottles contain the original medications, and ask additional questions when the contents are not consistent with expectations. For example, if the label indicates that the original prescription was for 30 pills, but it has not been refilled for 1 year, the nurse might inquire about the reason. Patients may explain that they cannot afford the prescription or they cannot manipulate the childproof lid.

Cultural Considerations 8-2

Culturally Specific Health Care Sources and Practices

Cultural Group	Sources of Care*	Health Practices*
African Americans	Home remedies, faith and root healers (herbalists)	Folk remedies (e.g., teas, herbs); magic or voodoo (especially in rural areas)
Native Americans/ Alaskan Natives	Native practitioners	Roots, herbs, physical modalities (e.g., purification rituals), sacred objects
Cambodians (Khmer)	Vietnamese or Cambodian practitioners	Herbs, medicated strips of adhesive tape, and physical modalities
Chinese	Herbalists, acupuncturists	Herbs, food, beverages, and other remedies to balance yin and yang
East Indians	Homeopathic or Ayurvedic doctors, spiritual healers	Yoga, diet, fasting, prayer, rituals
Japanese	Herbalists	Herbs, prayer at temple, church, or small shrines at home
Mexicans	Folk healer (*curandero*) or spiritualist (*espirituista*)	Herbs, teas, soups, rituals, physical modalities (massage, manipulation), prayer, candles
Puerto Ricans	Healers (*espiritistas* and *santeros*)	Tea, herbs, folk remedies, liquid astringent
Russians	Folk remedies	Herbal teas, sweet liquor, physical modalities (oils, ointments, enemas, mud baths)

*In the United States, Western practitioners and medicine often are used in conjunction with these sources of care and health practices.

From Lipson, J. G., & Dibble, S. L. (2005). *Culture & clinical care*. San Francisco: UCSF Nursing Press.

Another purpose for examining medication containers is to discover information about sources of care and duplication of medications. It is not unusual to find that patients are getting prescriptions from more than one health care practitioner. Sometimes patients have the same or similar medications from different sources or under more than one name (e.g., generic and brand names).

Linking the Medication Assessment to the Overall Assessment

The nurse uses information from the medication interview in conjunction with the overall health assessment in several ways. First, information about past and present medication patterns can provide clues to identified problems or complaints. For example, if the person complains of nervousness or difficulty sleeping, the nurse can inquire about the use of caffeine-containing medications. Information about recent medication-taking behaviors can also shed light on current problems, such as the recurrence of symptoms that once were controlled by medications. For example, if someone stopped taking an antiarrhythmic medication, symptoms of dizziness may be a result. Recent medication-taking behaviors also may account for health problems that are residual or latent adverse medication effects. Examples of residual adverse effects include diarrhea occurring after a course of antibiotics and gastrointestinal symptoms arising from the administration of anti-inflammatory medications.

Second, nurses use the overall health assessment as a base of information to determine the expected and actual outcomes of medications. These outcomes are evaluated through subjective and objective assessment information. For example, analgesic effectiveness is measured according to reported level of pain relief, and the effectiveness of antihypertensive medications is judged according to lowered blood pressure readings.

Third, the overall assessment, including functional aspects, helps answer the question "*Can the person or caregivers safely and effectively administer medications?*" This complex question involves an assessment of all aspects of medication-taking behaviors, as described in the section on Age-Related Changes and Risk Factors. The environment also should be assessed in relation to certain conditions, such as the accessibility of water and the availability of a refrigerator (if necessary for medication storage), that can affect medication-taking behaviors. The overall assessment also might provide information about financial limitations, mobility, or transportation problems that interfere with obtaining medications.

Fourth, if the home environment can be observed as part of the overall assessment, important clues to health problems and medication-taking behaviors may be disclosed. For example, observing that nitroglycerin is stored on a window sill may explain why the medication is not effective in relieving angina. An assessment of the home environment also may lead to additional pertinent information, such as when the nurse notices over-the-counter preparations and folk remedies in a conspicuous place and asks about these items.

Finally, the overall health assessment serves as the basis for identifying the many factors that can increase the risk for nonadherence, altered therapeutic effects, and adverse medication effects. For example, the nursing assessment of the older adult's cognitive abilities and abilities to perform daily activities provides valuable information about factors that can significantly influence medication-taking behaviors. Similarly, the nursing assessment of depression and other psychosocial aspects of functioning can provide important information about motivational and behavioral factors that can influence medication-taking behaviors.

Identifying Adverse Medication Effects

The first, and sometimes most difficult, step in alleviating adverse medication effects is to recognize their existence. Because many adverse effects are subtle and superimposed on one or more symptoms of illness, they often are attributed to pathologic conditions rather than to the treatment of the condition. Nurses often are the first to recognize adverse medication effects because they generally spend more time with patients than do primary care practitioners. Nurses also are more attentive to long-term monitoring of changes in day-to-day function, in contrast to the medical practitioner's focus on acute illness. Especially in long-term care and home settings, the nurse is the health professional most likely to notice subtle changes in function that may be attributable to adverse medication effects.

Health care practitioners may hesitate to discuss adverse medication effects with patients for any of the following reasons: (1) they may be uncertain about the potential adverse effects of a prescribed drug, especially when newer medications are prescribed; (2) they may assume that the power of suggesting possible adverse effects will become a self-fulfilling prophecy; or (3) they may fear that the patient will choose not to take the medication. The nurse can serve as an "interpreter" between the prescribing practitioner and the patient by emphasizing the medication's benefits, as well as pointing out the problems that are most likely to arise. The nurse also can provide health education about ways to avoid adverse effects. For example, if a medication is likely to cause stomach irritation, taking the medication after meals or with milk may prevent this effect. Nurses do not automatically initiate a discussion of all the potential adverse effects of a medication, but when a change in health status is potentially related to adverse medication effects, nurses can raise that possibility.

Changes in mental status are a potentially devastating adverse medication effect that is often overlooked as such, especially when superimposed on existing dementia. Medication-induced mental status changes (e.g., confusion, lethargy, depression, or agitation) can be sudden and obvious, or subtle and gradual. For example, delirium or hallucinations usually are very obvious, but they may be attributed mistakenly to pathologic processes rather than to medication effects. Thus, whenever an older person experiences an alteration in mental status, medication intake must be assessed carefully. In addition to considering all prescription drugs, alcohol and over-the-counter medications (especially those with anticholinergic agents) must be considered as potential contributing factors. When medications are a potential cause of altered mental status, consideration must be given to discontinuing or lowering the dose of the medication. Assessment also addresses the possibility that the altered mental state interferes with proper dosing (e.g., when memory impairment contributes to overdosing or underdosing). Another aspect of assessing the relationship between mental changes and medications is to recognize that it may take days or even months after discontinuation of the medication before the mental status returns to baseline. The resolution time depends on the particular medication involved, the length of time it was consumed, and the person's general health status.

NURSING DIAGNOSIS

When the nursing assessment identifies factors that interfere with safe and accurate medication self-administration (e.g., cognitive or functional impairments affecting medication-taking ability), an applicable nursing diagnosis is Instrumental Self-Care Deficit. This term is defined as "a state in which the individual experiences an impaired ability to perform certain activities or access certain services essential for managing a household" (Carpenito-Moyet, 2006, p. 789).

The nursing diagnosis of Noncompliance is defined as "the state in which an individual or group desires to comply but factors are present that deter adherence to agreed-upon health-related advice given by health professionals" (Carpenito-Moyet, 2006, p. 290). Related factors that might be identified include complex medication regimens, inadequate social supports, adverse effects of medication(s), lack of money or transportation, and lack of understanding of instructions.

If the nursing assessment identifies adverse effects of medications, particularly those that affect one's safety or quality of life, the nurse might address these through a nursing diagnosis that is specific to the adverse effect. Examples of these diagnoses include Confusion, Constipation, Urinary Incontinence, Imbalanced Nutrition, Impaired Memory, Ineffective Thermoregulation, Sexual Dysfunction, Sleep Pattern Disturbance, Impaired Physical Mobility, and Risk for Injury because of medication-related falls and postural hypotension. These nursing diagnoses are discussed in other chapters of this text.

Wellness Opportunity

Nurses can use the wellness nursing diagnosis of Readiness for Enhanced Therapeutic Regimen Management when caring for older adults who are interested in addressing potential adverse effects.

PLANNING FOR WELLNESS OUTCOMES

Wellness outcomes pertinent to medications and older adults include Adherence to Therapeutic Regimens and Identification and Prevention of Adverse Effects. Nurses can use any of the following Nursing Outcomes Classification (NOC) terminology in their care plans: Compliance Behavior, Health Promoting Behaviors, Knowledge: Medication, Medication Response, Risk Detection, and Self-Care: Non-Parenteral Medication.

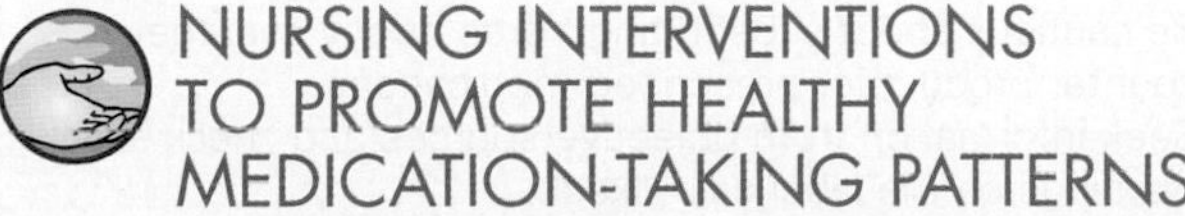

Participation in Health Care Decisions is an outcome that is applicable when nurses empower older adults to make responsible decisions about the use of over-the-counter products, such as herbs and medications.

NURSING INTERVENTIONS TO PROMOTE HEALTHY MEDICATION-TAKING PATTERNS

Nursing interventions for older adults who are taking medications focus on teaching about both the therapeutic and potential adverse effects and on addressing any factors that interfere with adherence to the therapeutic regimen. In addition, when appropriate, nurses teach older adults how to communicate with prescribing practitioners, and they provide information about the use of other bioactive substances, such as herbs and homeopathic remedies. Nurses can consider using any of the following Nursing Interventions Classification (NIC) terminology in care plans: Health Education, Medication Management, Risk Identification, Self-Care Assistance: IADL, and Teaching: Prescribed Medication.

Teaching About Medications

Medications are safest and most therapeutic when they are taken as prescribed and when the regimen is periodically reevaluated for maximum effectiveness and minimal risk of adverse reactions. Because most community-living older adults take medications with little advice or supervision from health care practitioners, health education about medications that addresses all prescription and nonprescription agents is an important and effective intervention for promoting responsible medication-taking behaviors (Neafsey & Shellman, 2002).

An easy and nonthreatening way to initiate health education about medications is to have the person write a list of all medications and over-the-counter agents taken, and to list the history of medication allergies and adverse effects. Nurses can emphasize that this information should be available to health care practitioners during all interactions because it is a convenient way of keeping track of the person's medications. This list is especially important when more than one health care practitioner is involved. Nurses should explain that a medication list facilitates communication and reminds the health care practitioner periodically to reevaluate the medication regimen. Nurses can discuss each medication on the list and provide appropriate information based on assessment of the person's knowledge and understanding.

Because older adults may be reluctant to question their health care practitioners, nurses can suggest pertinent questions for discussion with prescribing practitioners. In addition, nurses can teach older adults and their caregivers about obtaining medication-related information from knowledgeable sources, such as pharmacists. People need to understand that prescribing practitioners are skilled in diagnosing illnesses and deciding the most appropriate interventions, and that pharmacists are the health care practitioners who are most knowledgeable about the specific actions and interactions of medications. Nurses can use Box 8-8 to teach older adults about which medication questions are best answered by prescribing practitioners and which are best addressed by pharmacists.

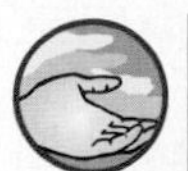

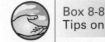

Box 8-8
Tips on Safe and Effective Medication Use

- Carry an up-to-date list of all your medications, including herbs and over-the-counter preparations, and show the list to your health care practitioner(s).
- When your health care practitioner suggests a medication, ask if there is any way to take care of the problem without medication.
- Ask your health care practitioner the following questions about each new, regularly scheduled medication:
  - What is the reason for taking the medication?
  - How will I know if it's doing what it's meant to do?
  - How soon can I expect to feel the beneficial effects?
  - What will happen if I don't take it?
  - How often am I supposed to take it?
  - How long should I continue taking it?
  - What should I do if I miss a dose?
  - When will you want to see me again, and what will you want me to tell you so that you can determine whether the medication is effective?
- Ask your health care practitioner the following questions at follow-up visits:
  - Do I still need to take this medication?
  - Can the dosage be reduced?
- Ask your health care practitioner the following questions about each medication that is prescribed on an "as-needed" (PRN) basis:
  - What is the reason for taking the medication, and how should I determine whether I need the medication?
  - How often can I take it? Is there a range of frequency?
  - What is the maximum dose I can take within 24 hours?
  - What should I do if the medication does not relieve the symptoms (e.g., if chest pain continues after taking several nitroglycerin tablets)?
- Ask your pharmacist the following questions:
  - What are the generic and brand names for this medication?
  - Is it likely to interact with the other medications I'm taking?
  - Is it likely to interact with herbs, cigarettes, alcohol, or any nutrient?
  - What is the best time of day to take it?
  - Does it matter if I take it before or after meals?
  - Are there any side effects I should watch for?
  - Is there anything I can do to minimize the risk of side effects (e.g., taking the medication with milk or meals to reduce stomach irritation)?
  - Is there anything I should avoid while I'm taking this medication (e.g., milk, certain foods, driving)?
  - Are there any special instructions for storing this medication?

Because good communication skills are essential to obtaining answers to the questions listed in Box 8-8, nurses can suggest ways of communicating effectively with pharmacists and other health care practitioners. For example, nurses can help older adults develop a list of questions about specific medications that they can discuss with pharmacists or health care practitioners. In home settings, nurses can serve as role models of appropriate communication by calling the pharmacist or prescribing practitioner to discuss medications in the presence of the older adult or caregiver.

Wellness Opportunity

Nurses find opportunities to empower older adults by teaching them effective ways of communicating with health care providers so that they can knowledgeably observe for therapeutic and adverse medication effects.

Teaching About Herbs and Other Bioactive Substances

As discussed in the Assessment section, nurses need to ask about the use of herbs and other bioactive substances so that they can observe for and teach about interactions and adverse effects, when appropriate. Although nurses are expected to ask if their patients are using complementary and alternative therapies, they are not expected to know all the details about all products and therapies. At a minimum, however, they need to educate health care consumers about these remedies, just as they teach about pharmacologic and medical interventions. Nurses can use Box 8-9 as a tool to teach their patients about general precautions, such as being aware of potential interactions and adverse effects and making sure that all health care practitioners are aware of all over-the-counter products (including herbs and dietary supplements) that are used.

Another important nursing role—and a way of promoting personal responsibility—is teaching patients about reliable sources of information on which they can base decisions about self-care practices. The National Institutes of Health (NIH) established an Office of Alternative Medicine to fund research and provide evidence-based information about complementary and alternative practices. Nurses can keep up to date on developments and find reliable information that is pertinent to the care of older adults by periodically checking the NIH website at www.nccam.gov. In addition, the FDA web site (www.fda.gov) provides a wealth of evidence-based information about prescription and over-the-counter products, and also publishes a consumer-oriented guide to evaluating internet-based health information.

Box 8-9
Tips on the Use of Herbs and Homeopathic Remedies

- Before treating any symptom with a nonprescription product, make sure you are not overlooking a condition that requires medical attention.
- Discuss the use of any nonprescription product with your primary health care provider(s).
- Be cautious about substituting herbs or any over-the-counter product for prescribed medications.
- Seek information from objective sources and check any warnings on the label or package.
- Observe for beneficial and harmful effects.
- Report any possible side effects to your primary health care provider for evaluation.
- Keep in mind that some products, such as herbs, are not required to meet FDA standards for safety and efficacy.
- Introduce only one new substance at a time.
- Start with a low dose and increase the dose gradually.
- Doses may need to be lowered when combining two or more herbs or an herb and a medication.
- Some herbs are for short-term use only.
- Some herbs need to be taken for 1 to 3 months before effects are noticed (e.g., ginkgo biloba, St. John's wort).
- Herbs can interact with all of the following: other herbs, food, beverages, caffeine, nutrients, prescription medications, and over-the-counter medications.
- Some herbs are contraindicated in people with the following conditions: stroke, glaucoma, diabetes, hypertension, heart disease, thyroid disorder, and any bleeding disorder or condition requiring anticoagulation.
- Some herbs are most effective when taken on an empty stomach.
- Many herbs can cause gastrointestinal effects (e.g., anorexia, nausea, diarrhea).
- Some herbs, especially those that are applied externally, can cause skin rashes.
- Herbs can cause allergic reactions.
- Some herbs are extremely toxic, or fatal, if ingested.
- A few herbs, or ingredients in herbs, can be toxic when taken in large doses or for a long time. (For example, Oregon grape, used for prostatitis, may cause heart failure.)
- A few herbs are thought to be carcinogenic.
- Herbs that are used for anxiety or insomnia should not be taken before driving a car.
- Be skeptical about exaggerated claims; if it sounds too good to be true, it probably is!

FDA, U.S. Food and Drug Administration.

Addressing Factors That Affect Adherence

When older adults have trouble adhering to their medication regimen, nurses can work with them and their caregivers to identify methods of improving adherence. For example, "unit-dose" medication systems, which have been widely used in institutional settings, are becoming more available for use in home settings, and may be helpful in improving medication adherence, especially when medication regimens are complex. A variety of simple "pill organizers" (i.e., containers with separate compartments designated for each day of the week and with one to four compartments for each day) are widely available in stores. In addition, more sophisticated devices to enhance independence and improve adherence are available and may be particularly helpful for people with cognitive or functional impairments. For example, human voice recordings, telephone-computer services, and beeping watches or key chains can be used to remind the person to take medications at designated times. Medication-dispensing systems, which can be filled monthly and programmed to dispense medications at specific times, also are available. Internet sites that provide information about these more technologically advanced systems include www.epill.com, www.ontimerx.com, and www.medprompt.com. Nurses can encourage older adults and their caregivers to investigate different types of devices and systems (such as those depicted in Fig. 8-1) that can be used to improve medication adherence.

Wellness Opportunity

Nurses promote self-responsibility by addressing factors that interfere with adherence and, at the same time, supporting independence.

Even with the availability of Medicare Part D, older adults and people with chronic conditions are burdened by the high and increasing cost of prescription medications. Thus, nurses often need to address financial barriers that affect adherence to medication regimens because even a person who has an adequate income may decide that a medication is not worth the high cost, especially on an ongoing basis. Many of the newer medications are developed because they are safer or more effective than older medications; however, they usually are more expensive. Nurses can encourage older adults to be candid with their health care practitioners and ask about the availability of less costly but equally safe and effective medications.

One way of addressing high costs is to use generic medications. The FDA authorizes the manufacture of generic drugs when the patent on a brand-name drug expires, and they require these drugs to be bioequivalent (i.e., identical)

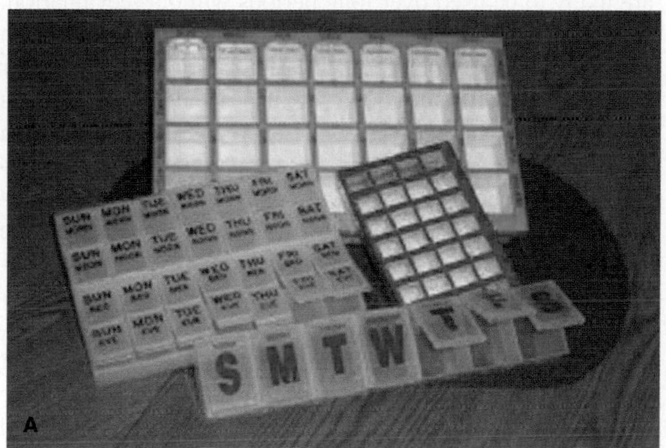

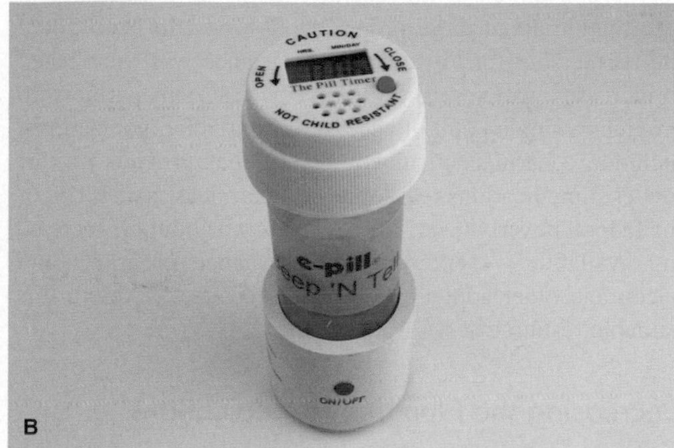

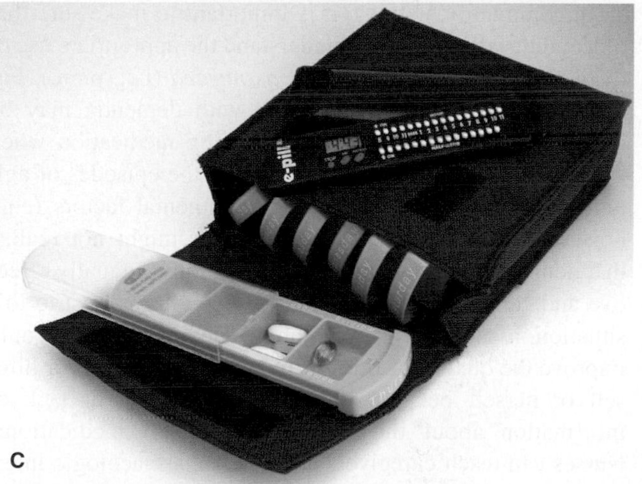

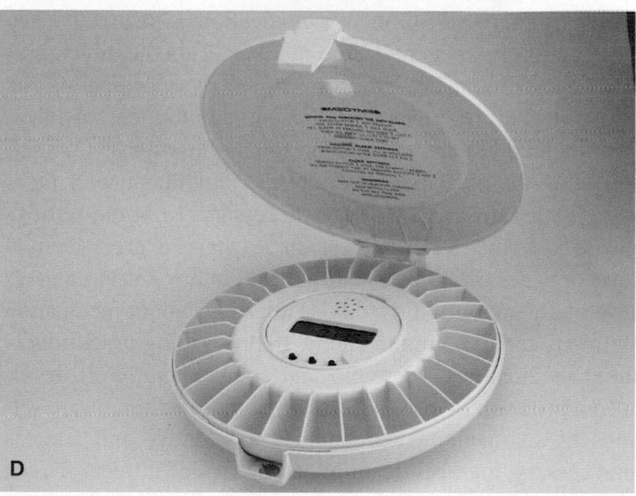

FIGURE 8-1 A sampling of the many devices and systems that are available to improve medication adherence. **(A)** Many simple pill organizers are available in drugstores. **(B)** The Beep 'N Tell pill bottle can be programmed to sound a beeping alarm or play a recorded message. **(C)** The 7-Day Organizer & Reminder has daily pill containers with four large compartments and a multi-alarm electronic reminder system. **(D)** The Automatic Medication Dispenser can be filled with 28 doses of pills and programmed to move the compartments for opening at a predetermined time. It also has a lock and audible alarm with three different sounds. (**A** courtesy of Tracey Moulton. **B**, **C**, and **D** courtesy of www.e-pill.com, e-pill Medication Reminders, 70 Walnut Street, Wellesley, MA 02481, [800] 549-0095.)

to their brand-name counterparts in dosage form, safety, purity, strength, quality, intended use, performance characteristics, and route of administration. About half of all prescriptions are available in generic form, and about half of these are manufactured by the same brand-name companies that developed the original drug. The FDA and other organizations estimate that generics cost 30% to 80% less than their brand-name equivalents. With the exception of drugs that have a very narrow therapeutic range, the use of generic drugs is a safe and effective way of reducing costs. Examples of drugs that should not be used in generic form are digoxin, lithium, phenytoin, warfarin, quinidine, theophylline, carbamazepine, and valproic acid. The FDA provides complete and up-to-date information about the equivalency of all generic drugs at www.fda.gov/cder.

Additional ways of decreasing the cost of medications include obtaining free samples of medications from prescribing practitioners and enrolling in **prescription assistance programs**, which provide medications at little or no cost to consumers. Until recently, it was difficult to obtain information about these programs; however, in April 2005, the Partnership for Prescription Assistance was established to increase awareness and improve access. This partnership provides a single point of access to about 500 organizations, including pharmaceutical companies that provide free or low-cost medications to people who earn less than 200% of the federal poverty level. Nurses can teach about the increasing availability of prescription assistance programs and encourage older adults and their caregivers to explore this valuable resource at www.pparx.org.

Decreasing the Number of Medications

Because the chance of adverse medication effects increases in proportion to the number of medications consumed, a key intervention is to decrease the number of medications to as few as possible. This is accomplished by coordinating the efforts of the prescriber(s) to discontinue duplicate medications or medications that are no longer appropriate, and by educating the older person about the judicious use of medications that are not medically necessary. In home settings and long-term care facilities, nurses have a great deal of autonomy regarding medications, and in any setting, nurses have many opportunities to raise questions about medication regimens and to communicate with prescribing practitioners about medications. Meredith and colleagues (2002) developed a program to improve medication use in home care settings by using home care nurses to identify and address unnecessary therapeutic duplication (which affects 4% of home care patients) and the use of medications that have high potential for adverse effects. This intervention can be implemented with minimal use of outside resources and within the context of routinely provided care.

When older adults are admitted to the hospital, they often are under the care of primary care practitioners who were not the ones who prescribed the medications taken before the admission. Nurses usually obtain the medication history, and the prescribing practitioner may automatically order the medications that are listed on the admission assessment. Because the hospital admission is an ideal time to reevaluate the safety, efficacy, and necessity of medications, nurses should ask older adults or their caregivers about the purpose and potential adverse effects of each medication. This assessment may provide important clues to medications or interactions that contributed to or directly caused the problem for which the patient is hospitalized.

When medications are prescribed for behavioral reasons rather than for a medical condition, nurses can teach older adults and their caregivers about these medications and about nonpharmacologic alternatives. For example, caregivers of people with dementia may use medications to address behaviors that might respond equally well to nonpharmacologic interventions that do not have any risk of adverse effects. Once these medications are prescribed, they are likely to be used over long periods without reevaluation. Nurses need to recognize that the efficacy may diminish (e.g., with hypnotics), the underlying reason may resolve or change (e.g., with situational anxiety), and adverse effects may develop gradually and not be recognized (e.g., with anticholinergic agents). Thus, it is imperative to review periodically all medications and to consider whether nonpharmacologic approaches could be used to address the symptoms or behaviors. Behavioral problems are one example of the types of symptoms that can be managed medically but might be managed just as well, and with fewer risks, through nonpharmacologic interventions. Other types of problems that can often be managed without pharmacologic agents are those related to sleep, comfort, anxiety, and chronic illnesses.

In community settings, it is important to make sure that older adults and caregivers understand the appropriate use of medications that are prescribed *as needed* (i.e., p.r.n.). For example, a caregiver of someone with dementia may be instructed to give a behavior-modifying medication when the person becomes agitated. Although the episodes of agitation may be precipitated by environmental factors (e.g., noise or overstimulation), the caregiver might not realize that nonpharmacologic interventions could be equally effective and carry no risk of adverse effects. In contrast to this situation, a caregiver may withhold medications that could improve the quality of life for the older person and for himself or herself because of misunderstandings or lack of information about the appropriate use of medications. Nurses can teach caregivers about nonpharmacologic interventions, as well as the appropriate use of medications for behavior management, particularly for people with dementia (discussed in Chapter 14).

In institutional settings, nurses must establish clear criteria for administering medications for behavior management. These criteria must be based primarily on the patient's needs, rather than those of the staff. In home settings, different criteria for behavioral medication might be justified, and the needs of the caregivers may take precedence over the needs of the dependent older adult. For example, if nighttime wakening of a dependent older person interferes with the caregiver's sleep, medication intervention might be warranted. In an institutional setting, however, the nursing staff paid to provide around-the-clock care might try nonpharmacologic interventions, or allow the person to be awake at night, rather than immediately turning to the use of medications.

Wellness Opportunity

Nurses promote wellness by talking with older adults and their caregivers when appropriate about choosing interventions, such as relaxation techniques, that can improve health and quality of life, rather than using medications.

EVALUATING EFFECTIVENESS OF NURSING INTERVENTIONS

Nurses evaluate interventions related to medication management according to the degree to which the older adult follows a safe and effective medication regimen. This process involves an evaluation of medication-taking behaviors, as well as an evaluation of the therapeutic effects of the medication. Another evaluation criterion is the extent to which negative functional consequences, such as interactions and adverse effects, are prevented, alleviated, or controlled. In home settings nurses can evaluate the effectiveness of their interventions by observing the medication-taking patterns of the older adult. In any setting, nurses can evaluate the knowledge of safe and effective use of prescription and over-the-counter medications. Another measure of effectiveness is the degree to which barriers to adherence are eliminated or addressed.

Mrs. M., who is 76 years old, is being discharged to her home after a stay in a nursing home for rehabilitation after a stroke. Residual problems from the stroke include left-sided weakness and visual–perceptual difficulties. In addition to the stroke, Mrs. M.'s medical problems include glaucoma, depression, and congestive heart failure. Her medications include the following: Centrum Silver, 1 tablet daily; furosemide, 20 mg, 2 tablets twice a day; Lanoxicaps, 0.1 mg daily except Mondays and Thursdays; Ecotrin, 81 mg, 1 tablet daily; Transderm-Nitro, 0.2 mg/hour daily; Zoloft, 50 mg daily; Cardizem, 60 mg three times a day; and Timoptic, 0.25% twice daily. The nursing home regimen for administering the medications is as follows:

7:30 AM:	Lanoxicaps (except Mondays and Thursdays)
	Cardizem, 60 mg
	Furosemide, 20 mg, 2 tablets
	Timoptic, 0.25% in each eye
9:00 AM:	Transderm-Nitro, 0.2 mg/hour
1:00 PM:	Centrum Silver, 1 tablet
	Ecotrin, 81 mg, 1 tablet
	Cardizem, 60 mg
3:30 PM:	Furosemide, 20 mg, 2 tablets
7:30 PM:	Timoptic, 0.25% in each eye
	Cardizem, 60 mg
9:00 PM:	Zoloft, 50 mg

NURSING ASSESSMENT

Your assessment reveals that, before her hospitalization and nursing home stay, Mrs. M. administered her medications independently, but the only medications she took were the eye drops, furosemide (20 mg once daily), and Lanoxicaps. The functional assessment indicates that Mrs. M. has weakness and limited use of her left arm and hand, causing difficulty performing tasks that require fine motor movements. She has full use of her right upper extremity, and she is right-hand dominant. She ambulates independently, but slowly, with a walker. A mental status assessment reveals that Mrs. M. is alert, oriented, and has no memory deficits; however, her abstract thinking and time perception have been impaired by the stroke. She has some expressive aphasia, but she seems to understand instructions, especially if ideas are reinforced by using concrete examples and demonstrations.

(case study continues on page 142)

Mrs. M. expresses motivation to take her medications, but she admits to being overwhelmed by the complexity of the regimen, stating that at the nursing home they administered her medications at six different times. She is also concerned about self-administering her eye drops because she used to use her left hand to hold her eyelids open. With regard to furosemide, she says she does not like taking it twice a day because it makes her go to the bathroom too much. While at the nursing home, she has not had any trouble with incontinence, but she worries about what she'll do at home because there is no bathroom on the first floor. She asks whether she can take the entire dose of furosemide at night so that she will only have to get up during the night to go to the bathroom, which is located near the bedroom.

In response to your questions about medication management routines before her stroke, Mrs. M. reports using a compartmentalized medication container and taking her two medications and the eye drops after breakfast, around 9:30 AM. She would administer the second dose of eye drops around 9:30 PM, before getting ready for bed. She had no difficulty remembering the medications because she kept the pill container and one bottle of eye drops near the toaster, and she kept a second bottle of eye drops on her nightstand. Now, however, she expresses concern about the number of times she must take medications if the regimen remains the same as in the nursing home, and she thinks she will need six pill containers, but is not sure where she should put all of them. She also worries about the cost of all the medications.

Mrs. M. lives with her husband, who is physically healthy but has early-stage Alzheimer's disease. Their daughter lives nearby and visits two or three times weekly to assist with grocery shopping, laundry, and household chores. She also provides transportation to stores and appointments.

NURSING DIAGNOSIS

You decide on a nursing diagnosis of Noncompliance because Mrs. M. expresses a desire to take her medications, but several factors deter adherence to the current regimen. Related factors include functional impairments, complex medication regimens, negative side effects of furosemide, and concern about the cost of medications.

NURSING CARE PLAN FOR MRS. M

Expected Outcome	Nursing Interventions	Nursing Evaluation

Mrs. M.'s medication routine will be simplified.	• Work with the pharmacist and the prescribing practitioner to simplify the medication regimen.
	  • Discuss with Mrs. M.'s prescribing practitioner the problem of the complexity of the regimen and the cost of medications. Ask Mrs. M.'s prescribing practitioner if she can take Cardizem CD, 180 mg daily, rather than Cardizem, 60 mg three times a day. (This will be less expensive and will eliminate two doses of medication daily.)
	  • Ask the pharmacist about combining medications to allow twice-daily administration.
	• Assist Mrs. M. in establishing a routine for self-administering medications that will fit in with her usual activities.
	• At least 3 days before discharge from the nursing home, arrange for Mrs. M. to assume responsibility for her own medication management, using pill containers that she herself fills.
		• Mrs. M. will be able to follow a twice-daily medication dosing schedule.

Mrs. M.'s concerns about furosemide will be addressed.	• Explain the importance of taking furosemide, as ordered, to control congestive heart failure effectively. • Suggest that Mrs. M. obtain a portable commode for use downstairs during the day.	• Mrs. M. will take furosemide as ordered and will not experience difficulty with urinary incontinence.

(case study continues on page 143)

Expected Outcome	Nursing Interventions	Nursing Evaluation
Mrs. M.'s concerns about the cost of medications will be addressed.	• Encourage Mrs. M. to talk with her primary care practitioner about her concerns over the cost of the prescribed medications. • Suggest that Mrs. M. consider using the pharmacy services provided by AARP (American Association of Retired Persons) to obtain her prescriptions.	• Mrs. M. will be able to afford her prescribed medications.
A system for self-administering eye drops will be identified.	• Ask an occupational therapist to evaluate Mrs. M.'s ability to self-administer her eye drops and to identify any assistive devices that may increase her independence and reliability in performing this task. • Have Mrs. M. practice self-administering her eye drops before she is discharged from the nursing home, with staff providing whatever assistance is necessary. • Talk with Mrs. M. about the possibility of her husband assisting with the eye drop procedure if she is unable to do this independently. • Ask Mrs. M.'s ophthalmologist whether the eye drop regimen can be simplified to once-daily dosing by prescribing an extended-action eye drop formula.	• Mrs. M. will self-administer her eye drops or will receive the assistance she needs for eye drop administration from her husband.

THINKING POINTS

- What are the factors that influence Mrs. M.'s ability to manage her medications independently?
- What additional assessment information would be helpful in establishing a plan for Mrs. M. to manage her medications independently?
- What health education would you provide to address Mrs. M.'s concerns about the cost of her medications?
- What steps would you take to ensure that expected outcomes are achieved after Mrs. M. is back in her own home?

CHAPTER HIGHLIGHTS

Introduction to Bioactive Substances

- Effects of medications in the body are usually considered in relation to pharmacokinetics and pharmacodynamics
- Herbs and medications that are similar in bioactivity (Table 8-1)
- Potential adverse effects of herbs (Table 8-2)
- Herbs commonly used by older adults: uses, actions and precautions, standardization and dose (Table 8-3)
- Homeopathic remedies

Age-Related Changes That Affect Bioactive Substances in Older Adults

- Decreased clearance due to changes in the kidneys and liver (Box 8-1)
- Metabolism by the cytochrome P-450 system (Table 8-4)
- Effects of changes in body composition (Box 8-2)
- Medications affected by serum albumin levels (Box 8-3)
- Effects of changes in receptor sensitivity (Box 8-4)
- Changes that affect medication-taking behaviors

Risks Factors That Affect Bioactive Substances

- Pathologic processes and functional impairments (medication–disease interactions, effects on the ability to take substances)
- Behaviors based on myths and misunderstandings (attitudes about and expectations for bioactive substances)
- Communication barriers between older adults and prescribing practitioners
- Lack of information about bioactive substances and older adults
- Inappropriate prescribing practices (Beers criteria)
- Polypharmacy and inadequate monitoring
- Medication nonadherence (including financial factors, Medicare Part D)
- Insufficient recognition of adverse effects (Table 8-5)

Medication Interactions

- Medication–medication interactions (Table 8-6)
- Medication–herb interactions (Table 8-3)
- Medications and nutrients (Table 8-7)
- Medications and alcohol (Table 8-8)
- Medications and caffeine (Table 8-9)
- Medications and nicotine (Table 8-10)

Functional Consequences Associated With Bioactive Substances in Older Adults

- Altered therapeutic effects (less predictable)
- Increased potential for adverse effects (Box 8-5)
- Adverse effects of anticholinergic medications (Box 8-6)

- Increased potential for altered mental status (Table 8-11)
- Increased potential for tardive dyskinesia

Nursing Assessment of Medication Use and Effects

- Communication techniques for obtaining accurate information (open-ended, nonjudgmental)
- Scope of a medication assessment (all bioactive substances, older adult's understanding of regimen, preferences) (Box 8-7)
- Cultural considerations (factors that influence medication-taking behaviors, culturally specific health care sources and practices) (Cultural Considerations 8-1, 8-2)
- Patterns of medication use
- Medication assessment as it relates to the overall assessment
- Factors in identifying adverse medication effects

Nursing Diagnoses

- Readiness for Enhanced Therapeutic Regimen Management
- Instrumental Self-Care Deficit
- Noncompliance

Planning for Wellness Outcomes

- Knowledge: Medication
- Self-Care: Non-Parenteral Medication
- Compliance Behavior

Nursing Interventions to Promote Healthy Medication-Taking Patterns

- Teaching about medications (Box 8-8, patient teaching tool)
- Teaching about herbs and other bioactive substances (Box 8-9, patient teaching tool)
- Addressing factors that affect adherence (Fig. 8-1)
- Decreasing the number of medications

Evaluating Effectiveness of Nursing Interventions

- Medication-taking behaviors that are safe and effective
- Prevention, alleviation, or control of negative functional consequences (e.g., interactions, adverse effects)

Critical Thinking Exercises

1. You are asked to give a half-hour presentation on "Medications and Aging" to a local senior citizens group. Describe the following:
   - What points would you cover about age-related changes?
   - How would you address the risk factors that affect medication action and medication-taking behaviors?
   - What tips would you give about taking medications?
   - What educational materials would you use?
   - How would you involve the group participants in the discussion?
2. Carefully read the interview questions in Box 8-7 and decide which questions you would use and how you would phrase the questions in your own words for each of the following situations:
   - You are doing an admission interview for a 78-year-old man who lives alone and has been admitted to the hospital for the third time in 18 months for congestive heart failure.
   - You are working in a Senior Wellness program in an urban setting with a large number of older adults who were born in Mexico. You are preparing for 15-minute interviews with older adults who have agreed to participate in an educational session to which they must bring all their pills in a bag and ask the nurse about them.
3. Carefully read the information in Boxes 8-8 and 8-9 and describe what information you would be likely to use in each of the following situations.
   - Discharge planning for the 78-year-old man described in Exercise 2, bullet 1
   - Health education for the people described in the Senior Wellness program in Exercise 2, bullet 2

Clinical Tool Resources

Hartford Institute for Geriatric Nursing
Try This: Best Practices in Nursing Care to Older Adults
Issue Number 16, Beers' Criteria for Potentially Inappropriate Medication Use in the Elderly
Issue Number 17 (Revised 2007), Alcohol Screening and Assessment for Older Adults
www.hartfordign.org/resources/education/tryThis.html

Educational Resources

AARP (American Association of Retired Persons)
www.aarp.org

American Botanical Council
www.herbalgram.org

ConsumerLab
www.consumerlabs.com

Food and Drug Administration
www.fda.gov

Herb Research Foundation
www.herbs.org

Institute for Safe Medication Practices
www.ismp.org

National Center for Complementary and Alternative Medicine
http://nccam.nih.gov

National Council on Patient Information and Education
www.talkaboutrx.org

Partnership for Prescription Assistance
www.pparx.org

Peter Lamy Center for Drug Therapy and Aging
www.pharmacy.umaryland.edu/lamy

Therapeutic Products Directorate (Canada)
www.hc-sc.gc.ca

United States Pharmacopoeia (USP)
http://www.usp.org/USPVerified/

REFERENCES

Ancelin, M. L., Artero, S., Portet, F., Dupuy, A., Touchon, J., & Ritchie, K. (2006). Non-degenerative mild cognitive impairment in elderly people and use of anticholinergic drugs: Longitudinal cohort study. *British Medical Journal, 322*, 455–459.

Beers, M. H., Oslander, J. G., Rollingher, J., Brooks, J., Reuben, D., & Beck, J. C. (1991). Explicit criteria for determining potentially inappropriate medication use by the elderly. *Archives of Internal Medicine, 151*, 1825–1832.

Beyth, R. J., & Shorr, R. I. (2002). Principles of drug therapy in older patients: Rational drug prescribing. *Clinics in Geriatric Medicine, 18*, 577–592.

Blalock, S. J., Byrd, J. E., Hansen, R. A., Yananis, T. J., McMullin, K., DeVellis, B. M., et al. (2005). Factors associated with potentially inappropriate drug utilization in a sample of rural community-dwelling older adults. *American Journal of Geriatric Pharmacotherapy, 3*, 168–179.

Blanda, M. P. (2006). Pharmacologic issues in geriatric emergency medicine. *Emergency Medicine Clinics of North America, 24*, 449–465.

Briesacher, B. A., Limcangco, M. R., Simoni-Wastila, L., Doshi, J. A., Levens, S. R., Shea, D. G., et al. (2005). The quality of antipsychotic drug prescribing in nursing homes. *Archives of Internal Medicine, 165*, 1280–1285.

Carnahan, R. M., Lund, B. C., Perry, P. J., & Chrischilles, E. A. (2004). The concurrent use of anticholinergics and cholinesterase inhibitors: Rare event or common practice? *Journal of the American Geriatrics Society, 52*, 2082–2087.

Carnahan, R. M., Lund, B. C., Pollock, B. G., & Culp, K. R. (2006). The Anticholinergic Drug Scale as a measure of drug-related anticholinergic burden: Associations with the serum anticholinergic activity. *Journal of Clinical Pharmacology, 46*, 1481–1486.

Carpenito-Moyet, L. J. (2006). *Handbook of nursing diagnosis* (11th ed.). Philadelphia: Lippincott Williams & Wilkins.

Chew, M. L., Mulsant, B. H., & Pollock, B. G. (2005). Serum anticholinergic activity and cognition in patients with moderate-to-severe dementia. *American Journal of Geriatric Psychiatry, 13*, 535–538.

Chou, K. L., & Friedman, J. H. (2006). Tardive syndromes in the elderly. *Clinics in Geriatric Medicine, 22*, 915–933.

Espino, D. V., Bazaldua, O. V., Palmer, R. F., Mouton, C. P., Parchman, M. L., Miles, T. P., et al. (2006). Suboptimal medication use and mortality in an older adult community-based cohort: Results from the Hispanic EPESE Study. *Journals of Gerontology: Series A, Biological Sciences and Medical Sciences, 61*, 170–175.

Families USA. (2006). The Medicare Drug Program fails to reach low-income seniors: More than three out of every four low-income seniors eligible for special subsidies are still without drug coverage. Families USA special report. Available at www.familiesusa.org/assets/pdfs/Medicare-Enrollment-report-May-2006.pdf.

Families USA. (2007). No bargain: Medicare drug plans deliver high prices. Families USA report. Available at www.familiesusa.org/assets/pdfs/no-bargain-medicare-drug.pdf.

Federal Interagency Forum on Aging-Related Statistics. (2006). *Older Americans update 2006: Key indicators of well-being*. Washington, DC: U.S. Government Printing Office.

Fick, D. M., Cooper, J. W., Wade, W. E., Waller, J. L., Maclean, J. R., & Beers, M. H. (2003). Updating the Beers criteria for potentially inappropriate medication use in older adults: Results of a US consensus panel of experts. *Archives of Internal Medicine, 163*, 2716–2724.

Goulding, M. R. (2005). Trends in prescribed medicine use and spending by older Americans, 1992–2001. Aging Trends no. 5. Hyattsville, MD: National Center for Health Statistics.

Gurwitz, J. H., Field, T. S., Harrold, L. R., Rothschild, J., Debellis, K., Seger, A. C., et al., (2003). Incidence and preventability of adverse drug events among older persons in the ambulatory setting. *Journal of the American Medical Association, 289*, 1107–1116.

Gurwitz, J. H., Field, T. S., Judge, J., Rochon, P., Harrold, L. R., Cadoret, C., et al. (2005). The incidence of adverse drug events in two large academic long-term care facilities. *American Journal of Medicine, 118*, 251–258.

Hohl, C., Dankoff, J., Colacone, A., & Afilalo, M. (2001). Polypharmacy, adverse drug-related events, and potential adverse drug interactions in elderly patients present to an emergency department. *Annals of Emergency Medicine, 38*, 666–671.

Holbrook, A. M., Pereira, J. A., Labiris, R., McDonald, H., Douketis, J. D., Crowther, M., et al. (2005). Systematic overview of warfarin and its drug and food interactions. *Archives of Internal Medicine, 165*, 1095–1105.

Insel, K., Morrow, D., Brewer, B., & Figueredo, A. (2006). Executive function, working memory and medication adherence among older adults. *Journals of Gerontology: Series B, Psychological Sciences and Social Sciences, 61*, 102–107.

Jacobs, L. G. (2006). Warfarin pharmacology, clinical management, and evaluation of hemorrhagic risk for the elderly. *Clinics in Geriatric Medicine, 22*, 17–32.

Kyle, U. G., Genton, L., Hans, D., Karsegard, V. L., Michel, J.-P., Slosman, D. O., et al. (2001). Total body mass, fat mass, fat-free mass, and skeletal muscle in older people: Cross-sectional differences in 60-year-old persons. *Journal of the American Geriatrics Society, 49*, 1633–1640.

Lau, D. T., Kasper, J. D., Potter, D. E., Lyles, A., & Bennett, R. G. (2005). Hospitalization and death associated with potentially inappropriate medication prescriptions among elderly nursing home residents. *Archives of Internal Medicine, 165*, 68–74.

Lechevallier-Michel, N., Gautier-Bertrand, M., Alperovitch, A., Berr, C., Belmin, J., Legran, S., et al. (2005). Frequency and risk factors of potentially inappropriate medication use in a community-dwelling elderly population: Results from the 3C Study. *European Journal of Clinical Pharmacology, 60*, 813–819.

Lee, A., Chui, P. T., Aun, C. S. T., Lau, A. S. C., & Gin, T. (2006). Incidence and risk of adverse perioperative events among surgical patients taking traditional Chinese herbal medicines. *Anesthesiology, 105*, 454–461.

Lee, P. E., Sylora, K., Gill, S. S., Mamdani, M., Marras, C., Anderson, G., et al. (2005). Antipsychotic medications and drug-induced movement disorders other than Parkinsonism: A population-based cohort study in older adults. *Journal of the American Geriatrics Society, 53*, 1374–1379.

Lipson, J. G., & Dibble, S. L. (2005). *Culture & clinical care.* San Francisco: UCSF Nursing Press.

Ludwick, R. E., Sedlak, C. A., Doheny, M. O., & Martsolf, D. S. (2000). Alcohol use in elderly women: Nursing considerations in community settings. *Journal of Gerontological Nursing, 26*(2), 44–49.

Marti, J., Anton, E., & Ezcurra, I. (2005). An unexpected cause of delirium in an old patient [letter]. *Journal of the American Geriatrics Society, 53*, 545.

Meredith, S., Feldman, P., Grey, D., Giammaro, L., Hall, K., Arnold, K., et al. (2002). Improving medication use in newly admitted home healthcare patients: A randomized controlled trial. *Journal of the American Geriatrics Society, 50*, 1584–1941.

Metz, C. N., Gregersen, P. K., & Malhotra, A. K. (2004). Metabolism and biochemical effects of nicotine for primary care providers. *Medical Clinics of North America, 88*, 1399–1413.

Molony, S. L. (2003). Beers' criteria for potentially inappropriate medication use in the elderly. *Journal of Gerontological Nursing, 29*(11), 6–7.

Moss, J., & Yuan, C.-S. (2006). Herbal medicines and perioperative care. *Anesthesiology, 105*, 441–442.

Neafsey, P. J., & Shellman, J. (2002). Interactions of prescription medicines. *Journal of Gerontological Nursing, 28*(9), 30–39.

Niwata, S., Yamada, Y., & Ikegami, N. (2006). Prevalence of inappropriate medication using Beers criteria in Japanese long-term care facilities. *Boston Medical Center Geriatrics, 6*(1), 1–4.

Noyes, K., Liu, H., & Holloway, R. G. (2006). What is the risk of developing parkinsonism following neuroleptic use? *Neurology, 66*, 941–943.

Ownby, R. L. (2006). Medication adherence and cognition: Medical, personal and economic factors influence level of adherence in older adults. *Geriatrics, 61*(2), 30–35.

Perri, M., Menon, A. M., Deshpande, A. D., Shinde, S. B., Jiang, R., Cooper, J. W., et al. (2005). Adverse outcomes associated with inappropriate drug use in nursing homes. *Annals of Pharmacotherapy, 39*, 405–411.

Petrone, K., & Katz, P. (2005). Approaches to appropriate drug prescribing for the older adult. *Primary Care: Clinics in Office Practice, 32*, 755–775.

Pugh, M. J., Fincke, B. G., Bierman, A. S., Chang, B. H., Rosen, A. K., Cunningham, F. E., et al. (2005). Potentially inappropriate prescribing in elderly veterans: Are we using the wrong drug, wrong dose, or wrong duration? *Journal of the American Geriatrics Society, 53*, 1282–1289.

Raivio, M. M., Laurila, J. V., Strandberg, T. E., Tilvis, R. S., & Pitkala, K. H. (2006). Use of inappropriate medications and their prognostic significance among in-hospital and nursing home patients with and without dementia in Finland. *Drugs and Aging, 23*, 333–343.

Schlenk, E. A., Dunbar-Jacob, J., & Engberg, S. (2004). Medication non-adherence among older adults: A review of strategies and interventions for improvement. *Journal of Gerontological Nursing, 30*(7), 33–43.

Simon, S. R., Chan, K. A., Soumerai, S. B., Wagner, A. K., Andrade, S. E., Feldstein, A. C., et al. (2005). Potentially inappropriate medication use by elderly persons in U.S. health maintenance organizations, 2000–2001. *Journal of the American Geriatrics Society, 53*, 227–232.

Soumerai, S. B., Pierre-Jacques, M., Zhang, F., Ross-Degnan, D., Adams, A. S., Gurwitz, J., et al. (2006). Cost-related medication nonadherence among elderly and disabled Medicare beneficiaries: A national survey 1 year before the Medicare drug benefit. *Archives of Internal Medicine, 166*, 1829–1835.

Terrell, K. M., Heard, K., & Miller, D. K. (2006). Prescribing to older ED patients. *American Journal of Emergency Medicine, 24*, 468–478.

Wold, R. S., Lopez, S. T., Yau, C. L., Butler, L. M., Pareo-Tubbeh, S. L., Waters, D. L., et al. (2005). Increasing trends in elderly persons' use of nonvitamin, nonmineral dietary supplements and concurrent use of medications. *Journal of the American Dietetic Association, 105*, 54–63.

Zuckerman, I. H., Hernandez, J. J., Gruber-Baldini, A. L., Hebel, J. R., Stuart, B., Zimmerman, S., et al. (2005). Potentially inappropriate prescribing before and after nursing home admission among patients with and without dementia. *American Journal of Geriatric Pharmacotherapy, 3*, 246–254.

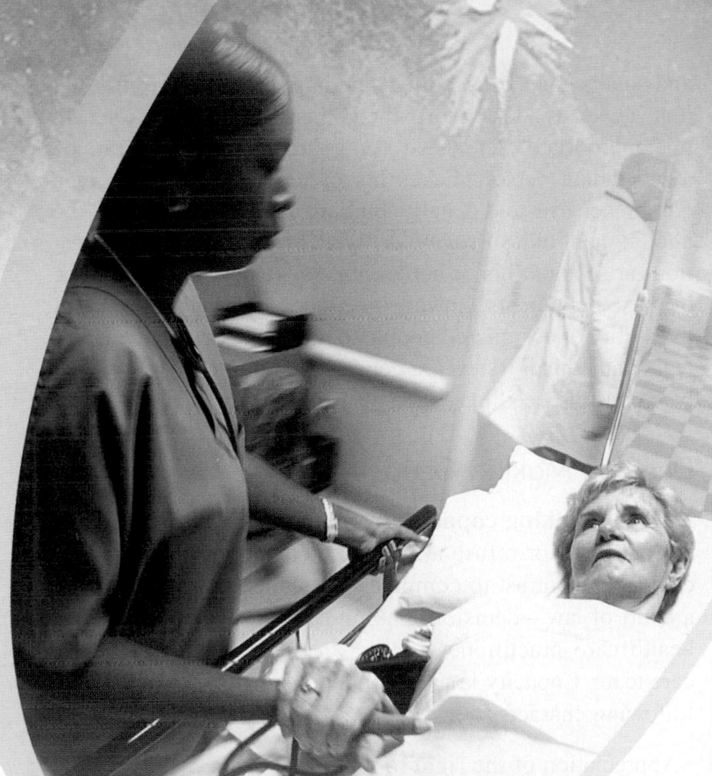

CHAPTER 9

Legal and Ethical Concerns

Learning Objectives

After reading this chapter, you will be able to:

1. Define the following terms: autonomy, competency, and decision-making capacity.
2. Describe the following advance directives: living wills, medical directives, and durable power of attorney for health care.
3. Discuss ethical issues that nurses commonly address when caring for older adults.
4. Describe cultural considerations that affect autonomy, decision making, and advance directives.
5. Describe nursing responsibilities regarding advance directives and decisions about care.

Key Terms

advance directives
autonomy
competency
conservatorship
decisional autonomy
decision-making capacity
Do Not Resuscitate (DNR) order
durable power of attorney for health care
executional autonomy
executive control functions
guardianship
health care proxy
incompetent
living wills
proxy decision maker

In the past several decades, various legislative efforts have addressed the rights of older adults and their quality of life. For example, during the early 1980s state and federal governments began addressing issues related to vulnerable elders. Later in that decade, legislative efforts focused on issues related to end-of-life decisions, the rights of patients and nursing home residents, and the quality of care provided under Medicaid and Medicare programs. Many of these legislative and policy initiatives have created ethical issues for gerontological health care practitioners. For example, nurses commonly address questions about the extent to which an older person is able to make decisions about his or her health care. Although legislation can provide legal guidelines for these questions, laws do not resolve ethical dilemmas that arise when no advance directive was provided or when conflicts exist about how an advance directive should be interpreted or implemented. The next sections review some of the pertinent legal and ethical issues that are relevant to nursing care of older adults. Additional legal and ethical considerations regarding vulnerable elders are addressed in Chapter 10.

AUTONOMY AND RIGHTS

Autonomy is the personal freedom to direct one's own life as long as it does not infringe on the rights of others. An autonomous person is capable of rational thought and is able to recognize the need for problem solving. The person can identify the problem, search for alternatives, and select a solution that allows his or her continued personal freedom, as long as it does not cause any harm to another's rights or property. Loss of autonomy and, therefore, loss of independence, is a very real fear among the elderly. Moreover, for older adults with dementia and other conditions that affect decision-making abilities, loss of autonomy is an inevitable reality that is addressed by families and health care professionals. Because autonomy is so highly valued and there is no easy way to evaluate decision-making abilities—which can fluctuate from day to day—questions often arise about medical interventions and health care decisions. Thus, nurses need to be familiar with legal and ethical guidelines related to competency and decision-making capacity. Nurses have a responsibility to assist older adults and their families, often as impartial mediators, when issues concerning personal autonomy arise. However, if the safety of the older person is threatened because of risky behaviors arising from impaired decision-making abilities, nurses must refer older people to the appropriate community agencies (e.g., Adult Protective Services) for further evaluation (see Chapter 10).

Competency

Competency is a legal term that refers to the ability to fulfill one's role and handle one's affairs in an adequate manner. All adults are presumed to be competent, and state laws designate the age of competency—usually 18 years—for participating in legally binding decisions. Because competent people are guaranteed all the rights granted by the Constitution and state laws, all adults who have not been declared incompetent by a judge have the legal right to make their own decisions about medical treatment and health care. However, families or health care providers often raise questions about an older person's ability to make reasonable decisions, particularly when the person is cognitively impaired.

When questions are raised about a person's ability to participate in medical care decisions, a legally appointed, surrogate decision maker, if one has been designated, assumes decision-making responsibility (see the discussion of "health care proxy" in the section on Advance Directives). In the absence of one, or when conflicts exist among the people involved with making and implementing decisions, a petition can be filed with probate court to determine whether the person is competent. Often, these petitions are filed because a health care provider (usually a physician) is concerned that appropriate decisions be made for a person who does not seem able to make reasonable medical decisions for himself or herself. Usually a family member files the petition, but if no qualified family member is available, or if family members are in conflict about the petition, an attorney or other person may file. If the court determines that the person is **incompetent** (i.e., incapable of making decisions on his or her own behalf), the judge assigns either a partial or a full **guardianship** (also called a **conservatorship**). With a partial guardianship, the incompetent person is permitted to make limited decisions; with a full guardianship, the person loses all of his or her rights to make such decisions. Although court action can revoke or reverse a guardianship, it typically remains in place until the incompetent person dies. Because guardianship is a drastic legal measure that takes away rights and entails court proceedings and ongoing court monitoring, it is viewed as a last resort when other legal interventions are not appropriate. The need for guardianship often can be avoided if a person makes his or her wishes known in a comprehensive and legally binding manner, including the appointment of a surrogate decision maker, before any questions arise about his or her mental capacities. In the absence of these documents, however, or when conflict arises about the ability of designated people to honor the person's wishes, legal and ethical issues are generally addressed through probate court proceedings, such as guardianship.

Decision-Making Capacity

Decision-making capacity refers to the ability of a person to consent to or refuse a specific medical treatment or procedure. In contrast to competency—which is determined by a court of law—decision-making capacity is determined by health care practitioners or by an interdisciplinary health care team. Capacity is based on a person's possession of the following characteristics:

- Appreciation of the right to make a choice
- Understanding of the risks and benefits of the medical intervention and lack of intervention
- Ability to communicate about the decision
- Stability over time
- Consistency with the person's usual beliefs and values

Determination of decision-making capacity should not be based on a particular diagnosis or the person's chronologic age. Rather, it should be based on a careful evaluation of his or her ability to understand the issues involved in a specific decision-making situation and to communicate about them. For example, a person with dementia may be able to participate in a decision about the appointment of a surrogate decision maker, but may not be able to participate in one about medical interventions for prostate cancer. In this situation, it might be reasonable for the person to designate his wife or one of his children to make the treatment decision for him. Nurses have dual roles in helping surrogate decision makers involve the older adult as much as possible, while at the same time supporting him or her in assuming responsibility for decisions. Some questions that health care professionals can ask to assess decision-making capacity are (Dalinis, 2005):

- What values, goals, and preferences does the patient hold?
- Is the patient able to understand and communicate information?
- Does the patient demonstrate the ability to reason and deliberate about choices?

Determination of decision-making capacity also takes into consideration that cognitive abilities can fluctuate from day to day and hour to hour and may be significantly influenced by factors such as medications, dementia, depression, and many acute and chronic medical conditions. Thus, an important role of nurses is to identify and address the factors that influence cognitive functioning (e.g., sensory impairments, medication effects) so that the person's decision-making abilities are at their best level. For example, even such a relatively simple measure as ensuring that a hearing-impaired person uses his or her hearing aid may improve communication and thereby have a positive effect on decision-making abilities. Similarly, if a person with dementia has better cognitive abilities in the morning or when he or she is rested, then efforts can be made to discuss health care decisions during this time, rather than when the person is more confused.

The phrases *decisional autonomy* and *executional autonomy* are sometimes used in relation to the concept of decision-making capacity. **Decisional autonomy** is the ability and freedom to make decisions without external influence, and **executional autonomy** (also called *executive autonomy*) is the ability to implement the decisions (Collopy, 1988). These concepts call attention to the complexity of assessing decision-making capacity and the importance of evaluating a person's ability not only to make reasonable decisions, but to carry out all of the actions necessary for implementing them. Medical ethicists point out that the traditional narrow focus on decisional autonomy is inadequate because it ignores the importance of evaluating a person's capacity to make, adapt, and implement plans (McCullough et al., 2001). This point is particularly important in relation to people with impaired **executive control functions**, which are the cognitive skills involved in successfully planning and carrying out goal-oriented behavior, such as self-care tasks. Conditions that are likely to cause impaired executive control functions include dementia, major depression, Parkinson's disease, and traumatic brain injury. These situations are particularly difficult to evaluate because the person may retain the capacity to understand and make decisions (decisional autonomy), but may not have the capacity to carry them out (executive autonomy). Therefore, assessment of both decisional and executive autonomy is essential (McCullough et al., 2001). Chapter 13 discusses guidelines for nursing assessment of executive control functions.

ADVANCE DIRECTIVES

Advance directives (also called *advance medical directives*) are legally binding documents that allow competent people to document what medical care they would or would not want to receive if they were not capable of making decisions and communicating their wishes. Advance directives also enable people to appoint a **proxy decision maker**, who is a person responsible for communicating his or her wishes if he or she becomes incompetent or unable to communicate them.

Advance directives are implemented on the basis of the Patient Self-Determination Act (PSDA), which was enacted by Congress in 1990 and became effective on December 1, 1991. The primary intent of this congressional legislation is to protect health care consumers by requiring that providers do all of the following:

- Inform patients of their right to refuse treatments and make health care decisions.
- Provide written information about their state's provisions for implementing advance directives.
- Ask each person whether an advance directive has been completed.
- Include documentation of patients' advance directives in their medical records.
- Provide education for their staff and the community on advance directives.

The PSDA applies to all hospices, hospitals, home health agencies, extended care facilities, and health maintenance organizations that receive federal funds. Because of this legislation, nurses in all settings routinely inquire about advance directives and facilitate communication about patients' wishes.

Many advocacy groups encourage all adults to establish advance directives and to make their wishes known to their families and health care providers regarding health care decisions, particularly end-of-life care issues. For example, Aging With Dignity promotes the use of the *Five Wishes* document (available in English or Spanish) for use as an advance directive document (see Educational Resources section). The *Five Wishes* document addresses the following questions (Aging With Dignity, 2001):

- Who do I want to make care decisions for me when I cannot make them for myself?
- What kind of medical treatment do I want or not want when I am very sick and unable to speak for myself?
- What would help me feel comfortable while I am dying?
- How do I want people to treat me?
- What do I want my loved ones to know about me and my feelings after I am gone?

Advance directive documents must be drawn up when the person is capable of understanding their intent, and they become effective only when the person lacks the capacity to make a particular health-related decision. These conditions are particularly relevant to people who are in early-stage dementia, because although loss of decisional capacity is a predictable outcome of this progressive condition, most people in early-stage dementia are capable of executing advance directives. For people with dementia, advance directives are essential tools for respecting patient rights and wishes when families and health care providers make decisions about care issues such as hospitalization, resuscitation, tube feeding, renal dialysis, antibiotic use, and end-of-life treatment care (Welie & Med, 2004). Feinberg and Whitlach (2002) found that people with mild to moderate cognitive impairment are able to communicate their wishes about daily care and to choose a surrogate decision maker.

In the absence of written advance directives, oral advance directives are often respected, but they may be challenged legally if family members do not agree with each other or have conflicts about the person's wishes. Oral advance directives are more likely to be accepted if the statements were (1) made known on a serious occasion, (2) repeated and consistent with the person's usual values, (3) made by a mature person who understood the underlying issues, or (4) made shortly before the need for a treatment decision or with some specificity to the actual conditions of the person (Bottrell, 2001).

Although all states and the District of Columbia have laws requiring all adults to have advance directive documents, only 10% to 20% of people in the United States have them (Brody, 2005). Most states require a periodic update of the advance directives (e.g., every 5 to 7 years). State laws vary regarding the scope and other details (e.g., type of document included, conditions under which it applies) of advance directives, and not all states honor out-of-state advance directives. This policy is particularly problematic for older adults who travel between or reside in more than one state. Gerontologists and lawmakers have called for standards and more uniformity among states regarding advance directives and recommend the use of one document that comprehensively addresses all of the issues related to health care decisions (Gunter-Hunt et al., 2002). Nurses need to have up-to-date information about their own state's legal requirements for advance directives, which is widely available in health care institutions. Common types of advance directives are discussed in the following sections.

Living Wills and Do Not Resuscitate (DNR) Orders

Living wills are legal documents whose purpose is to allow people to specify what type of medical treatment they would want or not want if they become incapacitated as a result of terminal illness. They evolved as a component of the first right-to-die statute, which was enacted in 1976 in California. People must be competent to initiate a living will, and they can revoke or change it at any time. A major goal of living wills is to affirm the right of a person to refuse treatment, but they do not always specify the particular type of treatment that can be refused. In addition to expressing wishes about refusal of treatment, living wills may express the person's preferences about pain management, organ donation, place of death, and specific treatments he or she would want to receive. A limitation of living will directives is that they apply only to situations in which the person is considered terminally ill, whereas advance directives apply to a broader range of circumstances (e.g., irreversible brain damage) that do not meet criteria for being a terminal illness, as previously discussed. Definitions of terminal illness are not always clear, and there may be disagreement about whether the person is terminally ill. In general, someone is considered to be terminally ill when a physician determines that his or her predictable life expectancy is 6 months or less. Some laws or policies require that two physicians document that the person is terminally ill.

Most states and the District of Columbia recognize the validity of living wills, but the scope and details of living wills differ from state to state. For example, some states require that living wills specifically address certain procedures, such as the withholding or withdrawal of artificial sustenance. Advocacy groups and health care professionals are encouraging all adults to draw up living wills and to take steps to ensure that all their health care providers have copies of these documents. For example, the United States Living Will Registry (listed in the Educational Resources section) electronically stores living wills and health care proxy documents and provides immediate access to living will documents for a small fee.

A **Do Not Resuscitate (DNR) order** is a very specific type of medical directive that compels health care providers to refrain from cardiopulmonary resuscitation if the person is no longer breathing and has no heartbeat. Sometimes families, as well as health care professionals, mistakenly associate DNR orders with directives to withhold other medical treatments. For example, they may raise questions about sending the person to a hospital or not requesting certain diagnostic or treatment procedures simply because a DNR order is in place. Thus, nurses have important roles in clarifying this document with the patient and the health care proxy so that additional and appropriate advance medical directives are in place to cover the circumstances that are most likely to arise.

In addition to focusing on the right to refuse treatments, medical directives address the person's desire for medical treatment that should be provided in certain circumstances. These directives can provide instructions about specific interventions, such as antibiotics, food and nutrition, and admission to the hospital. These documents afford reassurance to people who fear that medical treatments or pain control and comfort measures will not be provided when they are sick and cannot express their own wishes. Medical directives cannot guarantee that a medical intervention will be provided regardless of the circumstances; however, they provide legal assurance that the person's preferences will be considered. Because of the inability to predict medical treatments that might become available, and because of the changing health condition of the person executing the document, medical directives should be reviewed and updated periodically. Given the restrictions of living wills and the complexity of medical directives, older people who wish to use them should be encouraged to consult their attorneys and to fill out a durable power of attorney for health care, as well. In this way, the person will have legally recognized advance directives that facilitate decision making about end-of-life issues.

Durable Power of Attorney for Health Care

A **durable power of attorney for health care** is an advance directive that takes effect whenever someone cannot, for any reason, provide informed consent for health care treatment decisions. It allows a surrogate health care decision maker, also called a **health care proxy** or *proxy decision maker* (as previously discussed), to represent the person who is incapacitated. Like other powers of attorney, the durable power of attorney for health care must be initiated when the person is competent, and it takes effect only when the person is incapacitated. The document usually provides the proxy with written guidelines stating the person's wishes on issues such as the termination of life support. It is imperative that the health care proxy have a copy of all advance directives and periodically discuss the person's wishes about medical treatments and end-of-life issues. Because language in advance directive documents can sometimes be vague, nurses should encourage older adults to discuss their wishes with their primary care provider, other health care workers, and their designated surrogate before a crisis develops.

LEGAL ISSUES SPECIFIC TO LONG-TERM CARE SETTINGS

As the regulator of Medicare and Medicaid programs, Congress is responsible for ensuring that dollars expended for health care are well spent. In response to public concern about the quality of care in nursing homes during the 1960s, Congress mandated an Institute of Medicine study entitled *Improving the Quality of Care in Nursing Homes*, which was published in 1986. Recommendations of the study included the increased use of registered nurses, the use of standardized resident assessments, and the implementation of training and certification for nurse's aides. Subsequently, the Nursing Home Reform Act was included as part of the Omnibus Budget Reconciliation Act (OBRA) of 1987. It has had far-reaching consequences since its implementation during the early 1990s. For example, it established regulations for care of nursing home residents with particular emphasis on residents' rights and quality of life, and it established requirements for institutional staffing, training, and evaluation (Meyers, 2002). The provisions of OBRA that apply to nursing homes were developed through joint efforts of the Health Care Financing Administration, the National Citizens Coalition for Nursing Home Reform, the American Association for Retired Persons, representatives from the long-term care industry, and health care professionals.

OBRA states that each resident in a long-term care facility is to be at his or her highest practicable level of physical, mental, and psychosocial well-being, and that the long-term care facility is to accomplish this goal in an atmosphere that emphasizes residents' rights. To assist facilities in accomplishing this task, OBRA mandates that all Medicaid- and Medicare-funded facilities use a standardized form, known as the Minimum Data Set (MDS) for Resident Assessment and Care Planning. This form includes a Resident Assessment Instrument (RAI), which is a structured, multidimensional resident assessment and problem identification system. OBRA requires that within 14 days of admission, and at least annually thereafter, nursing facility staff performs a comprehensive, interdisciplinary assessment of every resident. Also, a care plan must be developed from that assessment, with the goal of continually evaluating the resident's highest functional level and preventing any deterioration unless it is assessed and clearly documented as unavoidable. A primary responsibility of nurses is to ensure that the comprehensive assessment is done at the appropriate times. Also, the nurse must ensure that the assessment tool is used as a basis for planning care that addresses the changing needs of the resident. By October of 1991, the RAI was being used in all Medicaid- and Medicare-funded nursing homes; in 1995, a second version of the MDS was developed to replace the first version.

In addition to addressing the development and documentation of care plans in nursing homes, OBRA strengthened the government oversight of nursing homes and addressed the many issues related to quality of care in nursing, which had been a focus of consumer advocacy groups since the 1970s. Improvements in nursing home care that have been attributed to the enactment of OBRA include decreased use of indwelling catheters, decreased prevalence of dehydration and pressure ulcers, increased presence of geriatricians and nurse practitioners, and reduced use of physical restraints and psychotropic drugs (Kane, 2001; Mitty, 2001; Sirin et al., 2002; Weintraub & Spurlock, 2002).

The Nursing Home Residents' Bill of Rights is one of the components of OBRA that has had the most far-reaching consequences for nursing home staff and residents. Federal law requires that all residents of long-term-care facilities are informed of their rights and that all long-term care facilities must have a mechanism in place for addressing complaints if residents think that their rights have been compromised. Moreover, facilities must post the Residents' Bill of Rights and the resources for investigating complaints in a prominent place. According to this law, "the resident has a right to a dignified existence, self-determination, and communication with and access to persons and services inside and outside the facility" (Code of Federal Regulations, Title 42, Section 483.10). Box 9-1 lists some of the rights explicitly defined by this bill. The National Long-Term Care Ombudsman program advocates for rights of residents of nursing homes, assisted-living facilities, and board and care homes, and investigates complaints. This program is established under the Older American Act and is available in every part of the United States (see the Educational Resources section for additional information).

ETHICAL ISSUES COMMONLY ADDRESSED IN GERONTOLOGICAL NURSING

Ethical Issues in Everyday Care of Older Adults

Health care professionals frequently encounter ethical dilemmas in relation to quality-of-life concerns because these issues involve choices and values that cannot be legislated. Nurses are increasingly recognizing that daily care issues involving patient preferences and quality of life frequently involve ethical dilemmas. For example, nurses

Box 9-1
Some Rights of Nursing Home Residents

The Right to Be Fully Informed

- The right to daily communication in their language
- The right to assistance if they have a sensory impairment
- The right to be notified in advance of any plans to change their room or roommate
- The right to be fully informed of all services available and the charge for each service

The Right to Participate in Their Own Care

- The right to receive adequate and appropriate care
- The right to participate in planning their treatment, care, and discharge
- The right to refuse medications, treatments, and physical and chemical restraints
- The right to review their own record

The Right to Make Independent Choices

- The right to make personal choices, such as what to wear and how to spend their time
- The right to reasonable accommodation of their needs and preferences
- The right to participate in activities, both inside and outside the nursing home
- The right to organize and participate in a Resident Council

The Right to Privacy and Confidentiality

- The right to private and unrestricted communication with any person
- The right to privacy in treatment and in personal care activities
- The right to confidentiality regarding their medical, personal, or financial affairs

The Right to Dignity, Respect, and Freedom

- The right to be treated with the fullest measure of consideration, respect, and dignity
- The right to be free from mental and physical abuse
- The right to self-determination

The Right to Security of Possessions

- The right to manage their own financial affairs
- The right to be free from charge for services covered by Medicaid or Medicare

Rights During Transfers and Discharges

- The right to remain in the facility unless a transfer or discharge is necessary, appropriate, or required
- The right to receive a 30-day notice of transfer or discharge

The Right to Complain

- The right to present grievances without fear of reprisal
- The right to prompt efforts by the nursing home to resolve grievances

The Right to Visits

- The right to immediate access by their relatives
- The right to reasonable visits by organizations or individuals providing health, social, legal, or other services

(Adapted from the U. S. Code of Federal Regulations, Title 42, Section 483.10, with permission.)

holistically address ethical questions such as the following in their usual care of patients (Keegan, 2005):

- Am I wise and courageous enough to perceive and respect others' differences and honor them as I honor my own beliefs?
- What does the patient want?
- Does the patient understand his or her choices?
- Is the patient being coerced?
- What does quality of life mean for this patient?
- How are others responding to the patient's perceptions of quality of life?

Nurses caring for older adults address these kinds of questions in the context of daily decisions that significantly affect quality of life. A recent study funded by the American Nurses Foundation identified "everyday ethics" concerns of older adult health care consumers. Nurse researchers identified the following types of characteristics that are particularly relevant to providing ethical nursing care of older adults (Smith, 2005):

- Being attentive and focusing on the patient (e.g., being available, actively listening, using good communication skills)
- Respecting a patient's likes and dislikes, worth and individuality, and choices about how he or she spends time
- Providing care services that are competent, adequate, necessary, and accountable (i.e., health care professionals take responsibility for their actions)

Because these everyday concerns are mundane, they are likely to be ignored in discussions of ethical issues, which more commonly focus on dramatic life-and-death decisions. However, these care issues are the ones that can have a significant impact on the quality of life for older adults. More important, they are the ethical issues that nurses can readily address through their own actions by being attentive and respectful in all their care (Smith, 2005).

Ethical Issues Specific to Long-Term Care Settings

The focus on quality of *care* in long-term care settings that was addressed through OBRA and other legislative mandates has been broadened to also address quality of *life* for nursing home residents (Calkins, 2002; Kane, 2001). Rosalie Kane, a prominent gerontologist, proposed that "a good quality of life should be elevated to a priority goal for long-term care rather than a pious afterthought to quality of care"

(2001, p. 297). In 2001, Kane identified the following 11 quality-of-life domains for nursing home residents: security, comfort, meaningful activity, relationships, enjoyment, dignity, autonomy, privacy, individuality, spiritual well-being, and functional competence. She further recommended that rules and regulations for long-term care place less emphasis on "the best quality of life *as is consistent with health and safety*" and place more emphasis on "the best health and safety outcomes possible *that are consistent with a meaningful quality of life*" (Kane, 2001, p. 296).

The increasing emphasis on autonomy, individual rights, and quality of life for residents of long-term care settings can lead to ethical issues because it is not always easy to balance needs of individual residents with those of others and the institution itself. Ethical issues also are associated with questions about safety versus freedom. For example, conflicts arise when a resident with a history of falls desires to walk freely around the facility, but staff members want to limit that person's activity to reduce the risk of falls. Additional examples of ethical decisions that nurses in long-term care settings commonly address include

- Using physical restraints
- Restricting cigarette smoking
- Allowing residents to refuse treatments, social activities, and food or fluid
- Providing more care assistance than necessary because it is more time-efficient for the staff
- Accommodating residents who wish to express sexual interests and activities

Ethical Issues in Chronic and Terminal Illness

Gerontologists and health care practitioners currently are addressing ethical issues related to the care of older adults with chronic illnesses, particularly during later stages and the end-of-life period. For example, much attention is paid to issues related to care and comfort during the later stages of conditions such as dementia, chronic renal disease, congestive heart failure, and chronic obstructive pulmonary disease. Ethical issues are inherent during the middle and later stages of dementia because families and health care professionals address numerous questions about autonomy, competency, decision making, and implementation of advance directives (Pinch, 2004). In these situations, nurses often address ethical questions such as, "Is the *length* of life the ultimate value, or is the *quality* of life the ultimate value?" (Matzo & Sherman, 2001). Health care professionals are increasingly addressing these kinds of questions by using palliative and hospice models of holistic care, as discussed in Chapters 27 and 29.

Nurses who care for older adults who have little or no ability to chew and swallow frequently address ethical issues about artificial nutrition and hydration, and these issues have become more controversial in recent years. During the 1980s, percutaneous endoscopic gastrostomy (PEG) tubes were developed for use in children with swallowing difficulties, and they have been found to be useful for people recovering from acute episodes such as stroke (Post, 2001). During the next decades, feeding tubes became a usual intervention for older patients with chronic or progressive conditions, and by the early 2000s, over one third of severely cognitively impaired residents of nursing homes in the United States had feeding tubes (Mitchell et al., 2003).

Feeding tubes have been viewed as an extension of ordinary care in the form of sustenance, and since the early 1990s they have been legally recognized as life-sustaining medical treatments (Derse, 2005). Because of this legal status, consideration of inserting a PEG tube is required when patients with severe dementia are transferred from hospitals to nursing homes (Detweiler et al., 2004). Thus, proxy decision makers for people in middle and late stages of dementia often face decisions about the placement of a feeding tube. These decisions are fraught with legal, ethical, and emotional dilemmas and often it is the nurse who assumes a dominant role in providing information and support.

There is increasing evidence that people with dementia do not benefit from long-term tube feeding (Carey et al., 2006; Detweiler et al., 2004; Gillick & Mitchell, 2002). In fact, research does not support the common perception that the use of feeding tubes in patients with advanced dementia maintains weight, improves function, prolongs survival, provides comfort, prevents aspiration pneumonia, or reduces risks of pressure sores or infections (Daly, 2000; Finucane et al., 1999; Post, 2001). Moreover, feeding tubes may contribute to discomfort rather than relieve suffering, and they are associated with the increased use of physical restraints (Gillick, 2000; Mitchell et al., 2003; Pasman, et al., 2005). Another detrimental effect is that people who are still able to enjoy the sensation of food are deprived of that simple pleasure.

Sometimes, the discussion about tube feeding is initiated because caregivers must provide considerable and time-consuming assistance with oral hydration and nutrition. Another reason for initiating discussion about tube feeding is concern about hunger and discomfort, which is typically associated with poor intake. However, it is important to recognize that when patients with chronically declining conditions are impaired to the extent that they have significant difficulty maintaining adequate intake, they are usually in the terminal stage. There is much research to support the view that the withholding of artificial hydration and nutrition at this stage is not associated with suffering as long as good oral care and desired sips of water are provided (Daly, 2000; Pasman et al., 2005; Post, 2001). In fact, studies indicate that diminished fluid and nutrition stimulates the release of natural endorphins that provide an analgesic effect and protect the person from discomfort (Critchlow & Bauer-Wu, 2002; Daly, 2000; Post, 2001). There is increasing evidence that the risks of artificial nutrition and hydration with feeding tubes outweigh the benefits (Detweiler et al., 2004).

Despite the evidence to the contrary, families who make the decisions for cognitively impaired patients often have high, but unrealistic, expectations about longevity and improved functioning after insertion of a feeding tube (Carey et al., 2006). Studies indicate that families base decisions about treatments such as feeding tubes on their perception of suffering, realization of futility, and understanding of patient preferences (Furlong, 2004). Thus, when families face complex decisions about feeding tubes, nurses are responsible for providing up-to-date information and answering questions about the advantages and disadvantages of artificial fluid and nutrition. For example, they can teach families that assisting with feeding and providing the benefits of social interaction and enjoyment of food may be a more compassionate approach than using feeding tubes, even if caloric intake is reduced (Detweiler et al., 2004). In addition, nurses can explain about patient behaviors and teach families about comfort measures and various aspects of suffering (Furlong, 2004).

CULTURAL ASPECTS OF LEGAL AND ETHICAL ISSUES

One major area of concern relative to the cultural aspects of legal and ethical issues is the need to accommodate people who do not speak English. Language barriers can significantly increase the difficulty of understanding advance directives and participating in complex decisions about medical treatments and other aspects of care. For example, legal experts have questioned the validity of advance directive documents when they are signed by people who do not receive sufficient information to give informed consent (Jones, 2005). Even when advance directives are available in the person's primary language, it is difficult to communicate the intent of these documents when there are conflicting cultural views on decisions about health care choices. For example, health care providers need to be aware of the strong Anglocentric bias of certain laws, such as the PSDA. The concept of individual autonomy may be unfamiliar or irrelevant to people in cultural groups such as Korean Americans, Mexican Americans, and Native Americans because they value a family-centered model of decision making (Furlong, 2004).

There are many significant cultural differences with regard to patterns of decision making about medical interventions and health care services. For example, some families may believe it is a sign of respect to protect an elder from the burdens of receiving information about his or her health status, or from making decisions about medical interventions and long-term care plans. This attitude may be in conflict with health care professionals who believe that all competent adults are entitled to information about their own health. Thus, nurses need to identify culturally influenced patterns of decision making by asking questions such as the following (Jenko & Moffitt, 2006):

- Some people want to know everything about their conditions and others do not. What do you prefer?
- Do you prefer to make your own decisions about medical care or would you prefer that someone else make them?
- To whom do you talk about your health care decisions?
- Who will help you decide where you are going to live?

In some situations, it may be appropriate to ask a family member about decision-making patterns.

It is especially important to be sensitive to cultural differences when discussing not only advance directives, but all end-of-life issues, including hospice care. For example, because some Hispanic traditions place a high value on family caregiving, people from this group may prefer to provide personal care to dying elders, but they may be willing to accept help from hospice agencies with technical skills, such as pain management and symptom relief (Adams et al., 2005). Another example of cultural differences in the use of services is the underutilization of hospice services by African Americans. One study identified the following factors that may affect the use of hospice by African American people (Taxis, 2006):

- Emphasis of hospice programs on the acceptance of death, in contrast to some African American traditions that value aggressive life-sustaining treatments

A Student's Perspective

In working with "G," an 82-year-old Chinese woman, I have learned a lot about her background. She and her three brothers, two sisters, and parents were all born in China. Her parents moved the children to Jakarta, a city in Indonesia, which was a Dutch colony at the time, to get a better education. Chinese culture emphasizes respect for elders, especially the father, who is head of the family. G giggles and comments "when father said 'eat that,' we ate it, whether we liked it or not." As an adult, she worked for a time in the front lobby of the U.S. embassy as a translator. Her position led her on many journeys throughout the world, working in Russia, Germany, France, and eventually to the United States. G didn't marry until she was 70, when she married an American. She now lives in a quiet neighborhood with her husband.

A difficulty in learning more about G and her culture regarding health care has been her acceptance of her disease process. Her cultural background taught her to view authority figures such as physicians with incredible esteem. Until I learned more about her culture, I wasn't always certain she understood what was being said because she would sit with her head down and only nod, or simply say, "yes." I now realize those behaviors are her way of showing respect to an authority figure. She seldom looks you in the eye, another form of showing respect. She is also hesitant to ask questions so as not to appear disrespectful. G looks to her husband many times to make decisions for her.

Deborah L.

- Preference to avoid discussion related to end-of-life planning
- Mistrust of the health care system in general, which leads to fears of unfair treatment and the withholding of potentially life-saving measures
- Preference to trust close family members to make end-of-life decisions and therefore not to seek outside medical care
- Perception that hospice is equated with inadequate care and the giving up of hope
- Lack of information about services, which leads to misgivings, misconceptions, and fears

Cultural Considerations 9-1 summarizes some cultural considerations related to legal and ethical aspects of gerontological nursing care.

ROLE OF NURSES REGARDING LEGAL AND ETHICAL ISSUES

Nurses frequently address legal and ethical concerns with regard to implementing advance directives and facilitating decisions about care. Although these issues are often addressed within the context of a multidisciplinary team and always in conjunction with the primary care practitioner, nurses have unique and important responsibilities, which are reviewed in the following sections.

Implementing Advance Directives

In recent years, organizations such as the Agency for Healthcare Research Quality (AHRQ) have increasingly recognized and emphasized the important role of nurses and health care professionals in communicating with older adults about advance directives (Black & Emmet, 2006). Studies have identified the following roles of nurses in working with older adults with regard to advance care planning (Black & Emmet, 2006; Jezewski & Meeker, 2005):

- Improving the ability of older adults to better plan for the future
- Discussing plans for care, which increases older patients' satisfaction with plans
- Taking time to explain advance directives and answer patients' questions
- Increasing comfort level and decreasing fear and anxiety about advance care
- Engaging in conversations about hopes, wishes, values, and goals of care
- Facilitating the completion of advance care documents

In addition to working directly with older adults, nurses are responsible for informing other members of the health care team about advance care directives and for ensuring that documents are readily accessible. All caregivers should know what advance directives cover and, when they care for people over long periods, they should periodically review and discuss the documents with the older adult or his

Cultural Considerations 9-1

Cultural Considerations Related to Legal and Ethical Aspects of Care

Autonomy and Decision-Making Patterns

Decision-making patterns in many non-Western cultures are centered on the good of the group rather than the good of the individual, and are based on the social framework paradigm rather than the autonomy paradigm. Family and kinship patterns delineate the different roles, status, and power of each member of the group, and the social hierarchy governs decision making. For example, according to some Japanese traditions, group members are expected to honor and obey the male elder because he is accorded higher status and authority and carries a sense of responsibility for the entire group (Pacquiao, 2003).

In many non-Western cultures (Lipson & Dibble, 2005):

- Patients may prefer not to be informed about medical conditions or involved with decisions about their care.
- Decisions about medical care may be based on the good of the family, rather than the good of the individual.
- Families may expect that medical information will be given to the designated family authority figure, who then will decide what to do with the information.
- Decisions are likely to be made by a designated authority figure, although the opinions of all adult family members are acknowledged.
- As a sign of respect, elders may be protected from the burden and responsibility of making decisions about their own health care.
- The primary health care provider may be seen as the authority figure who should make decisions without discussing options with patients or their families.

Advance Directives

- Cultures with strong family ties may not see the need for advance directives because they expect the family members to make decisions, and advance directives may represent a conflict between individual autonomy and family solidarity (Pacquiao, 2003).
- Cultures that see the cycle of birth, life, and death as natural (e.g., Native American people) may see no need for advance directives.
- Cultures that believe in fatalism (e.g., Filipino) are likely to resist any discussion about planning for events that are beyond one's control, such as illness or death, because it is viewed as tempting fate and will likely bring the potential event into reality (Pacquiao, 2003).
- African American people may be suspicious of advance directives and equate these with abandonment by health care practitioners based on the legacy of slavery and past experiences with medical research (e.g., the Tuskegee experiments) (Crawley et al., 2002; Dupree, 2000).

continued on following page

Continued

- Filipino and Chinese nurses may be uncomfortable discussing advance directives because they see their role as caregivers; they may prefer that clergy or pastoral care service representatives discuss advance directives with hospitalized patients (Pacquiao, 2001).

or her proxy. In addition, nurses should encourage people to provide copies of advance directives to their family members, designated surrogate, and anyone likely to be involved with decisions about their medical care. When written advance directives do not exist, nurses can initiate a discussion of relevant medical care and end-of-life treatment preferences and document any statements made that express a patient's wishes.

Another role of nurses is addressing barriers to effective implementation of advance directives, such as the following (Meyers et al., 2004):

- Advance directives are not valid in health care institutions until they take the form of a physician's orders.
- Many institutions honor only their own specific forms, especially for DNR orders.
- Advance directive forms frequently do not accompany patients when they are transferred between settings.
- Information in advance directives is not always communicated or honored.

One way of conveying the wishes of a patient when he or she is transferred between health care settings is to develop a form that documents choices about specific end-of-life care and gives these choices the power of a physician's orders (Meyers et al., 2004).

Facilitating Decisions About Care

Older adults generally prefer that family members, rather than health care providers, be surrogate decision makers, and they trust that family members will make appropriate choices. Although most older people are willing to discuss their wishes about medical treatments, they usually expect health care professionals to initiate the topic. A study of preferences for care at the end of life found that 88% of respondents wanted health care providers to ask them about feelings related to their illness and dying, 85% wanted nurses to attend to emotional and spiritual needs in addition to physical needs, and 80% wished to have the opportunity to discuss fears about approaching death (Schirm & Sheehan, 2005). In light of this information, nurses have an obligation to older adults and their surrogate decision makers to assist them in decision-making processes by providing accurate information on rights and statutes, addressing questions about their care, listening to their needs, attending to concerns about end-of-life care, and acting as liaisons with primary care providers when necessary.

Another important role of nurses is to provide information and support to proxy decision makers. When complex decisions must be made, an interdisciplinary team—composed of a social worker, a religious leader, therapists, nurses, and a primary care provider—may provide information and support to proxy decision makers. Decision-making assistance from professionals may relieve families and proxy decision makers of some of the guilt they could experience when making and implementing decisions, particularly difficult end-of-life decisions. Hospitals and long-term care facilities that are accredited by the Joint Commission (formerly the Joint Commission on Accreditation of Healthcare Organizations [JCAHO]) are required to have ethics committees that provide a formal mechanism for addressing medical ethical dilemmas within their institutions. Nurses are encouraged to initiate the development of ethics committees in long-term care facilities and to use the facility's ethics handbook or policies and procedures as a guide for discussion and education (Hogstel et al., 2004).

Nurses also take a strong role in supporting and facilitating decisions about care during chronic conditions and end-of-life care. In addition to addressing concerns about hydration and nutrition (discussed previously), nurses provide information about the best types of services (e.g., hospice programs, palliative care) or place of care (e.g., hospital admission for nursing home residents when medical problems arise). Guidelines and recommendations for these decisions are available from nursing organizations such as the National League for Nursing (NLN) and the American Nurses Association (ANA). For example, in 1992 the ANA published a position statement on foregoing nutrition and hydration with specific recommendations about the role of nurses. Some of the many excellent educational resources that are available for nurses and consumers about end-of-life decisions are listed in the Educational Resources section.

CHAPTER HIGHLIGHTS

Autonomy and Rights

- Adults have the right to make health-related decisions unless they have been declared incompetent by a judge.
- If an adult's decision-making capacity is questionable, his or her rights can be protected through legal documents, such as advance directives.

Advance Directives

- Legal documents (e.g., living wills, Do Not Resuscitate orders) make a person's wishes relative to medical treatments known to care providers and surrogate decision makers.
- Nurses play an important role in making sure these documents are available and their instructions being followed.

Legal Issues Specific to Long-Term Care Settings

- Since the federal government enacted OBRA legislation in the 1980s, nursing homes are required to meet certain standards of care, and to document assessments and care plans.

- Positive consequences of OBRA in nursing homes include decreased use of indwelling catheters, reduced use of physical and chemical restraints, and fewer cases of dehydration and pressure ulcers.
- The Nursing Home Bill of Rights states that residents are entitled to dignity, self-determination, and the opportunity to communicate.
- Autonomy issues are frequently addressed by nurses in long-term care settings; balancing the rights of residents with institutional needs often poses a challenge.

Ethical Issues Commonly Addressed in Gerontological Nursing

- Nurses are often involved in decisions about artificial hydration and nutrition.
- Assisting with care decisions during chronic illness is one of the most challenging aspects of nursing.

Cultural Aspects of Legal and Ethical Issues

- Language barriers are important to consider when discussing advance directives.
- Nurses should identify culturally influenced patterns of decision making when discussing advance directives and end-of-life care with patients and their families.

Role of Nurses Regarding Legal and Ethical Issues

- Nurses communicate with older adults about advance directives, inform other members of the health care team about advance directives, and address barriers to implementing advance directives.
- Nurses facilitate decision making about advance directives by providing information about advance directives and care options to older adults and to proxy decision makers.

Critical Thinking Exercises

1. You have been assigned to work with Mrs. M., an 85-year-old, white, widowed woman who is in the hospital with congestive heart failure. Her son and daughter tell you they would like to arrange for her to be discharged to a nursing home because they don't think she takes her medications correctly and they are tired of her being admitted to the hospital every couple of months "to get her straightened out." The son and daughter live in another state and visit only when their mother is in the hospital. Mrs. M. has told you that she thinks her son and daughter would like to have her "put away in one of those homes" but she is adamantly opposed to leaving her home. She also has told you that they think she is "senile" and that she should stop driving her car, but she thinks she is quite capable of living alone, driving her car, and taking care of herself. Your observations are that she needs a lot of direction to take medications and participate in self-care activities, and she seems to be somewhat confused later in the day. What steps would you take to address her competency and decision-making abilities?
2. A Mexican American woman, 78 years old, is being admitted to the hospital with hemiplegia after a stroke. There are no advance directives on her chart. What information would you want to know before you approached her about a living will and durable power of attorney for health care? How would you explain these documents to her?
3. Mr. S. is 78 years old and has been admitted for hip surgery after a fall-related fracture. He has had dementia for 5 years and his family provides care for him in his home. His son is designated as his durable power of attorney for health care, but he will not make any decisions unless his three sisters agree to them. Mr. S. does not have any other advance directives and the family says he never talked much about what medical care services he would want. He always told his family that they could make whatever decisions are best for him. The physician has asked the family to consider placement of a PEG tube because Mr. S.'s food and fluid intake are inadequate to meet his needs and one pressure area is beginning to develop on his buttocks. Mr. S.'s son and one daughter think that their father would have wanted to have every intervention possible in such a situation, and they think the PEG tube will improve his comfort and prevent the pressure ulcer. The other two daughters adamantly state that their father would never agree to such an invasive procedure and they are not sure it will make him any more comfortable. They also worry that he will need to be restrained to keep him from pulling the tube out. You are a member of the multidisciplinary team that is meeting with the family to help them come to a decision about a PEG tube. What points would you want to make during this family conference?

Educational Resources

AARP (American Association of Retired Persons)
www.aarp.org

Aging With Dignity
www.agingwithdignity.org

American Association of Colleges of Nursing (AACN)
End-of-Life Nursing Education Consortium Project
www.aacn.nche.edu/elnec

American Bar Association Commission on Law and Aging
www.abanet.org/aging

American Bar Association, Senior Lawyers Division
www.abanet.org/srlawyers

American Nurses Association (ANA)
Center for Ethics & Human Rights
www.nursingworld.org/ethics

National Long-Term Care Ombudsman Program
www.ltcombudsman.org

National Senior Citizens Law Center
www.nsclc.org

U.S. Living Will Registry
www.uslivingwillregistry.com

REFERENCES

Adams, C. E., Horn, K., & Bader, J. (2005). A comparison of utilization of hospice services between Hispanics and whites. *Journal of Hospice and Palliative Nursing, 7*, 328–335.

Aging With Dignity. (2001). *Five wishes*. Tallahassee, FL: Author.

Black, K., & Emmet, C. (2006). Nurses' advance care planning communication: An investigation. *Geriatric Nursing, 27*, 222–227.

Bottrell, M. M. (2001). Advance directives. In M. D. Mezey (Ed.), *The encyclopedia of elder care* (pp. 21–24). New York: Springer.

Brody, H. (2005). Shared decision making and determining decision-making capacity. *Primary Care: Clinics in Office Practice, 32*, 645–658.

Calkins, M. C. (2002). The nursing home of the future: Are you ready? *Nursing Homes/Long Term Care Management, 51*(6), 42–47.

Carey, T. S., Hanson, L, Garrett, J. M., Lewis, C., Pfifer, N., Cox, C. E., et al. (2006). Expectations and outcomes of gastric feeding tubes. *American Journal of Medicine, 119*, 527.e11–527.e16.

Collopy, B. J. (1988). Autonomy in long term care: Some crucial distinctions. *The Gerontologist, 28*(Suppl.), 10–17.

Crawley, L. M., Marshall, P. A., Lo, B., & Koenig, B. A. (2002). Strategies for culturally effective end-of-life care. *Annals of Internal Medicine, 136*, 673–678.

Critchlow, J., & Bauer-Wu, S. M. (2002). Nurses' perceptions of dehydration. *Journal of Gerontological Nursing, 28*(12), 31–39.

Dalinis, P. M. (2005). Informed consent and decisional capacity. *Journal of Hospice and Palliative Nursing, 7*, 52–57.

Daly, B. J. (2000). Special challenges of withholding artificial nutrition and hydration. *Journal of Gerontological Nursing, 26*(9), 25–31.

Derse, A. R. (2005). Limitation of treatment at the end-of-life: Withholding the withdrawal. *Clinics in Geriatric Medicine, 21*, 223–238.

Detweiler, M. B., Kim, K. Y., & Bass, J. (2004). Percutaneous endoscopic gastrostomy in cognitively impaired older adults: A geropsychiatric perspective. *American Journal of Alzheimer's Disease and Other Dementias, 19*, 24–30.

Dupree, C. Y. (2000). The attitudes of black Americans toward advance directives. *Journal of Transcultural Nursing, 11*(1), 12–18.

Feinberg, L. F., & Whitlach, C. J. (2002). Decision-making for persons with cognitive impairment and their family caregivers. *American Journal of Alzheimer's Disease and Other Dementias, 17*, 237–244.

Finucane, T. E., Christmas, C., & Travis, K. (1999). Tube feeding in patients with advanced dementia: A review of the evidence. *Journal of the American Medical Association, 282*, 1365–1370.

Furlong, E. (2004). The role of nurses and nursing education in the palliative care of patients and their families. In R. B. Purtilo & H. tenHave (Eds.), *Ethical foundations of palliative care for Alzheimer's disease* (pp. 243–260). Baltimore: The Johns Hopkins University Press.

Gillick, M. R. (2000). Rethinking the role of tube feeding in patients with advanced dementia. *New England Journal of Medicine, 342*, 206–210.

Gillick, M. R., & Mitchell, S. L. (2002). Facing eating difficulties in end-stage dementia. *Alzheimer's Care Quarterly, 3*, 227–232.

Gunter-Hunt, G., Mahoney, J. E., & Sieger, C. E. (2002). A comparison of state advance directive documents. *The Gerontologist, 2*, 51–60.

Hogstel, M. O., Curry, L. C., Walker, C. A., & Burns, P. G. (2004). Ethics committees in long-term care facilities. *Geriatric Nursing, 25*, 364–368.

Jenko, M., & Moffitt, S. R. (2006). Transcultural nursing principles: An application to hospice care. *Journal of Hospice and Palliative Nursing, 8*, 172–180.

Jezewski, M. A., & Meeker, M. A. (2005). Constituting advance directives from the perspective of people with chronic illnesses. *Journal of Hospice and Palliative Nursing, 7*, 319–327.

Jones, C. J. (2005). Say what? How the Patient Self-Determination Act leaves the elderly with limited English proficiency out in the cold. *The Elder Law Journal, 13*, 490–518.

Kane, R. A. (2001). Long-term care and a good quality of life bringing them closer together. *The Gerontologist, 41*, 293–304.

Keegan, L. (2005). Holistic ethics. In B. M. Dossey, L. Keegan, & C. E. Guzetta (Eds.), *Holistic nursing: A handbook for practice* (4th ed., pp. 93–106). Boston: Jones and Bartlett.

Lipson, J. G., & Dibble, S. L. (2005). *Culture & clinical care*. San Francisco: UCSF Nursing Press.

Matzo, M. L., & Sherman, D. W. (2001). Palliative care nursing: Ensuring competent care at the end of life. *Geriatric Nursing, 22*, 288–293.

McCullough, L. B., Molinari, V., & Workman, R. H. (2001). Implications of impaired executive control functions for patient autonomy and surrogate decision making. *Journal of Clinical Ethics, 12*, 397–405.

Meyers, E. M. (2002). Physical restraints in nursing homes: An analysis of quality of care and legal liability. *The Elder Law Journal, 10*, 217–262.

Meyers, J. L., Moore, C., McGrory, A., Sparr, J., & Ahern, M. (2004). Physician orders for life-sustaining treatment form: Honoring end-of-life directives for nursing home residents. *Journal of Gerontological Nursing, 30*(9), 37–46.

Mitchell, S. L., Teno, J. M., Roy, J., Kabumoto, G., & Mor, V. (2003). Clinical and organizational factors associated with feeding tube use among nursing home residents with advanced cognitive impairment. *Journal of the American Medical Association, 290*, 73–80.

Mitty, E. L. (2001). Nursing homes. In M. D. Mezey (Ed.), *The encyclopedia of elder care* (pp. 452–455). New York: Springer.

Pacquiao, D. F. (2001). Addressing cultural incongruities of advance directives. *Bioethics Forum, 17*(1), 27–31.

Pacquiao, D. F. (2003). Cultural competence in ethical decision-making. In M. M. Andrews & J. S. Boyle (Eds.), *Transcultural concepts in nursing care* (4th ed., pp. 503–532). Philadelphia: Lippincott Williams & Wilkins.

Pasman, H. R. W., Onwuteaka-Philipsen, B. D., Kriegsman, D. M. W., Ooms, M. E., Ribbe, M. W., & van der Wal, G. (2005). Discomfort in nursing home patients with severe dementia in whom artificial nutrition and hydration is forgone. *Archives of Internal Medicine, 165*, 1729–1735.

Pinch, W. J. E. (2004). Advance directives and end-of-life decision making in Alzheimer disease. In R. B. Purtilo & H. tenHave (Eds.), *Ethical foundations of palliative care for Alzheimer's disease* (pp. 181–199) Baltimore: The Johns Hopkins University Press.

Post, S. G. (2001). Tube feeding and advanced progressive dementia. *Hastings Center Report, 31*(1), 36–42.

Schirm, V., & Sheehan, D. K. (2005). Conversations about choices for end-of-life care: Knowing and understanding preferences. *Journal of Hospice and Palliative Nursing, 7*, 91–97.

Sirin, S. R., Castle, N. G., & Smyer, M. (2002). Risk factors for physical restraint use in nursing homes: The impact of the Nursing Home Reform Act. *Research on Aging, 24*, 513–527.

Smith, K. V. (2005). Ethical issues and health care. *Journal of Gerontological Nursing, 31*(2), 32–39.

Taxis, J. C. (2006). Attitudes, values, and questions of African Americans regarding participation in hospice programs. *Journal of Hospice and Palliative Nursing, 8*, 77–85.

Weintraub, D., & Spurlock, M. (2002). Change in the rate of restraint use and falls on psychogeriatric inpatient unit: Impact of the Health Care Financing Administration's new restraint and seclusions standards for hospitals. *Journal of Geriatric Psychiatry and Neurology, 15*, 91–94.

Welie, J. V. M., & Med, M. (2004). The tendency of contemporary decision-making strategies to deny the condition of Alzheimer disease. In R. B. Purtilo & H. tenHave (Eds.), *Ethical foundations of palliative care for Alzheimer's disease* (pp. 164–180). Baltimore: The Johns Hopkins University Press.

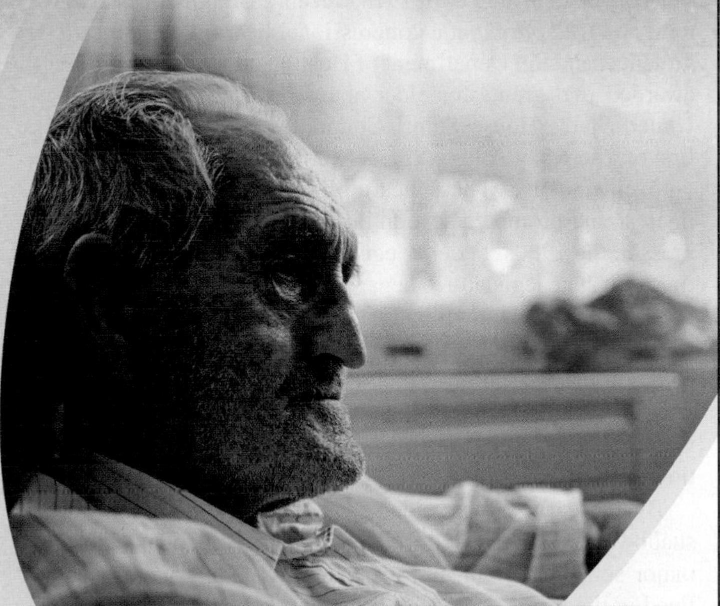

CHAPTER 10

Elder Abuse and Neglect

Learning Objectives

After reading this chapter, you will be able to:

1. Define the various types of elder abuse.
2. Describe risk factors that contribute to elder abuse and neglect.
3. Describe nursing assessment aimed toward identifying elder abuse and neglect, as well as risks for abuse and neglect.
4. Describe the nurse's opportunities for interventions for elder abuse in different practice settings.
5. Discuss the range of nursing and legal interventions directed toward preventing and alleviating elder abuse.

Key Terms

emotional (psychological) abuse
exploitation
neglect
physical abuse
self-abuse
self-neglect
sexual abuse

Because elder abuse is a very complex and serious negative functional consequence that affects vulnerable older adults, these situations challenge gerontological nurses to apply their highest level of nursing skills. This chapter presents elder abuse as a serious impairment of overall function and discusses it in the framework of the functional consequences theory.

OVERVIEW OF ELDER ABUSE AND NEGLECT

Certain members of any population are vulnerable to abuse and neglect by virtue of being physically or psychosocially impaired or subjugated. In industrialized societies today, vulnerable groups are protected and cared for through legislative mandates and social programs. For example, children and people with mental retardation have been protected for many decades in the United States and many other countries. More recently, two additional groups have been recognized as being in need of protection: victims of domestic violence and abused or neglected older people. Although the problem of abused or neglected older adults is not new, elder abuse has received increased attention as a social problem in recent decades.

Definitions

There are many definitions of elder abuse, and these have changed over time in response to shifts in political climate, public sentiment, available funding, and increasing knowledge and professional interest. This section presents several widely recognized definitions, and the following section provides an overview of the historical recognition of elder abuse.

The National Research Council (2003) defines elder mistreatment as: "(a) Intentional actions that cause harm or create a serious risk of harm, whether or not intended, to a vulnerable elder by a caregiver or other person who stands in a trust relationship to the elder, or (b) failure by a caregiver to satisfy the elder's basic needs or to protect the elder from harm." This definition was developed to address the historic ambiguities over what constitutes elder abuse and to foster empirical investigation of the subject using comparable research design. Although an admirable goal, the definition falls short of capturing the many elder abuse variations identified by clinicians and evident in state statutes (Hamp, 2003).

The National Center on Elder Abuse (2003b) recognizes three basic categories of elder abuse (i.e., domestic elder abuse, institutional elder abuse, and self-neglect or self-abuse) and seven major types or forms (i.e., physical abuse, sexual abuse, emotional or psychological abuse, neglect, abandonment, financial or material exploitation, and self-neglect). Self-neglect in this classification includes behaviors of older adults that threaten their health or safety (National Center on Elder Abuse, 2003a).

Recently, elder abuse has evolved into a concept with almost unlimited boundaries, as evidenced by the United Nations Second World Assembly on Aging (United Nations Economic and Social Council, 2002). This World Assembly viewed elder abuse as encompassing virtually anything that causes harm or distress to an older person and that occurs in a relationship with a trust expectation. This definition includes acts as wide ranging as scapegoating elders to small-scale warfare where older people are victimized. Other examples of an ever-expanding conceptualization of elder abuse include newspaper articles depicting older disaster victims as suffering from elder abuse and legal services advertisements labeling compromised quality of care in long-term care facilities as elder abuse.

Historical Recognition of a Social Problem

Awareness of elder abuse as a social problem began in the 1950s and 1960s as the writings of Geneva Mathiasen and Gertrude Hall introduced the concept of protecting vulnerable adults. Centers like the Benjamin Rose Institute in Cleveland, Ohio, developed the concept in the early 1970s through initial demonstration projects, usually specifically related to self-neglect. Awareness of physical abuse, however, did not surface until the late 1970s, and awareness of other types of elder abuse (e.g., domestic violence against elders) followed. The late 1980s witnessed the growing criminalization of elder abuse, a movement that peaked during the late 1990s. During this phase, consumer fraud aimed at older adults, including scams and con games, was subsumed under elder abuse.

During the late 1970s, domestic elder abuse was first brought to public attention when congressional hearings on child abuse suggested that the entire scope of family violence be considered. In 1978, Suzanne Steinmetz used the term *battered parent* at a congressional hearing on domestic violence, and the Department of Health and Human Services awarded two grants for elder abuse research. In 1979, the United States House Select Committee on Aging held the first of a series of congressional hearings dealing exclusively with elder abuse. These hearings stimulated much public interest and prompted several bills to be introduced in Congress in the 1980s. Federal legislation was not passed at that time, but state legislatures began addressing the issue and, by the mid-1990s, all states had passed some form of adult protective services or abuse-reporting laws. A major step was taken on the federal level in 1989 with the establishment of what is now called the National Center on Elder Abuse, which operates under the auspices of the National Association of State Units on Aging.

By the early 1990s, elder abuse had emerged from the shadows of child and spousal abuse and was recognized as a major social problem. Stories of abused elders were headlined in the print media and discussed on popular news programs and television talk shows. In addition, elder abuse and neglect emerged as topics at every major aging-related conference and in public policy agendas. For example, federal government agencies, including the Departments of Justice and Health and Human Services, have sponsored several national forums on elder abuse since 2000. These forums are indicative of increasing federal activity and interagency collaboration related to both service and criminal justice approaches to elder abuse.

Reports of elder abuse are increasing, and it is now recognized as a major social problem and a significant aspect of family violence. This increasing attention can be attributed to reasons such as the following:

- The older adult population has been increasing rapidly, with the most vulnerable groups of older people (i.e., those who are 85 years of age and older) increasing at the fastest rate.
- Adult children increasingly are called upon to care for their elderly parents; however, some do not have the skills, resources, availability, or physical proximity to undertake this responsibility successfully.
- Researchers and clinicians are directing more attention to the problems that affect the most vulnerable older adults, leading to more information and publications.
- Educational efforts have made professionals and the public more aware of reporting laws and adult protective services.
- Congressional hearings and educational programs have stimulated public and professional interest in the issue.
- Organizations such as the National Committee for the Prevention of Elder Abuse and the National Adult Protective Services Association have promoted professional

networking and advocated for public policy addressing elder abuse.

In 1975, gerontological practitioners became aware of elder abuse through a letter to the editor of the *British Medical Journal* referring to "granny-battering" (Burston, 1975). That same year, Robert Butler discussed the battered older person syndrome in his Pulitzer Prize–winning book *Why Survive? Being Old in America* (Butler, 1975). By the late 1970s, articles on the subject began appearing in the gerontological literature in both England and the United States. In 1979, the first published study on elder abuse revealed that nearly 10% of 404 clients of the Chronic Illness Center in Cleveland, Ohio, had suffered abuse or neglect during the previous year (Lau & Kosberg, 1979).

Gerontological nurses have been in the forefront of research and publications on elder abuse. Beginning in the late 1970s, nursing journals began publishing articles on elder abuse, and by the 1980s nurses had coauthored the first clinically oriented texts on elder abuse (Fulmer & O'Malley, 1987; Quinn & Tomita, 1986). Since the mid-1990s, nursing has been represented in the field of elder abuse through the research of such scholars as Terry Fulmer (Fulmer et al., 2004, 2005), Linda Phillips (2000; Phillips, et al., 2000), and Elizabeth Podnieks (2006).

Incidence and Causes

Elder abuse is neither a rare nor an isolated phenomenon in the United States. Rather, all indicators suggest that maltreatment of vulnerable older adults is widespread and occurs among all subgroups worldwide. Although estimates of elder abuse range from 1% to 10%, it is widely agreed that it is difficult to be confident about the accuracy of these estimates because of significant underreporting of cases and differing definitions of elder abuse and neglect. Studies suggest that most maltreatment is repeated, is seldom reported to authorities, and represents more than one form of abuse. Although the problem can affect any older person, the typical abuse victim is a socially isolated and physically or cognitively impaired woman of advanced age who lives alone or with the abuser and depends on the abuser for care.

A recent survey of elder abuse cases reported to adult protective services indicates that reporting increased by nearly 20% between 2000 and 2004 (Teaster et al., 2005). Additional statistics from the study of Teaster and colleagues include the following:

- Types of abuse
  - Self-neglect: 29%
  - Neglect by caregiver: 26%
  - Exploitation: 19%
  - Psychological or emotional abuse: 12%
  - Physical abuse: 12%
  - Sexual abuse: less than 1%
- Characteristics of abused elder
  - Female: 66%
  - Age 70 years or older: 57%, with 31% age 80 years and older
  - White: 77%
  - Living in a domestic setting: 89%
- Characteristics of abuse perpetrator
  - Female: 53%
  - Middle aged: 30%
  - Adult child of the victim: 33%
  - Other family member: 22%
  - Spouse or intimate partner: 10%

Additional results from this study and the National Elder Abuse Incidence Study are available at www.elderabusecenter.org.

Other studies have identified profiles of abused elders by type of abuse. For example, victims of self-neglect are more likely to be older, living alone, and isolated from family, and to have dementia, mental illness, or substance abuse (Tierney et al., 2004; Payne & Gainey, 2005). Many self-neglecters also exhibit hoarding behavior (Franks et al., 2004; Ramsey-Klawsnik, 2006). Finally, there may be some association between type of abuse and the sex of the perpetrator, with men being more likely to exploit or physically abuse elders and women being more likely to physically neglect or psychologically abuse elders.

Studies of specific types of maltreatment indicate that elder abuse results from multiple, interrelated variables. Lachs and Pillemer (2004) summarized the characteristics associated with victims and perpetrators (Box 10-1). In summary, research on the causes of elder abuse is pointing in the following directions:

- Causation varies by form of abuse.
- The etiology of any form of abuse is a composite of several interrelated variables.
- The origins of elder abuse are found in both the victim and the perpetrator, as well as in the relationship between the two.
- The etiology of elder abuse differs from that suggested for other abused populations in important ways (e.g., elder abuse is uniquely associated with ageism).

Box 10-1
Elder Abuse Profiles

Characteristics of the Perpetrator

- Alcohol abuse
- Mental illness
- History of violence or hostility
- Dependence on the victim
- Stress

Characteristics of the Victim

- Social isolation
- Chronic illness or functional limitation
- Cognitive impairment
- Shared living arrangement with the perpetrator

Cultural Considerations

As a worldwide issue, elder abuse is being addressed in the context of the basic human right to be free from violence in the home. Much of the focus is on cultural variations in definitions of elder abuse, and many studies in the United States center on attitudes toward elder abuse across different ethnic communities (Malley-Morrison et al., 2006) (Cultural Considerations 10-1).

Cultural Considerations 10-1

Studies of Cultural Variation and Commonality With Regard to Elder Abuse

- Korean American elders were found to be more tolerant of elder abuse in general and financial exploitation in particular than either white or African American elders (Moon & Benton, 2000).
- Korean Americans were more likely to blame the victims for their abuse and more resistant to seeking outside help than whites or African Americans (Moon & Benton, 2000).
- The only study of Native American elders in an urban setting found that 10% definitely or probably and an additional 7% possibly had been abused, with women nine times more likely to be physically abused than men, and elder abuse victims four times more likely to be dependent on others for food than nonvictims (Buchwald et al., 2000).
- Older African Americans were likely to emphasize physical abuse when giving examples of extremely abusive behavior (Tauriac & Scruggs, 2006).
- A study of four ethnic groups in two urban areas found comparability among European Americans, African Americans, Puerto Ricans, and Japanese Americans in the importance placed on psychological abuse and neglect as forms of mistreatment (Anetzberger et al., 1996).
- Asian Indians were found to consider ignoring and not visiting the worst things that family members can do to elderly people (Nagpaul, 1997).
- An investigation of two geographically distinct Plains Indian reservations revealed that elder abuse was more common in the reservation that had the higher unemployment and substance abuse rates and little potential income from the land (Krassen Maxwell & Maxwell, 1992).
- Financial abuse was the most prevalent form of mistreatment among African Americans in rural North Carolina (Griffin, 1994).
- In studies examining within-group differences among two Native American groups and five white American groups in North Carolina, differences were noted with regard to perceptions of the boundaries of elder abuse (Hudson et al., 1998, 2000).

Diversity Note

Strong family ties and respect for others that are inherent values in the Hispanic culture may minimize the incidence of elder abuse, but strong family ties and male/female roles may reduce the incidence of reporting it in the Hispanic community (Montoya, 1997).

Cultural variation extends beyond race and ethnicity, of course. Although research in this area is minimal, early explorations suggest differences among such other minority groups as older gays and lesbians. For instance, Cook-Daniels (1997) proposed that older gays and lesbians may be more vulnerable to elder abuse, especially self-neglect, because of social isolation stemming from living in a homophobic social environment. For many, this has resulted in a history of hiding, value of independence, and fear of encountering homophobia, particularly from senior service providers.

Although understanding cultural variations in the incidence and interpretations of elder abuse is important, nurses should also remember that individuals vary. Not all members of a cultural, religious, or minority group behave according to reported trends.

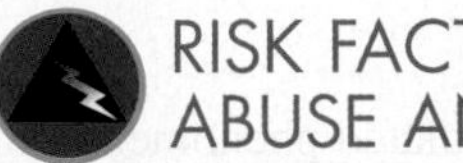

RISK FACTORS FOR ELDER ABUSE AND NEGLECT

Identification of risk factors for elder abuse is complex because risk often results from a combination of characteristics and circumstances in the victim and perpetrator. Perhaps the most accurate conclusion is that several risk factors must be present and these generally develop over a long period. The two characteristics that tend to be common to all elder abuse situations are the invisibility of the problem and the vulnerability of the older person. Psychosocial and caregiver risk factors are also common.

Invisibility

In contrast to most problems affecting older adults, one of the major risk factors for elder abuse is its invisibility. Despite the increasing attention given to elder abuse, only about 7% of cases are reported, even in states with good reporting and intervention models (Dong, 2005). Factors that contribute to this invisibility include the following:

- Older people generally have less contact with the community than do other segments of the population.
- Older people are reluctant to admit to being abused or neglected because they fear reprisal or believe that alternative situations may be worse than the abusive one.
- The myths and negative stereotypes associated with old age foster a strong denial of aging and an even stronger denial of the social problems associated with vulnerable older people.

Vulnerability

Abused elders are vulnerable because of a combination of social, personal, situational, and environmental factors. As a result, they require protective services because of the following characteristics (Anetzberger, 2002):

- Inability to maintain minimal social standards of care
- Inability to meet their own needs for food, shelter, or warmth
- Inability to manage their own financial affairs
- Psychosocial impairments (e.g., dementia, depression, long-term dependent personality) that cause them to be a danger to themselves or others
- Lack of relatives or others able and willing to provide adequate and appropriate assistance
- Inability to seek services for themselves

Wellness Opportunity

By sensitively communicating care and concern, nurses encourage vulnerable older adults to talk about conditions that can be addressed to prevent abuse or neglect.

Psychosocial Factors

Impaired cognitive function is one of the most common characteristics of abused older adults. Considerable attention has been focused on dementia as a risk factor for self-neglect and physical abuse (e.g., Dyer et al., 2000; Flannery, 2003; Hansberry et al., 2005). Impaired judgment, inability to make safe decisions, and loss of contact with reality are specific impairments that can lead to abuse and neglect. Conditions that impair cognitive abilities include dementia, delirium, or depression, or a combination of pathologic processes. When the older adult denies the cognitive impairment or refuses help or evaluation, the risk for elder abuse increases. Older people who live alone and are aware of their impairments may be afraid of acknowledging them because they fear that they have an untreatable problem that will require a move to a long-term care facility. This fear may lead to social isolation, the overlooking of treatable or reversible causes of impairment, or a progressive but unnecessary decline in function.

Long-term mental illness also may predispose an older adult to abuse or neglect, especially in combination with other factors, such as dementia or the loss of a significant social support. Characteristics of depression that contribute to its role in self-neglect include social isolation, a negative outlook, and lack of interest in self-care.

Additional risk factors arise from social and environmental sources. The absence of a support system is one of the most common contributing factors to self-neglect, especially in people in their 80s, 90s, or older who may have outlived most of the people who once provided support and tangible services. This is especially problematic for people who have been lifelong recluses or who have no children or extended family.

Caregiver Factors

Caregiving itself is not the cause of elder abuse. Rather, it can provide a context for abuse to occur when those assuming the caregiving role are incapable of doing so because of life stresses, pathologic characteristics, or personality characteristics. The potential volatility of caregiving can be exacerbated when the caregiver sees the older adult's behavior as being difficult or provocative (Anetzberger, 2000). Caregivers who perpetrate abuse often exhibit some of the same psychosocial risk factors associated with abused elders, particularly if the caregivers themselves are older adults. These factors include physical limitations, cognitive impairment, dependence and co-residence, a perception of social isolation, a recent decline in health, an external locus of control, and poor interpersonal relations with the dependent elder (Anetzberger, 1987; Beach et al., 2005). It is not unusual to have a mutually neglectful or abusive situation when an older married couple has several of the psychosocial risk factors just identified and is, in addition, socially isolated. For example, a couple who both have dementia may unintentionally abuse each other and neglect themselves.

Mrs. B. is an 82-year-old divorced and widowed mother of four. She lives in a senior citizens' apartment located in the downtown area of a large city. The building is regularly serviced by subsidized transportation to grocery stores and shopping malls, and has a nutrition center on the ground floor. Mrs. B.'s eldest son died in an accident 12 years ago. Her daughter lives 65 miles away but visits once a week to do the grocery shopping and other errands. Two sons live within 4 miles of their mother's apartment. Mrs. B. lived in the home of one son and his wife until they argued 1 year ago. The other son lives alone in a small apartment and visits his mother two or three times weekly and frequently takes her to lunch or dinner. Mrs. B. has been hospitalized for major depression eight times since her eldest son's death. She also has been diagnosed as having hypertension, rheumatoid arthritis, and type 2 diabetes.

Mrs. B. was referred to a home health agency for follow-up after her last hospital stay because her medication regimen, which she had followed for 6 years, had been changed while she was in the hospital. At the time of discharge, Mrs. B. was given a 30-day supply of medications set out in daily-dose medication containers for her. She was to take Dia-Beta, 2.5 mg once a day; Inderal, 40 mg twice a day; Paxil, 20 mg once a day; folic acid, 1 mg once a day;

(case study continues on page 164)

and methotrexate, 2.5 mg four tablets each Wednesday. Scheduled medication times were 8 AM and 8 PM. The home health nurse was to instruct Mrs. B. in her medication regimen, including what medications she was to take, how she was to take them, what each medication was expected to do, and possible side effects. The nurse was also to assess Mrs. B.'s ability to follow instructions and her adherence to the medication regimen.

Because Mrs. B.'s vision was impaired from diabetes, she had difficulty managing her complex medication regimen. The visiting nurse arranged for unit-dose packaging for Mrs. B.'s prescriptions and visited twice a day for 2 days to observe Mrs. B.'s ability to take her medications accurately. On the third morning, the nurse telephoned Mrs. B. at 8:15 AM and asked if Mrs. B. had any problems taking her pills. Mrs. B. happily reported that she had taken all the pills, including the four methotrexate tablets, without any difficulty. The nurse then scheduled Mrs. B. to be seen three times a week for ongoing assessment for several weeks.

THINKING POINTS

- What are the factors that contribute to the risk of Mrs. B. becoming abused or neglected?
- What are the factors that protect Mrs. B. from becoming abused or neglected?
- As the visiting nurse, what concerns would you have about Mrs. B. when you discharge her from home care, and how would you address these concerns?

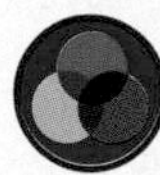

FUNCTIONAL CONSEQUENCES ASSOCIATED WITH ELDER ABUSE AND NEGLECT

Older people who have several risk factors are likely to become the knowing or unknowing victims of elder abuse, as illustrated by the following case examples:

1. A middle-aged alcoholic man hit his aged father during an argument. In turn, both were beaten by their sons/grandsons, who wanted money for drugs.
2. An elderly woman never left home because she feared her memory lapses would prevent her from finding the way back. When she did venture out, she fell on the porch, and the local office on aging was called. Outreach workers found she had no food in the house and was malnourished.
3. An unemployed couple kept their impaired grandparents confined to the house, refusing them visitors, abandoning them for days without adequate food, and denying them help for fear of losing access to their Social Security checks.
4. A son visited his mother in the nursing home and sexually assaulted her when staff members were not present.
5. A depressed elderly woman refused to take a needed medication with the result that her legs became so swollen that she could not leave her chair.
6. A woman in her 80s—who was weak, incontinent, and had hypertension—was abandoned in an emergency department with a note reading "Totally dependent! Handle with care."

These situations illustrate various forms of abuse, which are commonly classified as follows (Daley & Jogerst, 2005; National Center on Elder Abuse, 2003b):

- **Neglect**: intentional or unintentional refusal or failure to provide goods or services that are necessary to avoid physical harm, mental anguish, or mental illness
- **Physical abuse**: deprivation of a basic need; or, actual or threatened infliction of physical pain, injury, or violence
- **Emotional (psychological) abuse**: infliction of mental pain, distress, or anguish through verbal or nonverbal acts
- **Exploitation** (financial or property abuse): illegal taking, misuse, or concealment of funds, property, or assets
- **Sexual abuse**: nonconsensual sexual activity, contact, injury, or violence

In addition, some state laws address the following types of elder abuse: abandonment, unreasonable confinement, violation of rights, denying privacy or visitors, and undue influence (i.e., the substitution of one person's will for the true desires of another) (Brammer, 2003; Quinn, 2002; Roby & Sullivan, 2000).

Although rape and other sexual violence perpetrated against older people received some attention during the late 1970s, the focus at that time was on sexual assault by strangers. During the 1990s, sexual assault by family members and paid caregivers became a widely recognized aspect of elder abuse. Reports of sexual assault against older people are not common, but the resulting physical and emotional consequences can be severe and long lasting. Research on reported sexual abuse found the typical victim to be an older woman residing in a nursing facility. Her abuser tends to be a man who is another resident. The most common examples of sexual abuse involved sexualized kissing, fondling, or unwelcome sexual interest in the victim's body. Although sexual abuse usually is an isolated incident, it was ongoing in 16% of cases. Most cases are never prosecuted because of insufficient evidence or because victims are unable to participate in the prosecution (Teaster & Roberto, 2004).

Self-neglect and **self-abuse** are forms of elder abuse that differ from other types in that they have no perpetrator other than the older person himself or herself. In cases of self-neglect, the older person fails to meet essential needs, usually because of such factors as serious functional impairments or the desire to die. In cases of self-abuse, the older person causes injury or pain to herself or himself, including body mutilations.

Although until recently the elder abuse literature usually did not address situations that were mutually abusive or neglectful, nurses working in home settings have long encountered situations in which two people, often a married couple, abuse each other or are both neglected. These situations may be rooted in a long-term, mutually abusive relationship, but usually evolve because of gradual declines in the functional abilities of both people. They also may be associated with the poor coping skills of a spouse or caregiver who is faced with increasing demands and little or no outside help. Many of these situations are now being recognized as aspects of domestic violence.

Since the late 1980s, domestic violence against older adults has been recognized as another aspect of elder abuse. Attention has grown as feminists who formed the battered women's movement of the 1970s have aged and as AARP and other national organizations have focused attention on the issue (France, 2006). Recent research suggests that domestic violence against older women may be more common than suspected. For example, a cross-sectional study of 842 community-dwelling elderly women found that nearly half had experienced physical, psychological, or sexual abuse since turning 55 years of age, many repeatedly (Fisher & Regan, 2006). Very few viable programs address domestic violence and elders, and those that do tend to focus on screening tools and protocols for abuse identification and referral, hotlines, legal advocacy, peer and individual counseling, safety planning procedures, emergency shelter arrangements, and support groups for older victims (Anetzberger, 2001; Wolf, 2001). Multiple barriers can exist to the use of these resources, including the handicap inaccessibility of some shelters and the reluctance of many older victims to leave abusive relationships because of long-term attachment to the perpetrators, health challenges, and cohort effects (Zink et al., 2003).

When Mr. P.'s wife died, this frail man sought care in the home of a neighbor who offered both board and care in exchange for his monthly Social Security check. In reality, the neighbor provided neither, but locked Mr. P. in the basement and gave him little food. If he complained about the treatment or refused to sign over the income or property, the caregiver hit or kicked him. After 4 years, the situation was discovered and reported to the county protective services agency. Mr. P. later sat in the social worker's office and sadly commented, "So this is what it's like to be a protective case."

THINKING POINTS

- What type(s) of abuse does this case represent?
- What are some of the psychosocial consequences that Mr. P. is likely to have experienced in the past 4 years?
- What are some factors that contribute to this situation going on for 4 years?

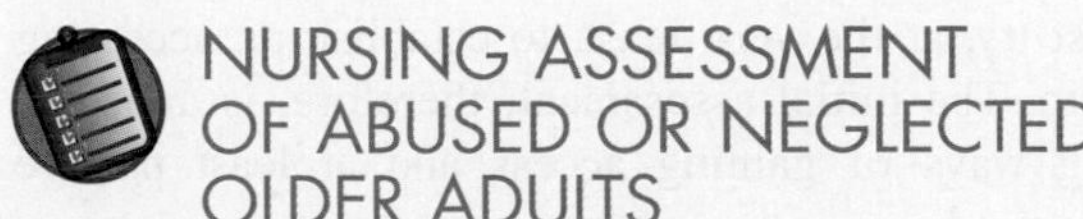

NURSING ASSESSMENT OF ABUSED OR NEGLECTED OLDER ADULTS

Elder abuse is not so much assessed as it is detected, so nurses often must assume the role of detective. Because elder abuse by its very nature is a hidden problem, assessment begins with a suspicion about its existence. Information may be purposefully withheld, and it is rarely volunteered, except in situations in which the older person or caregiver is desperate for help. Clues to elder abuse might first be noted when an older person is seen in an emergency department or admitted to a hospital. Most often, a home visit is an essential component of the assessment process, and gaining admission to the home usually is the first assessment challenge. Many times, the situation deteriorates so gradually that it is hard to determine the onset of abuse. In questionable situations, people who suspect that elder abuse is occurring may ignore the clues in hopes that the situation will resolve by itself.

Wellness Opportunity

Nurses pay particular attention to the older adult's relationships with others so they can detect clues to elder abuse.

Unique Aspects of Elder Abuse Assessment

Assessment of elder abuse differs from usual nursing assessment in several respects. First, a major focus is to determine whether legal interventions are appropriate or necessary, in contrast to situations in which a major goal is to identify broader health needs. In situations in which abuse is suspected, the primary concern usually is a determination of the safety of the older person. This approach is similar to emergency department nursing, in which basic life-sustaining needs are addressed immediately and other needs are considered later.

Second, realistic goals for elder abuse situations often are quite limited. Health care professionals sometimes have to accept basic safety as the only goal, especially when the elder and caregiver insist on choices that are not consistent with those recommended by health care workers. An assessment of risks to safety is essential, therefore, because legal interventions can be made only in high-risk situations. Because the determination of safety often is based on medical and nursing information, the role of the nurse is especially important. In home settings in particular, the nurse may be the only health care professional who directly assesses the situation, and the nursing assessment may be the major determinant of recommendations for legal intervention.

Third, cases of elder abuse generally involve some element of resistance from the older person or caregiver(s). Only in rare situations do abused elders or their caregivers seek assistance from health care professionals. Although it might be impossible to establish a trusting relationship, the nurse must try, at the very least, to establish an accepting relationship. The initial assessment, therefore, is aimed at identifying ways of gaining access and at least passive acceptance.

Fourth, in contrast to most health care situations, the nurse may be viewed as a threat rather than a help. Nurses are not accustomed to being viewed as the "bad guy," and often must identify a way to minimize the perceived threat, even before the initial contact. Nurses can accomplish this by identifying someone who acknowledges that a problem exists and is willing to assist with gaining access. Any of the following people can be helpful in gaining access and acceptance:

- Neighbors or friends
- Relatives (especially family members who do not live in the problematic home setting)
- Staff from senior centers, offices on aging, or health care or community agencies
- Physicians or any other health professionals
- Church-based people (e.g., clergy).

Fifth, when legal interventions are being considered, the legal rights of the person and the caregivers must be addressed. Nurses and other workers involved in elder abuse cases usually are uncomfortable making decisions that involve the rights of other adults. In institutional settings, legal and ethical decisions are guided by medical information and institutional policies, and the role of the physician usually is the most important. In home settings, however, there are few clear guidelines and little or no physician input.

Finally, the personal safety of the nurse is an assessment consideration in many elder abuse situations, especially when the nurse visits homes where the caregiver is a known or suspected perpetrator. In any situation that places a nurse at risk, an essential component of the assessment is assuring that protections are in place for the nurse. For example, nurses can arrange their visits in conjunction with protective service workers or, if warranted, law enforcement officers. Some communities have law enforcement officers who are specially trained to deal with elder abuse situations. Whenever nurses visit patients in places where their safety may be threatened, they need to be vigilant about potential risks and always be attentive to an escape route.

Wellness Opportunity

When making home visits, nurses pay particular attention to self-wellness by protecting themselves from risks.

Physical Health

The nursing assessment of physical abuse and neglect focuses on the following: nutrition, hydration, bruises and injuries, degree of frailty, and presence of pathologic conditions.

Nutrition and Hydration

Nutrition and hydration are important in determining not only the existence of physical neglect but the seriousness and urgency of the situation. In community settings, nutrition and hydration status are often crucial in determining if time allows for working with the elder in the home setting. The guidelines discussed in Chapter 18, particularly in Table 18-2 (Causes and Consequences of Nutrient Deficiencies), can be applied to the detection of malnutrition and dehydration.

Skin turgor over the extremities is not necessarily a reliable indicator of hydration, especially for very old people or for people who have lost weight. Examination of the mucous membranes and an assessment of skin turgor over the sternum or abdomen provide more accurate clues to dehydration. The absence of thirst sensation is not necessarily an indicator of adequate hydration because older people may have a diminished thirst response. On the other hand, the presence of thirst sensation is a definite indicator of dehydration, a physiologic disturbance, or an adverse medication effect. If a urine sample can be obtained, a measurement of specific gravity will provide information about hydration. When a urinometer is not available, a visual examination of urine concentration provides some clues about hydration.

When any indicators of malnutrition or dehydration are identified, the next step is to determine whether the hydration or nutritional status can be improved adequately without removing the person from the setting. The role of the nurse can be especially important in assessing not only the nutrition and hydration status, but the measures required to alleviate these risks immediately. Sometimes, the provision of water and food is the most important intervention in neglect situations. In addition, this intervention is inexpensive and readily available, and can be quite effective in establishing a relationship with a hungry or thirsty person!

Injuries, Bruises, and Other Physical Harm

Assessment of indicators of physical harm is an important aspect of the detection of neglect or physical abuse. Any of the following conditions can be indicators of abuse or self-neglect: leg ulcers; pressure ulcers; dependent edema; poor wound healing; burns from stoves, cigarettes, or hot water; and bruises, swelling, or injuries from falls, especially repeated falls. The presence of more than one of these indicators at the same time, or over a short period of time, should raise high levels of suspicion about neglect. The possibility of drug or alcohol abuse also should be considered when any of these indicators is identified, especially if the person is also depressed or socially isolated. To detect physical abuse, the nurse should look for any indication of injury caused by people who live with or visit a vulnerable older adult. Examples are marks from cuts, bites, burns, or punctures; bruises or injuries, especially of the face, head, or trunk; bruises on both upper arms, as would result from being grabbed or shaken harshly; or bruises that reflect the shape of objects, like belts or hairbrushes. If evidence of injuries from falls is present, the nurse must consider the possibility that the person was shoved or otherwise caused to fall by someone else.

Nurses routinely assess the presence and characteristics of bruises, with particular attention to the onset of new bruises and the progression of bruises. Changes in color have traditionally been considered indicators of the age of bruises, with the expectation that they progress from blue/black, to green, then yellow, with red appearing at any time. A few studies have addressed progression of accidental bruises in relation to child abuse, but there is little research on bruises in older adults. In 2002, Mosqueda and colleagues conducted a landmark study on the life cycle of bruises in older adults (Mosqueda et al., 2005). Trained research assistants performed daily head-to-toe examinations of 101 older adults during the initial 14-day inspection period to identify the onset of new bruises. Seventy-three subjects had 108 bruises, which were documented and examined daily for up to 6 weeks. Researchers screened subjects to exclude any possibility of abuse and they considered variables such as medications, fall history, and medical conditions. The following findings from this study are pertinent to nursing assessment of bruises in older adults (Mosqueda et al., 2005):

- Accidental bruises occur in a predictable pattern in older adults, with nearly 90% appearing on extremities.
- No accidental bruises were observed on the neck, ears, genitalia, buttocks, or soles of the feet.
- Bruise duration varied from 4 to 41 days, with 81% resolving by day 11.
- Red, yellow, and purple are the most common discolorations during the early phase, but they can last throughout the life of the bruise.
- Yellow discoloration can begin within the first 24-hours after onset, tends to increase over time, and was the most common color in bruises after 3 weeks.
- Subjects were more likely to know the cause when the bruises occurred on their trunks than when it was on their extremities.
- The most commonly reported cause was bumping into something.
- Subjects with compromised function and those on medications known to affect coagulation were more likely to have multiple bruises, with no differences in size, color, or location.

Nurses can use the illustration of most common sites of accidental bruising (Fig. 10-1) to help identify bruises that are more likely to be associated with abusive situations. In addition, nurses can review the photographs of elder abuse victims that the National Center on Elder Abuse posts on their website for educational purposes (www.elderabusecenter.org).

Nurses also assess for indicators of abuse caused indirectly, as by a caregiver who gives the person excessive amounts of alcohol or drugs, especially psychoactive

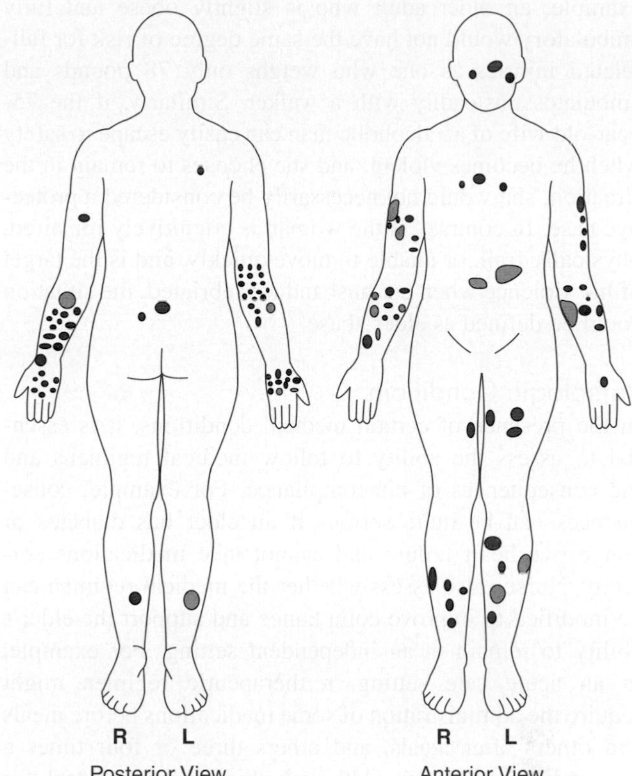

FIGURE 10-1 Most common sites of accidental bruises in older adults. (From Mosqueda, L., Burnright, K., & Liao, S. [2005]. The life cycle of bruises in older adults. *Journal of the American Geriatrics Society, 53*, 1339–1343. Used with permission from Wiley-Blackwell.)

medications. Sometimes caregivers who abuse drugs or alcohol will give these substances to the people for whom they care, especially if the dependent person is not able or willing to refuse. Another sign of abuse is excessive use of psychoactive medications solely for the caregiver's benefit so the elder is more easily managed. Nurses are likely to observe any of the following indicators of overmedication in an elder: ataxia, somnolence, clouded mentation, slurred speech, staggering gait, or extrapyramidal manifestations.

Aspects of physical neglect may include withholding therapeutic medications or interfering with medical care. For example, caregivers may decide not to purchase prescriptions or provide nursing care, medical equipment, or comfort items because they do not want to spend the money, even though this care is necessary. If the older adult has not freely chosen to forego treatments, medications, or assistance, then this may constitute physical neglect. If the caregiver is likely to inherit the money that is being saved, this may represent financial exploitation as well.

Degree of Frailty

The degree of frailty of the older adult is another consideration in assessing actual or potential abuse or neglect. For example, an older adult who is slightly obese and fully ambulatory would not have the same degree of risk for fall-related injuries as one who weighs only 78 pounds and ambulates unsteadily with a walker. Similarly, if the 75-year-old wife of an alcoholic man can easily escape to safety when he becomes violent, and she chooses to remain in the situation, she would not necessarily be considered a protective case. In contrast, if the woman is cognitively impaired, physically frail, or unable to move quickly, and is the target of his violence when her husband is inebriated, the situation could be defined as elder abuse.

Pathologic Conditions

In the presence of certain medical conditions, it is essential to assess the ability to follow medical regimens and the consequences of noncompliance. For example, consequences can be quite serious if an elder has diabetes or congestive heart failure and cannot take medications correctly. Nurses also assess whether the medical regimen can be modified to improve compliance and support the elder's ability to remain in an independent setting. For example, in an acute care setting, a therapeutic regimen might require the administration of some medications before meals and others after meals, and others three or four times a day at different times. Although this might be ideal for optimal effectiveness, elders or caregivers in a home setting may not be able to comply. A thorough nursing assessment can lead to interventions, such as patient education or simplification of the regimen, to achieve adequate compliance.

Activities of Daily Living

A major focus of assessment in elder abuse situations is to determine the necessity for legal interventions. Therefore, a nursing assessment of the person's potential for safe performance of activities of daily living (ADLs) is extremely important. For community-living older adults, it is essential to assess the home environment and the elder's level of functioning in that environment. In addition, nurses often need to obtain information from caregivers. Home care workers provide valuable information, and they usually are more objective than family members. In some circumstances, it may be appropriate to involve occupational or physical therapists in the home assessment. When a difference of opinion exists, or when it is difficult to determine the safety of the situation, it may be helpful to have a team conference that includes all of the people who function in assessment or caregiving capacities and who have some degree of objectivity. In cases of suspected elder abuse, the assessment team may include many informal sources of help, such as family and neighbors, as well as formal sources of help, such as nurses and social workers.

Personal dress, hygiene, and grooming are among the most visible and commonly appraised aspects of daily function. People often are viewed as neglected when they do not comply with socially defined standards of cleanliness, particularly when an unpleasant odor is noted. In elder abuse situations, nurses need to consider that poor hygiene and grooming are important reflections of many underlying problems, but they are not necessarily indicators of safety concerns. When families and health care or social service workers initially work with a neglected older person who is in need of much personal care, they often are tempted to begin by assisting the person with bathing and grooming. Although the workers may view this as a socially acceptable way to begin, this may be very threatening to the elder. Thus, nurses assess the impact of poor hygiene on the elder's health and they assess the consequences of imposing assistance when the elder is unwilling to accept help or acknowledge a hygiene problem. The nurse may determine that efforts to deal with personal hygiene would interfere with the short-term goal of establishing a relationship and the long-term goal of assisting with other aspects of daily function. Thus, nurses may need to begin by addressing nutrition, hydration, and safety, while deferring attention to personal care issues associated with the most resistance.

Adequate nutrition, hydration, and an ability to obtain help in an emergency are the basic human needs that are most often called into question in cases of elder abuse. Other basic needs may also be compromised, usually in relation to specific functional impairments and environmental circumstances. For instance, it is imperative to address bowel and bladder elimination for people who are confined to bed or a chair. For people with mobility limitations or serious vision impairments, safe ambulation and the ability to avoid falls are important considerations. Table 10-1 summarizes some of the specific functional and environmental conditions that present risks to basic needs.

TABLE 10-1 Risks to Safety Associated With Functional Limitations

Functional Limitation	Risks to Safety
Any mental or physical impairment, especially in combination with social isolation and lack of a support system	Nutrition and hydration
Mobility limitations or seriously impaired vision, especially in combination with poor judgment	Falls
Cognitive impairments in ambulatory people	Wandering, getting lost
Compromised mobility	Pressure sores
Cognitive impairment, especially poor judgment	Inability to get help
Poor judgment, especially when living in an unsafe neighborhood	Basic safety and security

Psychosocial Function

Information in Chapters 13 (Psychosocial Assessment), 14 (Delirium and Dementia), and 15 (Depression) is pertinent to assessing psychosocial function in relation to elder abuse. In addition, the most important aspect of psychosocial function for abuse situations is assessment of the elder's capacity for reasonable judgments about self-care. This is difficult because the determination of someone's ability to make appropriate judgments is based, at least in part, on subjective criteria and opinions. People whose judgment is impaired to the point that they are at serious risk, especially if they do not acknowledge the risk, are usually considered incompetent or incapacitated. Thus, the crucial element of psychosocial assessment for elder abuse cases is a determination of risk (i.e., danger to the person) rather than a determination of whether other people would judge the decision as *good* or *appropriate*. When the competence of an older adult to make safe decisions regarding self-care is in doubt, nurses may be legally bound to make reports or consider other legal interventions. There are no federal guidelines for determining the mental capacity of abused or neglected older adults, and the legal criteria differ from state to state. The ethical and legal considerations related to elder abuse are discussed later in this chapter and more extensively in Chapter 9.

Wellness Opportunity

Nurses promote self-determination for older adults by respecting their rights to make decisions about their care, as long as their actions do not jeopardize safety for themselves or others.

Support Resources

Support resources include those people, such as caregivers and friends, who influence a person's physical and psychosocial function. Some or all of the support people may directly cause the abusive situation or may actively or passively contribute to it. Therefore, nurses assess the support resources in terms of both helpful and detrimental effects. In addition, support resources not currently being used are identified as potential sources of help.

When the caregivers who perpetrate the abuse are also the support resources, nurses assess the potential for working with them to alleviate the negative consequences. Although it is not always easy to work with abusive caregivers, it may be even more difficult to eliminate their influence over an older adult. During the assessment, therefore, nurses identify any strengths of the caregiver and any willingness to change the situation voluntarily. If the caregiver is extremely stressed, then respite, along with individual or group support and counseling, may be effective interventions. In mutually abusive situations in which the designated caregiver also is abused or neglected, the nurse tries to identify any outside sources of support that have not been tapped. For example, in a mutually abusive situation involving a socially isolated married couple, the nurse might identify a relative or friend who is willing to assist with caregiving or decision-making responsibilities.

Because a caregiver's lack of knowledge can be an underlying factor in elder abuse, nurses assess the caregiver's understanding of the elder's needs. For example, caregivers may have good intentions when they use adult briefs for the control of incontinence and do not change them frequently, but they may not understand the potential for skin breakdown. Caregivers may administer excessive amounts of psychoactive medications because they do not understand the correct dosing schedule or the potential adverse effects. This is especially common when medications are ordered on an as-needed basis and the caregiver has not been given clear guidelines for determining when the medication is needed, or what the most effective dosage is. In these situations, nursing assessment of the caregiver's knowledge is especially important because educational interventions, role modeling, or the provision of additional services may alleviate the abuse.

In situations of neglect, there usually are very few support services to assess, and the task of the nurse is to identify potential sources of help and the barriers that interfere with the use of these resources. The assessment of barriers to the use of resources is discussed in Chapter 13 and is summarized in Box 13-9. It is especially important to identify these barriers because simple interventions, such as provision of information or assistance with transportation, may be effective in eliminating them. Cultural influences also must be assessed in relation to the use of support resources, as discussed in Chapter 4.

Environmental Influences

As with other aspects of elder abuse, the primary purposes of assessing the environment are to identify the factors that create risks and to determine which of these factors can be alleviated through interventions. With regard to the immediate living conditions, the nurse assesses whether minimal standards of safety and cleanliness are being maintained. When nurses assess home environments that are terribly cluttered, they must make some determination of both the meaning and the consequences of the clutter. A massive collection of clutter reflects an underlying disorder and may or may not be a risk factor that needs to be addressed. Consequences of clutter range from socially unacceptable appearances to serious risks to health and safety. Therefore, the nurse must assess the person's ability to maneuver in the environment during daily activities, as well as the person's safety in emergency situations, such as a fire. When nurses and other workers are initially exposed to massive amounts of clutter, their first inclination may be to think of a way to eliminate some of it. If this reaction is communicated to the resident of the cluttered home, however, it may become impossible to establish an accepting relationship, and the older adult may reject any further interventions. In assessing the home environment, therefore, nurses must be nonjudgmental, except in circumstances in which the risks are so great that immediate action must be taken.

Nurses also assess the neighborhood environment for its impact on the safety of the person. This is especially important when the older person lives in an area of high crime or extreme isolation and is vulnerable by virtue of impaired judgment, physical frailty, or a combination of physical and psychosocial impairments. People who are only moderately forgetful may be safe in an apartment or a suburban neighborhood where neighbors watch out for them. In a high-crime neighborhood, however, forgetting to lock the doors or to take other precautions may place the person at increased risk for physical harm, financial exploitation, or other serious abuses. Likewise, in a rural environment, social isolation may increase the risks for vulnerable elderly people.

Finally, seasonal conditions can influence the degree of risk for self-neglect in people who have dementia and live in climates characterized by extreme heat or cold. For example, a person who does not pay utility bills may not be in any danger as long as the weather is mild, but when the temperature turns cold, that person would be at risk for hypothermia. The same is true for people who occasionally wander outside without dressing appropriately. As long as the neighborhood is safe and the weather mild, they may be relatively safe; however, they may be at increased risk during the cold months, especially if they do not wear proper foot covering. Nurses also assess any of the risk factors for hypothermia or heat-related illness discussed in Chapter 25.

Threats to Life

The most immediate consideration in determining whether legal interventions are necessary is the assessment of threats to life. Situations often are viewed as being of crisis proportions when they are first discovered, and the immediate reaction of the person who discovers the situation may be to remove a person from the environment. Many times, however, the person may not want to leave, or there may be no better setting in which the person can receive care immediately. In these situations, the nurse may be asked to assess the urgency and seriousness of the situation and to provide an opinion about whether legal interventions are justified. The nurse often is the person who can either convince the elder to accept help or convince the caregivers and social workers that the present situation is tolerable. For instance, when nurses determine that the situation is not life-threatening, they can assure the person that they are trying to improve the situation and support the person remaining as safe and independent as possible.

Examples of threats that nurses commonly assess in elder abuse situations include the following:

- History of physical violence on the part of the caregiver, especially when the elder is unable to escape or otherwise be protected
- Untreated wounds or infections
- Inability to administer insulin correctly
- Progressive gangrene or ulcerated conditions
- Inability to adhere to therapeutic regimens
- Consistent wandering in unsafe neighborhoods or in very cold weather
- Misuse (usually unintentional) of certain medications, such as digitalis or insulin
- Excessive use of drugs or alcohol, either self- or caregiver-induced.

In situations in which the caregiver is the abuser, the nurse and other team members must assess whether the caregiver presents a threat to the life of the dependent older person.

When nurses do not have firsthand knowledge of the abused or neglected older person before being notified of a crisis situation, the first consideration is whether this is objectively a crisis, or is merely a crisis in the eyes of the person who just discovered the situation. Situations that appear the most appalling may actually represent a gradual deterioration over several months or years. Therefore, the initial assessment is aimed at determining the presence of any immediate threats to the life of the abused elder, such as malnutrition, dehydration, or an untreated medical condition. Finally, suicide potential must be assessed, especially in self-neglected elders who also are depressed and expressing feelings of hopelessness. Nurses can apply all of the principles of suicide assessment, discussed in Chapter 15, to abused and neglected elders.

Cultural Aspects

Definitions and perceptions of elder abuse and neglect are influenced to a great extent by cultural norms. For example, Asian Indians may consider not visiting an older family member to be a form of psychological neglect, but Anglo Americans may consider it a way of respecting privacy and autonomy. Cultural factors also have a strong influence on caregiver roles and responsibilities. Most families have culturally influenced expectations about which family members should provide care to dependent older adults and about whether it is acceptable to enlist the aid of paid caregivers. In some families, there may be conflicts about these expectations, particularly between older and younger generations. Sometimes these conflicts may need to be identified and addressed before elder abuse or neglect can be resolved.

Nurses must identify cultural factors that influence the care that is provided—or not provided—to older adults. Cultural Considerations 10-2 lists some of the assessment questions that should be considered in identifying cultural influences. When assessing family caregiver relationships, nurses should be sensitive to cultural variations

Cultural Considerations 10-2

Cultural Considerations in Assessing Elder Abuse and Neglect

- What are the family and cultural expectations concerning family caregivers? (For example, is it acceptable to employ paid caregivers, or are family members expected to provide all the care?)
- Do family members differ in their perceptions about caregiving responsibilities?
- What are the family and cultural perspectives on autonomy and independence?
- Do family members differ in their perspectives on autonomy and independence?
- How are decisions made about care of the older adult? (For example, is it a patriarchal or matriarchal family?)
- Who are the acceptable sources of social support and personal assistance?
- Who are the acceptable sources of health care (e.g., herbalists, spiritual healers, Native American practitioners)?
- What are the acceptable health care practices (e.g., herbs, homeopathy, acupuncture, faith healing, folk remedies)?
- Are there language barriers that influence the care that is provided or that limit the number of care providers?
- How does skin color affect assessment of bruises, pressure sores, and other skin changes?

in perspectives on family caregiving and respect differences, but they also must address abusive situations. In addition, cultural assessment information on the following topics should be considered: communication and psychosocial assessment (see Chapter 13), nutrition (see Chapter 18), dementia (see Chapter 14), and depression (see Chapter 15).

Mrs. K. is 80 years old and had resided in a nursing facility for 1 year until she recently was discharged at her request but "against medical advice" with no prescriptions for her medications or medical referral for home care. She has complex health conditions, including osteoarthritis, coronary artery disease, congestive heart failure, chronic obstructive pulmonary disease (COPD), depression, and insulin-dependent diabetes. Although alert and oriented, Mrs. K. has major deficits in her ability to perform daily living tasks. She also depends on a walker for ambulation and has a history of falling, including a fall that resulted in a hip fracture and her admission to a nursing facility.

Mrs. K.'s support system is limited. Her son lives in another state but functions as power-of-attorney and provides some telephone reassurance. Her daughter is estranged from Mrs. K., and at their last meeting was verbally abusive to her. Mrs. K.'s older brother visits a few times weekly to help with meal preparation, grocery shopping, transportation, and medication pick-ups; however, his own health problems prevent him from providing more help.

Shortly after returning home, Mrs. K.'s precarious health status rapidly deteriorated. She became severely short of breath, requiring continuous oxygen. She began to hallucinate in the evening, believing that she alone had the responsibility of feeding all of the children in the neighborhood. As her fears increased, so too did the calls to her brother. Eventually she made several calls every night, overwhelming and exhausting him.

THINKING POINTS

- What form(s) of elder abuse is (are) represented?
- What are signs or indicators of abuse that you as a nurse would be able to identify?
- What factors contribute to Mrs. K.'s current risks?
- How will you proceed in conducting a nursing assessment of Mrs. K.?
- What barriers might you encounter in conducting the assessment? How will you overcome them?

NURSING DIAGNOSIS

Because elder abuse and neglect is so broad and complex, various nursing diagnoses are applicable, depending on the situation. A nursing diagnosis that would apply to many elder abuse situations where family members are caregivers is Disabled Family Coping. This is defined as "the state in which a family demonstrates, or is at risk to demonstrate, destructive behavior in response to an inability to manage internal or external stressors due to inadequate resources (physical, psychological, or cognitive)" (Carpenito-Moyet, 2006, p. 117). Related factors include changes in family roles, unrealistic expectations about caregiving, and changes in the health status of the older adult. If the nursing assessment identifies several stressors primarily related to family caregiving, the nursing diagnosis of Caregiver Role Strain might be used. This is defined as "a state in which an individual is experiencing physical, emotional, social, and/or financial burden(s) in the process of giving care to another" (Carpenito-Moyet, 2006, p. 161). Related caregiver factors include ineffective coping patterns, functional or cognitive impairments, and insufficient resources (e.g., respite, financial assets, assistance with care). Related factors involving the dependent older adult include increased dependence and the presence of difficult or unsafe behaviors (e.g., paranoia, wandering, incontinence).

The nursing diagnosis of Risk for Injury might be used for older adults who are in self-neglecting situations, especially if the person lives alone and is physically and psychosocially impaired. The nursing diagnosis of Decisional Conflict might apply to abused or neglected older adults who live in an environment that places them at risk for harm because they are unable to make decisions about alternative environments. Related factors include fear, lack of information about alternatives, and impaired decision-making ability.

Wellness Opportunity

Nurses address body–mind–spirit interrelatedness by identifying nursing diagnoses that address fear and other psychosocial consequences of abuse or neglect.

PLANNING FOR WELLNESS OUTCOMES

Nurses direct care for abused or neglected older adults toward addressing the complex needs of the elder as well as those of the family caregivers. Some Nursing Outcomes Classification (NOC) terminology that is likely to pertain to the abused older adult includes Abuse Cessation, Abuse Protection, Abuse Recovery Status, Neglect Cessation, Risk Control, Self-Care Status, and Social Support. Outcomes related to abusive caregivers or family members include Abusive Behavior Self-Restraint, Caregiver Emotional Health, Caregiver-Patient Relationship, Caregiver Stressors, Caregiver Endurance Potential, Family Coping, Family Social Climate, Knowledge: Health Resources, Role Performance, and Stress Level.

Wellness Opportunity

Quality of Life is a wellness outcome that is applicable to older adults and their caregivers when conditions contributing to abuse or neglect are alleviated.

NURSING INTERVENTIONS TO ADDRESS ELDER ABUSE AND NEGLECT

From a health care perspective, abused elders can be described as the intensive care patients of the community because they require the highest level of skill from a variety of professionals. Unlike intensive care patients in hospitals, however, the team members are not specialized health care professionals, but rather are community-based workers and people who provide informal support. Nurses often assume the role of coordinator or team leader in implementing interventions that address the older adults, the caregivers, and the environment for these inherently complex and challenging situations.

Because of the extensive scope of elder abuse, there are numerous Nursing Interventions Classification (NIC) terms that could be applicable to both the abused or neglected elder and the caregiver. Some that would be appropriate in most situations are Abuse Protection Support: Elder, Crisis Intervention, Referral, and Risk Identification for the elder; and Caregiver Support, Coping Enhancement, Referral, Role Enhancement, and Teaching for caregivers.

Interventions in elder abuse situations often include legal actions because decision-making abilities of the older adult may be impaired. Many situations also involve caregivers who are not competent decision makers or are not acting in the best interest of the elder. Thus, many cases of elder abuse involve legal and ethical questions about the competency of the elder and the caregivers. Nurses often have a key role in advocating for the older adult and may feel unprepared or uncomfortable either making or participating in decisions that affect the rights of others. Similarly, nurses may feel torn between the right of the person to refuse treatment and the obligation to report abuse and neglect situations, as discussed later in this chapter.

Interventions for elder abuse are implemented in community settings, over a long period of time, by a team of formal and informal care providers. Nurses working in home and community settings have the most direct opportunities for both the prevention of and interventions for elder abuse. Home care services, including home-delivered meals and nursing and medical strategies, have been identified as the most accepted and effective intervention strategies for abused older adults in community settings (Heath et al., 2005; Nahmiash & Reis, 2000). Nurses in institutional settings, however, have many opportunities for detecting elder abuse, working with caregivers, and facilitating referrals to appropriate community agencies. Because the opportunities for intervention in institutional settings are quite different from those in community settings, each of these areas is discussed separately in the following sections.

Interventions in Institutional Settings

Nurses in acute and long-term care settings can intervene in cases of elder abuse when they interact with caregivers, who often seek advice from nurses about ways of providing care. For example, nurses can encourage caregivers to use a period of institutionalization to reevaluate the demands of the situation and to consider resources for support and assistance. Family may express ambivalence about managing the older adult's care at home, or they may be unsure or unrealistic about their own ability to provide appropriate care or to cope with the stress of the situation. In some cases, caregivers may be seeking approval for not providing care at home. In these situations, nurses can facilitate communication among all the decision makers, including the primary care provider, the older adult (if appropriate), and the various family members who are responsible for care. Sometimes it is appropriate to suggest individual counseling or support groups or make referrals for social services, particularly when caregivers are very stressed about care-related decisions.

When elder abuse is rooted in the caregiver's lack of information, nurses can role model and teach about appropriate caregiving measures. When caregivers need additional health education or support services, nurses can initiate a referral to a home care agency for follow-up. Nurses also try to identify needs for skilled nursing care because health insurance usually covers these services. When nurses have serious questions about the adequacy of a discharge plan, they can refer to a protective service agency for further assessment and ongoing services.

Wellness Opportunity

When vulnerable older adults are in an acute or long-term care setting, nurses address psychosocial needs of family caregivers by providing support and education; these are effective tools for preventing elder abuse.

Interventions in Community Settings

Nurses in home settings have many opportunities for teaching caregivers about adequate care through role modeling and verbal and written instruction. For example, if caregivers have trouble managing complex medication regimens, nurses can use charts and organizers to facilitate compliance. Nurses also can educate caregivers about basic care needs, such as nutrition, exercise, and elimination. For example, nurses may suggest innovative ways of meeting the nutritional requirements of an elderly person who does not eat adequately. Home care nurses have the advantage of observing many creative and effective techniques used by caregivers that have never been described in any nursing texts. Thus, experienced home care nurses are continually expanding their repertoire of techniques for physical care and behavioral management, and these techniques can then be passed on to other family caregivers. When elder abuse is rooted in caregiver stress, nurses can suggest services and help find ways of providing care so the caregiver can use these resources for self-care. The following are examples of services aimed at reducing caregiver stress or dealing with caregiver problems:

- Alcoholics Anonymous for caregivers who are alcoholic
- Individual counseling to learn coping skills
- Alzheimer's Association for support and education groups
- In-home or day care for respite

Home health aides are the service providers who are most likely to care for abused elders in home settings, but they often are ill-prepared to detect or address elder abuse. Nurses who provide home-based services, therefore, have a tremendous responsibility to help home care workers recognize and intervene in elder abuse situations. For example, nurses can teach about detecting clues to elder abuse, and they can address concerns about questionable conditions. If nurses cannot openly discuss the situation during home visits, they may have to arrange for a phone conversation with the home care worker. In situations in which the older adult requires a significant degree of physical care or supervision, the services of a home health aide may be the most effective means of preventing elder abuse. Often, however, the retention of a home health aide in challenging situations depends largely on the degree of support and guidance provided by a professional nurse.

Nurses in other community settings, such as clinics or senior centers, have opportunities to intervene in elder abuse. For example, parish nurses may be the only contact for older adults who neglect themselves or care for a dependent spouse and are not aware of the many resources to address their needs. Nurses can prevent or alleviate elder abuse by facilitating referrals for appropriate community-based resources, such as adult day care or group or home-delivered meals. Even if nurses are not familiar with specific community services, they can discuss the advantages of various types of services and encourage older adults to call their local office on aging. At a minimum, however, nurses need to be familiar with the phone number for the area agency on aging that serves as an information center about local resources in every geographic area of the United States. Information about local agencies on aging also is available by calling the Eldercare Locator at (800) 677-1116.

Wellness Opportunity

Nurses help caregivers maintain self-wellness by identifying ways of alleviating stress associated with the demands of caregiving.

Interventions in Multidisciplinary Teams

Nurses often implement interventions as part of multidisciplinary teams, which have been established in a variety of health care settings. For example, hospitals have elder abuse teams, and agencies offer protective or case management services to older people and their families. In either instance, multidisciplinary teams include professionals who offer the perspectives of law, nursing, medicine, psychiatry, social work, and rehabilitation therapy. Additional disciplines are included if the situation requires. When legal interventions are being considered, the multidisciplinary team must conduct a complete assessment, including assessment of the person's ability to function safely in the home environment, the involvement of the family and significant others in meeting basic needs, and the ability of the older person to participate in developing a safe and realistic plan of action.

If nurses are not part of a multidisciplinary team, they sometimes need to be creative in finding other professionals with whom they can work. For example, when nurses work with people who are homebound, they may need to identify resources for an initial medical evaluation or for ongoing monitoring. In many areas of the country, primary care providers are resuming the practice of making home visits. In addition, with the growing demand for home health services, an increased number of diagnostic tests are performed in the home (e.g., radiographs, blood tests, and electrocardiograms). In many situations, these diagnostic tests are essential for determining whether involuntary care measures are justified. For instance, if the older adult refuses to go out of the home, blood tests or radiographs done in the home may provide the evidence needed to determine whether a hospitalization is warranted.

Referrals

Nurses often facilitate referrals for services that decrease the burden of caregiving responsibilities and improve an older adult's self-esteem and level of independence. For instance, speech, physical, and occupational therapies may be useful in improving the older person's ability to communicate, ambulate, and perform ADLs. Referrals for skilled home care services usually are made at the time of discharge from an institution; however, the older adult or family may have refused the services at that time. Older adults who are not admitted to health care facilities may not know they qualify for skilled home care services, and a nurse making a home visit may be the first health professional to suggest these resources. Although older adults or their families may not know about or may have refused such services, nurses need to assess their willingness to accept help as conditions change. Nurses also assess whether recent changes in the elder qualify the person for skilled home care services. For example, a change in medications might qualify a person for skilled nursing care, and a fall might qualify a person for skilled physical therapy. Nurses in home care agencies usually are happy to discuss skilled care services with anyone who calls for information. Nurses also can advise about the possibility of having services covered by health insurance, and they can obtain orders from the primary care provider for those services that are covered under Medicare or other health insurance programs.

Another important role for nurses is suggesting types of medical equipment, disposable supplies, and assistive devices to improve function and safety for the elder and ease caregiver burden. For example, caregivers may respond positively to suggestions from the nurse about obtaining and using grab bars for preventing falls in the bathroom. Some durable medical equipment is covered by health insurance, and medical supply companies usually are quite helpful in advising people about specific equipment.

Prevention and Treatment Interventions

Abused elders and their caregivers or abusers typically need a wide range of interventions, which can be categorized according to basic function:

- Core, or essential, integrative services
- Emergency services, during crises or just before or after abuse or neglect occurs
- Support services for managing the problem and improving the situation
- Rehabilitative services to address problems of either the victim or the perpetrator
- Preventive services, including programs directed toward changing society in ways that diminish the likelihood of maltreatment or self-neglect

Figure 10-2 identifies some of the specific types of services, arranged by function, that may be needed in elder abuse situations. Intervention models identify nurses as having primary responsibility for implementing the most successful interventions directed toward both the caregivers and abused or neglected older person(s). Not only are nurses highly qualified as health professionals to address the complex issues involved with elder abuse, they are highly accepted by older adults (Nahmiash & Reis, 2000).

Financial exploitation is an aspect of elder abuse that can be prevented through relatively simple and widely available measures to protect assets. For example, nurses can suggest that a trusted family member establish a joint account with the older adult and keep track of all transactions. Out-of-town families can oversee financial transactions through online banking. Nurses also can suggest referrals for local programs directed toward prevention of financial abuse and exploitation. The National Center on Elder Abuse has identified the following programs as Promising Practices to Prevent Financial Abuse:

- Arizona Money Management Program: Daily money management services for low-income older or disabled adults who have difficulty budgeting, paying routine bills, or keeping track of financial matters
- Seniors Against Investment Fraud: Enlists and trains California volunteers at the grassroots level to give presentations on investment and telemarketing fraud targeting older people
- Sage Services: Works with area agencies on aging in Connecticut to recruit and train volunteer guardians and court visitors
- Project Reach: Provides help in the form of legal assistance, financial counseling, and home visits for at-risk older Hawaiians who are ineligible for state protective services
- Check It Out: Provides an 800 number older adults in Maine can call for advice before making potentially risky financial decisions
- Health Care Fraud Education Project: Uses retired professionals or volunteers to teach other Pennsylvanian older people about health care fraud and their rights to quality care
- Wisconsin Financial Abuse Specialist Team: Offers quick multidisciplinary response to identify, investigate, and prevent financial abuse involving elderly and dependent adult victims

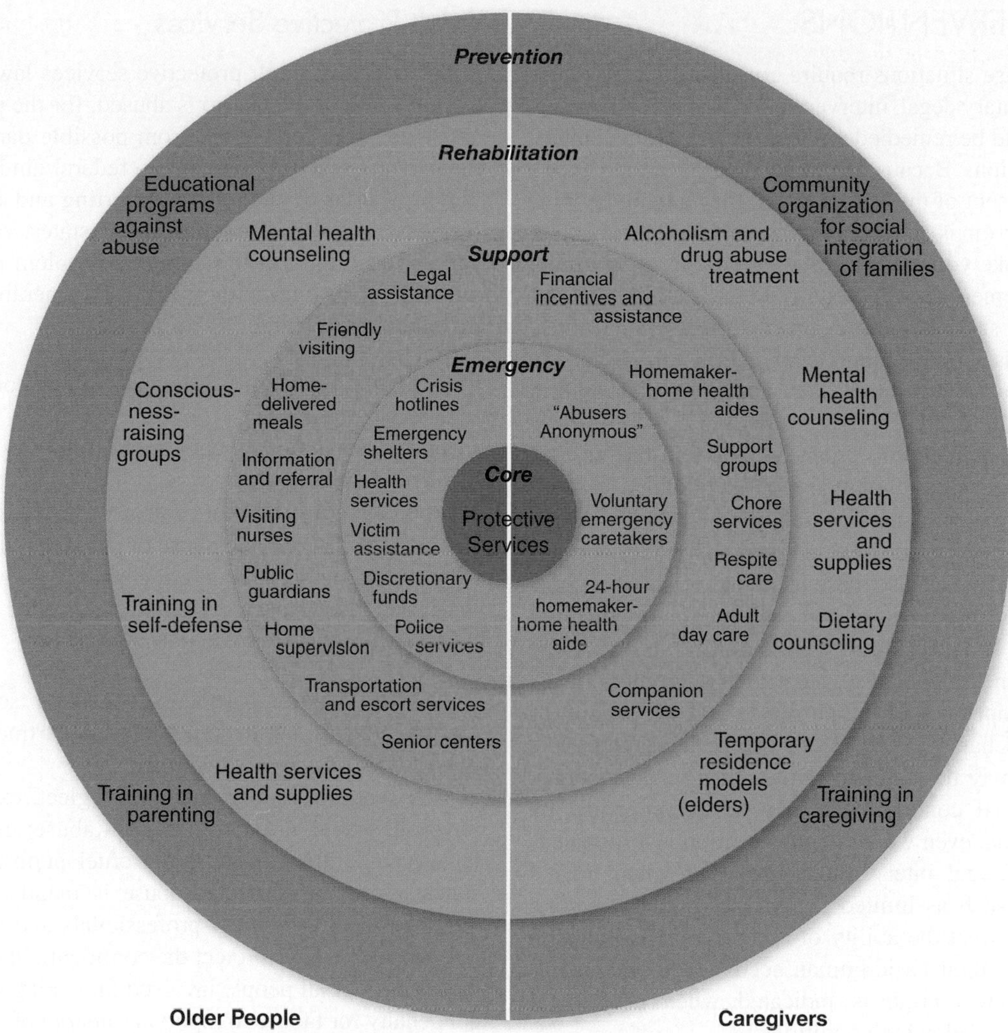

FIGURE 10-2 Types of services needed by abused older adults and their caregivers. (From Anetzberger, G. J. [1982]. *Report of the Elder Abuse Project: Recommendations for addressing the problem of elder abuse in Cuyahoga County.* Cleveland, OH: Federation for Community Planning. Used with permission.)

Mr. and Mrs. G. have been married for over 50 years and have six children, four of whom live in their area. Because of Mrs. G.'s memory loss in recent years, Mr. G. has allowed home care workers into the house to help her with eating and to perform personal care. The workers report that Mr. G. yells at his wife when she forgets things. On more than one occasion, they witnessed him attempting to force feed her when she failed to eat an entire meal. After the couple has gone to their bedroom in the evening, the night workers have reported hearing screams, crying, and slapping sounds coming from behind the closed bedroom door. In the morning, Mrs. G. had bruises on her body and bumps on her head. When asked, Mr. G. denied hitting his wife. Mrs. G. cried when questioned, never providing an explanation for her injuries.

Mr. G. is reluctant to consider additional services, like adult day care, fearing that the couple's savings will evaporate. He had Mrs. G. change doctors several times in recent years because "they don't do anything to really help her." The children who live nearby have said that they do not want to get involved in their parents' situation. They describe years of their father physically and verbally abusing their mother, and fear what might happen if any action is taken now.

THINKING POINTS

- What interventions might be helpful in addressing the elder abuse evident in this situation?
- What is the role of the home care nurse in introducing and implementing these interventions?
- What barriers might be encountered in acceptance of the interventions?
- As the home care nurse in this situation, how will you help to overcome these barriers?

LEGAL INTERVENTIONS

Most elder abuse situations require consideration of voluntary or involuntary legal interventions; whenever feasible, problems should be remedied without the use of involuntary legal intervention. Because voluntary legal interventions require the consent of the older person, they cannot be initiated if the person is not mentally competent. Competent adults can revoke voluntary legal interventions at any time. Money management, power of attorney, and various types of bank accounts, such as joint or direct deposit, are all interventions of this nature. Other legal interventions that are useful for mentally competent older adults are discussed in Chapter 9.

Some legal interventions, such as guardianship or civil commitment, are either voluntary or involuntary, but are most commonly used on an involuntary basis when others in the community believe that the older person's safety or property is in jeopardy. Because these legal interventions involve a much more extensive loss of personal freedom than voluntary ones, they should be used with extreme caution. A key consideration in the choice of legal interventions is determining the competency of the person to make decisions, as discussed in Chapters 9 and 13. Some measures, like guardianship, may be easier to initiate than to discontinue. Others, like civil commitment, may be accompanied by long-term stigma, even when the intervention is terminated.

Involuntary legal interventions are used when mental impairments—such as limited insight, judgment, memory, or cognition—affect the ability of older people to function safely and meet their basic human needs. Generally, involuntary legal intervention is indicated when assessment reveals all of the following conditions:

- Decisions must be made about the older person's health, living arrangements, money, or property.
- The older person is not capable of making reasonable decisions.
- There is a risk to the older person's health, safety, money, or property.
- The risk would be reduced or eliminated if someone else were empowered to make and implement decisions.

Legal interventions that address the abuser include domestic violence law and the criminal code. Adult protective services law is particularly limited when considerable property needs protection, the maltreatment is significant and repeated, the older person's mental impairment is substantial and permanent, or the goal is to prevent maltreatment rather than to treat it. Under these conditions, other legal interventions should be considered in conjunction with, or as alternatives to, adult protective services.

Wellness Opportunity

Nurses support autonomy for older adults by identifying the least invasive legal interventions, while also ensuring the least amount of endangerment.

Adult Protective Services

Philosophically, adult protective services law provides protection for the person who is abused, for the person offering assistance, and for society from possible dangers posed by the person. Because there are no federal guidelines or funding, provisions of elder abuse reporting and adult protective services laws differ among the 50 states. Although states vary in dealing with the complex problem of elder abuse, purposes of state laws for protecting vulnerable older people include the following:

- Facilitating the identification and referral of abuse or neglect
- Conveying public and centralized authority for addressing protective matters
- Establishing a system of protective services to prevent, correct, or discontinue abuse or neglect
- Permitting, under certain circumstances, involuntary access to the suspected victim of abuse for the purpose of investigation and service delivery

Usually local departments of social services receive reports of abuse, but in some states, departments of aging or prosecutors' offices receive them.

The scope of reports includes neglect, exploitation, and physical, sexual, and psychological abuse; in several states, laws include abandonment and cruel punishment. In most states, reporting suspected abuse is mandatory for health, social service, and safety professionals and paraprofessionals. Most state laws protect the confidentiality of reports and the identity of all people involved in making them. The typical penalty for failure to report is a charge of a misdemeanor, with or without financial penalty. In some states, however, failure to report can result in imprisonment, civil liability for damages, or notification of the state licensing board.

The public authority responsible for implementation must investigate promptly; sometimes, the law mandates a response within 24 to 72 hours. Investigation generally includes a home visit with the alleged victim and consultation with people knowledgeable about the situation. Service intervention for endangered older people often includes health care, support services, protective placement, emergency services, or financial management. Most laws emphasize due process, self-determination, least restrictive interventions, and voluntary acceptance of services by mentally competent adults. Although protective service workers have the primary responsibility for implementing elder abuse laws, nurses have essential roles in reporting and collaborating, assessing, consulting, testifying in court, and providing care. Nursing responsibilities associated with each of these roles are discussed in the next sections.

Reporting and Collaborating

Nurses are the health care workers most commonly identified as mandatory reporters in adult abuse and protective services laws. Personnel in long-term care facilities and mental health professionals are the second and third most commonly cited in state law as mandatory reporters (Roby & Sullivan, 2000). This is appropriate because the usual duties assumed by nurses place them in a critical position for witnessing the consequences of abuse and neglect. In addition, a primary role of nurses is to foster collaboration between health care professionals as abuse reporters and adult protective service or law enforcement officials as abuse investigators or service providers.

Mandatory reporting laws do not require reporters to *know* whether abuse or neglect has occurred, but merely to report it if they *suspect* its occurrence. The responsibility for problem verification rests with the public agency charged with law implementation, not with the reporter or referral source. Suspecting elder abuse means detecting signs of violence, such as bruises, welts, or fractures. It also means recognizing conditions associated with neglect or deprivation, such as frostbite, malnutrition, dehydration, oversedation, mental changes, or uncontrolled medical conditions.

Because most reporting laws provide immunity for mandatory reporters, nurses who act in good faith and without malicious intent can report suspected cases without fear of liability. Some laws offer immunity in the workplace; in these cases, nurses cannot be fired, transferred, or demoted for making a report. In all states, responsibility for making the report rests with the individual nurse, so nurses cannot delegate reporting to anyone else. The nurse alone has the responsibility for reporting, and for the consequences—both legal and moral—of failing to do so. Even though individual nurses are responsible for reporting, most agencies and hospitals have established protocols to clarify roles and enhance the credibility of the report. Excellent examples of elder abuse detection protocols are available, and they should be considered for use by nurses in all health care settings involving multiple professions and levels of authority. Box 10-2 illustrates a typical protocol for hospital- or agency-based nurses.

Assessing

Protective service workers often call upon nurses to assess their clients, especially when there is concern about endangerment or questions about the effects of neglect or abuse. Nurses commonly are involved with assessments of clients who are newly referred or experiencing a change in health status. Nurses are the preferred health care worker for such assessments because of their holistic approach, their availability through nursing agencies, their willingness to make home visits, and the relative ease with which older people usually accept nurses.

Because assessment was discussed earlier in this chapter, only one aspect requires further examination here. Formal elder abuse assessment instruments are used to collect and organize all pertinent information, summarize observations, and provide a base for planning referrals, services, or legal actions. These tools assess and document all of the following:

- Background data (e.g., client's name and address)
- Signs of maltreatment or self-neglect according to type (e.g., bruises or welts in cases of suspected physical abuse)
- Severity of signs (e.g., an immediate life threat)
- Indicators of maltreatment intentionality (e.g., a caregiver who will not allow the nurse to be alone with the client)
- Symptoms of acute or chronic illness or impairment (e.g., incontinence)
- Functional incapacity (e.g., an inability to dress or toilet without assistance)

Box 10-2
Sample Protocol for Nurses Wih Regard to Elder Abuse

Perform an Initial Assessment

- Gather data on the client's clinical presentation; observe the client and interview the client, caregivers, or both.
- Analyze data that raise a suspicion of abuse, neglect, or exploitation; consider objective findings and whether these fit the explanations; consider client–caregiver interactions.

If There Is Reason for Suspicion, Use an Assessment Guide

If There Is Continued Suspicion, Consult the Abuse Detection Team

- Report pertinent findings to the primary nurse.
- Summarize findings from the assessment guide on progress notes.
- Discuss the information with the assigned primary care provider and social worker as soon as possible.
- Determine the need to report abuse or neglect to authorities charged with investigation under law.
- Document additional facts, and whether a report was made, in the progress notes.

Meet With the Client and Caregivers to Inform Them of the Intent to Report

- Include representatives from at least two health care, social service, or other professional disciplines in the meeting.
- Document the interaction and the results of the meeting in the progress notes.

Follow-up Actions

- Provide a report to the appropriate abuse detection team member for handling and distribution.
- Identify any security measures that must be taken to protect the client.
- Implement appropriate interventions.

Source: Cleveland Metropolitan General/Highland View Hospital. (1987). *Statement of policy and procedure: Abuse/neglect cases, reporting of suspected elder abuse* (unpublished manuscript).

- Aggravating social conditions (e.g., a client who lives alone and is socially isolated)
- Source of information (e.g., agency referral)
- Recommended action (e.g., referral of the case to home health care service providers)

Fulmer and colleagues (1984) developed an Elder Assessment Instrument (Fig. 10-3) that currently is recommended as a *Try This: Best Practices in Nursing Care to Older Adults* tool by the Hartford Institute for Geriatric Nursing.

Consulting

In addition to providing direct assessment, nurses often provide phone or e-mail consultation when questions arise regarding the health status of clients. Typical questions relate to medications, continence, nutrition and hydration, and disease signs. Consultation services are often part of networks among service providers in a given community; sometimes, they are formally organized through clinical consultation teams that are integral parts of protective services coalitions. Another role for nurses is in staff education for protective services workers on topics such as health assessment, recognition of endangerment, and disease prevention and detection.

Testifying in Court

Although very few cases of elder abuse involve court actions, adult protective service workers may need legal assistance to gain access, deliver services, or obtain a comprehensive assessment. In these situations, the older person usually is mentally impaired and unable to make decisions that would alleviate or eliminate the neglect or abuse. Legal intervention may also be appropriate when older adults in life-endangering circumstances refuse help. Before legal interventions are permitted, the protective service worker must present evidence to a judge or referee about all of the following:

- Abuse or neglect
- Need for protective services
- Inability to gain voluntary cooperation
- No other way to alleviate the problems

Most of the evidence is provided by physicians, mental health providers, and protective service workers; however, nurses are sometimes asked to testify or submit reports about their assessments or services.

Testimony provides two types of evidence: direct observation and opinion. Direct observation is an eyewitness account of the health status or function of the older person. Expert opinion represents conclusions about the situation based on the training and experience of the expert witness. To be effective, opinion must never be overstated or relate to areas outside the nurse's scope of practice or expertise. Medical records are useful as evidence because they are maintained in the regular course of client care by people who understand the facts being documented. Characteristics of good documentation include timeliness, legibility, thoroughness, and objectivity. In addition, corrections to medical records must be obvious and clear, removing any doubt about the destruction of relevant evidence.

Providing Care

As discussed in the nursing interventions section of this chapter, nurses provide essential care and treatment for abused and neglected older people. They help correct conditions caused by maltreatment and self-neglect, and they prevent their recurrence through such activities as treating injuries, monitoring medication, educating caregivers, obtaining assistive devices, and facilitating service referrals. In this role, as in others, nurses work cooperatively with other professionals and with paraprofessionals, using their knowledge and expertise to help the victims of elder abuse.

Ethical Issues

Ethical issues related to abused and neglected elders are similar to ethical issues in medicine and other fields. Rather than having clear answers and absolute rights and wrongs, there are usually differing perspectives and different implications, depending on what course of action is taken. Law, community pressures, and personal concepts of professionalism lead to the erroneous assumption that a problem, such as maltreatment or self-neglect, can be easily or simply resolved. However, protective situations involving older people are rarely easily resolved.

One dilemma surrounding ethical issues in adult protective services is the fact that all adults in American society have rights—including freedom from intrusion, the right to fair treatment, freedom from unnecessary restraint, and the right to self-determination—but these rights can be taken away through the use of legal measures. Professionals often are reluctant to initiate legal measures that take away the rights of other adults. For example, unless an older adult has been judged to be incompetent by a court of law, he or she has the right to be protected from intrusion, even by well-intentioned professionals. In adult protective service situations, this right is threatened and services can be imposed on an older person who does not willingly agree to assistance.

Another dilemma involves the characteristics of protective situations that sometimes make respecting personal rights so difficult. The following are examples of situations that present ethical dilemmas in relation to respecting personal rights:

- In situations that are urgent or dangerous, it is hard to walk away, even when the older person asks to be left alone.
- Public pressure to do something, no matter what, places pressure on care providers who are trying to resolve the situation while respecting the rights of the older person.
- Contradictory societal values may pit individual rights against other values, such as paternalism and protectionism.

ELDER ASSESSMENT INSTRUMENT (EAI)

	Very Good	Good	Poor	Very Poor	Unable to Assess
I. General Assessment					
1. Clothing					
2. Hygiene					
3. Nutrition					
4. Skin integrity					
5. Additional Comments:					

	No Evidence	Possible Evidence	Probable Evidence	Definite Evidence	Unable to Assess
II. Possible Abuse Indicators					
6. Bruising					
7. Lacerations					
8. Fractures					
9. Various states of healing of any bruises or fractures					
10. Evidence of sexual abuse					
11. Statement by elder re: abuse					
12. Additional Comments:					
III. Possible Neglect Indicators					
13. Contractures					
14. Decubiti					
15. Dehydration					
16. Diarrhea					
17. Depression					
18. Impaction					
19. Malnutrition					
20. Urine burns					
21. Poor hygiene					
22. Failure to respond to warning of obvious disease					
23. Inappropriate medications (under/over)					
24. Repetitive hospital admissions due to probable failure of healthcare surveillance					
25. Statement by elder re: neglect					
26. Additional Comments:					
IV. Possible Exploitation Indicators					
27. Misuse of money					
28. Evidence of financial exploitation					
29. Reports of demands for goods in exchange for services					
30. Inability to account for money/property					
31. Statement by elder re: exploitation					
32. Additional Comments:					
V. Possible Abandonment Indicators					
33. Evidence that a caretaker has withdrawn care precipitously without alternate arrangements					
34. Evidence that elder is left alone in an unsafe environment for extended periods of time without adequate support					
35. Statement by elder re: abandonment					
36. Additional Comments:					
VI. Summary					
37. Evidence of abuse					
38. Evidence of neglect					
39. Evidence of exploitation					
40. Evidence of abandonment					
41. Additional Comments:					

VII. Comments and Follow-up

Adapted from Fulmer, T., & Cahill, V. M. (1984). Assessing elder abuse: A study. Journal of Gerontological Nursing, 10*(12), 16–20; Fulmer, T., Street, S., & Carr, K. (1984). Abuse of the elderly: Screening and detection.* Journal of Emergency Nursing, 10*(3), 131–140.*

FIGURE 10-3 Elder Assessment Instrument (EAI) recommended as a *Try This. Best Practices in Nursing Care to Older Adults* tool by the Hartford Institute for Geriatric Nursing. (Available at www.hartfordign.org/publications/trythis/issue15.pdf.)

- Nursing is directed toward helping others. This presents difficulties for nurses when others do not accept their help, especially when the lack of help has detrimental consequences.
- Serious decisions often have to be made without an adequate base of information. Older adults may be too impaired to provide accurate information, the situation may not allow time for a good assessment, or pertinent information may be withheld by the older person or the caregivers.
- The questionable mental status of many abused or neglected elders places decision-making responsibility in the hands of other people. Involuntary legal interventions may unnecessarily deprive the person of certain rights, but inaction can mean that basic human needs are not being met adequately, or at all.
- The intrusive nature of legal interventions, including protective services law, robs older adults of fundamental rights. Mandatory reporting provisions, for example, by their very nature, invade privacy. Likewise, the sharing of information among agencies involved in case planning infringes on confidentiality.

Ethical dilemmas about particular situations sometimes can be resolved by applying practice guidelines (Anetzberger et al., 1997) or a hierarchy of principles, such as the one in Box 10-3 (Anetzberger, 1999). The principles of adult protective services, which were developed from long-term experience with abused elders, are arranged from the most to the least important considerations with regard to interventions for abused or neglected elders.

Adult protective services are fraught with ethical dilemmas. Some of these dilemmas are related to the five basic roles—reporter, investigator, service provider, administrator, and planner—assumed by professionals. Each role has a particular sphere of responsibility in addressing elder abuse and neglect. The reporter detects the situation and describes it to someone authorized by law to deal with it. The investigator is the legal agent who assesses the situation and determines the need for protective services. The service provider offers interventions for correcting or discontinuing maltreatment or self-neglect. The administrator manages a protective services program. Finally, the planner develops policies and programs, as well as community education initiatives, aimed at preventing or treating the problem.

Professional workers in each of these roles face different ethical issues. Issues of the reporter role include questions about whether to make a report and the consequences of doing so. The role of the investigator involves confronting questions about privacy, openness, and confidentiality. The service provider deals with issues about the rights of the elder, the rights of the caregivers, and the degree of risk for the elder. Program planners and administrators face dilemmas about service priorities and the lack of funds, staff, and other critical resources. Nurses most often deal with ethical issues in their roles as reporters, investigators, and service providers. Table 10-2 identifies some of the ethical problems, as well as related solutions, that nurses may encounter in their roles in adult protective services.

EVALUATING EFFECTIVENESS OF NURSING INTERVENTIONS

Nursing care of abused or neglected older adults is evaluated by the extent to which nursing goals are achieved. If a nursing goal is to alleviate the contributing factor of unnecessary dependence, the care is evaluated by whether the older adult is functioning at a higher level of independence. If a nursing goal is to address caregiver stress, the nursing care might be

Box 10-3
Principles of Adult Protective Services

I. **Freedom Over Safety.** The client has a right to choose to live at risk of harm, providing she or he is capable of making that choice, harms no one, and commits no crime.

II. **Self-Determination.** The client has a right to personal choices and decisions until such time that she or he delegates, or the court grants, the responsibility to someone else.

III. **Participation in Decision Making.** The client has a right to receive information to make informed decisions and to participate in all decision making affecting her or his circumstances to the extent that she or he is able.

IV. **Least Restrictive Alternative.** The client has a right to service alternatives that maximize choice and minimize lifestyle disruption.

V. **Primacy of the Adult.** The worker has a responsibility to serve the client, not the community people concerned about appearances, the landlord concerned about crime, or the family concerned about finances.

VI. **Confidentiality.** The client has a right to privacy and secrecy.

VII. **Benefit of Doubt.** If there is evidence that the client is making a reasoned choice, the worker has a responsibility to see that the benefit of doubt is in her or his favor.

VIII. **Do No Harm.** The worker has a responsibility to take no action that places the client at greater risk of harm.

IX. **Avoidance of Blame.** The worker has a responsibility to understand the origins of any maltreatment and to commit no action that would antagonize the perpetrator and so reduce the chances of terminating the maltreatment.

X. **Maintenance of the Family.** The worker has a responsibility to deal with the maltreatment as a family problem, if the perpetrator is a family member, and to try to find the necessary family services to resolve the problem.

Anetzberger, G. J. (1999). Ethical issues in personal safety. In T. F. Johnson (Ed.), *Handbook on ethical issues in aging* (pp. 187–219). Westport, CT: Greenwood Press.

TABLE 10-2 Ethical Questions and Suggested Solutions Regarding Abused Elders

Ethical Question/Implications	Suggested Solution
When do I report elder abuse? (If I report too soon, I may needlessly invade someone's privacy. If I wait, the situation may worsen.)	Report elder abuse when you believe that, without intervention, the situation will deteriorate or endanger the elder.
What if my report places the elder in more danger, or labels someone inaccurately? What if it causes the elder to shy away from me and my agency?	Report elder abuse if you believe that the protective services system can reduce the risk better than the current interventions.
How do I decide if the elder or the caregiver receives priority? (If my priority is the elder, I may alienate his or her family members, who serve as the primary sources of care. If my priority is the family, then the care plan may be contrary to the elder's wishes and may not adequately respect his or her rights.)	With certain exceptions, the elder should receive priority. These exceptions are limited to circumstances in which the elder has been judged to be incompetent by a court of law or is endangering others by his or her behavior.
Is it more important to maintain standards of confidentiality than to comply with a reporting law?	State law takes precedence over professional standards.
Does the right of an elder to refuse services extend to total self-neglect and intentional suicide? How can I know that endangered elders clearly understand the consequences of their self-neglect? How can I accept abandoning the situation?	Ethical dilemmas such as these often can be resolved through the use of a hierarchy of values or principles, such as those summarized in Box 10-3.
Can emergency services be thrust upon an elder who would have refused them under ordinary circumstances? If the elder's life is endangered, then is it not my primary responsibility to use my nursing skills in life-saving ways, no matter what the elder chooses? Even if the elder might have refused services in the past, does that mean he or she absolutely would refuse them now?	If the elder is incapable of deciding whether to accept or reject emergency services, then these services should be provided, subject to the constraints of the protective services law. This offers the elder essential protection, but recognizes his or her right to refuse ongoing services when the emergency has subsided and he or she is capable of making decisions on his or her own behalf.

evaluated by the caregiver accepting help with the care, attending caregiver support groups, and expressing less stress about his or her caregiving responsibilities. When the nursing goal is to protect an incompetent older adult from harm, nursing care might be evaluated by the extent to which the least restrictive legal interventions are implemented. In such cases, nursing care is evaluated in terms of protecting the older adult from harm while also protecting his or her rights.

Recall that Mrs. B. is 82 years old and lives in a senior citizens apartment. After 2 months of receiving skilled nursing visits, Mrs. B. was discharged from the home care agency because she was successfully managing her medications and other aspects of functioning adequately. Several months after she was discharged, the nurse in the wellness clinic at the senior citizens apartment noted a change in her mannerisms, accompanied by slurred speech and an unbalanced gait. Mrs. B. had bruises on her arms, knees, and forehead, but insisted that she had not fallen. After further investigation, the nurse found that her blood pressure was 210/104 mm Hg and that her blood glucose level was 410 mg/dL on the glucometer that the nurse kept in the clinic. A pill count revealed that Mrs. B. had not taken her medications for $2^1/_2$ days. After a consultation with her primary care provider, Mrs. B. was admitted to the hospital. Tests revealed that she had suffered a stroke, resulting in left-sided weakness and short-term memory loss.

Mrs. B. left the hospital against medical advice and returned to her apartment, initially refusing visits from the home health nurse. She insisted that her children come and administer her medications and prepare her meals because she was unable to do this for herself. Mrs. B. reasoned that she had cared for her children when they were young, so they should come when she needed them. The children tried to assist Mrs. B. for 4 days, but were unable to meet both her demands and those of their jobs and families. Mrs. B. reluctantly agreed to a visit from the home health nurse who had visited her before. She expected that she would see the nurse once and that the nurse would "make my children do right."

Mrs. B.'s children were present for the initial assessment. Mrs. B. was unable to stand or transfer to the commode without help. She could not use her chart and color-coded boxes to take her pills. Mrs. B. flatly refused to consider admission to a nursing facility to receive therapy to regain her strength, and she would not consider living with her daughter or either son. The family told the nurse that they were exhausted and on the "verge of a breakdown" and could not continue to provide the care that Mrs. B. needed. The nurse explained to Mrs. B. that it was

(case study continues on page 182)

not safe for her to remain in her apartment without assistance. She suggested that she hire an aide until other arrangements could be made, because her children were not obligated to lose their jobs or jeopardize their family relationships to care for her. Mrs. B. accused her children of being greedy and caring only about themselves. She said that children have a duty to care for their parents and that she wasn't going to "have strangers doing the things that decent children should be doing." She directed her concluding remarks at the nurse, stating, "What's more, I don't need you to come back either, because all you want to do is side with my children."

THINKING POINTS

- What strategies would you use to establish a relationship with Mrs. B.?
- What additional assessment information would you want to obtain, and how would you obtain it?
- What would your next steps be in working with Mrs. B.?
- How would you work with the family?
- What other resources would you involve in planning and providing care for Mrs. B.?
- What criteria would you use for making a referral for adult protective services?

Chapter Highlights

Overview of Elder Abuse and Neglect (Box 10-1)

- Types of elder abuse include self-neglect, physical or psychological abuse or neglect by others, exploitation, sexual abuse, violation of rights, and abandonment.
- Awareness of elder abuse as a social problem began in the 1950s and 1960s. Elder abuse is receiving increasing attention because of the increase in reports of abuse, the growing elder population, research on the topic, and public policy action.
- Characteristics of victim: female, older, socially isolated, living alone or with abuser, functionally dependent
- Characteristics of abuser: stress, psychosocial impairment, history of violence, dependent on victim
- Cultural differences in family and caregiver roles affect definitions of elder abuse (Cultural Considerations 10-1).

Risk Factors That Contribute to Elder Abuse and Neglect

- Elder abuse causation is extremely complex, with many variables associated with both the victim and the perpetrator.
- Invisibility
- Vulnerability
- Psychosocial factors (impaired cognition, long-term mental illness)
- Caregiver factors (psychosocial impairments)

Functional Consequences Associated With Elder Abuse and Neglect

- Neglect
- Physical abuse
- Emotional (psychological) abuse
- Exploitation (financial or property abuse)
- Sexual abuse

Nursing Assessment of Abused or Neglected Older Adults

- Unique aspects of elder abuse assessment: safety, limited goals, resistance, nurse viewed as threat, legal and ethical considerations, safety of nurse
- Physical health: indicators of harm, dehydration, malnutrition, bruises, medical conditions, caregiver abilities
- Activities of daily living: assess in relation to safety, basic needs, vulnerability (Table 10-1)
- Psychosocial function: impaired cognition, judgments about self-care
- Support resources: caregivers who also are perpetrators, lack of resources, barriers to using services
- Environmental influences: home, neighborhood, seasonal factors
- Threats to life: degree of endangerment and ability to alleviate risks
- Cultural aspects: family and cultural expectations, perspectives on caregiving, barriers to assessment (Cultural Considerations 10-2)

Nursing Diagnosis

- Disabled Family Coping
- Caregiver Role Strain
- Risk for Injury
- Decisional Conflict

Planning for Wellness Outcomes

- Quality of Life
- Abuse Cessation, Protection, Recovery Status
- Neglect Cessation
- Risk Control
- Caregiver Stressors, Emotional Health, Endurance Potential
- Family Coping
- Social Support

Nursing Interventions to Address Elder Abuse and Neglect

- Role of the nurse in institutional settings (teaching caregivers, discharge planning, addressing caregiver stress)
- Role of the nurse in community settings (teaching, supervising, providing direct care, working with home health aides, facilitating referrals)
- Role of the nurse in multidisciplinary teams
- Facilitating referrals (services for older adults and caregivers, medical equipment)
- Prevention and treatment interventions (types of core services, programs for preventing financial abuse; Fig. 10-2)

Legal Interventions
- Voluntary and involuntary
- Adult protective services (Box 10-2): reporting and collaborating, assessing (Fig. 10-3), consulting, testifying in court, providing care
- Ethical issues: principles of adult protective services (Box 10-3)
- Ethical questions and suggested solutions (Table 10-2)

Evaluating Effectiveness of Nursing Interventions
- Higher level of functioning of older adult
- Alleviation of caregiver stress
- Use of least restrictive legal interventions
- Protection of the older adult

Critical Thinking Exercises

1. Identify factors in each of the following categories that currently contribute to elder abuse and neglect in the United States:
   - Demographic statistics
   - Changes in families
   - Health care systems
   - Health status and other characteristics of older adults
   - Social awareness
2. What is different about the nursing assessment of abused or neglected elders compared with the nursing assessment of other older adults?
3. What do you believe about family caregiving responsibilities? How would you deal with a family whose values about caregiving differ significantly from yours?
4. What are your beliefs about the degree of risk a frail elder should be allowed to take?
5. Under what circumstances should an elder be denied the right to remain in his or her own home?

Clinical Tool Resources

Hartford Institute for Geriatric Nursing
Try This: Best Practices in Nursing Care to Older Adults
Issue Number 15 (Revised 2007), Elder Mistreatment and Abuse Assessment
www.hartfordign.org/resources/education/tryThis.html

Educational Resources

National Center on Elder Abuse and the Clearinghouse on Abuse and Neglect of the Elderly (CANE)
www.elderabusecenter.org

National Clearinghouse on Family Violence, Health Canada
www.phac-aspc.gc.ca/ncfv-cnivf/familyviolence/

National Committee for the Prevention of Elder Abuse
www.preventelderabuse.org

National Eldercare Locator
www.eldercare.gov

References

Anetzberger, G. J. (1987). *The etiology of elder abuse by adult offspring*. Springfield, IL: Charles C Thomas.

Anetzberger, G. J. (1999). Ethical issues in personal safety. In T. F. Johnson (Ed.), *Handbook on ethical issues in aging* (pp. 187–219). Westport, CT: Greenwood Press.

Anetzberger, G. J. (2000). Caregiving: Primary cause of elder abuse? *Generations, 24*(11), 46–51.

Anetzberger, G. J. (2001). Elder abuse identification and referral: The importance of screening tools and referral protocols. *Journal of Elder Abuse & Neglect, 13*(2), 3–22.

Anetzberger, G. J. (2002). Adult protective services. In D. J. Ekerdt (Ed.), *The Macmillan encyclopedia of aging*. New York: Macmillan Reference USA.

Anetzberger, G. J., Dayton, C., & McMonagle, P. (1997). A community dialogue series on ethics and elder abuse: Guidelines for decision-making. *Journal of Elder Abuse & Neglect, 9*(1), 33–50.

Anetzberger, G. J., Korbin, J. E., & Tomito, S. K. (1996). Defining elder mistreatment in four ethnic groups across two generations. *Journal of Cross-Cultural Gerontology, 11*, 187–211.

Beach, S. R., Schulz, R., Williamson, G. M., Miller, L. S., Weiner, M. F., & Lance, C. E. (2005). Risk factors for potentially harmful informal caregiver behavior. *Journal of the American Geriatrics Society, 53*, 255–261.

Brammer, A. (2003). Undue influence? *Journal of Adult Protection, 5*(1), 40–44.

Buchwald, D., Tomita, S., Hartman, S., Furman, R., Dudden, M., & Manson, S. M. (2000). Physical abuse of urban Native Americans. *Journal of General Internal Medicine, 15*, 562–564.

Burston, G. R. (1975). Granny-battering. *British Medical Journal, 3*, 592.

Butler, R. N. (1975). *Why survive? Being old in America*. New York: Harper & Row.

Carpenito-Moyet, L. J. (2006). *Handbook of nursing diagnosis* (11th ed.). Philadelphia: Lippincott Williams & Wilkins.

Cook-Daniels, L. (1997). Lesbian, gay male, bisexual and transgendered elders: Elder abuse and neglect issues. *Journal of Elder Abuse & Neglect, 9*(2), 35–49.

Daly, J. M., & Jogerst, G. J. (2005). Definitions and indicators of elder abuse: A Delphi survey of APS caseworkers. *Journal of Elder Abuse & Neglect, 17*(1), 1–19.

Dong, X. (2005). Medical implications of elder abuse and neglect. *Clinics in Geriatric Medicine, 21*, 293–313.

Dyer, C. B., Pavlik, V. N., Murphy, K. P., & Hyman, D. J. (2000). The high prevalence of depression and dementia in elder abuse or neglect. *Journal of the American Geriatrics Society, 48*, 205–208.

Fisher, B. S., & Regan, S. L. (2006). The extent and frequency of abuse in the lives of older women and their relationship with health outcomes. *The Gerontologist, 46*, 200–209.

Flannery, R. B., Jr. (2003). Domestic violence and elderly dementia sufferers. *American Journal of Alzheimer's Disease and Other Dementia, 18*(1), 21–23.

France, D. (2006, January/February). "And then he hit me." *AARP Magazine*, 81–85, 112–113, 118.

Franks, M., Lund, D. A., Poulton, D., & Caserta, M. (2004). Understanding hoarding behavior among older adults: A case study approach. *Journal of Gerontological Social Work, 42*(3/4), 77–107.

Fulmer, T., Guadagno, L., Dyer, C. B., & Connolley, M. T. (2004). Progress in elder abuse screening and assessment instruments. *Journal of the American Geriatrics Society, 52*, 297–304.

Fulmer, T., Paveza, G., Vandeweerd, C., Guadagno, L., Fairchild, S., Norman, R., et al. (2005). Neglect assessment in urban emergency departments and confirmation by an expert clinical tea. *Journals of Gerontology: Series A, Biological Sciences and Medical Sciences, 60*, 1002–1006.

Fulmer, T., Street, S., & Carr, K. (1984). Abuse of the elderly: Screening and detection. *Journal of Emergency Nursing, 10*, 131–140.

Fulmer, T. T., & O'Malley, T. A. (1987). *Inadequate care of the elderly: A health care perspective on abuse and neglect*. New York: Springer.

Griffin, L. W. (1994). Elder maltreatment among rural African-Americans. *Journal of Elder Abuse & Neglect, 6*(1), 1–27.

Hamp, L. F. (2003). Analysis of elder abuse and neglect definitions under state law. In National Research Council (Ed.), *Elder mistreatment: Abuse, neglect, and exploitation in an aging America* (pp. 181–237). Washington, DC: The National Academies Press.

Hansberry, M. R., Chen, E., & Gorbien, M. J. (2005). Dementia and elder abuse. *Clinics in Geriatric Medicine, 21*, 315–332.

Heath, J. M., Kobylarz, F. A., Brown, M., & Castano, S. (2005). Interventions from home-based geriatric assessments of adult protective service clients suffering elder mistreatment. *Journal of the American Geriatrics Society, 53*, 1538–1542.

Hudson, M. F., Armachain, W. D., Beasley, C. M., & Carlson, J. R. (1998). Elder abuse: Two Native American views. *The Gerontologist, 38*, 538–548.

Hudson, M. F., Beasley, C., Benedict, R. H., Carlson, J. R., Craig, B. F., Herman, C., et al. (2000). Elder abuse: Some Caucasian-American views. *Journal of Elder Abuse & Neglect, 12*(1), 89–114.

Krassen Maxwell, E., & Maxwell, R. J. (1992). Insults to the body civil: Mistreatment of the elderly in two Plains Indian tribes. *Journal of Cross-Cultural Gerontology, 7*, 3–23.

Lachs, M. S., & Pillemer, K. (2004). Elder abuse. *Lancet, 364*, 1263–1272.

Lau, E., & Kosberg, J. (1979). Abuse of the elderly by informal care providers. *Aging, 299–300*, 10–15.

Malley-Morrison, K., Nolido, N. E.-V., & Chawla, S. (2006). International perspectives on elder abuse: Five case studies. *Educational Gerontology, 32*, 1–11.

Moon, A., & Benton, D. (2000). Tolerance of elder abuse and attitudes toward third-party intervention among African American, Korean American, and white elderly. *Journal of Multicultural Social Work, 8*, 283–303.

Montoya, V. (1997). Understanding and combating elder abuse in Hispanic communities. *Journal of Elder Abuse & Neglect, 9*(2), 5–17.

Mosqueda, L., Burnright, K., & Liao, S., (2005). The life cycle of bruises in older adults. *Journal of the American Geriatrics Society, 53*, 1339–1343.

Nagpaul, K. (1997). Elder abuse among Asian Indians: Traditional versus modern perspectives. *Journal of Elder Abuse & Neglect, 9*(2), 77–92.

Nahmiash, D., & Reis, M. (2000). Most successful intervention strategies for abused older adults. *Journal of Elder Abuse & Neglect, 12*(3/4), 53–70.

National Center on Elder Abuse. (2003a). Elder abuse/mistreatment defined. Available at www.elderabusecenter.org/default.cfm?p=mistreatment.cfm. Retrieved August 23, 2006.

National Center on Elder Abuse. (2003b). Major types of elder abuse. Available at www.elderabusecenter.org/default.cfm?p=basics.cfm. Retrieved August 23, 2006.

National Research Council. (2003). *Elder mistreatment: Abuse, neglect, and exploitation in an aging America*. Washington, DC: The National Academies Press.

Payne, B. K., & Gainey, R. R. (2005). Differentiating self-neglect as a type of elder mistreatment: How do these cases compare to traditional types of elder mistreatment? *Journal of Elder Abuse & Neglect, 17*(1), 21–36.

Phillips, L. (2000). Domestic violence and aging women. *Geriatric Nursing, 21*, 188–198.

Phillips, L. R., Torres de Ardon, E., & Briones, G. S. (2000). Abuse of female caregivers by care recipients: Another form of elder abuse. *Journal of Elder Abuse & Neglect, 12*(3/4), 123–143.

Podnieks, E. (2006). Social inclusion: An interplay of the determinants of health—new insights into elder abuse. *Journal of Gerontological Social Work, 46*(3/4), 57–79.

Quinn, M. J. (2002). Undue influence and elder abuse: Recognition and intervention strategies. *Geriatric Nursing, 23*, 11–15.

Quinn, M. J., & Tomita, S. K. (1986). *Elder abuse and neglect: Causes, diagnosis, and intervention strategies*. New York: Springer.

Ramsey-Klawsnik, H. (2006). Dynamics of self-neglect: Part 1. *Victimization of the Elderly and Disabled, 8*(5), 69–70, 76.

Roby, J. L., & Sullivan, R. (2000). Adult protective service laws: A comparison of state statutes from definition to case closure. *Journal of Elder Abuse & Neglect 12*(3/4), 17–51.

Tauriac, J. J., & Scruggs, N. (2006). Elder abuse among African Americans. *Educational Gerontology, 32*, 37–48.

Teaster, P. B., Dugar, T. A., Mendiondo, M. S., & Otto, J. M. (2005). *The 2004 survey of state adult protective services: Abuse of adults 60 years of age and older*. Washington, DC: National Center on Elder Abuse.

Teaster, P. B., & Roberto, K. A. (2004). Sexual abuse of older adults: APS cases and outcomes. *The Gerontologist, 44*, 788–796.

Tierney, M. C., Charles, J., Naglie, G., Jagial, S., Kiss, A., & Fisher, R. H. (2004). Risk factors for harm in cognitively impaired seniors who live alone: A prospective study. *Journal of the American Geriatrics Society, 52*, 1435–1441.

United Nations Economic and Social Council. (2002, February 25–March 1). *Abuse of older persons: Recognizing and responding to abuse of older persons in a global context*. Document of the Commission for Social Development presented at the Second World Assembly on Aging, New York.

Wolf, R. S. (2001). Support groups for older victims of domestic violence. *Journal of Women & Aging, 13*(4), 71–83.

Zink, T., Regan, S., Jacobson, C. J., Jr., & Pabst, S. (2003). Cohort, period, and aging effects: A qualitative study of older women's reasons for remaining in abusive relationships. *Violence Against Women, 9*, 1429–1441.

Promoting Wellness in Psychosocial Function

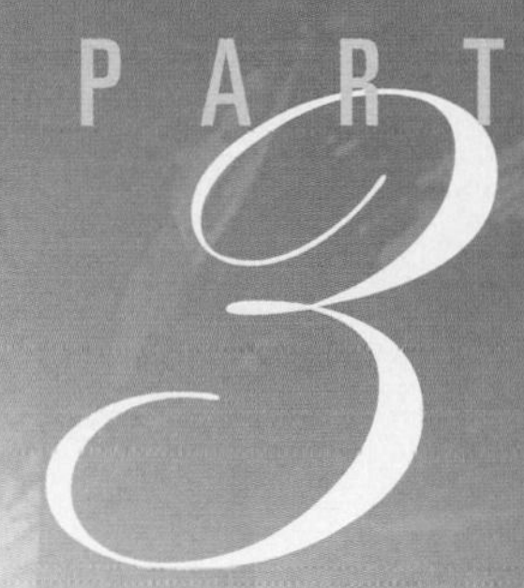

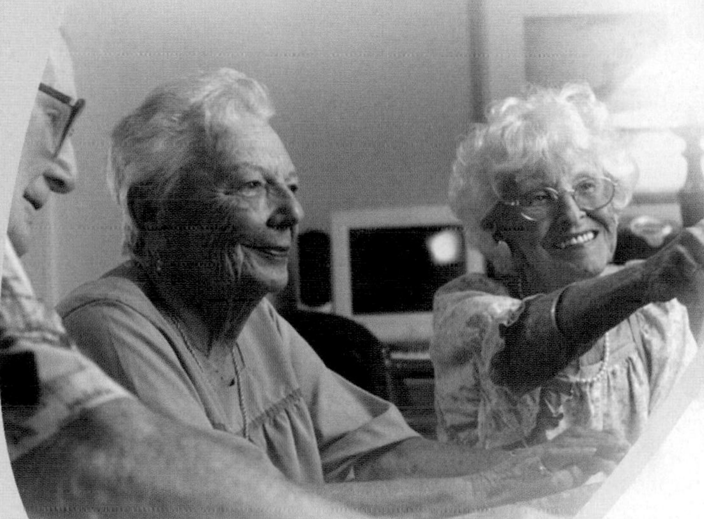

CHAPTER 11

Cognitive Function

Learning Objectives

After reading this chapter, you will be able to:

1. Describe age-related changes that affect cognitive abilities.
2. List risk factors that influence cognitive function in older adults.
3. Discuss the functional consequences associated with cognition in older adults.
4. Identify nursing interventions to help older adults maintain or improve cognitive abilities.

Key Terms

age-associated memory impairment
automatic and effortful processing theory
benign senescent forgetfulness
contextual theories
continuum of processing
crystallized intelligence
developmental intelligence
empowering model
everyday problem solving
fluid intelligence
metamemory
paradox of aging
plasticity
primary memory
recall memory
recognition memory
secondary memory
socioemotional selectivity
stage theories
wisdom

Cognition is the process of thinking, learning, and remembering. Myths about cognitive aging are pervasive and long-standing in society and can be detrimental to older adults. Indeed, the adage that "you can't teach an old dog new tricks" underlies some of the most widely held—and inaccurate—perspectives on older adults' cognition. Research in recent decades, however, consistently supports a more optimistic view of cognitive aging. One of the most

Promoting Cognitive Wellness in Older Adults

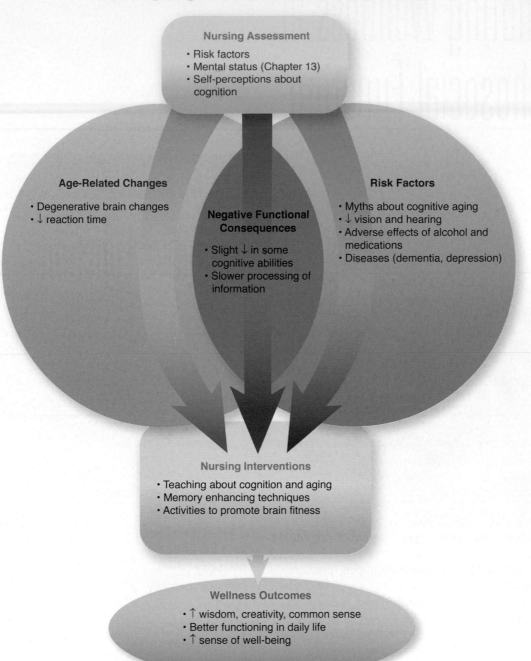

Nursing Assessment
- Risk factors
- Mental status (Chapter 13)
- Self-perceptions about cognition

Age-Related Changes
- Degenerative brain changes
- ↓ reaction time

Negative Functional Consequences
- Slight ↓ in some cognitive abilities
- Slower processing of information

Risk Factors
- Myths about cognitive aging
- ↓ vision and hearing
- Adverse effects of alcohol and medications
- Diseases (dementia, depression)

Nursing Interventions
- Teaching about cognition and aging
- Memory enhancing techniques
- Activities to promote brain fitness

Wellness Outcomes
- ↑ wisdom, creativity, common sense
- Better functioning in daily life
- ↑ sense of well-being

significant ways in which nurses can promote wellness for older adults is by correcting myth-based views and encouraging older adults to engage in activities that foster cognitive fitness.

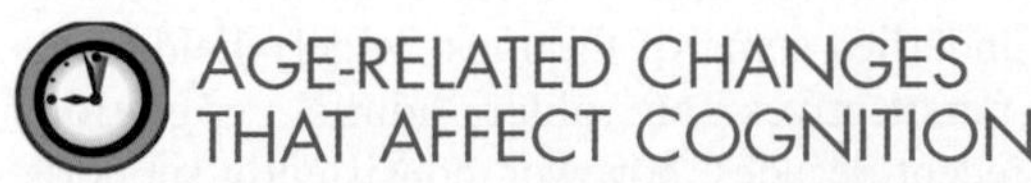

AGE-RELATED CHANGES THAT AFFECT COGNITION

Current theories about aging and cognition differ significantly from those that were first developed during the 1960s. Initial cross-sectional studies, which were based on tests designed to predict school performance in children, led to the conclusion that a decline in cognitive abilities was a normal part of the aging process. By the mid-1980s, results of longitudinal studies began showing that intellectual function remained the same or improved up to the age of 50 or 60 years, after which it gradually declined. In recent decades, researchers have addressed the influence of environment, life experiences, and socioemotional factors such as attitudes, expectations, and motivation (Carstensen et al., 2006). Researchers currently are developing theories that explain how variables such as health, emotion, cognition, personality, and other psychological characteristics affect cognitive abilities (Hofer & Sliwinski, 2006). Gerontologists are particularly interested in identifying interventions that improve cognitive abilities in older adults. For example, studies suggest that interventions to improve cardiovascular fitness have positive effects on cognitive function (Kramer et al., 2006).

As with many other aspects of function in older adults, gerontologists are trying to distinguish between the cognitive changes that occur in healthy older adults and those that are associated with pathologic processes such as dementia (discussed in Chapter 14). Age-related changes affecting cognition can be understood in terms of changes in the central nervous system and theories about intelligence, memory, and psychological development that attempt to explain the relationship between aging and cognition.

Central Nervous System

Knowledge about brain aging is gleaned from clinical, neuropsychological, neuropathologic, and neurochemical investigations. Initial studies of brain aging relied on autopsy findings, but recent major advances in noninvasive neuroimaging techniques (e.g., functional magnetic resonance imaging) have significantly broadened the knowledge base. Thus, the findings from more recent studies sometimes differ from earlier studies. For example, studies continue to find evidence for age-related decline in some aspects of cognition, but there is no evidence of widespread neuronal loss that causes general and progressive cognitive decline during older adulthood (Albert & Killiany, 2001). Some of the age-related changes in the brain that are likely to affect cognition in healthy older adults are as follows (Backman et al., 2001; Simensky & Abeles, 2002; Vinters, 2001):

- A gradual reduction in brain weight of 2 to 3 g per year (from an average of 1400 g in adult men and 1250 g in adult women) beginning around the age of 60 years, due primarily to loss of white matter, particularly in the frontal lobes
- Diminished ratio of brain to skull volume, from 95% around the age of 60 years to 80% in nonagenarians
- Enlarged ventricles, with average ventricle volume increasing from 15 mL in teens to 55 mL in people older than 60 years of age
- Widening of the sulci
- Shrinkage of larger neurons and possibly some neuronal loss, particularly in frontal and temporal lobes
- Loss of neurotransmitters or their binding sites
- A gradual decrease in dopaminergic function of 6% to 10 % per decade from early to later adulthood
- Diminished cerebral blood flow, particularly in the prefrontal cortex
- Accumulation of lipofuscin in nerve cell bodies

Slower reaction time is the age-related central nervous system change most commonly associated with declines in cognitive function; however, gerontologists are emphasizing that speed of processing is one variable among many factors that affect cognitive aging (Hartley, 2006). Diminished sensory ability and other age-related variables are discussed in the section on Risk Factors.

Much of the current research focuses on differentiating between normal and pathologic brain changes that affect cognitive abilities, with emphasis on the importance of considering the influence of variables such as prior mental ability (Deary et al., 2006). Gerontologists also are exploring the potential relationship between brain changes associated with dementia and memory complaints or subtle memory impairments (Bennett et al., 2006; Saykin et al., 2006). Another area of intense research is in identifying effects of normal and pathologic brain changes on specific cognitive abilities. For example, studies suggest that age-related changes in the frontal lobe explain diminished executive control processes in healthy older adults (Hedden & Gabrieli, 2005). (Refer to Chapter 13 for information related to assessment of executive control and other cognitive abilities.)

Despite age-related degenerative changes, research of the past two decades indicates that "healthy older brains are often as good as or better than younger brains in a wide variety of tasks" (Cohen, 2005, p. 4). Studies have identified the following characteristics of the brain that support an optimistic view of cognitive aging (Cohen, 2005):

- New brain cells form throughout life.
- Experience and learning enable the brain to "resculpt" itself.
- Emotional circuitry of the brain matures and becomes more balanced during older adulthood.
- Functions of the left and right hemispheres of the brain become more integrated in older adults.

Although research on brain aging provides the biologic base of information, psychological theories explain differences in cognitive abilities, as discussed in the following sections.

Fluid and Crystallized Intelligence

Cattell and Horn's theory of fluid and crystallized intelligence, first proposed in the late 1960s, is one of the first theories that attempted to explain age-related changes in some cognitive abilities. **Fluid intelligence** depends primarily on a person's inherent abilities, such as memory, pattern recognition, and the central nervous system. Fluid intelligence is associated with integration, inductive reasoning, abstract thinking, and flexible and adaptive thinking. This cognitive characteristic enables people to identify and draw conclusions about complex relationships. **Crystallized intelligence** refers to cognitive skills, such as vocabulary, information, and verbal comprehension, that people acquire through culture, education, informal learning, and other life experiences. This cognitive characteristic is strongly associated with wisdom, judgment, and life experiences.

According to this theory, fluid and crystallized intelligence develop concurrently during infancy and childhood and, in fact, are indistinguishable as the central nervous system is maturing. During early adulthood, age-related changes in neural structures cause a decline in fluid intelligence (Horn & Hofer, 1992). By contrast, crystallized intelligence continues to develop throughout adulthood because of accumulated experiences and learning. Crystallized intelligence, except for those processes that depend on speed of response, does not decline with age, and it may even increase because of experiences that improve wisdom. Many studies support this theory; however, they also indicate that older adults are likely to have greater differences in crystallized intelligence (Thompson & Foth, 2005).

Memory

Memory is often conceptualized as a computer-like information-processing system in which information is first perceived, then stored, and finally retrieved when needed or wanted. **Primary memory** has a short duration and a very small capacity, and serves as a holding tank for events of the immediate past few seconds rather than as a true memory storage system. Information in the primary memory either can be recalled for a brief time or be transmitted to long-term storage. **Secondary memory** is longer-term and therefore is more important in terms of the retrieval, as well as storage, of information. Retrieval of information from storage is referred to as remote, tertiary, or very–long-term memory processing, and skills involved are classified as **recall memory** and **recognition memory**. Theories associated with this conceptualization of memory suggested that older people remember events of long ago better than recent events. This conclusion is not supported by studies, which indicate that both types of memory decline equally in older adulthood, but older adults have a larger store of information about events of long ago (Botwinick, 1984).

More recently, gerontologists have come to view the information-processing model as too simplistic because it ignores the milieu in which the memory operates. Newer theories, called **contextual theories**, address some of the variables that can affect memory, including motivation, expectations, experiences, education, personality, task demands, learning habits, intellectual skills, sociocultural background, physical and mental health, and style of processing information.

Because processing speed is a contextual factor that most consistently affects memory, older adults will have better memory skills when they have more time to process information.

Another theoretical approach emphasizes encoding and analyzing rather than storage and retrieval aspects of memory. According to this perspective, memory is a **continuum of processing**, ranging from shallow to deep levels; the deeper the level at which information is stored, the longer the memory will last. Any of the following variables can affect the depth of storage (Botwinick, 1984):

- Processing techniques, ranging from the shallowest levels used for sensory information to the deepest levels used for highly abstract information
- Elaboration, or quality, of processing carried out at any depth level
- Distinctiveness of the information, which depends partially on how well it is learned
- Depth and elaboration of retrieval processes

Several studies based on this framework have concluded that older adults have decreased memory function because of faulty processing mechanisms (Botwinick, 1984).

Another theoretical perspective that views memory as a continuum is the **automatic and effortful processing theory** (Hasher & Zacks, 1979). At one end of the continuum is automatic processing, or those tasks that do not require attention or awareness and do not improve with practice. At the other end is effortful processing, or those tasks that demand high levels of attention and cognitive energy. With practice, effortful tasks require less attention and become more automatic. According to this theory, aging does not affect automatic memory because these tasks require little or no cognitive energy. Effortful memory, however, declines with age because only a limited amount of cognitive resources are available for memory functions, and these resources begin to decline in early adulthood. Many studies have confirmed declines in effortful processes including selective attention, mental imagery, verbal fluency, language production, and verbal and visuospatial working memory. Studies also have confirmed no declines in automatic cognitive functions such as picture recognition and implicit and procedural memory (Carstensen et al., 2006).

Metamemory refers to self-knowledge and perceptions about memory, cognitive function, and development of memory. Gerontologists study metamemory because they believe that metacognitive processes enable a person to influence memory consciously by using compensatory strategies (DeFries et al., 2003). Metamemory is important in everyday activities because if people know what they can remember and how much effort they will need to remember certain things, they can plan efficient and effective strategies for remembering. Older adults tend to perceive themselves as less competent than younger adults or less competent than they actually are in many cognitive tasks.

A current focus of research is on identifying interventions to improve memory functioning, particularly in relation to health status and health-related behaviors. For example, many studies show a "robust effect of fitness training" on many measures of cognitive function (Hoyer & Verhaeghen, 2006, p. 222). Older adults benefit from memory-enhancing techniques such as mnemonic training; however, health and mental status significantly affect outcomes (Hoyer & Verhaeghen, 2006). Studies suggest that memory-enhancing methods must include both internal (e.g., imagery) and external (e.g., calendars and notes) memory aids (Thompson &

Foth, 2005). Gerontologists also emphasize the importance of addressing ageist attitudes that contribute to detrimental self-stereotypes about cognitive abilities.

Wellness Opportunity

Nurses can influence attitudes by conveying positive beliefs about the ability of older adults to improve memory skills.

Adult Psychological Development

Theories about psychological development postulate that the thinking of older adults becomes increasingly complex and shows progressive reorganization of intellectual skills (Labouvie-Vief & Blanchard-Fields, 1982). For example, a recent focus of these theories is on cognitive abilities associated with decision making and **everyday problem solving**. Conclusions from studies of decision-making skills are as follows (Mariske & Margrett, 2006):

- Affect and motivation are strong predictors of decision making in older adults.
- Older adults are more selective in the information they use for decision making (i.e., they base decisions on less information).
- Older adults require more time to make decisions that are equal in quality to those of younger adults, but they may choose to spend the same or less time.
- Increased task complexity is associated with greater error and more inconsistencies for both older and younger adults.
- Task expertise and prior experience contribute to better decisions for both older and younger adults.

Nurses can apply conclusions from these studies when they involve older adults in decisions about self-care.

Stage theories of adult cognitive development were first developed during the 1970s as an extension of Piaget's theory of intellectual development in children and adolescents. One such theory postulated that children and adolescents focus on acquiring knowledge, and adults focus on applying knowledge in the following stages (Schaie, 1977-1978):

- *Achieving stage* (early adulthood): adults apply acquired knowledge to demands and commitments, such as career and family; they use their intellectual abilities to establish their independence and develop goal-oriented behaviors.
- *Responsible stage* (late 30s to early 60s): adults integrate long-range goals and attend to the needs of their family and society.
- *Executive stage* (a subset of the Responsible stage): applies to people who have high levels of social responsibilities.
- *Reintegration stage* (later adulthood): intellectual tasks are to simplify life and select only those responsibilities that have meaning and purpose; older adults ask "Why should I know?" rather than "What should I know?"

More recently, Cohen (2005) developed an **empowering model**, based on studies of more than 3000 older adults. This model describes the following four phases of mature aging:

- *Midlife reevaluation* (early 40s to late 50s): people confront their sense of mortality; plans and actions are shaped by a quest or crisis; brain changes spur developmental intelligence.
- *Liberation* (late 50s to early 70s): people feel a new sense of inner liberation; development in information-processing part of the brain increases desire for novelty; plans and actions are shaped by personal freedom; retirement allows time for new experiences.
- *Summing up* (late 60s through 80s): people are motivated to share wisdom; plans and actions are shaped by a desire to find meaning; brain development improves capacity for autobiographical expression; people may feel compelled to attend to unfinished business and unresolved conflict.
- *Encore* (late 70s to end of life): plans and actions are shaped by the desire to restate and reaffirm major themes and to explore novel variations on those themes; brain changes promote positive emotions and morale; the desire to live well to the very end has a positive impact on others.

Gerontologists currently are focusing on questions about the "**paradox of aging**," which describes the phenomenon of older adults suffering significant loss with age but experiencing life more positively (Carstensen et al., 2006). The **socioemotional selectivity** theory addresses this question in the context of motivation. According to this theory, older adults do not have the expanded time perspective of youth; rather they recognize that time is limited, so they are motivated to pursue emotional satisfaction. Thus, they "invest in sure things, deepen existing relationships, and savor life" (Carstensen et al., 2006, p. 347). According to theory, older adults allocate a larger portion of cognitive resources to both negative and positive emotional information and devote their attention and memory capacity to information that enhances their mood.

Another current focus is on **wisdom** as an aspect of cognitive function, which is viewed as "a body of expert knowledge about the meaning and conduct of life" (Brugman, 2006). A similar concept is **developmental intelligence**, defined as "the maturing of cognition, emotional intelligence, judgment, social skills, life experience, and consciousness and their integration and synergy" (Cohen, 2005, p. 35). Cohen's view of cognitive aging, which is both optimistic and research based, emphasizes that many older adults display the age-dependent quality of wisdom because they integrate all the components of developmental intelligence.

A Student's Perspective

The residents at Heritage continue to amaze me with their stories. There is so much one can learn just by listening, and the residents just want to share their stories and have our company more than anything—at least that is the impression I continually receive from them. They are all friendly, open people who are no different than the rest of us, but they have gained a large amount of knowledge over the years that many of us who are students probably have not acquired yet.

Megan S.

Wellness Opportunity

Nurses acknowledge the wisdom of older adults by asking questions such as "Do you have some words of wisdom to share about that valuable experience?"

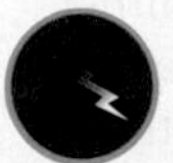

RISK FACTORS THAT AFFECT COGNITIVE WELLNESS

Cognitive function in people of all ages is affected by a multitude of internal and external conditions. It is especially important to identify risk factors that affect cognition in older adults because age-related changes increase their vulnerability to negative functional consequences. Nurses pay particular attention to identifying the risk factors that they can address through health promotion interventions.

Personal and Social Influences

Numerous personal characteristics affect cognitive abilities in people of any age, and researchers have tried to identify those that most significantly affect older adults. Years of formal education is the factor most consistently associated with cognitive performance in older adults, and this association is independent of race and sex and cultural, geographic, or other variables. Other personal characteristics that affect cognitive function include past and current socioeconomic status, the content of the educational material, mental stimulation in the workplace, or a combination of these factors (Cagney & Lauderdale, 2002; Turrell et al., 2002). Self-perceptions and expectations also significantly affect cognitive skills and performance on intelligence tests. Low self-efficacy (i.e., the belief in one's ability to perform at a given level) is associated with persistent emotional stress and poor cognitive performance (Ball & Birge, 2002).

Diversity Note

In developing countries such as China, socioeconomic disparities are a major variable contributing to higher prevalence of cognitive impairment in older women (Zhang, 2006).

Ageism and diminished expectations of older adults in modern societies can negatively affect cognitive function. Studies indicate that modern societies view memory decline as an inevitable and normal process; moreover, older adults internalize these negative beliefs, which then lead to self-doubts (Dark-Freudeman et al., 2006). These perceptions contribute to further decline in cognitive abilities; however, memory training can change false beliefs and improve performance (Hess, 2006).

Wellness Opportunity

Nurses assess their own attitudes about cognitive aging and identify the effects of myths and negative beliefs on their perceptions of older adults.

Sensory Function and Health Factors

All cognitive processes are affected when hearing or vision impairments limit the quantity and quality of information received from the environment. Although this holds true for all people, studies indicate that hearing and vision changes may account for most, if not all, of the variance in cognitive abilities in older adults (Hoyer & Verhaeghen, 2006). Because sensory input significantly influences learning, nurses need to ensure optimal visual and hearing conditions when teaching older adults. For example, studies indicate that background noise can interfere with listening comprehension even in older adults with apparently normal hearing (Thornton & Light, 2006).

Many chronic conditions and other aspects of physical health are correlated with cognitive abilities in older adults. Examples of chronic conditions associated with impaired cognitive function include the following (Backman et al., 2001):

- Thyroid disorders
- Diabetes and impaired glucose tolerance
- Dementia (e.g., Alzheimer's disease, vascular dementia)
- Cardiovascular disorders (e.g., stroke, hypertension, transient ischemic attacks)

Studies indicate that both physical and psychological stress, especially if prolonged, can suppress the development of new neurons (Cohen, 2005). Anxiety is consistently identified as a condition that impairs cognitive abilities by causing excessive worry and self-doubts. Depression and even subclinical variations in depressive symptoms are strongly associated with impaired cognitive function (especially memory), as discussed in Chapter 15 (Backman et al., 2001). Depression contributes to negative self-expectations and interferes with attention and concentration, which are two cognitive skills that significantly affect memory.

Researchers also are examining risk factors such as smoking and exposure to lead. One longitudinal study found that current smoking was associated with marked declines in memory skills in subjects who were 75 years of age and older (Reitz et al., 2005). Studies have found an association between occupational exposure to lead and progressive declines in cognitive function, even after an average of 16 years after the exposure ended (Stewart et al., 2006). A current question for research is whether environmental exposure to toxins such as solvents, mercury, pesticides, and cigarette smoke causes progressive and long-term damage that mimics the aging process (Rowland & McKinstry, 2006).

Nutritional and Chemical Factors

Nutritional status can affect cognitive function, particularly memory performance, regardless of a person's age. For example, low levels of beta-carotene, B vitamins, and vitamin C can negatively affect cognitive function. Even subclinical deficiencies of B vitamins can have a detrimental effect on memory (Backman et al., 2001; Calvaresi & Bryan, 2001). Studies have found that higher intake of vitamin E, in food or supplements, is associated with improved cognitive function in older adults (Morris, 2002; Ortega, 2002). Interest in the role of choline and lecithin stems from the theory that cognitive and memory deficits may be caused by a disruption of normal acetylcholine transmission in the brain. Although the consumption of foods rich in choline or lecithin can increase plasma choline levels, the effectiveness of these interventions on cognitive function has not been determined.

Much of the research on the relationship between alcohol consumption and cognitive function is not age specific, but conclusions can be applied to older adults as well as younger adults. For example, moderate consumption of alcohol is likely to interfere with short-term memory, but not with immediate or long-term memory, and long-term consumption of alcohol in excessive amounts is likely to interfere with memory performance, even during periods of abstention from alcohol.

Medication Effects

Prescription and over-the-counter medications can interfere with memory and other cognitive functions in a variety of ways. For example, anticholinergic ingredients, contained in numerous prescription and over-the-counter medications, significantly affect memory and other cognitive functions and are a common cause of changes in mental status in older adults. Older adults are particularly susceptible to development of adverse cognitive effects from the anticholinergic medications that cross the blood–brain barrier (e.g., atropine, benztropine, dicyclomine, flavoxate, and trihexyphenidyl). Because many medications have direct anticholinergic effects or increase the effects of anticholinergic medications, researchers and geriatric clinicians have paid particular attention in recent years to drug interactions and the cumulative effects of these medications on acetylcholine (a neurotransmitter that directly affects cognitive function) (Tune, 2001). The risk for medication-induced cognitive impairment from anticholinergic medications is greater in people who have dementia because they already experience a deficit of acetylcholine. Mechanisms of medication action that can interfere with cognitive function are described in detail in Chapter 8.

Wellness Opportunity

From a holistic perspective, nurses help older adults identify risk factors, such as nutrition, alcohol, and over-the-counter medications, that can be addressed through self-care actions.

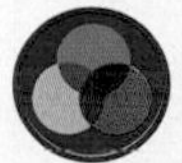

FUNCTIONAL CONSEQUENCES AFFECTING COGNITIVE FUNCTION

It is widely agreed that some cognitive decline occurs in later adulthood, with subtle, but noticeable, effects occurring after the age of 60 or 70 years. However, gerontologists emphasize that there is a great deal of individual variation in cognitive changes, with some older adults showing no decline and a small percentage even showing improvement in cognitive abilities. At any point in their life cycle, all adults have some cognitive abilities that are declining, some that are stable, and others that are improving (Thompson & Foth, 2005). In healthy, active, and mentally stimulated older adults, the deficits are generally minimal and do not interfere with daily functioning. Moreover, gerontologists have identified ways of improving cognitive abilities, as discussed in the section on Nursing Interventions.

The terms **benign senescent forgetfulness** or **age-associated memory impairment** refer to memory deficits that are thought to occur in older adults, even in the absence of any risk factors. These deficits are minor and nonprogressive, and they are most noticeable in stressful conditions. In actuality, they are not much different from the kind of forgetfulness that all people experience at times. A major difference, however, is that when these memory deficits occur in older people, they are likely to be viewed incorrectly as evidence of progressive cognitive decline.

Box 11-1 summarizes some of research-based conclusions about cognitive aging that are most relevant for identifying appropriate health education interventions. It is important to keep in mind that conclusions about cognitive aging do not address cultural factors, and therefore are limited by the factors cited in Cultural Considerations 11-1.

Wellness Opportunity

Nurses promote wellness by encouraging older adults to identify ways in which their cognitive abilities have improved.

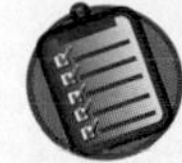

NURSING ASSESSMENT OF COGNITIVE FUNCTION

Formal assessment of intellectual performance involves administering psychometric tests, but nurses can informally assess memory and cognitive skills. In addition to assessing the intellectual performance of older adults, nurses can

Box 11-1
Functional Consequences Affecting Cognition in Older Adults

Cognitive Abilities in Healthy Older Adults

- Skills that stay the same or improve: wisdom, judgment, creativity, common sense, coordination of facts and ideas, and breadth of knowledge and experience
- Skills that decline slightly and gradually: abstraction, calculation, word fluency, verbal comprehension, spatial orientation, inductive reasoning, and short-term memory
- Word finding may be more difficult (i.e., "tip-of-the-tongue" experiences), but total vocabulary increases.
- Remote memory remains intact and holds a large store of information about the past.
- Factors that interfere with cognitive function: anxiety, depression, diminished sensory input, poor health, negative beliefs, ageist attitudes
- Factors that improve cognitive function: physical exercise, mental stimulation, challenging leisure activities, strong social networks, and activities that provide a sense of control and mastery

Learning Abilities

- Older adults are as capable of learning new things as younger people, but the speed with which they process information is slower.
- Older adults are more cautious in their responses and make more errors of omission.
- Potential barriers to learning in older adults include distractions, sensory deficits, lack of relevance, teacher–learner age differences, and values that are incongruent with new knowledge.

assess for risk factors that are likely to interfere with cognitive function. Because nursing assessment of cognition is an integral part of the psychosocial assessment, it is addressed comprehensively in Chapter 13, rather than in this chapter. Nursing assessment of impaired cognitive function is addressed in Chapter 14 (Delirium and Dementia).

NURSING DIAGNOSIS

Because age-related changes in cognitive function do not significantly affect healthy older adults, an applicable nursing diagnosis is Health-Seeking Behaviors. This diagnosis is defined as "the state in which an individual in stable health actively seeks ways to alter personal health habits and/or the environment in order to move toward a higher level of wellness" (Carpenito-Moyet, 2006, p. 208). Nurses can use this diagnosis for older adults who are aware of some decline in their intellectual abilities and who wish to preserve specific cognitive abilities, such as memory. Nursing diagnoses related to cognitive impairment associated with confusion or serious memory problems are discussed in Chapter 14.

Cultural Considerations 11-1

Cultural Factors and Cognitive Function

- It is important to recognize that the standards of intellectual performance used in the United States have been developed for English-speaking white Americans.
- It is important to recognize that cognitive abilities are highly influenced by health, education, and socioeconomic status and that these factors and cultural factors are interrelated.
- Cultural and language factors may influence an older adult's perception and description of memory problems.

Wellness Opportunity

Nurses can use the wellness nursing diagnosis of Readiness for Enhanced Knowledge for older adults who are motivated to improve their cognitive skills.

PLANNING FOR WELLNESS OUTCOMES

An outcome criterion for older adults with health-seeking behaviors related to cognitive function would be that the person takes responsibility for maintaining cognitive abilities or compensating for age-related cognitive changes. An indicator of achievement would be that the person participates in activities that address risk factors (e.g., participation in physically and mentally stimulating activities) or compensates for age-related changes (e.g., use of memory-enhancing techniques). Nurses can apply the following Nursing Outcomes Classification (NOC) terminology for outcomes related to cognitive wellness: Cognition, Concentration, Health Beliefs, Health-Seeking Behavior, Information Processing, Knowledge: Health Promotion, Leisure Participation, Hearing Compensation Behavior, and Vision Compensation Behavior.

Wellness Opportunity

Personal Well-Being is a wellness outcome that nurses can promote by supporting personal responsibility for actions that improve cognitive abilities.

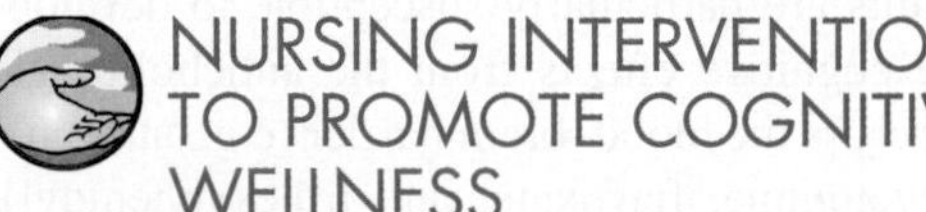

NURSING INTERVENTIONS TO PROMOTE COGNITIVE WELLNESS

Studies indicate that the following types of activities are effective for improving "brain fitness" in older adults (Cohen, 2005):

- Mental exercise: engaging in new learning experiences that are appealing and challenging
- Physical exercise: regular exercise, including aerobic
- Challenging leisure activities (listed in order of most to least effective): dancing, playing board games, playing a musical instrument, doing crossword puzzles, reading

- Activities in which there is a sense of control and mastery: learning computer skills, a new language, or how to play a musical instrument
- Strong social networks: maintaining social relationships with family and friends

Wellness Opportunity

Nurses promote personal responsibility for wellness by helping older adults identify ways of incorporating "brain fitness" activities into their daily lives.

Many of the health promotion interventions discussed throughout this text provide specific examples of these types of activities. For example, interventions for cardiovascular wellness (see Chapter 20) are particularly relevant to promoting optimal cognitive function. Also, because vision and hearing impairments can interfere with cognitive abilities, any interventions directed toward improving sensory function (discussed in Chapters 16 and 17) may also be effective in improving cognitive function.

Nurses can apply the following Nursing Interventions Classification (NIC) terminology for interventions related to cognitive wellness: Activity Therapy, Communication Enhancement: Hearing Deficit, Communication Enhancement: Visual Deficit, Exercise Promotion, Health Education, Learning Facilitation, Learning Readiness Enhancement, Meditation Facilitation, Progressive Muscle Relaxation, Role Enhancement, Self-Awareness Enhancement, Self-Responsibility Enhancement, and Teaching: Individual.

Encouraging Educational Opportunities

There is strong support for the idea that the educational process itself is a major underlying factor for maintenance of cognitive health in older adults. Since the mid-1960s, gerontologists have been studying **plasticity**, which refers to the ability of the brain to change physically in response to learning. Studies have found that learning links neurons in new patterns and stimulates the growth of new synapses (Cohen, 2005). Thus, nurses promote cognitive wellness by providing health education and encouraging older adults to participate in adult learning activities. In some settings, nurses can address health-related concerns of older adults through group health education programs, which have the additional benefit of providing social support. Nurses also can actively promote the use of computers by older adults for mental stimulation and practical benefits, such as increased communication with others and the acquisition of information that is relevant to their health and daily functioning. Hendrix and Sakauye (2001) have developed an excellent nursing model for teaching older adults about using computers.

Nurses also can help older adults identify educational opportunities in their local communities. For example, some universities and colleges (particularly community colleges) offer reduced-rate or no fee courses for students 60 years of age and older. Some programs also offer associate degrees, certification programs, or a General Equivalency Diploma (GED). The Institutes for Learning in Retirement (ILR) is a community-based organization for retirement-age learners that develops and implements educational programs in affiliation with a college or university. These sessions typically involve homework and usually are held for a few hours weekly for several months. Less formal education programs often are available through local senior centers and adult education programs affiliated with local school districts.

Some programs provide opportunities for travel and education. For example, Elderhostel is a national organization that provides numerous opportunities for individuals 55 years of age and older to become involved in educational and social action groups in the United States and worldwide. These educational activities involve short-term residential programs that usually last 4 to 5 days in the United States and 2 to 4 weeks in other countries (see the Educational Resources section for information about Elderhostel and ILR).

Wellness Opportunity

Nurses promote personal responsibility by helping older adults identify activities that address their unique learning needs based on their life experiences and current interests.

Teaching About Memory and Cognition

The concept of metacognition suggests that an understanding of one's own cognitive processes can influence performance. For example, someone who wants to remember a list of names needs both the intent to remember and knowledge about techniques for remembering. Because self-efficacy beliefs also affect one's ability to learn, health education needs to include all the following aspects:

- Correcting myths and misinformation
- Providing accurate information about age-related changes
- Communicating positive expectations
- Identifying goals for self-learning
- Providing information about techniques to enhance cognitive abilities.
- Identifying the techniques that are most effective for the individual

In community and long-term care settings, group sessions can effectively and efficiently address many psychosocial aspects of aging, including cognitive function. For example, the Healthy Aging Class (described in detail in Chapter 12) can be used as a model for health education about age-related cognitive changes. Nurses can use the model developed by Turner Geriatric Services at the University of Michigan for either single- or multiple-session programs for older adults. A training manual provides information about developing memory training programs, and it includes lesson plans and handouts for group leaders (Fogler & Stern, 1994). Box 11-2, which outlines a sample presentation for older adults based on the material from the Turner Geriatric Clinic,

Box 11-2
Memory Training for Older Adults

Introduction

- Forgetting is a normal part of life for all people, but memory skills can be learned. The purposes of this program are to look at some reasons people forget things and to discuss ways of improving memory skills.
- When older adults are forgetful, they may blame it on old age, rather than seeing it as something that happens to everyone, regardless of age.
- Memory problems can be viewed as a challenge. Anyone can improve his or her memory, but as with any other skill, an effort must be made.

Stages of Memory

- *Sensory memory* lasts only a few seconds. It involves the awareness of information obtained through vision, hearing, smell, taste, and touch.
- *Short-term memory* is your working memory, or what's in your conscious thoughts. This, too, is very brief and contains small amounts of information. For example, this type of memory allows you to recall a telephone number as you dial it.
- *Long-term memory* is the memory bank, or what you depend on whenever you need to retrieve information. This memory bank is almost limitless and contains information you just learned, as well as information from long ago.

Memory Changes and Aging

- Aging is blamed for a lot of memory problems, but very few changes occur solely because of aging.
- In older adulthood, the processes of learning new information and recalling old information slow down a little. The overall ability to learn and remember, however, is not significantly affected in healthy older people.

Factors That Interfere With Memory

As people grow older, an increasing number of factors may interfere with their ability to remember, including the following:

- Not being attentive to the situation. This might be attributable, for example, to the fact that the situation is not relevant to you.
- Being distracted by a lot of things that interfere with your ability to concentrate. For example, this might be the result of worry or anxiety.
- Feeling stressed
- Having a physical illness or being tired
- Having vision, hearing, or other functional impairments that interfere with the ability to obtain information
- Feeling sad or depressed, or coping with loss or grief
- Not being intellectually stimulated (principle of "use it or lose it!")
- Not having cues to help you remember
- Not organizing information for easy retention; not being organized in daily life
- Taking medications or alcohol that interfere with mental abilities
- Not being physically fit (e.g., as a result of poor nutrition or lack of exercise)

Ways of Improving Memory Skills

- Write things down (e.g., use lists, calendars, and notebooks).
- Use auditory cues (e.g., timers, alarm clocks) in conjunction with written cues.
- Use environmental cues. (For instance, you might remove something from its usual place, then return it to its normal location after it has served its purpose as a reminder.)
- Assign specific places for specific items and keep the items in their proper place (e.g., keep keys on a hook near the door).
- Put reminders in appropriate places (e.g., place shoes that need to be repaired near the door).
- Use visual images. ("A picture is worth a thousand words.") Create a picture in your mind when you want to remember something; the more bizarre the picture, the more likely it is that you will remember.
- Use active observation: pay attention to details of what's going on around you and be alert to the environment.
- Make associations, or mental connections. (For example, the phrase "spring ahead, fall back" can be recalled to ensure accuracy in changing clocks for seasonal time changes [from daylight savings time to standard time and vice versa].)
- Make associations between names and mental images (e.g., Carol and Christmas carol).
- Rehearse items you want to remember by repeating them aloud or writing the information on paper.
- Use self-instruction; say things aloud (e.g., "I'm putting my keys on the counter so I remember to turn off the stove before I leave").
- Divide information into small parts that can be remembered easily. (For instance, to remember an address or a zip code, divide it into groups [seven hundred sixty, fifty-five].)
- Organize information into logical categories (e.g., shampoo and hair spray, toothpaste and mouthwash, soap and deodorant).
- Use rhyming cues (e.g., "In 1492, Columbus sailed the ocean blue.").
- Use first-letter cues and make associations. (For example, to remember to buy carrots, apples, radishes, pickles, eggs, and tea bags, remember the word CARPET.)
- Make word associations. (For instance, to remember the letters of your license plate, make a word, such as camel, out of the letters CML.)
- Search the alphabet while focusing on what you're trying to remember. (For example, to remember that someone's name is Martin, start with names that begin with A and continue naming names through the alphabet until your memory is jogged for the correct one.)
- Make up a story to connect things you want to remember. (For instance, if you have to go to the cleaners and the post office, create a story about mailing a pair of pants.)

(Continued on following page)

Box 11-2
Memory Training for Older Adults (continued)

Conclusion

- Don't try to remember all of these techniques—you'll need another method just to remember them all!
- Select a few techniques that you like, and use these whenever appropriate or needed.
- Minimize any distractions; pay attention to one thing at a time.
- Give yourself time to remember; forgetfulness is most likely to occur when you are in a hurry. Try to prepare in advance, when you have time to concentrate.
- Maintain some sense of organization in your daily life, and devise systems to organize routine tasks, like taking medications.
- Carry a note pad or calendar, and use written records so you don't have to rely entirely on mental cues.
- Relax and maintain a sense of humor. If you become anxious about your memory and are convinced you can't remember, then you will create a self-fulfilling prophecy.

(Adapted, with permission, from Fogler, J., & Stern, L. [1994]. *Improving your memory: How to remember what you're starting to forget.* Baltimore: Johns Hopkins University Press.)

can be used to educate older adults about techniques for memory enhancement. Examples of additional models for group educational programs to enhance cognitive abilities in older adults can be found in gerontological journals (e.g., Rapp et al., 2002; Weinstein & Sachs, 2000; Werner, 2000).

Wellness Opportunity

Nurses holistically address learning needs of older adults by encouraging participation in group programs, which have the additional benefit of offering social support.

Improving Concentration and Attention

When one's ability to attend to the environment and concentrate on visual and auditory cues is limited, the ability to learn and remember is also impaired. Thus, techniques such as relaxation, imagery, and meditation, which enhance attention and concentration, may also improve memory and learning. Likewise, any method that reduces environmental distractions may also improve one's cognitive abilities. Mindfulness, defined as a focused awareness of the environment and one's reactions to it, is a self-care practice that can improve cognitive function (Aldwin et al., 2006). Many self-help books describe techniques for meditation, mindfulness, and relaxation as ways of opening the mind to new learning. Nurses can teach the relaxation technique outlined in Chapter 24 to older adults for a variety of uses, including the enhancement of mental skills. Nurses also promote personal responsibility for cognitive wellness by encouraging older adults to identify self-care practices that improve attention.

Adapting Health Education Materials

Much of the research on cognitive aging has centered on factors that affect learning in older adulthood. For example, researchers have found that visual, rather than auditory, presentation of educational materials results in better recall, learning, and retrieval of information (Constantinidou, 2002). Because many nursing interventions include patient teaching or health education, information about cognitive aging can be used to adapt educational methods and materials to older adults. For example, nurses facilitate learning by emphasizing individualized health-related benefits because older adults remember information better when it is relevant and has practical application (Meyer & Pollard, 2006). The suggestions presented in this text for communicating with older adults and compensating for hearing and vision deficit (see Chapters 13, 16, and 17) can be applied to health education. Nurses can apply the guidelines in Box 11-3 to educational interventions for older adults. Examples of models of educational materials that have been adapted to meet the unique learning styles of older adults can be found in the

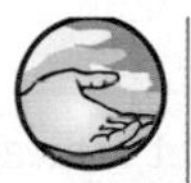

Box 11-3
Guidelines for Health Education for Older Adults

Conditions That Promote Learning

- Supportive and rewarding contexts (e.g., praise and positive feedback) in contrast to those that are neutral, challenging, or critical
- Environment that is pleasant, familiar, brightly lit, with little or no background noise and as few distractions as possible
- Personally relevant information that builds on prior experiences
- Information that is concrete rather than abstract
- Shorter, more frequent sessions

Presentation Methods Most Conducive to Learning

- Self-paced rate that allows time for assimilation
- Presentation of one idea at a time
- Emphasis on integration and application of knowledge and experience, rather than on acquisition of irrelevant information
- Visual methods for material that lends itself to thoughtful analysis
- Auditory methods, alone or with visual methods, for information that is factual
- Advance organizers, such as outlines, overviews, and written cues
- Reinforcement of the value of using organizing aids

nursing and gerontology literature (e.g., Conn et al., 2001; Rankin et al., 2005; Van Wynen, 2001).

Adaptations of health education materials may also be necessary to ensure they are culturally appropriate. Many teaching materials are available in languages other than English. For instance, many of the federal government sites listed in the Educational Resources section of Chapter 5 and other chapters provide health education materials in Spanish. Because there is growing emphasis on addressing needs of culturally diverse populations, nurses periodically need to check the resources and inquire about the availability of teaching materials for specific groups. Nurses can contact organizations, local hospitals, home care agencies, and long-term care facilities or check Internet sources to inquire about health education materials available to address learning needs of culturally diverse populations in their service area. For example, organizations and state governments have developed advance directive forms and teaching tools that address learning needs of specific cultural groups, as discussed in Chapter 9. Chapter 4 of this text further addresses the topic of culturally sensitive health education.

EVALUATING EFFECTIVENESS OF NURSING INTERVENTIONS

Nursing care of older adults who want to maintain high levels of cognitive function is evaluated by the degree to which these adults express satisfaction with their cognitive abilities, such as memory skills. Objectively, it is evaluated by the degree to which they use their cognitive abilities to meet their daily needs. For example, an older adult who forgets to keep appointments might learn to use a calendar or other organizational aids to remember the appointments. In this situation, the effectiveness of interventions would be measured by how well the person remembers to keep appointments. Subjectively, it is evaluated by the degree to which older adults express positive perceptions of their cognitive abilities and satisfaction with interventions, including self-care actions.

Mrs. C. is 71 years old and lives alone in her own home. She attends a local Senior Wellness clinic for blood pressure checks, health screenings (e.g., cholesterol levels), and her annual flu shot. During her monthly visit for a blood pressure check, she confides that she is embarrassed about missing a doctor's appointment last week. She says she has been noticing increased difficulties with memory, and one of her friends has told her that she probably has Alzheimer's disease. She asks if there's a place where she can get a test for Alzheimer's.

NURSING ASSESSMENT

Your nursing assessment indicates that Mrs. C. has missed a couple of health care appointments during the past year. She said she missed a dental appointment 6 months ago when she was very worried about her daughter, who was undergoing diagnostic tests for a lump in her breast. Last week, when she missed her doctor's appointment, she had been busy shopping for presents for her grandson's wedding. When you ask about additional problems with memory, Mrs. C. admits that she has more difficulty remembering people's names than she used to have. You do not identify any risk factors that might affect Mrs. C.'s cognitive abilities (e.g., depression, medication effects, poor nutrition). Mrs. C. has never used calendars, and she says she remembers her doctor's appointments by keeping the appointment cards in her desk drawer along with her bills and her checkbook. She says that she checks her appointment cards every month, but she had not noticed the cards for the two appointments she missed.

NURSING DIAGNOSIS

You use the nursing diagnosis of Health-Seeking Behaviors because Mrs. C. is interested in learning about memory training skills to assist her in remembering appointments. Mrs. C. has a poor understanding of age-related cognitive changes, and she indicates that she is interested in learning about ways to improve her memory.

(case study continues on page 197)

NURSING CARE PLAN FOR MRS. C.

Expected Outcome	Nursing Interventions	Nursing Evaluation
Mrs. C. will express an interest in improving her memory skills.	• Use information in Box 11-1 to teach Mrs. C. about age-related changes that affect cognitive abilities. • Discuss the difference between dementia and age-associated memory impairment. • Emphasize that memory skills can be developed through memory training techniques.	Mrs. C. will agree to participate in a discussion of memory training skills.
Mrs. C. will use memory training techniques to improve her functional level.	• Give Mrs. C. a copy of Box 11-2 and review the information. • Assist Mrs. C. in identifying one or two strategies for remembering appointments (e.g., begin using a calendar). • Assist Mrs. C. in identifying one or two strategies for remembering the names of people she meets (e.g., using visual images).	Mrs. C. will report success in using a method for remembering appointments. Mrs. C. will report success in using a method for remembering names of people.

THINKING POINTS

- What factors are likely to be contributing to Mrs. C.'s forgetting about her appointments?
- What is the most effective way of using information in Boxes 11-1 and 11-2 to facilitate learning for Mrs. C?
- What additional interventions would you suggest for Mrs. C?

Chapter Highlights

Age-Related Changes That Affect Cognition

- Central nervous system: degenerative changes in brain, slower reaction time
- Fluid intelligence (inductive reasoning, abstract thinking) declines, but crystallized intelligence (wisdom and judgment) improves
- Some memory functions decline (short-term and effortful processes), but some memory functions (long-term and automatic) remain the same
- Stage theories of adult psychological development describe phases of mature aging

Risks Factors That Affect Cognitive Wellness

- Personal and social influences: personality, socioeconomic factors, ageism
- Diminished hearing and vision
- Chronic conditions: dementia, diabetes, thyroid and cardiovascular disorders
- Nutrition, alcohol, and medications

Functional Consequences Associated With Cognitive Function (Box 11-1)

- Minor and nonprogressive declines in cognitive abilities (benign senescent forgetfulness)
- Any major or progressive declines are due to pathologic processes (e.g., dementia)
- Cultural factors and cognitive function (Cultural Considerations 11-1)

Nursing Assessment of Cognitive Function

- Refer to Chapter 13

Nursing Diagnosis

- Readiness for Enhanced Knowledge
- Health-Seeking Behaviors

Planning for Wellness Outcomes

- Cognition
- Concentration
- Health Beliefs
- Health-Seeking Behavior
- Information Processing
- Knowledge: Health Promotion
- Leisure Participation

Nursing Interventions to Promote Cognitive Wellness

- Activities to promote "brain fitness": mental exercise, physical exercise, challenging leisure activities, strong social networks, activities that foster a sense of control and mastery
- Encouraging educational opportunities (e.g., computers, classes, travel)

- Teaching about memory and cognition for individuals and groups (Box 11-2)
- Improving concentration and attention (mindfulness, imagery, relaxation)
- Adapting health education materials (Box 11-3)

Evaluating Effectiveness of Nursing Interventions

- Expresses satisfaction with improved cognitive abilities
- Able to use cognitive skills in daily activities

Critical Thinking Exercises

1. Identify the factors in your own life that interfere with cognitive function.
2. What memory aids do you use in your life? Are they effective? Would you like to develop additional memory aids?
3. You are working in a senior center and have suggested that the center sponsor a series of classes on the memory problems of older adults. This suggestion is based on your observation that many of the older adults have asked you questions about memory problems, and some are concerned about Alzheimer's disease. Address each of the following issues:
   - The center director is a firm believer in the adage, "You can't teach an old dog new tricks." How would you convince the director that the classes you wish to offer are worthwhile?
   - How would you structure the sessions (number and length of sessions, number of participants, and so forth)?
   - Describe the content you would cover and the approach you would use for each topic. Include information about normal cognitive aging, risk factors for impaired cognitive function, and techniques for improving memory and other aspects of cognition.
   - What audiovisual aids, including written materials, would you use?
   - How would you adapt your teaching method and materials for the group?
   - How would you evaluate the sessions?

Educational Resources

Elderhostel, Institute for Learning in Retirement
www.elderhostel.org

Turner Geriatric Clinic
Publications include *Improving Your Memory: How to Remember What You're Starting to Forget* and *Teaching Memory Improvement to Adults.*
www.med.umich.edu

References

Albert, M. S., & Killiany, R. J. (2001). Age-related cognitive change and brain-behavior relationships. In J. E. Birren & K. W. Schaie (Eds.), *Handbook of the psychology of aging* (5th ed., pp. 161–185). San Diego: Academic Press.

Aldwin, C. M., Spiro, A., & Park. C. L. (2006). Health, behavior, and optimal aging: A life span development perspective. In J. E. Birren & K. W. Schaie (Eds.), *Handbook of the psychology of aging* (6th ed., pp. 85–104). San Diego: Academic Press.

Backman, L., Small, B. J., & Wahlin, A. (2001). Aging and memory: Cognitive and biological perspectives. In J. E. Birren & K. W. Schaie (Eds.), *Handbook of the psychology of aging* (5th ed., pp. 349–377). San Diego: Academic Press.

Ball, L. J., & Birge, S. J. (2002). Prevention of brain aging and dementia. *Clinics in Geriatric Medicine, 18*, 485–504.

Bennett, D. A., Schneider, J. A., & Arvanitakis, Z. (2006). Neuropathology of older persons without cognitive impairment from two community-based studies. *Neurology, 66*, 1837–1844.

Botwinick, J. (1984). *Aging and behavior* (3rd ed.). New York: Springer.

Brugman, G. M. (2006). Wisdom and aging. In J. E. Birren & K. W. Schaie (Eds.), *Handbook of the psychology of aging* (6th ed., pp. 445–476.). San Diego: Academic Press.

Carpenito-Moyet, L. J. (2006). *Handbook of nursing diagnosis* (11th ed.). Philadelphia: Lippincott Williams & Wilkins.

Cagney, K. A., & Lauderdale, D. S. (2002). Education, wealth, and cognitive function in later life. *Journals of Gerontology: Series B, Psychological Sciences and Social Sciences, 57*, P163–P172.

Calvaresi, E., & Bryan, J. (2001). B vitamins, cognition, and aging: A review. *Journals of Gerontology: Series B, Psychological Sciences and Social Sciences, 56*, P327–P339.

Carstensen, L. L., Mikels, J. A., & Mather, M. (2006). Aging and the intersection of cognition, motivation, and emotion. In J. E. Birren & K. W. Schaie (Eds.), *Handbook of the psychology of aging* (6th ed., pp. 343–362). San Diego: Academic Press.

Cohen, G. D. (2005). *The mature mind: The positive power of the aging brain.* New York: Basic Books.

Conn, V. S., Armer, J. M., & Hayes, K. S. (2001). Knowledge deficit. In M. L. Maas, K. C. Buckwalter, M. D. Hardy, T. Tripp-Reimer, M. G. Titler, & J. P. Specht (Eds.), *Nursing care of older adults: Diagnoses, outcomes, and interventions* (pp. 503–515). St. Louis: Mosby.

Constantinidou, F. (2002). Stimulus modality and verbal learning performance in normal aging. *Brain and Language, 82*, 296–311.

Dark-Freudeman, A., West, R. L., & Viverito, K. M. (2006). Future selves and aging: Older adults' memory fears. *Educational Gerontology, 32*, 85–109.

Deary, I. J., Bastin, M. E., Pattie, A., Clayden, J. D., Whalley, L. J., Starr, J. M., et al. (2006). White matter integrity and cognition in childhood and old age. *Neurology, 66*, 505–512.

DeFries, C. M., Dixon, R. A., & Backman, L. (2003). Use of memory compensation strategies is related to psychosocial and health indicators. *Journals of Gerontology: Series B, Psychological Sciences and Social Sciences, 58*, P12–P22.

Fogler, J., & Stern, L. (1994). *Teaching memory improvement to adults* (rev. ed.). Baltimore: Johns Hopkins University Press.

Hartley, A. (2006). Changing role of the speed of processing construct in the cognitive psychology of human aging. In J. E. Birren & K. W. Schaie (Eds.), *Handbook of the psychology of aging* (6th ed., pp. 183–207). San Diego: Academic Press.

Hasher, L., & Zacks, R. T. (1979). Autonomic and effortful processes in memory. *Journal of Experimental Psychology: General, 108*, 356–388.

Hedden, T., & Gabrieli, J. D. E. (2005). Healthy and pathological processes in adult development: New evidence from neuroimaging of the aging brain. *Current Opinion in Neurology, 18*, 740–747.

Hendrix, C. C., & Sakauye, K. M. (2001). Teaching elderly individuals on computer use. *Journal of Gerontological Nursing, 27*(6), 47–53.

Hess, T. M. (2006). Attitudes toward aging and their effects on behavior. In J. E. Birren & K. W. Schaie (Eds.), *Handbook of the psychology of aging* (6th ed., pp. 379–406). San Diego: Academic Press.

Hofer, S. M., & Sliwinski, M. J. (2006). Design and analysis of longitudinal studies on aging. In J. E. Birren & K. W. Schaie (Eds.), *Handbook of the psychology of aging* (6th ed., pp. 17–37). San Diego: Academic Press.

Horn, J. L., & Hofer, S. M. (1992). Major abilities and development in the adult period. In R. J. Sternberg & C. A. Berg (Eds.), *Intellectual development* (pp. 44–99). New York: Cambridge University Press.

Hoyer, W. J., & Verhaeghen, P. (2006). Memory aging. In J. E. Birren & K. W. Schaie (Eds.), *Handbook of the psychology of aging* (6th ed., pp. 209–232). San Diego: Academic Press.

Kramer, A. F., Fabiani, M., & Colcombe, S. J. (2006). Contributions of cognitive neuroscience to the understanding of behavior and aging. In J. E. Birren & K. W. Schaie (Eds.), *Handbook of the psychology of aging* (6th ed., pp. 57–83). San Diego: Academic Press.

Labouvie-Vief, G., & Blanchard-Fields, F. (1982). Cognitive aging and psychological growth. *Ageing and Society, 2*, 183–209.

Mariske, M., & Margrett, J. A. (2006). Everyday problem solving and decision making. In J. E. Birren & K. W. Schaie (Eds.), *Handbook of the psychology of aging* (6th ed., pp. 315–342). San Diego: Academic Press.

Meyer, B. J. F., & Pollard, C. K. (2006). Applied learning and aging: A closer look at reading. In J. E. Birren & K. W. Schaie (Eds.), *Handbook of the psychology of aging* (6th ed., pp. 233–260). San Diego: Academic Press.

Morris, M. C. (2002). Vitamin E and cognitive decline in older persons. *Archives of Neurology, 59*, 1125–1132.

Ortega, R. M. (2002). Cognitive function in elderly people is influenced by vitamin E status. *Journal of Nutrition, 132*, 2065–2068.

Rankin S. H., Stallings, K. D., & London, F. (2005). *Patient education in health and illness* (5th ed.). Philadelphia: Lippincott Williams & Wilkins.

Rapp, S., Brenes, G., & Marsh, A. P. (2002). Memory enhancement training for older adults with mild cognitive impairment: A preliminary study. *Aging and Mental Health, 6*(1), 5–11.

Reitz, C., Luchsinger, J., Tang, M-X., & Mayeux, R. (2005). Effect of smoking and time on cognitive function in the elderly without dementia. *Neurology, 65*, 870–875.

Rowland, A., S., & McKinstry, R. C. (2006). Lead toxicity, white matter lesions, and aging. *Neurology, 66*, 1464–1466.

Saykin, A. J., Wishart, H. A., Rabin, L. A., Santulli, R. B., Flashman, L. A., West, J. D., et al. (2006). Older adults with cognitive complaints show brain atrophy similar to that of amnestic MCI. *Neurology, 67*, 834–842.

Schaie, K. W. (1977-1978). Toward a stage theory of adult cognitive development. *Journal of Aging and Human Development, 8*, 129–138.

Simensky, J. D., & Abeles, N. (2002). Decline in verbal memory performance with advancing age: The role of frontal lobe functioning. *Aging and Mental Health, 6*, 293–303.

Stewart, W. F., Schwartz, B. S., Davatzikos, C., Shen, D., Liu, D., Wu, X., et al. (2006). Past adult lead exposure is linked to neurodegeneration measured by brain MRI. *Neurology, 66*, 1476–1484.

Thompson, G., & Foth, D. (2005). Cognitive-training programs for older adults: What are they and can they enhance mental fitness? *Educational Gerontology, 31*, 603–626.

Thornton, R., & Light, L. L. (2006). Language comprehension and production in normal aging. In J. E. Birren & K. W. Schaie (Eds.), *Handbook of the psychology of aging* (6th ed., pp. 262–287). San Diego: Academic Press.

Tune, L. E. (2001). Anticholinergic effects of medication in elderly patients. *Journal of Clinical Psychiatry, 62*(Suppl. 21), 11–14.

Turrell, G., Lynch, J. W., Kaplan, G. A., Everson, S. A., Helkala, E-L., Kauhanen, J., et al. (2002). Socioeconomic position across the lifecourse and cognitive function in late middle age. *Journals of Gerontology: Series B, Psychological Sciences and Social Sciences, 57*, S43–S51.

Van Wynen, E. A. (2001). A key to successful aging: Learning-style patterns of older adults. *Journal of Gerontological Nursing, 27*(9), 6–15.

Vinters, H. V. (2001). Aging and the human nervous system. In J. E. Birren & K. W. Schaie (Eds.), *Handbook of the psychology of aging* (5th ed., pp. 135–160). San Diego: Academic Press.

Weinstein, C. S., & Sachs, W. (2000). Memory 101: A psychotherapist's guide to understanding and teaching memory strategies to patients and significant others. *Journal of Geriatric Psychiatry: A Multidisciplinary Journal of Mental Health and Aging, 33*(1), 5–26.

Werner, P. (2000). Assessing the effectiveness of a memory club for elderly persons suffering from mild cognitive deterioration. *Clinical Gerontologist, 22*(1), 3–14.

Zhang, Z. (2006). Gender differentials in cognitive impairment and decline of the oldest old in China. *Journals of Gerontology: Series B, Psychological Sciences and Social Sciences, 61*, S107–S115.

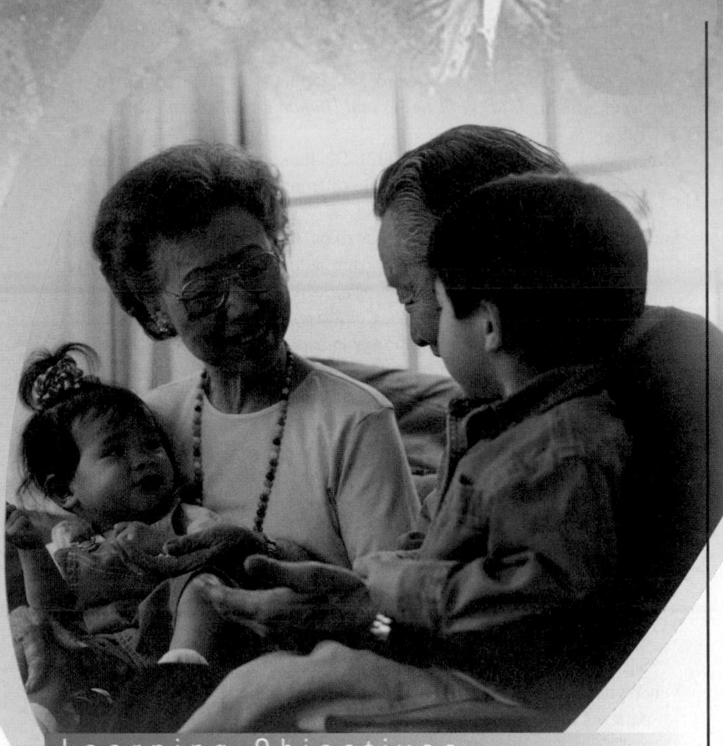

CHAPTER 12

Psychosocial Function

Learning Objectives

After reading this chapter, you will be able to:

1. Identify the life events that commonly occur in older adulthood.
2. Discuss theories related to stress and coping as they apply to older adults.
3. Identify the risk factors and cultural factors that influence psychosocial function in older adults.
4. Describe the functional consequences associated with psychosocial function in older adults.
5. Identify nursing interventions that promote psychosocial wellness in older adults.
6. Describe how to teach a Healthy Aging Class for a small group of older adults.

Key Terms

culture-bound syndrome
elderspeak
infantilization
learned helplessness
life events
self-esteem
stress
stressors
transfer trauma
transplantation shock

Although the physiologic changes and chronic illnesses associated with older adulthood may affect a person's functional abilities, the psychosocial changes are often the most challenging and demanding in terms of coping energy. Of course, some of the psychosocial challenges arise from physical changes, but many are attributable to changes in roles, relationships, and living environments. Because many of the psychosocial changes are inevitable and somewhat predictable, older adults can prepare for and respond to psychosocial changes by developing and using effective coping strategies. By focusing on functional consequences related to psychosocial function for the older adult, nurses can promote psychosocial wellness by supporting effective coping mechanisms and assisting in the development of new coping strategies.

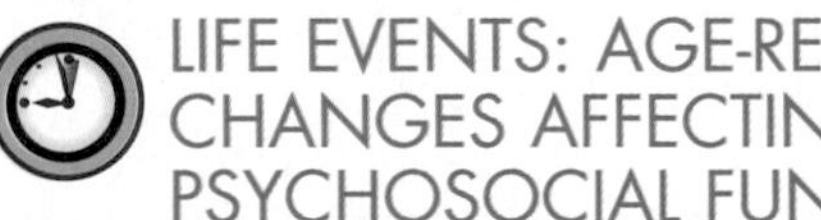

LIFE EVENTS: AGE-RELATED CHANGES AFFECTING PSYCHOSOCIAL FUNCTION

Life events are the major changes that occur at various times during the life cycle and significantly affect daily life, with certain ones commonly associated with different periods in one's life. For example, younger adults are likely to experience the following life events: establishing a career, moving away from the nuclear family, committing to a partner, buying a house, and beginning a family. The major life events of younger adulthood are familiar to us through either personal experiences or the shared experiences of friends. People usually view these events as positive gains and choose them purposefully. By contrast, life events of older adulthood might be unknown, unexpected, inevitable, and, in fact, unwanted or even feared. In addition, life events during older adulthood are likely to involve losses of significant others and objects that have been part of life for many decades. Moreover, they tend to occur close together, with less time available to adjust to each event, and they often evolve into chronic stresses. Life events that commonly occur during older adulthood are associated with the following experiences (Settersten, 2006):

- Losses in physical and cognitive capacities and an increased likelihood of having poor health and chronic conditions
- Shorter time horizon and concomitant need to come to terms with one's mortality
- Focus on achieving integrity and finding meaning in life
- Bereavement associated with death of parents, spouse, and friends
- More restricted but intense social networks and relationships
- Dealing with ageist attitudes and behaviors of others
- Greater acceptance of things that cannot be controlled, along with greater fear of losing control over one's life

Life events that are most likely to occur during older adulthood include retirement, relocation, chronic illness and functional impairments, decisions about driving a car, widowhood, death of friends and family, and confrontation of ageist attitudes. Figure 12-1 illustrates some of the major life events that are likely to occur in older adulthood, as well as

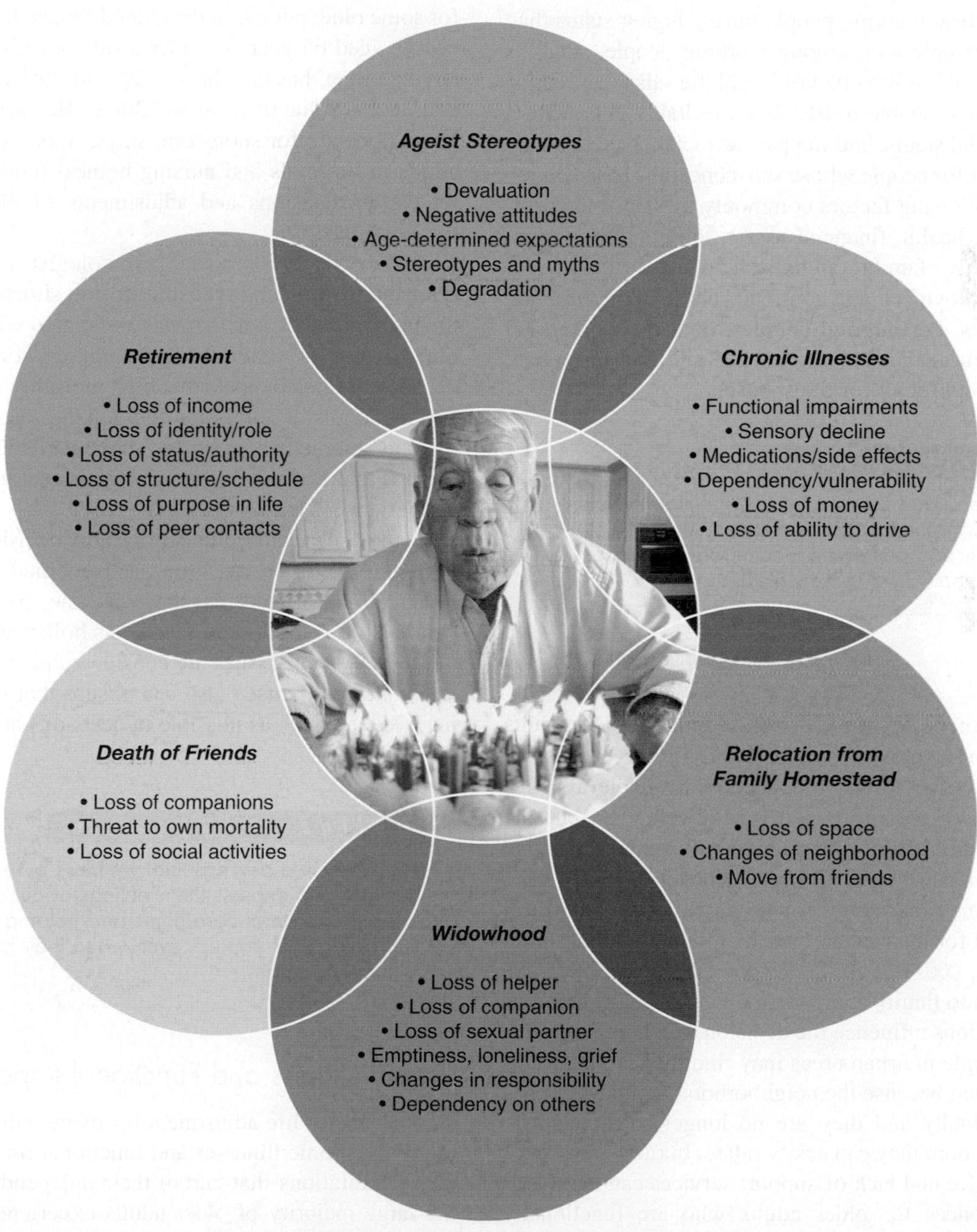
Ageist Stereotypes
• Devaluation
• Negative attitudes
• Age-determined expectations
• Stereotypes and myths
• Degradation
Retirement
• Loss of income
• Loss of identity/role
• Loss of status/authority
• Loss of structure/schedule
• Loss of purpose in life
• Loss of peer contacts
Chronic Illnesses
• Functional impairments
• Sensory decline
• Medications/side effects
• Dependency/vulnerability
• Loss of money
• Loss of ability to drive
Death of Friends
• Loss of companions
• Threat to own mortality
• Loss of social activities
Relocation from Family Homestead
• Loss of space
• Changes of neighborhood
• Move from friends
Widowhood
• Loss of helper
• Loss of companion
• Loss of sexual partner
• Emptiness, loneliness, grief
• Changes in responsibility
• Dependency on others

FIGURE 12-1 Psychosocial challenges of older adulthood.

the related consequences. The illustration attempts to show the interrelatedness among the life events of older adulthood.

Wellness Opportunity

Nurses promote wellness by asking older adults to talk about the meaning of life events that they have experienced.

Retirement

Retirement from a primary career is a milestone that marks the passage into later stages of adulthood (Kim & Moen, 2002). Societal attitudes can influence one's adjustment to retirement, particularly in societies with a strong work ethic. In these societies, working people have a higher status than unemployed people and, among working people, status is based on the kind of job one holds and the salary one earns. Therefore, when people retire, they inevitably cope with a change in social status, and the psychosocial challenge may be the greatest for people whose self-concept is based on job status. The following factors commonly influence the decision to retire: health, financial assets, job conditions, pension availability, family circumstances, opportunities for continued employment, and continued ability to perform job responsibilities. For married couples, both the worker and the spouse must adjust to retirement, and the adjustment might be more difficult for the spouse.

Diversity Note

When women retire they have higher initial levels of depressive symptoms and lower levels of morale, personal control, and perceived income adequacy compared with men (Kim & Moen, 2002).

Relocation

Another common psychosocial adjustment for older adults is the decision to move from the family home because of factors such as loss of spouse, lack of available assistive services, lack of a kinship network or caregiver, chronic conditions and declining functional abilities, and cognitive impairment or psychiatric illness. Relocation occurs more often for women than men, for urban residents than rural residents, and for married couples than widows (Johnson & Tripp-Reimer, 2001).

In addition to family and personal factors, many environmental conditions influence the decision to move. For example, older people in urban areas may find they are unsafe or socially isolated because the neighborhood around them has changed gradually and they are no longer surrounded by people with whom they can easily relate. In rural areas, geographic distance and lack of support services can have serious consequences for older adults who are functionally impaired, especially if they have few social supports. Problems also arise for older homeowners who find it more difficult to physically and financially maintain the house and pay for utilities.

Gerontologists have identified three types of moves that commonly occur during older adulthood (Longino & Bradley, 2006):

- "Amenity-driven moves," involving a voluntary move to a desirable geographic location shortly after retirement
- "Assistance moves" to be close to family members and medical care because of moderate disability and compounded by widowhood
- Institutional moves due to health problems that are too great to be met in the community

Relocation to a nursing home is a significant life event for some older adults. In the United States, fewer than 5% of people aged 65 years or older reside in nursing facilities at any one time, but they have a 39% to 49% chance of being admitted at some time (Stone, 2006). Because most of these admissions are for short-term stays, nurses caring for older adults in hospitals and nursing homes frequently deal with relocation decisions and adjustments of older adults and their families.

In the early 1960s, social gerontologists coined the terms **transfer trauma** and **transplantation shock** in reference to the high mortality rate that was associated with relocation to nursing homes (Aldrich & Mendkoff, 1963). In recent decades, studies indicate that high mortality rates within the first 6 months of admission to a nursing facility are related to many interacting health and social variables, such as willingness to move and degree of involvement in decision making (Tracy & DeYoung, 2004).

In the American health care system, decisions about long-term care are often based on a narrow medical perspective, rather than a broader psychosocial one. Nurses are in key positions to address these decisions holistically by ensuring that psychosocial issues are considered along with the medical concerns. Nurses also can ensure that older adults are involved as much as possible in decisions about this important life event.

Wellness Opportunity

Nurses promote psychosocial wellness by encouraging older adults to express their feelings about decisions related to long-term care plans and helping them identify effective ways of coping, even when they are not happy about the decision.

Chronic Illness and Functional Impairments

Another major life adjustment for many older adults is coping with chronic illnesses and functional limitations, particularly limitations that curtail their independence. Although the large majority of older adults experience one or more chronic conditions that affect their daily functioning, 80% to

90% of people aged 65 to 75 years and 60% of those aged 85 years and older perceive themselves as healthy (Østbye et al., 2006). Most functional limitations necessitate only minor adjustments in daily living, but some functional consequences, such as considerable cognitive, mobility, or visual impairments, significantly increase one's dependency on others. Other consequences of chronic illnesses include

- Threats to self-esteem and altered self-concept
- Changes in lifestyle
- Unpredictability about one's ability to do what one wants
- Expenditures for assistance, medications, and medical care
- Frequent trips to health care providers
- Adverse medication effects, which sometimes cause further functional impairments
- Increased vulnerability to personal crimes and fear of crime

Decisions About Driving a Car

Decisions about driving a car represent one of the most emotionally charged issues relating to functional impairment that older adults, their families, and health care professionals face. In the United States, access to an automobile and the possession of a valid driver's license not only provide transportation but also serve as significant indicators of autonomy. In fact, for many older adults, the ability to drive is synonymous with independence, and the possession of a driver's license, even one that goes unused, is a symbol of one's ability to shield oneself from dependence on others.

The loss of an independent means of transportation affects every aspect of an older person's life, from the acquisition of food and medicine to opportunities for social interaction. Because of this far-reaching impact, families and older persons may avoid dealing with driving-related issues. Family members may be reluctant to suggest that an older relative give up driving for a number of reasons. For example, family members may not want to assume an authority role, or they may lack acceptable alternatives for transportation. It is not surprising, then, that older adults and their families may avoid or resist the decision to stop driving. Neither is it surprising that when older adults give up or significantly curtail their driving, they face a difficult psychosocial challenge that may be viewed as a major life event.

Widowhood

The example of widowhood as a life event of older adulthood illustrates all of the characteristics listed earlier. For most older couples, widowhood is inevitable, and the chances are greater that the woman will be widowed rather than the man. When widowhood occurs, additional consequences follow. Common additional consequences include

- Loss of companionship and intimacy
- Loss of one's sexual partner
- Feelings of grief, loneliness, and emptiness
- Increased responsibilities
- Increased dependency on others
- Loss of income and less efficient financial management
- Changes in relationships with children, married friends, and other family members

When a marriage has lasted for many decades, as is common in people who are in their seventies and eighties, the impact of the loss can be tremendous, and the feelings of grief, loneliness, and emptiness may be overwhelming. Despite the major impact of widowhood, however, some studies have found that spousal bereavement is associated with higher risk of mortality among middle-aged, but not older, adults (Aldwin et al., 2006). Another study found that older women experienced a negative impact on health and well-being soon after the loss of their spouse, but that this was followed by a shift into a new and positive life phase of learning to live alone (Young & Cochrane, 2004).

Another characteristic of widowhood in older adulthood is that the chance of remarriage diminishes with advancing age, especially for women. Thus, there is little potential for resuming the married lifestyle. Last, if the married couple had clearly divided roles, as is common in the cohort of people who are old today, loss of the partner means an adjustment in important day-to-day tasks. For example, older couples often divide tasks so that only one of the two manages money, drives the car, cleans the house, shops for groceries, and does household repairs and maintenance. When the person responsible for a task no longer performs the role, the other person may be unable, unwilling, or unprepared to assume this role.

Wellness Opportunity

When applicable, nurses encourage older adults to talk about their experience of widowhood by opening the conversation with a question such as, "How is your life different since your husband passed away?"

Death of Friends and Family

Like other life events of older adulthood, the loss of friends and family becomes inevitable with each advancing year. Many people who are in their nineties have outlived most, if not all, of their friends and many of their relatives. Indeed, people who are in their nineties may not even know anyone who is older than they are. Moreover, as people are confronted with the death of others who are younger than or similar to them in age, they become increasingly aware of their own mortality. Older people may read obituaries and death notices in the newspaper as a daily activity. Although families may view this activity as a morbid preoccupation, it may, in fact, be an effective way for older people to learn what is happening to their friends. Because meaningful social relationships are an important predictor of well-being for older adults, loss of family and friends is likely to have a negative impact on psychosocial wellness (George, 2006; Litwin & Shiovitz-Ezra, 2006).

Ageist Attitudes

A life adjustment that, by its nature, is unique to older adulthood is the acceptance of being old. Because of the ageist attitudes common in modern industrialized societies, many older adults deny that they are old. Ageism can lead to prejudices, fear of aging, and feelings of devaluation and degradation (as discussed in Chapter 1) (Robinson & Umphery, 2006). Even if a person has a good self-acceptance of being old, the person may feel that it is socially unacceptable to admit that it is okay to be old.

Because of these societal attitudes, older adults may be confronted with age-determined expectations that dictate appropriate social behaviors. For example, public displays of affection are viewed as socially appropriate for teenagers and younger adults. However, when older adults hold hands or kiss in public, observers are likely to make comments like, "Isn't that cute, look at that old couple holding hands." Having sexual relationships outside of a marriage is another action that is generally overlooked when done by young adults, but that is likely to be criticized when done by older adults.

As an example of age-determined expectations, consider the following scene: a gray-haired man, who was clearly an older adult, was wearing headphones and listening to music on a portable radio. He was briskly moving along in a combination dance–walk tempo on a public sidewalk in an urban area. Observers remarked that the old man looked like he needed psychiatric care, whereas they ignored several teens nearby who were exhibiting the same type of behavior. The only apparent difference between the older adult and the teens was that the younger people were listening to louder music and demonstrated less control in their movements. The primary difference, however, was in the age-determined expectations in the eyes of the beholders!

Wellness Opportunity

Nurses can promote positive attitudes about aging by talking about friends and relatives who are examples of successful aging.

THEORIES ABOUT PSYCHOSOCIAL FUNCTION IN OLDER ADULTS

Theories about aging and psychosocial function address questions such as, *How do emotions develop over the life course? What influences the way older adults respond to life events? Are certain life events more stressful for older adults? How do coping patterns change in older adulthood?* The following sections address a few of the more widely accepted theories about emotional development, stress, and coping. In addition, some of the recent conclusions about the response of older adults to stressful events are discussed. In keeping with the perspective of this text, these theories are used to explain the age-related changes that can cause positive or negative functional consequences with regard to psychosocial function.

Theories About Emotional Development During Later Adulthood

For several decades, gerontologists have studied emotional development during later adulthood. Initial studies, which focused on institutionalized older adults, suggested that a blunting of emotions and an increase in negative affect occurred in older adulthood. However, gerontologists now emphasize that older adults vary significantly in emotional development, but they have a high capacity for emotional complexity (i.e., the ability to experience and reflect on both pleasant and unpleasant emotions) (Ong & Bergeman, 2004). Recent studies have found the following conclusions (Carstensen et al., 2006; Phillips et al., 2006):

- Emotion regulation and emotional experience are as good as, or even better than, they are in younger years.
- Older adults are at least as emotionally expressive as younger adults, and perhaps more so; however, their physiologic responses to emotional experiences may be less intense.
- Older adults report fewer negative emotions (e.g., less anger) and more positive affect.
- Older adults report more inner control over emotions such as anger and use more self-calming strategies compared with younger counterparts.
- Older adults report greater emotional control and more complex emotional experiences involving a combination of positive and negative emotions.

Theories About Stress

Hans Selye, who proposed the first major theory about stress in the mid-1950s, defined **stress** as the sum of all the effects of factors that act on the body (Selye, 1956). According to Selye's theory, **stressors** include normal activities as well as disease states, and all factors, whether pleasant or unpleasant, are equally important. Moreover, people respond to stressors in three stages: alarm, resistance, and exhaustion. Limitations of this theory include the broad conceptualization of stress, the lack of distinction between pleasant and unpleasant stressors, and the failure to address the meaning of events for the person.

Holmes and Rahe (1967) proposed that stress was a mediator between a life event and adaptation to that event. They define life events as discrete and identifiable changes in life patterns that create stress and that can lead to negative health outcomes. According to this theory, stress causes physical and psychological harm that is in proportion to the intensity of the impact on and duration of a disruption in one's usual life pattern. Holmes and Rahe developed the Social Readjustment Rating Scale (SRRS) as a tool for measuring the duration and intensity of specific life events. The SRRS is a checklist of 43 life events, with relative weights assigned to each according to the usual amount of adaptive effort required by each event.

Because one of the criticisms of the SRRS is its assumption that life events always have a negative impact, researchers have developed variations of the SRRS that account for the meaning of life events for the person. Lazarus (1966), for instance, proposed a scale based on his cognitive appraisal approach. According to Lazarus, people initially appraise the significance of an event according to the way it actually or potentially affects their well-being. Secondarily, they appraise the event according to the personal and social resources that are available for coping, as well as the cost of these resources in relation to positive and negative outcomes. Using these concepts, Folkman and Lazarus (1980) proposed the Ways of Coping Checklist to measure individual thoughts, feelings, and actions in response to specific stressful situations.

Because most stress scales focus on life events of younger and middle-aged adults, they are not as applicable to older adults. In 1988, two nurses developed the Stokes/Gordon Stress Scale (SGSS), a 104-item checklist for use with older adults (Stokes & Gordon, 1988). The SGSS can be self-administered and scored to identify the level of stress an older person is experiencing at a given time. Nurses identified the items included in this checklist through interviews with older adults, a literature review, and consultations with gerontological nurses. Nurses can address many of the significant stresses, such as decreasing eyesight and hearing, through interventions aimed at improving functional abilities. Other significant stresses, such as losses of or changes in relationships, can be addressed through the psychosocial interventions discussed in this chapter. Table 12-1 identifies some of the SGSS items and their corresponding relative weights. The SGSS and a user's guide can be obtained from the Stokes/Gordon Stress Study (listed in the Educational Resources section of this chapter).

In addition to addressing the impact of major life events (acute stress), studies address the impact of daily hassles (chronic stress). Gerontologists initially proposed that older adults experienced more stressors that are chronic; however, studies do not consistently support this. Rather, some recent studies suggest that older adults report less stress from daily hassles such as those associated with chronic illness, which become stressful only when there is a flare-up or acute episode. However, older adults are more likely to experience stress from problems such as bereavement or ill health (Aldwin et al., 2006). Gerontologists also are focusing on effects of chronic stress, such as long-term caregiving or financial problems. A review of literature suggests that chronic stress is particularly detrimental because it erodes social supports that are a major coping resource for older adults (Krause, 2006b).

TABLE 12-1 Stokes/Gordon Stress Scale (SGSS): Selected Items

Rank	Event or Situation	Weight
1	Death of a son or daughter (unexpected)	100
2	Decreasing eyesight	99
2	Death of a grandchild	99
3	Death of spouse (unexpected)	97
4	Loss of ability to get around	96
4	Death of son or daughter (expected, anticipated)	96
5	Fear of your home being invaded or robbed	93
5	Constant or recurring pain or discomfort	93
6	Illness or injury of close relative	92
7	Death of spouse (expected, anticipated)	90
7	Moving in with children or other family	90
7	Moving to an institution	90
8	Minor or major car accident	89
8	Needing to rely on cane, wheelchair, walker, hearing aid	89
8	Change in ability to do personal care	89
10	Loneliness or aloneness	87
11	Having an unexpected debt	86
11	Your own hospitalization (unplanned)	86
12	Decreasing hearing	85
13	Fear of abuse from others	84
13	Being judged legally incompetent	84
13	Not feeling needed or having a purpose in life	84
14	Decreasing mental abilities	84
15	Giving up long-cherished possessions	82
15	Wishing parts of your life had been different	82
16	Using your savings for living expenses	80
17	Change in behavior of family member	79
18	Taking a relative or friend into your home to live	78
19	Concern about elimination	77
19	Illness in public places	77
20	Feeling of remaining time being short	76
20	Giving up or losing driver's license	76
20	Change in your sleeping habits	76
21	Difficulty using public transportation system	75
23	Uncertainty about the future	73
25	Fear of your own or your spouse's driving	71
27	Concern for completing required forms	69
27	Death of a loved pet	69
29	Reaching a milestone year	67
32	Outstanding personal achievement	64
33	Retirement	63
35	Change in your sexual activity	59

(Adapted with permission from Stokes, S. A., & Gordon, S. E. [1988]. *User's manual,* SGSS. Pleasantville, NY: Pace University.)

Theories About Coping

Theories about age-related differences in coping often address the following types of internal mechanisms that people use to deal with stressful situations: seeking information; maintaining a hopeful outlook; using stress reduction techniques; denying or minimizing the threat; channeling energy into physical activity; creating fantasies about various outcomes; finding reassurance and emotional support;

identifying limited and realistic goals; identifying a positive purpose for the event; getting involved in other activities, such as work and family; and expressing oneself creatively, such as through music, art, or writing. These coping styles are categorized as problem-focused (i.e., directed toward altering the source of stress) or emotion-focused (i.e., directed toward regulating one's response). Within these categories, they are further characterized as active or passive. A similar schema categorizes coping styles as assimilation (i.e., actual and intentional efforts to change the stressful life circumstances) or accommodation (i.e., adjustment of goals and preferences to limitations of the situation). People first use assimilation coping efforts to overcome obstacles, and they use accommodation when initial attempts are unsuccessful.

Studies of age differences have found that older adults are more likely to use the following types of coping mechanisms (Marsiske & Margrett, 2006; Riediger et al., 2006):

- More passive emotion-focused strategies, such as denial, acceptance, or suppressing emotion
- A combination of emotion- and problem-focused strategies for interpersonal and emotionally charged situations
- More passive–dependent and avoidant–withdrawal solutions when faced with interpersonal problems and in situations in which they have the least self-confidence
- More problem-focused coping styles in situations involving everyday functioning
- Accommodative rather than assimilative coping when losses increase and they face more obstacles to goal achievement

Overall, studies also suggest that older adults who are not cognitively impaired use fewer coping styles but are just as skilled in coping as are midlife adults (Aldwin et al., 2006).

Before the 1980s, gerontologists assumed that life events of older adulthood had negative effects on older adults. Based on this assumption, researchers tried, but failed, to identify specific changes that adversely affect older adults. There is now much agreement that both the strength of the life event (i.e., the meaning of the event to the individual) and the coping resources available to the individual are the factors that determine whether the life event has a negative impact on health (George, 2006). Thus, researchers have focused on identifying the factors that affect one's ability to cope with life events, with much emphasis on the influence of social resources, such as economic resources and social support, which are particularly powerful resources for offsetting the effects of stress (Jopp & Smith, 2006; Stevens et al., 2006).

Gerontologists widely agree that older adults who are engaged in interaction with supportive social networks have better mental and physical health than those who do not maintain meaningful ties with others (Krause, 2006b). For example, researchers have found that older adults who had higher levels of social support after natural disasters experienced lower levels of depressive symptoms (Tyler, 2006). Social support is categorized as (Krause, 2001):

- Instrumental support, which provides tangible assistance (e.g., transportation, personal care)
- Informational support, which provides essential information about appropriate resources (e.g., information about community services)
- Emotional support, which provides comfort, self-validation, and companionship from intimate others (e.g., evidence that the person is loved, cared for, esteemed, valued, and part of a network of communication and mutual obligations)

Physical, mental, and emotional health status is another factor that significantly affects the coping abilities of older adults. Researchers have found a positive association between improved coping and the following characteristics in older adults (Blazer, 2002; DiBartolo, 2002; Steverink et al., 2001):

- Hardiness
- Self-esteem
- Good social skills
- Good cognitive abilities
- Good physical health and functioning
- Beliefs about self-efficacy
- Greater sense of mastery and personal control
- A sense of person and existential integrity

The timing of life events also can affect coping abilities because it is more difficult to cope with cumulative losses or losses that occur close together. Ability to anticipate life events as well as social supports are other factors that affect coping. For example, older adults who can anticipate having social supports feel a sense of hope because they have a "social safety net" (Krause, 2001, p. 274). Studies also have suggested that anticipated and predictable life events are less stressful than unexpected events, but this finding may not apply to death of a spouse for older adults. Carr and colleagues (2001) found that sudden spousal death does not have serious and far-reaching deleterious effects on mental health, and these researchers suggest that the impact of spousal death is affected by much more than the degree of anticipation.

FACTORS THAT INFLUENCE PSYCHOSOCIAL FUNCTION IN OLDER ADULTS

Religion and Spirituality

Gerontologists consistently identify religion and spirituality as major coping resources and significant aspects of psychosocial function for older adults (Birkenmaier et al., 2005). Nursing research identifies the following themes related to religion, spirituality, and aging (Spurlock, 2005; Weaver et al., 2001):

- The need for sensitivity to cultural differences in religious practices and beliefs

- The importance of recognizing and addressing the individual cognitive, emotional, physical, and spiritual needs of older adults
- The need to encourage support services for caregivers and community-dwelling older adults
- The importance of assessing spirituality and spiritual practices to identify potential strengths, supports, and areas of conflict

Religion and spirituality are closely related but distinct concepts. Religion and religiosity, which have a strong social component, refer to the beliefs, feelings, and behaviors that are associated with a faith community. Spirituality generally is conceptualized as broader and more personal than religion. In addition to religious practices associated with a formal church, other spiritual expressions include prayer, meditation, centering, forgiveness, creative activities, love and caring, storytelling and reminiscence, finding meaning in life, work in service to others, and rituals and other activities that nourish the spirit. Florence Nightingale viewed spirituality as intrinsic to human nature and emphasized that it was an individual's deepest and most potent resource for healing. Definitions of spirituality generally include the following concepts: healing; wholeness; social justice; personal growth; interpersonal relationships; a sense of meaning and purpose to life; a transcendent relationship with a higher being; an association with reverence, mystery, and inspiration; connectedness with nature, other people, and the universe; and feelings of and behaviors arising from love, faith, hope, trust, and forgiveness.

Studies consistently find that religion becomes increasingly salient with age and that it has beneficial effects on physical and mental health of older adults (Idler, 2006; Kirby et al., 2004; Krause, 2006b). The following specific health benefits are associated with religiousness in older adults (Aldwin et al., 2006; Armer & Conn, 2001; Crowther et al., 2002):

- Longer life expectancy
- Lower rates of cancer, alcoholism, hypertension, heart disease
- Better adaptation to medical illness
- Better immune system function
- Fewer hospitalizations and shorter hospital stays
- Greater well-being and life satisfaction
- Less anxiety and depression
- Lower rates of suicide
- Better adaptation to caregiving burden
- Faster recovery from depression
- Higher levels of hope and optimism
- Higher levels of participation in health promotion activities (e.g., increased exercise and smoking cessation)

One explanation for the strong health benefits of religiosity is that the buffering effect of participation in formal religious services is an important coping mechanism for meeting the challenges associated with stresses that commonly occur during older adulthood (George, 2006). This explanation is supported by research indicating that the health-enhancing or health-protecting effects of religiosity are due to the unique qualities of social support provided through church networks (Krause, 2006a).

Diversity Note

Hispanics, African Americans, and Native Americans are among the ethnic groups that report high levels of involvement of older adults in both organizational and nonorganizational religious activities.

Gerontologists address spirituality as an important aspect of psychosocial function in later adulthood, particularly as a component of successful aging. For example, a study of life-review narratives of creative older adults identified the following spiritual qualities as aspects of inner and outer empowerment (Bianchi, 2005):

- Participating in aesthetic ways of experiencing life
- Discovering a serene self-esteem
- Harvesting of memories, with emphasis on transformative turning points
- Fostering humor, playfulness, and gratitude
- Being committed to life-long learning
- Encountering one's own mortality
- Developing new purposes
- Welcoming possibilities and allowing the Spirit to lead one to further opportunities
- Looking at the last phase of life as a period of greater freedom from past problems and for new expression
- Sustaining family relationships and cultivating friendships
- Belonging to intentional communities (i.e., small groups of people who meet regularly for social and service-oriented goals)
- Embracing human causes (e.g., using skills and talents to foster a better world for future generations)

Wellness Opportunity

Nurses promote wellness by asking older adults about relationships that provide meaning in their lives.

Culture

Cultural considerations are important for addressing many aspects of function, but they are especially important in relation to psychosocial function because a person's cultural background significantly influences the way a person defines and perceives all aspects of psychosocial function. In assessing psychosocial function in older adults, for example, it is essential to recognize that every society has standards of "normal" or "abnormal" behaviors, and these standards provide guidelines for determining whether behaviors are healthy or unhealthy. Many societies, how-

A Student's Perspective

While I was caring for my client, she asked if she could tell me a story. She proceeded to tell me that, a few nights earlier, she was lying in bed unable to sleep because of various health issues. All of a sudden, she heard this calm yet intense chant moving down the hall. One of the residents is Native American and recently received news that his nephew had passed away. He was performing a traditional chant in mourning for the loss of a loved one. My client said that the sound was peaceful and soothing as she lay awake in bed. She wished she could have recorded it to play every night. She felt it was special that this man was able to maintain his culture in a place far from home and that people respected his need to express himself in this way. She was very touched—and so was I—as she told me this story. I believe that maintaining one's culture is a part of the healing process and should be respected and upheld.

Eliza T.

ever, do not have the rigid distinctions between health and illness that are part of Western cultures, and concepts such as mental health have little meaning in many non-Western societies (Kavanagh, 2003). Cultural perceptions determine all of the following aspects of psychosocial function:

- Definition of mental health and mental illness
- Belief about the causes of mental health and illness
- Expression of symptoms or clinical manifestations
- Criteria for labeling or diagnosing someone as mentally ill
- Decisions concerning appropriate healer(s)
- Choice of treatment(s) to cure mental illness
- Determination that mental health has been restored after an illness episode
- Relative degree of tolerance for abnormal behavior by other members of society

Cultural Considerations 12-1 identifies some of the cultural influences on psychosocial function and is particularly applicable to nursing care of older adults.

In some instances, people from diverse cultures may perceive or interpret physical symptoms and their interconnected psychological or emotional components in a manner that is unfamiliar to the nurse. For example, this is likely to occur with people who have a **culture-bound syndrome**, defined as a disorder that is "restricted to a particular culture or group of cultures because of certain psychosocial characteristics of those cultures" (Andrews, 2003, p. 42). Because these conditions are unique to a particular culture, they may be unrecognized as a disease condition in the biomedical health care system and by professionals who do not share the same cultural background. Anthropologists have identified approximately 150 culture-bound syndromes, and some

Cultural Considerations 12-1

Cultural Influences on Psychosocial Function

Cultural Influences on Beliefs About the Cause of Mental Disorders

- In traditional Chinese culture, many diseases are attributed to an imbalance of yin and yang.
- Many Native American groups embrace a belief system in which balance and harmony are essential for mental and physical health.
- For some Hispanics, mental illness may be viewed as a punishment by a supreme being for past transgressions.
- Some African Americans, especially those of circum-Caribbean descent, may attribute the cause of mental illness to voodoo, sorcery, or other spiritual forces.
- Some European Americans believe that mental illness has physiologic origins related to chemical disturbances, genetic disturbances, or both.

Cultural Influences on the Manifestations of Mental Illness

- Cultural norms determine whether behaviors such as any of the following are viewed as either normal or abnormal: dreams, fainting, visions, trances, sorcery, delusions, hallucinations, intoxication, suicide, speaking in tongues, communicating with spirits, and the use of certain substances (e.g., alcohol, tobacco, peyote, marijuana, and other drugs) (Kavanagh, 2003).
- Post-traumatic stress disorders are relatively common in immigrants and refugees (Boyle, 2003a).
- Hispanic older adults define mental health problems as alcohol and other drug abuse (American Association of Retired Persons, 1997).
- Filipino Americans consider forgetfulness and anger to be mental health problems (American Association of Retired Persons, 1997).
- Although psychotic disorders (i.e., loss of contact with reality) occur in every society and are characterized by similar primary symptoms (e.g., insomnia, delusions, hallucinations, flat affect, and social or emotional withdrawal), the secondary features are highly influenced by cultural factors (Kavanagh, 2003).
- Whereas sadness, joylessness, anxiety, tension, and lack of energy are common manifestations of depression across cultures, feelings of guilt and suicidal ideation occur only in some groups (Kirmayer & Groleau, 2001).

Cultural Influences on Stress and Coping

- Cultural factors often create barriers to the use of formal support services by ethnic elders, and these barriers may increase the feelings of burden experienced by caregivers.
- African American families tend to use religion and spirituality to help them cope with caregiving stress, and religious organizations are a major source of social support for them (Boyle, 2003b).

- In Latino families, the stress of caregiving may be appraised in relation to the degree of disruption to the family rather than the degree of interference with a person's perceived control over life circumstances (Aranda & Knight, 1997).
- In Chinese families, cultural ideals promoting filial piety, family interdependence, veneration of elderly family members, and acceptance of family caregiving roles may affect the way families experience and cope with stress related to their roles as caregivers.

of these are listed as diagnoses in official diagnostic manuals, such as the American Psychiatric Association's *Diagnostic and Statistic Manual of Mental Disorders, Fourth Edition, Text Revision* (*DSM-IV-TR*) and the *International Classification of Mental Disorders* (*ICD-10*), which was developed by the World Health Organization (Mezzich et al., 2001). Table 12-2 lists selected culture-bound syndromes found in specific cultural groups.

Professionals and folk or indigenous healers with the same cultural background usually are knowledgeable about interventions for culture-bound syndromes. Older adults may be reluctant to discuss culture-bound syndromes or folk treatments with health care professionals, especially if the care provider has a different cultural background. The reasons for withholding such information are complex and may include fears that the nurse or other health care provider will disapprove, ridicule, or fail to understand their folk or indigenous healing system. Because of these factors, nurses may consider asking the person's permission to include folk or indigenous healers in discussions about health-related issues. These healers frequently have considerable insight into the cultural and psychosocial aspects of human behavior, and they may be remarkably successful in treating culture-bound syndromes and other disorders that have psychological and emotional components. Because herbal remedies that sometimes are used to treat culture-bound syndromes may interact with prescription or over-the-counter medications, nurses need to make every effort to elicit information about such remedies as part of an assessment (see Chapter 8).

The following case study is based on an example from Andrews and Boyle (2003).

Mrs. Y. is a 79-year-old native of the Philippines. She moved to an urban area in California to be near her four children, who live in the same state. She had lived in the same town in the Philippines for her entire adult life and had stayed there to care for her

(case study continues on page 210)

TABLE 12-2 Selected Culture-Bound Syndromes

Group	Disorder	Remarks
Blacks, Haitians	Blackout	Collapse, dizziness, inability to move
	Low blood	Not enough blood or weakness of the blood that is often treated with diet
	High blood	Blood that is too rich in certain things because of the ingestion of too much red meat or rich foods
	Thin blood	Occurs in women, children, and old people; renders the individual more susceptible to illness in general
	Diseases of hex, witchcraft, or conjuring	Sense of being doomed by spell; gastrointestinal symptoms, e.g., vomiting; hallucinations; part of voodoo beliefs
Chinese, Southeast Asians	*Koro*	Intense anxiety that penis is retracting into body
Greeks	Hysteria	Bizarre complaints and behavior because the uterus leaves the pelvis for another part of the body
Hispanics	*Empacho*	Food forms into a ball and clings to the stomach or intestines, causing pain and cramping
	Fatigue	Asthma-like symptoms
	Mal ojo, "evil eye"	Fitful sleep, crying, diarrhea in children caused by a stranger's attention; sudden onset
	Pasmo	Paralysis-like symptoms of face or limbs; prevented or relieved by massage
	Susto	Anxiety, trembling, phobias from sudden fright
Japanese	*Wagamama*	Apathetic childish behavior with emotional outbursts
Koreans	*Hwa-byung*	Multiple somatic and psychological symptoms: "pushing up" sensation of chest, palpitations, flushing, headache, "epigastric mass," dysphoria, anxiety, irritability, and difficulty concentrating; mostly afflicts married women
Native Americans	Ghost	Terror, hallucinations, sense of danger
North India Indians	Ghost	Death from fever and illness in children; convulsions, delirious speech (or incessant crying in infants); choking, difficulty breathing; based on Hindu religious beliefs and curing practices
Whites	Anorexia nervosa	Excessive preoccupation with thinness; self-imposed starvation
	Bulimia	Gross overeating and then vomiting or fasting

(Andrews, M. M. [2003]. Cultural competence in the health history and physical examination [p. 43]. In M. M. Andrews & J. S. Boyle [Eds.], *Transcultural concepts in nursing care* [4th ed., pp. 36–72]. Philadelphia: Lippincott Williams & Wilkins.)

husband and her sister, who both required care for chronic conditions. Although she was a much-needed and highly esteemed member of her household in the Philippines, Mrs. Y., like many other immigrants, experienced role reversal when she lost her once-dominant position in the family and became financially dependent on her adult children after her relocation.

Like many older immigrants from the Philippines, Mrs. Y. had a more active social network before her relocation. She, like many of her peers, spoke a dialect and did not speak Tagalog, the language spoken by many younger residents of the Philippines. After her relocation to the United States, her communication and interaction with others became restricted to her extended family because she did not feel confident using her limited English and could not find other speakers of her dialect. To buffer the disequilibrium she felt as a result of her migration, Mrs. Y. sought comfort through prayer and regular attendance at the local Roman Catholic Church. She also began to care for her two daughters' children regularly.

You are the nurse at the local hospital who treated Mrs. Y. in the emergency department after she fractured her wrist. During your assessment, you noted that Mrs. Y.'s injury would place a strain on the family because they would temporarily be without their child care provider.

THINKING POINTS

- How would you involve the family members in the discharge plan for Mrs. Y. so that her recovery could be assured, she would not lose respect, and she would not feel responsible to assume her usual duties until she felt better?
- What problems would you anticipate with communicating with Mrs. Y. in the emergency department? How would you handle these problems?
- What psychosocial repercussions did Mrs. Y.'s move to the United States have? Did she cope with these effectively? Would you have had any other suggestions for helping her to cope?
- How did Mrs. Y's culture influence her coping mechanisms?

RISK FACTORS THAT AFFECT PSYCHOSOCIAL FUNCTION

Theories about stress and coping and research about causes of impaired mental health in older adults provide information about risks that can affect psychosocial function. The following factors contribute to high levels of stress and poor coping in older adults:

- Poor physical health
- Impaired functional abilities
- Weak social supports
- Lack of economic resources
- An immature developmental level
- Narrow range of coping skills
- The occurrence of unanticipated events
- The occurrence of several daily hassles at the same time
- The occurrence of several major life events in a short period of time
- High social status and feelings of high self-efficacy in situations that cannot be changed or in which control cannot be exerted over the environment

In addition, because the ability to determine the potential for change influences one's response to a stressful situation, people who cannot realistically appraise a situation may have more difficulty coping effectively. This is particularly pertinent with regard to health and functioning because older adults who view functional decline as an inevitable consequence of aging are less likely to seek help for treatable problems (Sarkisian et al., 2002). Thus, nurses have important roles in teaching older adults about risk factors and potential interventions for health problems. For example, older adults who experience urinary incontinence or difficulties with sexual function may consider these changes to be inevitable consequences of age. Based on this appraisal, they are likely to use passive, emotion-focused coping mechanisms, trying simply to accept the situation. In addition, they are more likely to experience an unnecessary and unfortunate functional impairment and a diminished quality of life. By contrast, if the situation is appraised more accurately as a potentially treatable condition, more active, problem-focused coping mechanisms are likely to be used. Even when older adults accurately appraise health problems as changeable, they must identify health professionals who understand the problem and who will attempt to find solutions. Thus, both the older adult and the health care professional must accurately appraise the situation so they can initiate interventions and achieve wellness outcomes.

Older adults who normally have a sense of high self-efficacy may be particularly susceptible to disturbed self-esteem and feelings of powerlessness when they are in situations where they have little control over their environment. For example, studies have found that a sense of mastery protects older adults against depression, fosters resilience under stressful situations, and promotes physical and emotional well-being (Jang et al., 2002). Studies also are addressing the effects of involvement or lack of involvement in decision making, particularly on older adults who are cognitively intact. For example, the degree of involvement in everyday decisions, such as routine health care, timing of meals, placement of furniture, and choice of seating in the dining room can significantly affect the well-being of nursing home residents and their adjustment to the institutional setting (Shawler et al., 2001).

The concept of **learned helplessness** has been used to explain the excess dependency that occurs in older adults in hospital or long-term care settings (Faulkner, 2001). Learned helplessness is the experience of uncontrollable events that leads to expectations that future events will also be uncontrollable. Thus, actions that increase dependency or disempower older adults (e.g., providing assistance because this is more time-efficient rather than allowing the older person to function independently or with only a little assistance) are risk factors for diminished self-esteem and feelings of powerlessness. In addition, learned helplessness may contribute to depression, as discussed in Chapter 15. Similarly, studies suggest that the provision of more assistance than is needed, especially with tasks such as daily activities, results in reduced self-esteem and well-being (Antonucci, 2001).

Wellness Opportunity

Nurses promote wellness by allowing older adults to function as independently as possible and providing the supports they need, even if this is not as time-efficient as doing things for them.

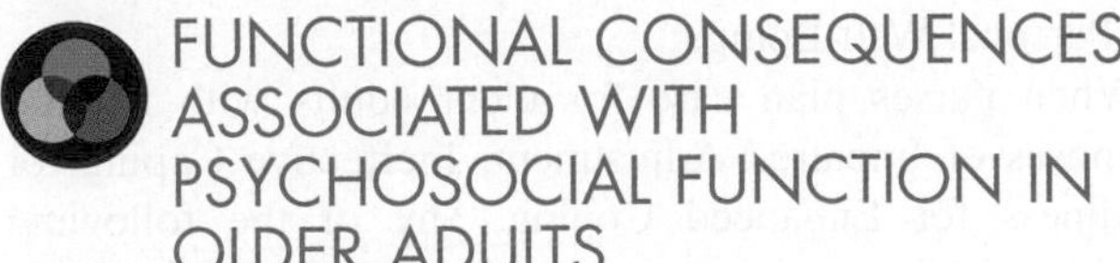

FUNCTIONAL CONSEQUENCES ASSOCIATED WITH PSYCHOSOCIAL FUNCTION IN OLDER ADULTS

Since the mid-1960s, many studies have used life-events scales to measure the negative impact of stressful events, with particular emphasis on physical health effects. Although some studies have found an association between high stress and the occurrence of certain diseases (e.g., heart attacks), most people who experience life events do not become ill (George, 2006). Because the impact of life events on health is significantly affected by many interacting factors, older adults experience a wide range of both negative and positive functional consequences with regard to psychosocial function.

Negative functional consequences include anxiety, loneliness, depression, and cognitive impairment. About 20% of older adults report clinically relevant symptoms of anxiety, which manifests in older adults as distress, exaggerated fears and concerns about their health, and a heightened awareness of physiologic arousal and discomfort (Frazier et al., 2002). Older adults who are homebound and chronically ill are likely to experience higher levels of worry, which is considered the cognitive component of anxiety (Fakouri & Lyon, 2005). Older adults who are widowed or who have few social contacts are likely to experience feelings of loneliness that have a negative impact on their quality of life (Borg et al., 2006). Negative functional consequences associated with cognitive function and depression are discussed in Chapters 11 and 15, respectively.

In addition to focusing on anxiety, depression, and other negative emotions, gerontologists also are addressing the relationship between positive emotions (e.g., happiness, life satisfaction, emotional well-being) and health in older adults. For example, a study of 125 older adults 85 years of age or older found equal or higher levels of a sense of coherence, resilience, self-transcendence, and purpose in life compared with younger adults (Nygren et al., 2005). Further research may examine whether there is a relationship between these positive psychosocial findings and physical health. Much of the current focus on psychosocial function in older adults is on identifying the factors that affect emotional well-being and thereby improve health and quality of life. The following characteristics of older adults are associated with emotional vitality and improved health (Aldwin et al., 2006; Krause, 2006b):

- Feeling happy, enjoying life
- Experiencing autonomy
- Experiencing personal growth
- Having a purpose in life
- Being extroverted and outgoing
- Feeling hopeful about the future
- Having positive relations with others
- Having a sense of self-acceptance
- Having a high sense of personal mastery
- Having a sense of hardiness and coherence
- Having low measures of anxiety and depression
- Having a sense of religious or spiritual connectedness
- Experiencing a sense of mastery over one's environment

An important aspect of promoting psychosocial wellness for older adults is focusing at least some attention on strengths that can be supported rather than addressing only the negative functional consequences.

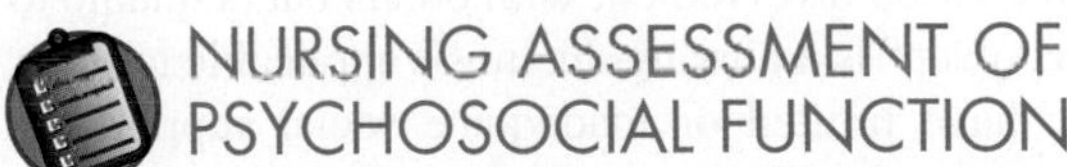

NURSING ASSESSMENT OF PSYCHOSOCIAL FUNCTION

Because psychosocial function encompasses a broad range of social, cognitive, and emotional aspects of functioning that are intertwined, the assessment of psychosocial function is addressed comprehensively in a separate chapter. Readers are directed to Chapter 13 for a thorough review of nursing assessment of psychosocial function.

NURSING DIAGNOSIS

The nursing diagnoses of Self-Esteem Disturbance or Situational Low Self-Esteem (or Risk for) are applicable in relation to some of the psychosocial adjustment issues of older adulthood. Situational Low Self-Esteem is defined as "the state in which an individual who previously had positive self-esteem experiences negative feelings about self in response to an event (loss, change)" (Carpenito-Moyet, 2006, p. 421). Related factors might be the internalization of ageist attitudes, the loss of roles or financial security, the need for a change to a more dependent living arrangement, and chronic illnesses that affect one's abilities and role identities.

If the nursing assessment identifies threats to the older person's sense of control, an appropriate nursing diagnosis is Powerlessness (or Risk for). This is defined as "the state in which an individual or group perceives a lack of personal control over certain events or situations, which affects outlook, goals, and lifestyle" (Carpenito-Moyet, 2006, p. 338). Common related factors for older adults are forced retirement, loss of the ability to drive a car, lack of involvement in decision making, chronic conditions that cause progressive functional declines (e.g., dementia), and institutional constraints, such as lack of privacy and the need to follow schedules that do not meet the needs of the individual.

Impaired Adjustment is another nursing diagnosis that addresses the psychosocial needs of older adults. This diagnosis is defined as "the state in which an individual is unable to modify his or her lifestyle or behavior in a manner consistent with a change in health status" (Carpenito-Moyet, 2006, p. 10). For example, this nursing diagnosis would be applicable to an older adult who is driving unsafely because of cognitive or other functional deficits, but who refuses to give up driving. Another nursing diagnosis that might be applied to the psychosocial needs of older adults is Ineffective Coping, which is defined as "the state in which the individual experiences or is at risk of experiencing an inability to manage internal or environmental stressors adequately because of inadequate resources (physical, psychological, behavioral, and/or cognitive)" (Carpenito-Moyet, 2006, p. 97).

Social Isolation, which is defined as "the state in which an individual or group experiences or perceives a need or desire for increased involvement with others but is unable to make that contact," is a nursing diagnosis applicable to older adults who have limited or inadequate social supports to address their needs (Carpenito-Moyet, 2006, p. 463). A closely related nursing diagnosis is Impaired Social Interaction, defined as "the state in which an individual experiences, or is at risk of experiencing, negative, insufficient, or unsatisfactory responses from interactions" (Carpenito-Moyet, 2006, p. 459). For example, nurses would use these diagnoses when they are making referrals for community resources to improve social supports for older adults.

Nurses can use any of the following diagnoses to address spiritual needs of older adults: Spiritual Distress (or Risk for) or Impaired Religiosity (or Risk for). In addition, nurses can use Readiness for Enhanced Spiritual Well-Being when they are addressing the older adult's sense of meaning and purpose. This wellness diagnosis is defined as the "ability to experience and integrate meaning and purpose in life through connectedness with self, others, art, music, literature, nature, or a power greater than oneself" (Johnson et al., 2006, p. 425).

Wellness Opportunity

Readiness for Enhanced Coping and Readiness for Enhanced Self-Concept are wellness nursing diagnoses that are applicable for many older adults.

PLANNING FOR WELLNESS OUTCOMES

Wellness outcomes related to psychosocial function focus on stress reduction, enhanced coping skills, and improved quality of life. When planning wellness outcomes pertinent to Situational Low Self-Esteem (or Risk for) or Readiness for Enhanced Self-Concept, nurses can apply any of the following Nursing Outcomes Classification (NOC) terminology: Psychosocial Adjustment: Life Change; Self-Esteem; Adaptation to Physical Disability; Body Image; Grief Resolution; Personal Autonomy; Depression Level; and Quality of Life (Johnson et al., 2006).

Outcomes for older adults who experience Powerlessness include Hope, Personal Autonomy, and Participation in Health Care Decisions. Outcomes related to the nursing diagnosis of Social Isolation include Loneliness Severity, Social Support, Social Involvement, Leisure Participation, and Personal Well-Being.

When nurses plan care for older adults with nursing diagnoses of Impaired Adjustment, Ineffective Coping, or Readiness for Enhanced Coping, any of the following NOC terminology might be pertinent: Psychosocial Adjustment: Life Change; Acceptance: Health Status; Adaptation to Physical Disability; Coping; Decision Making; Knowledge: Health Resources; Personal Well-Being; and Stress Level.

Wellness Opportunity

Hope and Quality of Life would be appropriate NOC terminology when nurses direct care toward improving psychosocial wellness.

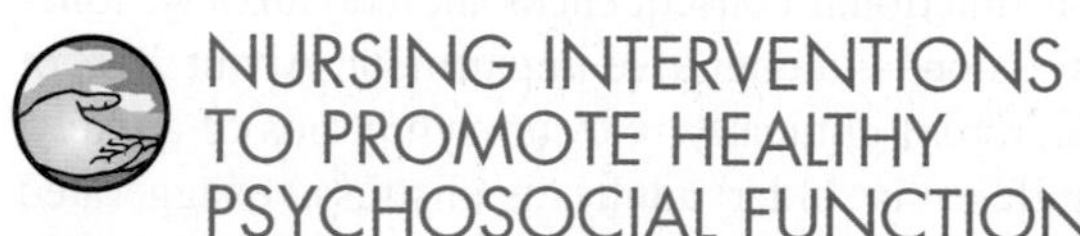

NURSING INTERVENTIONS TO PROMOTE HEALTHY PSYCHOSOCIAL FUNCTION

Nurses have many opportunities to promote healthy psychosocial function during the usual course of caring for older adults. For example, they can incorporate communication techniques and other interventions to enhance self-esteem, promote a sense of control, and address spiritual needs. They also can use life review and reminiscence interventions, especially in home and long-term care settings. In addition to incorporating interventions in usual care, nurses promote psychosocial wellness by facilitating referrals for social supports. In some settings, nurses can implement group interventions, such as healthy aging classes, to help older adults cope effectively with the life events of older adulthood. Studies support the significant role of nurses in promoting psychosocial wellness through interventions that improve social interaction, perceived control, and participation in decision making (Sparks et al., 2004).

The following Nursing Interventions Classification (NIC) terms relate to interventions discussed in this chapter: Active Listening; Anxiety Reduction; Caregiver Support; Coping Enhancement; Decision-Making Support; Emotional Support; Grief Work Facilitation; Hope Instillation; Presence; Religious Ritual Enhancement; Reminiscence Therapy; Resiliency Promotion; Role Enhancement; Self-Esteem Enhancement; Socialization Enhancement; Spiritual Growth Facilitation; Support System Enhancement; and Teaching: Group.

In addition to the interventions reviewed in this chapter, interventions that improve functional abilities promote psychosocial wellness because of the close relationship between physiologic and psychosocial aspects of health and function. Thus, interventions to improve functional abilities, which are discussed throughout this text, also promote psychosocial wellness. Participation in physical activity has many benefits, not only on physical but also on psychosocial function, including improved cognition and positive mood (McReynolds & Rossen, 2004).

Enhancing Self-Esteem

Self-esteem enhancement is an essential component of nursing care for older adults because self-esteem is an important coping resource and a factor that influences well-being. **Self-esteem** refers to the feelings one has about one's self, or the extent to which one perceives oneself to be worthy or significant. It is the emotional component of self-concept and is based on one's perceptions of other people's opinions about oneself. People with good self-esteem are happier, healthier, less anxious, more independent, more self-confident, and more effective in meeting environmental demands than people with low self-esteem (Reitzes & Mutran, 2006). Chapter 13 includes information on assessing self-esteem; this chapter focuses on nursing interventions that enhance self-esteem, with emphasis on addressing factors that threaten it (e.g., dependence, devaluation, depersonalization, and powerlessness).

Many factors that are threats to self-esteem are associated with staff and environments in institutional settings and can be addressed through relatively simple nursing interventions. This is particularly important in environments such as long-term care settings where the caregiving environment affects virtually every aspect of daily life for the residents. For instance, when older adults are admitted to institutional settings, nurses may be able to identify environmental or other factors that can quickly and easily be modified to promote a sense of control and minimize or eliminate a threat to self-esteem, as in the following examples:

- Ensuring easy access to his or her usual assistive devices (walkers, eyeglasses, hearing aids)
- Asking about food preferences and ensuring as much choice as possible
- Asking open-ended questions, such as, "Is there anything that we can do to help you manage better while you're here?"
- Asking, "Is there anything you're worried about that I can help you with?"
- Ensuring that staff address the person by the preferred name

Threats to self-esteem also arise when caregivers promote unnecessary dependence for their own convenience. For example, using incontinence products and telling a bedridden person to wet the bed because it is easier to change the disposable pad or brief than to assist with toileting is a tremendous blow to the person's self-esteem. Thus, interventions that improve independent function, which are discussed throughout this text, are important for enhancing self-esteem.

Because self-esteem depends to some extent on the perceived appraisal of significant others, nurses can use communication interventions to increase the older adult's perception of self-worth. Nurses must be aware of their ageist attitudes and avoid reflecting these attitudes in verbal statements. For example, even a remark such as "You certainly look good for 85 years old," although said with good intentions, can reinforce ageist attitudes. Hidden messages in this statement may be that it is better to look younger, and that when you are old, you generally do not look good. Nurses can address ageism by avoiding even subtle messages that communicate negative attitudes. For instance, a statement such as the following might enhance an older person's self-esteem and challenge ageist attitudes: "At 85 years old, you must have a lot of wisdom. What advice can you give about successful aging?"

Nonverbal communication may influence the person's perception of self-worth even more than verbal communication. For example, if a nurse walks past an older person sitting in a hallway without acknowledging his or her presence, this may be perceived as an indicator that the nurse does not value the older person. Even though the nurse may have been attending to responsibilities and had not intended to communicate this negative message, this action may negatively affect that older person's self-esteem. Thus, nurses must keep in mind that the perception of their actions is often more important than their intent, and they must use verbal and nonverbal messages to communicate feelings of positive regard whenever possible.

For dependent older adults, the negative impact of disability and functional impairments on self-esteem is heightened by behaviors of others that convey attitudes of **infantilization** (i.e., treating an adult in a way that is similar to the way infants are treated). For example, remarks such as "He acts just like a baby" or "Now, now, dear, let's be a good girl" convey infantilization. The term **elderspeak**—also called "baby talk"—describes speech that is modified when addressed to older adults, usually by younger adults. This communication style is characterized by slower rate, fewer clauses, more repetitions, longer pauses, shorter utterances, exaggerated intonation, more fillers (e.g., you know), more sentence fragments, elevated pitch and volume, and fewer words with more than two syllables (Thornton & Light, 2006; Williams et al., 2004). Older adults perceive this type of communication as demeaning, patronizing, and implying incompetence, and it can inadvertently promote depression, social withdrawal, lowered self-esteem, and unnecessary dependency (Williams et al., 2004). Moreover, it can reflect ageist attitudes or negative and inaccurate stereotypes. Thus, nurses need to monitor their communication with older adults to ensure that they avoid inappropriate terminology and elderspeak. Box 12-1 summarizes nursing interventions for enhancing self-esteem in older adults.

Wellness Opportunity

Nurses can enhance self-esteem by pointing out positive qualities of an older adult during routine care activities.

Promoting a Sense of Control

Because perceived control is a factor that significantly affects psychosocial wellness, nursing interventions are directed toward promoting a sense of control and involving older adults in decisions. Researchers have found that a sense of control contributes to positive affect and improved well-being for older adults, particularly in cultures that value independent functioning (Ashman et al., 2006). Nursing interventions to promote a sense of control for older adults in acute care settings include involving patients in organizing their schedule and providing information about their plan of care (Jacelon, 2004).

Many studies have confirmed the importance of modifying the way people perceive and explain events, shifting attention to factors that can be changed or controlled. In the classic study by Rodin and Langer (1980), whenever a nursing home resident attributed a problem to being old, the staff provided another explanation and identified a causative factor that was amenable to change. For instance, when residents attributed feelings of fatigue to being old, they were reminded that they were awakened at 5:30 AM (Rodin & Langer, 1980). Nurses can listen for opportunities to challenge older adults' perceptions that promote a sense of hopelessness and rephrase the situation in a context that is empowering. For example, they can help older adults develop problem-focused coping mechanisms rather than passively, and sometimes inaccurately, accepting the negative functional consequences of aging.

Nursing interventions also address factors that can threaten perceived control, such as lack of privacy and loss of individuality, which commonly occur in institutional settings. Nurses can show respect for privacy by knocking on bedroom doors and asking permission before entering, by closing doors when privacy is desired, by asking permission before pulling bed curtains open, and by being careful about moving personal belongings without permission from the older person. Encouraging the person to have personal belongings and to arrange these belongings in whatever fashion is desired also shows concern for individuality.

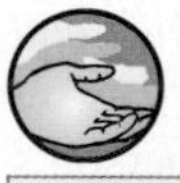

Box 12-1 Nursing Interventions to Promote Self-Esteem

Communication Techniques

- Acknowledge a person by using his or her preferred name and title.
- When talking with older people, use the same tone of voice you use for your colleagues.
- Provide positive feedback for individual accomplishments, even in daily self-care tasks that require effort.
- Focus conversations on the person's strengths and positive attributes, rather than on their limitations. (For example, for people who have physical impairments, focus on nonphysical attributes, such as personality characteristics or interpersonal relationships.)
- When negative functional consequences are attributed to old age, offer an alternative explanation and identify a contributing factor that is amenable to change. (For example, when someone attributes weakness "simply" to being old, remind them that they are recovering from hip surgery and should expect to improve with therapy.)
- Be cautious about communicating ageist attitudes, even inadvertently, in conversations.

Verbal Communication to Observe for and Avoid

- Do not use names or phrases that reflect ageist attitudes (e.g., "little old lady," "dirty old man"), even in jest.
- Do not raise your voice except when necessary to facilitate communication with someone who has impaired hearing.
- Do not use terms that are associated with babies (e.g., *diapers, baby food*).
- Do not use *we* or *us* unless the term is accurate. (For example, do not say "Let's take our medicine now.")
- Do not use the term *senile*.

Nonverbal Communication Techniques and Additional Nursing Actions

- When labeling clothing, put the person's name in an inconspicuous place.
- Use actions consciously to communicate positive regard (e.g., recognize the presence of someone as you walk past).

Wellness Opportunity

Nurses show concern for individuality by asking an older adult about a family photo or greeting card that is in view.

Involving Older Adults in Decision Making

Older people frequently are left out of the decision-making process, even for those decisions that most profoundly affect their lives, such as moving to a long-term care facility. This lack of involvement occurs for a variety of reasons, related both to the older adult and to the decision makers. Some of the barriers within the older adult may be dementia, depression, long-term passivity regarding decisions, or hearing impairments or other communication barriers. Some of the barriers within the decision makers that may thwart the decision-making process include stereotypes of older people as incompetent, perceptions that the older adult is not interested in or capable of making decisions, and an unwillingness to deal with the older person's anticipated resistance to the desired outcome.

Many of the reasons for excluding older adults from the decision-making process are related to the attitudes of the family and of professional caregivers, so one nursing intervention is to challenge these attitudes. For example, in acute care settings, nurses can facilitate communication between older patients and their primary care provider to ensure that the older person is included in decisions about medical treatment and discharge plans. In long-term care settings, nurses have numerous opportunities to involve older adults in decisions about their daily care, medical interventions, and discharge plans. In home settings, nurses might work with family members as well as older adults to ensure that the latter are involved in decisions about their care and that their rights are respected. In any setting, nurses may have to remind health professionals, as well as family members and other caregivers, that although people may gain rights by virtue of being a certain age, they do not lose their rights just because they reach a certain age. For a comprehensive discussion of the nurse's role in decisions regarding long-term care for people with dementia, refer to Chapter 14.

Other aspects of decision making that can be addressed in nursing interventions are one's verbal interactions and choice of terminology. With regard to verbal communication, health professionals often talk *about* older adults when in their presence rather than addressing questions *to* them and focusing the conversation *on* them. This commonly occurs when family members or other caregivers are discussing situations with a nurse or other professional and the conversation takes place in the presence of the older person without directly involving him or her. In working with older adults, nurses need to pay particular attention to including older adults in conversations when the topic is directly related to them. When it is not appropriate to include the older adult in the conversation, the nurse can take steps to facilitate the conversation outside the presence of the older person. In these situations, the nurse can ask the older person's permission to discuss his or her situation with family member or caregivers and then report back to the older person, in language that the person can understand, about any discussions that take place or decisions that are made or pending.

With regard to terminology, the word "placement" often is used in reference to an older adult's admission to a nursing home. This term denotes passivity on the part of the older adult; it is closer to the terminology used when objects are placed on a shelf than to words normally used in reference to human beings. Nurses would communicate more positive feelings and a greater sense of control if they referred to an "admission" to a nursing home. The term admission suggests that certain criteria have been met and that an active decision has been made to determine whether the person meets these criteria. Even more important than using the correct terms, nurses must ensure that older adults are, in fact, actively involved in the decision-making process, rather than passively being "placed." Nurses can help older adults and their families with decisions about long-term care by helping them assess their situation and by correcting misinformation and providing accurate information about specific resources and the range of services available (as described in Chapter 6).

Addressing Role Loss

Meaningful roles (e.g., spouse, caregiver, volunteer) are important determinants of feelings of worth, efficacy, and self-esteem. Although role loss is a common occurrence in later adulthood, studies indicate that the development of new roles is an effective coping strategy for older adults (George, 2006). In addition to helping older adults develop new roles, nurses can focus on past as well as current achievements as an intervention for enhancing self-esteem, especially for older adults who are dependent on others and have difficulty feeling a sense of accomplishment, or even a sense of basic usefulness. Nurses implement this intervention, which may be especially helpful for older adults who have difficulty identifying meaningful roles, in a group setting or on an individual basis.

Wellness Opportunity

Nurses can ask older adults about their accomplishments in areas such as work and family and give positive feedback about meaningful roles.

Encouraging Life Review and Reminiscence

Life review and reminiscence are two closely related processes that are used to promote psychosocial health in older adults. Butler (2001) describes life review as a progressive return to consciousness of past experiences, particularly unresolved conflicts, for reexamination and reintegration. If the reintegration process is successful, the process gives new significance and meaning to life and prepares the person for death by alleviating fear and anxiety (Butler, 2001). Positive effects of life review include accepting one's mortality, righting of old wrongs, taking pride in accomplishments, gaining a sense of serenity, and feeling that one has done one's best (Butler, 2001). Nursing home residents who participated in life review therapy showed significant improvement over a 3-year period on measures of depression, life satisfaction, and self-esteem (Haight, 2000).

Reminiscence is based on the same theoretical framework as life review; however, it can be done outside the life review process, and it is more informal and less intense. Another difference is that life review addresses both pleasant and unpleasant issues of the past, whereas reminiscence focuses primarily on pleasant and positive experiences. Reminiscence therapy as a nursing intervention is defined as "using the recall of past events, feelings, and thoughts to facilitate pleasure, quality of life, or adaptation to present circumstances" (Johnson et al., 2006, p. 661). As a group therapy, the reminiscence group is one of the most widely used interventions for older adults, and it may be particularly effective for improving self-esteem in long-term care settings (Chao et al., 2006). Although life review interventions require the involvement of a person with advanced mental health skills, nurses can incorporate reminiscence interventions in their usual care (Borglin et al., 2005).

Fostering Social Supports

Although many of the important social supports that serve as coping resources, such as financial assets, usually are not addressed through nursing interventions, nurses have many opportunities to foster the development of social networks for older adults, and this is an appropriate intervention for addressing social isolation. In some situations, particularly in home and long-term care settings, nurses are an integral part of the older person's social network. Social isolation is likely to occur because of any of the following factors that commonly occur in older adulthood:

- Hearing impairments and other communication barriers
- Chronic illnesses that limit activity or energy
- Lack of social opportunities because of caregiving responsibilities
- Mobility limitations, including inability to drive a car
- Mental or psychosocial impairments that interfere with relationships
- Loss of spouse, friends, or family through death, illness, or physical distance

Thus, nursing interventions that address these risk factors (e.g., improved mobility or sensory function) also are likely to have the positive consequence of improved social supports.

In long-term care settings, nurses can foster positive social interactions in group settings, such as dining and activity rooms. Sometimes, a very simple intervention, such as positioning chairs (including wheelchairs) so people can interact with each other, can significantly influence social contacts, either positively or negatively. Whenever possible, nurses should arrange room assignments to encourage opportunities for positive social interactions. In addition, nurses can facilitate referrals for social and therapeutic activities in long-term care facilities.

In home settings, nurses can identify community resources, such as volunteer friendly visitor and meal programs, to decrease social isolation. Support and education groups that primarily focus on coping with a chronic illness (e.g., stroke clubs, or better breathing groups) also provide excellent opportunities for social contact and the development of friendships with people who are in similar situations. For people who are socially isolated because of caregiving responsibility, caregiver support groups can enhance coping abilities and provide social support.

Selected nursing interventions to promote psychosocial wellness are described in Box 12-2.

A Student's Perspective

I had a special experience with a man at the nursing and rehab center. "Mort" and I had great conversations, and he quickly became a friend. Mort was suffering from cardiovascular failure, and I knew he did not have long to live. I interviewed Mort and then wrote a paper about his life. I wrote the paper early so that I could read it to Mort before his health declined any more. I read my paper to Mort one morning, and he listened with a seeming sense of sacredness about the words being read. This was his life, and I could tell that it meant a lot to him that I wrote it all down. When I finished, Mort simply said, "I thank you... I thank you." He asked me to put the paper in a safe place so it would not get ruined. Mort and I had a special connection; he was a hero to me. The following week, I came to clinical and found out that Mort had passed away. I am grateful that I had the opportunity to know Mort and to grow and learn from his good life. I am glad that I could serve him at this final time and help him reflect on his life.

Amy C.

Wellness Opportunity

Nurses can talk with older adults about the benefits of support groups and provide a list of local resources that address specific needs of older adults and their caregivers.

Addressing Spiritual Needs

Addressing spiritual needs of patients is within the scope of nursing, as exemplified in the following interventions that are commonly included in nursing care:

Box 12-2
Nursing Interventions to Promote Psychosocial Wellness

Facilitating Maximum Independence

- Make sure that the person has access to all necessary assistive devices and personal accessories (e.g., wigs, canes, dentures, walkers, and hearing aids).
- Allow enough time for the person to perform tasks at her or his own pace, and avoid unnecessary dependence that results from an overemphasis on time efficiency.
- Make sure that the environment has been adapted as much as possible to compensate for sensory losses and other functional impairments.

Promoting a Sense of Control

- Make a conscious effort to involve older adults in decisions regarding their care, both in small daily matters as well as in major health care concerns.
- Ask about likes and dislikes and try to address personal preferences.
- Whenever possible, allow the person to choose between two alternatives, even if the options are in a very narrow range (e.g., "Would you prefer to wear the yellow sweater or the pink one today?").
- Ensure as much privacy, or perceived privacy, as possible.
- Knock on the door and ask permission before entering a bedroom, even in institutional settings.
- Allow as much expression of individuality as possible in the personal environment (e.g., use personal furniture when possible and display family pictures in full view).
- Make sure that the call light is accessible for people who are confined.
- Do not talk about someone in his or her presence as if he or she does not exist.
- Avoid referring to nursing home *placement*. Refer instead to an *admission*, and include the person in the decision-making process.

Addressing Role Loss

- Identify new roles for people and acknowledge those past and present roles that are viewed positively.
- Encourage participation in reminiscence groups and other group therapies.
- Find opportunities to create meaningful roles, such as helper or assistant, by involving older adults in useful tasks, such as folding laundry.
- When older adults volunteer to assist others, acknowledge their contribution with a remark such as, "You certainly help us a lot when you help take Mrs. Smith to the dining room in her wheelchair."
- Acknowledge an older adult's nonphysical assets and attributes, such as family relationships or a good sense of humor.
- Focus on positive relationships by acknowledging or asking about the receipt of flowers, greeting cards, and other visible signs of concern expressed by others.
- Ask older adults about their responsibilities as parents, grandparents, or roommates and point out their positive contributions.
- Ask older adults about family photos, initiate a discussion of positive relationships, and remind them that others care about them (e.g., encourage them to talk about grandchildren and great-grandchildren).
- Ask older adults about accomplishments in areas such as work, family, hobbies, and volunteer activities.
- Respond with comments such as, "You must be proud of your children," or "You certainly have accomplished a lot."

Fostering Social Supports

- Use interventions to address hearing impairments and other communication barriers (see Chapter 16).
- Encourage participation in group activities.
- For people in wheelchairs, especially those who cannot move independently, position the chair in a way that promotes social interaction.
- For nursing home residents, plan table and room arrangements in a way that fosters social relationships.

- Intentionally communicating caring and compassion
- Facilitating reminiscence
- Honoring a person's integrity
- Providing active and passive listening
- Making referrals for spiritual care
- Caring for someone who feels hopeless
- Arranging for participation in religious services
- Encouraging or facilitating participation in activities such as prayer and meditation

Nursing interventions to address the spiritual needs of older adults need to be individualized and offered only if the person is receptive to the interventions. In addition, nurses need to be nonjudgmental about religion and spirituality and avoid imposing their personal beliefs. Moreover, because cultural factors significantly influence a person's spirituality and religious beliefs, interventions must be culturally sensitive. Andrews and Hanson (2003) provide an excellent overview of specific cultural influences on religion and spirituality, including details about health-related beliefs and practices of selected religious groups in North America.

In addition to addressing spiritual needs as a routine part of psychosocial nursing care, nurses often address spiritual needs during times of spiritual distress (Tuck et al., 2006). For example, older adults are likely to express spiritual needs when they are coping with the loss of a significant relationship or dealing with news about a serious or terminal illness. Older adults who are caregivers for others, especially a spouse, are likely to express spiritual needs in relation to decisions about the care of the other person. For example, they may experience feelings of guilt about not being able to meet the needs of a dependent loved one, or feelings of "playing God" with regard to decisions about mentally incompetent loved ones. In these circumstances, the provision of support, information, and reassurance from a nurse who has dealt with these decisions in professional experiences may be an effective counseling intervention. At times, information from the primary care provider may be helpful in alleviating spiritual distress associated with end-of-life decisions or decisions about long-term care. In these cases, the nurse may be able to facilitate communication between the primary care provider and the family to alleviate the spiritual distress. Some nursing interventions that address spiritual needs of older adults are listed in Box 12-3.

Promoting Wellness Through Healthy Aging Classes

When older adults need assistance in coping with specific functional consequences, or when they need education to clarify myths and misunderstandings about age-related changes, individual counseling may be the best intervention. When older adults need counseling about psychosocial adjustments, however, educational groups may be more effective. For example, nurses can develop groups that focus on education and psychological growth to teach older adults new skills and behaviors (Schneider & Cook, 2005). Common themes that nurses can address through group education include resources, independence, loss of family and friends, and physical and cognitive impairments (Toseland & Rizzo, 2004).

An example of a nurse-led group intervention that allows for sharing of experiences among peers is the healthy aging class, developed by this author and used successfully during two decades in a variety of settings with older adults at various functional levels. This model is based on the belief that older adults who are beginning to recognize age-related physical and psychosocial changes or who are already dealing with such changes can benefit from sharing their experiences with their peers. Nurses can use this model, which is described in detail, to enhance the coping skills of older adults who are adjusting to any of the challenges of older adulthood.

Goals

Goals for older adults who participate in healthy aging classes are as follows:

- Recognize the impact of common age-related physical and psychosocial changes.
- Support and encourage any effective coping mechanisms already being used.
- Develop new skills that could be effective for coping with current stressors.
- Obtain information that will facilitate problem-focused coping mechanisms for stressful situations that are amenable to change.
- Provide an opportunity for the sharing of similar experiences with peers.

Setting

Nurses in any setting can initiate healthy aging classes, but long-term care institutions are perhaps the most conducive setting for the following reasons:

- Nurses have many opportunities to establish and lead groups.
- Residents of long-term care facilities provide a captive audience from which to select group members.

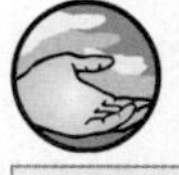

Box 12-3
Nursing Interventions to Address Spiritual Needs

Therapeutic Communication Interventions

- Use verbal and nonverbal communication to establish trust and convey empathic caring.
- Use active supportive listening.
- Convey nonjudgmental attitudes.
- Communicate respect for individuality.
- Provide a supportive presence.
- Be open to expressions of feelings such as fear, anger, loneliness, and powerlessness.
- Honor a person's integrity.
- Support the person in his or her feeling of being loved by others and by a higher power (e.g., God, Allah, Jehovah).
- Encourage verbalization of feelings about meaning of illness.
- Provide positive feedback about faith, courage, sense of humor, and other such feelings and experiences.
- Encourage discussion of events and relationships that provide spiritual support.

Actions to Foster Religious and Spiritual Activities

- Facilitate referrals for visits from religious care providers and sources of spiritual care (clergy, rabbis, church members, spiritual directors).
- Facilitate participation in religious services or activities (e.g., tapes, readings, videos, observations of "holy days").
- Assist with obtaining requested religious items (books, music, statues).
- Provide quiet and private time for individual spiritual or religious activities (e.g., prayer, reflection, meditation, guided imagery).
- Provide necessary support for religious rituals (e.g., lighting candles, receiving communion, praying the rosary).
- Encourage participation in relaxing and enjoyable activities (art, music, nature).

Interventions for Specific Circumstances

- Provide support and care during times of suffering.
- Assist in the process of dying.
- Assist a person who is fearful of the future.
- Provide care for the person who feels hopeless.
- Facilitate reconciliation among family members.
- Encourage participation in support groups.

- Residents of long-term care institutions usually are not acutely ill, and they are dealing with psychosocial adjustments that are readily identified.
- Residents of long-term care settings have in common at least one major life event, which is a temporary or permanent move to a more dependent setting.

Community settings also are conducive to successful healthy aging classes, but nurses may have to be more creative in gathering the group members. Nurses who provide health services or education programs for senior centers or assisted-living facilities might be able to establish ongoing healthy aging classes as part of their responsibilities. In these settings, a healthy aging class may be an efficient, as well as effective, way of providing health education using a format that has the additional advantage of enhancing coping mechanisms.

In acute care settings, nurses usually do not plan and implement group therapies, but in rehabilitative settings, nurses may have the opportunity to initiate healthy aging classes. In psychiatric units, often there are enough older adults among the patients to warrant the implementation of healthy aging classes as a form of group therapy.

Membership Criteria

The primary criteria for group membership are that the person be willing to acknowledge age-related changes and be capable of acquiring insight into his or her adjustment to these changes. This author has led groups ranging from highly functional older adults in community settings to seriously impaired older adults in a hospital-based medical geropsychiatric unit. Group members may be coping with similar psychosocial stresses, but this is not necessarily a criterion for participation. For example, a healthy aging class can comprise older adults who all have some degree of depression or who are coping with a particular stressful event, such as widowhood. An ideal group includes members who are coping with various life events commonly associated with older adulthood and who are motivated to learn effective coping styles.

The group works best if the membership is stable and closed, but this is not always possible. A disadvantage of an open group is that it is very difficult to develop cohesiveness. If the membership is open and changing, the leader must be more directive, and the group as a whole will not be able to establish ongoing priorities for discussion topics. In addition, with changing membership, the leader has to focus more attention on the exchange of information about group members at the beginning of each session.

Size of Group and Length, Duration, and Frequency of Sessions

Although group size can range from 5 to 12 members, the ideal is about 8 members. Groups can be either ongoing or time-limited. When the membership is changing, such as in acute or rehabilitative settings, sessions can be an ongoing mode of therapy. In long-term care or community settings, it is best to schedule group meetings for a predetermined length of time, such as 8 to 10 weeks, and allow for changes in membership at the end of each period. One-hour sessions are held at weekly intervals, at a consistent time and place. In community settings, it can be helpful to convene the groups in conjunction with a meal program because participants will already have social relationships. As in institutional settings, a community center offers an audience from which to select the group members. Other potential community-based sites include assisted-living facilities and group settings, such as adult care homes (also called board-and-care homes).

Criteria for and Responsibilities of Group Leaders

One nurse can lead group sessions, but it is often helpful to have a co-leader who has had social service training. An older adult who has made a positive psychosocial adjustment and who can serve as a role model also can be a good co-leader. The nurse must be able to clarify myths and misunderstandings about age-related changes and be skilled in group dynamics. As with the reminiscence group, the healthy aging class is not an intense psychotherapy session; therefore, the group leader is not required to be specially trained in mental health. To lead a healthy aging class, however, a good understanding of both the physiologic and psychosocial aspects of aging is essential.

The primary responsibilities of the group leaders are to facilitate the discussion of psychosocial adjustments of older adulthood and to provide feedback and clarification to the members. As with other groups, the leader must ensure that all members have an opportunity to participate and that the members attend to the identified topic. The leaders also must ensure that the group reaches some conclusions before the end of each session so that members leave with a feeling of accomplishment relating to at least one psychosocial challenge of older adulthood.

Format

As in all educational groups, the leader begins with an explanation of the purpose of the group and an introduction of the leaders and members. The leader also reviews the details of the sessions, such as their length, the duration of the group, the role of the leader, and the expectations of the members. After addressing questions and introductory material, the leader introduces the concepts of life events and adjustments to the challenges of older adulthood. The leader can use a statement similar to the following: "Throughout life, certain events are likely to occur that affect us emotionally. These events may involve our health, our personal relationships, the place where we live, our job or career responsibilities and opportunities, or other events that require an adjustment on our part. These are called major life events, and they often occur at certain points of life. To begin our discussion today, let's look at some of the major life events that are likely to occur in younger adulthood, around the age of 20 to 30 years." The group then identifies various life events, such as finding a job, moving from the family home, finding a partner, and starting a family. The leader then asks members to identify life adjustments that are likely to occur between 30 and 50 years of age.

After the members have identified these life events, the leader emphasizes that one purpose of the healthy aging class is to identify effective ways of addressing the challenges inherent in the life events of older adulthood. The term *challenges* is used to communicate an active mode of addressing issues. The leader may want to discuss the phrase "challenges of older adulthood" and allow the group members to comment on what they see as challenges in their lives. As the members identify the life events of older adulthood, the leader writes the events on a board or paper so all the members can see the list. The leader can then ask about life events that the members think they are likely to experience in the next few years. As events are identified, the members also are asked to identify the consequences of the events that require an adjustment. Examples of these life events and consequences have been discussed earlier in this chapter, and they are summarized in Figure 12-1. If group members do not identify all the life events, the leader may ask about a certain event, such as coping with one's own or a spouse's retirement. This discussion should continue until all the events and consequences in Figure 12-1 have been identified.

If the group is ongoing and has a stable membership, the leader may devote the majority of the first meeting to this discussion. The leader should emphasize that the rest of the meetings will be devoted to discussions of the identified issues, and that the first meeting will set the stage for future sessions. If the group is open and has a changing membership, the leader may need to be more directive during this first phase in order to limit the time spent on this topic. With changing membership, this initial identification of issues would be limited to the first 20 to 30 minutes. The group can then discuss coping mechanisms for one specific issue during the latter half of the meeting.

After the issues are identified, the leader summarizes the discussion, referring to the list of challenges written for the members to see. The members then share ideas about coping strategies that they have found to be helpful in adjusting to these changes. The leader may begin this part with a statement such as, "Now that we've identified the challenges of older adulthood, let's look at what things are helpful in responding to these challenges. I'd like each of you to share with the group one thing you do to help yourself face difficult challenges." After members have identified general coping mechanisms, the leader can suggest that the group choose one specific life event of older adulthood and discuss coping mechanisms that are helpful for addressing this challenge. Examples of coping strategies that might be discussed in relation to specific life events are summarized in Table 12-3. As these coping strategies are identified, they should be written on a board, and members should be encouraged to relate their personal experiences.

As the cohesiveness and trust level among members increase, particularly in closed groups, the sharing of experiences may become very open and revealing. The task of the leader, then, is to keep the discussion focused on appropriate coping mechanisms. In cohesive groups with highly functional members, the leader might have an opportunity to discuss the difference between emotion-focused and problem-focused mechanisms. The depth of discussion will depend on the degree of group cohesiveness and trust, the functional level of the members, and the comfort level and willingness of the leader to deal with the identified issues.

During the last 10 minutes of each session, the leader should attempt to bring the discussion to some closure on at least one issue. This may be accomplished by summarizing the issues and coping mechanisms that were identified. In open groups, the leader would end by encouraging those members who do not return to the group to look at coping

TABLE 12-3 Coping Strategies for the Psychosocial Challenges of Older Adulthood

Psychosocial Adjustment	Coping Strategy
Ageist stereotypes	Develop a firm self-identity, challenge the myths, question any behaviors that are based on age-determined expectations.
Retirement	Develop new skills, use time for hobbies and personal pursuits, become involved with meaningful volunteer activities.
Reduced income	Take advantage of discounts for seniors.
Declining physical health	Maintain good health practices (nutrition, exercise, rest).
Functional limitations	Adapt the environment to ensure safety and optimal functional status, take advantage of assistive devices and equipment, accept help when necessary.
Changes in cognitive skills	Take advantage of educational opportunities, enroll in classes, keep mentally stimulated, join a discussion group, use the library, avoid dwelling on the things you cannot do and focus on your abilities, take advantage of increased potential for wisdom and creativity.
Death of spouse, friends, and family members	Allow yourself to grieve appropriately, take advantage of opportunities for group or individual counseling and support, establish new relationships, renew old friendships, cherish the happy memories of the past, realize new freedoms.
Relocation from family home	Look into the broad range of options for housing, appreciate the relief from the responsibilities of home ownership, take advantage of new services and opportunities for socialization.
Other challenges to mental health	Maintain a sense of humor, use stress-reduction techniques, learn assertiveness skills, participate in support groups.

mechanisms for their own specific issues, either by themselves or with a friend or confidant(e). For ongoing groups, the leader would end the session by facilitating agreement about the issues that will be discussed during the next session. The leader also can encourage members to think about the identified issues in the interim.

EVALUATING EFFECTIVENESS OF NURSING INTERVENTIONS

Nurses evaluate the effectiveness of interventions for older adults with Self-Concept Disturbance by determining the extent to which older adults express positive views of themselves. Another measure of effective nursing care is that older adults no longer verbalize ageist attitudes. Nursing care of older adults who express a sense of Powerlessness is evaluated by the extent to which they become involved in decisions that affect them and the degree to which they express feelings of control over their lives. Nurses evaluate care for older adults with Ineffective Individual Coping by observing behaviors that reflect the use of a variety of coping strategies. For example, an older adult might learn to use problem-focused coping strategies for a situation he or she previously viewed as hopeless and unchangeable.

Mr. P. is 86 years old and has recently been admitted to a nursing facility for long-term care. His medical diagnoses are diabetes, glaucoma, retinopathy, and dementia of Alzheimer's type. Mr. P. lived with his wife until 6 months ago, when she died after a brief illness. After her death, he needed help with all his activities of daily living, and his daughter arranged home care assistance for 6 hours a day. About 1 month ago, he started getting up and wandering outside at night. Once, he wandered off at 3:00 AM, and the police had to take him home. After this episode, he was afraid to be alone, and he agreed to go to a nursing facility because he could not afford to pay for 24-hour assistance at home.

During the first week in the nursing facility, Mr. P. was cooperative with the staff and sociable with the other residents. He was resistant to the morning schedule of getting up at 6:00 AM and eating breakfast in the dining room at 7:30 AM, but he passively complied when the staff firmly directed him. His daughter visited him daily and accompanied him to social and recreational activities with other residents. Mr. P. has been in the nursing facility for 10 days, and he is becoming very resistant to staff efforts to get him dressed for breakfast. When he attends group activities, he is disruptive, yelling about being a hostage in a monastery. Mr. P. tells other residents that he was tricked into coming to this place, and that the only reason he has to stay is because his daughter has taken over his house and is living there with her family. He frequently paces up and down the corridors and says he has to find his daughter to take him home because his wife is sick and she needs him to take care of her. You walk with him in the hallway and he says, "I don't know why they keep me locked up here. I can't do anything like I used to do at home. It's like a monastery where you have to get up in the middle of the night and they make you get cleaned up and eat breakfast when it's still dark out."

NURSING ASSESSMENT

Your nursing assessment shows that Mr. P. needs supervision in all activities of daily living because of poor vision and memory impairment. He needs some assistance with personal care, but he can dress himself if staff set his clothes out for him. When Mr. P. was admitted to the nursing facility, he was assigned to the "night shift wakers" group, which means that the night shift is responsible for waking him and getting him ready for breakfast by 7:30 AM. The night shift nursing assistants help him with showering, shaving, and dressing.

During the admission interview, Mr. P.'s daughter, Jane, said that his typical morning routine at home was to get up around 8:30 AM and get dressed independently, using the clothes that were set out for him by the home health aide. He ate breakfast around 9:30 AM and then spent the day "working on his papers." Jane, who lives out of town, would call her father four times a week. When Jane talked with him on the phone, he

(case study continues on page 222)

always told her how busy he was working on his papers. Although Jane was paying all his bills from a joint bank account, Mr. P. would spend hours and hours with bill stubs, old bank statements, and an inactive checking account, thinking he was paying his bills.

Jane was staying at her father's house for the 2 weeks before his admission and for 1 week after admission to the nursing facility. She plans to return to town for a couple of days every other month and will visit her father at those times. The only nearby relative is a sister-in-law who comes to visit Mr. P. every 2 weeks.

NURSING DIAGNOSIS

You use the nursing diagnosis of Powerlessness related to relocation to a nursing facility and lack of control over activities of daily living. You select this diagnosis, rather than Impaired Adjustment or Ineffective Individual Coping, because Mr. P. focuses on a theme of loss of control. Your assessment identifies several factors that contribute to his powerlessness, and you address these factors in your nursing care plan.

NURSING CARE PLAN FOR MR. P.

Expected Outcome	Nursing Interventions	Nursing Evaluation
Mr. P. will feel he has greater control over his morning schedule.	• Take Mr. P. off the "night-shift wakers" list and allow him to sleep until 8 AM. • Allow Mr. P. to wear his pajamas and robe to breakfast and to shower, bathe, and dress after breakfast.	• Mr. P. will no longer verbalize feelings of being locked up in a monastery or a prison.
Mr. P. will function as independently as possible.	• The staff will set out Mr. P.'s clothing and allow him to dress himself. • The staff will give Mr. P. positive feedback for dressing himself.	• Mr. P. will dress himself with minimal supervision. • Mr. P. will carry out his personal care activities at a pace that is comfortable for him.
Mr. P. will engage in a familiar activity that gives him a meaningful role.	• Ask Jane to send a set of bill stubs, old bank statements, and the inactive checkbook so that Mr. P. can do his "work." • Encourage Mr. P. to "work with his papers" in the activity room, where he can interact with other residents. • Give Mr. P. positive feedback when he interacts with other residents. • Compliment Mr. P. about doing his paperwork.	• Mr. P. will resume his former routine of working with his papers and will interact with other residents.

Chapter Highlights

Life Events: The Age-Related Changes Affecting Psychosocial Function (Fig. 12-1)

- Retirement
- Relocation
- Chronic illness and functional impairments
- Decisions about driving a car
- Widowhood
- Death of family and friends
- Ageist attitudes

Theories About Psychosocial Function in Older Adults

- High capacity for emotional complexity
- Stokes/Gordon Stress Scale (Table 12-1) can be used to identify stress level
- Coping styles vary depending on type of stress
- Social supports are an important resource for coping

Factors That Influence Psychosocial Function in Older Adults

- Religion and spirituality are increasingly important resources for older adults
- Cultural differences influence definitions of health and illness and normal and abnormal behaviors (Cultural Considerations 12-1)
- Culture-bound syndromes: culturally specific disorders associated with psychosocial characteristics of a particular group (Table 12-2)

Risks Factors That Affect Psychosocial Wellness

- Physical, functional, and psychosocial health significantly affect coping skills

- The ability accurately to appraise a situation affects psychosocial function
- Learned helplessness results when uncontrollable events reinforce the idea that future events will also be uncontrollable

Functional Consequences Associated With Psychosocial Function
- Negative functional consequences include anxiety, loneliness, depression, cognitive impairment
- Positive emotions and characteristics are associated with emotional well-being (e.g., joy, happiness, satisfaction, purpose in life, sense of mastery)

Nursing Assessment of Psychosocial Function (refer to Chapter 13)

Nursing Diagnosis
- Self-Esteem Disturbance
- Situational Low Self-Esteem (or Risk for)
- Powerlessness
- Impaired Adjustment
- Social Isolation
- Readiness for Enhanced Coping
- Readiness for Enhanced Self-Concept

Planning for Wellness Outcomes
- Psychosocial Adjustment: Life Change
- Adaptation to Physical Disability
- Personal Autonomy
- Self-Esteem
- Quality of Life

Nursing Interventions for Psychosocial Wellness
- Enhancing self-esteem: improving functioning, using verbal and nonverbal communication, avoiding elderspeak
- Promoting a sense of control: providing information, rephrasing events, addressing threats such as lack of privacy and loss of individuality
- Involving older adults in decision making: challenging attitudes, facilitating communication, using verbal and nonverbal communication techniques
- Addressing role loss: identifying meaningful roles
- Encouraging life review and reminiscence
- Fostering social supports
- Addressing spiritual needs: communicating caring and compassion, instilling hope, referring for spiritual care, encouraging participation in religious activities
- Leading Healthy Aging classes

Evaluating Effectiveness of Nursing Interventions
- Positive self-perceptions
- Involvement in decisions
- Effective coping strategies

Critical Thinking Exercises

1. Take a sheet of paper and draw two vertical lines to make three equal columns. Think of someone you know in your personal life or professional practice who is 80 years old or older. In the left column, list three or more life events that this person has experienced in later adulthood. In the center column, describe the impact of the life event on the person's daily life. In the right column, list the coping mechanisms the person has used to deal with the life event. You can guess at the information, as needed, to complete the information in the center and right columns.
2. Think of a recent life event in your own life and answer the following questions: How close in time was the life event to other stressful events in your life? What impact did the life event have, and what were the manifestations of stress in your life (e.g., in your work, your health, your personal life, your relationships with other people)? What coping mechanisms did you use? Were the coping mechanisms effective? What coping mechanisms would you like to develop to prepare yourself for older adulthood?
3. You are asked to lead a 1-hour discussion titled "Mental Health and Aging" for a group of 10 people at a senior citizen center. Describe your approach to this topic. What would your goals for the class be? How would you involve the participants? What visual aids would you use?

Educational Resources

National Senior Service Corps
www.seniorcorps.org

Stokes/Gordon Stress Scale
Pace University, Leinhard School of Nursing
(914) 773–3200
www.pace.edu

References

Aldrich, C., & Mendkoff, E. (1963). Relocation of the aged and disabled: A mortality study. *Journal of the American Geriatrics Society, 11*, 185–194.

Aldwin, D. F., Hofer, S. M., & McCammon, R. J. (2006). Modeling the effects of time: Integrating demographic and developmental perspectives. In R. H. Binstock & L. K. George (Eds.), *Handbook of aging and the social sciences* (6th ed., pp. 20–40). San Diego: Academic Press.

American Association of Retired Persons (AARP). (1997). *Mental health issues for minority seniors*. Washington, DC: Author.

Andrews, M. M. (2003). Cultural competence in the health history and physical examination. In M. M. Andrews, & J. S. Boyle (Eds.), *Transcultural concepts in nursing care* (4th ed., pp. 36–72.). Philadelphia: Lippincott Williams & Wilkins.

Andrews, M. M., & Boyle, J. S. (Eds.). (2003). *Transcultural concepts in nursing care* (4th ed.). Philadelphia: Lippincott Williams & Wilkins.

Andrews, M. M., & Hanson, P. A. (2003). Religion, culture, and nursing. In M. M. Andrews & J. S. Boyle (Eds.), *Transcultural concepts in nursing care* (4th ed., pp. 432–502). Philadelphia: Lippincott Williams & Wilkins.

Antonucci, T. C. (2001). Social relations: An examination of social networks, social support, and sense of control. In J. E. Birren & K. W. Schaie (Eds.), *Handbook of the psychology of aging* (5th ed., pp. 427–453). San Diego: Academic Press.

Aranda, M. P., & Knight, B. G. (1997). The influence of ethnicity and culture on the caregiver's stress and coping process: A sociocultural review and analysis. *The Gerontologist, 37*, 342–354.

Armer, J. M., & Conn, V. S. (2001). Exploration of spirituality and health among diverse rural elderly individuals. *Journal of Gerontological Nursing, 27*(6), 28–37.

Ashman, O., Shiomura, K., & Levy, B. R. (2006). Influence of culture and age on control beliefs: The missing link of interdependence. *International Journal of Aging and Human Development, 62*, 143–157.

Bianchi, E. (2005). Living with elder wisdom. *Religion, Spirituality, and Aging: A Social Work Perspective, 45*, 319–329.

Birkenmaier, J., Behrman, G., & Berg-Weger, M. (2005). Integrating curriculum and practice with students and their field supervisors: Reflections on spirituality and the aging (Rosa) model. *Educational Gerontology, 31*, 745–763.

Blazer, D. G. (2002). Self-efficacy and depression in late life: A primary prevention proposal. *Aging & Mental Health, 6*, 315–324.

Borg, C., Hallberg, I. R., & Blomquist, K. (2006). Life satisfaction among older people (65+) with reduced self-care capacity: The relationship to social, health and financial aspects. *Journal of Clinical Nursing, 15*, 607–618.

Borglin, G., Edberg, A.-K., & Hallberg, I. R. (2005). The experience of quality of life among older people. *Journal of Aging Studies, 19*, 201–220.

Boyle, J. S. (2003a). Culture, family, and community. In M. M. Andrews & J. S. Boyle (Eds.), *Transcultural concepts in nursing care* (4th ed., pp. 315–360). Philadelphia: Lippincott Williams & Wilkins.

Boyle, J. S. (2003b). Transcultural perspectives in the nursing care of adults. In M. M. Andrews & J. S. Boyle (Eds.), *Transcultural concepts in nursing care* (4th ed., pp. 181–208). Philadelphia: Lippincott Williams & Wilkins.

Butler, R. N. (2001). Life review. In M. D. Mezey (Ed.), *The encyclopedia of elder care* (pp. 401–402). New York: Springer.

Carpenito-Moyet, L. J. (2006). *Handbook of nursing diagnosis* (11th ed.). Philadelphia: Lippincott Williams & Wilkins.

Carr, D., House, J. S., Wortman, C., Nesse, R., & Kessler, R. C. (2001). Psychological adjustment to sudden and anticipated spousal loss among older widowed persons. *Journals of Gerontology: Series B, Psychological Sciences and Social Sciences, 56*, S237–S248.

Carstensen, L. L., Mikels, J. A., & Mather, M. (2006). Aging and the intersection of cognition, motivation, and emotion. In J. E. Birren & K. W. Schaie (Eds.), *Handbook of the psychology of aging* (6th ed., pp. 343–362). San Diego: Academic Press.

Chao, S.-Y., Liu, H.-Y., Wu, C.-Y., Jin, S.-F., Chu, T.-L., Huang, T.-S., et al. (2006). The effects of group reminiscence therapy on depression, self esteem, and life satisfaction of elderly nursing home residents. *Journal of Nursing Research, 14*, 36–45.

Crowther, M. R., Parker, M. W., Achenbaum, W. A., Larimore, W. L., & Koenig, H. G. (2002). Rowe and Kahn's model of successful aging revisited: Positive spirituality— the forgotten factor. *The Gerontologist, 42*, 613–620.

DiBartolo, M. C. (2002). Exploring self-efficacy and hardiness in spousal caregivers of individuals with dementia. *Journal of Gerontological Nursing, 28*(4), 24–33.

Fakouri, C., & Lyon, B. (2005). Perceived health and life satisfaction among older adults: The effects of worry and personal variables. *Journal of Gerontological Nursing, 31*(10), 17–24.

Faulkner, M. (2001). The onset and alleviation of learned helplessness in older hospitalized people. *Aging & Mental Health, 5*, 379–386.

Folkman, S., & Lazarus, R. S. (1980). An analysis of coping in a middle-aged community sample. *Journal of Health and Social Behavior, 21*, 219–239.

Frazier, L. D., Waid, L. D., & Fincke, C. (2002). Coping with anxiety in later life. *Journal of Gerontological Nursing, 28*(12), 40–47.

George, L. K. (2006). Perceived quality of life. In R. H. Binstock & L. K. George (Eds.), *Handbook of aging and the social sciences* (6th ed., pp. 320–336). San Diego: Academic Press.

Haight, B. K. (2000). The extended effects of life review in nursing home residents. *International Journal of Aging and Human Development, 50*, 151–168.

Holmes, T. H., & Rahe, R. H. (1967). The social readjustment rating scale. *Journal of Psychosomatic Research, 11*, 213–218.

Idler, E. (2006). Religion and aging. In R. H. Binstock & L. K. George (Eds.), *Handbook of aging and the social sciences* (6th ed., pp. 277–300). San Diego: Academic Press.

Jacelon, C. S. (2004). Older adults and autonomy in acute care: Increasing patients' independence and control during hospitalization. *Journal of Gerontological Nursing, 30*(11), 29–36.

Jang, Y., Haley, W. E., Small, B. J., & Mortimer, J. A. (2002). The role of mastery and social resources in the associations between disability and depression in later life. *The Gerontologist, 42*, 807–813.

Johnson, M., Bulechek, G. M., Dochterman, J. M., Maas, M. L., Moorhead, S., Swanson, E., et al. (2006). *NANDA, NOC, and NIC linkages* (2nd ed.). St. Louis: Mosby Elsevier.

Johnson, R. A., & Tripp-Reimer, T. (2001). Relocation among ethnic elders. *Journal of Gerontological Nursing, 27*(6), 22–27.

Jopp, D., & Smith, J. (2006). Resources and life-management strategies as determinants of successful aging: On the protective effect of selection, optimization, and compensation. *Psychology and Aging, 21*, 253–265.

Kavanagh, K. H. (2003). Transcultural perspectives in mental health nursing. In M. M. Andrews & J. S. Boyle (Eds.), *Transcultural concepts in nursing care* (4th ed., pp. 272–314). Philadelphia: Lippincott Williams & Wilkins.

Kim, J. E., & Moen, P. (2002). Retirement transitions, gender, and psychological well-being: A life course, ecological model. *Journals of Gerontology: Series B, Psychological Sciences and Social Sciences, 57*, P212–P222.

Kirby, S. E., Coleman, P. G., & Daley, D. (2004). Spirituality and well-being in frail and nonfrail older adults. *Journals of Gerontology: Series B, Psychological Sciences and Social Sciences, 59*, P123–P129.

Kirmayer, L. J., & Groleau, D. (2001). Affective disorders in cultural context. *Psychiatric Clinics of North America, 24*, 465–478.

Krause, N. (2001). Social support. In R. H. Binstock & L. K. George (Eds.), *Handbook of aging and the social sciences* (5th ed., pp. 272–294). San Diego: Academic Press.

Krause, N. (2006a). Exploring the stress-buffering effects of church-based and secular social support on self-rated health in late life. *Journals of Gerontology: Series B, Psychological Sciences and Social Sciences, 61*, S35–S43.

Krause, N. (2006b). Religion and health in late life. In J. E. Birren & K. W. Schaie (Eds.), *Handbook of the psychology of aging* (6th ed., pp. 499–518). San Diego: Academic Press.

Lazarus, R. S. (1966). *Psychological stress and the coping process.* New York: McGraw-Hill.

Litwin, H., & Shiovitz-Ezra, S. (2006). The association between activity and wellbeing in later life: What really matters? *Ageing and Society, 26*, 225–242.

Longino, C. F., & Bradley, D. E. (2006). Internal and international migration. In R. H. Binstock & L. K. George (Eds.), *Handbook of aging and the social sciences* (6th ed., pp. 76–93). San Diego: Academic Press.

Marsiske, M., & Margrett, J. A. (2006). Everyday problem solving and decision making. In J. E. Birren & K. W. Schaie (Eds.), *Handbook of the psychology of aging* (6th ed., pp. 315–342). San Diego: Academic Press.

McReynolds, J. L., & Rossen, E. K. (2004). Importance of physical activity, nutrition, and social support for optimal aging. *Clinical Nurse Specialist, 18*, 200–205.

Mezzich, J. E., Berganze, C. E., & Ruiperez, M. A. (2001). Culture in DSM-IV, ICD-10, and evolving diagnostic systems. *Psychiatric Clinics of North America, 24*, 407–419.

Nygren, B., Alex, L., Jonsen, E., Gustafson, Y., Norberg, A., & Lundman, B. (2005). Resilience, sense of coherence, purpose in life and self-transcendence in relation to perceived physical and mental health among the oldest old. *Aging & Mental Health, 9*, 354–362.

Ong, A., D., & Bergeman, C. S. (2004). The complexity of emotions in later life. *Journals of Gerontology: Series B, Psychological Sciences and Social Sciences, 59*, P117–P122.

Østbye, T., Krause, K. M., Norton, N. C., Tschanz, J., Sanders, L., Hayden, K., et al. (2006). Ten dimensions of health and their relationship with overall self-reported health and survival in a predominantly religiously active elderly population: The Cache County Memory Study. *Journal of the American Geriatrics Society, 54*, 199–209.

Phillips, L. H., Henry, J. D., Hosie, J. A., & Milne, A. B. (2006). Age, anger regulation and well-being. *Aging & Mental Health, 10*, 250–256.

Reitzes, D. C., & Mutran, E. J. (2006). Self and health: Factors that encourage self-esteem and functional health. *Journals of Gerontology: Series B, Psychological Sciences and Social Sciences, 61*, S44–S51.

Riediger, M., Li, S.-C., & Lindenberger, U. (2006). Selection, optimization, and compensation as developmental mechanisms of adaptive resource allocation: Review and preview. In J. E. Birren & K. W. Schaie (Eds.), *Handbook of the psychology of aging* (6th ed., pp. 289–313). San Diego: Academic Press.

Robinson, T., & Umphery, D. (2006). First- and third-person perceptions of images of older people in advertising: An inter-generational evaluation. *International Journal of Aging and Human Development, 62*, 159–173.

Rodin, J., & Langer, E. (1980). Aging labels: The decline of control and the fall of self-esteem. *Journal of Social Issues, 36*(2), 12–29.

Sarkisian, C. A., Hays, R. D., & Mangione, C. M. (2002). Do older adults expect to age successfully? The association between expectations regarding aging and beliefs regarding healthcare seeking among older adults. *Journal of the American Geriatrics Society, 50*, 1837–1843.

Schneider, J. K., & Cook, J. H. (2005). Planning psychoeducational groups. *Journal of Gerontological Nursing, 31*(8), 33–38.

Selye, H. (1956). *The stress of life*. New York: McGraw-Hill.

Settersten, R. A. (2006). Aging and the life course. In R. H. Binstock & L. K. George (Eds.), *Handbook of aging and the social sciences* (6th ed., pp. 3–19). San Diego: Academic Press.

Shawler, C., Rowles, G. D., & High, D. M. (2001). Analysis of key decision making incidents in the life of a nursing home resident. *The Gerontologist, 5*, 612–622.

Sparks, M., Zehr, D., & Painter, B. (2004). Predictors of life satisfaction. *Journal of Gerontological Nursing, 30*(8), 47–53.

Spurlock, W. R. (2005). Spiritual well-being and caregiver burden in Alzheimer's caregivers. *Geriatric Nursing, 26*, 154–161.

Stevens, N. L., Martina, C. M. S., & Westerhof, G. J. (2006). Meeting the need to belong: Predicting effects of a friendship enrichment program for older women. *The Gerontologist, 46*, 495–502.

Steverink, N., Westerhof, G. J., Bode, C., & Dittmann-Kohli, F. (2001). The personal experience of aging, individual resources, and subjective well-being. *Journals of Gerontology: Series B, Psychological Sciences and Social Sciences, 56*, P364–P373.

Stokes, S. A., & Gordon, S. E. (1988). Development of an instrument to measure stress in the older adult. *Nursing Research, 37*, 16–19.

Stone, R. I. (2006). Emerging issues in long term care. In R. H. Binstock & L. K. George (Eds.), *Handbook of aging and the social sciences* (6th ed., pp. 397–418). San Diego: Academic Press.

Thornton, R., & Light, L. L. (2006). Language comprehension and production in normal aging. In J. E. Birren & K. W. Schaie (Eds.), *Handbook of the psychology of aging* (6th ed., pp. 261–287). San Diego: Academic Press.

Toseland, R. W., & Rizzo, V. M. (2004). What's different about working with older people in groups? *Group Work and Aging: Issues in Practice, Research, and Education, 44*, 5–23.

Tracy, J. P., & DeYoung, S. (2004). Moving to an assisted living facility: Exploring the transitional experience of elderly individuals. *Journal of Gerontological Nursing, 30*(10), 26–33.

Tuck, I., Alleyne, R., & Thinganjana, W. (2006). Spirituality and stress management in healthy adults. *Journal of Holistic Nursing, 24*, 245–253.

Tyler, K. A. (2006). The impact of support received and support provision of changes in perceived social support among older adults. *International Journal of Aging and Human Development, 62*,,21–28.

Weaver, A. J., Flannelly, L. T., & Flannelly, K. J. (2001). A review of research on religious and spiritual variables in two primary gerontological nursing journals. *Journal of Gerontological* Nursing, *27*(9), 47–54.

Williams, K., Kemper, S., & Hummert, M. L. (2004). Enhancing communication with older adults. *Journal of Gerontological Nursing, 30*(10), 17–25.

Young, H. M., & Cochrane, B. B. (2004). Healthy aging for older women. *Nursing Clinics of North America, 39*, 131–143.

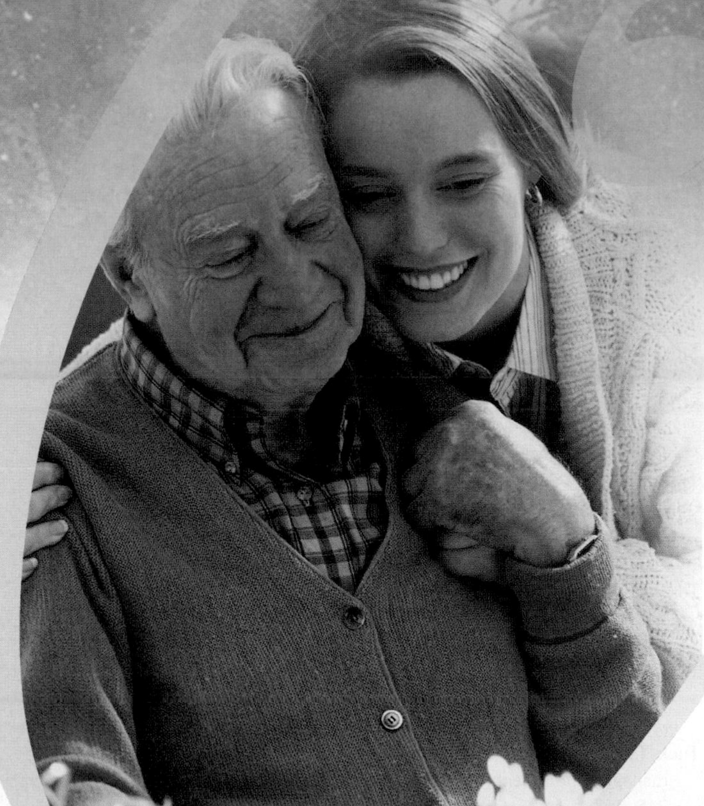

CHAPTER 13

Psychosocial Assessment

Learning Objectives

After reading this chapter, you will be able to:

1. Describe the psychosocial assessment of older adults in terms of purpose, procedure, and scope.
2. Describe barriers to communication and communication techniques that are helpful for conducting a psychosocial assessment.
3. Describe how to assess each of the following specific components of mental status: physical appearance, motor function, social skills, response to the interview, orientation, alertness, memory, speech characteristics, calculation and higher language skills, and decision making.
4. Explain how to perform a nursing assessment of skills involved with decision-making capacity and executive function of older adults.
5. Describe how to assess each of the following components of affective function: mood, anxiety, self-esteem, depression, happiness, and well-being.
6. Discuss distinguishing characteristics of delusions, hallucinations, and illusions as they relate to the underlying conditions common in older adults.
7. Explain how to perform a nursing assessment of the following aspects of social supports: social network, barriers to services, and economic resources.
8. Explain how to perform a nursing assessment of spiritual needs of older adults, including factors that cause spiritual distress as well as those that promote spiritual wellness.

Key Terms

abstract thinking
affect
akathisia
anxiety
circumstantiality
confabulation
delusions
denial
emotional lability
executive function
hallucinations
illusions
insight
judgment
paranoia
problem-solving abilities
social supports

Psychosocial assessment is a complex and challenging—but essential—aspect of nursing care of older adults. Although psychosocial impairments are often attributed to factors relating to normal aging or to untreatable conditions, a careful psychosocial assessment can identify the underlying cause(s) of mental changes, many of which can then be reversed or addressed through interventions. Thus, nurses can use assessment skills to improve quality of life for older adults by ensuring that psychosocial issues are identified and addressed. This chapter provides information on the assessment component of the nursing process related to cognitive and psychosocial function (Chapters 11 and 12). In addition, it is intended to supplement assessment information in other chapters of this text, particularly the chapters on elder abuse (Chapter 10), dementia (Chapter 14), and depression (Chapter 15).

OVERVIEW OF PSYCHOSOCIAL ASSESSMENT OF OLDER ADULTS

In contrast to physical and functional assessment procedures, which are viewed as routine measures to identify causes of troublesome symptoms, psychosocial assessment procedures are commonly perceived as formal psychological tests that analyze personality traits or identify the need for psychiatric treatment. Consequently, health care professionals may overlook the psychosocial component of assessment or relegate it to the realm of psychiatry. However, an assessment of psychosocial function is an essential component of holistic nursing care that addresses the body–mind–spirit needs of older adults.

This chapter focuses on those aspects of psychosocial function that are pertinent to caring for older adults from a wellness perspective. This comprehensive perspective is like the emergency cart that is available in every hospital unit. The cart stands ready at all times and is equipped with any items that would be needed to handle medical emergencies. When a serious medical problem arises, health care professionals quickly pull the cart to the patient's bedside and select the needed items. Similarly, nurses must have access to an array of skills for assessing psychosocial function as the need arises. In a few situations, their entire array of skills will be called into play, but in most situations, only a few of the examination tools will be necessary. Nurses can use the material in this chapter to "fill their mental status assessment carts" so they are prepared to select the appropriate tools for each situation.

The first sections of this chapter cover the purposes, procedures, and scope of a psychosocial assessment and are applicable to nursing care of all older adults. The second major section reviews unique aspects of communicating with older adults, and applies the concepts to psychosocial assessment. Each of the following components, which nurses would selectively assess depending on the individual situation, are discussed in separate sections: mental status, decision making and executive function, affective function, contact with reality, and social supports. Nurses can use the assessment boxes as a guide to observations and communication techniques pertinent to each aspect of psychosocial assessment.

Purposes of the Psychosocial Assessment Process

From a wellness perspective, purposes of psychosocial assessment include the following:

- Detecting asymptomatic or unacknowledged health problems at an early stage
- Identifying signs or symptoms of psychosocial dysfunction (e.g., anxiety, depression, memory problems, depression, change in mental status)
- Identifying stressors and other risk factors (especially those that are amenable to interventions) that affect cognitive, emotional, or social function
- Obtaining information about the person's usual personality, coping mechanisms, and cognitive abilities
- Identifying social supports and other coping resources that could be supported or strengthened
- Identifying the older adult's personal goals for psychosocial wellness

As with other types of assessment, nurses use this information to plan interventions that are based on realistic expectations.

When the nursing assessment identifies mental changes in an older adult, a multidisciplinary approach is important for further assessment and implementation of effective interventions. A common mistake is to label the changes as "normal for the person's age." This not only is unfair to the older adult, but can be detrimental, especially if a treatable underlying condition is overlooked or appropriate interventions to improve functional abilities are neglected. As should be clear from the discussion of cognitive function in Chapter 11, age-related cognitive changes are rarely brought to the attention of health care professionals. For example, an older adult would be unlikely to describe the following complaint: "I know I can learn new information, but I don't seem to be able to comprehend information as quickly as I used to." When mental changes are noted by other people or brought to the attention of health care professionals it is more likely that they arise from a pathologic process than from age-related processes. Therefore, whenever changes in psychosocial function are identified, health care professionals must make every effort to identify the underlying cause.

Procedure for the Psychosocial Assessment

Nurses obtain psychosocial assessment information by interviewing older adults and their caregivers and by observing older adults in their environments. Opportunities for performing psychosocial assessments vary in different health care settings, and nurses obtain much of the assessment information informally during the course of their usual care. In acute care settings, nurses perform an assessment at the time of admission to establish a baseline for planning nursing care. Although the initial nursing assessment focuses on the patient's immediate needs, nurses should not overlook the psychosocial assessment because it often provides clues to the causes of existing medical problems. Thus, as soon as the patient's condition is medically stable, the nurse begins addressing psychosocial issues as an important component of holistic care and discharge planning. In long-term care settings, psychosocial assessment information is obtained as an ongoing part of care and is commonly addressed in team conferences. When nurses provide care in home and community settings, they can obtain valuable psychosocial assessment information by observing the interactions between older adults and their caregivers and environments.

In addition to interviewing and observing older adults, nurses obtain psychosocial assessment information from other sources. For example, when the older person's cognitive function is compromised, it is essential to obtain information from family members and others who can provide a reliable history of the mental changes. In long-term care settings, nursing assistants, who are usually the health care workers who spend the most time with residents, are an important source of psychosocial information. Nursing assistants generally are not included in team discussions when psychosocial problems are addressed, but nurses can obtain information from them and incorporate it in the care plans.

The tools for an effective psychosocial assessment are a trusting relationship, a listening ear, an intuitive mind, a sensitive heart, and good communication skills. Although nurses routinely provide patient care involving physically intimate activities, such as bathing, they may be less confident about having the skills to discuss psychosocial function, especially if it involves emotionally charged issues that would not normally be discussed with strangers. Moreover, older adults may feel threatened by psychosocial assessment questions, especially if they are trying to cover up cognitive deficits. Thus, both the nurse and the older adult initially may feel uncomfortable during a psychosocial assessment. Because increased awareness of one's own attitudes is an important first step in becoming comfortable in performing a psychosocial assessment, nurses can use a self-assessment guide (Box 13-1) to examine their own attitudes about older adults and identify areas of discomfort.

The nurse begins a psychosocial assessment by explaining the purpose of the questions with a statement like one of the following:

- "I'd like to get to know you better so we can make the best plans for follow-up after you leave the hospital."
- "I'd like to ask you some questions about your interests so we can plan for your care while you're here at the nursing facility."
- "I'd like to ask some questions about how you manage from day to day so we can identify any community services that might be helpful to you."

Nurses can ask initially about events of the remote past, such as where the person was born and grew up, as a nonthreatening way of leading into further questions about psychosocial function. Nurses may believe that it is unprofessional to talk about themselves, but incorporating some personal information in conversations can facilitate the establishment of a trusting relationship. Offering a little information about their own pets or family, for instance, might encourage the older adult to share feelings that they might not mention otherwise and may help to establish a framework of mutual interest. Sharing information about ethnic background also can be an effective and nonthreatening way of obtaining information about possible cultural influences.

If formal mental status assessment questions are asked, they can be introduced after the older adult is more comfortable discussing psychosocial issues. Because questions about memory can be very threatening, the topic might be introduced as follows: "I notice you have a hard time remembering dates. Have you noticed any other problems with your memory? Is it okay with you if I ask some questions about your memory?" If no evidence of cognitive impairment is evident, but other people have expressed concern about the person's memory, a statement such as the following might be used: "Your daughter is concerned that you don't remember to keep appointments. Have you noticed any problems with your memory? Is it okay with you if I ask some questions about your memory?"

Scope of the Psychosocial Assessment

Nurses holistically address psychosocial needs of older adults by identifying the unique meaning of events, with

Box 13-1
Self-Assessment of Attitudes About Psychosocial Aspects of Aging

What is my level of comfort in discussing psychosocial issues with older adults?

- How comfortable am I discussing emotional, cultural, spiritual, and psychosocial subjects?
- Are there certain topics with which I am uncomfortable (e.g., death, suicide, alcoholism, sexuality, spirituality, terminal illness, abusive relationships)?
- Does the person's age influence my degree of comfort (e.g., Am I more comfortable discussing issues with someone who is in their 60s than with someone who is in their 90s?)
- Does the person's gender influence my degree of comfort?
- To what groups of older adults do I find it easy or difficult to relate?
- How do I feel about older adults who are single, divorced, widowed, separated, or living together in a same-sex or heterosexual but unmarried relationship?

When I was growing up …

- How were older adults treated?
- How were people with mental or emotional disorders viewed?
- What language was used to describe aging, old age, and older adults with disturbed mental function?
- What words did my family use, and what was the connotative meaning of the words used, to describe older adults? Was it positive, negative, or mixed?

What experiences have I had with older adults …

- From different racial, ethnic, and religious backgrounds?
- With functional impairments or mental, psychological, or emotional disorders?

particular emphasis on the impact of health changes, for each older adult. Nurses can focus initial questions on events that occurred many years ago because the person is likely to be quite comfortable discussing such topics. For example, a question such as "What kind of work did you do?" may prompt a discussion of feelings about retirement. Because changes in living arrangements can precipitate feelings of loss, a nonthreatening question such as "What were the circumstances of your moving here?" might lead to further discussion of the meaning of the living arrangement for that person. A question such as "Do you ever think about moving from this house?" encourages a discussion of concerns about living arrangements. People who have experienced the loss of a pet may be reluctant to acknowledge the depth of their feelings. When an older person asks the nurse a question, such as "Do you have a dog?", he or she may be indirectly testing the nurse's feelings about pets. The astute nurse will use this opportunity to explore the person's feelings about the subject, perhaps responding, "No, but I have a cat. Have you ever had any pets?" Pets may be especially significant for older adults, and, indeed, may be the only meaningful relationships that remain in their life. In planning for hospital admissions and long-term care arrangements, consideration also must be given to the person's responsibilities for and relationship with pets. Therefore, even if the person does not initiate the topic, at least one question about pets is included in the psychosocial assessment of older adults.

Diversity Note

Older adults from some Asian and African cultures may not approve of keeping dogs, cats, and other domestic animals indoors because they are considered unclean carriers of fleas, ticks, rabies, and other disease-causing organisms.

People usually are very receptive to discussing concerns about their health with a nurse because they view the nurse as someone who is knowledgeable about health problems and committed to helping people deal with these problems. For the purposes of the psychosocial assessment, however, it is important to address not only the physical aspects of health problems but also to assess the meaning of medical conditions for the person, because adjusting to and coping with medical problems and functional limitations is a common and very challenging task for many older adults. Nurses also try to identify the person's concerns about the functional consequences that are likely to be associated with illness and disability, which may be more significant to the person than the immediate medical diagnosis. For example, older adults with diabetes may be less interested in knowing how the pancreas functions than in learning to cope with the attendant visual impairment or their fear of increasing dependence on others. Therefore, rather than focusing the assessment on medically labeled problems, the nurse begins with open-ended questions about the person's self-perceptions of health and function. Rather than asking specifically about the identified problem of diabetes, the nurse might begin with a question such as "If you had to rate your health on a scale of 0% to 100%, what rating would you give it today?" After the person responds to this question, the nurse might ask additional questions, such as "What would have to be changed for you to feel 100% healthy?" or "What rating would you have given yourself a year ago?" Answers to these questions assist the nurse in assessing the impact of the illness on the person's life and in establishing realistic goals for interventions.

A Student's Perspective

I found the most successful strategy with E.H. was to ask open-ended questions and just let him go. He needed very little leading to get him to talk about what I wanted to know. I found him to be very open and willing to talk in detail about surgeries, and so forth, that I never thought he would talk about with me. I remembered to ask him how he felt during the described events, as men often leave out emotional comments in my experience. E.H. was very able to express his feelings of fear, anger, and happiness at different times when I made it clear that knowing his state of mind was important.

Charlotte L.

COMMUNICATION SKILLS FOR PSYCHOSOCIAL ASSESSMENT

Analogous to the use of a stethoscope and other tools for assessing physiologic function, nurses use skillful communication techniques as an essential tool for the psychosocial assessment. When caring for older adults, however, nurses encounter many communication barriers that make it more difficult to discuss personal information, such as feelings and life events. Thus, to perform an effective psychosocial assessment, nurses need to identify and address the barriers that commonly affect communication with older adults.

Identifying Communication Barriers

Nonverbal communication techniques are particularly important when discussing sensitive issues, but visual impairments can interfere with the older adult's ability to perceive nonverbal messages. Similarly, hearing impairment can cause discomfort for both the nurse and the older adult if they need to speak loudly about sensitive topics such as adjusting to significant losses.

External and internal distractions can interfere with the ability to focus on the conversation, particularly for older adults who are cognitively impaired. These barriers can occur in any of the following circumstances:

- Too much information being requested at one time (e.g., responding to questions about social background, cognitive abilities, and emotional function during a single interview)
- Too many people trying to communicate at one time (e.g., family members, caregivers, or more than one professional)
- Environmental noise, especially for people who use hearing aids, which usually magnify background noises
- Physical discomfort (e.g., pain, thirst, hunger, fatigue, bladder fullness, or uncomfortable temperatures)

Communication barriers can also arise from pathologic disorders and adverse medication effects. For example, neurologic conditions (e.g., aphasia from strokes) often affect language and verbal skills, and cognitive impairments can interfere with a person's ability to listen, remember, and respond to questions. Similarly, people who are actively delusional or hallucinatory, or who are not fully in touch with reality for any reason, may have difficulty attending to the conversation. Adverse medication effects that can interfere with communication include dry mouth, clouded mentation, and tardive dyskinesia (discussed in Chapter 8).

Sometimes nurses inadvertently use communication methods that are perceived as insensitive, or even uncaring, offensive, or condescending, as in the following examples:

- Giving false reassurance (e.g., "Everything's going to be okay") when the person is facing overwhelming circumstances
- Offering trite responses (e.g., "Why cry over spilled milk?") when the person is seriously depressed
- Changing the subject to avoid sensitive issues
- Jumping to conclusions
- Giving unwanted advice
- Minimizing the person's feelings
- Addressing older adults by any title other than their preferred name (e.g., using generic titles such as "dear," "honey," or "grandma")

These communication methods may interfere with the ability to develop the sense of trust that is necessary for discussing psychosocial issues.

Other verbal barriers include inarticulate speech or obstructive mannerisms, such as covering one's mouth or turning one's head away while talking. In institutional settings, much verbal communication takes place while nurses are walking down the hall, pushing a wheelchair, assisting with personal care, or performing other activities. During these activities, nurses can listen and engage in social conversation, but these are not the best times for asking personal questions or giving important information. Not only are the activities a distraction, but also they interfere with the face-to-face positioning that enhances communication and might even be essential for communication with people who are hearing impaired.

Cultural differences can create communication barriers that are difficult, and sometimes impossible, to overcome. For example, it is difficult to establish a trusting relationship when either the older adult or the nurse holds stereotypes or prejudices about the other person. Foreign-born people who have a condition that drains their energy or affects their cognitive function may revert to their native language, even if they previously spoke English well. In these situations, family members may be able to facilitate communication, or it may be appropriate to use interpreters, as discussed in Chapter 4. However, the nurse should consider the impact of the older adult's relationship with the interpreter on his or her willingness to discuss psychosocial issues openly.

Enhancing Communication With Older Adults

Because the initial tone of conversations influences further communication, nurses can use a simple introduction, if done effectively, to establish rapport. A verbal introduction is especially important for patients who have difficulty reading name tags or remembering names and for those who need assistance because it is easier to ask for help when they can address someone by name. Although checking a wristband or other identifier is an efficient and reliable way of confirming a patient's identity, it is not a substitute for exchanging names because people sometimes feel at a disadvantage if someone else knows their name when they do not know the other person's name. Rather, a more personal approach is to introduce yourself, explain your role, then ask the person his or her preferred name, and use the wristband to confirm information. The following example illustrates this kind of introduction: "Good morning, my name is Carol Miller and I'm the charge nurse today. Are you Señor Juan Garcia? You can call me Carol. What do you like to be called? I have your morning pills for you to take. Do you mind if I check your wristband first?" This approach is more likely to foster a trusting relationship than a scenario in which the nurse walks into a room, silently checks the wristband to confirm that the person is Juan Garcia, and says, "Here are your morning pills."

Touch is widely recognized as an important communication tool and is an intervention for many nursing diagnoses that are applicable to older adults, including Hopelessness, Relocation Stress Syndrome, and Sensory/Perceptual Alterations: Kinesthetic. Although older adults generally are quite receptive to touch, especially by a nurse whose responsibilities naturally entail much physical contact, cultural and gender factors can influence perceptions of touch and other nonverbal modes of communication. Nursing research indicates that the nurse's use of hand massage and other modes of touch with older adults in long-term care settings can promote comfort and facilitate communication (Gleeson & Timmins, 2004; Kolcaba et al., 2006). In home and community settings, nurses can purposefully use a handshake to facilitate communication, especially during an initial interaction with older adults. Although not all people are receptive to this form of nonverbal communication, no harm is done as long as a response has not been forced. In addition, a handshake or similar form of touch can provide assessment information about skin temperature, the presence or absence of tremors, and other characteristics of one upper extremity. It also can provide clues about the person's social skills and awareness of others.

Attentive listening is an important communication skill, and it can be particularly effective as a psychosocial assessment tool. In addition, listening is a nursing intervention that can be used effectively to enhance quality of life, especially for older adults in long-term care settings (Jonas-Simpson et al., 2006). Usually, the best communication occurs when the nurse is verbally quiet and nonverbally responsive. Asking open-ended questions and nonverbally responding to indicate interest in what the person is saying is usually effective in obtaining important information. Nonverbal responses, such as sustained eye contact, and short verbal responses such as, "And then what happened?" will encourage the person to elaborate on the information they consider most important.

Nurses have many opportunities to identify psychosocial issues by listening for pertinent concerns and asking appropriate questions to obtain further information. For example, consider the case of Mrs. P. who, during an admission interview, gave the following response to a question about where she lives:

> *I moved to Sunnybrook Retirement Village after my last stroke. I couldn't stay in my own home because the bedrooms were on the second floor. The doctor told me I had to live where I could get help, and my daughter didn't want me with her. Now that I've fallen and broken my wrist, I'm not sure what the doctor will tell me. My daughter doesn't want to be bothered with me.*

This response gives clues to several potential issues, which the nurse can explore with any of the following questions:

- "What do you miss most since you moved?"
- "You mentioned that your daughter didn't want you living with her. Is that something you had hoped you could do?"
- "Do you worry that the doctor will suggest that you go to a nursing home?"
- "Do you see your daughter as often as you'd like?"

Answers to these questions might uncover psychosocial concerns that need to be addressed as a part of discharge planning.

When communicating about psychosocial issues, it is important periodically to clarify the messages. One clarification technique is to repeat part of a prior answer when asking further questions. For example, saying to Mrs. P., "You mentioned that your daughter doesn't want you living with her…" gives feedback about what the nurse heard and leads into further questions about underlying feelings. Feedback can also be helpful when discrepancies between verbal and nonverbal communication are observed. For example, Mrs. P. might begin to cry and clench her fists as she says, "My daughter has her own life to worry about. I can take care of myself. It doesn't bother me that I can't live with her." A statement like, "You look awfully sad. Are you sure it doesn't bother you?" might lead to an acknowledgment of feelings such as anger, rejection, and loneliness.

When communicating with older adults, nurses might hear information that is contrary to their own values or cultural expectations, such as the following examples:

- Expressions of racial prejudice, including use of derogatory labels
- Attitudes of extreme passivity about decisions involving their care
- Situations in which older adults are abused or exploited by friends, family, or others
- Attitudes about women or other groups that are judgmental or not in accordance with the nurse's beliefs

When dealing with these kinds of experiences, it is important to be aware of one's own feelings and to address them appropriately. For example, during the psychosocial assessment nurses must communicate a nonjudgmental attitude, but afterwards they can share their feelings with colleagues. In some situations, however, it is appropriate for

A Student's Perspective

My communication with patients is something that I am always aware of. I have continued to learn something new each week. Silence during a conversation is something that is always uncomfortable for me. When talking with my client last week, I was trying to get a better sense of his level of family support. I began by asking him if he had any children. He indicated that he had two daughters, but they lived in Florida. Normally I would have had a follow-up question for this response, but I decided to give the client some time to see if he would expand on his original response. It was an awkward few minutes—okay, it was probably just a few seconds that seemed like minutes—but he did open up tremendously. He went on to explain to me that he felt like they have abandoned him since their mother passed away. He began to tear up as he went on to explain that he has grandchildren he has only seen in pictures in Christmas cards. I was able to talk with him about his feelings about these issues and offer him some encouragement. Had I chosen to guide the conversation I would have most likely never had this opportunity. I continue to enjoy confronting uncomfortable communication situations so that I can overcome them and foster better therapeutic communication between myself and clients.

Amanda A.

nurses to acknowledge their feelings or opinions during the assessment. For instance, if the person describes an episode of extreme exploitation and expresses feelings of anger about the situation, the nurse can show empathy and understanding by a statement such as, "That sounds like a terrible situation to have been in."

Creating an Environment That Supports Good Communication

Face-to-face positioning facilitates verbal as well as nonverbal communication and is particularly important when visual or hearing impairments interfere with communication. Moreover, people usually feel more comfortable talking with others when they are at the same level of eye contact. Therefore, when conversing with someone in a bed or wheelchair, the nurse should sit in a chair. If possible, remove any physical barrier that interferes with direct face-to-face contact. For example, putting side rails down when talking with someone confined to bed, or moving a walker that is in the line of vision, can improve face-to-face communication. Before moving walkers or side rails, however, ask the older person's permission to do so; this demonstrates respect for the wishes of the individual.

Each person has his or her own "comfort zone" for communication, which is the physical space required for the person to feel at ease when communicating with others. This space varies according to the type of interactions and has been conceptualized as follows:

- Intimate distance is 0 to 18 inches.
- Personal distance is 1.5 to 4 feet.
- Social distance is 4 to 12 feet.

The provision of nursing care often requires that interactions take place in the intimate or personal zones, even though the relationship would normally dictate that interactions take place in the social distance zone. Thus, nurses need to be aware of the influence of personal space on the comfort level of the older person and consider this during communication interactions. Because cultural factors strongly influence perception of appropriate distance zones and many other aspects of nonverbal communication (e.g., touch, eye contact), it is essential to be sensitive to cultural differences that may affect communication. Cultural Considerations 13-1 identifies some cultural influences on expressions of nonverbal communication.

During conversations with older adults, especially when discussing psychosocial issues, nurses must provide as much privacy as possible. This may be difficult in institutional settings, particularly when patients or residents share rooms with others. Even in these situations, however, closing the door and pulling the bed curtain will increase the perception of privacy. In addition, nurses can take advantage of times that the roommate is out of the room; or, it may be appropriate for the nurse to ask the roommate to allow private use of the room. Eliminating distracting noises is also

Cultural Considerations 13-1

Cultural Influences on Expressions of Nonverbal Communication

Perception of Personal Space

- Cultural groups that are likely to have a narrower comfort space for personal distance include Arabs, Hispanics, Japanese, East Indian, Latin Americans, and Middle Easterners.
- British, Canadians, and European North Americans are likely to require the most personal space.
- Men usually have larger personal space than women.

Touch

- Cultural groups that are likely to be most comfortable with physical touch are Jews, French, Spanish, Italians, Indonesian, and Latin Americans.
- Cultural groups that are likely to be uncomfortable with touch are British, Germans, and North Americans.
- Asians may believe that it is disrespectful to touch the head because it is thought to be a source of the person's strength.
- Vietnamese view the human head as the seat of life and highly personal; they may feel anxious if touched on their head or shoulders; if any orifice of the head is invaded, they may fear these procedures could provide an escape for the essence of life.
- Mexican Americans and Native Americans may view touch as a means for healing, preventing harm, or removing an evil spell.

Touch Between Men and Women

- Middle Eastern men and women do not touch outside the marital relationship.
- In many Hispanic and Middle Eastern cultures, male health care providers may be prohibited from touching or examining part or all of the female body.
- In some Asian cultures, touching between persons of the same sex (but not between those of the opposite sex) is common and acceptable.

Hand Shaking

- Middle Eastern women may not shake hands with men.
- Asian women may not shake hands with each other or with men.
- Native Americans may interpret vigorous handshaking as an aggressive action and are offended by a firm, lengthy handshake.

Eye Contact

- People from some Asian, Hispanic, Indochinese, Appalachian, Middle Eastern, and African American cultures may consider direct eye contact impolite, immodest, or aggressive, and they may avert their eyes when talking with health care professionals or when women are talking with men.

- Native Americans may direct their eye contact to the floor during conversations as an indication that they are paying close attention to the speaker.
- Hispanic cultures dictate appropriate deferential behavior in the form of downcast eyes toward others on the basis of age, sex, social position, economic status, and position of authority (e.g., elders expect respect from younger people).

Facial Expression

- Italians, Jews, Hispanics, and African Americans smile readily and use many facial expressions along with words and gestures to communicate pain, happiness, or displeasure.
- Irish, English, and northern Europeans generally do not use facial expressions or other nonverbal expressions.

Data based partially on information from Andrews, M. M., & Boyle, J. S. (2003). *Transcultural concepts in nursing care* (4th ed.). Philadelphia: Lippincott Williams & Wilkins; and Giger, J. S., & Davidhizer, R. E. (1999). *Transcultural nursing: Assessment and intervention* (4th ed.). St Louis: Mosby.

essential for establishing an environment that supports good communication. In institutional settings, closing the door to bedrooms not only increases privacy, but eliminates noises from the hallway. Before closing a door or bed curtains, however, the nurse should ask permission from the older person. Asking permission shows respect for the person's territory and may be especially important when talking with people who become anxious when they are in closed spaces. Likewise, if a radio or television is on, the nurse can ask permission to turn it off.

All the environmental modifications related to improving hearing and vision (discussed in Chapters 16 and 17, respectively) may be appropriate interventions for enhancing communication during a psychosocial assessment. One particularly easy and important consideration is the avoidance of background glare. In hospital or long-term care settings, people often stand in front of a window when talking to a patient/resident in a bed near the window. When the sun is shining or lights are reflected in the window, the background glare may interfere with the older person's ability to see the person in front of the window. In these situations, simply closing the window curtains or sitting on the other side of the bed may significantly improve communication. In home settings, lack of lighting is a more common problem than glare. Asking the person's permission to turn on lights can be a very effective and easy way of improving communication. After finishing the conversation, the nurse must remember to ask whether the person wants the environment returned to the way it was before. Turning on radios and televisions, replacing walkers and side rails, and leaving bed curtains and doors the way they were found shows respect for the person's preferences. Box 13-2 summarizes verbal and nonverbal strategies to enhance communication with older adults and includes some strategies that are specific to communication during a psychosocial assessment.

Nurses need to consider all the communication techniques discussed here during any interactions with older adults. This is especially important before beginning any type of psychosocial assessment because of the sensitivity of the topics and the importance of establishing a trusting relationship. With good communication skills on hand, nurses can successfully assess psychosocial function in older adults using the tools that are discussed in the following sections.

MENTAL STATUS ASSESSMENT

A mental status assessment is an organized approach to collecting data about a person's psychosocial function. Although the mental status assessment is very broad in scope, the discussion in this section focuses on cognitive abilities; other aspects of psychosocial function (i.e., affective function, contact with reality, and social supports) are discussed in separate sections. Some indicators of psychosocial function that are included in this section on a mental status assessment are physical appearance, psychomotor behavior, social skills, orientation, alertness, memory, and speech characteristics. Mental status assessments are performed by various health care professionals, with each discipline specializing in various components. For example, psychiatrists are skilled in assessing affective and cognitive components, whereas social workers are skilled in assessing family relationship components. In the framework of this text, nurses assess the aspects of psychosocial function that most directly influence the day-to-day activities of older adults.

The Mini-Mental State Exam (MMSE) is widely used as a screening tool for cognitive impairment, with specific focus on orientation, word recall, language skills, and attention and concentration (see Educational Resources section). Although 23 or fewer of 30 points is often considered the cut-off score for dementia, gerontologists have suggested that scores of 25 or 27 or fewer points more accurately identify people who have dementia (Salmon & Lange, 2001). Limitations of this tool include its inability to detect some of the cognitive deficits that occur early in dementia and the fact that it can be significantly influenced by cultural characteristics and level of education. Despite these limitations, the MMSE is useful for identifying and measuring cognitive abilities over time, and it is responsive to short-term changes for monitoring mental status in hospitalized older adults (O'Keefe et al., 2005). However, it is important to recognize that the MMSE is primarily a screening tool and does not provide a broad perspective on psychosocial function.

Physical Appearance

Physical appearance is readily observed and reveals many aspects of psychosocial function. Clothing, grooming, cos-

Box 13-2
Strategies to Enhance Communication With Older Adults

Communication Strategies for Good Communication With Older Adults

- Arrange for face-to-face positioning whenever possible.
- Ensure as much privacy as possible.
- Provide good lighting and avoid background glare.
- Eliminate as much background noise as possible.
- Compensate as much as possible for vision or hearing impairments (e.g., make sure the person is using eyeglasses and hearing aid if appropriate).
- Begin contacts with an exchange of names and, if appropriate, a handshake.
- Use culturally appropriate titles of respect, such as Señor, Señora, Señorita, Mr., Mrs., Ms., Dr., Reverend, Elder, Bishop, and so forth.
- Before calling a person by his or her first name, obtain permission or wait until you have been invited to use this familiar form of address. In some cultures, it is considered inappropriate or disrespectful for anyone but family or close friends to use first names.
- Be sure to pronounce names correctly. When in doubt, ask the older adult to say his or her name. Names that are difficult to pronounce may be written phonetically on the chart for later reference.
- Be aware of subtle linguistic messages that may convey bias or inequality (e.g., using Mr. and the last name to call a white man but addressing an African American woman by her first name).
- Avoid slang expressions, such as "Pop," "Grandma," "dear," "chief," or similar terms, unless the older adult suggests that you do so.
- Never use slang, pejorative, or derogatory terms to refer to ethnic, racial, religious, or any other group (e.g., gays or lesbians).
- Use touch purposefully—providing the person is open to this—to reinforce verbal messages and as a primary method of nonverbal communication.
- In all interactions, be aware of cultural differences that influence the perception and interpretation of verbal and nonverbal communication.

Communication Strategies Specific to a Psychosocial Assessment

- Explain the purpose of the psychosocial assessment in relation to a nursing goal. Begin with questions about remote, nonthreatening topics.
- Use open-ended questions and learn to use silence effectively and comfortably.
- Periodically clarify the messages.
- Maintain good eye contact, use attentive listening, and encourage the person to elaborate on information.
- Remain nonjudgmental in your responses, but show appropriate empathy.
- Ask formal mental status questions, or the most threatening questions, toward the end of the interview.
- Gain the person's permission before asking formal assessment questions regarding memory and other cognitive abilities.

metics, and hygiene provide many clues to psychological function, but they are only clues, and questions must be asked before any conclusions are drawn. For example, the presence of body odor, poor hygiene, and tattered clothing may be associated with any of the following conditions: depression, incontinence, impaired cognitive abilities, limited financial resources, overwhelming caregiving responsibilities, impaired vision or sense of smell, or lack of access to or inability to use bathing facilities.

Observations about how clothing fits provide clues to weight changes (e.g., if clothing is too tight or loose, especially in the waist). A history of weight loss may provide clues to depression, cognitive impairment, medical status, or other barriers to adequate nutrition.

Observations about grooming practices such as hair being dyed can suggest any of the following questions about psychosocial function: Is this a reflection of positive or negative self-esteem? Does she want to appear younger than her age because she believes that old age is not as socially acceptable as youth? Does she want to deny her age because she associates old age with negative images? Similarly, an older woman's preference for wearing high-heeled shoes may be an indicator of self-image and of a desire to appear youthful. This is an important assessment issue because of the potential risk for falls and fractures.

Motor Function and Psychomotor Behaviors

Assessment of motor function, which includes posture, movement, and body language, can provide clues to broader aspects of psychosocial function. For example, stooped posture may be a clue to depression, whereas erect posture may indicate positive self-esteem. A shuffling, staggering, or uncoordinated gait could indicate neurologic deficits secondary to a disease process or adverse effects from alcohol or medications. Gait disturbances, as well as other abnormal movements, are possible signs of tardive dyskinesia or extrapyramidal symptoms. Evidence of tardive dyskinesia raises the question of past or present use of psychotropic medications (discussed in Chapter 8) and may give clues to psychiatric history.

Body language also provides clues to affective illnesses. Slouching and head hanging are common manifestations of withdrawal and depression. Poor eye contact, especially looking at the floor, may be indicative of depression or the inability to answer questions, but nurses assess this in relation to cultural factors that influence the type and amount of eye contact considered to be appropriate. Depression is usually associated with slowed psychomotor function, but excessive activity can be a clue to agitated depression. Agitation can be symptomatic of cognitive, affective, or other psychiatric disturbances; it also may be an adverse medication effect or an indicator of a physiologic disturbance (e.g., dehydration, electrolyte imbalance) or a pathologic condition (e.g., pneumonia, urinary tract infection), especially in older adults with dementia.

Similarly, psychomotor behaviors are part of the mental status assessment because the ability to purposefully carry out simple motor skills is highly influenced by cognitive status. For example, observations of how someone navigates and avoids obstacles in the environment provide clues to the person's judgment (providing that the person has good vision). Nurses can assess psychomotor behaviors by asking the person to perform a simple activity of daily living (e.g., combing hair) and observing the person's ability to comprehend and perform the request.

Social Skills

Assessment of social skills provides information about many aspects of psychosocial function. For example, friendly and cooperative people with good conversational skills may use social skills to hide their cognitive deficits, especially if they are motivated to do so. By contrast, people with longstanding patterns of hostility, social isolation, poor social skills, and lack of ambition may be less motivated to perform well. In addition, people sometimes use the following social skills to cover up cognitive deficits: humor, evasiveness, leading the conversation, and making up answers to questions. Some older adults with dementia maintain very good social skills, even in the later stages of dementia when other skills have long since declined. Nurses also need to be aware of cultural factors that influence social skills and consider the cultural context of the relationship between the interviewer and the interviewee.

Response to the Interview

The older adult's initial response to the interview, as well as changes that occur during the interview, can provide important assessment information. For example, an older adult may initially be very receptive to the questions, but become defensive or sarcastic when he or she is uncomfortable with the line of questioning. In addition, nurses assess the amount of time and effort expended in answering questions. This is especially important when trying to differentiate between dementia and depression because cognitively impaired people may exert great effort in responding to questions, but depressed people may lack energy or motivation to answer correctly. Thus, two people may score the same on a formal mental status questionnaire, but one may miss the questions because of dementia and the other may miss them because of depression. When nurses suspect that lack of motivation is a reason for incorrect or missing answers, they might clarify this by asking, "Is it that you don't know the answers, or that you just don't feel like answering the questions?"

Nurses are likely to encounter attitudes of hostility, resistance, and defensiveness during the interview for a variety of reasons. For example, a person who is depressed may be apathetic and may not want to expend the energy to answer the questions. A cognitively impaired person may be angry, hostile, or defensive, especially if he or she is trying to hide or deny cognitive deficits. A person who has always been reclusive or suspicious may be unwilling to answer questions or may feel very defensive. Assessing the person's underlying attitude is as important as assessing the accuracy of responses to questions.

Assessing for **confabulation**, which is the process of making up information, is difficult when the nurse does not know the correct information. For example, questions about the person's place of birth or childhood experiences are not effective for assessing cognitive function unless the accuracy of the answers can be confirmed. **Circumstantiality**, another cover-up technique, involves the use of excessive details and roundabout answers in responding to questions.

Finally, nurses assess all information in relation to the person's usual personality traits. For example, highly sociable people might always use humor, whereas talkative people might naturally use circumstantiality. The use of humor and circumstantiality by people who are normally quiet and serious might indicate a great effort to cover up cognitive deficits. On the other hand, people who are normally quiet and withdrawn may be perceived falsely as being depressed. Finding out about the usual personality of an individual is difficult; however, nurses can ask a question such as, "would you describe what you were like when you were 40 years old?" Family members and caregivers who have known the person for a long time are good sources of information about lifelong personality characteristics. Box 13-3 summarizes guidelines for assessing physical appearance, motor function, social skills, and response to the interview in relation to the person's psychosocial function.

Orientation

Orientation to person, place, and time is the indicator of mental status that is most frequently assessed and documented. Often, however, orientation is viewed as the primary indicator of cognitive function, rather than as one small piece of a larger picture. For example, the following questions are the gold standard for assessing orientation: "What is your name?" "Where are you?" and "What time is it?" Based on accuracy of each answer, the person is then labeled as "oriented times one," "oriented times two," or "oriented times three." The superficial use of orientation questions and the subsequent labeling of the person as oriented times one, two, or three, ignores important considerations such as:

- Do sociocultural factors influence the person's response to these questions?
- Can the person name familiar people, such as a spouse or children, even if he cannot state his own name?
- If the person cannot give specific names of other people, can he describe the correct role of the other person?

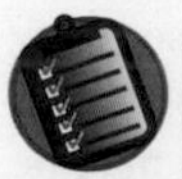

Box 13-3
Guidelines for Assessing Physical Appearance, Motor Function, Social Skills, and Response to the Interview

Observations Regarding Physical Appearance and Motor Function

- What is the person's apparent age in relation to his or her chronologic age?
- How do the following factors reflect psychological function: hygiene, grooming, clothing, cosmetics?
- Does the person's physical appearance provide clues to dementia or depression, or to other impairments of psychosocial function?
- What do the person's gait, posture, and body language indicate about his or her psychological function?
- Is there any evidence of tardive dyskinesia or other adverse medication effects?
- How does the person maneuver in the environment, and what does this reflect regarding judgment, vision, and other skills?

Observations Regarding Social Skills and Response to the Interview

- What are the person's lifelong patterns of social skills, and how do these influence the assessment process?
- How do the person's social skills influence the interviewer's interpretation of other aspects of psychosocial function?
- Is the person motivated to answer questions?
- What is the person's attitude about the interview?
- If the person does not answer the questions, or gives incorrect answers, is it because of inability, cultural factors, or lack of motivation?
- Does the person use any of the following in an attempt to hide possible cognitive deficits: humor, sarcasm, avoidance, evasiveness, confabulation, circumstantiality, or leading the conversation?
- Does the person manifest any of the following characteristics: anger, hostility, resistance, defensiveness, or suspiciousness?
- Do the person's underlying attitudes reflect his or her usual personality, or are they manifestations of cognitive or affective disturbances?

- If the person cannot state the exact time, can she give the general time of day?
- Are any environmental clues available to the person to orient him to the time or place?
- Has the person been at the institution long enough to have learned its name?
- If the person cannot state the exact name of the facility, can she describe the type of facility it is or its general location?
- Does the person have medical problems that interfere with cognition?
- Is the person taking medications that can influence mental function?

A good assessment extends beyond the three classic questions and describes levels of orientation that are meaningful for the person in a particular setting. For example, the following description is far more useful than simply noting that the person is "oriented times one":

> *Mrs. S. could state her name, but did not remember the name of this hospital. She could not give her daughter's name, but was able to introduce her daughter to me, without stating her name. She thought that the month was December because of the Chanukah decorations in her room. She could not state the time because she did not have her watch with her, but she thought that it was afternoon because lunch had recently been served.*

If the nurse had used only the standard questions of "What is your name?" "Where are you?" and "What time is it?" Mrs. S. would be judged to be "oriented times one." Most health care providers, after reading the results of that assessment, would have assumed that Mrs. S. had serious cognitive impairment, especially if she were 85 years of age or older. Mrs. S.'s actual responses, however, reflected various cognitive skills involved in organizing information, making associations, and using judgment. The more detailed description shows that Mrs. S. is probably a quite logical person who has not yet learned the name of the hospital and who might have some temporary memory impairment because of anxiety, medications, or acute medical problems.

Alertness and Attention

Besides orientation, level of alertness is the mental status indicator that health care providers most frequently assess and document. Level of alertness is measured along a continuum, which includes stupor, drowsiness, somnolence, intermittent alertness/drowsiness, and hyperalertness. An important aspect of assessing the person's level of alertness is the identification of any factors that can either increase or decrease alertness, with particular attention to those factors that can be addressed. For example, excessive daytime drowsiness can be associated with any of the following factors: medical problems, electrolyte imbalances, adverse medication effects (e.g., narcotics, anticholinergics, psychoactive medications), depression, dementia, excessive alcohol intake, or lack of sleep at night because of a variety of reasons (e.g., caregiver responsibilities).

In addition to assessing level of alertness, nurses also assess attention. Attention includes the ability to focus on a task, resist distractions, and shift or divide attention between tasks (Cole & Tak, 2006).

Memory

Formal memory testing assesses memory of remote events, recent past events, and immediate memory, which is further divided into retention, recall, and recognition. Nurses can assess memory during usual conversations because all verbal communication depends to some degree on memory function. Nurses pay particular attention to assessing memory in relation to activities that are important in daily life, such as remembering to pay bills, take medications, and shop for groceries. This assessment is made in relation to the expectations and demands of the person's usual environment. For example, if the person lives alone and manages finances independently, the ability to pay bills is quite important. By contrast, if the person lives with a daughter and her family, remembering the birth dates of grandchildren may be an important memory task.

Assessment of memory is especially challenging because memory complaints are common among older adults, but they are not necessarily based on actual deficits in memory function. For example, memory complaints are often prominent in people who are depressed, even though their memory skills are good. In contrast to this situation, older adults with dementia may not even be aware of memory impairment or they may deny the memory deficit as a self-protective response (Cetinski, 2004; Kazui et al., 2006). Thus, the question "Do you ever have trouble remembering things?" may elicit a positive response, but the response is likely to tell you more about the person's perception of memory than about his or her actual memory function. Although this question may be quite useful in identifying any concerns that the older adult might have, it is not very useful in assessing memory function.

In addition to assessing memory directly, the nurse assesses the person's use of memory aids by posing a question like, "Is there anything you do to help you remember appointments or other things?" Assessment of the extent to which the person depends on memory aids is useful in setting goals and planning for improved memory function. For example, if the person's memory function is barely adequate and is based heavily on memory aids, then the potential for further improvement is minimal. In contrast, if the person has some memory deficits but does not use any memory aids, then the potential for improvement is increased. Observations about the use of memory aids also may provide clues to unacknowledged memory deficits. For example, if the person denies any problems with memory, but repeatedly refers to written notes during an interview, then he or she may be compensating for an impaired memory. In this situation, the person is quite willing to use memory aids, but is unwilling to acknowledge the need for such aids. Box 13-4 summarizes guidelines for nursing assessment of orientation, alertness, and memory, and includes examples of appropriate questions for assessing the different types of memory. Examples of direct questions are identified by quotation marks to distinguish them from the questions that are answered indirectly through observations.

Speech and Language Characteristics

Speech and language characteristics provide important information about many aspects of psychosocial function, such as the ability to organize and communicate thoughts. In addition, a good assessment of language skills helps the nurse identify words and language patterns that are most appropriate for use with the older person. Because speech

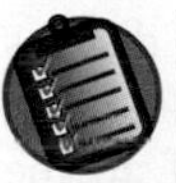

Box 13-4
Guidelines for Assessing Orientation, Alertness, and Memory

Interview Questions to Assess Orientation

- *Person:* "What is your name?" "What is your wife's name?" If names can't be given, can the person describe roles?
- *Place:* "What is your address?" "What is the name of this place?" "What kind of place is this?" "What is the name of this city?" "What is the name of this state?"
- *Time:* "What time is it?" "What day of the week is today?" "What month and date is it today?" "What season is it?"

Observations to Assess Alertness

- What is the person's level of alertness on the following continuum: hyperalert, alert, drowsy, somnolent, stuporous?
- Does the person's level of alertness fluctuate? If so, is there any pattern to the fluctuations?
- Are there physiologic factors that might influence the person's level of alertness, such as medical conditions or effects of chemicals or medications?
- Are there psychosocial factors that might influence the person's level of alertness, such as anxiety, depression, nighttime caregiving responsibilities, or any other factor that might disrupt nighttime sleep?

Interview Questions to Assess Memory

- *Remote events:* "Where were you born?" "Where did you go to grade school?" "What was your first job?" "When were you married?"
- *Recent past events:* "Do you live with anyone?" "Do you have any grandchildren?" "What are the names of your grandchildren?" "When was the last time you went to the doctor?"
- *Immediate memory, retention:* State three unrelated words and ask the person to repeat the information, both immediately and again after 5 minutes.
- *Immediate memory, general grasp and recall:* Ask the person to read a short story and then to summarize the information presented in the story.
- *Immediate memory, recognition:* Ask a multiple-choice question and then ask the person to choose the correct answer.

and language skills are highly dependent on cultural, educational, and socioeconomic factors, it is important to consider these influences, especially when assessing foreign-born older adults.

During any verbal interaction, nurses can assess all of the following speech and language characteristics: pace, tone, volume, articulation, ability to organize and communicate thoughts, and any abnormal speech or language characteristics. The following examples describe some common speech variations and associated conditions:

- Rapid pace: anxiety, agitation, or mental illness
- Slow-paced or excessively brief verbal communication: depression, cognitive impairment, or simple cautiousness
- Tone of voice: indirectly expressed feelings, such as anger, hostility, and resentment
- Hypophonia (i.e., abnormally low speech volume): depression, physical illness, low self-esteem, or long-standing speech habits
- Abnormally loud volume: impaired hearing or long-term experience communicating with someone who is hearing impaired
- Poor articulation or slurred speech: hearing impairment, ill-fitting dentures, lack of teeth or dentures, nervous system disorder, effects of alcohol or medications
- Phonemic errors (i.e., incorrect pronunciation): hearing impairment, cognitive deficits, educational and cultural influences
- Semantic errors (i.e., misinterpretation of the meaning of words): hearing impairment, cognitive deficits
- Neologisms (i.e., self-created and meaningless words): dementia, psychotic disorder (e.g., schizophrenia), repetition of a word that was not heard accurately
- Incoherent speech: dementia, aphasia, psychiatric disorders, alcohol or medication effects
- Perseveration (i.e., a repetitive or stuttering pattern of verbal or written communication) and agnosia (i.e., difficulty finding the correct words, or the inability to name an object accurately, especially if it is unfamiliar): dementia

Aphasia is a communication disorder that is associated with neurologic conditions such as stroke or vascular dementia. In contrast to the speech characteristics summarized in the preceding list, aphasia is not primarily associated with conditions such as dementia, sensory deficits, or psychiatric disorders (Ashley et al., 2006). Expressive aphasia occurs when comprehension abilities are not affected but word retrieval or word-finding abilities are impaired. Receptive aphasia occurs when verbal and comprehension abilities are impaired but some language skills are retained. Global aphasia, which is a combination of receptive and expressive aphasia, results from more extensive neurologic damage and is manifested by inconsistent and poorly controlled language skills.

Higher Language Skills

Reading, writing, spelling, and arithmetic are calculation and higher language skills that are assessed as indicators of cognition. As with assessment of other indicators, the person's education, occupation, and other influencing factors must be considered. Nurses can informally assess these skills in relation to how the person performs important daily activities. For example, for an older adult who lives alone, an assessment of the ability to pay utility bills and use money to purchase groceries is more valuable than a measurement of mathematical skills using a psychometric test. Likewise, a person's ability to read the daily newspaper or the markings on a thermostat may be a more valid gauge of functional ability than a score on a formal reading test.

Nurses can use written health education materials to assess reading and comprehension skills informally, and this method serves a practical purpose. For example, when collecting a urine sample, the nurse can give the person a list of instructions and ask him or her to read the instructions aloud. An observation of how well the person comprehends the instructions provides an assessment of reading skills that are important in daily life. Another opportunity for assessing reading comprehension may arise if the nurse observes that an older adult has a newspaper nearby. A nonthreatening question, such as "What's new in the paper today?" can provide information about the person's interests in outside events and his or her ability to comprehend and remember written information.

Nurses can assess writing and other higher language skills by observing older adults during interactions that pertain to their care. For example, nurses can observe the way an older adult signs his or her name on documents, such as permission forms. Nurses can also observe the older adult during performance of more complex tasks, such as compiling a written medication list or a list of questions to discuss with the primary care provider. Difficulty with writing skills is a common sign of early stages of dementia. Of all the higher language skills, spelling is the least important in terms of daily function, but it is a good indicator of changes in mental abilities.

With traditional psychometric testing, calculation is measured with the "7s" test: the person is asked to subtract 7 from 100 and to continue subtracting 7s. Because this test is highly influenced by level of education, it is not necessarily the most appropriate test for older adults. It may be more appropriate to ask the older person to add 3 plus 3, and to continue adding 3s. Older adults who are depressed may not answer correctly because they do not want to expend the energy to calculate serial sevens. Older adults who have dementia may be able to perform well on this task if they try hard and if they previously had highly developed mathematical skills. Box 13-5 summarizes the considerations that are important in assessing speech characteristics and calculation and higher language skills.

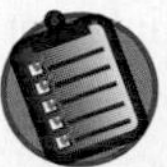

Box 13-5
Guidelines for Assessing Speech Characteristics and Calculation and Higher Language Skills

Observations to Assess Speech Characteristics

- Is the pace of speech normal, slow, or fast?
- Is the tone of voice suggestive of underlying feelings, such as anger, hostility, or resentment?
- Is the volume abnormally soft or loud?
- Do the sentences flow coherently and smoothly?
- Is there evidence of any problem with integrating speech sounds into words (e.g., neologisms, or phonemic or semantic errors)?
- Do any of the following factors affect the person's speech: dry mouth, poorly fitting dentures, absence of teeth or dentures, alcohol or medication effects, or neurologic or other pathologic processes?
- Does the person exhibit any of the following: agnosia; perseveration; or expressive, receptive, or global aphasia?

Observations to Assess Calculation and Higher Language Skills

- What is the person's ability to comprehend written materials encountered in the course of routine activities, such as the daily newspaper or instructions for medications?
- What is the quality of the person's handwriting (e.g., his or her signature)?
- Is the person able to perform mathematical computations necessary for daily activities?

DECISION MAKING AND EXECUTIVE FUNCTION

Decision making, one of the most important and complex of all cognitive abilities, is an important aspect of psychosocial function because all legally competent older adults, including those with dementia, have the right to be involved in decisions about their care. Moreover, most people in mild to moderate stages of dementia want to be involved with treatment decisions (Hirschman et al., 2005). Insight, learning, memory, reasoning, judgment, problem solving, and abstract thinking are some of the cognitive skills that are involved with decision making. Although no one assessment tool focuses specifically on decision making, nurses assess this aspect of psychosocial function by observing the abilities of older adults to solve problems during the course of daily activities and by asking assessment questions such as the ones in Box 13-6.

Abstract thinking is difficult to assess because it is strongly influenced by other factors, such as education, personality, and affective state. People who are very anxious or depressed may lack the attention or motivation required to respond to the questions typically used for the assessment of abstract thinking patterns. Similarity questions, such as "How are apples and oranges alike?" are used to assess the person's ability to think abstractly. Asking someone to explain the meaning of an adage, such as "People who live in glass houses shouldn't throw stones," is another way to assess the person's level of abstract thinking.

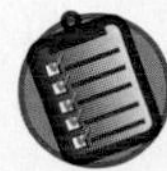

Box 13-6
Guidelines for Assessing Decision-Making Skills and Executive Functions

Abstract Thinking

- "How are apples and oranges alike?"
- "How are a table and chair alike?"

Reasoning and Judgment

- "What would you do if you woke up in the middle of the night and smelled smoke?"
- "If you received $100 as a gift, how would you spend it?"

Insight

- "What's the reason for your hospitalization?"
- "What kind of help do you think you might need when you leave the hospital?"

Cognitive Flexibility

- "Say as many words as you can that begin with the letter 'T' without using people's names."

During an interview, opportunities for assessing abstract thinking may arise, and the nurse listens for clues to the person's level of abstract, versus concrete, thinking. The following exchange is an example of an unsolicited opportunity this author had to assess one older adult's concrete thinking pattern:

Nurse: How did you feel about having to move from your home in Texas to live with your daughter and her family here in Ohio?

Mr. L.: I don't know; how would you feel?

Nurse: I'm not sure how I'd feel; that's never happened to me. I'm not in your shoes.

Mr. L.: Well, here, put them on [stated emphatically while taking off his shoes to give to the nurse].

One interpretation of Mr. L.'s response is that his thinking pattern is very concrete, rather than abstract.

Nurses assess **problem-solving abilities** through observations about how older adults meet their needs in a particular situation. For instance, the nurse observes the way older adults use call lights to meet their needs when confined to bed, or the way they engage in the complex decisions related to discharge planning. Similarly, a very important problem-solving task for an older adult who lives alone may be meeting basic safety needs. Therefore, a question such as "What would you do if you woke up at night and smelled smoke?" might be an appropriate way of assessing judgment related to safety. For an older adult who lives in a nursing home, a very important but complex problem-solving task may involve dealing with a disruptive roommate. In this situation, the answer to a question such as "What would you do if your roommate started taking your belongings?" might provide the most pertinent information for assessing problem-solving skills.

Assessment of **judgment** is based on observations such as the following:

- Does the person pay bills on time?
- Does the person have enough food in the house?
- What resources does the person use in dealing with illness?
- Are the person's clothing and grooming appropriate for the situation?
- Does the person use memory aids to compensate for cognitive deficits?
- Does the person know how to find phone numbers when help is needed?
- Can the person prepare food, or use resources such as a home-delivered meals program, to meet nutritional needs?

Insight is the ability to understand the significance of the present situation. This skill is an important component of the problem-solving process because it establishes a basis for planning care. Insight is influenced by psychosocial factors such as feelings, personality, and coping mechanisms. **Denial** is a defense mechanism that is often used to protect oneself from unpleasant realities; the stronger the denial, the more limited the insight. It is important to assess for denial because if the person refuses to acknowledge that he or she has a condition, it will be very difficult to plan interventions. Nursing assessment of insight concentrates on those areas of function that are pertinent to the care plan. For example, in assessing the insight of an older adult who has been brought to the hospital with malnutrition and uncontrolled hypertension, the nurse may ask questions such as the following:

- What's the reason your daughter brought you to the hospital?
- How do you manage with grocery shopping and getting your meals?
- Do you take any medications?
- What are the medications for?
- What kinds of things does your daughter do for you?

Answers to questions such as these facilitate care planning because they help the nurse assess the person's understanding of the present situation.

When the person has little or no understanding of his or her health situation, the nurse tries to identify the factors that interfere with insight. In the example just described, insight may be absent or limited because of feelings of depression and hopelessness, lack of information about the medication regimen, denial of a reality that is too threatening, inability to remember information, or fear of losing independence. An essential component of discharge planning is identifying both the level of insight and the factors that interfere with insight. In addition, the nurse attempts to identify factors that may improve the person's insight. For example, if insight is lacking because of denial that stems from exaggerated fears, then alleviating the fears may facilitate insight.

In recent years, nurses have recognized the importance of assessing **executive function** abilities in conjunction with determining a patient's capacity to participate in decisions about health care and discharge planning (Kennedy, 2003). The following cognitive abilities are identified as components of executive function:

- Insight
- Judgment
- Reasoning
- Attention
- Concept formation
- Cognitive flexibility
- Problem-solving skills
- Abstraction
- Self-evaluation
- Ability to plan and initiate activity with future goals in mind
- Ability to think, plan, initiate, sequence, monitor, and stop complex behavior

Executive function deficits, which can occur during the earliest stage of dementia, can precede memory deficits, especially if the frontal lobes are affected. Because people with executive cognitive dysfunction may perform well on the MMSE but still not be able to perform essential daily activities independently, it is imperative that health care professionals assess executive function skills (Juby et al., 2002; Kennedy, 2003). The following behaviors are indicative of executive function deficits (Piquet et al., 2002):

- Reduced mental flexibility
- Inability to solve problems
- Decline in ability to conceptualize
- Difficulty adapting to new situations
- Diminished ability to think abstractly
- Increased time required to shift thought processes from one idea to another

Because it is important to assess these skills in relation to previous level of function, it may be necessary to ask family members, or the person being assessed, if they have noticed changes in these abilities in recent years. When families or health care providers have serious questions about the decision-making abilities of an older person, or when a major decision must be made and there is disagreement about it, a more comprehensive assessment using neuropsychological tests may be warranted. For example, if a cognitively impaired older person expresses a strong desire to live alone but family members question the person's ability to function safely, a comprehensive geriatric assessment with emphasis on decision-making and executive function skills will provide useful information. Nurses can use Box 13-6 as a guide to assessing decision-making skills and identifying deficits in executive functions.

AFFECTIVE FUNCTION

A person's **affect** refers to his or her mood, emotions, and expressions of emotions. Happiness and sadness are feelings commonly associated with affective states, but all of the following have been identified as primary affects (also called *discrete emotions*): joy, awe, hope, fear, pain, rage, pride, guilt, shame, anger, regret, relief, hatred, surprise, interest, boredom, elation, confusion, jealousy, depression, suspicion, frustration, anxiety, bewilderment, amorousness, and lack of feelings. Contrary to what many people believe, older adults experience a wide range of positive emotions, such as happiness, contentment, and gratitude, more commonly than negative emotions such as sadness and frustration (Chipperfield et al., 2003).

The components of affective state that are reviewed in this section are general mood, anxiety, self-esteem, depression, and happiness. These five aspects were selected for the following reasons:

- An assessment of general mood assists the nurse in determining appropriate goals based on the person's usual affective state.
- Anxiety is a common factor in older adults that can often be alleviated or minimized through nursing interventions.
- Self-esteem is a major determinant of feelings, especially depression and happiness.
- Self-esteem is particularly important because older adults face many conditions that threaten their self-esteem.
- Depression and happiness are two primary affects that have been the target of much of the research regarding affective states in older people.

Nursing interventions are directed toward all of these affective components to improve the quality of life of older adults.

Guidelines for Assessing Affective Function

Affective function is assessed both quantitatively and qualitatively in relation to expectations about appropriate expressions of emotions. For example, people are expected to show some expression of sadness when talking about sad events. When the person's expression of feelings is not consistent with the external event, however, the affect is considered inappropriate. Affect also is assessed in relation to the personal meaning and the nearness in time of an event. People are expected to show greater feelings of sadness in response to tragic news than in response to neutral events. Likewise, people are expected to show a deeper affective response soon after experiencing a sad event than they would years after the event occurred.

The depth and duration of affect, which are important considerations in differentiating between dementia and depression in older adults, also are assessed. The affect of depressed people generally is sad and negativistic and is not influenced by external circumstances. By contrast, the affect of people who have dementia fluctuates more and changes in response to distractions. **Emotional lability** (i.e., emotional instability or fluctuation) is a characteristic of vascular dementia that is often seen in people who have had strokes.

Nonverbal behaviors, such as those indicating anxiety, sadness, and happiness, provide a wealth of useful information about a person's affective state. During a mental status assessment, nonverbal behaviors provide information that the person may not offer verbally. For example, despite a person's denial of feeling sad, he or she may exhibit the following nonverbal cues: crying, slouching over, looking at the ground, and having a mournful facial expression. The nurse uses this information as the basis for a leading comment, such as "You look like you're feeling sad."

Expressions of emotions are strongly determined by cultural norms and personality characteristics. In most Western societies, crying is more acceptable for women and children than for men and older boys, and showing anger and rage is more acceptable for men than for women. Cultural expectations also influence the way a person expresses feelings in certain circumstances. For example, a person may be expected to cry and loudly proclaim mournful feelings at a funeral, but may be prohibited from expressing any feelings in front of strangers or in a public place, such as a hospital. Because some emotions, such as anger or depression, are viewed as less acceptable than others, such as happiness, people learn to deny and hide feelings that may be judged as unacceptable. Older adults, especially, may have learned that certain feelings should not be expressed directly or verbally. Thus, it is especially important to observe for any indirect or nonverbal clues of anger, depression, and other less socially acceptable feelings.

In assessing the affective state of older adults, it is important to identify the terminology that is most acceptable. Many people will not admit to feeling anxious or depressed because they associate these terms with a serious mental illness or with a socially unacceptable state. Therefore, the nurse begins the assessment of affective state by focusing on feelings that are viewed positively or neutrally. If the person initiates the topic of feeling anxious or depressed, the nurse responds to those feelings and pursues a related line of questioning. In most circumstances, however, it is best to begin with open-ended questions. A simple question, such as "How are you feeling today?" when asked with sincerity, is a familiar and comfortable way of eliciting information.

Mood

Mood is closely associated with emotions, but differs from them in that it is more pervasive, less intense, and longer lasting. People are usually quite comfortable describing their mood as either bad or good, and are more likely to offer information about their mood than their emotions. Thus, during a mental status examination, a question such as "How would you describe your usual mood?" may be perceived as less threatening than the question, "How do you feel most of the time?" Nonverbal behaviors provide many clues about a person's mood and may be more accurate than verbal responses as an indicator of affective state. Joy, anger, anxiety, sadness, happiness, and depression are examples of moods that are expressed in nonverbal behaviors in everyday life by most people.

Anxiety

Anxiety is defined as a feeling of distress, subjectively experienced as fear or worry and objectively expressed through autonomic and central nervous system responses. Moderate anxiety is beneficial because it motivates protective behaviors, but extreme anxiety is detrimental because it channels personal energy into defensive behaviors. Therefore, it is important to assess the degree of anxiety and the extent to which the anxiety is beneficial or detrimental. In recent years, increasing attention has been given to generalized anxiety disorder, which has a significant negative impact on health, functioning, and quality of life for many older adults, especially those who are homebound or in long-term care facilities (Wetherell et al., 2005). Generalized anxiety disorder is characterized by excessive and uncontrollable worry accompanied by physiologic symptoms, including fatigue, irritability, restlessness, sleep disturbances, and difficulty concentrating.

In assessing anxiety, nurses must identify the terminology that is most acceptable to the older adult. Words like "worries" and "concerns" are readily understood and usually elicit responses about sources of anxiety. Older adults also often use the phrases "nerve trouble" or "trouble with my nerves" in reference to anxiety states. Asking questions such as "Do you ever have nerve trouble?" or "What kinds of things give you trouble with your nerves?" may elicit a response filled with information about sources of anxiety.

Nurses observe for nonverbal manifestations of anxiety to supplement the information obtained from verbal communication. In any adult, anxiety may be manifested in the following nonverbal ways: pacing, shakiness, restlessness, irritability, fidgeting, diaphoresis, tachycardia, hyperventilation, dry mouth, voice changes, smoking habits, urinary frequency, increased muscle tension, poor eye contact, poor attention span, inability to sit still, changes in eating patterns, rapid or disconnected speech, or repetitive motions of facial muscles or any extremities. Although any of these indicators may be observed in older adults, the presence of mobility limitations or pathologic conditions can interfere with some of them. For example, older adults who are confined to bed cannot pace, but may experience subtle changes in eating or sleeping patterns because of anxiety. Older adults may be reluctant to report that they are worried or anxious; instead, they may focus on physiologic symptoms (e.g., pain, fatigue, anorexia, insomnia, or stomach distress).

Because anxiety is always a response to real or perceived threats, the nurse tries to identify sources of anxiety, even though they may not be readily apparent. Potential sources of anxiety (i.e., real or perceived threats) include health, assets, values, environment, self-concept, role function, needs fulfillment, goal achievement, personal relationships, and sense of security. People do not always recognize the source of their anxiety because it may arise from unconscious conflicts, unacknowledged fears, maturational crises, or developmental challenges. Even when people recognize the source of anxiety, they may be reluctant to discuss it, or they may refer to the threat only indirectly. For example, an older adult may have the perception that other people have the power to "put him away" in a nursing home simply because of a slight memory impairment. If the person knows other older adults who have been admitted unwillingly to a nursing home, this fear may be exacerbated. Further anxiety might arise from the person's fear of discussing the subject because of the perception that initiating the topic might precipitate actions leading to nursing home admission. Rather than directly talking about the fears, the person might provide vague clues, such as by stating, "I felt so sorry for Mildred when her son put her in the nursing home."

Nurses must phrase questions aimed at identifying sources of anxiety in the least threatening way possible. When older adults express concerns about other older people, it may be appropriate to ask questions aimed at determining whether they have the same worries about themselves. For example, in response to the statement "I felt so sorry for Mildred," the nurse might ask, "Do you ever worry that you'll have to go to a nursing home?" Nurses use open-ended questions that allow for a wide range of answers to identify sources of anxiety that might not otherwise be revealed. For example, nurses in institutional settings can ask, "What is your biggest worry about going home?" or "Do you have any worries about how you'll manage at home after you leave here?" In home settings, the nurse might ask an even broader question, such as "Do you have any concerns about the future?" or "What kinds of things do you worry about?" Answers to these questions usually are filled with clues to sources of anxiety and lead to many additional questions.

Anxiety can be caused or exacerbated by physiologic conditions arising from disease processes or adverse effects of bioactive substances, as in the following examples:

- Herbs, caffeine, nicotine, and medications (both prescription and over-the-counter) can cause physiologic anxiety reactions.
- Anxiety may be associated with withdrawal from nicotine or alcohol.
- Anxiety is often an indicator of pathologic processes that diminish cerebral oxygen, such as pulmonary or cardiovascular diseases.
- Endocrine disorders, such as hyperthyroidism, may be manifested primarily by anxiety or other psychosocial symptoms.
- People with dementia may show signs of excessive anxiety when they are experiencing pain or physical discom-

fort, especially if their verbal communication skills are impaired.
- Pacing is a commonly observed manifestation of anxiety in ambulatory older adults who have dementia.

Therefore, information about medical conditions and the person's use of herbs, caffeine, and medications, is an essential component of the assessment of anxiety.

Chemicals or medications that stimulate the central nervous system or act on the autonomic nervous system may precipitate or exacerbate anxiety. **Akathisia** is a frequently reported extrapyramidal effect of some neuroleptics that may subjectively or objectively be interpreted as anxiety. Akathisia is defined as an inner sense of restlessness that is worsened by inactivity and is manifested by motor restlessness. It is more common in women and older adults, and it can occur any time during the course of treatment with psychotropic medications. Therefore, if an older adult who is taking neuroleptics complains of certain feelings, such as "shaking on the inside," the possibility of adverse medication effects must be considered as a cause.

In addition to identifying sources and manifestations of anxiety, it is important to identify acceptable methods for reducing anxiety. Even if the sources of anxiety are not identified or cannot be changed, the experience of anxiety can be addressed through psychosocial and educational interventions that facilitate effective coping for management of anxiety (Frazier et al., 2002). To this end, the nurse asks questions about usual coping methods. Questions such as "What do you do when you have trouble with your nerves?" or "What do you find helpful when your nerves are bad?" can pave the way for a discussion about coping with anxiety. If the person cannot identify effective coping mechanisms, the nurse offers suggestions in a nonjudgmental way and assesses the person's response to them. For example, nurses can ask any of the following questions:

- "Does it help to talk to someone about your worries?"
- "Have you ever tried any relaxation methods when you're nervous?"
- "Do you find that taking a walk helps you when your nerves are bad?"

Self-Esteem

Self-esteem cannot be measured numerically, but nurses can observe for verbal and nonverbal indicators. For example, a statement such as "You're wasting your time on me, you have more important things to do" is a clue to poor self-esteem. Nonverbal indicators of self-esteem include the way people dress, care for themselves, and present themselves to others. Although interpreting behaviors in relation to self-esteem must be done with caution, the following behaviors may be associated with low self-esteem: rigidity, procrastination, unnecessary apologies, lack of confidence, expectations of failure, exaggeration of deficits, disappointment in self, self-destructive behaviors, constant approval-seeking, overemphasis on weaknesses, inability to accept compliments, minimizing personal capabilities, disregarding one's own opinions, inability to form close relationships, inability to accept help from others, and inability to say "no" when appropriate. It may be appropriate to ask some questions, however, especially about the person's perception of positive qualities.

In addition to observing for indicators of self-esteem, nurses can ask questions that give insight into the older adult's self-perceptions. For example, a question such as "What is the quality in yourself that other people admire the most?" is nonthreatening. Moreover, this kind of question helps identify strengths that can be supported and it provides clues to self-esteem.

Nursing assessment also is directed toward identifying actual and potential threats to self-esteem, so they can be addressed through interventions (discussed in Chapter 12). Examples of threats to self-esteem that are within the realm of nursing are:

- Referring to patients by anything other than their preferred salutation
- Environmental factors that interfere with optimal independence (i.e., not having items such as eyeglasses, hearing aids, walkers, and assistive devices)
- Lack of privacy
- Not involving patients or residents in decisions affecting their care
- Staff attitudes and behaviors that foster unnecessary dependency (i.e., having to use a bed pan or incontinent products when one is capable of going to the bathroom with assistance)

Because self-esteem is influenced by the person's perception of the opinions held by significant others, it is important to identify who the significant others are for any particular person (e.g., peers; spouse or partner; authority figures; and people in the work, church, and social environments). Culture often defines who is the significant other. Some Chinese American older adults, for example, expect their oldest son to look after their affairs and make key decisions about their health and well-being. Widows in some Middle Eastern and African cultures expect one of their husband's brothers to take care of them, an arrangement that fosters social and economic security for women who have lost a spouse. Being cared for by a family member (rather than by strangers) enhances self-esteem for older adults from all cultural backgrounds and increases the likelihood that their needs will be met as they age.

Depression

Depression is discussed as a general component of a psychosocial assessment in this chapter and it is covered more comprehensively as an aspect of impaired psychosocial function in Chapter 15. Nurses can apply information in this chapter when assessing all older adults, and use information in Chapter 15 as a guide to caring for older adults who are depressed.

Nurses assess for depression by identifying verbal and nonverbal cues. Direct questions such as "Are you depressed?" usually are not effective in eliciting information because people may associate the word "depressed" with states of overwhelming grief. Older adults may be more comfortable responding to questions about whether they feel "sad," "blue," or "down in the dumps." Therefore, unless the older adult uses the term "depressed" to describe his or her feelings, other terminology is more likely to elicit an accurate response. As with other aspects of the mental status assessment, it is best to start with open-ended questions, such as "How are you feeling right now?" or "How have you been feeling this week?"

One of the purposes of an assessment of depression is to identify the person's usual patterns of coping with losses. For this reason, the nurse encourages older adults to express their feelings about significant changes in their lives. For instance, when an older adult talks about a change that might be experienced as a loss, nurses can ask nonthreatening questions that might lead to a discussion of feelings, such as: "What's it like to live alone after 50 years of being married?" "How is life different since your friend moved away?" "Are there people you miss seeing since you retired?" "Are there any activities you miss doing since you no longer drive?" If the open-ended questions do not elicit information about feelings, the nurse can comment on specific feelings that the person is likely to be experiencing. For example, a remark such as, "It seems like it would be pretty sad and lonely being here all by yourself after 55 years of marriage" allows the person to agree, disagree, or offer an alternative to the suggested feelings. Be aware that, for older adults from some Asian, Native American, and other cultures, expressing one's emotions overtly or discussing them with a stranger may be considered inappropriate.

Happiness and Well-Being

Happiness in relation to aging is often equated with morale, contentment, well-being, life satisfaction, successful aging, quality of life, and "the good life." Although these terms often are used interchangeably, happiness is an affective quality, whereas well-being and life satisfaction are cognitive qualities. Gerontologists also focus on the concept of quality of life, which includes both affective and cognitive qualities (Ryff & Kwan, 2001). Studies have identified the following key dimensions of psychological well-being in older adults (Blazer, 2002b; Ostbye et al., 2006; Ryff & Kwan, 2001):

- Positive relations with others
- A sense of identity
- Self-acceptance
- Self-efficacy
- Autonomy, self-determination, and the capacity to follow one's own convictions
- A unifying outlook and sense of meaning and purpose in life
- An accurate perception of reality and sensitivity to situations of others
- An investment in living and in realizing one's potential
- Personal growth
- Mastery of the environment, including the ability to solve problems, manage the demands of daily life, and create living contexts suitable to one's needs and capacities

Although nurses cannot address all these characteristics in a psychosocial assessment, they can include a few questions about happiness and well-being. Psychologists sometimes use the following question to assess happiness: "Taking all things together, how would you say things are today—would you say you're very happy, pretty happy, or not too happy these days?" Nurses can ask a similar question such as "If you had to rate your present level of happiness on a scale of 0% to 100%, what rating would you give it?" Nurses can use the person's response as a base for additional questions such as "What would have to change to increase the rating by 10%?" "What kinds of things interfere with your happiness?" "If you could change one thing to be happier, what would it be?" Older adults usually will respond to these questions in a realistic manner, and their answers will provide information for establishing appropriate goals.

Box 13-7 summarizes the considerations involved in assessing affective function in older adults. Examples of direct questions are identified by quotation marks to distinguish them from the questions that are answered indirectly through observations.

CONTACT WITH REALITY

Although a certain amount of fantasy is acceptable in everyday patterns of thinking, people are expected to remain in contact with the world around them and to respond appropriately to the same realities that others perceive. People lose contact with reality for numerous reasons, including dementia, delirium, psychotic disorders, and a transient denial of a threatening reality. Many of these underlying conditions are treatable; however, when older adults lose contact with reality, they are likely to be labeled as "senile." Thus, because of stereotypes about older people, as well as the broad array of potential causes for loss of contact with reality, the assessment of an older person's contact with reality is especially challenging.

Loss of contact with reality includes a wide range of behaviors, ranging from simple and harmless misperceptions of reality to unyielding delusions or disturbing hallucinations. For example, people who are in early stages of dementia may actively conceal or not acknowledge memory deficits, and those in later stages of dementia may experience delusions that lead to behaviors that are inappropriate or even dangerous. For instance, if someone believes that his

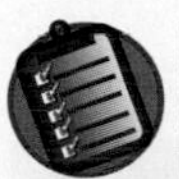

Box 13-7
Guidelines for Assessing Affective Function

General Affective Function

- Are the quantity and quality of emotions appropriate for the objective reality?
- What is the depth and duration of emotions regarding a particular event?
- What are the nonverbal cues to the person's affective state?
- How do sociocultural or environmental factors influence the person's expression of emotions?
- What terminology is acceptable to this person, especially with regard to feelings such as anger, anxiety, and depression?
- Does the person have any pets, or has he or she lost any pets?

Observations/Questions to Assess Mood

- What is the person's usual affective state?
- What are the nonverbal indicators of the person's mood?

Observations/Questions to Assess Anxiety

- What are the nonverbal indicators of anxiety?
- What real or perceived threats are present that might be sources of anxiety for the person?
- Might any of the following factors be contributing to the person's anxiety: caffeine, pathologic conditions, medications, herbs, or interventions by folk or indigenous healers that act on the central or autonomic nervous systems?
- What methods of coping has the person tried, and what have been the effects of these interventions?
- "What kinds of things do you worry about?"
- "Do you have any worries that you'd be willing to discuss with me?"
- "Do you ever have trouble with your nerves?"

Observations/Questions to Assess Self-Esteem

- What verbal and nonverbal clues to self-esteem can be detected?
- What are the factors that influence self-esteem for this person?
- Does the environment present any real or potential threats to self-esteem?
- How are my actions as a nurse influencing the self-esteem of the older adults to whom I relate?
- Are caregiver attitudes, such as infantilization or the promotion of unnecessary dependence, influencing the person's self-esteem?

Observations/Questions to Assess Depression

- What are the verbal and nonverbal clues to depression?
- "Do you ever feel blue or down in the dumps?"
- "How has your life changed since your husband died?"
- "What do you miss the most since you moved from your family home?"

Observations/Questions to Assess Happiness and Life Satisfaction

- How is the person's happiness and life satisfaction influenced by the following: functional abilities, personal relationships, and socioeconomic resources?
- "On a scale of 0% to 100%, how happy would you say you are right now?"
- "If you could change one thing to increase your happiness rating, what would it be?"

belongings have been stolen, he may report the theft to the police or insist on going out to look for the robber. Three types of loss of contact with reality are delusions, hallucinations, and illusions, which are defined as follows:

- **Delusions**: Fixed false beliefs that have little or no basis in reality and cannot be corrected by appealing to reason.
- **Hallucinations**: Sensory experiences that have no basis in an external stimulus. Visual and auditory hallucinations are most common, but tactile, olfactory, and gustatory hallucinations also occur.
- **Illusions**: Misperceptions of an external stimulus. They may be mistaken for hallucinations, but differ in having some basis in reality, whereas hallucinations do not.

Just as a fever is one manifestation of a physical illness, loss of contact with reality is one manifestation of a psychiatric imbalance. Common manifestations of loss of contact with reality in people with dementia include delusions, hallucinations, misidentification, accusatory behaviors, and persecutory ideation (Nagaratnam et al., 2006; Piccininni et al., 2005). Certain characteristics of delusions, hallucinations, and illusions are associated with specific conditions, such as delirium, dementia, and depression. In addition, loss of contact with reality typically occurs in combination with other manifestations of an underlying condition. Thus, an astute nursing assessment of contact with reality can provide essential information for identifying underlying causes. The following sections address delusions, hallucinations, and illusions in relation to associated conditions that are most common in older adults.

Delusions

Delusions are a psychological mechanism that helps people preserve their egos, maintain control over threatening situations, and organize information that is difficult to process. **Paranoia**, defined as an extreme degree of suspiciousness, is one of the most common types of delusions in older adults. The following are typical paranoid complaints or behaviors of older adults:

- The accusation that others are stealing their money or belongings
- The perception that they are being cheated, observed, attacked, persecuted, or sexually harassed

- The accusation that others are coming in and taking things, or messing up their belongings; and the belief that they have been injured by medical interventions, such as pills or radiation

Although the terms *paranoia* and *delusions* are sometimes used interchangeably in geriatric practice and references, this is inaccurate because there are many types of delusions.

In older adults, delusions can arise from pathologic conditions such as delirium, dementia, depression, and paranoid disorder. Delusions associated with each of these disorders are characterized in unique ways and occur in combination with other manifestations of the underlying condition, as discussed in the following sections.

Delusions Associated With Delirium

Delusions arising from delirium—also referred to as an *acute confusional state*—are only one manifestation of a complex pathologic process that is further characterized by physiologic disturbances, diminished attention, a clouded state of consciousness, and possibly hallucinations. Assessment of such delusions is relatively easy because they are commonly accompanied by other manifestations of delirium and disappear once the delirium is resolved. Another characteristic of delusions associated with delirium is that they are likely to be poorly organized and persecutory in nature. Delusions as a manifestation of delirium are not unique to older adults, and they often accompany delirium in people of any age. Older adults, however, are more susceptible to delirium because the older brain is less able to adapt to metabolic disturbances, and the older person is more likely to have precipitating conditions, such as physiologic disturbances and adverse medication reactions. In addition to being associated with delirium, delusions may be the sole or primary manifestation of pathologic conditions (e.g., strokes, hypothyroidism, hyperthyroidism) and functional impairment (e.g., disability in daily life) (Ostling, 2002; Talbot-Stern et al., 2000). Some of the physiologic disorders that are likely to cause delusions in older adults are listed in Table 13-1.

TABLE 13-1 Physiologic Disorders Causing Delusions

Type of Disorder	Specific Examples
Metabolic disorders	Uremia, dehydration, electrolyte imbalance
Endocrine disorders	Hypoglycemia, hypothyroidism, hyperthyroidism
Neurologic disorders	Stroke, cerebral trauma
Deficiency states	Vitamin deficiencies (B_{12}, folate, niacin, thiamine)
Infections	Septicemia, pneumonia, urinary tract infections, subacute bacterial endocarditis
Adverse medication effects	Anticholinergics, anticonvulsants, antidepressants, antiparkinson agents, benzodiazepines, cimetidine, clonidine, corticosteroids, digitalis toxicity, propranolol

Delusions Associated With Dementia

Studies indicate that delusions occur in up to 70% of people with dementia, with most studies reporting prevalences of between 30% and 40% (Mizrahl et al., 2006; Scarmeas et al., 2005). Delusions associated with dementia may be caused by impaired memory and an inability to integrate information. The psychiatric literature usually does not differentiate between delusions that are typical of people with dementia and those that are characteristic of people with psychotic disorders but without dementia. Despite the lack of published studies, however, nurses and other professionals who care for people who have dementia can describe many examples of delusions that are not typical psychotic delusions. In contrast to delusions arising from psychotic states, delusions arising from dementia are not fixed and well organized, and are readily changed or forgotten. Common themes of delusions associated with dementia are fearfulness, theft of property, and concern about deprivation. Nurses may be reluctant to label these behaviors as delusions because they are probably misinterpretations of reality, rather than fixed false beliefs. Until the geropsychiatric literature suggests a better term, however, delusion is the most accurate label.

In one of the early studies addressing delusions associated with dementia, Cummings (1985, p. 190) described the categories of complex delusions and simple persecutory delusions:

> *Simple persecutory delusions consisted of elementary, loosely structured, usually transient beliefs, such as believing that possessions or money were being stolen or that one's spouse was unfaithful. Complex delusions were characterized by a more complicated and intricate structure, rigidity, and stability and were supported by substantial, though distorted, "confirmatory" observations.*

The terms *simple delusion* and *complex delusion* are not widely used, but they are applicable for distinguishing delusions associated with dementia from those that are associated with psychosis. This distinction could be quite helpful because nursing interventions differ for people with psychosis or dementia. For example, a typical psychiatric nursing approach for dealing with delusions in people who are psychotic is to talk with the client about the delusional thoughts as a problem in his or her life. In contrast, appropriate interventions for people with dementia include avoidance of arguing and provision of distractions.

Delusions regarding theft of personal belongings are one of the most common behavioral manifestations of dementia, and are particularly problematic in home and long-term care settings. These delusions occur because the person with dementia forgets where an article is kept or was placed, then, in an attempt to deny the memory impairment, or as a defense against acknowledging the deficit to others, comes to believe that the article has been stolen and accuses someone else of stealing it. Caregivers, roommates, and family members are often the targets of such accusations for those who live with others. For people living alone, the accusations may be directed toward "strangers who come in when I'm gone." In these situations, nurses often deal not only with the delusional person but also with the family, caregivers, and nursing staff who are the target of the accusations.

Delusions associated with dementia commonly involve misidentification of, or false beliefs about, people or environments. These misidentifications arise from the person's inability to match his or her perceptions with the memory or recognition of people or environments that were once familiar. This type of delusion can lead to behaviors that are quite challenging. For example, in home settings, this false belief is especially problematic when a spouse or other devoted caregiver is accused of being a stranger intent on harming the person. Another common misidentification delusion is the belief that the person is not in his or her own home. These delusions can lead to troublesome behaviors such as wandering and agitation, with the person insisting on going out to "find my home." Another delusion associated with dementia is the belief that deceased parents or other close relatives are still alive. Delusions such as this precipitate agitation and searching behavior, typified by the person who insists that he or she "has to go take care of Mother." Another common type of delusion that is similar to the misidentification type is a false belief about spousal infidelity. In these situations, the person with dementia may firmly believe that his or her spouse is having sexual relationships with other people.

People with dementia will readily talk about delusions, whereas those who do not have dementia typically withhold or are secretive about information. The challenge in assessing these delusions, however, is to identify the possible reality of the situation. Nurses cannot assume that all accusations are unfounded just because people have serious cognitive impairments. Thus, nurses must be sure there is no basis in reality before labeling the thoughts as delusional, because even the most bizarre-sounding assertions may be based partially or entirely on reality.

Delusions Associated With Depression

Persecutory and other delusions can be a manifestation of a major depression, but they are often overlooked or attributed to other factors, especially in older adults living in community or long-term care settings. For example, when dementia and depression coexist, the delusions may be attributed to the dementia, rather than considered as possible indicators of a treatable affective disorder. Likewise, when a person with a paranoid personality becomes depressed, the delusions may be falsely attributed to the personality, especially if the delusions are persecutory in nature. When delusions arise from depression, other manifestations of depression usually are identified in a thorough depression assessment, as discussed in Chapter 15.

Delusional themes may provide clues to an affective disorder, especially if the focus is on a recent loss. Therefore, carefully listening to the content of the delusions is essential to an accurate assessment. In depressed older adults, delusional themes often revolve around an exaggerated emphasis on guilt, money, illnesses, self-reproach, gloomy foreboding, diminished self esteem, or feelings of worthlessness. Although some basis may exist in reality, the feelings of being persecuted and deserving of punishment are grossly exaggerated. The following are some examples of delusions arising from depression:

- Mrs. N. believes that she is responsible for her husband's death; therefore, she believes she does not deserve help for her own illness.
- Mr. A. believes that his Medicare insurance has been canceled as punishment for his not cashing his Social Security check, and insists that he cannot go to a doctor because he has no insurance.
- Ms. K. has an unshakable belief that she has undiagnosed cancer and begins to plan for her funeral, even though numerous doctors have not found any disease process.
- Mr. M., who recently had surgery for prostate cancer, is convinced that his house is going to explode from a gas leak and repeatedly calls the gas company to come check it.

Delusions Associated With Paranoid Disorder

Paranoid disorder—also called *paranoid ideation*—refers to a delusional disorder that is not associated with schizophrenia and is characterized by the tendency to view individuals or agencies with suspicion or as having harmful intentions (Bazargan et al., 2001). Studies have found that the following factors increase the risk for developing a late-life paranoid disorder (Bazargan et al., 2001; Ostling, 2002):

- Depression
- Social isolation
- Medical illness
- Cognitive or sensory impairments
- A sense of injustice and deprivation
- A greater number of stressful life events
- A sense of loss of control over the environment

Common themes of delusions include spies, noises, threats, obscenities, lethal gases, bodily harm, stolen belongings, sexual infidelity or molestation, poisoned food or water, and having people enter living quarters by mysterious means at night. The delusions may occur more often when the person is socially isolated or in a particular environment, such as the home. If the person takes action based on the delusions, such as moving to another apartment or living with a family member, the delusions may subside temporarily.

Many people who have a paranoid disorder function well in the community, with the exception of one or two functional areas that are influenced by the delusions. Sometimes, a delusional state that was previously well hidden may surface when the person is admitted to a long-term care facility, and the staff may think that the problem is new. In other situations, nurses will identify a paranoid disorder on making a home visit or interviewing an older person who has been admitted to the hospital. If the person also suffers from dementia, the delusions may be interpreted mistakenly as evidence of advancing dementia. When this occurs, a recommendation for long-term institutional care may be made when other recommendations might be more appropriate.

Identifying a paranoid disorder in the psychosocial assessment is important so that the symptoms can be alleviated with appropriate interventions. When left unattended or written off as eccentricities, these disorders may progress to a point at which they seriously disrupt functional abilities. Therefore, when delusions and cognitive impairments coexist, it is essential to determine whether the delusions existed before the dementia and to what extent, if any, they interfered with daily activities. If the delusions are part of a long-term pattern that has not interfered with the person's ability to function in daily life, the person may be able to remain in the community with support services and treatment directed toward the cognitive impairment. When delusions interfere with daily activities, however, medical intervention (e.g., psychotropic medications) may be effective in eliminating the delusions or minimizing their effects so the person can maintain an independent level of function. When interventions are directed toward both the delusions and the cognitive impairment, the older person may be able to remain independent.

Hallucinations and Illusions

In older adults, hallucinations and illusions are associated most often with dementia, depression, sensory deprivation, and physiologic disturbances, including adverse medication effects. Nurses deal less frequently with hallucinations than with delusions, but this is partially because hallucinations are more easily overlooked or hidden. People experiencing hallucinations may know that their behavior is not socially acceptable. They may not offer information about hallucinations; in fact, they may try to hide their hallucinatory experiences. Older adults who are socially isolated are especially successful in hiding hallucinatory experiences. As with delusions, it is important to identify the underlying cause of hallucinations and illusions because the selection of appropriate interventions depends on an accurate assessment.

Nurses assess hallucinations by making astute observations and asking nonthreatening questions. Although older adults usually do not know they are having hallucinations, sometimes they are aware, especially if the hallucinations are caused by adverse effects of medications (e.g., anticholinergics) or a chronic condition such as Parkinson's disease. Any of the following behaviors are clues to auditory or visual hallucinations:

- Reaching out for objects that are not there
- Stepping over objects on the ground that are not visible to others
- Conversing with people who are not there
- Reporting noises, such as knocking or ringing sounds, that have no environmental source

An appropriate assessment technique is to elicit information from family and caregivers with a statement such as, "Sometimes people see or hear things that others don't perceive. Do you notice any evidence of that happening to your father?"

Because hallucinations and illusions are abnormal sensory experiences, it is essential to assess for environmental influences and to make sure that sensory deficits are compensated for as much as possible. For example, an older adult with visual impairment may look at a chair and misperceive it as someone sitting. In this case, it would be inaccurate to label this person as having hallucinations or illusions, and it would be more effective to ensure that he or she is wearing eyeglasses if appropriate.

Hallucinations and Illusions Associated With Delirium

As with delusions associated with delirium, hallucinations and illusions arising from delirium are assessed within the context of other manifestation of a complex process. In addition to being accompanied by other signs and symptoms, hallucinations arising from delirium are brief, vivid, visual, colorful, threatening, and poorly organized. Occasionally, hallucinations or illusions are the earliest sign of delirium and they may be overlooked or attributed to another condition (e.g., dementia). Hallucinations arising from drug or alcohol withdrawal may occur during the first days of admission to an acute care setting, or in any circumstance in which the person suddenly does not have access to their usual drugs or alcohol. Auditory hallucinations associated with alcohol withdrawal typically are accusatory and threatening, and they are sometimes organized into a complete paranoid system. Table 13-2 summarizes the physiologic disorders, including some adverse medication effects, that are most likely to cause hallucinations.

The detection of alcohol-induced delirium is especially important in acute care settings because people who are dependent on alcohol are more likely to acknowledge the problem and agree to appropriate interventions when they are in a crisis. The following example illustrates such a situation.

Mr. K. is 73 years old and has been caring for his wife, who has Alzheimer's disease, for several years. He is a very proud man who has difficulty accepting help. One morning, Mr. K. begins vomiting coffee-ground emesis and is admitted to an acute care setting with the diagnosis of gastrointestinal bleeding. On admission, Mr. K. is

TABLE 13-2 Physiologic Disorders Causing Hallucinations

Type of Disorder	Specific Examples
Adverse medication effects	Alcohol, anticholinergics, clonidine, corticosteroids, digitalis toxicity, levodopa, propranolol
Endocrine disorders	Thyrotoxicosis
Neurologic disease	Brain tumor or cortical ischemia
Deficiency state	Niacin deficiency
Drug or alcohol withdrawal	Alcohol, barbiturates, meprobamate

very pleasant and expresses concern about his wife's care. The next morning, Mr. K. complains angrily to the nurses about the bars on the windows and is very belligerent about the fact that he has been put in jail. He develops additional manifestations of delirium and is treated for alcohol withdrawal.

When the delirium has subsided, the nurse initiates a conversation about the care of his wife and asks him how he copes with the responsibility. Mr. K. admits that he has difficulty coping with his and his wife's declining health and his increasing loneliness and responsibilities. He has always been a social drinker, but he has gradually increased his consumption of alcohol to three six-packs of beer a day. As part of the discharge plan, Mr. K. agrees to talk with a sponsor from Alcoholics Anonymous.

Visual hallucinations may occur in older adults who are visually impaired and have no additional functional or cognitive impairments (Silber et al., 2005). Hallucinations also are common in people with Parkinson's disease, and may be related not only to the disease itself but to the medications used to treat it (Biousse et al., 2004; Swick & Walling, 2005).

Hallucinations and Illusions Associated With Dementia

Hallucinations and illusions may occur at any time in the course of a dementing illness and also are likely to occur during a transient ischemic attack, a condition associated with vascular dementia. Although hallucinations occur less commonly than delusions, studies indicate that they occur in up to 18% of people with dementia and are more likely to be visual rather than auditory (Chung & Cummings, 2000; Ropacki & Jeste, 2005). When illusions occur, they often are related to environmental conditions that can be modified. For example, poor lighting or reflections from glass or mirrors can cause visual illusions, and background noise can contribute to auditory illusions, especially for people with hearing aids.

The psychiatric literature usually addresses illusions only with regard to misperceptions of visual or auditory stimuli, but an illusion, by definition, is a misinterpretation of any external stimulus. Nurses who care for people with dementia can cite numerous examples of behaviors that fit this broader definition of an illusion, such as the following:

- Mistaking the identity of caregivers, family members, or other familiar people
- Perceiving an object as something other than what it really is
- Taking an object under the mistaken belief that it belongs to them
- Refusing to believe that they are in their home when they really are

These experiences might be labeled as delusions or disorientation, but they are more accurately defined as illusions because they involve a misinterpretation of reality rather than a false perception that has no base in reality.

Hallucinations Associated With Depression

Severely depressed older adults are more likely to experience delusions rather than hallucinations, but visual and auditory hallucinations of deceased loved ones commonly occur during periods of bereavement. When hallucinations occur as a manifestation of depression, they are likely to be auditory and derogatory, or they may involve visual perceptions of dead people. They also may take the form of false perceptions of smell, taste, touch, movement, or body sensation (Blazer, 2002a). The following examples are typical of hallucinations arising from depression:

- Ms. C. reports that at night she hears the people in the next apartment saying that she has cancer.
- Mr. T. reports hearing younger men say that he is sexually impotent and that he was not a good provider to his wife (who died within the past year).
- Ms. F. looks down from her second-floor window and sees a man, dressed in black, lying injured on the sidewalk.
- Mr. S. insists that there is a pervasive smell of skunk coming from his basement and he believes he will be contaminated if he goes downstairs.

Hallucinations Associated With Paranoid Disorder

If hallucinations are a symptom of paranoid disorder, they are likely to be closely related to the theme of the delusions. The following examples are characteristic of hallucinations arising from paranoid states:

- Mr. F. says that he hears people in the next apartment talking about him. These are the same people whom he believes will come in and steal things when he leaves the apartment.
- Ms. J. reports seeing men observing her when she undresses or takes a bath. Moreover, when she goes to the grocery store, the man at the checkout always offers her money in exchange for sexual favors.

TABLE 13-3 Distinguishing Features of Delusions, Hallucinations, and Illusions

Underlying Cause	Accompanying Manifestations	Characteristics
Delirium	Diminished attention, a clouded state of consciousness, and other typical manifestations of delirium; metabolic disturbance, adverse medication effect, or other underlying cause	*Delusions:* poorly organized, persecutory. *Hallucinations:* vivid, visual, colorful, threatening; accusatory auditory hallucinations induced by alcohol withdrawal. *Illusions:* brief, poorly organized.
Dementia	Cognitive impairment (especially memory deficits); alert level of consciousness. Agitation, anxiety, or wandering may be associated with loss of contact with reality. Neurologic manifestations may accompany hallucinations, particularly when the underlying cause is vascular dementia.	*Delusions:* not fixed, loosely organized, readily changed or forgotten. Themes may include theft, fears, misidentification of places or people, and spousal infidelity. *Illusions:* occur more commonly than hallucinations; may be partially attributable to environmental factors. *Hallucinations:* more often visual than auditory; may be partially attributable to environmental factors.
Depression	Typical depressive symptoms, including anorexia, lack of energy, sleep disturbances, and weight loss	*Delusions:* Themes may include death, guilt, money, illnesses, self-reproach, gloomy foreboding, diminished self-esteem, and feelings of worthlessness. There may be some basis in reality, but perceptions are exaggerated. *Hallucinations:* typically auditory and derogatory.
Paranoid disorder	Absence of cognitive deficits or affective disorders; long-term social isolation or suspicious personality; may be well hidden for years	*Delusions:* fixed and well organized; may subside temporarily in different environments. Themes usually involve plots, noises, threats, obscenities, or sexual assaults. *Hallucinations:* If present, these are related to the delusional themes.

Table 13-3 summarizes the characteristics that distinguish delusions, hallucinations, and illusions according to their underlying causes.

Special Considerations for Assessing Contact With Reality in Older Adults

Assessment of contact with reality presents a special assessment challenge for nurses for a variety of reasons:

- People often try to conceal delusions and hallucinations.
- When delusions and hallucinations arise from social isolation, opportunities for assessment are extremely limited.
- To determine whether a reported experience is delusional, the nurse needs information about the reality, which is difficult to obtain if a reliable and objective observer is not available.
- Even after delusions or hallucinations are identified as such, the underlying factors may be difficult to identify.
- Older adults often have more than one underlying condition, such as a delirium superimposed on a dementia.

Delusions usually are more readily acknowledged than hallucinations, and the most effective tools for assessing delusions are asking leading questions and listening attentively. Most older adults will confide their delusions to a nurse who they perceive as interested, sympathetic, and nonjudgmental, especially if a trusting relationship has been established. Difficulty arises, however, when nurses hear information that may be interpreted as delusional but in fact is based wholly or partially in reality. For example, financial exploitation, violation of rights, and other aspects of elder abuse are not uncommon, especially in older adults who are cognitively impaired or who live with family members who are psychosocially impaired. When older adults who have cognitive impairments or a lifelong suspicious personality describe abusive or exploitative situations, they are likely to be considered delusional or not to be taken seriously. In these situations, the assessment challenge is to determine what is real, what is distorted, and what is not based at all in reality.

Nurses also consider the potential effects of environmental and interpersonal factors in contributing to delusions, illusions, or hallucinations. For example, the reflection of fluorescent lights on a highly polished floor can produce the illusion of water on the floor, and an older adult might walk around the reflection. Stressful interpersonal relationships may contribute to the development of paranoid ideations, especially in the context of past or present exploitation or abuse. Another important assessment consideration is whether a lack of assistive devices, such as eyeglasses and hearing aids, is contributing to altered perceptions. For example, if someone usually depends on eyeglasses, contact lenses, or a hearing aid for adequate visual or auditory function, the absence of these items may contribute to the development of illusions or hallucinations.

During the assessment, nurses consider cultural factors that are likely to influence perceptions of reality and manifestations of mental illness, as discussed in Chapter 12. Studies indicate that cultural and socioeconomic factors contribute to the higher prevalence of hallucinations among Hispanic populations (Geltman & Chang, 2004). Religious background is a common cultural factor that can influence the content of delusions or hallucinations. For example, delusions and hallucinations in Irish Catholics are likely to focus on Jesus, a saint, or the Virgin Mary. Similarly, Mus-

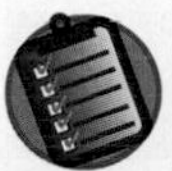

Box 13-8
Guidelines for Assessing Contact With Reality

General Principles

- In assessing any loss of contact with reality, the effects of alcohol, medications, and physiologic disturbances must always be considered as potential causative influences.
- People who are not cognitively impaired are usually more reluctant to talk about delusions and hallucinations than people who have dementia.
- When people talk about things that might be delusional, it is important to determine, through information provided by a reliable and objective observer, whether their perceptions have any basis in reality.
- When delusions are initially identified, it is important to determine whether they are of recent onset or have been long-standing but only recently discovered.
- When delusions are identified in someone who has dementia, it is especially important to consider the influence of treatable causative factors, such as depression or physiologic disturbances.
- People who have dementia are likely to have illusions rather than hallucinations.
- People who are socially isolated are usually quite successful in concealing hallucinations.
- In assessing hallucinations and illusions, it is especially important to consider the influence of the environment.

Interview Questions to Assess Delusions, Hallucinations, and Illusions

- "Do you have any thoughts that you can't seem to get rid of?"
- "People sometimes have thoughts that they're afraid to talk about because they believe others will think they're 'crazy.' Do you ever have thoughts like that?"
- "Do you sometimes hear voices when you're alone?"
- "Do you sometimes think you see things that other people don't see?"

Nonverbal Clues to Hallucinations

- Extreme withdrawal and isolation
- Contentment with social isolation, especially if the person previously had many social contacts
- Gestures and other actions that normally occur in response to perceived stimuli

lims with African, Near Eastern, or Middle Eastern cultural heritage may focus on the Prophet Mohammed.

Box 13-8 summarizes guidelines for assessing an individual's contact with reality. Examples of direct questions are identified by quotation marks to distinguish them from questions that are answered indirectly through observation.

SOCIAL SUPPORTS

Social supports, which are categorized as *informal* and *formal*, refer to the services provided to address functional and psychosocial needs. Even the most independent people receive social supports (e.g., emotional support from family and friends), but social supports are usually discussed in relation to meeting the needs of people who depend on others in some way for assistance. Whereas friends, family, clergy, neighbors, or coworkers provide informal social support, workers who are paid by the older person or their family or by health and social service agencies or institutions provide formal social support.

Social supports significantly influence psychosocial function in older adults because they affect the person's ability to cope with stressful life experiences. Researchers have consistently found that social supports protect older people against harmful effects of stress and promote physical and emotional well-being (Jang et al., 2002). Because the importance of social supports increases in relation to the degree of impairment of the older adult, it is essential to assess social supports for any older adults who have conditions that affect their functional abilities. Nursing assessment of social supports identifies not only the resources that are needed, available, or being used to support highest level of functioning, but the barriers to the use of appropriate resources. Specific aspects of social supports that nurses assess include social network, economic resources, and religion and spirituality. Box 13-9 summarizes important questions and considerations involved in assessing social supports.

Social Network

Nursing assessment of the social network addresses the social supports that are important for day-to-day functioning as well as those that affect the person's quality of life. The nurse can initiate the assessment by asking a broad question such as, "Whom do you rely on for help?" The nurse can then ask more specific questions about how the person accomplishes tasks that are most important for day-to-day function. For example, in discussing a follow-up appointment for medical care, the nurse may ask, "How do you get to your doctor appointments?" Because a relationship with a confidant(e) is a significant predictor of quality of life for older adults, at least one question relating to this factor should be posed, such as "Is there anyone you can talk to about your worries?" The answer to this question may also be important if the nurse or health care team is assisting the older adult with a decision about long-term care because the older adult may want the confidant(e) to be involved in the decision-making process. In addition, the response to this question may provide important information about whether the older person has recently experienced a loss, or change in the availability, of a confidant(e).

After identifying existing social network, the nurse identifies the resources that might be helpful in addressing unmet

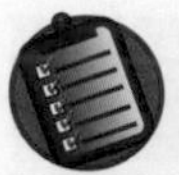

Box 13-9
Guidelines for Assessing Social Supports

Interview Questions to Assess Social Supports

- "On whom do you rely for help?"
- "Is there anyone who helps you with grocery shopping? Getting to doctor appointments? Getting prescriptions filled? Managing your money and paying bills?"
- "Is there anyone you can talk to when you have worries or difficulties?"
- "Is there anything you would like help with that you don't have help with now?"
- "Is there anyone in the family who could help with grocery shopping?"
- "Have you ever received information about the transportation services (or meals, or other services) that are available through the senior center?"

Potential Barriers to the Use of Formal Supports

- Unwillingness to acknowledge, or lack of insight to recognize, the need for services
- Expectation that family members will provide the needed care
- Unwillingness to admit that family members cannot or will not provide the needed care
- Lack of financial resources to purchase services, or unwillingness to spend money for services
- Perceived correlation between formal services and "welfare"
- Lack of transportation to access services
- Mistrust of service providers, or an unwillingness to allow outsiders into the home
- Bad experiences with service providers, or hearsay about the bad experiences of others
- Fear that the home situation will be judged as socially unacceptable, or embarrassment because it is socially unacceptable
- Fear that having outsiders in the house will lead to admission to a nursing home
- Lack of time, energy, or problem-solving ability to obtain information about and select the appropriate services
- Fear that the service will be provided by someone about whom the care recipient holds prejudices
- Language and cultural barriers

Interview Questions to Assess Financial Resources

- "Do you have any money worries?"
- "Do you have any concerns about paying for services that you might need?"
- "Would you liko to talk to someone about any financial concerns?"
- "Do you think you can afford the kind of help that your doctor recommended?"
- "Have you received any advice about financial planning for nursing home care?"

Interview Questions to Assess Religious Affiliation

- "Do you belong to any church, synagogue, or mosque?"
- "Are you aware of any programs available at your church, synagogue, or mosque that might be helpful to you?"

needs. Such questions as "Do you have any grandchildren or neighbors who could help with shoveling the snow?" are aimed at identifying informal supports that may be available but are not currently being used. A question such as "Are you aware that the senior center has a van that takes people to doctor appointments?" is aimed at identifying the person's awareness of formal supports that might not be in use.

Barriers to Obtaining Social Supports

In addition to assessing the number and types of social supports available, nurses try to identify the barriers that interfere with the use of social supports. Only 20% of older adults who are eligible for service programs use these resources, which are viewed as costly, impersonal, overly structured, and hard to arrange (Anetzberger, 2002). Because older adults prefer to receive help from family and friends, negative attitudes about the use of formal social supports may be a source of resistance to their use. In the absence of adequate informal supports, or when conflicts exist between older adults and their informal supports, an increase in dependence can trigger less effective coping mechanisms. The following example is typical of such a situation:

Mr. and Mrs. S. always expected their children to care for them, but the children have moved to other cities and visit only several times a year. Mr. and Mrs. S. refuse to accept any of the formal services that are available because of their cost, and also because they expect their children to provide the services out of filial responsibility. Furthermore, Mrs. S. cared for her parents when they were old, so she expects her daughter to do the same for her.

Mr. and Mrs. S. frequently call their daughter and son-in-law to complain about their inability to get groceries and go to doctors' appointments. Rather than making use of transportation or other services available from the community, they neglect themselves. During the children's visit over the Christmas holiday, they find that their parents have not been eating adequately and are not taking their prescribed medications. When they mention these observations to their parents, Mr. and Mrs. S. tell their children, "If you loved us, you'd be taking care of us, and this wouldn't be happening."

In addition to some older people's preference for obtaining services from families rather than outside agencies, there are many other barriers to the use of formal services. Fears about outsiders coming into the home rank high among the barriers to the provision of in-home services. Financial barriers also often exist, either because of an inability or an unwillingness to pay for services. Additional barriers include unwillingness to accept help, lack of knowledge about types of services available, and not knowing where to go for specific services. The identification of these barriers is essential because counseling and educational interventions (e.g., providing information about services that are available) can address many of these issues. Issues that are not amenable to intervention may represent impenetrable barriers to the provision of social supports.

Assessing barriers to support services is particularly challenging because direct questions about these issues often are inappropriate and usually are very threatening. Rather, identification of these barriers is best accomplished by carefully listening to older people and their caregivers and by asking nonthreatening questions. For example, a caregiver might talk about a friend who had a home health aide who did nothing but watch television all day and got paid 12 dollars an hour. In response to this, the nurse might ask, "Do you think that might happen if we arrange for a home health aide to care for your father?" Other attitudinal barriers, such as prejudices, may be identified through statements made by the caregiver about prior experiences.

Economic Resources

Financial issues are generally within the purview of social workers, and nurses usually prefer to avoid discussing money with older adults or their families. In planning for formal services for older adults, however, some assessment of financial assets is necessary, and the nurse is often the health care professional who obtains this information, especially in home or other community settings. If no long-term care or community-based services are needed, the nurse can forego the financial assessment.

Many older adults and their families are shocked to find out that Medicare does not cover the costs of long-term care, with the exception of skilled care. In addition, people are often appalled by the restrictive definition of skilled care, as well as many other restrictions that are applied to determine eligibility for services. Even if a social worker has explained these facts, it is usually the nurse who deals with the related anxiety and other emotional reactions of the older adult and their families. Because nurses are in a position to help older adults and their families address and cope with the financial issues of long-term care, they frequently become involved in assessing the financial resources of the person and family.

It is not always necessary to ask details about monthly income or the exact amount of savings and assets, but questions must be asked about the resources available for the purchase of services. Asking a question such as "Do you have any money worries?" might reveal some anxieties that can be dealt with or allayed through counseling or the provision of accurate information. When the nurse reviews with the older adult or caregiver the services that are available, information also can be provided about the cost of these services, at which time a question such as "Do you think you could afford this kind of help?" can be posed.

RELIGION AND SPIRITUALITY

The biopsychosocial–spiritual model of care emphasizes that everyone has a spiritual history, and for many people, "this spiritual history unfolds within the context of an explicit religious tradition" (Sulmasy, 2002, p. 27). As discussed in Chapter 12, religion and spirituality become more important in older adulthood, and they are resources that should be identified as a part of a comprehensive psychosocial assessment. The person's religious affiliation is assessed as a component of his or her social supports, whereas spirituality is assessed as a separate component of the psychosocial assessment.

Identification of religious affiliation is a simple but important part of the psychosocial assessment because available religion-based programs for older adults may be perceived as more acceptable than those provided by a public or nonreligious agency. For example, an older Jewish person might be willing to go to the Jewish Community Center for a senior meal program, and an older Roman Catholic adult might be willing to accept mental health services from Catholic Social Services, but these people might refuse to avail themselves of the same kinds of services when they are offered by another organization. Often, religion-based services are viewed by the older adult as services that they deserve as a reward for years of attendance at or service to a church or synagogue. Although most religion-based programs serve older adults regardless of their religious affiliations, the programs often are perceived as more acceptable if the person is of the same faith.

In addition to being perceived as more acceptable, some religion-based services are not available elsewhere, and they often are provided by trained volunteers free of charge. Examples of programs or services that may be available to members of a particular church, synagogue, or mosque include transportation, respite care, peer counseling, chore assistance, friendly visiting, and telephone reassurance. Older adults also can take advantage of any church-, synagogue-, or mosque-based program that is available for people of all ages. The Stephen Ministries, founded in 1975, is an example of a volunteer program that is available in many Christian denominations throughout the United States. This program offers peer counseling and other services, provided by volunteers with special training in ministering to older, depressed, shut-in, and grieving persons.

Identification of a specific place of worship is also important because attendance at religious services may be a significant factor in the older adult's social life. For many older adults, especially those with limited mobility or those who have full-time caregiving responsibilities, attendance at religious services is their only opportunity for social interaction and personal support. Most people who are unable to attend religious services can arrange for home visits by a clergy person or lay minister; indeed, these visits may be the only source of outside contact and emotional support that is acceptable to a home-bound older adult. Moreover, for people who are socially isolated, a visitor from their place of worship may be the only person monitoring the home situation. In these situations, health professionals who are concerned about home-bound older adults may be able to monitor their status through these visitors, as in the following example:

Mr. S. was admitted to the hospital after a syncopal episode that resulted in a minor car accident. On admission, Mr. S. was slightly unkempt and showed some memory deficits, but his self-care abilities improved during his 2-day hospitalization. The nurse suggested that Mr. S. consider home-delivered meals and the use of other community resources, but he refused these services. His situation did not warrant a report to a protective services agency.

The nurse was concerned because Mr. S. lived alone and had no outside contacts other than Ms. C., a lay minister who had visited weekly for 2 years. The nurse asked for and received permission from Mr. S. to contact Ms. C. to inform her of available community services. Ms. C. was grateful for the information and said that she would contact the appropriate agencies if Mr. S.'s condition declined or if he agreed to accept help.

In this situation, information about the church affiliation enabled the nurse to implement a discharge plan that otherwise would not have been possible.

Nursing assessment of spiritual needs is not routinely included in an assessment because it is not always relevant to the health issues being addressed. There are times, however, when a nursing assessment of the spiritual needs of older adults is warranted. When an older person provides clues about spiritual distress or discomfort, the nurse must be willing to respond to the older person, rather than simply ignore the clues, as discussed in Chapter 12. Moreover, when a nurse is addressing quality-of-life issues, it is important to include questions about spirituality (O'Connell & Skevington, 2005). For example, when planning long-term care, it is especially important to assess and address spiritual needs. Assessment of spiritual needs is directed toward a discussion of sources of power and meaning in the older person's life and is not intended to evaluate whether a person is more or less spiritual or beholden to doctrinaire beliefs (Delaney, 2005; Ortiz & Langer, 2002). Nurses can ask a simple but concrete question about an older adult's engagement in family or personal prayer to open a discussion of religious beliefs (Campesino & Schwartz, 2006). As with all aspects of care, nurses need to be particularly aware of cultural influences on religious practices and expressions of spirituality. At the same time, however, they need to be cautious about generalizations with regard to any cultural group.

Nurses, like many people, may not be comfortable discussing spirituality, but they can increase their comfort level by recognizing their own feelings and acknowledging that spirituality is a universal human need. Nurses might avoid discussion of spiritual needs because they believe that they are not skilled in meeting these needs. However, nurses routinely identify many needs that they are not trained to meet directly. If nurses view the assessment of spiritual needs as one aspect of overall health, they may become comfortable addressing the spiritual needs of the older adults to whom they provide care. As with other broad health problems, nurses address the nursing aspects of those problems and refer the person to the appropriate resource for interventions that address the non-nursing aspects. In addition to providing direct nursing interventions to address spiritual needs, nurses suggest referrals to appropriate clergy or spiritual practitioners. Involvement with support groups can also be effective in dealing with spiritual distress when it arises from feelings of guilt, anger, or inadequacy.

Box 13-10 presents guidelines for assessing spiritual needs. Assessment of spiritual needs includes not only the factors that cause spiritual distress but the factors that are essential to spiritual growth, even in the absence of spiritual distress.

CHAPTER HIGHLIGHTS

Overview of Psychosocial Assessment of Older Adults

- Psychosocial assessment is a very complex process that involves the use of good communication skills, appropriate interview questions, purposeful observations, and relevant assessment tools.
- Nurses can assess their own attitudes to increase their comfort level in performing a psychosocial assessment of older adults (Box 13-1).

Communication Skills for Psychosocial Assessment (Box 13-2)

- Barriers to communication include visual and hearing impairments, internal and external distractions, pathologic disorders, adverse medication effects, poor communication methods, and cultural differences.
- Establishing rapport, using touch, listening, asking questions, and giving feedback, can enhance communication during psychosocial assessment.
- Nurses create an environment for communication by speaking face to face at eye level, respecting the person's comfort zone, ensuring privacy, eliminating distractions, and facilitating optimal vision and hearing functioning.

Mental Status Assessment (Boxes 13-3, 13-4, and 13-5)

- An assessment of mental status involves an assessment of all of the following: physical appearance, motor function, social skills, response to the interview, orientation, alertness and attention, memory, speech characteristics, and calculation and higher language skills.

Decision Making and Executive Function (Box 13-6)

- Assessment of cognitive skills, such as executive function, is particularly important for determining

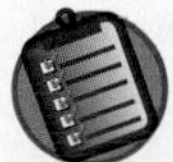

Box 13-10
Guidelines for Assessing Spiritual Needs

Guidelines for Nursing Assessment

- Be aware of your own feelings about spirituality so you can recognize and respond to the spiritual needs of others.
- Recognize that spiritual needs are a universal human phenomenon. Although not all people experience spiritual distress, all people have spiritual needs and the potential for spiritual growth.
- Recognize that it is within the realm of holistic nursing care to identify and plan interventions for spiritual growth as well as for spiritual distress.
- Convey a nonjudgmental, open-minded attitude when eliciting information about a person's spirituality and religious beliefs.

Questions to Assess Spiritual Health

- "What in your life is meaningful and important?"
- "What do you hope to accomplish in your life?"
- "What do you do that gives you pleasure and satisfaction?"
- "Who are the people you can turn to when you need someone to listen to you or to help you?"
- "Do you believe in a higher being?" (examples: God, Goddess, Divinity) "How do you describe this being?"
- "Do you participate in any activities (rituals) that foster a connection with a higher being?" (examples: prayer or other religious activities)
- "What activities are helpful in bringing you inner peace and relieving stress?" (examples: meditation, walking in the woods)
- "What are your beliefs about death?"
- "Do you see a connection between your body, your mind, your emotions, and your soul?"
- "Is there anything you need or would like to have to support your beliefs and your spiritual needs?" (example: Bible, sacred or revered object)
- "Would you like to arrange a visit from a spiritual leader?"
- "Are there any health practices that you would like to consider, even though our society may not consider them to be conventional?" (examples: therapeutic touch, guided imagery)

Observations/Questions to Assess Spiritual Distress

- During the psychosocial interview, listen for clues to spiritual distress, such as the following: suicidal ideation; anger toward God; inability to forgive others; feelings of hopelessness, uselessness, or abandonment; questions about the meaning of life, losses, or suffering.
- "Are there any conflicts between your beliefs or values and actions that you feel you should be taking?" (example: feeling entitled to some time to oneself, which may be in conflict with the demands of caregiving for a spouse)
- "Are there any conflicts between what you believe in and what society or health care professionals are encouraging or suggesting you do?" (example: questioning the wisdom of using a feeding tube for a spouse who is chronically and severely impaired and unable to participate in the decision)
- "Do you have any special religious considerations that are not being addressed?" (examples: dietary practices, observance of religious holidays)
- *For people in institutional settings:* "Is there anything here that interferes with your spiritual needs?" (examples: noisy environment, lack of privacy)

the ability of the older adult to participate in decision making.

- Insight, learning, memory, reasoning, judgment, problem solving, and abstract thinking are some of the cognitive skills that are involved with decision making.

Affective Function (Box 13-7)

- An assessment of affective function includes consideration of mood, anxiety, self-esteem, depression, and happiness and well-being.

Contact With Reality (Box 13-8)

- Nurses assess contact with reality within the context of behavioral indicators to identify potential underlying causes of any loss of contact with reality.
- Three types of loss of contact with reality are delusions, hallucinations, and illusions.

Social Supports (Box 13-9)

- Psychosocial assessment identifies social supports and economic resources as well as barriers to obtaining services.

Religion and Spirituality (Box 13-10)

- A holistic nursing assessment addresses religious affiliation and spirituality.

Critical Thinking Exercises

1. Complete the psychosocial self-assessment in Box 13-1.
2. Think of several different situations in the past few weeks in which you worked with older adults and answer the following questions:
   - What aspects of psychosocial function did you observe?
   - What questions did you ask that would give you information about their psychosocial function?
   - What information did you obtain about their social supports?
3. Name at least three things you would observe or determine in order to assess each of the following when you are working with older adults: physical appearance, social skills, orientation, alertness and attention, memory, speech characteristics, calculation and higher language skills, decision-making skills, anxiety, self-esteem, depression, and contact with reality.
4. What questions would you ask an older adult to identify social supports and barriers to the use of services?
5. What approach would you use to assess an older adult's spiritual health and identify spiritual distress?

Clinical Tool Resources

Hartford Institute for Geriatric Nursing

Try This: Best Practices in Nursing Care for Hospitalized Older Adults With Dementia

Issue Number D3 (Revised 2007): Brief Evaluation of Executive Dysfunction: An Essential Refinement in the Assessment of Cognitive Impairment

www.hartfordign.org/resources/education/tryThis.html

Refer also to all tools listed in Chapter 14 for assessment of older adults with delirium or dementia.

The Mini-Mental State Examination

www.minimental.com

References

Anetzberger, G. J. (2002). Community resources to promote successful aging. *Clinics in Geriatric Medicine, 18*, 611–626.

Ashley, J., Duggan, M., & Sutcliffe, N. (2006). Speech, language, and swallowing disorders in the older adult. *Clinics in Geriatric Medicine, 22*, 291–310.

Bazargan, M., Bazargan, S., & King, L. (2001). Paranoid ideation among elderly African American persons. *The Gerontologist, 41*, 366–373.

Biousse, V., Skibell, B. C., Watts, R. L., Loupe, D. N., Drews-Botsch, C., & Newman, N. J. (2004). Ophthalmologic features of Parkinson's disease. *Neurology, 62*, 177–180.

Blazer, D. G. (2002a). *Depression in late life* (3rd ed.). New York: Springer.

Blazer, D. G. (2002b). Self-efficacy and depression in late life: A primary prevention proposal. *Aging & Mental Health, 6*, 315–324.

Campesino, M., & Schwartz, G. E. (2006). Spirituality among Latinas/os: Implications of culture in conceptualization and measurement. *Advances in Nursing Science, 29*, 69–81.

Cetinski, G. (2004). Patients' expressions of awareness of memory problems in early stage Alzheimer's disease reflected varying combinations of self maintaining and self adjusting styles of responding. *Evidence-Based Nursing, 7*(3), 96.

Chipperfield, J. G., Perry, R. P., & Weiner, B. (2003). Discrete emotions in later life. *Journals of Gerontology: Series B, Psychological Sciences and Social Sciences, 58*, P23–P34.

Chung, J. A., & Cummings, J. F. (2000). Neurobehavioral and neuropsychiatric symptoms in Alzheimer's disease: Characteristics and treatment. *Neurology Clinics, 18*, 829–846.

Cole, C. S., & Tak, S. H. (2006). Assessment of attention in Alzheimer's disease. *Geriatric Nursing, 27*, 238–243.

Cummings, J. L. (1985). Organic delusions: Phenomenology, anatomical correlations, and review. *British Journal of Psychiatry, 146*, 184–197.

Delaney, C. (2005). Development and psychometric testing of a holistic instrument to assess the human spiritual dimension. *Journal of Holistic Nursing, 23*, 145–167.

Frazier, L. D., Waid, L. D., & Fincke, C. (2002). Coping with anxiety in later life. *Journal of Gerontological Nursing, 28*(12), 40–47.

Geltman, D., & Chang, G., (2004). Hallucinations in Latino psychiatric outpatients: A preliminary investigation. *General Hospital Psychiatry, 26*, 153–157.

Gleeson, M., & Timmins, F. (2004). The use of touch to enhance nursing care of older persons in long-term mental health care facilities. *Journal of Psychiatric and Mental Health Nursing, 11*, 541–545.

Hirschman, K. B., Joyce, C. M., James, B. D., Xie, S. X., & Karlawish, J. H. (2005). Do Alzheimer's disease patients want to participate in a treatment decision, and would their caregivers let them? *The Gerontologist, 45*, 381–388.

Jang, Y., Haley, W. E., Small, B. J., & Mortimer, J. A. (2002). The role of mastery and social resources in the association between disability and depression in later life. *The Gerontologist, 42*, 807–813.

Jonas-Simpson, C. M., Mitchell, G. J., Fisher, A., Jones, G., & Linscott, J. (2006). Being listened to: A qualitative study of older adults in long-term care settings. *Journal of Gerontological Nursing, 32*(1), 46–53.

Juby, A., Tench, S., & Baker, V. (2002). The value of a clock drawing in identifying executive cognitive dysfunction in people with a normal Mini-Mental State Examination score. *Canadian Medical Association Journal, 167*, 859–864.

Kazui, H., Hirono, N., Hashimoto, M., Nakano, Y., Matsumoto, K., Takatsuki, Y., et al. (2006). Symptoms underlying unawareness of memory impairment in patients with mild Alzheimer's disease. *Journal of Geriatric Psychiatry and Neurology, 19*, 3–12.

Kennedy, G. J. (2003; revised 2007). Brief evaluation of executive dysfunction: An essential refinement in the assessment of cognitive impairment. *Try This: Best Practices in Nursing Care for Hospitalized Older Adults With Dementia*, Issue D3. New York University, Hartford Institute for Geriatric Nursing. Available at www.hartfordign.org/resources/education/tryThis.html.

Kolcaba, K., Schirm, V., & Steiner, R. (2006). Effects of hand massage on comfort of nursing home residents. *Geriatric Nursing, 27*, 85–91.

Mizrahl, R., Starkstein, S. E., Jorge, R., & Robinson, R. G. (2006). Phenomenology and clinical correlates of delusions in Alzheimer disease. *American Journal of Geriatric Psychiatry, 14*, 573–581.

Nagaratnam, N., Keen, R., & Gayagay, G. (2006). The accusers in dementia. *American Journal of Alzheimer Disease and Other Dementias, 21*, 164–168.

O'Connell, K. A., & Skevington, S. M. (2005). The relevance of spirituality, religion and personal beliefs to health-related quality of life: Themes from focus groups in Britain. *Journal of Health Psychology, 10*, 379–398.

O'Keefe, S. T., Mulkerrin, E. C., Nayeem, K., Varughese, M., & Pillay, I. (2005). Use of serial Mini-Mental State Examinations to diagnose and monitor delirium in elderly hospital patients. *Journal of the American Geriatrics Society, 53*, 867–870.

Ortiz, L. P. A., & Langer, N. (2002). Assessment of spirituality and religion in later life: Acknowledging clients' needs and personal resources. *Journal of Gerontological Social Work, 37*(2), 5–21.

Ostbye, T., Krause, K. M., Norton, M. C., Tschanz, J., Sanders, L., Hayden, K., et al. (2006). Ten dimensions of health and their relationships with overall self-reported health and survival in a predominately religiously active elderly population: The Cache County Memory Study. *Journal of the American Geriatrics Society, 54*, 199–209.

Ostling, S. (2002). Psychotic symptoms and paranoid ideation in a nondemented population-based sample of the very old. *Archives of General Psychiatry, 59*, 53–59.

Piccininni, M., DiCarlo, A., Baldereschi, M., Zaccara, G., & Inzitari, D. (2005). Behavioral and psychological symptoms in Alzheimer's disease: Frequency and relationship with duration and severity of the disease. *Dementia and Geriatric Cognitive Disorders, 19*, 276–281.

Piquet, O., Grayson, D. A., Broe, A., Tate, R. L., Bennett, H. P., Lye, T. C., et al. (2002). Normal aging and executive functions in "old-old" community dwellers: Poor performance is not an inevitable outcome. *International Psychogeriatrics, 14*, 139–159.

Ropacki, S. A., & Jeste, D. V. (2005). Epidemiology of and risk factors for psychosis of Alzheimer's disease: A review of 55 studies published from 1990 to 2003. *American Journal of Psychiatry, 162*, 2022–2030.

Ryff, C. D., & Kwan, C. M. L. (2001). Personality and aging: Flourishing agendas and future challenges. In J. E. Birren & K. W. Schaie (Eds.), *Handbook of the psychology of aging* (5th ed., pp. 477–499). San Diego: Academic Press.

Salmon, D. P., & Lange, K. L. (2001). Cognitive screening and neuropsychological assessment in early Alzheimer's disease. *Clinics in Geriatric Medicine, 17*, 229–254.

Scarmeas, N., Brandt, J., Albert, M., Hadjigeorgiou, G., Papadimitriou, A., Dubois, B., et al. (2005). Delusions and hallucinations are associated with worse outcome in Alzheimer disease. *Archives of Neurology, 62*, 1601–1608.

Silber, M. H., Hansen, M. R., & Girish, M. (2005). Complex nocturnal visual hallucinations. *Sleep Medicine, 6*, 363–366.

Sulmasy, D. P. (2002). A biopsychosocial-spiritual model for the care of patients at the end of life. *The Gerontologist, 42*(Special Issue III), 24–33.

Swick, B. L., & Walling, H. W. (2005). Drug-induced delusions of parasitosis during treatment of Parkinson's disease. *Journal of the American Academy of Dermatology, 53*, 1086–1087.

Talbot-Stern, J. K., Green, T., & Royle, T. (2000). Psychiatric manifestations of systemic illness. *Emergency Medicine Clinics of North America, 18*, 199–209.

Wetherell, J. L., Lenze, E. J., & Stanley, M. A. (2005). Evidence-based treatment of geriatric anxiety disorders. *Psychiatric Clinics of North America, 28*, 871–896.

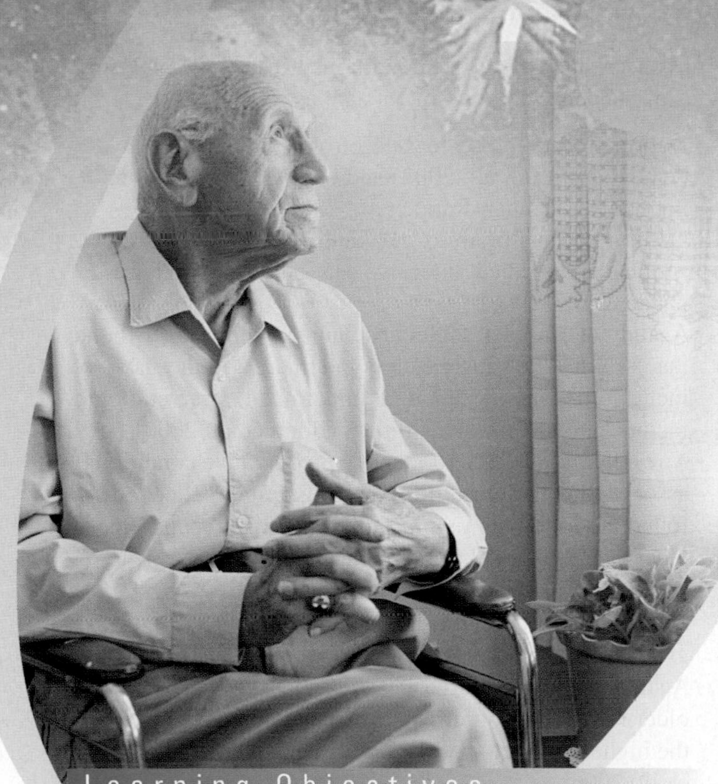

CHAPTER 14

Impaired Cognitive Function: Delirium and Dementia

Learning Objectives

After reading this chapter, you will be able to:

1. Describe delirium and discuss nursing assessment and interventions related to delirium.
2. Explain appropriate use of terminology that describes impaired cognitive function in older adults.
3. Describe characteristics of Alzheimer's disease, vascular dementia, frontotemporal dementia, and dementia with Lewy bodies.
4. List the factors that affect the risk for development of dementia.
5. Discuss the functional consequences of impaired cognitive function.
6. Describe guidelines for initial and ongoing assessment of cognitively impaired older adults.
7. Identify nonpharmacologic interventions for addressing dementia-related behaviors, including environmental modifications and communication techniques.
8. Discuss medications for slowing the progression of dementia and for managing dementia-related behaviors.

Key Terms

Alzheimer's disease
anosognosia
behavioral and psychological symptoms of dementia (BPSD)
beta-amyloid
catastrophic reaction
cerebrovascular brain injury
cognitive reserve
delirium
dementia
dementia with Lewy bodies
frontotemporal dementia
hardening of the arteries
hyperactive delirium
hypoactive delirium
mild cognitive impairment (MCI)
organic brain syndrome (OBS)
reality orientation
senility
vascular dementia

Healthy older adults experience only minor changes in cognitive abilities (as described in Chapter 11), but as people age, they are increasingly more likely to experience pathologic conditions that have a major impact on cognitive function. When impaired cognitive functioning causes a progressive loss of abilities that affects all aspects of functioning, it is one of the most devastating losses that older adults and their caregivers must confront. Nurses in all settings frequently care for older adults who have dementia or delirium—the two main causes of significant cognitive impairment in older adults. Nurses are responsible for identifying factors that contribute to impaired cognitive functioning in older adults. In addition, nurses and the other people who care for people with dementia must meet the challenge of preserving as much of the person's dignity and quality of life as possible, despite the serious and progressive losses the person with dementia experiences.

DELIRIUM

Overview and Types

Researchers and practitioners are increasingly addressing delirium as a serious, preventable, treatable, commonly occurring, and often unrecognized condition affecting older adults. **Delirium** is a syndrome characterized by the following (Peterson et al., 2006; Rigney, 2006):

- Fluctuating levels of altered mental status with reduced ability to focus, sustain, or shift attention
- Confusion, memory loss, disorientation
- Disorganized thinking, disordered speech
- Fatigue, sleep disturbances
- Fearfulness, excessive energy
- Altered perceptions, including hallucinations and delusions
- Personality changes
- Behavioral changes (e.g., loud vocalizations, hitting caregivers, attempts to remove clothing or medical equipment)

Three behavioral subtypes of delirium are hyperactive, hypoactive, and mixed. Patients with **hyperactive delirium** are overly alert, have increased psychomotor activity, and are acutely responsive to their environments (Rigney, 2006). In contrast, patients with **hypoactive delirium,** which also is called the *quiet delirium*, have low levels of psychomotor activity and may appear to be sedated or depressed (Peterson et al., 2006). Patients with mixed type fluctuate between hypoactive and hyperactive delirium over brief or long periods.

Although hypoactive delirium is considered to be the less common type, recent studies are challenging this perception, particularly with regard to older adults (Pandharipande & Ely, 2006). For example, a study of delirium in 112 medical intensive care patients found that 41% of patients aged 65 years and older but only 22% of the younger patients had hypoactive delirium, and none of the older patients experienced the purely hyperactive type (Peterson et al., 2006). Manifestations of either form of delirium develop over a short time (hours or days), fluctuate over the course of the day (usually affecting the sleep–wake cycle), and are not directly caused by a dementia or depression.

Prevalence and Risk Factors

Because 50% to 60% of all hospitalized older adults experience delirium, it is often cited as the most frequent complication of hospitalization. Factors that most commonly are cited as increasing the risk for delirium include advanced age, pain, dementia, surgery, medications, physiologic disturbances, and pathologic conditions. Results of some studies of incidence and risk factors are as follows:

- Delirium occurs in up to 89% of older adults who have dementia (Fick et al., 2002) and in 40% to 60% of nursing home residents (Rapp et al., 2001).
- Delirium occurs in up to 70% and 80%, respectively, of surgical and medical intensive care patients (Pandharipande & Ely, 2006).
- A study of 76 older adults hospitalized with cancer found that 57% had delirium; factors that increased the risk included increased functional impairment, more etiologic factors, and more serious illness (Bond et al., 2006).
- A review of literature to identify preoperative conditions associated with delirium in noncardiac surgical patients found the following risk factors: cognitive impairment, older age, functional impairment, sensory impairment, depression, preoperative psychotropic drugs, psychopathologic symptoms, institutional residence, and greater comorbidity (Dasgupta & Dumbrell, 2006).
- A study of 603 hip surgical patients age 70 years and older found that cognitive impairment on admission was the highest predictor of postoperative delirium (Kalisvaart et al., 2006).
- A 1-year study of 156 patients with stroke age 65 years and older identified the following independent risk factors: older age, intracerebral hemorrhage, metabolic factors, prestroke dementia, initial Glasgow Coma Scale score less than 15, and inability to lift both arms on admission (Sheng et al., 2006).
- A study of 71 hospitalized older adults with delirium superimposed on dementia found that the severity of prior cognitive impairment was predictive of the severity of most symptoms of delirium (Voyer et al., 2006).

Researchers and practitioners also are trying to determine the most common time frame for the onset and duration of delirium symptoms. For older adults, the onset is likely to occur during the first 2 days of hospitalization; it occurs only occasionally after the sixth day (Rapp et al., 2001). After discharge to rehabilitation or skilled nursing, the duration is likely to be prolonged in older adults and may last for up to 6 months after discharge (Marcantonio et al., 2003).

Functional Consequences of Delirium

Researchers have identified the following serious functional consequences of delirium in older adults (Leslie et al., 2005; McAvay et al., 2006; Pandharipande & Ely, 2006; Pitkala et al., 2006; Sheng et al., 2006):

- Longer hospital stays
- Increased mortality
- Increased nursing care
- Development of dementia
- Immediate and long-term functional impairment
- Higher rates of permanent residency in long-term care facilities

Nursing Assessment of Delirium

Researchers and clinicians also are focusing on the very common occurrence of clinicians failing to recognize delirium in up to 84% of older adults (Lemiengre et al., 2006; Pandharipande & Ely, 2006). Nurse-related factors that contribute to this failure are lack of knowledge about assessment methods and lack of communication among nursing staff. Patient-related contributing factors include older age, preexisting dementia, vision impairment, and having the hypoactive type (Inouye et al., 2005; Rigney, 2006). The Hartford Institute for Geriatric Nursing recommends the Confusion Assessment Method and the use of a delirium algorithm for assessing and managing delirium (see Clinical Tool Resources). The Hospital Elder Life Program also has published a protocol for assessing and managing delirium in older adults (Fig. 14-1) (Sandhaus et al., 2006). Studies have found that the serial use of the Mini-Mental State Examination (MMSE) is a reliable way of detecting delirium, particularly in people who also have dementia, because it measures fluctuations in cognition (O'Keeffe et al., 2005).

Nursing Diagnosis and Outcomes

The nursing diagnosis of Acute Confusion is applicable when the onset of mental changes is abrupt or caused by risk factors such as medical conditions and adverse medication effects. To address this diagnosis, nurses can use the following Nursing Outcomes Classification (NOC) terms in their care plans: Anxiety Level, Cognition, Cognitive Orientation, Concentration, Distorted Thought Self-Control, Identity, Information Processing, Memory, Mood Equilibrium, Neurologic Status, Psychomotor Energy. In addition, the following NOC terms may be applicable to address causative factors: Electrolyte & Acid/Base Balance, Hydration, Infection Severity, Nutritional Status, Risk Control, and Sensory Function Status.

Wellness Opportunity

Nurses can use the NOC Comfort Level in their care plans to address holistically the needs of older adults with delirium.

Nursing Interventions for Delirium

Because of the complexity of delirium, it requires a multidisciplinary approach to management, with nurses having a key role in detection, ongoing assessment, and management. Models of management typically are multifactorial and include the following components: staff education, comprehensive geriatric assessment and treatments for all contributing factors, appropriate use and discontinuation of medications, orientation, environmental modification, physical and occupational therapies, nutritional interventions (e.g., calcium and vitamin D supplements), measures for preventing complications (e.g., falls, injuries, sleep problems, pressure ulcers, aspiration), and comprehensive discharge planning (Bergmann et al., 2005; Lundstrom et al., 2005; Pitkala et al., 2006). The following are examples of specific interventions that nurses can include in care plans:

- Provision of aids to orientation (e.g., clock, watch, calendar) and aids to improve sensory function (e.g., eyeglasses, hearing aids)
- Environmental modification (e.g., noise reduction, familiar objects)
- Psychological support (e.g., cognitive and social stimulation)
- Identification of adverse medication effects and discussion of medication regimen with prescribing practitioners
- Interventions to promote physiologic stability (e.g., low-dose oxygenation, maintenance of fluid and electrolyte balance)
- Adequate pain management (refer to Chapter 28)
- Physical activity (e.g., ambulation, physical therapy).

Figure 14-1 lists examples of research-based nursing interventions that address physical needs of hospitalized older adults with delirium (Sandhaus et al., 2006).

The following Nursing Interventions Classification (NIC) terms are examples of interventions that can be used in care plans for acute confusion: Anxiety Reduction, Behavior Management, Cognitive Stimulation, Delirium Management, Energy Management, Environmental Management, Fluid/Electrolyte Management, Hallucination Management, Medication Management, Mood Management, Nutrition Management, Pain Management, Reality Orientation, Sedation Management, and Surveillance: Safety.

Wellness Opportunity

Nursing interventions to address holistically the needs of older adults during confusional states include Calming Technique, Emotional Support, Music Therapy, Presence, and Touch.

OVERVIEW OF DEMENTIA

Terminology to Describe Dementia

An understanding of impaired cognitive function is complicated by the many terms that have been used interchangeably—and often inaccurately—to describe dementia. Major progress in evidence-based research has greatly improved the ability of clinicians to diagnose and treat different types of dementia, but it has also led to the proliferation of dementia-related terminology. Perhaps more than any other terms used in reference to older adults, those associated with cognitive impairments are the most misused, misunderstood, and emotionally charged. The following are some of the terms that health care professionals use in reference to cognitive impairment in older adults: confusion, dementia,

CARING FOR YOUR PATIENT WITH DELIRIUM

Features of delirium

- Acute onset of confusion with a fluctuating course
- Inattention: highly distractible, with difficulty focusing
- Disorganized thinking, altered level of consciousness, or both

Rule out physiologic causes

NEURO EVENT

- Check level of consciousness.
- History of recent head injury (subdural hematoma)
- Neurologic check, noting motor deficit, pupil changes
- Diagnostic testing as ordered
- Lab studies (vitamin B_{12}, folate, blood chemistries, thyroid-stimulating hormone)

MEDICATION

- Check recent medication changes. Check drug levels. Avoid these medications: benzodiazepines, anticholinergics (diphenhydramine [Benadryl], oxybutynin [Ditropan], metoclopramide [Reglan]), steroids, $histamine_2$ blockers (famotidine [Pepcid], ranitidine HCI [Zantac]), drugs with high toxicity (digoxin [Lanoxin], phenytoin sodium [Dilantin]), psychotropics.

INFECTION

- Consider urinary tract infection or pneumonia.
- Check temperature and vital signs.
- Lab work
- Chest X-ray
- Urinalysis (culture and sensitivity)
- Blood culture
- Sputum culture

DEHYDRATION

- Monitor intake and output.
- Check serum glucose.
- Give I.V. fluid as needed.
- Review lab work.
- Ensure adequate nutrition and hydration.
- Check for electrolyte imbalance.

HYPOXIA

- Pulse oximetry
- Respiratory rate
- Sputum
- Arterial blood gases
- Chest X-ray

Address physical needs

SAFETY

- Glasses
- Hearing device
- Orientation or reorientation
- Gentle reassurance
- Family at bedside
- Early mobilization
- Fall-prevention protocol
- Consult physical therapy, occupational therapy.

PAIN

- Provide comfort, supportive measures.
- Give medication as ordered and assess pain control.
- Avoid meperidine (Demerol) and propoxyphene/acetaminophen (Darvocet), which may cause seizures, delirium in elderly.
- Use acetaminophen (Tylenol) around the clock as first-line analgesic.
- Add a laxative to any opioid regimen.

ELIMINATION

- Frequent toileting
- Bowel regimen
- Remove urinary drainage catheter as soon as possible.
- Treat constipation.

SLEEP

- Use comfort measures, back rub.
- Allow for long intervals of uninterrupted sleep.
- Avoid sedative-hypnotic medications.

NUTRITION

- Assist or feed.
- Give supplements as required.
- Consult speech pathologist for swallow evaluation, nutritionist.
- Skin assessment

SOURCE: Adapted from a delirium algorithm developed at Moses Taylor Hospital.

FIGURE 14-1 Protocol for assessing and managing delirium in older adults published by the Hospital Elder Life Program. (Reprinted with permission from Sandhaus, S., Harrell, F., & Valenti, D. [2006]. Healthier aging: Here's help to prevent delirium in the hospital. *Nursing 2006, 36*[7], 60–62.)

senility, Alzheimer's disease, small strokes, memory problems, "old-timer's disease," organic brain syndrome, and "hardening of the arteries." Because labels that describe cognitive impairments are associated with fear and stigma, gerontologists in many countries (e.g., Japan, Canada, the United States) are trying to identify less stigmatizing and more accurate terminology (Whitehouse, 2006).

Different terms are more or less acceptable to different people, and the selection of a term often is based on emotional preferences or lack of accurate information. Because cognitive impairment is an emotionally charged subject, nurses must understand the correct terminology and then choose the most appropriate term based on an understanding of the underlying causes for the impairment and an assessment of what term is most acceptable to the older adult and his or her caregivers.

By definition, **senility** means old age, or pertaining to old age, and originally it was a neutral term. Over the past two centuries, however, it has become associated with infirmity, diseases, and feeblemindedness. As recently as the 1970s, senility was the explanation given for any condition associated with "aging" that was viewed as needing no further investigation or treatment. Unfortunately, current usage implies that the impairments are a necessary consequence of being old. Two decades ago, nurses were advised never to use the word *senile* because it is an archaic, negative, prejudicial, and unprofessional term that should never be used to describe an older person (Hogstel, 1988).

During the early 1900s, the phrase "**hardening of the arteries**" was the common diagnostic label for cognitive impairment in older adults. Although this term suggested that there was a pathologic cause, the condition was still viewed as an inevitable consequence of aging. This label, therefore, did nothing to challenge the myth that cognitive impairments were an integral part of aging. Like *senility*, this term is now considered outdated and is not used in reference to cognitive impairments.

By the 1950s, the phrase **organic brain syndrome (OBS)** had become the commonly used term for cognitive impairment in older adults. This term described a constellation of acute or chronic neurologic effects of underlying pathologic conditions. The term *acute organic brain syndrome* (also called *delirium*) referred to conditions that would resolve after the underlying cause was treated. By contrast, the term *chronic organic brain syndrome* (COBS) referred to an irreversible condition that was closely associated with underlying vascular pathology. With the use of the terms OBS and COBS, cognitive impairments were no longer viewed as inevitable, but they still were considered untreatable.

In the 1960s, autopsy examination of brain specimens provided the first scientific evidence about the underlying causes of cognitive impairments. Based on these findings, researchers and practitioners concluded that as many as 25% of the changes previously attributed to COBS or untreatable vascular diseases actually were manifestations of treatable conditions. During the 1970s, *pseudodementia* was used in reference to cognitive impairments caused by physiologic conditions, but this term is no longer used.

Dementia is the term that most accurately describes progressive declines in cognitive function. Dementia is "a syndrome of impaired cognition caused by brain dysfunction" and characterized by multiple cognitive deficits, such as memory impairment, aphasia, apraxia, agnosia, or impaired executive functions (Morris, 2000, p. 774). In addition, noncognitive characteristics, such as changes in personality and behavior, are manifestations of dementia. Unfortunately, this medical term is associated with the lay term "demented," which has a long history of pejorative use in popular language and is even more derogatory than the word "senile." Thus, nurses can use phrases such as "a person with dementia" or a "person with a dementing illness" to accurately refer to the medical syndrome of impaired cognitive function while avoiding pejorative connotations.

An additional point must be emphasized with regard to the term *dementia*. Dementia is not a single disease but a syndrome, and the term refers to a combination of manifestations that arise from different and sometimes interacting causes. Because **Alzheimer's disease** is the most common type of dementia, and the type with the longest history of recognition, *Alzheimer's disease* and *dementia* are often used interchangeably. In this chapter, theories about dementia are discussed in the following section, and the four most widely recognized types of dementia are described (see section on Types of Dementia). The term *dementia* is used throughout the chapter, except when the information is pertinent to a particular type. The text refers to Alzheimer's disease when a source used that term; however, readers need to recognize that many of the citations in the literature on Alzheimer's disease refer to dementia in the broader sense.

An important consideration regarding terminology is that there are significant overlaps in manifestations of different types of dementia and that two (or more) types of dementia can coexist in the same person. Researchers now acknowledge that even Alzheimer's disease is not a single entity, but, like dementia, it also is a syndrome that cannot be clearly defined (Whitehouse, 2006). There is increasing recognition that advances in research and technology have caused the boundaries of dementia terminology to become fuzzier rather than clearer (Whitehouse & Moody, 2006).

Theories to Explain Dementia

The evolution of dementia terminology just described is indicative of the significant developments in theories to explain dementia during the past century. Gerontologists have made major progress in identifying pathologic changes and behavioral manifestations that characterize different types of dementia, and some progress has been made in identifying various causes of dementia. However, despite more than 100 years of research on causes of impaired cognitive function in older adults, theories to explain dementia are still evolving.

During the 1800s, European physicians discovered neuritic plaques in the brains of older adults and identified these changes as the cause of senility, or senile dementia. Around that same time, medical scientists discovered that arteries throughout the body lose their elasticity and become hardened during later adulthood and they theorized that this was the underlying cause of the brain changes in older adults. In 1906, Alois Alzheimer, a German physician, discovered neuritic plaques in the autopsied brain specimens from a woman who was 55 years old when she died and had initially manifested cognitive and behavior changes around the age of 50 years. Based on these findings, physicians and researchers concluded that neuritic plaques caused presenile dementia, hardening of the arteries caused senile dementia, and Alzheimer's disease and senile dementia were distinct diseases differentiated by age at onset. Simply stated, if the onset of the cognitive impairment occurred before the age of 65 years, it was called Alzheimer's disease, whereas if the onset took place after the age of 65 years, it was called senility or hardening of the arteries.

This chronologic distinction between senile and presenile dementia was not challenged until the 1960s, when autopsy studies found no association between the degree of arteriosclerotic brain changes and the clinical manifestations of dementia during the person's lifetime. These landmark studies by Tomlinson and colleagues (1968, 1970) led to the theory that the neuropathologic changes of Alzheimer's disease represent a single disease process, regardless of the age at onset. Furthermore, autopsy studies of brain specimens from subjects with and without dementia revealed that Alzheimer's disease was the underlying cause of progressive dementia in most cases.

In 1974, the conclusions of Tomlinson and associates were supported by a landmark study of Hachinski and colleagues, which found that cerebral atherosclerosis was both a major cause of cognitive impairments and the most common medical misdiagnosis. Moreover, these scientists denounced the use of the phrase "hardening of the arteries" and introduced the term "multi-infarct dementia" to describe dementias of cerebrovascular origin. Their rationale was that dementia was not caused by atherosclerosis or chronic ischemia, but by the occurrence of multiple cerebral infarcts. More recent studies suggest that the term *vascular dementia* is more accurate, as discussed in the section on Types of Dementia.

Since the 1990s, theories about dementia have expanded, due largely to brain imaging techniques that can provide information about different aspects of brain function. For example, computed tomography (CT) and magnetic resonance imaging (MRI) provide information about structural brain changes and lesions that can cause cognitive impairment. Single photon emission computed tomography (SPECT) and positron emission tomography (PET) scans provide specific information about metabolism rates for glucose and oxygen in the brain. Researchers currently use information from imaging techniques to supplement information from autopsies, clinical records, mental status tests, and other sources. In addition, many longitudinal studies provide valuable information about lifestyle patterns and cognitive function during adulthood, and some studies are designed to evaluate this information in relation to autopsy findings.

TYPES OF DEMENTIA

This chapter reviews current information about the four most commonly recognized types of dementia, but it is important to realize that despite the increasing research, the knowledge base about dementia is still very weak. In addition, older adults commonly have more than one type of dementia, and as the pathologic process progresses, it becomes more difficult to distinguish one type of dementia from another. Information that is clinically important in relation to a specific type of dementia is discussed in this chapter; however, information about functional consequences, assessment, and interventions applies to all types.

Alzheimer's Disease

Various figures on the prevalence of Alzheimer's disease have been quoted, with many estimates indicating that 50% of people aged 85 years or older and up to 80% of nursing home residents have Alzheimer's disease. Although studies about the rates of Alzheimer's disease at specific ages vary, gerontologists agree that the chance of having Alzheimer's disease increases with increasing age. Figure 14-2 shows percentages of community-residing men and women according to age categories who had moderate or severe memory impairment, which was defined as the ability to recall 4 or fewer words out of 20 on a simple test or per report of proxy responders (Federal Interagency Forum, 2006). Data from the 2000 census indicates that 4.5 million people in the United States have Alzheimer's disease, with the following distribution by age category: 7% age 65 to 74 years, 53% between 75 and 84 years, and 40% age 85 years and older (Morris, 2005).

Pathologic Changes Associated With Alzheimer's Disease

The hallmark pathologic criterion for Alzheimer's disease is the presence of neuritic plaques and neurofibrillary tangles, as identified by Alzheimer in 1907 (Alzheimer, 1907) and confirmed by numerous autopsy studies done since the 1960s (Fig. 14-3). Although these pathologic alterations also occur in normal aging and other neurodegenerative diseases, the combination of a higher density in specific regions (e.g., the neocortex) and a clinical history consistent with Alzheimer's disease confirms the diagnosis of Alzheimer's disease with a high degree of accuracy (Morris, 2005). Loss or degeneration of neurons and synapses, particularly in the neocortex and hippocampus, is another cen-

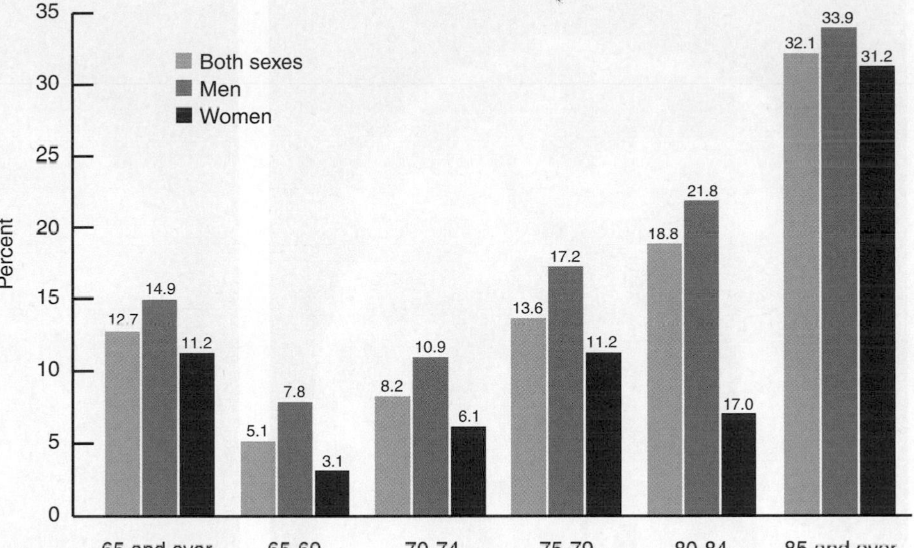

FIGURE 14-2 Percentage of people age 65 years of age and older with moderate or severe memory impairment (i.e., recall of 4 or fewer words of 20 on delayed recall test) by age group and sex, 2002. (Source: Federal Interagency Forum on Aging-Related Statistics. [2006]. *Older Americans update 2006: Key indicators of well-being* [p. 26]. Washington, DC: U.S. Government Printing Office.)

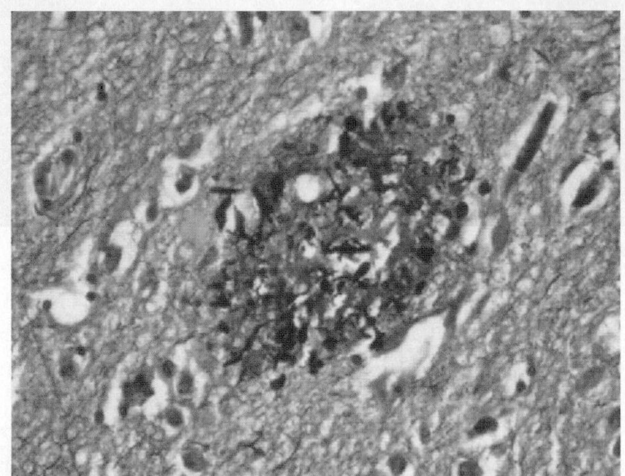

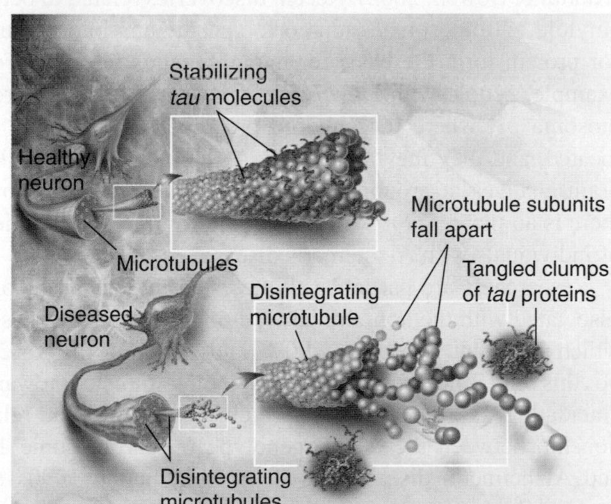

FIGURE 14-3 The hallmark neuropathologic findings in Alzheimer's disease. **(A)** Amyloid plaque. **(B)** Neurofibrillary tangle. (Images courtesy of the Alzheimer's Disease Education and Referral Center, a service of the National Institute on Aging.)

tral feature of the brain changes associated with Alzheimer's disease (Fig. 14-4). In addition, Alzheimer's disease is associated with a marked reduction in brain weight.

Alzheimer first described **beta-amyloid** as a "peculiar substance" in 1907, but this substance was not named or defined until 1984. By the early 1990s, scientists had identified the presence of beta-amyloid in the plaques and blood vessels as another pathologic hallmark of Alzheimer's disease. The discovery that beta-amyloid was a normal substance produced by many cells in the body laid the groundwork for much of the current research on the role of beta-amyloid and its precursor protein. Scientists now know that beta-amyloid is a tiny, insoluble protein fragment of a much larger protein called the *amyloid precursor protein*. The exact functions of the amyloid precursor protein have not been identified, but researchers recognize that this protein has multiple essential roles in cells throughout the body. What is known is that excessive amounts of beta-amyloid are found in the neuritic plaques and the walls of the blood vessels in the brains of people with Alzheimer's disease and Down syndrome. Current research is addressing the following questions about the relationship between beta-amyloid and Alzheimer's disease: does the abnormal accumulation of beta-amyloid result from excessive production or insufficient removal; and is beta-amyloid the cause or effect of pathologic processes? Researchers also are examining the potential cause–effect relationship between increased deposits of tau proteins in cerebrospinal fluid and in the damaged regions of the brain (Haroutunian et al., 2007; Morris, 2005).

Pathologic brain changes of Alzheimer's disease trigger changes in neurotransmitters that lead to the degeneration of healthy neurons and, eventually, to cell death. Specific effects on neurotransmitters include loss of serotonin receptors and decreased production of acetylcholine, acetylcholinesterase, and choline acetyltransferase. The greatest

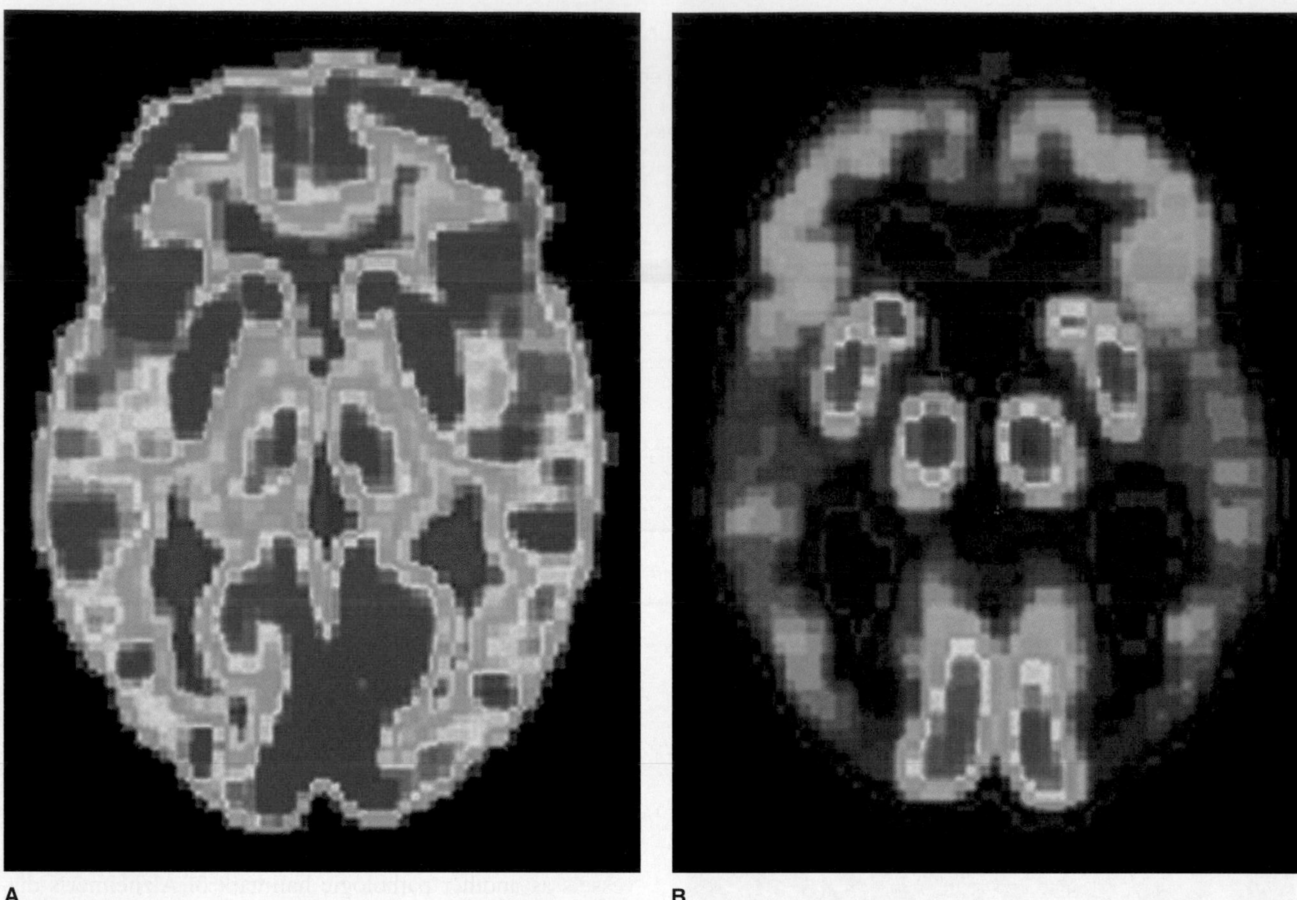

FIGURE 14-4 (A) A positron emission tomography (PET) scan of a brain of a healthy person. **(B)** A PET scan of a brain of a person with Alzheimer's disease. The blue areas indicate reduced brain activity. (Images courtesy of the Alzheimer's Disease Education and Referral Center, a service of the National Institute on Aging.)

reduction in transmitters occurs in the areas most affected by plaques and tangles, and these changes cause both cognitive and behavioral symptoms. These research findings have led to the development of cholinesterase inhibitor drugs that prevent or slow the breakdown of acetylcholine (e.g., tacrine, donepezil, rivastigmine, and galantamine).

Causes of and Risks for Alzheimer's Disease

Researchers first raised questions about genetic factors as a cause of Alzheimer's disease in the mid-1930s, but it was not until the late 1970s that the phrase "familial Alzheimer's disease" appeared in the literature. Research indicates that an identifiable genetic mutation is found in 5% to 10% of cases of Alzheimer's disease (Rogan & Lippa, 2002). In familial Alzheimer's disease, the children of an affected parent have a 25% to 50% chance of having Alzheimer's disease if they live to be old enough for the disease to manifest itself. The risk is higher if the disease occurs in more than one generation and when the onset of the disease is before the age of 65 years (Tsuang & Bird, 2002). Abnormalities on chromosomes 1, 14, and 21 are associated with early-onset, or familial, Alzheimer's disease, but researchers have yet to identify one fourth to one half of the genes for this disease (Kukull & Bowen, 2002). Recent discoveries related to beta-amyloid, chromosomal mutations, and the amyloid precursor protein form the basis for much genetics research. For example, people with Down syndrome have an extra chromosome 21, where the amyloid precursor protein gene is located, and they inevitably show Alzheimer's disease–like brain changes at around the age of 40 years. In addition, there is an increased risk of Down syndrome in the families of individuals with Alzheimer's disease.

Researchers are particularly interested in genetic factors associated with the nonfamilial type of Alzheimer's disease, which constitutes between 90% and 95% of the cases. To this end, intensive efforts are being directed toward elucidating the role of apolipoprotein E (APOE). The relationship between the APOE genotype on chromosome 19 and Alzheimer's disease was discovered in the 1990s as a spin-off of studies on triglyceride metabolism and cholesterol levels in cardiovascular disease (Roses, 1995). There are three variants of the APOE gene, designated as APOE-$_{E}$2, APOE-$_{E}$3, and APOE-$_{E}$4. Each person inherits one APOE gene from each parent, so there are six possible combinations (2/2, 2/3, 2/4, 3/3, 3/4, and 4/4). The inherited combination may be at least partially predictive of the risk for and age at onset of Alzheimer's disease. For example, an increased risk for and younger age at onset is associated with APOE-$_E$4, particularly in women (Choi et al., 2003; Tsuang & Bird, 2002). By contrast, APOE-$_E$2 is associated with both a decreased risk for Alzheimer's disease and a later age at onset if the disease does develop. Current research is focusing on the practical implications of the role of APOE in causing or preventing Alzheimer's disease. Another area of research is the role of APOE-$_E$4 as a risk factor for longer duration of delirium in older adults (Ely et al., 2007).

In addition to studying genetic factors, researchers are focusing on the following factors:

- Inflammatory processes
- Vascular risk factors (e.g., smoking, hypertension, diabetes, serum lipids, dietary fat intake, and abnormal insulin metabolism)
- The role of nerve growth factors (i.e., proteins that regulate nerve cell maturation)
- Diverse causative factors such as head trauma, environmental toxins, the flow of calcium in and out of brain cells, and the possibility that Alzheimer's disease is a systemic metabolic disorder with some specificity for brain tissue
- Early-life risk factors, including perinatal conditions, growth patterns, socioeconomic conditions, and environmental influences (Borenstein et al., 2006)
- Psychosocial factors (e.g., depression, loneliness, social isolation) (Morris, 2005; Wilson et al., 2007)

Some theories have been studied for many decades and are inconclusive but still being investigated. For example, researchers are still investigating viral origins of dementia, based on the discovery in the 1920s of viral causes of some types of dementia. Questions about aluminum were first raised in the 1960s when abnormally high levels were found in the brains of people with Alzheimer's disease. Although a few studies have confirmed this finding, there is no evidence of a cause–effect relationship, nor is there evidence that high levels in the brain are related to the amount of aluminum ingested through the diet. Studies also are addressing potential effects of other minerals, including zinc, calcium, and fluoride.

Theories About the Stages of Alzheimer's Disease

Gerontologists are addressing questions about stages of Alzheimer's disease because longitudinal studies indicate that pathologic changes affect the brain years before the manifestation of symptoms. Thus, the concept of preclinical Alzheimer's disease (or a predementia syndrome) has emerged and researchers and practitioners have been using the term **mild cognitive impairment (MCI)** to describe a transitional stage between normal cognitive aging and diagnosable dementia (Panza et al., 2005). People with MCI have short-term memory impairment and some difficulty with complex cognitive skills (e.g., written arithmetic). Studies indicate that people with MCI are more impaired in daily activities than healthy control subjects (Farias et al., 2006). Longitudinal studies have consistently found that MCI is associated with a higher risk for Alzheimer's disease, a more rapid decline, and higher mortality (Boyle et al., 2006; Gualtieri & Johnson, 2005; Joshi & Morley, 2006). Other diagnostic labels that are used to describe preclinical stages of dementia include age-associated memory impairment, age-associated cognitive decline, and cognitive impairment not dementia (Feldman & Jacova, 2005; Serrano et al., 2007). Pathologic brain changes can be correlated with stages of disease as illustrated in Figure 14-5. Cognitive and behavioral changes associated with each of these stages are discussed in the section on Functional Consequences.

Vascular Dementia

Vascular dementia has been identified as a common and distinct type of dementia for several decades. However, recent studies, particularly those based on autopsies, indicate that cerebrovascular damage most often occurs concurrently with the neuropathologic changes of other types of dementia. One study found that only 3% of 382 autopsied brains showed pure vascular dementia, and another study found that vascular lesions coexisted with Alzheimer's pathology in 77% of the cases of presumed vascular dementia (Morris, 2005). Despite these questions, there is agreement that vascular dementia is caused by the death of nerve cells in the regions nourished by the diseased vessels. The concept of **cerebrovascular brain injury** addresses underlying pathologic processes, which include the following conditions (Chui, 2005):

- Single or multiple emboli or atherosclerotic occlusions of large blood vessels
- Microinfarcts (lacunar strokes of the small arteries)
- Diffuse lesions involving the white matter (e.g., Binswanger's disease)
- Hemorrhage of large or small blood vessels
- Hypoxic lesions
- Hypoperfusion secondary to global brain ischemia after cardiac arrest or profound hypotension
- Hypoperfusion from chronic conditions such as orthostatic hypotension, cardiac arrhythmias, congestive heart failure
- Narrowing of the lumen associated with diabetes, hypertension, or arteriosclerosis

Because of the broader understanding of vascular dementia, the term *multi-infarct dementia* is considered inaccurate.

Clinical manifestations of vascular dementia vary according to the area of brain that is affected. Common manifestations include cognitive impairments (e.g., aphasia, memory impairment), behavior changes (e.g., apathy, depression,

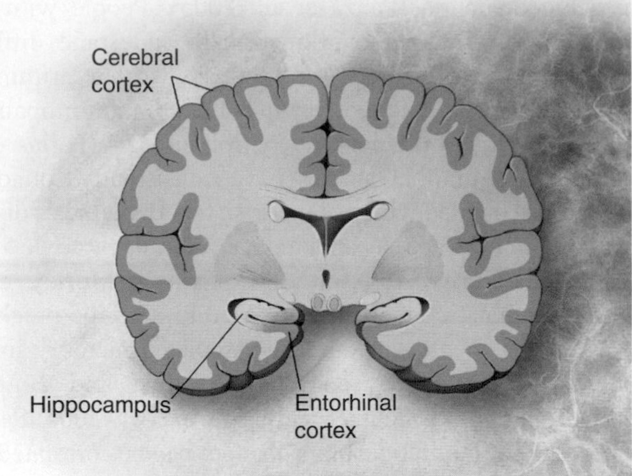

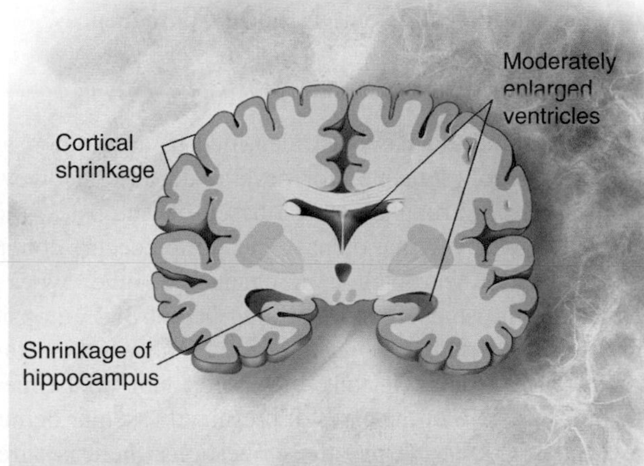

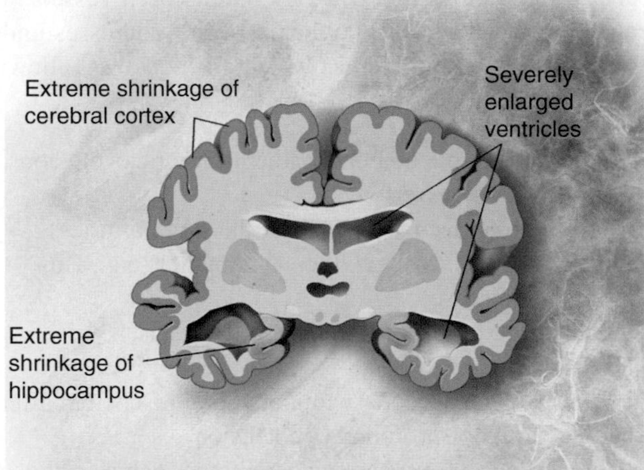

FIGURE 14-5 **(A)** Preclinical Alzheimer's disease. Subtle degenerative changes begin to occur in the cortex, and the person develops mild cognitive impairment. **(B)** Mild Alzheimer's disease. Degenerative changes affect the areas of the brain that control memory, language, and reasoning. **(C)** Severe Alzheimer's disease. Degenerative brain changes have caused significant atrophy in many areas. (Images courtesy of the Alzheimer's Disease Education and Referral Center, a service of the National Institute on Aging.)

emotional lability), and sensory-motor deficits (e.g., hemiparesis, gait disturbances, hemisensory loss, urinary incontinence). Many references state that vascular dementia is characterized by an abrupt onset and a stepwise progression, but this is not always obvious because it can occur in combination with other types of dementia. Studies indicate that clinically silent presentations are more common and that the classic presentation of sudden onset with stepwise deterioration occurs less than half the time (Ross & Bowen, 2002).

Dementia With Lewy Bodies

Dementia with Lewy bodies (i.e., spherical, cytoplasmic inclusions that are formed by a protein called alpha-synuclein) is now recognized as the second most common type of dementia (Morris, 2005). Gerontologists do not agree on whether dementia with Lewy bodies is a subtype of Alzheimer's disease, a form of Parkinson's disease, or a distinct pathologic entity with characteristics of both Alzheimer's and Parkinson's (Chartier-Harlan et al., 2004; Morris, 2005). Autopsy studies have confirmed that many people who have dementia with Lewy bodies also have Alzheimer's disease, with one study finding a co-occurrence rate of 66% (Johnson et al., 2005; Morris, 2005).

Practitioners can identify dementia with Lewy bodies according to the following characteristics, which are based on guidelines established by an international consortium (Morris, 2005; Mosimann et al., 2006; Neef & Walling, 2006):

- Impaired cognition, especially executive functioning and visuospatial skills (less memory impairment than with Alzheimer's disease)
- Widely fluctuating cognition over minutes, hours, or days
- Increased sensitivity to neuroleptic medications
- Recurrent visual hallucinations, which typically are vivid and colorful and involve complex images of humans, animals, or objects
- Parkinsonism, with motor symptoms occurring within 1 year of the cognitive symptoms
- Additional common symptoms include falls, apathy, syncope, depression, sleep disorders, and urinary incontinence

Nurses and primary care practitioners need to be alert to the clinical implications of the increased neuroleptic sensitivity that is characteristic of dementia with Lewy bodies. People with this type of dementia are likely to have extreme, idiosyncratic, or fatal reactions to even low doses of cholinergic-type medications, such as antipsychotics. For example, sedatives may cause extreme agitation, somnolence, or sleeplessness. Likewise, antipsychotic medications or medications for Parkinson's disease may cause or exacerbate delusions and visual hallucinations. Anticholinergic medications, including over-the-counter products, should be avoided.

Another clinically important characteristic is that people with dementia with Lewy bodies are medically frail and may decompensate rapidly and significantly when they have a medical condition (e.g., minor infection) or when their environment is changed (Rogan & Lippa, 2002). Because of the serious clinical implications of this type of dementia and because it is difficult to diagnose, nurses need to be alert to the possibility that someone may have undiagnosed dementia with Lewy bodies.

Diversity Note

Studies indicate that the prevalence of dementia with Lewy bodies is higher in men than in women (Johnson et al., 2005).

Frontotemporal Dementia

Frontotemporal dementia describes a group of neurodegenerative conditions associated with disorders of *tau* (a type of protein in neurons) that cause atrophy in the frontal and temporal lobes. Several decades of research have led to the conclusion that frontotemporal dementia is as common or only slightly less so than Alzheimer's disease as a cause of dementia in people younger than 65 years of age (Grossman, 2005; Morris, 2005). The mean age at onset is between 52 and 56 years, but it has been reported in people between the ages of 21 and 85 years (Boxer & Miller, 2005; Farmer & Grossman, 2005). Gerontologists now recognize that there are many forms of frontotemporal dementia, with Pick's disease being the first type identified, in 1892 (Kertesz, 2005). Researchers have linked frontotemporal dementia to abnormalities on chromosome 17, and 30% to 40% of people with this type of dementia have other family members with a neurodegenerative condition (Farmer & Grossman, 2005).

Clinical manifestations of frontotemporal dementia differ significantly from those of other types of dementia during early stages, but as the disease progresses they are similar to other dementias. Gerontologists have developed criteria for frontotemporal dementia and emphasized the importance of recognizing this condition as a dementia rather than a psychiatric disorder (McKhann et al., 2001). The following are commonly occurring characteristics of frontotemporal dementia (Boxer & Miller, 2005; Farmer & Grossman, 2005; Langmore et al., 2007):

- Initial onset: personality changes, progressive aphasia, impaired judgment and problem-solving skills
- Behavioral manifestations: apathy, self-neglect, disinhibition, blunted affect, lack of insight, insensitivity to others, perseverative activity (e.g., repetitive clapping, humming, or singing)
- Orolingual manifestations: language impairment (e.g., using words incorrectly, echoing what others say), hyperorality (e.g., excessive or compulsive eating or drinking)
- Later-stage manifestations: mutism, dysphagia, incontinence

FACTORS ASSOCIATED WITH DEMENTIA

From a wellness perspective, it is important to recognize not only the factors that increase the risk for dementia but those that protect against cognitive impairment. Thus, this section addresses both those aspects, with emphasis on those factors that nurses can address through health education. In addition, this section addresses factors that interfere with assessment and interventions, because dementia is a condition that is common in older adults but is very complex and difficult to diagnose and manage.

Factors That Increase the Risk for Development of Dementia

Epidemiologic studies of people who are cognitively impaired are flourishing, and researchers are trying to identify conditions that increase the risk for development of dementia. Although some studies focus on dementia in general, most focus on a particular type of dementia, and still others focus on preclinical dementia (e.g., MCI). Thus, conclusions about risk factors are clouded by differing scopes of studies and overlapping and poorly defined terminology. Current information about risk factors for the four most widely studied types of dementia is described in the corresponding sections under Types of Dementia. Nurses need to keep in mind that because our understanding of different types of dementia has changed significantly in the past two decades, information about risks also will continue to evolve rapidly.

Factors That Protect Against Dementia

In recent years, researchers have focused increasingly on preventive strategies to protect against dementia. A consistent finding is that the same behaviors that have positive outcomes for overall wellness also have a positive effect on preventing cognitive decline. For example, engaging in regular physical exercise is one of the most commonly identified preventive strategies (Larson et al., 2006). Nutritional interventions for preserving cognitive function include consuming foods that are high in antioxidants (e.g., vitamins C and E) and in omega-3 polyunsaturated fatty acids (e.g., fish and fish oil) (Morris, 2005). As discussed in Chapter 11, there is increasing evidence that engaging in socially and cognitively stimulating and meaningful activities is beneficial for preventing cognitive decline. Studies also indicate that higher educational levels can protect from dementia by increasing a person's **cognitive reserve**, which is defined as the ability to cope with brain pathology without experiencing cognitive decline (Roe et al., 2007). Longitudinal studies also are focusing on potential preventive effects of medications such as statins. Estrogen and nonsteroidal anti-inflammatory drugs (NSAIDs) are medical interventions that are no longer being investigated because of concern about adverse effects (Morris, 2005).

Wellness Opportunity

Nurses can teach all adults that engaging in social, mental, and physical activity is a risk-free way of promoting cognitive wellness and may also prevent dementia.

Factors That Interfere With Assessment of and Interventions for Dementia

Attitudes, myths, and lack of information are risk factors that interfere with appropriate assessment of, and interventions for, dementia. In recent years, gerontologists have made tremendous progress in understanding and identifying causes of impaired cognitive function, so health care providers are increasingly less likely to attribute serious cognitive impairments to "normal aging." However, many older adults and their families and caregivers still falsely believe that "senility" is an expected and normal concomitant of aging. When this happens, treatable conditions are likely to be overlooked and older adults are denied the appropriate interventions to treat or manage their conditions. Even in the absence of curative treatments, many interventions are effective in delaying the progression of the condition, managing symptoms, and assisting with long-term planning.

Wellness Opportunity

Nurses have many opportunities to teach older adults and their caregivers about the importance of evaluating any significant cognitive impairment.

Cultural factors that influence perceptions about aging and illness can significantly affect both the evaluation and treatment of dementia. For example, some cultural groups accept cognitive impairment as "normal aging," whereas others view dementia-related behaviors as shameful. Gerontologists are just beginning to study various aspects of cultural influences on perception of mental changes and acceptance of interventions.

FUNCTIONAL CONSEQUENCES ASSOCIATED WITH DEMENTIA IN OLDER ADULTS

As with other aspects of dementia, functional consequences are discussed in reference to Alzheimer's disease because these have been studied since the 1950s and gerontologists are just beginning to identify the unique manifestations of different dementias. Moreover, many functional consequences are common to all of the dementias, and as pathologic processes progress, manifestations of all types of dementia become more similar. It is important to recognize, however, that during all stages and in all types of dementia, functional consequences vary tremendously among individuals because of unique personality characteristics, coexisting conditions (e.g., depression, functional impairments), and other influencing factors.

Fifty years ago, Sjögren, a Scandinavian psychiatrist, described the stages of Alzheimer's disease as (1) memory loss; (2) impairment of language, motor ability, and object recognition; and (3) the terminal stage, which is marked by loss of continence, ambulation, and all language skills. This three-stage classification was widely used until the 1980s, when an American psychiatrist, Reisberg, proposed a more detailed approach based on seven specific stages of Alzheimer's disease. Reisberg subdivided the last two stages (six and seven) to reflect the loss of functional abilities in reverse order from that in which they were acquired during development—a process he refers to as *retrogenesis* (Reisberg, 1986; Reisberg et al., 2002). Reisberg's staging schema, which has been updated and refined, is referred to as the Global Deterioration Scale/Functional Assessment Staging, or GDS/FAST (Auer & Reisberg, 1997). This staging system is widely used and has been found to be valid and reliable for staging Alzheimer's disease in diverse settings. Table 14-1 summarizes the functional consequences associated with each of the seven stages of the GDS/FAST. According to this framework, the diagnosis of Alzheimer's disease is made retrospectively because it is based on a progression of manifestations.

Gerontologists, clinicians, people with dementia, and families and caregivers are intensely interested in identifying factors that influence not only the course of the disease but the person's survival time. Although many variables have been identified (e.g., age, depression, family history), findings are inconsistent. One consistent finding, however, is that the rate of decline in people with dementia is slower during early stages and accelerates during later stages (Morris, 2005). Dementia is now widely recognized as a terminal illness because death is the ultimate functional consequence.

One of the myths associated with dementia is that people with dementia deny their symptoms or have no awareness of their deficits. Unfortunately, this fallacy has led to serious misunderstandings on the part of some health care professionals as exemplified by statements such as, "If they can ask if they have Alzheimer's disease, then they don't have it." In recent years, this perception of a high prevalence of so-called denial in people with dementia has diminished, and gerontologists are researching **anosognosia** (i.e., the lack of awareness of cognitive deficit) and insight in people with dementia. Some studies suggest that the degree of insight and awareness is associated with damage to specific areas of the brain (e.g., damage to the right hemisphere causing emotional unawareness) (Spalletta et al., 2006). Recent studies, however, also indicate that unawareness is influenced by many interacting factors, such as coping skills and personality characteristics (Clare, 2002a; Kazui et al., 2006). In contrast to the common perception that insight and awareness diminish as the disease progresses, studies indi-

TABLE 14-1 Global Deterioration Scale/Functional Assessment Staging (GDS/FAST) of Alzheimer's Disease

Stage	Effects on Functioning
1: Normal adult	No deficits or complaints
2: Age-associated memory impairment	Deficits consistent with normal aging (i.e., no objective findings, difficulty with word finding, forgets location of objects)
3: Mild cognitive impairment	Some deficits in performing complex tasks, especially in demanding social and employment settings; diminished organizational skills; deficits noted by others for the first time
4: Mild dementia	Diminished ability to perform complex tasks (e.g., meal planning, financial management); decreased knowledge of current and recent events; flattened affect and withdrawal from challenging situations
5: Moderate dementia	Obvious cognitive deficits; unable to manage complex daily tasks without some supervision or assistance; difficulty remembering names of familiar people
6: Moderately severe dementia	Increasingly obvious cognitive deficits (e.g., disorientation, significant short-term memory impairment); personality and emotional changes (e.g., anxiety, delusions) Loss of abilities in the following order: (a) Difficulty putting clothing on properly without assistance (b) Unable to bathe independently (c) Unable to handle all aspects of toileting (e.g., does not wipe properly) (d) Occasional or frequent urinary incontinence (e) Occasional or frequent fecal incontinence
7: Severe dementia	Progressive loss of all verbal and psychomotor abilities: (a) Verbal abilities limited to six or fewer different words (b) Verbal abilities limited to a single intelligible word (c) Unable to walk without assistance (d) Unable to sit without assistance (e) Unable to smile (f) Unable to hold up head independently

(Reisberg, B. [1986]. Dementia: A systematic approach to identifying reversible causes. *Geriatrics, 41*[4], 30–46.)

cate that it fluctuates during the course of the disease and only the ability to verbalize it diminishes steadily with progression of the disease (Arkin & Mahendra, 2001).

During the early stages, only the people who live, work, or have close contact with a person with dementia notice the initial changes, such as impaired judgment and short-term memory. When the changes are noticed, numerous explanations may be applicable, and the deficits may be attributed to such factors as depression or the occurrence of a major life event (e.g., retirement, widowhood). People in the early stages of dementia may withdraw from complex tasks as a way of protecting themselves from the effects of diminishing cognitive abilities. For example, employed people may retire without acknowledging cognitive impairments as the reason. People who do not have to perform complex intellectual or psychomotor tasks may be able to conceal or compensate for the cognitive losses until the deficits seriously interfere with activities of daily living (ADLs). As the disease progresses, however, the person with dementia is less able to cover up the changes, and people with less intimate contact will begin to question the underlying cause of the deficits.

Common emotions and behaviors of people with dementia during the early stages include fear, shame, anger, anxiety, frustration, loneliness, depression, sense of uselessness, self-blame, diminished affect, and withdrawal from challenging activities. Very commonly, people with dementia try to cover up their deficits to protect themselves and their families. These behaviors are not necessarily associated with denial, unawareness, or lack of insight; rather, they may reflect acceptance and positive coping (Clare, 2002a).

Clare (2002b) interviewed people in the early stages of Alzheimer's disease and their partners to identify coping mechanisms they used to adjust to the onset of this disease. The most commonly identified coping mechanisms can be categorized as follows:

- *Holding on* (e.g., trying harder, taking medications, sticking to routine)
- *Compensating* (e.g., using memory aids, relying on the partner)
- *Developing a fighting spirit* (e.g., obtaining information, talking about it, finding new roles, fighting it as long as possible)
- *Coming to terms* (e.g., finding a balance between hope and despair, accepting losses)

A common objective of all coping mechanisms was achieving a positive outcome for the self.

Feelings of fear, shame, anger, anxiety, and frustration may occur at any stage or last throughout the course of the disease, but they vary in their manifestations. Even in the later stages of dementia, when cognitive abilities are severely impaired, emotional response may be blunted or altered, but it is never absent. As dementia progresses, the person is likely to express emotions nonverbally and behaviorally. Thus, two important responsibilities of caregivers are to encourage and interpret nonverbal communication, which becomes the primary mode of communication during later stages of dementia (Hubbard et al., 2002).

Wellness Opportunity

Nurses holistically address psychosocial needs by recognizing that individuals vary significantly in their emotional responses, but people with dementia never lose the ability to respond to others.

People with dementia exhibit a wide range of behaviors that are superimposed on the cognitive impairments. Gerontologists and clinicians commonly refer to these as **behavioral and psychological symptoms of dementia (BPSD)**, and studies have found prevalence rates between 61% and 88% (Steffens et al., 2005). The common occurrence of BPSD has serious implications because it is strongly associated with increased caregiver burden and distress and is often cited as a factor that contributes to high rates of institutionalization (Fischer et al., 2006; Craig et al., 2005). The following manifestations are considered BPSD:

- Agitation, defined as inappropriate verbal, vocal, or motor activity that is not directly explained by needs or confusion (e.g., aggression, screaming)
- Psychiatric symptoms (e.g., delusions, hallucinations)
- Personality changes, inappropriate sexual behavior, disinhibition
- Mood disturbances (e.g., apathy, depression, euphoria, emotional lability)
- Aberrant motor movements (e.g., pacing, rummaging, wandering)
- Neurovegetative changes (e.g., appetite changes, sleep disturbances)

A Student's Perspective

There is a woman at my nursing home who has severe dementia, to the point where she often is not very kind to the nurses, PTs, OTs, and other staff. For most of our clinical rotation, I only heard reports of her being angry and sometimes insulting. This can be comical at times, and we all know not to take it personally because we know her attitude is a result of her disease. Understanding the chance I was taking, I went to talk to her during breakfast because she was just staring off into space. Kneeling at her eye level and placing my hand on her shoulder, I began by asking how her morning was. She complained about the cold weather and about how aggressive the OTs were in dressing her. I let her vent, I made some positive remarks, and I complimented her on how beautiful she looked that day.

As I rose to my feet to leave her a few minutes later, she reached for my arm and said, "You're such a sweetheart; you're so kind." My first internal reaction was to be blown away! I had never heard of this woman delivering compliments! But throughout the rest of the day I couldn't keep the smile off my face. This encounter helped me realize that this woman's beautiful personality is still with her and will always be a part of her. Yes, right now it's being masked most of the time by her dementia, but she still has feelings of kindness and a desire for happiness that fight past her disease every once in a while. I'm just glad I got to be part of that moment and discover that she's still there and needs to be treated like it always. One day she'll have the opportunity and power to express her thanks for those who showed her love and patience.

Shannon H.

Not all behavioral changes are problematic for caregivers, but the geriatric literature tends to focus on those behaviors that cause management problems. This is unfortunate because it reinforces fears and anxieties about functional consequences of dementia that may never occur. This author has heard such remarks as, "I know he doesn't have Alzheimer's disease because he doesn't hallucinate," or "I know she doesn't have Alzheimer's disease because she's not violent." These comments reflect a false belief that certain difficult behaviors are an inevitable consequence of dementia. Another caregiver recently asked, "Can you tell me if my mother will be the 'nice kind' or the 'mean kind' as her Alzheimer's gets worse?" This question at least acknowledges that not all people with dementia are difficult, but it reflects another negative and false belief about categorical types of behaviors in people with dementia. Environmental influences and perceptions of caregivers determine whether behaviors are viewed as problematic. For example, in a locked institutional unit, wandering behaviors might not be problematic, whereas in a home setting, wandering may be both unsafe and otherwise problematic. Likewise, nighttime restlessness creates more problems for a spouse who is the sole caregiver than for nursing staff who are paid to provide 24-hour care.

The term **catastrophic reaction** has been used for several decades in reference to a wide range of behaviors that occur in people with brain damage and are disproportionate to the reactions that would normally be expected in a situation (Mace & Rabins, 2006). These behaviors involve a sudden and exaggerated response to a situation that the person with dementia perceives as threatening. The onset of a catastrophic reaction may be signaled by a sudden change in mood, increased restlessness, stubbornness, or wandering. In addition, any of the following behaviors may be a component of the catastrophic reaction: anger, crying, shouting, anxiety, irritability, combativeness, and physical or verbal aggression. Caregivers may interpret the overreaction as intentional and think the person is being obstinate, critical, or overemotional. Caregivers sometimes can identify specific precipitants of these episodes (e.g., assistance during bathing), but at other times, they may be unable to identify any precipitating factor. Catastrophic reactions resolve when the perceived threat is removed, or when the person with dementia again feels safe and secure.

Gerontologists are addressing questions about the meaning of behaviors for both the person with dementia and their caregivers. For example, Johansson and colleagues (2002) found that caregivers interpreted "picking behavior" in people with dementia as a means of diminishing anxiety and striving for control, normalization, and a sense of staying in contact with others. Gerontologists and clinicians are increasingly recognizing that people with dementia communicate their needs and feelings through behaviors that may be perceived as problematic (Cohen-Mansfield & Mintzer, 2005; Talerico et al., 2002). Thus, it is imperative to assess all BPSD and try to identify and address underlying factors, as discussed in the sections on Assessment and Interventions.

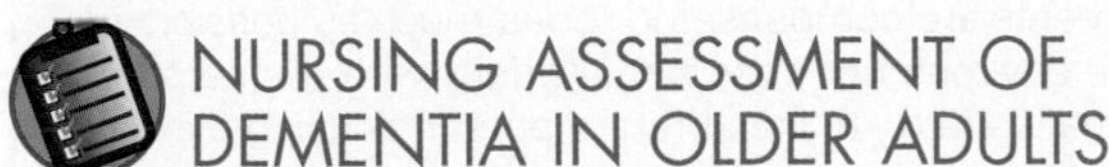

NURSING ASSESSMENT OF DEMENTIA IN OLDER ADULTS

Despite the tremendous evolution of information about dementia, many questions remain unanswered. There is consensus among researchers and clinicians that dementia is a most complex syndrome that usually involves a combination of distinct features and coexisting conditions. Although geriatric assessment programs and research settings have significantly improved the ability to identify dementia and other conditions that impair cognition, specific types of dementia can be identified with certainty only on autopsy.

Initial Assessment

With the exception of delirium and poststroke dementia, impaired cognitive function is a slowly progressive process that requires careful assessment to correctly identify underlying causes. Often, the changes occur slowly over a period of years, and an assessment is delayed until the changes significantly interfere with normal functioning. The assessment process usually takes place over weeks or months and involves the compilation of information about both medical and psychosocial functioning. Because progressive cognitive impairment is a very complex phenomenon, it is quite difficult for a single health care professional to obtain and evaluate all the information necessary to accurately determine the causes. Thus, the assessment process generally is multidisciplinary, requiring input from primary care providers, psychiatrists, nurses, social workers, and rehabilitation therapists. Members of the assessment team must work with the family and other caregivers to obtain information and determine the appropriate level of involvement of the cognitively impaired person with regard to discussing assessment results and planning care. The major nursing focus is to determine the person's level of function, to identify the factors that affect the person's level of function, and to identify the person's response to his or her illness. Frequently, the nurse serves as the team leader and is responsible for coordinating information and facilitating communication among team members and with the older adult and his or her family or other caregivers. Nurses can use Box 14-1 as a guide for assessing progressive cognitive impairments in older adults.

Ongoing Assessment of Consequences

Because dementia is a progressive condition that commonly coexists with other conditions, all people with dementia require ongoing assessment of all of the following:

- Changes in cognitive and psychosocial function related to the dementia (e.g., a decline in cognitive abilities, the onset of anxiety or depression)
- Changes in mental status related to concurrent conditions (e.g., delirium due to a medical condition or adverse medication effects)
- Changes in functional abilities
- Causes of behavioral changes related to treatable conditions (e.g., anxiety, physical discomfort, environmental factors)

A major goal of ongoing assessment is to identify factors that interfere with the person's level of functioning or quality of life so that interventions can be initiated to alleviate these contributing factors. Even though dementia is a progressive condition that gradually affects all levels of functioning, some of the changes that occur are caused by concurrent conditions rather than by the dementia itself. Thus, ongoing assessment to identify all factors that affect level of functioning is essential. Another goal of ongoing assessment is to identify both strengths and limitations in the person's abilities in order to plan individualized interventions to improve the person's functioning and quality of life. Because of the progressive and fluctuating nature of impaired cognitive function, the person's strengths and limitations will change periodically, so care plans must be updated frequently.

Nurses can use Table 14-1 as a guide to assessing the progression of dementia from early to later stages. The following guides in this text are pertinent for ongoing assessment of the many aspects of functional consequences associated with the progression of dementia: functioning and safety (Chapter 7), psychosocial function and depression (Chapters 12 and 15), hearing and vision (Chapters 16 and 17), urinary function (Chapter 19), fall risks (Chapter 22), and sleep and rest (Chapter 24). Nurses also can use the assessment tools in the chapters on medications (Chapter 8) and pain (Chapter 28) to address those aspects of care that are particularly important for people with dementia. In addition, the assessment tools available from the Hartford Institute for Geriatric Nursing that are listed in the Clinical Tool Resources section of this and other chapters are applicable to assessing aspects of functioning and care for people with dementia.

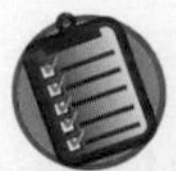

Box 14-1
Guidelines for Assessing Progressive Cognitive Impairment in Older Adults

General Principles

- Assessment of impaired cognitive function usually takes place during several visits, and it might include a home assessment.
- Recognize that the person with impaired cognitive function may not be a reliable reporter and that health care professionals may need to check the accuracy of information.
- Health care professionals must respect the person's rights and ask permission before obtaining information from others, including family members.
- Do not assume that the family has drawn accurate conclusions about events of the past (e.g., family members may state that the person retired and then showed cognitive deficits when, in reality, the person retired because of an inability to cope with job demands).

Focus of the Assessment

- The primary purpose of the assessment is to identify causes of the cognitive impairment.
- An assessment of a person with impaired cognitive function is multidisciplinary and includes the following components: complete medical history and physical examination, including a review of all medications; a functional assessment; a comprehensive psychosocial and formal mental status assessment; and an assessment of environmental and caregiver influences, with particular emphasis on those factors that affect functional abilities.
- The assessment includes an interview with caregivers, family members, and other people who can describe the progression of the manifestations of impairment.
- Information about lifelong patterns of personality, coping, and performance characteristics is considered in relation to the person's current functional level.
- It may be necessary to ask probing questions to help family members recognize clues to cognitive deficits retrospectively.

Considerations in Assessing Risk Factors That Contribute to Impaired Cognitive Function

- Never assume that all cognitive impairments and behavioral manifestations stem from a dementing illness.
- Because risk factors can either cause the initial cognitive impairments or develop later, causing additional impairments, they must be reassessed periodically.
- The following categories of risk factors must be assessed, both initially and on an ongoing basis: depression, physiologic alterations, functional impairments, adverse medication effects, and environmental and psychosocial influences.
- Early in the assessment, ensure that vision and hearing impairments are compensated for as much as possible and that the environment does not interfere with the person's performance (e.g., make sure the person is using eyeglasses and a hearing aid if needed, and make sure the lighting is optimal).
- A priority is to identify and treat those factors that are reversible before deciding on a long-term management plan.

Wellness Opportunity

Nurses promote wellness by identifying factors that support optimal functioning rather than focusing only on those that are problematic.

NURSING DIAGNOSIS

A nursing diagnosis most often applied to older adults who have dementia is Chronic Confusion, defined as "a state in which an individual experiences an irreversible, longstanding, and/or progressive deterioration of intellect and personality" (Carpenito-Moyet, 2006, p. 82). Additional nursing diagnoses that are applicable to functional consequences associated with psychosocial responses to dementia include Fear, Anxiety, Hopelessness, Impaired Memory, Social Isolation, Self-Esteem Disturbance, and Ineffective Individual Coping. During the later stages when dementia affects the person's functional abilities, applicable nursing diagnoses include Wandering, Imbalanced Nutrition, Urinary Incontinence, Self-Care Deficit, Impaired Verbal Communication, Risk for Falls, Risk for Injury, Disturbed Sensory Perception, and Disturbed Sleep Pattern. If cognitive deficits interfere with the person's ability to accurately take medications, the nurse might apply the diagnosis of Ineffective Therapeutic Regimen Management.

Nursing diagnoses also address the needs of caregivers because much of the care of people with dementia focuses on helping the family and other caregivers address the day-to-day needs and issues of the person with dementia. Nursing diagnoses that might be used to address caregiver needs include Family Coping and Caregiver Role Strain (or Risk for Caregiver Role Strain). During the later stages of dementia, the nursing diagnosis Anticipatory Grieving may be appropriate, particularly for spousal caregivers.

Wellness Opportunity

Readiness for Enhanced Coping is a wellness nursing diagnosis that nurses can apply for people with dementia as well as their caregivers.

PLANNING FOR WELLNESS OUTCOMES

During all stages of dementia, nursing care is directed toward promoting the highest level of functioning, while also supporting the highest quality of life. Nurses can apply the following Nursing Outcomes Classification (NOC) terminology to address the needs of people with dementia: Anxiety Level, Cognition, Cognitive Orientation, Comfort Level, Communication, Coping, Leisure Participation, Memory, Mood Equilibrium, Nutritional Status, Quality of Life, Self-Care Status, Sleep, Social Interaction Skills, and Symptom Control.

When friends, family members, or paid caregivers care for the person with dementia, nurses plan outcomes to promote caregiver wellness. In the early stages of dementia, the caregiver's foremost need might be for information about the disease and about resources that address the changing needs of the person with dementia and the caregiver's own needs. As the dementia progresses, caregivers are likely to need emotional support and practical assistance. Some NOC terms that are pertinent to caregivers include Caregiver Adaptation to Patient Institutionalization, Caregiver Emotional Health, Caregiver Lifestyle Disruption, Caregiver Physical Health, Caregiver Stressors, Caregiver Well-Being, Caregiving Endurance Potential, Coping, Grief Resolution, and Quality of Life.

Wellness Opportunity

Hope is a NOC that would be applicable when nurses plan wellness outcomes to address body–mind–spirit needs of both people with dementia and their caregivers.

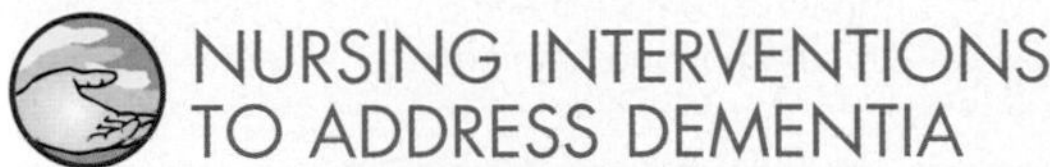

NURSING INTERVENTIONS TO ADDRESS DEMENTIA

Information about interventions to address dementia is evolving at a rapid pace, and research by nurses and other health care professionals is shedding light on appropriate interventions for treating the disease and managing the functional consequences. Most of the research on interventions has focused on Alzheimer's disease, but studies are expanding to address other types of dementia. For example, all the initial research on drug development focused on Alzheimer's disease, but recent studies address the use of these medications for other types of dementia, such as vascular dementia and dementia with Lewy bodies. Regardless of underlying causes, however, many interventions are applicable to all people with dementia and are individualized according to specific manifestations (e.g., reassurance for anxiety and confusion, redirection for unsafe or inappropriate behaviors). Similarly, health promotion interventions (e.g., exercise and nutrition) are applicable for primary and secondary prevention for all types of dementia.

The approach to diagnosing and treating dementia can be likened to the approach taken when diagnosing and treating an infection. An infection is a generic diagnosis indicating the presence of a constellation of signs and symptoms (e.g., malaise, elevated temperature), but it does not indicate the causative factor. As additional information is collected, the specific type of infection is identified (e.g., pneumonia, urinary tract infection), and sometimes more than one infection is discovered. Until the specific causative agent is identified, generic measures are taken (e.g., antipyretics, broad-spectrum antibiotics). After the specific causative agent is identified (e.g., through culture and sensitivity tests), the infection is treated with very specific antimicrobial agents. At all stages, comfort measures are used.

Analogously, dementia is a generic diagnosis indicating the presence of a constellation of signs and symptoms (e.g., memory impairment, personality changes), but initially little or no information is available about the cause. Because there are no clear indicators during early stages of most types of dementia, the cause is difficult to identify until the condition progresses. As further information evolves (e.g., patterns of cognitive and behavioral changes emerge, or the person has strokes or transient ischemic attacks), and clues are considered (e.g., the person's mother and father both had Alzheimer's disease), one or more causative factors is likely to be identified. As these factors are recognized, specific interventions can be used (e.g., cholinesterase inhibitors for Alzheimer's disease). Unfortunately, there are no "culture and sensitivity" tests for dementia, and sophisticated diagnostic procedures are not widely available, so it is difficult to distinguish between different types of dementia until the condition progresses or unless specific risk factors are identified. Similarly, there currently are no pharmaceutical agents to cure dementia, although some medications can delay the progression of the disease. Continuing the analogy, scientific developments for treating dementia are still in the "pre-antibiotic" phase. At any phase of dementia, and regardless of the cause, numerous interventions can be used to address comfort, functioning, and quality of life.

As anyone who has cared for a person with dementia knows, interventions must be highly individualized and frequently modified. An intervention that works for one person may not work for others, and interventions that are effective one day will not necessarily be effective the next day. A dominant theme of both research and practice is the implementation of person-centered interventions that are based on a comprehensive and ongoing assessment of the person's unique and changing needs. Thus, caring for people with dementia is a creative and most challenging process.

A comprehensive discussion of interventions for specific behaviors associated with dementia is beyond the scope of this chapter, but there are many practical references available on the management of dementia. Table 14-2 lists examples of nursing studies of nonpharmacologic interventions for dementia-related behaviors. In addition to professional nursing references, numerous books have been written by highly qualified and experienced caregivers that are excellent references for any nurse caring for people with dementia. The Alzheimer's Association and other resources listed at the end of this chapter provide health education materials and additional reliable information about interventions for people with dementia and their caregivers. This text

TABLE 14-2 Studies of Interventions for Dementia-Related Behaviors

Reference	Intervention	Dementia-Related Behavior Addressed
Brush et al., 2002	Enhanced lighting in the dining room	Poor nutritional intake
Cohen-Mansfield, 2003	Various nonpharmacologic interventions	Psychotic behaviors
Cohen-Mansfield et al., 2006	Communication and assistance techniques	Dressing
Cohen-Mansfield & Mintzer, 2005	Nonpharmacologic interventions	Behavior problems
DeYoung et al., 2002	Music therapy and management strategies such as encouraging independence, using time-outs, providing consistency in routines, and knowing the residents as unique individuals	Aggressive, agitated, disruptive behaviors
Dunn et al., 2002	Modified bed bath (thermal bath)	Agitation during bathing
Futrell & Melillo, 2002; Peatfield et al., 2002	Environmental modification; devices for safety; physical and psychosocial interventions; support and education of caregivers	Wandering
Gigliotti & Jarrott, 2005	Horticulture therapy	Affect and engagement
Hicks-Moore, 2005	Music at mealtime	Agitation during meals
Kolanowski et al., 2002	Diversional activities (e.g., games, sing-alongs, objects for tactile and visual stimulation)	Physical aggression, disruptive vocalization, nonaggressive physical behavior
Kovach & Wells, 2002	Pacing of sensory stimulation and sensory calming activity	Agitation
Lim, 2003	Systematic prompting and social reinforcement, using a series of one-step commands	Grooming behaviors
Lucero, 2002	Participation in structured recreational group activity and engagement in purposeful work-related activities	Wandering
McCurry et al., 2005	Sleep hygiene education, daily walking, increased light exposure	Sleep disturbances
Mickus et al., 2002	Privacy, Reassurance, Information, Distraction, and Evaluation (PRIDE)	Agitation during bathing
Miller et al., 2001	Audio presence intervention	Agitation
Moss et al., 2002	Reminiscence group activities	Impaired communication
Perry et al., 2005	Communication techniques	Impaired communication
Rader & Barrick, 2000	Person-centered, rather than task-centered, focus	Agitation during bathing
Roberts & Durnbaugh, 2002	Modifications of dining room milieu	Poor nutritional intake
Sloane et al., 2004	Towel bath technique	Agitation during bathing
Somboontanont et al., 2004	Caregiver education	Assaultive behavior toward assistants during bathing

addresses nursing interventions by reviewing theoretical frameworks, applying general principles in different clinical settings, and giving an overview of nursing interventions that are applicable in all settings.

Examples of Nursing Interventions Classification (NIC) terminology that may be applicable to caring for people with dementia include Active Listening, Activity Therapy, Anxiety Reduction, Behavior Management, Calming Technique, Dementia Management, Elopement Management, Emotional Support, Environmental Management, Exercise Promotion, Fall Prevention, Humor, Memory Training, Milieu Therapy, Mood Management, Music Therapy, Presence, Reality Orientation, Reminiscence Therapy, Self-Care Assistance, Spiritual Support, and Touch. Nurses can use the following NIC terms when they address caregiver needs: Anticipatory Guidance, Caregiver Support, Consultation, Coping Enhancement, Counseling, Decision-Making Support, Humor, Referral, Respite Care, Simple Relaxation Therapy, Spiritual Growth Facilitation, and Teaching.

Wellness Opportunity

Hope Instillation is a NIC that nurses address when they help people with dementia and their caregivers identify a positive meaning for their situation.

Theoretical Frameworks for Nursing Interventions

Hall and Buckwalter (1987) first proposed a theoretical framework for nursing interventions for people with dementia called the *progressively lowered stress threshold* (PLST) model. Briefly stated, this model posits that dysfunctional behaviors indicate a progressive lowering of the stress threshold, which, in turn, interferes with the person's functioning and ability to interact with the environment. The goal of nursing care, then, is to maximize the person's function by relieving stressors that cause excess disability. The choice of interventions is based on an ongoing assessment

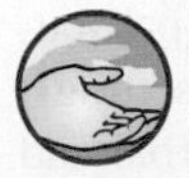

Box 14-2
Nursing Interventions for People With Dementia Based on the Progressively Lowered Stress Threshold Model (PLST)

- Maximize safety by modifying the environment to compensate for cognitive losses.
- Control any factors that increase stress, such as fatigue; physical stressors; competing or overwhelming stimuli; changes in routine, caregiver, or environment; and activities or demands that exceed the person's functional ability.
- Plan and maintain a consistent routine.
- Implement regular rest periods to compensate for fatigue and loss of reserve energy.
- Provide unconditional positive regard.
- Remain nonjudgmental about the appropriateness of all behaviors except those that present threats to safety
- Recognize individual expressions of fatigue, anxiety, and increasing stress, and intervene to reduce stressors as soon as possible.
- Modify reality orientation and other therapeutic interventions to incorporate only that information needed for safe function.
- Use reassuring forms of therapy, such as music and reminiscence.

(Hall, G. R., & Buckwalter, K. C. [1987]. Progressively lowered stress threshold: A conceptual model for care of adults with Alzheimer's disease. *Archives of Psychiatric Nursing, 1,* 399–406.)

of anxiety "as a barometer to determine how much activity and stimuli the anxious person can tolerate at any point during their illness. As anxious behaviors occur, activities and environmental stimuli are modified and simplified until the anxiety disappears" (Hall & Buckwalter, 1987, p. 403). This approach is highly individualized, and from a nursing perspective, it is analogous to adjusting insulin doses for people with diabetes according to serum glucose levels. Box 14-2 summarizes the principles of this approach.

In recent years, researchers have developed many additional theoretical frameworks to explain behavioral problems in people with dementia. These theoretical frameworks, which are not mutually exclusive, focus on the following causes of dementia-related behaviors (Cohen-Mansfield, 2003):

- The neuropathologic changes inherent in the disease itself
- Unmet needs of the person with dementia
- Behavioral patterns that are controlled by antecedents and consequences
- Environmental effects

Health care professionals are increasingly recognizing that dementia-related behaviors reflect an attempt to communicate needs that the person may not consciously recognize and cannot express verbally. Models based on this "informed care" approach focus on improving overall well-being and addressing the needs of the person with dementia through best efforts to identify underlying causes (Cohen-Mansfield & Mintzer, 2005).

General Principles of Nursing Interventions in Different Settings

Long-Term Care Settings

The current direction of care has seen the increasing implementation of multifaceted interventions for people with dementia in nursing home settings. For example, many long-term care facilities are developing specially designed special care units (SCUs) for people with dementia. Essential features of these units for cognitively impaired residents include environmental modifications, family involvement, individualized care plans, dementia-specific activity programs, and specially trained and selected staff. Many long-term care facilities incorporate these features into all nursing care units and address the individualized needs of the residents, as discussed in Chapter 6.

Acute Care Settings

Older adults are rarely hospitalized for an initial evaluation of dementia, but they frequently are admitted to acute care settings for evaluation and treatment of medical problems that are superimposed on the dementia. Consequently, nurses in hospital settings usually deal not only with the acute illness but also with the dementia-related behaviors, which are exacerbated by the medical problem, the hospital environment, the unfamiliar caregivers, and the change in routines. Thus, nurses in acute care settings face a tremendous challenge in caring for people with dementia.

One of the most important initial interventions is to involve at least one of the older adult's usual caregivers in planning and implementing care for the cognitively impaired person. Although the person with dementia is likely to exhibit different behaviors in the hospital than at home, nurses must begin by identifying any interventions that were effective in the home environment. During the admission process, nurses may save a lot of time and frustration by interviewing the caregivers about specific methods that help or hinder care. For example, if nurses know that the person eats only sandwiches or needs assistance with a specific toileting routine, they can incorporate appropriate interventions in their care plans. Because many people with dementia have lost the ability to express their needs verbally, nurses need to obtain information from family caregivers who understand how the person expresses needs. The Hartford Institute for Geriatric Nursing recommends tools for assessing family preferences and working with families of hospitalized older adults with dementia (see Clinical Tool Resources).

In addition to obtaining information from one of the usual caregivers, nurses may consider involving the caregiver in the person's care or asking him or her to provide a familiar presence during the hospitalization. Although family members and other caregivers deserve a respite from caregiving responsibilities, they may be willing to provide assistance and guidance. This may be particularly helpful during the first few days of hospitalization, and with patients who are especially difficult to manage.

Community Settings

In community settings, the role of nurses typically involves working with family members or paid caregivers, rather than directly implementing the interventions for the person with dementia. Thus, they serve as role models and also teach caregivers about interventions that improve functioning for the person with dementia, alleviate the burden for the caregivers, and improve quality of life for both the person with dementia and his or her caregivers. An intervention that might be most effective, as well as efficient, is to encourage caregivers to participate in educational or support groups. Caregiver support groups are widely available and have been found to be successful in diminishing caregiver stress and helping caregivers cope with challenging situations (Hébert et al., 2003). The number of groups addressing the needs of caregivers is increasing rapidly, and information about these groups is available from the Alzheimer's Association or local hospitals. Nurses also can encourage caregivers to purchase one of the many caregiver guides that are available in bookstores or through the Internet and to contact the Alzheimer's Association and other resources for information.

In addition to educating caregivers about specific management problems, nurses in community settings must be ready to discuss resources for medical care, home services, and other community-based services for people with dementia and their caregivers. As the number and range of services increase, it is becoming more and more difficult to keep up to date on the resources in one's own community. Although nurses cannot be expected to know all the details about all available community services, they should know about the general types of services available. In addition, they must be able to suggest at least one information and referral resource from which caregivers can obtain specific information. A good rule of thumb is to suggest that caregivers call the local area agency on aging because this type of organization serves every part of the United States. Information about these services can be obtained from the national Alzheimer's Association and the Eldercare Locator (see Educational Resources).

Improving Safety and Function Through Environmental Modifications

Environmental modifications are important interventions for people with dementia because environmental factors profoundly affect their safety, functioning, and quality of life. During the 1960s, gerontologists initially emphasized the importance of cognitive stimulation and suggested that reality orientation programs be widely implemented, particularly in nursing homes and other residential care settings. **Reality orientation** involves the repeated use of verbal and nonverbal indicators of time, place, and person in the context of the individual, group, and environment. Reality orientation interventions include frequent verbal reminders about the time of day from all staff and "reality orientation boards" that display large print information about the day, date, and weather. The goals are to improve the person's self-esteem and sense of control and to reduce his or her confusion, anxiety, and disorientation. Reality orientation may be effective for some people with dementia, especially when combined with other strategies, but this intervention must be tailored to individual needs rather than being universally applied.

Currently, gerontologists emphasize the important role of the total physical and psychosocial environment as a therapeutic tool (Werezak & Morgan, 2003). Lighting and sensory stimulation are two specific aspects of environmental interventions that researchers have addressed recently. For example, Ancoli-Israel and colleagues (2003) found that morning exposure to bright light (from sun or artificial sources) improved sleep patterns and diminished agitation in people with dementia, and this effect may be particularly beneficial during the mild or moderate stages. Long-term care facilities are increasingly using multisensory environments that include aromatherapy, soft music, favorite foods, and colored lighting effects. Studies of one widely used model, called the Snoezelen, indicate that multisensory interventions can provide pleasure and improve well-being not only for people with dementia but for their visitors and caregivers (Chitsey et al., 2002; Cox et al., 2004). A review of studies on nonpharmacologic interventions for dementia found promising results for the following types of environmentally based interventions in reducing dementia-related behaviors: music, aromatherapy, bright light, pet therapy, simulated presence, and multisensory stimulation (Forbes et al., 2005).

Wellness Opportunity

Nurses promote emotional wellness by encouraging older adults with dementia to talk about happy memories of earlier years and by affirming the pleasant feelings the person experiences when recalling these events.

In addition to improving quality of life, environmental interventions are essential for ensuring safety, fostering independence in ADLs, and preventing and addressing problematic behaviors (e.g., wandering). Examples of environmental factors that significantly affect the safety, functioning, and well-being of people with dementia are

- Noise
- Floor surfaces
- Colors and color contrast
- Lighting (e.g., glare, shadows, brightness)
- Design and placement of exits and bathrooms

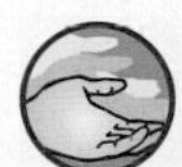

Box 14-3
Environmental Adaptations and Techniques for Improving Safety and Functioning in People With Dementia

General Environmental Modifications

- Modify the environment to compensate as much as possible for sensory deficits and other functional impairments. (Refer to interventions in Chapters 16 through 19 and 22.)
- Use clocks, calendars, daily newspapers, and simple written cues for orientation (e.g., day, date, names, place, and events).
- Use simple pictures, written cues, or color codes for identifying items and places (e.g., toilet, bedroom).
- Use simple written cues to clarify directions for operating radios, televisions, appliances, and thermostats (e.g., on, off, directional arrows).
- Place pictures of familiar people in highly visible places, but use nonglossy pictures and nonglare glass in picture frames.
- Turn lights on as soon as or before it begins to get dark.
- Use nightlights, or leave dim lights on during the night.
- Provide adequate environmental stimuli while avoiding overstimulation.

Techniques to Ensure Safety

- Make sure the person carries some form of identification, along with the phone number of someone to call.
- Adapt the environment for safety (e.g., use alarm devices for doors to prevent wandering).
- Keep the environment uncluttered.
- Keep medications, cleaning solutions, and any poisonous chemicals in inaccessible places.
- Enroll the person in a protective program, such as the Safe Return program sponsored by the Alzheimer's Association.

Techniques to Facilitate Independent Performance of Activities of Daily Living (ADLs)

- Keep all activities as simple and routine as possible.
- Establish routines that allow for maximum independence and the least amount of frustration.
- While keeping the routines as consistent as possible, recognize that they will have to be changed as the person's level of function changes.
- Lay out one set of clothing in the order in which the items are to be donned.
- If the person needs assistance with hygiene, use matter-of-fact statements, such as "It's time for your bath."
- Arrange personal care items, such as grooming and hygiene aids, in a visible and uncluttered place, in the order in which the items are to be used.
- Leave a toothbrush on the bathroom sink with toothpaste already on it.
- Establish an individualized toileting plan that allows for maximum independence but minimal risk for incontinence episodes.
- Offer finger foods and nutritious snacks if the person will not sit at the table to eat a meal.

- Presence of living things (e.g., plants, birds, fish, pets)
- Furniture (seating, placement, heights of tables and chairs)
- Use of safety devices (e.g., rails, grab bars)
- Provisions for privacy and social interaction
- Presence of items that improve comfort and homeyness (e.g., decorative items, textured items, meaningful personal belongings)
- Absence of potentially harmful items (e.g., clutter, obstacles, sharp knives, cleaning solutions and other potentially toxic products)

Box 14-3 summarizes environmental interventions and techniques to address safety and independence in ADLs.

Communicating With Older Adults With Dementia

Verbal and nonverbal communication techniques are widely recognized as essential interventions for people with dementia throughout the entire course of the disease. Nurses need to pay particular attention to the effects of touch, facial expressions, tone of voice, and body language on communication. Box 14-4 summarizes techniques for facilitating communication with people with dementia. Nurses also can use the guides to assessment and interventions for people with dementia available from the Hartford Institute for Geriatric Nursing (see Clinical Tool Resources at the end of this chapter).

Teaching About Medications

Nurses have important roles in teaching caregivers about medications for dementia. Medications are becoming increasingly important in treating dementia because recent studies and guidelines support and encourage the medications to slow the progress of the disease. In addition, many types of medications are being investigated for treatment of dementia, and some over-the-counter products are being promoted for prevention and treatment of dementia. Nurses also are frequently involved with decisions about medications for managing dementia-related symptoms.

Medications for Slowing the Progression of Dementia

Since 1993, when the first medication was approved for the treatment of Alzheimer's disease, much progress has been made in our knowledge about pharmaceutical treatment and prevention strategies for Alzheimer's disease as well as other types of dementia. By 2001, the U.S. Food and Drug Administration (FDA) had approved four cholinesterase inhibitors for the treatment of Alzheimer's disease. Although tacrine (Cognex), the first medication approved, is still available, the other three medications—donepezil (Ari-

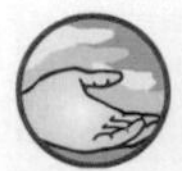

Box 14-4
Facilitating Communication With People Who Have Dementia

Verbal Communication

- Adapt your level of communication to the abilities of the person with dementia.
- Use very simple sentences.
- Present only one idea at a time.
- Allow enough time for processing.
- Avoid infantilization (e.g., do not talk baby talk or use a demeaning or condescending tone of voice).
- Assist with word finding (e.g., supply missing words, repeat the person's sentence with the correct word).
- Avoid shaming the person (e.g., do not emphasize deficits).
- Paraphrase what the person says and ask for clarification about the meaning.
- If the person does not understand a statement, repeat the statement using the same words, or simplify the wording.
- Do not argue with the person, unless it is a matter of safety.
- Avoid complex or sarcastic humor.
- Use positive statements (i.e., avoid using statements containing the word "don't" or other negative commands).
- Involve the person with decisions to the best of his or her ability by offering simple and concrete choices (e.g., "Do you want chicken or steak?" rather than "What do you want to eat?").
- Do not ask questions that you know the person cannot answer correctly.
- Do not test the person's memory unnecessarily.
- Listen to the feelings the person is trying to express and respond to the feelings, rather than the statement.
- When discussing activities of daily living (ADLs), avoid statements such as "You need a bath now," which may be interpreted as judgmental.

Nonverbal Communication

- Attract and maintain the person's attention (e.g., through eye contact, pleasant facial expressions).
- Use a relaxed and smiling approach.
- Reinforce verbal communication with appropriate nonverbal communication (e.g., demonstrate what you are asking the person to do).
- Use simple pictures rather than written cues.
- Use appropriate touch for communication (e.g., to gain the person's attention or reinforce feelings of concern), unless the person responds negatively to touch.
- Be aware of your own nonverbal communication.
- Keep in mind that your nonverbal cues will probably communicate more than your spoken words and will not necessarily be interpreted correctly.
- Closely observe all nonverbal cues exhibited by the person, especially those that express feelings.
- Assume that all nonverbal expressions of the person with dementia are attempts to communicate needs or feelings.

cept), rivastigmine (Exelon), and galantamine (Reminyl)—are the standards for mild to moderate Alzheimer's disease because they have fewer adverse effects. Reviews of studies consistently find that these medications exert modest positive effects in improving or delaying the progression of functional decline and cognitive and behavioral symptoms (Standridge, 2006).

In late 2003, memantine (Namenda) became the first medication approved for treatment of moderate to severe Alzheimer's disease. The physiologic action of this medication, which differs from that of cholinesterase inhibitors, blocks the neural toxicity associated with excess release of glutamate. Studies consistently show that memantine improves symptoms and slows the rate of decline in patients in moderate to later stages of Alzheimer's disease (Bullock, 2006). The usual pharmacologic approach is to begin a cholinesterase inhibitor before or during the moderate stage and to add memantine during the moderate or later stages.

In the early 2000s, researchers began publishing studies of the effects of cholinesterase inhibitors on types of dementia other than Alzheimer's disease. A recent research review identified donepezil and galantamine as the most effective evidence-based treatments for vascular dementia and vascular cognitive impairment (Demaerschalk & Wingerchuk, 2007). Because of the increasing evidence that these medications are effective for other types of dementia, and the increasing evidence that two or more types of dementia coexist, cholinesterase inhibitors and memantine are commonly used for all types of dementia. Moreover, memantine is likely to be approved for earlier stages of dementia. Nurses can use Box 14-5, which summarizes current information about medications to slow the progression of dementia, to teach older adults and their families about these medications.

Medications for Managing Dementia-Related Symptoms

Although psychotropic medications are commonly used for dementia-related disruptive behaviors, decisions about the use of these medications are very complex for several reasons. First, because difficult behaviors are often precipitated by factors, including medical conditions, environmental influences, and adverse medication effects (e.g., anticholinergic medications), initial interventions should always address any contributing factors. For example, if behaviors are adverse effects of medications, initial interventions should focus on eliminating or reducing the dose. Second, there is always a risk that medications will further interfere with function and perhaps even cause serious harm. A third consideration is whether the behaviors justify the risks associated with medications. Bothersome or socially inappropriate behaviors might better be ignored or tolerated than treated with medications. However, if the behavior is unsafe,

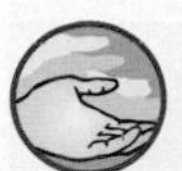

Box 14-5
Health Education About Medications for Slowing the Progression of Dementia

Cholinesterase Inhibitors for Mild to Moderate Dementia

- Cholinesterase inhibitors commonly used in the United States include
  - Donepezil (Aricept)
  - Rivastigmine (Exelon)
  - Galantamine (Reminyl)

Effectiveness of Cholinesterase Inhibitors for Dementia

- There is increasing support for starting a cholinesterase inhibitor early in the course of dementia and continuing the treatment during the early and middle stages.
- Cholinesterase inhibitors delay the progression of symptoms and stabilize or improve all of the following: memory, language skills, functional abilities, and behaviors such as pacing, delusions, and uncooperativeness.
- Because the effectiveness of a cholinesterase inhibitor is significantly diminished if it is stopped and then restarted, it is important to ensure regular administration.

Dosing and Adverse Effects

- The usual dosing schedule for the commonly used drugs is once daily for donepezil and twice daily for rivastigmine and galantamine.
- Nausea, vomiting, diarrhea, and loss of appetite are common adverse effects, but these effects can be prevented or reduced by starting with a low dose and gradually increasing to the maximum dose.
- Less common adverse effects include sleep disturbances, extrapyramidal symptoms, and cardiorespiratory events.
- Rivastigmine may be more likely than donepezil or galantamine to cause gastrointestinal adverse effects but less likely to interact with other medications.

Memantine (Namenda) for Moderate to Severe Dementia

- Memantine, which was approved by the U.S. Food and Drug Administration in October 2003, is the first medication authorized for patients in moderate to severe stages of dementia.
- Pharmacologic action of memantine differs from that of cholinesterase inhibitors and it usually is prescribed in addition to a cholinesterase inhibitor, which typically is prescribed earlier in the course of the disease.
- Studies have found the following benefits of memantine: less decline in global, functional, behavioral, and cognitive measures; improvements in degree of agitation and in performance of activities of daily living.
- Usual initial dose is 5 mg once daily, with gradual titration up to 10 mg twice daily.
- Adverse effects include dizziness, headache, constipation, hypertension, dyspnea, somnolence, hallucinations, and gastrointestinal symptoms.

uncomfortable, or interferes with the function of the person with dementia or the rights or safety of others, then pharmaceutical intervention may be appropriate, but only if other interventions are not successful. In any situation, health care professionals should view behavior-modifying medications as one component of a comprehensive management plan that addresses the complex nature of dementia-related behaviors. Nurses can use information in Box 14-6 to guide decisions about behavior-modifying medications for people with dementia.

Antipsychotics are the most commonly used type of medication for BPSD (e.g., agitation, delusions, hallucinations, and physical aggression), and many studies focus on both the beneficial and adverse effects of this approach. In recent years, concern about adverse effects of the older antipsychotics (e.g., haloperidol) has led to increased use of the so-called atypical antipsychotics, including olanzapine (Zyprexa), quetiapine (Seroquel), and risperidone (Risperdal). Researchers have not identified any medication that is both safe and consistently more effective than nonpharmacologic interventions, and there is increasing concern about adverse effects of antipsychotics. A recent Cochrane review concluded that atypical antipsychotics show modest efficacy but are associated with increased risks for mortality, edema, extrapyramidal symptoms, upper respiratory infections, and cerebrovascular adverse events (Ballard et al., 2007). There is much support for nonpharmacologic approaches (e.g., activities and sensory-based modalities), whenever possible, and using antipsychotics very cautiously and only when necessary (Bharani & Snowden, 2005). Antidepressants and mood stabilizers (e.g., valproate, carbamazepine) may be effective for people with dementia who also have mood disturbances.

Wellness Opportunity

Nurses holistically address behavioral symptoms by trying to identify nonpharmacologic interventions that improve quality of life for the person with dementia and his or her caregivers.

Teaching About Complementary and Alternative Care Practices

Nutrition, exercise, and general mental, physical, and spiritual health practices have long been considered essential components of maintaining optimal cognitive function in people with and without dementia. In addition, there is much support for the use of meditation and other relaxation techniques both for people with dementia and their caregivers (Pope et al., 2006; Sierpina et al., 2005). Recently, increasing attention has been given to the quest for remedies, such as "brain boosters," that can improve cognitive function (e.g., herbs, antioxidants, ginkgo biloba). The

Box 14-6
Guidelines for Decisions About Behavior-Modifying Medications for People With Dementia

Considerations Regarding Behavior-Modifying Medications

- Assess whether any of the following factors cause or contribute to the difficult behaviors: environmental conditions; psychosocial factors, such as anxiety or depression; or physiologic factors, such as pain, discomfort, or medical disorders. If any of these factors are implicated, interventions should be directed at the causative factor.
- Are the behaviors caused by adverse medication effects? In this case, the appropriate intervention might be to reduce the dose of or discontinue a medication, rather than begin a new medication.
- Treatment with medication should be implemented for behavior problems only after a trial of nonmedication interventions.
- Do the behaviors truly justify the use of medications, or are the caregivers requesting medications for their own comfort and convenience?

Considerations Regarding the Choice and Dose of Medications

- The specific goals of and expectations for the medication interventions should be clear to all caregivers.
- If the person is depressed, antidepressants may be effective in treating the depression, and some functional improvement may occur, as the depression is alleviated.
- Caregivers should not assume that, just because medications are necessary and appropriate during one stage of dementia, they will be necessary and appropriate on an ongoing basis.
- Medication regimens should be reevaluated as the dementia progresses or as other conditions, such as medical disorders, affect the person's functional level.
- People with dementia exhibit a wide range of responses to various medications, and the selection of a particular medication should be based on current manifestations as well as prior experiences with medications.
- Some people with dementia, especially those with dementia with Lewy bodies, are highly sensitive to even minute doses of psychotropic medications.
- Any behavior-modifying medication is likely to interfere with cognitive function.
- The type of behavior-modifying medication should be appropriate for the type of behavioral manifestations (e.g., antipsychotics for delusions and hallucination, antianxiety agents for anxiety).
- The initial dose should be one half to one third the normal adult dose.
- Dosage should be increased gradually until therapeutic effects are achieved, all the while observing the person for adverse effects.
- Medications with long half-lives (e.g., flurazepam, diazepam, chlordiazepoxide) should be avoided.
- The half-life of a medication should be considered in determining the frequency of doses.

physiologic effects of some of these products are similar to those of medications that currently are used or under investigation for dementia. For example, willow bark has anti-inflammatory effects; ginkgo biloba has antioxidant effects; and sage and rosemary affect acetylcholine levels. Several traditional Chinese herbal remedies (e.g., huperzine, *Corydalis ternata*) mimic the effects of the FDA-approved cholinesterase inhibitors and are commonly used for improving memory (Truscott-Brock, 2006). The National Institutes of Health (NIH), many medical institutions, and Alzheimer's research centers in the United States are studying these herbs and other alternative care practices that are widely used in other countries. Nurses can use Box 14-7 for health education about complementary and alternative approaches to management of dementia.

Facilitating Decisions About Care for People With Dementia

Nurses are frequently asked to facilitate decisions about care for people with dementia because families face complex decisions and assume uncomfortable levels of responsibility for people who once were able to make their own decisions. Although some families take on too much decision-making power, most are reluctant to make decisions about dependent older adults. Decision making is especially difficult when the older adult is physically healthy but mentally impaired, or when the person voices strong opinions about unwise or unsafe actions. For example, families of people with dementia often deal with decisions about the person driving a car. Decisions about specific behaviors, like driving, may be relatively easy, however, compared with decisions about long-term or end-of-life care, decisions that most families of people with progressively declining conditions must confront. In addition to basic safety and medical concerns, these decisions involve complex emotional and financial issues. Because several people are involved in these decisions, differing opinions and interests may complicate the process.

The role of the nurse in facilitating decision making varies in different settings. For example, if decisions about long-term care are made during a hospitalization, much of the decision-making responsibility may be assumed by or relegated to the primary care provider, and the decision may be based primarily on medical concerns. When the person is being cared for at home, however, the decision-making process is more nebulous and the responsibility rests primarily with the family. When the dependent person primarily needs social activities or supervision of daily care, the decision is more psychosocial than medical. In many situations, especially in home or residential settings, nurses are the only health care professionals who maintain close and ongoing

Box 14-7
Health Education About Complementary and Alternative Care Practices for People With Dementia

Nutritional Interventions

- Although vitamin E supplements had been recommended, recent studies do not support this and in fact suggest that high doses of vitamin E can increase the risk of mortality in people with heart disease.
- Dietary intake of vitamins B-complex, C, and E and polyunsaturated fatty acids may be beneficial.

Herbal Therapies

- Ginkgo biloba (120–160 mg daily in two or three doses) increases blood supply to the brain and may improve cognitive function (especially memory and attention) to a small degree in some people with dementia. Ginkgo biloba may cause serious bleeding if taken with anticoagulants or nonsteroidal anti-inflammatory drugs (NSAIDs; e.g., ibuprofen).

Additional Therapies That May Be Effective for Managing Symptoms

- Physical exercise, including dancing, walking, and tai chi
- Bright-light therapy, 1/2 hour daily to reduce agitation and improve sleep
- Aromatherapy (inhaled or applied to the skin): rosemary for mental stimulation, lavender oil or lemon balm for calming effects
- Relaxation and stress reduction therapies for people with dementia and their caregivers: music, massage, meditation, touch therapy, deep breathing
- Prayer and other spiritual practices for people with dementia and their caregivers
- Acupuncture for anxiety and depression in people with dementia

relationships with dependent older adults and their caregivers. Thus, the nurse often becomes a support person or a care manager. Nurses can use the following six-step decision-making model as a guide to assisting families with this challenging process. Specific questions and considerations for each of the six steps are listed in Box 14-8. It is important to keep in mind that the identification of caregivers and decision makers should be done with a high degree of cultural sensitivity because decision-making and caregiving patterns are strongly influenced by cultural factors.

Step I: Assessing the Decision-Making Situation

To facilitate decisions about long-term care for cognitively impaired older adults, nurses begin by assessing all of the following: (1) physical and psychosocial function of the dependent person, (2) resources that can be used to meet identified needs, and (3) factors that influence the decision on the part of the caregivers and the dependent person. This assessment usually is very complex and time consuming. If this step is done well, however, the nurse will save time in the end, and the plan is increasingly likely to succeed.

Step II: Obtaining Consensus About Problems and Needs

After obtaining as much assessment information as possible, it usually is effective and efficient to gather all the decision makers together. The nurse then leads the conference of decision makers to obtain consensus about problems and needs. When caregivers do not have a broad perspective on the dependent person's needs, the nurse may provide additional input about the person's needs. For example, the nurse might point out that social activities and interactions with others are important ways of meeting psychosocial needs and helping cognitively impaired people maintain the highest level of function. Although group activities cannot be provided in home settings, they are available in residential facilities or community-based programs, such as adult day care centers.

Step III: Discussing Potential Resources

After summarizing the older person's needs, the nurse then initiates and guides a discussion about potential resources for addressing the problems. Attention is focused on the needs of the caregivers, as well as the needs of the dependent older person. Often, the needs of caregivers may be addressed through support groups or individual counseling. Many families are not aware of the range of housing options and community-based services that are available. Nurses who are not familiar with these resources should arrange for a social worker to participate in the conference. As resources are identified, advantages and disadvantages are discussed from various perspectives. The nurse can begin with a statement such as "As we identify different options, let's look at the good points and bad points of each. We need to look at the financial costs and emotional costs that affect each of you, as well as the person for whom we are planning the care." Because the financial aspects are the most objective, they often are a good starting point. Financial decisions, however, can involve many repercussions for spouses and for anyone who might inherit money from the dependent older adult. Sometimes, some of the decision makers may be more concerned about protecting their own financial interests than implementing a plan that is in the best interests of the dependent elder. Another pertinent question that may be asked regarding the advantages and disadvantages of various options is "What is the cost of not providing this service?" This approach is especially effective in broadening the caregivers' perspective when their viewpoint is very narrow. For example, the nurse may be able to use professional knowledge and experience to convince a family that the long-term benefits of a particular plan may far outweigh the immediate cost of services.

Step IV: Agreeing on a Plan of Action

After reviewing the options, the nurse then summarizes the information and eliminates those options that are

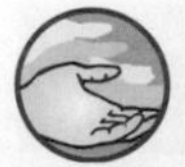

Box 14-8
Model for Facilitating Decisions About the Care of People With Dementia

Step I: Assess the decision-making situation.

- What are the typical decision-making patterns in the family?
- Who influences the decision making, either directly or indirectly?
- How do family relationships help or hinder the decision-making process?
- Are there patterns of passive nondecisions, as well as active decisions?
- What is each person's perception of the situation?
- How objective are the perceptions of the various decision makers?
- What does each person in the decision-making process have to gain or lose based on various decisions?

Step II: Obtain consensus about problems and needs.

- Have the most involved caregivers describe the problems first.
- After those who are most involved voice their opinions, those who are less involved can be asked to describe the problems.
- Provide objective information to ensure that the various needs of the dependent person are recognized.
- Address the needs of the caregivers as well as the needs of the person with dementia.
- Summarize the identified needs of the older adult and the caregivers.

Step III: Discuss potential resources.

- Ask caregivers to suggest potential solutions and resources.
- Identify resources for the caregivers' needs as well as for those of the person with dementia.
- Supplement the family's knowledge about resources and potential solutions.
- Discuss the positive and negative consequences of each option for the person with dementia and for the caregivers.
- As the family members discuss solutions, assess their attitudes about using various services and spending family resources to purchase services.
- Provide information about the long-range benefits that the caregivers might not perceive.
- Summarize important points on paper or a blackboard for all participants to review.

Step IV: Agree on a plan of action.

- Eliminate the least acceptable options.
- Agree on the two or three most acceptable alternatives.
- Emphasize the fact that any plan of action will be given a trial period and should not be viewed as a permanent decision.
- Suggest a time frame and criteria for evaluating the plan of action.
- Identify one or two people who will evaluate the plan and make appropriate changes.

Step V: Involve the person with dementia.

- Discuss the ability of the person with dementia to understand the decision.
- Identify the most realistic level of involvement for the person with dementia.
- Identify the best approach to take in involving the person with dementia.
- Identify the roles of caregivers and professionals in assisting the person with dementia to understand the decision.

Step VI: Summarize the plan and clarify roles.

- Review and summarize the plan of action.
- Have the caregivers state their roles in very specific terms.
- Clarify the role of the nurse and other professionals.
- Assure caregivers that you will be available for further discussion and problem solving, or provide the name of someone who can assume this role.

least acceptable. The nurse then tries to identify two options that are the best (or only) alternatives. There are always at least two final choices: to do nothing or to make a change. If caregivers are reluctant to accept any of the options identified, the nurse might review the consequences associated with doing nothing, as well as the consequences of implementing one or two of the possible action steps. When neither alternative is deemed acceptable initially, it may be helpful to say, "I realize that neither of these choices may seem desirable, but there are no other options." Families sometimes need to hear this kind of conclusion, and they may accept it more readily when it is based on professional experience and knowledge. Once the choices are defined, the decision makers must agree on what action to take. At this point it is helpful to emphasize that no decision is permanent, and to set a specific time frame for evaluating the decision after a trial period. If the caregivers understand that the decision can be altered after a fair trial period, they usually are more comfortable with a particular action.

Because this decision-making process can be very time-consuming, it is important to identify ways of streamlining the process as much as possible. Therefore, when many people are involved in the conference, one or two key people should be designated as the ones responsible for follow-up. Unless there is a major change in the situation, effective communication networks can eliminate the need for additional conferences with all the decision makers. The evaluation plan may even be carried out through phone contact, rather than in-person contact.

Step V: Involving the Person With Dementia

When the older adult cannot participate in the decision-making conference, the participants must determine the best way of involving that person in the decision. The decision-making process just described applies primarily to situations in which the dependent older person is not able to make decisions on his or her own behalf. In any situation, it is crucial to address the rights and wishes of the dependent older person at every step. In situations in which the person has serious cognitive impairments, the decision makers may simply need to identify the best way to gain acceptance and cooperation. In situations in which the person has some problem-solving abilities, the caregivers may identify the person who is best able to discuss the decision. When spouses are involved in the decision making, they usually assume the role of communicating the decision to the dependent older person. At times, the nurse, physician, or other professional person may assume the role of an authority figure to assist in explaining the decision to the dependent older adult.

Step VI: Summarizing the Plan and Clarifying Roles

The final step is to clarify the roles of various people. The nurse and other professionals who are part of the decision-making process should inform the caregivers about their ongoing roles. If several caregivers are involved with the plan, each person should state his or her understanding of his or her role.

EVALUATING THE EFFECTIVENESS OF NURSING INTERVENTIONS

Nurses can evaluate care of people with dementia according to the extent to which they receive needed supports and maintain their dignity and quality of life. Because a decline in function is an inherent part of dementia, nursing care is evaluated on an ongoing basis as the person's condition changes and in relation to appropriate and changing goals. Nurses evaluate the degree to which quality of life is maintained by obtaining feedback about life satisfaction, which people in the early and middle stages of dementia usually can express verbally or nonverbally. For example, nurses can evaluate the extent to which the person enjoys or participates in meaningful activities and interactions. As the dementia progresses, it becomes more difficult to obtain this kind of information and nurses rely more on feedback from caregivers and their own judgment about the person's quality of life. During the later stages of dementia, measures of quality of life focus more on comfort and basic physical needs. Throughout the course of dementia, care can be evaluated by the extent to which the person is free from pain, fear, and anxiety.

Another consideration in evaluating care for a person with dementia is the extent to which the needs of caregivers are met. An evaluation criterion is whether caregivers express satisfaction with their own quality of life, despite the demands of the situation. Other evaluation criteria may be a caregiver's attendance at support groups and the use of resources to assist with or guide care.

Mrs. D. is 85 years old and lives with her 86-year-old husband in a high-rise apartment for the elderly. Two years ago, Mrs. D. was diagnosed as having Alzheimer's disease, but she was able to participate in her usual activities until the past year. Now she is neglecting her personal care and is unsafe in meal preparation.

When she wakes up several times nightly to go to the bathroom, she sometimes goes to the apartment door rather than returning to the bedroom. Mr. D. worries that she will leave in the middle of the night, and his sleep is disrupted because he maintains a state of constant vigilance. Mr. D. has called a home care agency requesting home health aide assistance, and you are the nurse responsible for the initial assessment and for working with the home health aides.

NURSING ASSESSMENT

During your initial assessment, you find that Mrs. D. is pleasant and receptive, but has little insight into her need for help. She acknowledges that her doctor has told her she has "a memory problem." Mrs. D. reports that this problem doesn't affect her daily life, except that her husband has to remind her about things like turning the stove off after cooking meals. She acknowledges being lonely and says she misses being able to read books and talk to people. Mrs. D. takes Aricept and vitamin E, and is otherwise physically healthy.

With regard to her ADLs, Mrs. D. has not taken a bath or shower in several months, and she gets very angry if Mr. D. suggests that she take one. She gets confused about her clothing and sometimes wears her underwear over her regular clothes, or wears a skirt and slacks at the same time. She insists on doing the meal preparation, but she is unsafe using the stove and gets confused about ingredients in recipes (e.g., she may use salt instead of sugar). Mrs. D. always has done the laundry and housekeeping, but in the past months, she has "made a lot of mistakes," such as using powdered milk for laundry detergent.

(case study continues on page 286)

Mr. D. reports feeling very stressed about the full-time responsibilities of caring for his wife, and this stress has escalated in the past month because he no longer feels he can leave her alone. Mrs. D. "shadows" him and feels very insecure if he is out of her sight for more than a few minutes. Mr. D. has taken her everywhere with him for the past year, but in the last few months, this has become increasingly more difficult. For example, when they are in the grocery store, Mrs. D. gets very impatient and pushes the cart into other people. Also, while they are waiting in the checkout line, she insists on taking one of each of the tabloids and magazines near the counter, and she creates a big scene if he doesn't buy them for her.

Mr. D. confides that he expected to be able to care for his wife at home "until the end," but now he has doubts about his ability to keep her at home. He perceives her as being "senile" and feels he should be able to meet her needs. There are no nearby family members who can help with her care, but his son and daughter have offered to help pay for some services. Mr. D. is aware of support groups offered by the Alzheimer's Association, but he has not attended any because he cannot leave his wife alone. When asked about his health, Mr. D. says, "I see the doctor for my arthritis and heart problems, but I get along OK, except that I'm supposed to have cataract surgery and I don't know how I'll manage to get that done."

NURSING DIAGNOSIS

Your nursing diagnosis for Mrs. D. is Altered Thought Processes related to the effects of dementia. You use the nursing diagnosis of Caregiver Role Strain for Mr. D. because you recognize the need to address Mr. D.'s problems. Your immediate goal is to arrange for supportive services and assistance with Mrs. D.'s care because this will improve the quality of life for both Mr. and Mrs. D., and it will alleviate some of the caregiver stress for Mr. D. A long-term goal is to arrange for respite services so Mr. D. can undergo cataract surgery. You also recognize the need for educational and support services for Mr. D.

NURSING CARE PLAN FOR MR. AND MRS. D.

Expected Outcome	Nursing Interventions	Nursing Evaluation
Mrs. D. will function at her highest level of independence.	• Work with Mr. D. to identify ways to improve Mrs. D.'s ability to function safely and independently in performing her ADLs. (For instance, Mr. D. can involve Mrs. D. in selecting an outfit to wear and can set out the clothing in the order in which it should be donned.) • Arrange for an HHA to work with Mrs. D. and assist her with complex tasks, such as laundry, housekeeping, and meal preparation. • Teach the HHA to assume an "assistant" and "friend" role by providing only subtle supervision and minimal direct help with activities such as laundry.	• Mrs. D. will perform ADLs and IADLs with minimal assistance.
Mrs. D.'s quality of life will be maintained.	• Work with Mr. D. and the HHA to identify activities that are interesting, satisfying, and intellectually stimulating (e.g., "word find" games). • Explore the possibility of Mrs. D.'s attending an adult day care program for group activities. • Support Mrs. D. in carrying out familiar roles and meaningful activities.	• Mrs. D. will continue to engage in activities that are satisfying.
Mr. D. will use sources of support to alleviate caregiver-related stress.	• Arrange the HHA's schedule to enable Mr. D. to attend caregiver support groups and educational programs.	• Mr. D. will verbalize feelings of being able to cope effectively with caregiver responsibilities.

(case study continues on page 287)

Expected Outcome	Nursing Interventions	Nursing Evaluation
	• Help Mr. D. in identifying one activity per week that he could do to promote his own well-being (e.g., going to lunch with a friend). • Provide HHA assistance for 4-hour periods to allow Mr. D. time for grocery shopping and pursuing his own interests. • Provide Mr. D. with information about the "Caregiver Connection Hot Line" at the Alzheimer's Association, and suggest that he join this telephone support network.	• Mr. D. will participate in one activity per week that is focused on his own needs and interests.

THINKING POINTS

- Use the GDS/FAST in Table 14-1 to assess Mrs. D.'s stage of dementia.
- What would you identify as Mr. D.'s needs as a caregiver?
- What health education information would you plan for Mr. D.?
- What approaches would you suggest for Mr. D. and home care workers for communicating with Mrs. D.?
- What challenges would you anticipate having to address as you provide ongoing supervision of the home health aide and continue to work with Mr. and Mrs. D.?

ADLs, activities of daily living; IADLs, instrumental activities of daily living; HHA, home health aide.

CHAPTER HIGHLIGHTS

Delirium

- Characteristics: fluctuating levels of consciousness, confusion, disorganized thinking, altered perceptions, personality and behavioral changes
- Hyperactive delirium is easily recognized, and hypoactive delirium, which is common in older adults, is sometimes unrecognized
- Risk factors include advanced age, pain, dementia, surgery, medications, physiologic disturbances, and pathologic conditions
- Functional consequences include decline in functioning, increased mortality, and permanent residency in long-term care facilities
- Nursing assessment: identifying behavior changes by using assessment tools such as the MMSE
- Nursing Diagnosis: Acute Confusion
- Nursing Outcomes: Cognition, Concentration, Information Processing, Memory, Psychomotor Energy
- Nursing Interventions: addressing risk factors (Fig. 14-1)

Overview of Dementia

- Terminology (senility, hardening of the arteries, organic brain syndrome) reflects complexity of causes and types of dementia
- Dementia is a syndrome of impaired cognition caused by brain dysfunction
- Theories to explain dementia are still evolving

Types of Dementia

- Prevalence of dementia (Fig. 14-2)
- Alzheimer's disease: pathologic changes (Figs. 14-3 and 14-4), theories about causes and risk factors, theories about stages (Fig. 14-5)
- Vascular dementia, cerebrovascular brain injury
- Dementia with Lewy bodies
- Frontotemporal dementia

Risk Factors Associated With Dementia

- Factors that increase the risk for dementia include genetic factors, lifestyle factors, and health status
- Factors that protect against dementia include physical exercise, nutrition (antioxidants and omega-3 fatty acids), engaging in socially and cognitively stimulating and meaningful activities, and having cognitive reserve
- Factors that interfere with assessment and interventions include attitudes, myths, lack of information, and cultural influences on perceptions of dementia

Functional Consequences Associated With Dementia

- Stages of progression (early to severe; Table 14-1)
- Impact of dementia on the person: awareness, emotional response, behavioral and psychological symptoms (BPSD), catastrophic reactions

Nursing Assessment of Dementia

- Initial assessment: multidisciplinary, focus on level of function, response to illness (Box 14-1)
- Ongoing assessment of consequences (Table 14-1, assessment guides in other chapters, and Clinical Tool Resources)

Nursing Diagnosis

- Wellness nursing diagnosis for person with dementia and caregivers: Readiness for Enhanced Coping

- Person with dementia: Chronic Confusion, Anxiety, Impaired Memory, Risk for Injury, Self-Care Deficit, Disturbed Sleep Pattern, Imbalanced Nutrition, Wandering, Urinary Incontinence
- Caregivers: Family Coping and Caregiver Role Strain (or Risk for), Anticipatory Grieving.

Planning for Wellness Outcomes

- Person with dementia: Anxiety Level, Cognition, Cognitive Orientation, Comfort Level, Communication, Memory, Mood Equilibrium, Nutritional Status, Self-Care Status, Sleep, Symptom Control
- Caregivers: Caregiver Emotional or Physical Health, Caregiver Stressors, Caregiving Endurance Potential
- For both the person with dementia and his or her caregivers: Coping, Quality of life

Nursing Interventions to Address Dementia

- Nursing studies of nonpharmacologic interventions for dementia-related behaviors (Table 14-2)
- Theoretical frameworks for nursing interventions: progressively lowered stress threshold (PLST) model (Box 14-2)
- General principles in long-term care, acute care (Clinical Tool Resources from Hartford Institute for Geriatric Nursing), community settings
- Improving safety and functioning through environmental modifications (Box 14-3)
- Communicating with older adults who have dementia (Box 14-4, Clinical Tool Resources)
- Teaching about medications for slowing the progression of dementia (Box 14-5)
- Teaching about medications for managing dementia-related symptoms (Box 14-6)
- Teaching about complementary and alternative care practices (Box 14-7)
- Facilitating decisions about care for people with dementia (Box 14-8)

Evaluating Effectiveness of Nursing Interventions

- Maintenance of dignity and quality of life for the person with dementia
- Extent to which needs of caregivers are met

Critical Thinking Exercises

1. Define each of the following terms and describe the relevance of each term according to our current understanding of impaired cognitive function: senility, organic brain syndrome, hardening of the arteries, delirium, dementia, and Alzheimer's disease.
2. Describe the distinguishing features of the early stages of each of following types of dementia: Alzheimer's disease, vascular dementia, frontotemporal dementia, and dementia with Lewy bodies.
3. You are working in a nursing clinic at a senior center. How would you respond to the following questions, posed by a 74-year-old woman: "I've been having memory problems lately, but I know it's not Alzheimer's because I haven't done anything really stupid. What do you think I should do? My friend says ginkgo helps her a lot, and I was thinking of trying that. Do you know how much of it I should take?"
4. You are planning an in-service program to nursing home staff about medications used in the treatment of dementia and the management of dementia-related behaviors. What information would you present?

Clinical Tool Resources

Hartford Institute for Geriatric Nursing
Try This: Best Practices in Nursing Care to Older Adults
www.hartfordign.org/resources/education/tryThis.html
Issue Number 13 (Revised 2007), Confusion Assessment Method (CAM)
Issue Number 22 (Revised 2007), Assessing Family Preferences for Participation in Care in Hospitalized Older Adults
Issue Number D1 (Revised 2007), Avoiding Restraints in Older Adults with Dementia
Issue Number D4 (Revised 2007), Therapeutic Activity Kits
Issue Number D5 (Revised 2007), Recognition of Dementia in Hospitalized Older Adults
Issue Number D6 (Revised 2007), Wandering in the Hospitalized Older Adult
Issue Number D7 (Revised 2007), Communication Difficulties: Assessment and Interventions
Issue Number D8 (Revised 2007), Assessing and Managing Delirium in Persons with Dementia
Issue Number D10 (Revised 2007), Working with Families of Hospitalized Older Adults with Dementia

Educational Resources

Alzheimer's Association
www.alz.org

Alzheimer's Disease Education and Referral (ADEAR) Center
www.alzheimers.org

Alzheimer's Society of Canada
www.alzheimer.ca

Family Caregiver Alliance
www.caregiver.org

National Institute on Aging (NIA)
http://www.nih.gov/nia

National Institute of Neurological Disorders and Stroke
www.ninds.nih.gov

United States Agency for Healthcare Research and Quality
www.ahcrq.gov

References

Alzheimer, A. (1907). Uber eine eigenartige Erkrankung der Hirnrinde. *Assgemeine Zeitschrift fur Psychiatrie und Psychisch-Gerichtliche Medicin, 64*, 146–148.

Ancoli-Israel, S., Martin, J. L., Gehrman, P., Sochat, T., Corey-Bloom, J., Marler, M., et al. (2003). Effect of light on agitation in institutionalized patients with severe Alzheimer disease. *American Journal of Geriatric Psychiatry, 11*, 194–203.

Arkin, S., & Mahendra, N. (2001). Insights in Alzheimer's patients: Results of a longitudinal study using three assessments methods. *American Journal of Alzheimer's Disease and Other Dementias, 16*, 211–224.

Auer, S., & Reisberg, B. (1997). The GDS/FAST staging system. *International Psychogeriatrics, 9*(Suppl. 1), 167–171.

Ballard, C., Waite, J., & Birks, J. (2007). Atypical antipsychotics for aggression and psychosis in Alzheimer's disease. *The Cochrane Database of Systemic Reviews 2007*, Issue 1. Available at www.cochrane.org/reviews/en/ab003476.html. Accessed March 1, 2007.

Bergmann, M. A., Murphy, K. M., Kiely, D. K., Jones, R. N., & Marcantonio, E. P. (2005). A model for management of delirious postacute care patients. *Journal of the American Geriatrics Society, 53*, 1817–1825.

Bharani, N., & Snowden, M. (2005). Evidence-based interventions for nursing home residents with dementia-related behavioral symptoms. *Psychiatric Clinics of North America, 28*, 985–1005.

Bond, S. M., Neelon, V. J., & Belyea, M. J. (2006). Delirium in hospitalized older patients with cancer. *Oncology Nursing Forum, 33*, 1075–1083.

Borenstein, A. R., Copenhaver, C. I., & Mortimer, J. A. (2006). Early-life risk factors for Alzheimer disease. *Alzheimer Disease and Associated Disorders, 20*, 63–72.

Boxer, A. L., & Miller, B. L. (2005). Clinical features of frontotemporal dementia. *Alzheimer Disease and Associated Disorders, 19*(Suppl. 1), S3–S6.

Boyle, P. A., Wilson, R. S., Aggarwal, N. T., Tang, Y., & Bennett, D. A. (2006). Mild cognitive impairment: Risk of Alzheimer disease and rate of cognitive decline. *Neurology, 67*, 441–445.

Brush, J. A., Meehan, R. A., & Calkins, M. P. (2002). Using the environment to improve intake for people with dementia. *Alzheimer's Care Quarterly, 3*, 330–338.

Bullock, R. (2006). Efficacy and safety of memantine in moderate-to-severe Alzheimer disease: The evidence to date. *Alzheimer Disease and Associated Disorders, 20*, 23–29.

Carpenito-Moyet, L. J. (2006). *Handbook of nursing diagnosis* (11th ed.). Philadelphia: Lippincott Williams & Wilkins.

Chartier-Harlin, M. C., Kachergus, J., Roumier, C., Mouroux, V., Douay, X., Lincoln, S., et al. (2004). Alpha-synuclein locus duplication as a cause of familial Parkinson's disease. *Lancet, 364*, 1167–1169.

Chitsey, A. M., Haight, B. K., & Jones, M. M. (2002). A multisensory intervention. *Journal of Gerontological Nursing, 28*(3), 41–49.

Choi, Y.-H., Kim, J.-H., Kim, D.-K., Kim, J.-W., Kim, D.-K., Lee, M.-S., et al. (2003). Distributions of ACE and APOE polymorphisms and their relations with dementia status in Korean centenarians. *Journals of Gerontology: Series A, Biological Sciences and Medical Sciences, 58*, 227–231.

Chui, H. (2005). Neuropathology lessons in vascular dementia. *Alzheimer Disease and Associated Disorders, 19*, 45–52.

Clare, L. (2002a). Developing awareness about awareness in early-stage dementia. *Dementia, 1*, 295–312.

Clare, L. (2002b). We'll fight it as long as we can: Coping with the onset of Alzheimer's disease. *Aging & Mental Health, 6*, 139–148.

Cohen-Mansfield, J. (2003). Nonpharmacologic interventions for psychotic symptoms in dementia. *Journal of Geriatric Psychiatry and Neurology, 16*, 219–224.

Cohen-Mansfield, J., Creedon, M. A., Malone, T., Parpura-Gill, A., Dakheel-Ali, M., & Heasly, C. (2006). Dressing of cognitively impaired nursing home residents: Description and analysis. *The Gerontologist, 46*, 89–96.

Cohen-Mansfield, J., & Mintzer, J. E. (2005). Time for change: The role of nonpharmacological interventions in treating behavior problems in nursing home residents with dementia. *Alzheimer Disease and Associated Disorders, 19*, 37–40.

Cox, H., Burns, I., & Savage, S. (2004). Multisensory environments for leisure: Promoting well-being in nursing home residents with dementia. *Journal of Gerontological Nursing, 30*(2), 37–45.

Craig, D., Mirakhur, A., Hart, D. J., McIlroy, S. P., & Passmore, A. P. (2005). A cross-sectional study of neuropsychiatric symptoms in 435 patients with Alzheimer's disease. *American Journal of Geriatric Psychiatry, 13*, 460–468.

Dasgupta, M., & Dumbrell, A. C. (2006). Preoperative risk assessment for delirium after noncardiac surgery: A systematic review. *Journal of the American Geriatrics Society, 54*, 1578–1589.

Demaerschalk, B. M., & Wingerchuk, D. M. (2007). Treatment of vascular dementia and vascular cognitive impairment. *The Neurologist, 13*, 37–41.

DeYoung, S., Just, G., & Harrison, R. (2002). Decreasing aggressive, agitated, or disruptive behavior. *Journal of Gerontological Nursing, 28*(6), 22–31.

Dunn, J. C., Thiru-Chelvam, B., & Beck, C. H. M. (2002). Bathing: Pleasure or pain? *Journal of Gerontological Nursing, 28*(11), 6–12.

Ely, E. W., Girard, T. D., Shintani, A. K., Jackson, J. C., Gordon, S. M., Thomason, J. W. W., et al. (2007). Apolipoprotein E4 polymorphism as a genetic predisposition to delirium in critically ill patients. *Critical Care Medicine, 35*, 112–116.

Farias, S. T., Mungas, D., Reed, B. R., Harvey, D., Cahn-Weiner, D., & DeCarli, C. (2006). MCI is associated with deficits in everyday functioning. *Alzheimer Disease and Associated Disorders, 20*, 217–223.

Farmer, J., & Grossman, M. (2005). Frontotemporal dementia: An overview. *Alzheimer's Care Quarterly, 6*, 225–232.

Federal Interagency Forum on Aging-Related Statistics. (2006). *Older Americans update 2006: Key indicators of well-being*. Washington, DC: U.S. Government Printing Office.

Feldman, H. H., & Jacova, C. (2005). Mild cognitive impairment. *American Journal of Geriatric Psychiatry, 13*, 645–655.

Fick, D. M., Agostini, J. V., & Inouye, S. K. (2002). Delirium superimposed on dementia: A systematic review. *Journal of the American Geriatrics Society, 50*, 1723–1732.

Fischer, C., Ladowsky-Brooks, R., Millikin, C., Norris, M., Hansen, K., & Rourke, S. B. (2006). Neuropsychological functioning and delusions in dementia: A pilot study. *Aging & Mental Health, 10*, 27–32.

Forbes, D. A., Peacock, S., & Morgan, D. (2005). Nonpharmacological management of agitated behaviors associated with dementia. *Geriatrics Aging, 8*(4), 26–30.

Futrell, M., & Melillo, K. D. (2002). Evidence-based protocol: Wandering. *Journal of Gerontological Nursing, 28*(11), 14–22.

Gigliotti, C. M., & Jarrott, S. E. (2005). Effects of horticulture therapy on engagement and affect. *Canadian Journal on Aging, 24*, 367–377.

Grossman, M. (2005). Frontotemporal dementia. *Alzheimer Disease and Associated Disorders, 19*(Suppl. 1), S1–S2.

Gualtieri, C. T., & Johnson, L. G. (2005). Neurocognitive testing supports a broader concept of mild cognitive impairment. *American Journal of Alzheimer's Disease and Other Dementias, 20*, 359–366.

Hachinski, V. C., Lassen, N. A., & Marshall, J. (1974). Multi-infarct dementia: A cause of mental deterioration in the elderly. *Lancet, 2*, 207–209.

Hall, G. R., & Buckwalter, K. C. (1987). Progressively lowered stress threshold: A conceptual model for care of adults with Alzheimer's disease. *Archives of Psychiatric Nursing, 1*, 399–406.

Haroutunian, V., Davies, P., Vianna, C., Buxbaum, J. D., & Purohit, D. P. (2007). Tau protein abnormalities associated with the progression of Alzheimer disease type dementia. *Neurobiology of Aging, 28*, 1–7.

Hébert, R., Lévesque, L., Vézina, J., Lavoie, J. P., Ducharme, F., Gendron, C., et al. (2003). Efficacy of a psychoeducative group program for caregivers of demented persons living at home: A randomized controlled trial. *Journals of Gerontology: Series B, Psychological Sciences and Social Sciences, 58*, S58–S67.

Hicks-Moore, S. L. (2005). Relaxing music at mealtime in nursing homes: Effects on agitated patients with dementia. *Journal of Gerontological Nursing, 31*(12), 26–32.

Hogstel, M. O. (1988). Forget these three words. *Journal of Gerontological Nursing, 14*(12), 7.

Hubbard, G., Cook, A., Tester, S., & Downs, M. (2002). Beyond words: Older people with dementia using and interpreting nonverbal behaviour. *Journal of Aging Studies, 16*, 155–167.

Inouye, S. K., Leo-Summers, L., Zhang, Y., Bogardus, S. T., Leslie, D. L., & Agostini, J. V. (2005). A chart-based method for identification of delirium: Validation compared with interviewer ratings using the confusion assessment method. *Journal of the American Geriatrics Society, 53*, 312–318.

Johansson, K., Norberg, A., & Lundman, B. (2002). Family members' and care providers interpretations of picking behavior. *Geriatric Nursing, 23*, 258–261.

Johnson, D. K., Morris, J. C., & Galvin, J. E. (2005). Verbal and visuospatial deficits in dementia with Lewy bodies. *Neurology, 65*, 1232–1238.

Joshi, S., & Morley, J. E. (2006). Cognitive impairment. *Medical Clinics of North America, 90*, 769–787.

Kalisvaart, K. J., Vreeswijk, R., de Jonghe, J. F., van der Ploeg, T., van Gool, W. A., & Eikelenboom, P. (2006). Risk factors and prediction of postoperative delirium in elderly hip-surgery patients: Implementation and validation of a medical risk factor model. *Journal of the American Geriatrics Society, 54*, 817–822.

Kazui, H., Hirono, N., Hashimoto, M., Nakano, Y., Matsumoto, K., Takatsuki, Y., et al. (2006). Symptoms underlying unawareness of memory impairment in patients with mild Alzheimer's disease. *Journal of Geriatric Psychiatry and Neurology, 19*, 3–12.

Kertesz, A. (2005). Frontotemporal dementia: One disease, or many? Probably one, possibly two. *Alzheimer Disease and Associated Disorders, 19*(Suppl. 1), S19–S23.

Kolanowski, A. M., Richards, K. C., & Sullivan, S. C. (2002). Activity preferences of persons with dementia. *Journal of Gerontological Nursing, 28*(10), 12–15.

Kovach, C. R., & Wells, T. (2002). Pacing of activity as predictor of agitation. *Journal of Gerontological Nursing, 28*(1), 28–35.

Kukull, W. A., & Bowen, J. D. (2002). Dementia epidemiology. *Medical Clinics of North America, 86*, 573–590.

Langmore, S. E., Olney, R. K., Lomen-Hoeth, C., & Miller, B. L. (2007). Dysphagia in patients with frontotemporal lobar dementia. *Archives of Neurology, 64*, 58–62.

Larson, E. B., Wang, L, Bowen, J. D., McCormick, W. C., Teri, L., Crane, P., et al. (2006). Exercise is associated with reduced risk for incident dementia among persons 65 years of age and older. *Annals of Internal Medicine, 144*, 73–81.

Lemiengre, J., Nelis, T., Joosten, E., Braes, T., Foreman, M., Gastmans, C., et al. (2006). Detection of delirium by bedside nurses using the confusion assessment method. *Journal of the American Geriatrics Society, 54*, 685–689.

Leslie, D. L., Zhang, Y., Holford, T. R., Bogardus, S. T., Leo-Summers, L. S., & Inouye, S. K. (2005). Premature death associated with delirium at 1-year follow-up. *Archives of Internal Medicine, 165*, 1657–1662.

Lim, Y. M. (2003). Nursing intervention for grooming of elders with mild cognitive impairments in Korea. *Geriatric Nursing, 24*, 11–15.

Lucero, M. (2002). Intervention strategies for exit-seeking wandering behavior in dementia residents. *American Journal of Alzheimer's Disease and Other Dementias, 5*, 277–280.

Lundstrom, M., Edlund, A., Karlsson, S., Brannstrom, B., Bucht, G., & Gustafson, Y. (2005). A multifactorial intervention program reduces the duration of delirium, length of hospitalization, and mortality in delirious patients. *Journal of the American Geriatrics Society, 53*, 622–628.

Mace, N. L., & Rabins, P. V. (2006). *The 36-hour day* (4th ed.). Baltimore: The Johns Hopkins University Press.

Marcantonio, E. R., Simon, S. E., Bergmann, M. A., Jones, R. N., Murphy, K. M., Morris, J. N., et al. (2003). Delirium symptoms in post acute care: Prevalent, persistent, and associated with poor functional recovery. *Journal of the American Geriatrics Society, 51*, 4–9.

McAvay, G. J., Van Ness, P. H., Bogardus, S. T., Zhang, Y., Leslie, D. L., Leo-Summers, L. S., et al. (2006). Older adults discharged from the hospital with delirium: 1-year outcomes. *Journal of the American Geriatrics Society, 54*, 1245–1250.

McCurry, S. M., Gibbons, L. E., Logsdon, R. G., Vitiello, M. V., & Teri, L. (2005). Nighttime insomnia treatment and education for Alzheimer's disease: A randomized, controlled trial. *Journal of the American Geriatrics Society, 53*, 793–802.

McKhann, G. M., Albert, M. S., Grossman, M., Miller, B., Dickson, D., Trojanowski, J. Q., & Work Group on Frontotemporal Dementia and Pick's Disease. (2001). Clinical and pathological diagnosis of frontotemporal dementia: Report of the Work Group on Frontotemporal Dementia and Pick's Disease. *Archives of Neurology, 58*, 1803–1809.

Mickus, M. A., Wagenaar, D. B., Averill, M., Colenda, C. C., Gardiner, J., & Luo, Z. (2002). Developing effective bathing strategies for reducing problematic behavior for residents with dementia: The PRIDE approach. *Journal of Mental Health and Aging, 8*(1), 37–43.

Miller, S., Vermeersch, P. E. H., Bohan, K., Renbarger, K., Kruep, A., & Sacre, S., et al. (2001). Audio presence intervention for decreasing agitation in people with dementia. *Geriatric Nursing, 22*, 66–70.

Morris, J. C. (2000). The nosology of dementia. *Neurologic Clinics, 18*, 773–788.

Morris, J. C. (2005). Dementia update 2005. *Alzheimer Disease and Associated Disorders, 19*, 100–116.

Mosimann, U. P., Rowan, E. N., Partington, C. E., Phil, M., Collerton, D., Littlewood, E., et al. (2006). Characteristics of visual hallucinations in Parkinson disease dementia and dementia with Lewy bodies. *American Journal of Geriatric Psychiatry, 14*, 153–160.

Moss, S. F., Polignano, E., White, C. L., Minichiello, C. L., & Sunderland, T. (2002). Interaction in Alzheimer's disease. *Journal of Gerontological Nursing, 28*(8), 36–44.

Neef, D., & Walling, A. D. (2006). Dementia with Lewy bodies: An emerging disease. *American Family Physician, 73*, 1223–1229.

O'Keeffe, S. T., Mulkerrin, E. C., Nayeem, K., Varughese, M., & Pillay, I. (2005). Use of serial Mini-Mental State Examinations to diagnose and monitor delirium in elderly hospital patients. *Journal of the American Geriatrics Society, 53*, 867–870.

Pandharipande, P., & Ely, E. W. (2006). Sedative and analgesic medications: Risk factors for delirium and sleep disturbances in the critically ill. *Critical Care Clinics, 22*, 313–327.

Panza, F., D'Introno, A., Colacicco, A. M., Capurso, C., Del Parigi, A., Caselli, R. J., et al. (2005). Current epidemiology of mild cognitive impairment and other predementia syndromes. *American Journal of Geriatric Psychiatry, 13*, 663–644.

Peatfield, J. G., Futrell, M., & Cox, C. L. (2002). Wandering. *Journal of Gerontological Nursing, 28*(4), 44–50.

Perry, J., Galloway, S., Bottorff, J. L., & Nixon, S. (2005). Nurse-patient communication in dementia: Improving the odds. *Journal of Gerontological Nursing, 31*(4), 43–52.

Peterson, J. F., Pun, B. T., Dittus, R. S., Thomason, J. W. W., Jackson, J. C., Shintani, A. K., et al. (2006). Delirium and its motoric subtypes: A study of 614 critically ill patients. *Journal of the American Geriatric Society, 54*, 479–484.

Pitkala, K. H., Laurila, J. V., Strandberg, T. E., & Tilvis, R. S. (2006). Multicomponent geriatric intervention for elderly inpatients with delirium: A randomized, controlled trial. *Journals of Gerontology: Series A, Biological Sciences and Medical Sciences, 61*, 176–181.

Pope, S. K., Horne, M. T., Morris, M. C., Sano, M., Gwyther, L. P., Lombardo, N. E., et al. (2006). Complementary and alternative therapies for Alzheimer's disease: A conference summary. *Alzheimer's Care Quarterly, 7*(1), 13–31.

Rader, J., & Barrick, A. L. (2000). Ways that work: Bathing without a battle. *Alzheimer's Care Quarterly, 1*(4), 35–49.

Rapp, C. G., & Iowa Veterans Affairs Nursing Research Consortium. (2001). Acute confusion/delirium protocol. *Journal of Gerontological Nursing, 27*(4), 21–33.

Reisberg, B. (1986). Dementia: A systematic approach to identifying reversible causes. *Geriatrics, 41*(4), 30–46.

Reisberg, B., Franssed, E. H., Souren, L. E., Auer, S. R., Akram, I., & Kenowsky, S. (2002). Evidence and mechanisms of retrogenesis in Alzheimer's and other dementias: Management and treatment import. *American Journal of Alzheimer's Disease and Other Dementias, 17*, 169–174.

Rigney, T. S. (2006). Delirium in the hospitalized elder and recommendations for practice. *Geriatric Nursing, 27*, 151–157.

Roberts, S., & Durnbaugh, T. (2002). Enhancing nutrition and eating skills in long-term care. *Alzheimer's Care Quarterly, 3*(4), 316–329.

Roe, C. M., Xiong, C., Miller, J. P., & Morris, J. C. (2007). Education and Alzheimer disease without dementia: Support for the cognitive reserve hypothesis. *Neurology, 68*, 223–228.

Rogan, S., & Lippa, C. F. (2002). Alzheimer's disease and other dementias: A review. *American Journal of Alzheimer's Disease and Other Dementias, 17*, 11–17.

Roses, A. D. (1995). Apolipoprotein E and Alzheimer's disease. *Science and Medicine, 2*(5), 16–25.

Ross, G. W., & Bowen, J. D. (2002). The diagnosis and differential diagnosis of dementia. *Medical Clinics of North America, 86*, 455–476.

Sandhaus, S., Harrell, F., & Valenti, D. (2006). Healthier aging: Here's help to prevent delirium in the hospital. *Nursing 2006, 36*(7), 60–62.

Serrano, S., Domingo, J., Rodriguez-Garcia, E., Castro, M. D., & del Ser, T. (2007). Stroke. *Stroke 2007, 38*, 105–109.

Sheng, A. Z., Shen, Q., Cordato, D., Zhang, Y. Y., & Yin Chan, D. K. (2006). Delirium within three days of stroke in a cohort of elderly patients. *Journal of the American Geriatrics Society, 54*, 1192–1198.

Sierpina, V. S., Sierpina, M., Loera, J. A., & Grumbles, L. (2005). Complementary and integrative approaches to dementia. *Southern Medical Journal, 98*, 636–645.

Sloane, P. D., Hoeffer, B., Mitchell, C. M., McKenzie, D. A., Barrick, A. L., Rader, J., et al. (2004). Effect of person-centered showering and the towel bath on bathing-associated aggression, agitation, and discomfort in nursing home residents with dementia: A randomized, controlled trial. *Journal of the American Geriatric Society, 52*, 1795–1804.

Somboontanont, W., Sloane, P. D., Floyd, F. J., Holditch-Davis, D., Hogue, C. C., & Mitchell, C. M. (2004). Assaultive behavior in Alzheimer's disease: Identifying immediate antecedents during bathing. *Journal of Gerontological Nursing, 30*(9), 22–29.

Spalletta, G., Ripa, A., Bria, P., Caltagirone, C., & Robinson, R. G. (2006). Response of emotional unawareness after stroke to antidepressant treatment. *American Journal of Geriatric Psychiatry, 14*, 220–227.

Standridge, J. B. (2006). Current status and future promise of pharmacotherapeutic strategies for Alzheimer's disease. *Journal of the American Medical Directors Association, 7*, S46–S51.

Steffens, D. C., Maytan, M., Helms, M. J., & Plassman, B. L. (2005). Prevalence and clinical correlates of neuropsychiatric symptoms in dementia. *American Journal of Alzheimer's Disease and Other Dementias, 20*, 367–373.

Talerico, K. A., Evans, L. K., & Strumpf, N. E. (2002). Mental health correlates of aggression in nursing home residents with dementia. *The Gerontologist, 42*, 169–177.

Tomlinson, B. E., Blessed, G., & Roth, M. (1968). Observations on the brains non-demented old people. *Journal of Neurological Science, 7*, 331–356.

Tomlinson, B. E., Blessed, G., & Roth, M. (1970). Observation on the brains of demented old people. *Journal of Neurological Science, 11*, 205–242.

Truscott-Brock, E. (2006). Naturopathic medicine and its complementary role in the care of persons with Alzheimer's disease. *Alzheimer's Care Quarterly, 7*(1), 41–48.

Tsuang, D. W., & Bird, T. D. (2002). Genetics of dementia. *Medical Clinics of North America, 86*, 591–614.

Voyer, P., McCusker, J., Cole, M. G., & Khomenko, L. (2006). Influence of prior cognitive impairment on the severity of delirium symptoms among older patients. *Journal of Neuroscience Nursing, 38*(2), 90–101.

Werezak, L. J., & Morgan, D. G. (2003). Creating a therapeutic psychosocial environment in dementia care: A preliminary framework. *Journal of Gerontological Nursing, 29*(12), 18–25.

Whitehouse, P. J. (2006). The end of AD part 3. *Alzheimer Disease and Associated Disorders, 20*, 195–198.

Whitehouse, P. J., & Moody, H. R. (2006). Mild cognitive impairment. A "hardening of the categories?" *Dementia, 5*(1), 11–25.

Wilson, R. S., Krueger, K. R., Arnold, S. E., Schneider, J. A., Kelly, J. F., Barnes, L. L., et al. (2007). Loneliness and risk of Alzheimer disease. *Archives of General Psychiatry, 64*, 234–240.

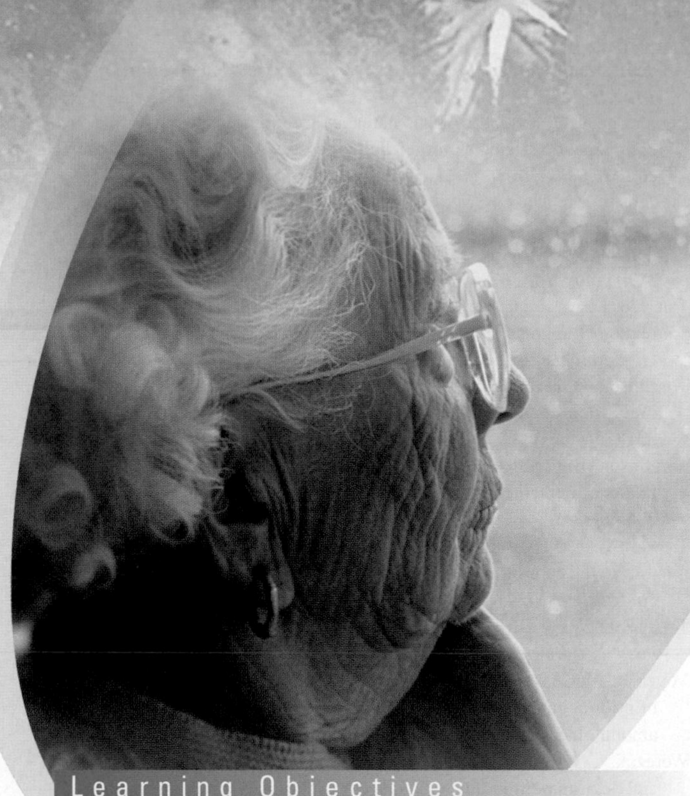

CHAPTER 15

Impaired Affective Function: Depression

Learning Objectives

After reading this chapter, you will be able to:

1. Describe theories that explain late-life depression.
2. Examine risk factors that cause or contribute to depression in older adults.
3. Discuss the functional consequences of late-life depression.
4. Describe the following aspects of assessment of late-life depression: unique manifestations of depression in older adults, cultural variations in the expression of depression, distinguishing features of dementia and depressive pseudodementia, and potential for suicide.
5. Identify interventions for alleviating risk factors for late-life depression, treating depression in older adults, and preventing suicide.

Key Terms

cognitive triad theory
cyclic antidepressants
depression
depressive pseudodementia
depressive symptoms
electroconvulsive therapy (ECT)
late-life depression
learned helplessness theory
monoamine oxidase inhibitors (MAOIs)
poststroke depression
psychomotor agitation
psychomotor retardation
reversible dementia
selective serotonin reuptake inhibitors (SSRIs)
vascular depression

Depression is the most common impairment of psychosocial function in older adulthood, yet it has the unfortunate distinction of being the most undetected and untreated of the treatable mental disorders in older adults. The term **depression** is difficult to define because it is considered a mood, a complaint, a syndrome, and a disease; however, gerontological references commonly use the term **depressive symptoms** to describe a constellation of symptoms that profoundly affect the quality of life of a significant number of older adults. Gerontologists have developed theories to explain depression in older adults, which is often called **late-life depression**, and health care practitioners have developed assessment tools to identify depression in older adults. Nurses have important roles in addressing depression because there is a range of nursing interventions that can have a significant positive impact on the quality of life of older adults.

THEORIES ABOUT LATE-LIFE DEPRESSION

Late-life depression is a multifaceted condition that is caused by complex relationships among many factors, as emphasized by Blazer (1993) and illustrated in Figure 15-1. Although no single theory can explain why older adults

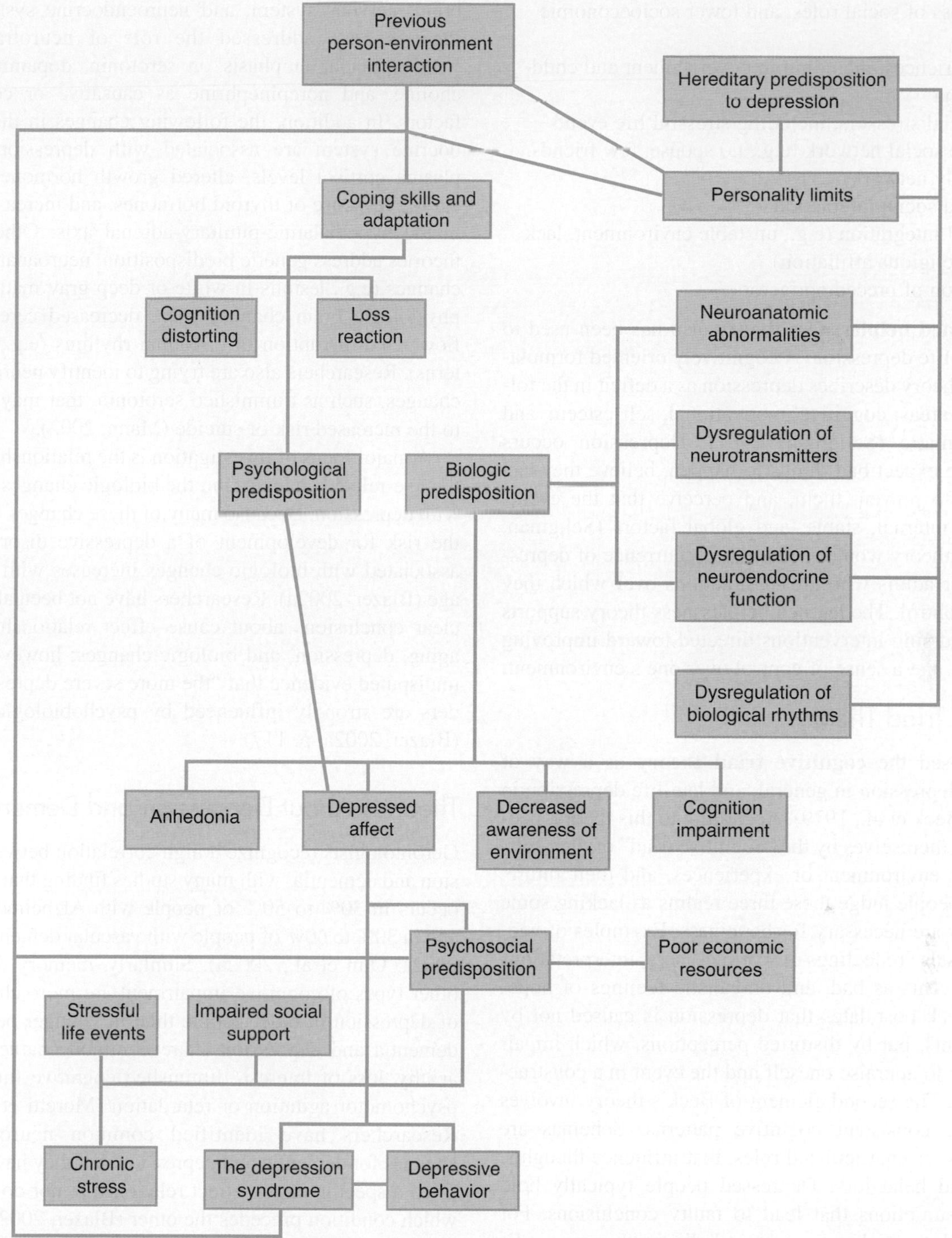

FIGURE 15-1 Possible etiologic factors contributing to depression in late life. (From Blazer, D. G. [1993]. *Depression in late life* [2nd ed.]. St. Louis: Mosby. Used with permission.)

are likely to become depressed, some of the more common psychosocial, cognitive, and biologic theories explain causative factors from various perspectives. A major focus of recent research is the relationship between dementia and depression, and studies are just beginning to address questions about the very common co-occurrence of these two conditions.

Psychosocial Theories

Psychosocial theories focus on the impact of loss as well as the buffering effects of social supports and the social network in protecting against depression. Blazer (2002a) reviewed psychosocial theories related to late-life depression and identified the following potential contributing factors:

- Ageism, loss of social roles, and lower socioeconomic status
- Early experiences, including impoverishment and childhood trauma
- Recent social stressors, including stressful life events
- Inadequate social network (e.g., no spouse, few friends, small family network)
- Diminished social interaction
- Poor social integration (e.g., unstable environment, lack of strong religious affiliation)
- Combination of preceding factors

The **learned helplessness theory** also has been used to explain late-life depression. A cognitively oriented formulation of this theory describes depression as a deficit in the following four areas: cognitive, motivational, self-esteem, and affective-somatic (Seligman, 1981). Depression occurs when people expect bad things to happen, believe they can do nothing to prevent them, and perceive that the events result from internal, stable, and global factors (Seligman, 1981). This theory would explain the occurrence of depression in older adults who are in situations over which they have little control. The learned helplessness theory supports the use of nursing interventions directed toward improving self-efficacy and a sense of control over one's environment.

Cognitive Triad Theory

Beck proposed the **cognitive triad theory** as a way of explaining depression in general, and late-life depression in particular (Beck et al., 1979). According to this theory, people appraise themselves by the "cognitive triad" of their self-image, their environment or experiences, and their future. Depressed people judge these three realms as lacking some features that are necessary for happiness. Examples of negative appraisals are feelings of worthlessness, interpretations of neutral events as bad, and unrealistic feelings of hopelessness. Beck postulates that depression is caused not by adverse events, but by distorted perceptions, which impair one's ability to appraise oneself and the event in a constructive manner. The second element of Beck's theory involves schemas, or consistent cognitive patterns. Schemas are assumptions, or unarticulated rules, that influence thoughts, feelings, and behaviors. Depressed people typically hold negative assumptions that lead to faulty conclusions. For instance, a depressed person might believe, "I must not be important because the nurse didn't stop to see me." The third component of Beck's theory is the existence of certain logical errors, such as personalization, minimization, magnification, and overgeneralization. This theory is supported by studies that have found a relationship between late-life depression and cognitive distortions or negative cognitions (Blazer, 2002a).

Biologic Theories

Biologic theories about late-life depression investigate the relationships among aging, depression, and changes in the brain, nervous system, and neuroendocrine system. Many theories have addressed the role of neurotransmitters, with particular emphasis on serotonin, dopamine, acetylcholine, and norepinephrine as causative or contributing factors. In addition, the following changes in the neuroendocrine system are associated with depression: elevated plasma cortisol levels, altered growth hormone secretion, altered response of thyroid hormones, and increased activity in the hypothalamic-pituitary-adrenal axis. Other biologic theories address genetic predisposition, neuroanatomic brain changes (e.g., lesions in white or deep gray matter), neurophysiologic brain changes (e.g., decreased cerebral blood flow), and disruption of circadian rhythms (e.g., sleep patterns). Researchers also are trying to identify neuroendocrine changes, such as diminished serotonin, that may contribute to the increased risk of suicide (Mann, 2002).

A major focus of investigation is the relationship between the age-related changes and the biologic changes associated with depression. Because many of these changes are similar, the risk for development of a depressive disorder that is associated with biologic changes increases with increasing age (Blazer, 2002a). Researchers have not been able to draw clear conclusions about cause–effect relationships among aging, depression, and biologic changes; however, there is undisputed evidence that "the more severe depressive disorders are strongly influenced by psychobiologic changes" (Blazer, 2002a, p. 117).

Theories About Depression and Dementia

Gerontologists recognize a high correlation between depression and dementia, with many studies finding that depression occurs in 30% to 50% of people with Alzheimer's disease and in 30% to 60% of people with vascular dementia (Blazer, 2002a; Olin et al., 2002a). Similarly, memory deficits and other types of cognitive impairment are more characteristic of depression in older people than in younger people. Both dementia and depression share common characteristics of apathy, loss of interest, diminished cognitive function, and psychomotor agitation or retardation (Moretti et al., 2002). Researchers have identified common neuropathologic changes for dementia and depression, but they have not identified a specific cause–effect relationship, nor do they know which condition precedes the other (Blazer, 2002a). Current theories address questions about depression as a causative factor for dementia and vice versa, and the implications of these relationships.

Depressive pseudodementia refers to a condition that appears to be a cognitive impairment—and may be labeled as a dementia—but whose underlying cause is depression. A similar concept, called **reversible dementia**, refers to a condition in which the remission of the depression causes a resolution of the cognitive deficits (Olin et al., 2002a). Long-term studies suggest that the type of depression that is accompanied by more severe cognitive deficits increases the risk for development of dementia in the future (Blazer,

2002a). Thus, from this perspective, depression is a risk factor for dementia.

In the mid-1990s, researchers started investigating the possible relationship between late-life depression and atrophy of brain cells, with particular attention on the relationship between vascular dementia and depression. Theories about **vascular depression** (also called **poststroke depression**) propose that major or minor depression can arise in late life from cerebrovascular damage, and that this type of depression has a distinct etiology and a different clinical presentation, which is described at the end of the following section (Miller et al., 2002; Simpson et al., 2000; Tateno et al., 2002).

TYPES OF DEPRESSION

Three of the mood disorders defined in the *Diagnostic and Statistical Manual of Mental Disorders, Fourth Edition, Text Revision* (*DSM-IV-TR*) are bipolar disorders, major depressive disorder, and dysthymic disorder (American Psychiatric Association, 2000). In addition, the *DSM-IV-TR* lists criteria for bereavement and adjustment disorder with depressed mood, which are closely associated with late-life depression. The majority of older adults who are admitted to hospitals for mood disorders are diagnosed with major depressive disorder, but dysthymic disorder and bereavement are much more common in community settings (Blazer, 2002a).

Because most early studies of mood disorders of later life focused primarily on major depression, which affects less than 3% of older adults, depression is likely to be unrecognized and untreated in the majority of older adults who have other types of depression. Terms such as *minor, subthreshold, subclinical*, and *subsyndromal depression* more accurately reflect depressive symptoms that occur on a continuum, ranging from no depression to major depression. This reconceptualization is based on studies indicating that minor and major depressions are not distinct disorders but are distinguished by severity of symptoms (Hybels et al., 2001; Lavretsky & Kumar, 2002; Oxman & Sengupta, 2002). Characteristics that most commonly occur, with varying degrees of severity, in any type of depression in older adults are discussed in the section on Functional Consequences.

Another recent trend in classifying depression in older adults is to identify the unique characteristics of depression with vascular dementia or Alzheimer's disease. In 2002, a group of researchers and clinicians with extensive experience related to both late-life depression and Alzheimer's disease proposed diagnostic criteria for "depression of Alzheimer's disease" (Olin et al., 2002b). Criteria for depression of Alzheimer's disease include the manifestations of depression discussed in the Functional Consequences section, all the criteria for the diagnosis of dementia of the Alzheimer's type (discussed in Chapter 14), and additional criteria such as "the symptoms cause clinically significant distress or disruption in functioning" (Olin et al., 2002a, p. 136). Specific diagnostic criteria have not been proposed for vascular depression, but studies have identified some unique characteristics of this type of depression (Miller et al., 2002; Tateno et al., 2002). Compared with other types of depression, vascular depression is characterized by poor insight, less agitation, increased disability, more cognitive impairment, more psychomotor retardation, and less depressive ideation (e.g., feelings of guilt).

RISK FACTORS FOR DEPRESSION IN OLDER ADULTS

Risk factors that are likely to cause or contribute to depression in older adults include demographic factors and psychosocial influences, medical conditions and functional impairments, and effects of medications and alcohol. Although these factors can increase the risk for depression in people of any age, older adults are more likely than younger people to have one or more of these variables. The following sections discuss each category of risk in relation to older adults. Additional risk factors for depression include cognitive impairments and dementia, as discussed in other sections of this chapter.

Demographic Factors and Psychosocial Influences

Demographic factors and psychosocial influences that are associated with depression in older adults include

- Female sex
- Personal or family history of depression
- Bereavement, loss of significant relationships
- Loneliness
- Chronic stress
- Recent social stressors
- Stressful social environment
- Loss of meaningful social interaction
- Lack of social supports
- Loss of significant roles
- Current or previous experiences of abuse or neglect
- Being a caregiver (including assuming primary care of a grandchild)

Although losses and stress can be risk factors for depression, the presence of social supports (e.g., having at least one close relationship) and the use of effective coping mechanisms can protect older adults from depression. Thus, the stressors alone are not the primary risk factor for depression; rather, it is the combination of the presence of stressors and the absence of social supports that increases the risk for depression. In addition to causing the onset of depression, psychosocial factors can affect the duration of depression. For example, a longitudinal study found that negative interactions with friends or family triggered higher levels of interpersonal stress and increased the risk for development of chronic or long-term depression (Moos et al., 2005).

Wellness Opportunity

During patient care activities, nurses have many opportunities to provide interactions that can have positive effects on depressed older adults.

Medical Conditions and Functional Impairments

The relationship between medical conditions and depression can be synergistic or cyclic, with depression contributing to medical illness and disability, and medical illness and disability contributing to depression. For example, cardiovascular disease is a risk factor for depression, and the risk is even greater in combination with a stressor such as the loss of a loved one. One explanation for this predisposition is that small vessel disease in the brain may disrupt the mood-regulating circuitry (Holley et al., 2006). Researchers also have found a synergy between the positive effects of interventions because treatment of depression can improve disability and rehabilitation can improve depression (Lenze et al., 2001). Similarly, the relationship between depression and functional impairments is complex and interactive. One way in which they are interactive is that medical conditions increase the risk for depression when they cause a decline in the person's level of functioning (Minicuci et al., 2002). In turn, the functional impairment, such as urinary incontinence, significantly increases the risk for depression (Nygaard et al., 2003). Examples of interrelationships between depression and medical conditions or functional impairments include the following:

- Depression is strongly associated through cause-and-effect relationships with numerous medical conditions (Box 15-1).
- Depression in medically ill older adults is associated with increased mortality, longer hospitalizations, and extended recovery time.
- Acute medical illnesses can threaten survival, independence, self-concept, role functions, economic resources, and sense of well-being.
- Depression in medically ill older adults can lead to other health problems, such as hip fracture and increased susceptibility to infection.
- Chronic pain is a common cause of depression, and it is sometimes a symptom of depression.
- Depression worsens pain, and pain worsens depression.
- Functional impairment is associated with depression as both a contributing factor and a consequence.
- Depression is a common cause of nutritional deficits in older adults.

Functional impairment is a risk factor for depression primarily because of the psychosocial impact of disability as a significant stressor. Researchers have found associations between physical disability and all of the following psychosocial risk factors for depression: social isolation, low self-esteem, restricted social activity, strained interpersonal relationships, loss of perceived control, and increased negative life events (Lenze et al., 2001). In addition, chronic illnesses create daily hassles (i.e., chronic stressors) that continually or frequently place demands on coping energy.

Another risk factor is that depression often goes unrecognized as a concomitant condition in older adults with medical conditions (Goldstein, 2002). For example, health care providers overlook depression in up to 86% of nursing home residents (McCurren, 2002). Although this is not a risk factor for causing depression, it is a risk factor for the progression of depression when it is untreated. Untreated depression leads to increased functional decline and increased morbidity and mortality (Fabacher et al., 2002).

Box 15-1
Medical Conditions That Can Cause Depression

Central Nervous System Disorders

Parkinson's disease
Dementia
Strokes
Hemorrhage or hematoma
Tumors
Neurosyphilis
Normal-pressure hydrocephalus

Nutritional Deficiencies

Folate or vitamin B_{12} deficiency
Pernicious anemia
Iron deficiency

Cardiovascular Disturbances

Myocardial infarction
Congestive heart failure
Subacute bacterial endocarditis

Miscellaneous

Rheumatoid arthritis
Cancer, particularly of the pancreas or intestinal tract
Tuberculosis
Tertiary syphilis

Metabolic and Endocrine Disorders

Diabetes
Hypothyroidism/hyperthyroidism
Hypoglycemia/hyperglycemia
Parathyroid disorders
Adrenal diseases
Hepatic or renal disease

Fluid and Electrolyte Disturbances

Hypercalcemia
Hypokalemia
Hyponatremia

Infections

Meningitis
Viral pneumonia
Hepatitis
Urinary tract infections

Effects of Medications and Alcohol

People of any age may experience depression as an adverse medication effect, but older adults are more likely than younger adults to be taking medication. Medications may be risk factors for depression in the following ways:

- Adverse medication effects can cause a depressive syndrome that improves or disappears when the medication is stopped.
- Adverse medication effects can induce a depression that does not remit when the medications are stopped.
- Adverse medication effects can simulate a depressive syndrome by causing lethargy, insomnia, and irritability.
- The withdrawal of certain medications, such as psychostimulants, can cause a depressive syndrome.

Depression as an adverse effect of medications is usually related to the use of prescription medications. For example, benzodiazepines—the type of medication that is most frequently abused by older adults—present a risk factor for depression. Box 15-2 lists some medications that may cause depression as an adverse effect.

Alcohol is the drug that is most commonly used by older people for its central nervous system effects as a sedative and antianxiety agent (Blazer, 2002a). Moreover, although people of any age may experience adverse effects from alcohol, older people are more sensitive to these adverse effects because of age-related changes. Alcohol and depression have a cyclic and synergistic relationship: alcohol causes depression, depression leads to alcohol abuse, which in turn exacerbates the depression. For example, depression is associated with higher alcohol intake, an increased risk for suicide, more frequent relapses in drinking, and a more severe course of alcoholism (Blow & Barry, 2000).

Box 15-2
Examples of Medications That Can Cause Depression

Analgesics

ibuprofen
indomethacin
narcotics
propoxyphene

Antihypertensives

clonidine
guanethidine
hydralazine
methyldopa
propranolol
reserpine

Antiparkinsonian Agents

levodopa

Cardiovascular Agents

digoxin
digitalis

Central Nervous System Agents

alcohol
barbiturates
benzodiazepines
fluphenazine
haloperidol
meprobamate

Histamine Blockers

cimetidine

Sterolds

corticosteroids
estrogen
progesterone

FUNCTIONAL CONSEQUENCES ASSOCIATED WITH DEPRESSION IN OLDER ADULTS

Depression has serious functional consequences for people of any age, but for frail and seriously depressed older adults, the effects can be life-threatening. Functional consequences range from a small negative impact on well-being and quality of life to the most serious consequence, which is suicide. In addition to focusing on specific functional consequences of depression, this section discusses types of depression that commonly affect older adults and terminology associated with depression in older adults.

Physical Health and Functioning

A decline in physical functioning is one of the most consistently identified functional consequences of depression in older adults (e.g., Blazer, 2002a; Mehta et al., 2002). Depression is more likely to interfere with daily functioning when the older person also is cognitively impaired (Kiosses et al., 2001). Additional functional consequences that affect health and functioning are a higher mortality rate, high number of physical complaints, perception of worse health, and inability to carry out important life functions such as managing money or medications (Callahan et al., 2005; Meyers, 2002; Rozzini et al., 2002; Unutzer et al., 2002). Moreover, the inability to manage money or medications may be a central factor preventing the person from living independently. Box 15-3 lists ways in which depression affects physical health and functioning.

Appetite disturbances, especially anorexia, are among the most common physical complaints of depressed older adults. Sometimes, the depressed person does not complain of anorexia and may even deny the problem, but a caregiver or family member may note that the person is not interested in food and is losing weight. Other gastrointestinal complaints that may be functional consequences of depression

Box 15-3
Functional Consequences of Late-Life Depression

Impact on Physical Function

- Loss of appetite
- Weight loss
- Digestive system complaints, especially dysphagia, flatulence, constipation, stomach distress, or early satiety
- Insomnia, hypersomnia, frequent awakening, early-morning awakening, and other sleep disturbances
- Fatigue, loss of energy
- Pain, discomfort, dyspnea, general malaise
- Slowed or increased psychomotor activities
- Loss of libido or other problems with sexual function

Impact on Psychosocial Function

- Affect: sad, low, "blue," worried, unhappy, "down in the dumps"
- Absence of feelings; feeling numb or empty
- Diminished life satisfaction
- Low self-esteem
- Loss of interest or pleasure
- Passivity, lack of motivation to do things
- Inattention to personal appearance
- Feelings of guilt, hopelessness, self-blame, unworthiness, uselessness, helplessness
- Anxiety, worry, irritability
- Slowed thinking, poor memory, inability to concentrate, poor attention span, inability to make decisions, exaggeration of any mental deficits
- Rumination about past and present problems and failures

include flatulence, constipation, early satiety, and attention to bowels. Any of these disturbances may be attributed to or actually caused by other factors, such as medical conditions or adverse medication effects, but depression must be considered as a possible underlying factor. Like weight loss and diminished appetite, sleep changes commonly occur in older adults, and they may or may not be caused by depression. Waking up more frequently during the night and early-morning awakening are two changes in sleep patterns that are characteristic of depression. Chronic fatigue and diminished energy are additional functional consequences of late-life depression that are likely to be attributed to or caused by other conditions.

Older adults, like seriously depressed people of any age, are likely to experience psychomotor agitation or retardation. **Psychomotor retardation** is manifested as slowed body movements and slowed verbal responses, sometimes to the point of muteness. A monotonous or whispering tone of voice might also be an indicator of psychomotor retardation. Affected people often complain of feeling extremely fatigued and having little or no energy. In contrast to people with psychomotor retardation, people with **psychomotor agitation** present an atypical picture of depression. These people manifest high levels of activity, such as pacing and hand wringing. They may be unable to sit still and may have verbal outbursts, such as shouting. Another activity associated with psychomotor agitation is compulsive behavior, such as frequent toileting or hand-washing.

Diversity Note

Older depressed women have more appetite disturbances and older depressed men have more agitation (Kockler & Heun, 2002).

Psychosocial Function and Quality of Life

Depression is inherently characterized by a depressed mood or sad affect, but older adults may not perceive or acknowledge these mood disturbances in themselves. Rather than acknowledging that they are depressed, older adults are more likely to talk about being "blue" or "down in the dumps." Depressed older people may feel like crying but may not be able to cry or identify the underlying reason for their sadness. Another psychosocial consequence of depression is the absence of life satisfaction even when the person has reasons to feel satisfied.

Anxiety, irritability, diminished self-esteem, and negative feelings about self are some of the more generalized affective consequences of depression. The absence of feelings, or a feeling of emptiness, also can be a functional consequence of depression. A loss of interest in social activities may be the depression-related psychosocial change that is most obvious to others. Similarly, other people are likely to observe that the depressed older person has little or no concern about personal appearance. In addition, the depressed person may be overly or unrealistically worried about illnesses, financial affairs, and family issues.

Cognitive impairments can occur because of depression, and in older adults, these deficits are likely to be viewed as a primary problem rather than as a consequence of another problem. Depressed older adults may, in fact, exaggerate cognitive deficits and make statements about global deficits, such as "I can't remember anything at all." In particular, they may emphasize memory deficits and attribute these to normal aging, when the underlying problem is actually a depression-related difficulty in concentrating. See Box 15-3 for a list of functional consequences of depression that affect psychosocial function.

Depression has a major negative impact on quality of life. For example, depressed older adults report unsatisfactory social functioning, lower levels of life satisfaction, and poor perceptions of physical and mental health (Doraiswamy et al., 2002; Meyers, 2002; Xavier et al., 2002). In addition, many of the symptoms of depression (e.g., worry, fatigue, sad affect, sleep disturbances, loss of interest) directly interfere with well-being and quality of life. Moreover, a sense of meaninglessness, which is a common symptom in late-life depression, can have a significant negative effect on quality of life because this causes the older adult to "view the structure and purpose of his or her life in negative ways" (Blazer, 2002a, p. 179).

Wellness Opportunity

Because someone who is depressed tends to have very low self-esteem, nurses can point out concrete examples of positive qualities that they see in the person.

Suicide

Despite the fact that suicide is the most serious functional consequence of late-life depression, nurses and other health care workers tend to overlook this risk. This tendency is partially attributable to the fact that old age is associated with passivity and nonviolence, whereas suicide is associated with aggressiveness and violence. In 2000, people aged 65 years and older constituted 13% of the population in the United States, but they committed 18% of all suicides. These rates do not reflect the "drastic underreporting" of suicides in older adults that occurs for reasons such as family efforts to conceal evidence and difficulty determining the actual cause of death in medically ill people (Roff, 2001). Nor do these rates reflect the unrecognized suicidal acts that older adults indirectly or subtly use to take their own lives, such as refusal to eat, failure to take medically necessary medications, and other means of self-neglect. In addition to having the highest rate of suicide, older people have the highest rate of completed suicides in proportion to unsuccessful attempts.

Diversity Note

In most countries, men have a higher rate of completed suicide, whereas women have a higher rate of attempted suicide (Mann, 2002).

Suicide rates among older adults in the United States vary significantly by sex and ethnicity, as illustrated in Figure 15-2. Across cultures, the suicide rate for men is four times higher than for women during younger adulthood, and it is even greater after the age of 75 years. Worldwide, the suicide rate increased by approximately 35% in men and 10% in women between 1950 and 1995 (Mann, 2002).

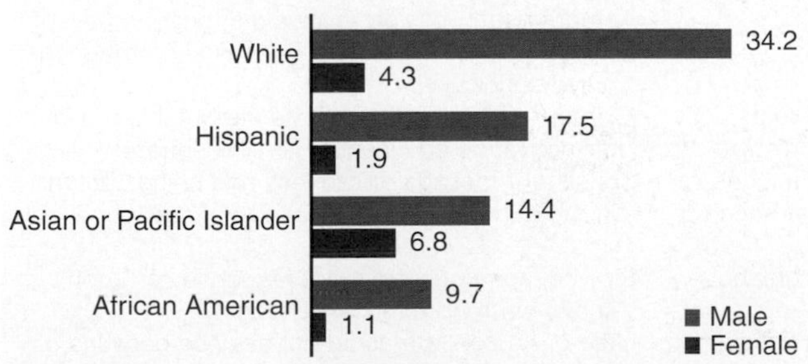

FIGURE 15-2 Differences in suicide rates for people 65 years and older in the United States according to race and sex (2002). Numbers shown are suicide deaths per 100,000 population. (Source: National Center for Health Statistics. [2005]. *Health, United States, 2005* [Table 46]. Hyattsville, MD: U.S. Department of Health and Human Services.)

Diversity Note

Studies have identified risk factors that are associated with higher suicide rates in specific groups. For example, among African Americans, being female and not having religious ties are risk factors for depression, and among whites, advanced age is a risk factor for depressive symptoms (Jang et al., 2005).

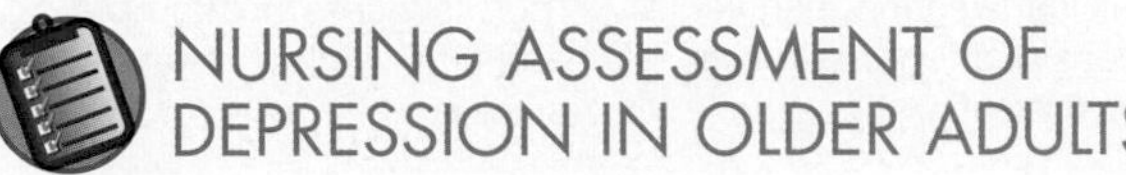

NURSING ASSESSMENT OF DEPRESSION IN OLDER ADULTS

Because Chapter 13 addresses all aspects of psychosocial assessment, this section is limited to the following specific aspects of late-life depression: identifying the unique manifestations of depression in older adults, differentiating between dementia and depressive pseudodementia, using screening tools to identify late-life depression, and assessing suicide risk in older adults. The assessment information in Chapter 13, particularly Box 13-7, can be used with the information in the following sections as a guide for assessing depression in older adults.

Wellness Opportunity

Nurses can ask a depressed older adult, "Can you think of one thing that we can do to improve your quality of life today?"

Identifying the Unique Manifestations of Depression

Assessment of late-life depression is complicated by a wide array of possible manifestations, as reviewed in the section on Functional Consequences. Moreover, manifestations of depression in older adults differ from those in younger adults. Although it is difficult to generalize about manifestations of depression according to age categories, some conclusions about the differences in younger and older adults are summarized in Table 15-1.

In assessing depression in any cognitively impaired older adult, it is often difficult to distinguish between manifestations of depression and dementia. Table 15-2, which identifies specific features that are most likely to be associated with either dementia or depression, can be used as a guide for nursing assessment to differentiate between these two conditions. It is important to keep in mind that older adults frequently have conditions that contribute to both depression and cognitive impairment, so manifestations will not always be clearly distinguished.

TABLE 15-1 Comparison of Depression in Younger and Older Adults

Depressed Younger Adults	Depressed Older Adults
More likely to report emotional symptoms	Report more cognitive and physical symptoms
Sense of hopelessness, uselessness, and helplessness	Apathy; exaggeration of personal helplessness
Negative feelings toward self	Sense of emptiness, loss of interest, withdrawal from social activities
Insomnia	Hypersomnia; early morning awakening
Eating disorders	Anorexia, weight loss
More verbal expressions of suicidal ideation than successful attempts; more passive means of suicide	Less talk about suicide, but more successful attempts and more violent means of suicide

Cultural factors can influence one's perception of depression, and nurses must consider these especially during their assessments. Nurses can use information in Cultural Considerations 15-1 to identify some of the cultural variations in expressions of depression.

Wellness Opportunity

Nurses respect individual preferences by listening carefully to identify acceptable terminology in older adults who do not want to acknowledge being "depressed."

Using Screening Tools

Concerns about depression being overlooked and underdiagnosed in older people have stimulated the development of very brief, two- or three-item screening tools that health care professionals can use in a variety of settings (e.g., Fabacher et al., 2002; National Institute of Mental Health, 2001; Thobaben, 2002). For example, the U.S. Preventive Services Task Force recently emphasized that there is sufficient research evidence to suggest that primary care practitioners should routinely screen for depression in all adults (Agency for Healthcare Research and Quality, 2002). The Task Force recommends that use of the following two questions may be as effective as using longer screening instruments (Agency for Healthcare Research and Quality, 2002):

1. During the past 2 weeks, have you felt down, depressed, or hopeless?
2. During the past 2 weeks, have you felt little interest or pleasure in doing things?

A positive response to either of these two questions warrants further assessment with a depression scale (e.g., the Geriatric Depression Scale). In addition to asking these two questions, depression screening should ascertain accurate information about past and current use of psychotropic medications (Norton et al., 2006).

The Geriatric Depression Scale (GDS) is a 30-question screening tool that has been widely used across health care settings for older adults who are healthy, medically ill, or mild to moderately cognitively impaired (Fig. 15-3). The Hartford Institute for Geriatric Nursing recommends the use of this screening tool—which is reliable, sensitive, and takes an average of 12 minutes to administer—to facilitate assessment of depression in older adults (Kurlowicz, 2003). Shorter forms of the GDS, consisting of 12 or 15 items, have been developed for use with residents in long-term care settings (McCurren, 2002; Sutcliffe et al., 2000).

Because of the high correlation between depression and medical illness, Piven (2001) developed a protocol to

TABLE 15-2 Distinguishing Features of Dementia and Depression

Parameter	Dementia	Depression
Onset of symptoms	Gradual onset, recognized only by hindsight	Abrupt onset, possibly involving a triggering event
Presentation of symptoms	Unawareness of symptoms, or attribution to nonpathologic causes	Exaggeration of memory problems and other cognitive deficits
Memory and attention	Impaired memory, especially for recent events; poor attention; strong attempts to perform well	Memory and attention deficits attributable to lack of motivation and inability to concentrate
Emotions	Labile affect that changes in response to suggestions; possible apathy owing to cognitive impairments	Consistent feelings of sadness and being "down in the dumps"; unresponsive to suggestions
Response to questions	Evasive, angry, sarcastic; use of humor, confabulation, or social skills to cover up deficits	Slowed, apathetic, frequent response of "I don't know," with no effort expended
Personal appearance	Inappropriate dress and actions owing to impaired perceptions and thought processes	Little or no concern about appearance because of lack of motivation or diminished self-esteem
Physical complaints	Vague fatigue and weakness; complaints are inconsistent and easily forgotten	Anorexia, weight loss, constipation, insomnia, decreased energy
Neurologic features	Aphasia, agnosia, agraphia, apraxia, perseveration	Complaints of dysphagia without any physical basis
Contact with reality	Denial of reality; illusions more predominant than hallucinations; if present, delusions are aimed at explaining deficits	Exaggerated sense of gloom; possible auditory hallucinations or self-derogatory delusions

Cultural Considerations 15-1

Cultural Variations in Expressions of Depression

Cultural Group	Common Expressions of Depression
African Americans	Fatigue and somatic complaints. "I sure have a lot of troubles."; "I know God won't give me more than I can handle."
Native Americans/ Alaskan Natives	Feeling "heavy" or "out of harmony"; may complain of heart problems
Caribbean blacks	Stress from a weakness or deficiency in character; influenced by fear of being ostracized by peers
Chinese Americans	Shameful to discuss; may be called "neurasthenia" (i.e., symptoms produced by social stressors)
Cubans	Attribute symptoms to "nerves," anxiety, or extreme stress; shameful
Filipinos	Shameful to discuss; may refer to *Lungknot* (i.e., sadness)
Japanese Americans	Because of shame and stigma, emotional distress may be expressed through physical symptoms and may become severe before help is sought
Koreans	Nonverbal expressions; *Chim-ool haumnida*
Mexican Americans	Sign of weakness, shameful to discuss, common response to stress
Puerto Ricans	Use *depresion* to convey sadness, grief, or anguish; use *nervios* (nervousness) or *ataque de nervios* (attack of nerves) to describe depressive symptoms
South Asians	References to *Dil uddas hona*, associated with spiritual unhappiness
White British	Associate depression with genetic predisposition, traumatic childhood, or poor relationship with mother
People from countries with a recent history of war, violence, or political upheaval	May be associated with posttraumatic stress disorder; feelings of helplessness; memories of war-related brutalities

Sources: Lipson, J. G., & Dibble, S. L. (2005). *Culture and clinical care.* San Francisco: UCSF Nursing Press; Lawrence, V., Murray, J., Banerjee, S., Turner, S., Sangha, K., Byng, R., et al. (2006). Concepts and causation of depression: A cross-cultural study of the beliefs of older adults. *The Gerontologist, 46,* 23–32; and Andrews, M. M., & Boyle, J. S. (2003). *Transcultural concepts in nursing care* [4th ed.]. Philadelphia: Lippincott Williams & Wilkins.)

improve detection of depression in medically compromised but cognitively intact older adults in health care facilities. This protocol advises the weekly use of the Folstein Mini-Mental State Examination (MMSE) and the short-form GDS to detect depression. The protocol includes a form to monitor detection of depression.

Diversity Note

A brief screening tool, which takes about 2 minutes to administer, is available for identifying Puerto Rican older adults who need further evaluation for depression (Robison et al., 2002).

Assessing the Risks for Suicide

Nursing assessment of suicide risk is especially important because most older people give clues, sometimes to many people, about potential suicide. These clues, however, may be subtle, and the person who hears them may not associate them with suicide risk, particularly in older adults. Although 70% of older people who commit suicide visit their primary care provider within 1 month before the act, fewer than 5% of depressed older adults directly express suicidal ideation to their primary care practitioner (Bartels et al., 2002). Even when older adults express suicidal ideation to primary care practitioners, they are less likely than younger adults to be viewed as having a serious and treatable condition (Uncapher & Arean, 2000). Thus, the nursing assessment of suicide risk must be based primarily on identification of potential risk factors for suicide in older adults, such as the following (Bartels et al., 2002; Turvey et al., 2002; Waern et al., 2002):

- Limited social support
- Poor impulse control
- Poor sleep quality
- Recent stressful life event (e.g., widowhood)
- Strong sense of hopelessness
- Lack of a reason for living
- Nonadherence to medical treatment
- Immediate access to a lethal method
- Serious medical illness (e.g., cancer, neurologic disorders)
- Moderate to severe functional impairment (e.g., visual impairment)
- Moderate to severe depression, often co-occurring with anxiety disorder

Because depression is the factor most consistently identified across studies as a risk factor for suicide, it is important to assess for suicidal ideation in any depressed older adult. In addition to these factors that alert the nurse to risk for suicide, the factors that are most strongly predictive of actual suicide are a history of previous attempts and current suicide ideation that includes a plan or evidence of preparation of a plan (Mann, 2002). Box 15-4 summarizes risk factors for suicide in older adults, verbal and nonverbal clues to suicide intent, and specific questions to assess immediate suicide risk.

When the assessment identifies risk factors or clues to potential suicide, the nurse must further assess the immediate potential for a suicide attempt. This assessment is multilevel, as outlined in Box 15-4, with each level of questions depending on the response to the previous level. The assess-

Geriatric Depression Scale (Short Form)

1.	Are you basically satisfied with your life?	Yes	No
2.	Have you dropped many of your activities and interests?	Yes	No
3.	Do you feel that your life is empty?	Yes	No
4.	Do you often get bored?	Yes	No
5.	Are you in good spririts most of the time?	Yes	No
6.	Are you afraid that something bad is going to happen to you?	Yes	No
7.	Do you feel happy most of the time?	Yes	No
8.	Do you often feel helpless?	Yes	No
9.	Do you prefer to stay at home rather than go out and do new things?	Yes	No
10.	Do you feel you have more problems with memory than most?	Yes	No
11.	Do you think it is wonderful to be alive now?	Yes	No
12.	Do you feel pretty worthless the way you are now?	Yes	No
13.	Do you feel full of energy?	Yes	No
14.	Do you feel that your situation is hopeless?	Yes	No
15.	Do you think that most people are better off than you are?	Yes	No

Score:___/15 One point for "No" to questions 1, 5, 7, 11, 13	Normal	3 ± 2
One point for "Yes" to other questions	Mildly depressed	7 ± 3
	Very depressed	12 ± 2

FIGURE 15-3 Geriatric Depression Scale (short form). (From Yesavage, J. A., Brink, T. L., Rose, T. L., Lum, O., Huang, V., Adey, M., et al. [1983]. Development and validation of a geriatric depression screening scale: A preliminary report. *Journal of Psychiatric Research, 17*, 37–49. Used with permission.)

ment begins with questions to determine the presence or absence of suicidal thoughts. Health care professionals may be reluctant to initiate questions about suicide because they fear that this line of questioning may "put ideas in the person's head." This fear is unfounded. People who do not have suicidal thoughts usually respect the necessity of the questions but do not begin thinking about suicide just because the topic was broached. Rather than asking a person "Do

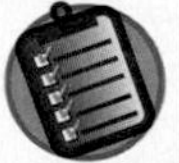

Box 15-4
Guidelines for Assessing Suicide Risk

Risk Factors for Suicide in Older Adults

- Demographic factors: white race, male gender, divorced or widowed, low socioeconomic status
- Depression, especially when accompanied by insomnia, agitation, and self-neglect
- Chronic illness with increasing dependence and helplessness; diagnosis of cancer or a terminal illness
- Poor social supports; social isolation, especially recent isolation
- History of psychiatric illness, especially major depression
- Onset of major depression within the past year
- Family history of suicide; personal or family history of suicide attempts
- Patterns of impulsive behavior
- Alcohol abuse
- Poor communication skills

Verbal Clues to Suicide Intent

- "Pretty soon you won't have to worry about me."
- "I would be better off dead."
- "I don't want to be a burden to others."
- Expressions of hopelessness
- Remarks about life being unbearable
- Reflections on the worthlessness of life

Nonverbal Clues to Suicide Intent

- Making a will; giving belongings away; preparing for own funeral
- Serious self-neglect, especially in people who have no cognitive impairments
- Frequent visits to primary care provider(s)
- Excessive use of medications or alcohol
- Accumulation of prescription medications
- Unusual preoccupation with self and withdrawal from others

Interview Questions to Assess the Immediate Risk of Suicide

Level 1

- "Do you ever think life is not worth living?"
- "Do you ever think about escaping from your problems?"

Level 2

- "Do you ever think about harming yourself?"
- "Do you ever think of taking your own life?"

Level 3

- "Do you have a plan?"
- "What would you do to take your life?"

Level 4

- "Have you ever started to act on a plan to harm yourself?"
- "Under what circumstances would you act on that plan?"

you ever think about committing suicide?," the nurse can phrase the question in such a way that the person will give clues to his or her intent if it exists, but will not be offended by the question if it does not.

If suicidal thoughts are suspected or identified at level 1, additional questions must be asked. Although level 1 questions are indirect, level 2 questions must be more direct and are aimed at determining the presence or absence of thoughts about self-harm. If the answer to any of these questions is positive, level 3 questions are asked to determine whether the person has a realistic suicide plan. Questions at level 3 must be very direct and specific because this information is crucial to assessing the immediate risk for suicide. If the person describes a detailed plan and has access to all the necessary implements, the potential for suicide is extremely high. By contrast, if the person has a plan that is vague or that cannot possibly be carried out, the immediate potential for suicide is lower. For example, if the plan involves a gun, but the person does not have a gun and cannot get out of the house, then the chance of a successful suicide is low. By contrast, if the person threatens to consume the bottle of barbiturates that is readily available in the medicine cabinet, then the chance of a successful suicide is quite high. Level 4 questions are asked to assess further the immediacy of the risk when the person has described a plan. When answers to levels 3 or 4 are positive, the nurse must plan immediate interventions to deal with the suicide risk.

In addition to using the guidelines in Box 15-4, nurses can refer to the evidence-based protocol described by Holkup and colleagues (2003) for recognizing and addressing suicidal behaviors in older adults.

Diversity Note

Researchers found that a Chinese version of the Geriatric Suicide Ideation Scale was effective for accurately identifying suicide ideation related to depression, loneliness, and hopelessness in older adults in Hong Kong (Chou et al., 2005).

NURSING DIAGNOSIS

Some nurses are advocating for the development of a nursing diagnosis of Depression, but in the absence of this specific nursing diagnosis, the following nursing diagnoses may be applicable: Ineffective Coping, Hopelessness, Chronic Low Self-Esteem, Social Isolation, Powerlessness, Caregiver Role Strain, Risk for Imbalanced Nutrition, and Adult Failure to Thrive. Related factors commonly found in older adults are relocation, ageist attitudes, financial concerns, social isolation, caregiving responsibilities, multiple social stressors, loss of significant roles or relationships, functional impairments (including cognitive deficits), and increased dependence (e.g., owing to the loss of the ability to drive).

If the nursing assessment identifies risk factors for suicide, an applicable nursing diagnosis would be Risk for Suicide, defined as "a state in which an individual is at risk for killing himself or herself' (Carpenito-Moyet, 2006, p. 433). Related factors would include any risk factors and verbal and nonverbal clues to suicide. An example is an 85-year-old widower who says his life is no longer worthwhile and who makes frequent visits to his doctor for complaints of weight loss and sleep disturbance.

Wellness Opportunity

Nurses can use the wellness nursing diagnosis of Readiness for Enhanced Coping for older adults who are interested in improving their coping skills to address depressive symptoms that are not severe.

PLANNING FOR WELLNESS OUTCOMES

When caring for older adults who are depressed, nurses identify outcomes as an essential part of the planning process. The following Nursing Outcomes Classification (NOC) terminology is applicable to depressed older adults: Coping, Hope, Self-Esteem, Social Support, Social Involvement, Role Performance, Caregiver Emotional Health, Caregiver Endurance Potential, Mood Equilibrium, Nutritional Status, and Physical Well-Being. Outcomes for older adults at risk for suicide include Suicide Self-Restraint and Personal Safety Behavior. Specific interventions to achieve outcomes related to depression and suicide are discussed in the following sections.

Wellness Opportunity

Quality of Life is a wellness outcome that is achieved by addressing the functional and psychosocial consequences of depression.

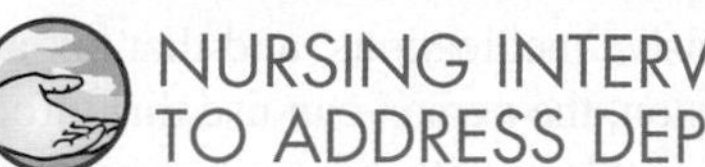

NURSING INTERVENTIONS TO ADDRESS DEPRESSION

Nurses in any setting are responsible for addressing depression in older adults. Particularly in long-term care settings, nurses are the health care providers most likely to identify manifestations of depression and to request further evaluation and treatment. In recent years, primary care physicians and nurse practitioners have been the health care professionals evaluating and managing depression, and referrals to psychiatrists and other mental health professionals for depression have become less common. This trend is due to the emphasis on cost-effectiveness and the availability of safer and more effective antidepressant medications. Nursing protocols for depression in elderly patients emphasize the important responsibility of nurses in reducing the negative consequences of depression through early recognition, intervention, and referral of patients with depression (Kurlowicz, 2003; Piven, 2005).

Nursing Interventions Classification (NIC) terminology pertinent to interventions for older adults who are depressed include the following: Caregiver Support, Coping Enhancement, Counseling, Crisis Intervention, Emotional Support, Exercise Promotion, Grief Work Facilitation, Hope Instillation, Mood Management, Music Therapy, Role Enhancement, Self-Esteem Enhancement, Suicide Prevention, and Teaching: Individual.

The next sections review the role of the nurse in planning and implementing interventions for late-life depression.

Alleviating Risk Factors

Nurses promote wellness for depressed older adults by addressing the many risk factors that are well within the realm of nursing, such as functional impairments, adverse medication effects, and excess alcohol use. Many nursing interventions that improve the level of functioning also are effective for alleviating or preventing depression. For example, dementia, sensory impairments, urinary incontinence, and mobility impairments are examples of conditions that can contribute to depression and will respond to the nursing interventions (refer to Chapters 14, 16, 17, 19, and 22).

Wellness Opportunity

Nurses promote wellness by challenging ageist stereotypes that falsely attribute functional impairments to inevitable consequences of aging.

If adverse medication effects are a risk factor for depression, nurses can educate the person about this potential relationship and identify problem-solving strategies to address the adverse effects. One such strategy, especially for older adults who are unaccustomed to raising questions about their medications, is to teach about communicating with the prescribing health care provider (as discussed in Chapter 8). For example, if the older person understands that there is a wide array of antihypertensive medications, and that not all of them will cause depression, the person can use this information in discussing the problem with his or her primary care provider. Nurses also can assure the older adult that it is acceptable to initiate this kind of problem-solving discussion with health care practitioners. When the nurse, rather than the patient, is the one who communicates with the primary care provider, the nurse can raise appropriate questions about depression as an adverse medication effect. This problem-solving approach is especially important when the primary care provider is considering adding an antidepressant medication to a regimen that includes a depression-inducing medication. In these situations, the solution may be to change medications, rather than to add another medication and increase the risk for adverse effects.

If excess alcohol use is a risk factor for depression, individual and group interventions can be effective, particularly when the alcohol abuse is a reaction to recent losses. Alcoholics Anonymous (AA) is the most widely used group program for alcoholics of any age, and in some areas, age-homogeneous groups have been established, including some for older adults. Nurses can encourage older adults to initiate contact with AA, or they might directly facilitate the referral if the person agrees to this. Individual and family counseling also may be effective, and nurses can suggest or facilitate referrals for these mental health services.

Improving Psychosocial Function

In addition to alleviating the risk factors for depression, health promotion interventions can improve psychosocial health and prevent depression from occurring or progressing. Blazer (2002b) emphasized the importance of primary prevention of late-life depression through interventions that enhance self-efficacy and alleviate sadness and loneliness. In addition to health promotion interventions for psychosocial health (discussed in Chapter 12), nurses can identify interventions to strengthen social supports and foster meaningful roles. For example, nurses have many opportunities to encourage participation in group meal or social programs. Most communities in the United States have some social programs for older adults, and many provide transportation. Many churches and religious organizations also have programs designed to meet the social needs of isolated older adults. Volunteer visitor or phone call programs, for example, are sometimes available to address the needs of people who have difficulty getting out of the house. Other programs, such as pet therapy or "Adopt a Grandparent," are available in some home, community-based, and long-term care settings, and they can be helpful in alleviating loneliness and depression.

Involvement in volunteer activities can enhance self-esteem and provide a meaningful role for older adults who are mildly depressed. Nurses can suggest that older adults explore opportunities for volunteer activities through organizations such as the National Senior Service Corps (previously called the Retired Senior Volunteer Program), which is one of the many programs in the United States that assists older adults in becoming involved in volunteer activities (see Educational Resources at the end of the chapter).

Wellness Opportunity

Nurses promote quality of life by encouraging an older adult to engage in activities that are meaningful to that person.

Promoting Health Through Exercise and Nutrition

The beneficial effects of exercise with regard to anxiety, depression, self-esteem, and other components of mental health are widely acknowledged. Researchers have identified the effects of physical exercise in both alleviating and preventing depression in older adults (e.g., Blazer, 2002b; Penninx et al., 2002; Singh et al., 2001; Strawbridge et al., 2002). Older adults, however, may not view exercise as important, or they may be reluctant to participate in exercise programs because of chronic illnesses, such as arthritis. If older adults understand the benefits of exercise for both their physical and mental health, and if an individually tailored program is developed for them, they may be more willing to become involved in exercise programs. In community and long-term care settings, nurses can facilitate the establishment of group exercise programs and encourage depressed older adults to participate in them.

Nutrition is an important consideration as an intervention for depression for three reasons. First, depression often negatively affects nutritional status, and this can cause additional negative consequences. Second, good nutrition has a positive effect on mental health and cognitive function. Third, constipation is both a consequence of depression and an adverse effect of some antidepressant medications, and it usually can be alleviated through nutritional interventions. During phases of serious depression, malnutrition can lead to medical problems, which may progress to the point of being life-threatening. Nutritional supplements, hyperalimentation, or tube feedings may be necessary interventions when depression seriously interferes with eating. When depression is severe enough to lead to malnutrition, the older person must be evaluated for psychiatric care. Interventions for less severely depressed older people are aimed at maintaining adequate hydration and nutrition and preventing or managing constipation (as discussed in Chapter 18).

Wellness Opportunity

Nurses address the body–mind–spirit interrelationship by incorporating interventions for optimal nutrition as an essential component of care for depressed older adults.

Providing Education and Counseling

Many types of individual and group psychosocial therapies are effective interventions for late-life depression. For example, when multiple stressors challenge the person's coping abilities and contribute to depression, individual or group therapy can be an important intervention for improving the person's psychosocial health and alleviating depression. Nurses provide counseling and emotional support for all depressed older adults, and in some situations, they providing specific psychosocial therapies. One psychosocial model for addressing depression includes the following components (Cole, 2005):

- Education about the significance of current risk factors for depression
- Skills training with emphasis on maintaining routines
- Identification and utilization of social support
- Adjustment to functional loss
- Bereavement counseling as needed and referral to a support group
- Information about sleep enhancement techniques

A nursing intervention that can be universally applied to care of depressed older adults is Emotional Support, defined as "provision of reassurance, acceptance, and encouragement during times of stress" (Johnson et al., 2005, p. 649). Counseling as a nursing intervention is defined as "the use of an interactive helping process focusing on the needs, problems, or feelings of the patient and significant others to enhance or support coping, problem solving, and interpersonal relationships" (Johnson et al., 2005, p. 646). Nursing activities listed under this Counseling intervention that are most applicable for depressed older adults include the following (Piven & Buckwalter, 2001):

- Establish a therapeutic relationship
- Encourage expression of feelings
- Demonstrate empathy, warmth, and genuineness
- Encourage new skill development, as appropriate
- Provide factual information, as necessary and appropriate
- Assist the patient to identify strengths and reinforce these

Nurses need to be at least minimally familiar with some of the individual therapies that have been found to be acceptable and effective for depressed older adults so they can encourage or facilitate referrals for these interventions. Therapies identified as effective and acceptable for depressed older adults include the following (Blazer, 2002a; Landreville et al., 2001; Piven & Buckwalter; 2001):

- Behavior therapy (e.g., problem solving, practicing assertiveness, setting up a daily schedule)
- Cognitive therapy (e.g., conscious restructuring of negative thought processes)
- Interpersonal therapy (e.g., modification of relationships or expectations about relationships)
- Supportive therapy (e.g., evaluating the person's strengths and weaknesses and facilitating choices that improve coping abilities)
- Dynamic psychotherapy (e.g., resolution of intrapsychic conflicts)
- Bibliotherapy (e.g., readings and exercises to assist the person in identifying and reducing dysfunctional thought processes)

Cognitive and behavior techniques may be especially useful in addressing the vicious cycle of negative feelings, lowered self-esteem, and helplessness associated with chronic illnesses and multiple personal losses (Cole, 2005).

In recent years, group therapies have been recognized as an effective and efficient intervention for depressed older adults. Group therapy is effective for depressed older adults because it imparts information, improves self-esteem, enhances social interaction, encourages attitudinal changes, and facilitates personal development (Blazer, 2002a). Support and self-help groups are commonly used interventions to improve psychosocial function and alleviate depression in older adults who are coping with life events, such as caregiving, widowhood, or grief reactions, and nurses can educate older adults about the availability of such groups. Numerous studies have found that support groups are particularly effective for caregivers of people with dementia.

Nurses generally do not lead psychotherapy groups as a primary responsibility, but they are increasingly assuming group leadership roles, particularly in community and long-term care settings. Other group models used as interventions for late-life depression include reminiscence, relaxation, art therapy, focused imagery, creative movement, and cognitive-behavioral strategies. In addition to groups specifically targeted for depression, groups such as the Healthy Aging Class (described in Chapter 12), which are directed toward developing coping skills, may be effective in alleviating depression.

Although adult day care programs are not primarily a group therapy for depressed older adults, they are a commonly available resource for providing structured social and therapeutic activities. Similarly, many community-based senior programs provide opportunities for group meals, exercise, and social interaction, and these can be quite effective in alleviating mild to moderate depression in older adults. Information about these and other group programs for older adults can be obtained from local offices on aging, and nurses can encourage older adults or their caregivers to seek out and take advantage of these programs.

Facilitating Referrals for Psychosocial Therapies

Nurses have important roles in facilitating referrals for appropriate psychosocial therapies, especially for older adults who are seriously depressed. Contrary to the common belief that older adults are not receptive to mental health services, most depressed older adults prefer counseling and are more likely to comply with depression treatment plans when counseling is included with medication treatment (Gum et al., 2006). In addition to relying on social workers for making referrals for mental health services, nurses often have opportunities to initiate discussion of psychosocial therapies during the course of their usual work with older adults. This is an important nursing responsibility because compliance and satisfaction with therapies for depression are most effective when older adults are involved in developing the plan (Gum et al., 2006). Hospital-based geropsychiatric programs offer assessment and treatment of late-life depression, and some community mental health centers have programs for depressed older adults. Nurses can either suggest or directly facilitate referrals to these programs.

Wellness Opportunity

Nurses promote wellness when they convince an older person that depression is not a necessary consequence of aging but is a condition that can respond to treatment.

Teaching About and Managing Antidepressant Medications

Types of Antidepressant Medications

Understanding the types of antidepressants available is important for nurses in order to educate older adults about their medications. Biochemical theories of depression have guided the development of various antidepressant medications. For example, the observation that depression was a common adverse effect of drugs that deplete the brain of catecholamine led to the development of tricyclic and other cyclic antidepressants, which block the reuptake of chemical messengers at neuronal synapses in the brain. As scientists have discovered more information about brain function and neurotransmitters, pharmaceutical companies have made major advances in developing safe and effective antidepressants.

Monoamine oxidase inhibitors (MAOIs) were the first medications used as antidepressants. After their use became widespread in the 1960s, it was discovered that medications in this category can cause dangerous and even fatal adverse effects (e.g., hypertensive crisis) when they interact with many other medications and with some types of food. Another disadvantage of using MAOIs is the common occurrence of confusion, restlessness, agitation, and paranoid ideation in older adults who are cognitively impaired (Blazer, 2002a). Because there are so many contraindications to the use of MAOIs in older adults, they are used with extreme caution and only when other therapies have been found to be ineffective. Thus, older adults who are taking an MAOI are usually very closely supervised and evaluated by a psychiatrist or other primary care practitioner. Examples of MAOIs are phenelzine, isocarboxazid, and tranylcypromine.

Cyclic antidepressants, used widely since the late 1950s, are considered particularly effective in alleviating the following depression-related symptoms: loss of libido, sleep and appetite disturbances, and loss of interest and pleasure in activities. Cyclic antidepressants are usually categorized as tricyclic antidepressants (which were the first ones developed), and second-generation agents (which have been widely used since the mid-1980s). Cyclic antidepressants differ more in their potential for adverse effects than in their therapeutic effects. Because cyclic antidepressants affect several neurotransmitters, they are associated with a variety of anticholinergic and other detrimental effects. Two particular areas of concern in geriatric care are the potential for adverse cardiovascular and anticholinergic effects. The most likely cardiovascular effects are orthostatic hypotension and altered cardiac rate and rhythm. Serious anticholinergic effects include blurred vision, urinary retention, and cognitive impairments. Additional common side effects are sedation, constipation, dry mouth, and weight gain. Because of these side effects, people with glaucoma, prostatic hyperplasia, or cardiac conduction abnormalities should not take cyclic antidepressants. In addition, cyclic antidepressants should be avoided in people with dementia or Parkinson's disease because of the potential adverse effect of cognitive impairment. Anticholinergic potency varies among the tricyclic antidepressants, with amitriptyline having the strongest anticholinergic effects and desipramine having the weakest. As a rule of thumb for older adults, cyclic agents with weaker anticholinergic effects should be prescribed over those with stronger anticholinergic effects.

During the late 1980s, pharmaceutical companies developed a class of antidepressant drugs that were more selective in their action than the cyclic antidepressants. Called **selective serotonin reuptake inhibitors (SSRIs)**, these drugs are chemically unrelated to cyclic or other types of antidepressants. The therapeutic effectiveness of SSRIs is similar to that of cyclic antidepressants, but they have minimal cholinergic, histaminic, dopaminergic, and noradrenergic effects. SSRIs currently are considered the first-line medications for depression because they are effective for most people, and their adverse effects are more tolerable and less dangerous (Blazer, 2002a; Snow et al., 2000; Williams et al., 2000). For example, an important consideration for older adults is that SSRIs are less likely than cyclics to cause orthostatic hypotension and anticholinergic effects. This is particularly important for mentally frail elderly who are susceptible to confusion and for physically frail elderly who are at high risk for falls.

Although SSRIs are safer than other types of antidepressants, nurses need to be aware of important adverse effects and drug interactions. For example, because SSRIs are metabolized in the liver and some of them are highly bound to plasma protein, SSRIs may interact with other drugs that are metabolized in the liver or are highly protein bound. In addition, when an SSRI is prescribed, special attention should be paid to potential interactions with nicotine, alcohol, and other medications (including some over-the-counter products). Drug interactions may occur even after an SSRI with a long half-life (e.g., fluoxetine) has been discontinued. Common adverse effects of SSRIs include nausea, vomiting, diarrhea, headache, nervousness, insomnia, tremor, dry mouth, and sexual dysfunction. Also, SSRIs can increase the risk for gastrointestinal bleeding, especially when used concurrently with nonsteroidal anti-inflammatory drugs or low-dose aspirin (Dalton et al., 2003). Withdrawal effects of SSRIs include nausea, tremor, anxiety, dizziness, palpitations, and paresthesias. Fluoxetine, the first available drug in this category, may cause agitation in as many as 20% to 30% of the patients taking it. Also, because of its long half-life, it may take 2 to 4 weeks to reach a steady state in older adults, and side effects may not resolve until 7 to 10 days after the drug is discontinued. Sertraline and paroxetine differ from fluoxetine in that they have shorter half-lives and no anticholinergic effects. Fluvoxamine, like fluoxetine, may have mild anticholinergic effects.

Several other antidepressants, each with a unique type of action on neurotransmitters, are available and are commonly used for older adults (Table 15-3). Special considerations in the use of some of these antidepressants are as follows: venlafaxine may cause an increase in blood pressure; mirtazapine can be helpful for stimulating appetite; trazodone and nefazodone are very sedating and may be useful in the treatment of depression with sleep disturbances; and bupropion has a stimulating effect, which sometimes can be therapeutic, but is contraindicated in people with a seizure disorder. Psychomotor stimulants (e.g., methylphenidate) have been used for decades for certain types of depression, but they are not commonly used for older adults.

TABLE 15-3 Antidepressants Commonly Used for Older Adults

Category	Examples	Trade Names
Selective serotonin reuptake inhibitors (SSRIs)	Citalopram Fluoxetine Fluvoxamine Paroxetine Sertraline	Celexa Prozac Luvox Paxil Zoloft
Serotonin and norepinephrine reuptake inhibitors	Mirtazapine Venlafaxine	Remeron Effexor
Serotonin modulators	Nefazodone Trazodone	Serzone Desyrel
Dopamine reuptake inhibitors	Bupropion	Wellbutrin
Cyclic antidepressants	Amoxapine Desipramine Imipramine	Asendin Norpramin Tofranil

Nursing Responsibilities Regarding Antidepressants

An important nursing responsibility regarding antidepressants is to educate older adults about the primary purpose of these medications, which is to alleviate depressive symptoms so that the person is able to respond to additional interventions, such as psychosocial therapy. For older adults who have both depression and dementia, antidepressant medications may improve the affective symptoms so that overall abilities are improved and the person is able to function more effectively and independently.

Nursing responsibilities regarding antidepressant medication therapy include observing for both adverse and therapeutic effects and educating the older adult about the unique aspects of these medication therapies. Another important responsibility is educating older adults about the need for ongoing evaluation and treatment of depression, including the monitoring of antidepressant medication use. Older adults who have been diagnosed with major depressive disorder are at high risk of recurrence, and this risk is increased if antidepressant medications are not maintained for at least 6 months (Geddes et al., 2003; Glick et al., 2001; Meyers et al., 2001). Older adults often want to discontinue medications when their depressive symptoms resolve, and nurses need to teach them about the importance of ongoing antidepressant therapy and periodic reevaluations after med-

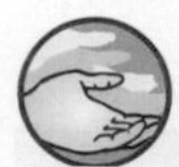

Box 15-5
Health Education About Antidepressant Medications

Information To Be Shared With the Older Adult

- Immediate improvement will not be evident, but a fair trial must be given to the medication as long as serious adverse effects are not noticed.
- The fair trial may take as long as 12 weeks, but some positive effects should be noticed within 2 to 4 weeks.
- If one type of antidepressant is not effective, another type may be effective.
- Antidepressants cannot be used on an "as needed" basis.
- Antidepressants should be viewed as part of a comprehensive approach to treating depression, and psychosocial therapies should be considered along with antidepressants.
- Antidepressants can interact with alcohol, nicotine, and other medications, including over-the-counter medications, possibly altering the effects of the medication or increasing the potential for adverse effects.
- The prescribing health care practitioner should be asked about potential adverse effects and drug–drug or food–drug interactions.
- The prescribing health care practitioner should be consulted before discontinuing an antidepressant.
- If postural hypotension occurs, the effects can be minimized through such interventions as changing position slowly and maintaining adequate fluid intake.
- If monoamine oxidase inhibitors (MAOIs) are prescribed, certain medications must be avoided, and a low-tyramine diet must be followed (i.e., avoidance of beer, yogurt, red wine, fermented cheese, and pickled foods, as well as excessive amounts of caffeine and chocolate).

Principles Regarding Dosage and Length of Treatment

- Older adults should be started at one-half to one-third the normal adult dose.
- Dosages can be increased gradually until maximal therapeutic levels are reached, while observing for adverse effects.
- Age-related changes may increase the time needed for medication to reach maximal effectiveness.
- A once-daily regimen usually is effective.
- Bedtime administration of an antidepressant may facilitate sleep as a result of the drug's hypnotic effects, but some antidepressants (e.g., fluoxetine) may be better taken in the morning because of side effects, such as agitation.
- The length of treatment is usually 6 months for a first-time depression, 1 to 2 years for people with a history of a prior depressive episode, and lifetime maintenance for people with a history of three or more depressive episodes.

ications are discontinued. This is especially important because a patient's beliefs about the use of medications affect adherence; therefore, beliefs need to be explored before and during medication therapy (Brown et al., 2005). Box 15-5 summarizes guidelines for the nursing responsibilities regarding antidepressant medications.

Teaching About Electroconvulsive Therapy

Electroconvulsive therapy (ECT) is increasingly being used as a low-risk treatment that has an efficacy rate of at least 80% for older depressed people, including patients as old as 102 years (Kelly & Zisselman, 2000; Manly et al., 2000). Studies have found that ECT is at least as effective, and perhaps more effective, as medications for older depressed patients, and it can be life-saving for seriously depressed older adults (Greenberg & Kellner, 2005; Kujala et al., 2002). Although ECT is usually recommended only after the person fails to respond adequately to a course of antidepressant medications, the American Psychiatric Association recommends it as a first-line treatment when a rapid and definitive response is needed for a severely depressed person or when patients have Parkinson's disease or cerebral vascular disease as comorbid conditions (Greenberg & Kellner, 2005; Shanmugham et al., 2005). ECT is contraindicated in certain medical conditions such as serious arrhythmias, acute myocardial infarction, uncompensated congestive heart failure, and increased intracranial pressure (Greenberg & Kellner, 2005). Older adults who respond to a course of ECT are likely to need maintenance ECT and medications to prevent a relapse (Shanmugham et al., 2005).

Prevalent negative attitudes about ECT are attributable, in part, to the alleged inhumane use of this procedure when it was first developed a half-century ago. In recent years, however, the technique for administering ECT has been refined, and the risks, discomfort, and side effects are now quite minimal. Most adverse effects—such as headache, nausea, bradycardia, memory impairment, and muscle pain—are transient. Occasionally, however, the adverse cognitive effects may be more extensive or even permanent, especially after several courses of ECT. Adverse cognitive effects can be described as follows (Greenberg & Kellner, 2005):

- Acute confusional state (disorientation), lasting for less than an hour and occurring after each treatment
- Anterograde amnesia (impaired ability to retain new memories), lasting for several weeks and occurring after a course of treatment
- Retrograde amnesia (forgetting events immediately before the treatment), lasting for several months and occurring after a course of treatment

Except in psychiatric settings, nurses will not be involved with the care of people who are undergoing ECT. Nurses caring for depressed people in any setting, however, need to maintain an open mind about this therapy. In addition, nurses may be in the position of encouraging older adults or their caregivers to seek advice about ECT from knowledgeable professionals.

Teaching About Alternative Health Care Practices

There has been increasing interest in the use of herbs and other natural remedies for depression. St. John's wort (*Hypericum perforatum*) is widely used in Europe and is the most commonly used antidepressant in Germany (Clement et al., 2006). Since 1998, the National Institutes of Health Office of Alternative Medicine has sponsored randomized, controlled, double-blinded studies in the United States to compare placebo, St. John's wort, and prescription antidepressants. A systematic review of recent studies concluded that St. John's wort, in doses as low as 300 mg daily, is a viable complementary treatment to traditional medical treatment for mild to moderate depression (Clement et al., 2006). St. John's wort is widely available and relatively inexpensive, but products are not standardized or regulated for quality. Although St. John's wort is not likely to cause any serious adverse reactions, precautions that apply to herbal products (discussed in Chapter 8) should be heeded. Common side effects include fatigue, headache, restlessness, anorgasmia, polyuria, hypothyroidism, pruritus, photosensitivity, dry mouth, and gastrointestinal effects. St. John's wort can interact with many medications, including digoxin, warfarin, amiodarone, theophylline, and antidepressants.

Bright-light therapy has been used to improve sleep in people with disturbed circadian rhythm, and it is an established therapy for treatment of seasonal affective disorder (Remick, 2002). Sumaya and colleagues (2001) explored the use of bright-light therapy as an intervention for depression in older nursing home residents and found that a half hour of exposure to 10,000 lux of bright light for 5 days produced clinically significant improvements in moderately to severely depressed subjects. Nurses can use Box 15-6 as a guide to teaching older adults about interventions that may be helpful for preventing or alleviating depression.

Preventing Suicide

Nurses do not routinely encounter suicidal older adults, but they need to be prepared to implement immediate interventions whenever they identify a patient at risk. The most important intervention is to seek out psychiatric resources and activate protective service agencies, rather than attempting to deal with potentially suicidal people without the help of specialized resources. All communities have some emergency psychiatric services, and nurses can either make referrals directly or discuss these resources with older adults and their caregivers. Some guidelines for working with people who are potentially suicidal are listed in Box 15-7.

EVALUATING THE EFFECTIVENESS OF NURSING INTERVENTIONS

Nursing care of depressed older adults is evaluated by documenting improved coping skills and diminished manifestations of depression. For example, the person may report diminished feelings of hopelessness and improved appetite and sleep. Another measure that would reflect improved quality of life would be that the older adult expresses interest in and participates in meaningful activities. Effectiveness of nursing interventions also could be evaluated by whether the older adult has begun taking antidepressant medications and participating in individual or group therapies.

Nursing care of older adults who are at high risk for self-harm would be evaluated by the prevention of harm. Another measure would be the degree to which the older adult develops coping skills to deal with the issues that underlie his or her suicidal thoughts. Nurses also can find out whether the older adult obtained suggested mental health services and ask about the effectiveness of any referrals that were made.

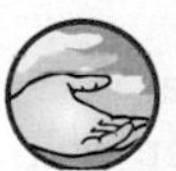

Box 15-6
Interventions Commonly Used for Preventing or Alleviating Depression

Health Promotion Interventions

- Participate in enjoyable exercise for a minimum of $^1/_2$ hour five times weekly.
- Do not smoke or use nicotine.
- Seek individual or group counseling to address stressful situations.
- If symptoms of depression affect daily functioning or quality of life, seek evaluation and treatment from a primary care practitioner.

Nutritional Considerations

- Ensure adequate intake of (or use supplements of) the following nutrients: vitamins B and C, magnesium, potassium, and selenium.
- Include foods that are high in tryptophan (e.g., eggs, milk, fish, nuts, turkey, bananas, soybeans, pumpkin seeds).
- Include food sources of phenylalanine (e.g., meat, fish, poultry, soybeans, chocolate, watercress, sunflower seeds, black beans).
- Avoid intake of large amounts of caffeine and artificial sweeteners (e.g., aspartame).

Complementary and Alternative Therapies

- St. John's wort, 300 mg three times daily, may be effective in reducing the symptoms of mild to moderate depression; however, do not take this with an antidepressant and be sure to talk with your primary care practitioner about using it.
- Bright-light therapy, $^1/_2$ hour daily
- Aromatherapy (inhaled or applied to the skin): rose, basil, jasmine, bergamot, lavender, chamomile, clary, sage
- Art, dance, music, drama, yoga, t'ai chi, quigong, massage, imagery, meditation, relaxation, stress management, spiritual healing

Box 15-7
Nursing Interventions for People Who Are Potentially Suicidal

Communicating With Someone Who Is Potentially Suicidal

- Be direct and honest; do not be afraid to ask direct questions, such as "Are you thinking of hurting yourself?"
- Express feelings of concern and confidence.
- Acknowledge the person's feelings of helplessness and hopelessness.
- Encourage the person to talk about the precipitating event, if there is one.
- Emphasize that suicide is only one of several options; then explore other options.
- Emphasize positive relationships; talk about the negative impact of suicide on survivors.
- Maintain a nonjudgmental attitude.
- Make a contract: ask the person to agree to do certain things for limited amounts of time and to call for help if he or she cannot keep the agreement.
- Discuss the problems openly with the family and caregivers.

Crisis Intervention

- Focus on the immediate precipitating event.
- Reduce the immediate danger by removing the implements, interfering with the plan, and providing constant supervision.
- Obtain psychiatric help; call a suicide hot line or activate emergency psychiatric services if necessary.

Mrs. D. is 81 years old and recently has been diagnosed with vascular dementia. She lives with her husband, who has diabetes, macular degeneration, and severe arthritis. Mrs. D. had managed all household and financial responsibilities until about 1 year ago, when she began having trouble with her memory. Mrs. D. was evaluated at the geriatric assessment program where you work, and she was advised to stop driving and to arrange for some help with complex tasks, such as bill paying and grocery shopping. Two months after the initial evaluation, Mrs. D. returns for follow-up and informs you that she limits her driving to short, daytime trips in familiar areas. When asked about getting help with complex tasks, she states, "I just don't have any energy to make all those calls you suggested. Besides, I don't want anyone else looking at my finances or going to the store for me."

NURSING ASSESSMENT

A mental status assessment indicates that Mrs. D.'s level of cognitive impairment is unchanged since her initial evaluation. She has prominent deficits in calculation, short-term memory, abstract thinking, problem solving, and language skills. Your psychosocial assessment reveals that Mrs. D. has a very sad affect and low self-esteem, and she expresses feelings of hopelessness and helplessness. She admits to being overwhelmed with feelings of responsibility for herself and her husband, and she says she feels "paralyzed because there's no light at the end of the tunnel."

When you ask about her daily life, Mrs. D. says she spends most of her time at home because she hasn't had the energy to go out. She admits that she doesn't sleep well and that she has difficulty falling asleep at night. She naps for a couple of hours in the morning and in the afternoon because "I feel tired all the time and I can't go out and do things anyway." Her appetite is poor, and in the past 2 months, her weight has declined from 140 pounds to 126 pounds (her height is 5′6″). She complains of constipation and "heartburn."

When you ask about meaningful activities, she tells you she no longer goes to her weekly bowling club because it meets in the evening and she doesn't want to drive at night. She also has given up her church activities (Thursday discussion club and Sunday service) because she does not want to inconvenience anyone by having them drive her. She feels it's "demeaning to have to tell my friends that I need a ride." She used to enjoy reading, but she hasn't felt like going to the library, and she's not interested in any of the books she has at home.

(case study continues on page 311)

NURSING DIAGNOSIS

You use the nursing diagnosis of Ineffective Individual Coping, related to depression and declining cognitive abilities. Evidence comes from Mrs. D.'s sad affect, low self-esteem, loss of interest in activities, feelings of hopelessness and helplessness, and inability to address her problems effectively. Physical manifestations are her poor appetite, weight loss, sleep disturbances, and complaints about constipation and heartburn.

NURSING CARE PLAN FOR MRS. D.

Expected Outcome	Nursing Interventions	Nursing Evaluation
Mrs. D. will be able to identify her coping patterns.	• Ask Mrs. D. to describe her prior experiences in dealing with her husband's illness. • Help Mrs. D. to identify coping strategies that have been helpful in the past.	• Mrs. D. will recognize and acknowledge the coping strategies that have been helpful in the past.
Mrs. D. will learn about depression and be encouraged to obtain further evaluation of her depression.	• Talk with Mrs. D. about her signs and symptoms of depression, emphasizing the fact that depression is a treatable condition. • Discuss the relationship between depression and the inability to cope effectively with stressful situations. • Ask Mrs. D. if she is willing to see a geropsychiatrist or talk to her primary care practitioner for further evaluation and treatment. • Explain that antidepressant medications can be very effective when used in conjunction with counseling.	• Mrs. D. will follow through with an appointment with a geropsychiatrist or talk with her primary care practitioner.
Effective coping strategies for addressing Mrs. D.'s declining abilities will be identified.	• Discuss with Mrs. D. several options for ongoing support and counseling to assist her in coping with her declining abilities (e.g., the "Something for You" support group for people with memory loss; or individual counseling sessions with the social worker who is affiliated with the geriatric assessment program). • Emphasize the importance of developing short-term goals that can be addressed through problem solving (e.g., suggest that Mrs. D. begin to address her lack of meaningful activities by going to the library for reading material).	• Mrs. D. will attend one support group on a trial basis and talk with you about the experience at her next appointment in 1 month. • Mrs. D. will make an appointment for counseling with the social worker. • Mrs. D. will participate in one meaningful activity each week for the next month.

THINKING POINTS

- What risk factors are likely contributing to Mrs. D.'s depression?
- What further assessment information would you obtain?
- If you applied the Geriatric Depression Scale (Fig. 15-3) to Mrs. D., what score do you think she would have?
- What additional interventions would you suggest for Mrs. D.?

CHAPTER HIGHLIGHTS

Theories About Late-Life Depression (Fig. 15-1)

- Psychosocial (impact of losses, effect of social supports)
- Cognitive triad (negative appraisals cause distorted perceptions and lead to faulty conclusions)
- Biologic (changes in the brain, nervous system, and neuroendocrine system interact with age-related changes)
- Depression and dementia (high correlation between depression and dementia related to neuropathologic changes)

Types of Depression

- Major depression
- Subclinical depression
- Vascular depression

Risk Factors for Depression in Older Adults (Boxes 15-1 and 15-2)

- Demographic and psychosocial (women, history of depression, losses, loneliness, stress)
- Medical conditions and functional impairment (synergistic relationship)
- Effects of alcohol and medications

Functional Consequences Associated With Depression in Older Adults

- Physical health and functioning
- Psychosocial function and quality of life
- Suicide (Fig. 15-2)

Nursing Assessment of Depression in Older Adults

- Cultural variations in expressions of depression (Cultural Considerations 15-1)
- Unique manifestations in older versus younger adults (Table 15-1)
- Differentiating between dementia and depression (Table 15-2)
- Screening tools (Fig. 15-3)
- Suicide risk (Box 15-4)

Nursing Diagnosis

- Readiness for Enhanced Coping
- Ineffective Coping
- Hopelessness
- Caregiver Role Strain
- Risk for Imbalanced Nutrition
- Adult Failure to Thrive
- Risk for Suicide

Planning for Wellness Outcomes

- Coping
- Hope
- Caregiver Emotional Health
- Nutritional Status
- Physical Well-Being
- Suicide Self-Restraint

Nursing Interventions to Address Depression (Table 15-3, Boxes 15-5 through 15-7)

- Alleviating risk factors (addressing functional limitations, teaching about adverse effects of medications and excessive alcohol)
- Improving psychosocial function (social supports, meaningful activities)
- Promoting health through exercise and nutrition
- Education and counseling (individual and group psychosocial interventions)
- Facilitating referrals for psychosocial therapies
- Teaching about antidepressant medications
- Teaching about ECT
- Teaching about alternative care practices (e.g., St. John's wort, bright-light therapy)
- Preventing suicide

Evaluating the Effectiveness of Nursing Interventions

- Improved coping skills
- Fewer manifestations of depression
- Expressed feelings of improved quality of life
- Reduced risk of self-harm
- Effective use of appropriate mental health services

Critical Thinking Exercises

1. Think of an older adult in your personal life or professional practice who is or has been depressed. What are (were) the risk factors in that person's situation that might play (have played) a part in the depression?
2. Describe at least four cultural variations in the way depression might be expressed.
3. What assessment observations would you make and what questions would you ask to differentiate between dementia and depression in older adults?
4. Make up a case example of someone who is potentially suicidal and who would require all four levels of suicide assessment. Describe how you would phrase the questions for each of the levels.
5. Describe a teaching plan for an 84-year-old woman for whom Paxil, 10 mg daily, has been prescribed.

Clinical Tool Resources

Hartford Institute for Geriatric Nursing
Try This: Best Practices in Nursing Care to Older Adults
Issue Number 4 (Revised 2007), The Geriatric Depression Scale (GDS)
www.hartfordign.org/resources/education/tryThis.html

Educational Resources

Depression and Bipolar Support Alliance (DBSA)
www.ndmda.org

National Center for Complementary and Alternative Medicine
NCCAM Clearinghouse
http://nccam.nih.gov/

National Institute of Mental Health
DEPRESSION Awareness, Recognition, and Treatment Program (D/ART)
www.nimh.nih.gov

Mental Health America
www.mentalhealthamerica.net

National Senior Service Corps
www.seniorcorps.org

U.S. Department of Health and Human Services
Agency for Healthcare Research and Quality
www.ahrq.gov

References

Agency for Healthcare Research and Quality. (2002, May 20). *U. S. Preventive Services Task Force now finds sufficient evidence to recommend screening adults for depression.* Available at www.ahrq.gov/news/press/pr2002/deprespr.htm.

American Psychiatric Association. (2000). *Diagnostic and statistical manual of mental disorders* (4th ed., text revision). Washington, DC: Author.

Bartels, S. J., Coakley, E., Oxman, T. E., Constantion, G., Oslin, D., Chen, H., et al. (2002). Suicidal and death ideation in older primary care patients with depression, anxiety, and at-risk alcohol use. *American Journal of Geriatric Psychiatry, 10*, 417–427.

Beck, A. T., Rush, A. J., Shaw, B., & Emery, G. (1979). *Cognitive therapy of depression*. New York: Guilford Press.

Blazer, D. G. (1993). *Depression in late life* (2nd ed.). St. Louis: C. V. Mosby.

Blazer, D. G. (2002a). *Depression in late life* (3rd ed.). New York: Springer.

Blazer, D. G. (2002b). The prevalence of depression symptoms. *Journals of Gerontology: Series A, Biological Sciences and Medical Sciences, 57*, M150–M151.

Blow, F. C., & Barry, K. L. (2000). Older patients with at-risk and problem drinking patterns: New developments in brief interventions. *Journal of Geriatric Psychiatry and Neurology, 13*, 115–123.

Brown, C., Battista, D. R., Bruehlman, R., Sereika, S. S., & Thase, M. E. (2005). Beliefs about antidepressant medications in primary care patients: Relationship to self-reported adherence. *Medical Care, 43*, 1203–1207.

Callahan, C. M., Kroenke, K., Counsell, S. R., Hendrie, H. C., & Perkins, A. J. (2005). Treatment of depression improves physical functioning in older adults. *Journal of the American Geriatrics Society, 53*, 367–373.

Carpenito-Moyet, L. J. (2006). *Handbook of nursing diagnosis* (11th ed.). Philadelphia: Lippincott Williams & Wilkins.

Chou, K. L., Jun, L. W., & Chi, I. (2005). Assessing Chinese older adults' suicidal ideation: Chinese version of the geriatric suicide ideation scale. *Aging & Mental Health, 9*, 167–171.

Clement, K., Covertson, C. R., Johnson, M. J., & Dearing, K. (2006). St. John's wort and the treatment of mild to moderate depression: A systematic review. *Holistic Nursing Practice, 20*, 197–203.

Cole, M. G. (2005). Evidence-based review of risk factors for geriatric depression and brief preventative interventions. *Psychiatric Clinics of North America, 28*, 785–803.

Dalton, S. O., Johansen, C., Lellemjaer, L., Norgard, B., Sorensen, H. T., & Olsen, J. H. (2003). Use of selective serotonin reuptake inhibitors and risk of upper gastrointestinal tract bleeding. *Archives of Internal Medicine, 163*, 59–64.

Doraiswamy, P. M., Khan, Z. M., Donahue, R. M. J., & Richard, N. E. (2002). The spectrum of quality-of-life impairments in recurrent geriatric depression. *Journals of Gerontology: Series A, Biological Sciences and Medical Sciences, 57*, M134–M137.

Fabacher, D. A., Raccio-Robak, N., McErlean, M. A., Milano, P. M., & Verdile, V. P. (2002). Validation of a brief screening tool to detect depression in elderly ED patients. *American Journal of Emergency Medicine, 20*, 99–102.

Geddes, J. R., Carney, S. M., Davies, C., Furakawa, T. A., Kupfer, D. J., Frank, E., et al. (2003). Relapse prevention with antidepressant drug treatment in depressive disorders: A systematic review. *Lancet, 361*, 653–661.

Glick, I. D., Suppes, T., DeBarrista, C., Hu, R. J., & Marder, S. (2001). Psychopharmacologic treatment strategies for depression, bipolar disorder, and schizophrenia. *Annals of Internal Medicine, 134*, 47–60.

Goldstein, M. Z. (2002). Depression and anxiety in older women. *Primary Care: Clinics in Office Practice, 29*(1), 69–80.

Greenberg, R. M., & Kellner, C. H. (2005). Electroconvulsive therapy: A selected review. *American Journal of Geriatric Psychiatry, 13*, 268–280.

Gum, A. M., Arean, P. A., Hunkeler, E., Tang, L., Katon, W., Hitchcock, P., et al. (2006). Depression treatment preferences in older primary care patients. *The Gerontologist, 46*, 14–22.

Holkup, P. A., Tang, J. H.-C., & Titler, M. G. (2003). Evidence-based protocol: Elderly suicide—secondary prevention. *Journal of Gerontological Nursing, 29*(6), 6–17.

Holley, C., Murrell, S. A., & Masst, B. T. (2006). Psychosocial and vascular risk factors for depression in the elderly. *American Journal of Geriatric Psychiatry, 14*, 84–90.

Hybels, C. F., Blazer, D. G., & Pieper, C. F. (2001). Toward a threshold for subthreshold depression: An analysis of correlates of depression by severity of symptoms using data from an elderly community. *The Gerontologist, 4*, 357–365.

Jang, Y., Borenstein, A. R., Chiriboga, D. A., & Mortimer, J. A. (2005). Depressive symptoms among African American and white older adults. *Journals of Gerontology: Series B, Psychological Sciences and Social Sciences, 60*, 313–319.

Johnson, M., Bulechek, G., Butcher, H., Dochterman, J. M., Maas, M., Moorehead, S., et al. (2005). *NANDA, NOC, and NIC linkages: Nursing diagnoses, outcomes, & interventions* (2nd ed.). St. Louis: Mosby Elsevier.

Kelly, K. G., & Zisselman, M. (2000). Update on electroconvulsive therapy (ECT) in older adults. *Journal of the American Geriatrics Society, 48*, 560–566.

Kiosses, D. N., Klimstra, S., Murphy, C., & Alexopoulos, G. S. (2001). Executive dysfunction and disability in elderly patients with major depression. *American Journal of Geriatric Psychiatry, 9*, 269–274.

Kockler, M., & Heun, R. (2002). Gender differences of depressive symptoms in depressed and nondepressed elderly persons. *International Journal of Geriatric Psychiatry, 17*, 65–72.

Kujala, I., Rosenvinge, B., & Bekkelund, S. I. (2002). Clinical outcome and adverse effects of electroconvulsive therapy in elderly psychiatric patients. *Journal of Geriatric Psychiatry and Neurology, 15*, 73–76.

Kurlowicz, L. H. (2003). Depression in older adults. In M. Mezey, T. Fulmer, I. Abraham, & D. A. Zwicker (Eds.), *Geriatric nursing protocols for best practice* (pp. 185–206). New York: Springer.

Landreville, P., Landry, J., Baillargeon, L., Guerette, A., & Matteau, E. (2001). Older adults' acceptance of psychological and pharmacological treatments for depression. *Journals of Gerontology: Series B, Psychological Sciences and Social Sciences, 56*, P285–P291.

Lavretsky, H., & Kumar, A. (2002). Clinically significant non-major depression. *American Journal of Geriatric Psychiatry, 10*, 239–255.

Lenze, E. J., Rogers, J. C., Martire, L. M., Mulsant, B. H., Rollman, B. L., Dew, M. A., et al. (2001). The association of late life depression and anxiety with physical disability. *American Journal of Geriatric Psychiatry, 9*, 113–135.

Manly, D. T., Oakley, S. P., & Bloch, R. M. (2000). Electroconvulsive therapy in old-old patients. *American Journal of Geriatric Psychiatry, 8*, 232–236.

Mann, J. J. (2002). A current perspective of suicide and attempted suicide. *Annals of Internal Medicine, 136*, 302–311.

McCurren, C. (2002). Assessment for depression among nursing home elders: Evaluation of the MDS mood assessment. *Geriatric Nursing, 23*(2), 103–107.

Mehta, K. M., Yaffe, K., & Covinsky, K. E. (2002). Cognitive impairment, depressive symptoms, and functional decline in older people. *Journal of the American Geriatrics Society, 50*, 1045–1050.

Meyers, B. S. (2002). Treatment and course of geriatric depression: Questions raised by an evolving clinical science. *American Journal of Geriatric Psychiatry, 10*, 497–502.

Meyers, B. S., Klimstra, S. A., Gabriele, M., Hamilton, M., Kakuman, T., Tirumalasetti, F., et al. (2001). Continuation treatment of delusional depression in older adults. *American Journal of Geriatric Psychiatry, 9*, 415–422.

Miller, M. D., Lenze, E. J., Dew, M. A., Whyte, E., Weber, E., Begley, A. E., et al. (2002). Effect of cerebrovascular risk factors on depression treatment outcome in later life. *American Journal of Geriatric Psychiatry, 10*, 592–598.

Minicuci, N., Maggi, S., Pavan, M., Enzi, G., & Crepaldi, G. (2002). Prevalence rate and correlates of depressive symptoms in older individuals: The Vento Study. *Journals of Gerontology: Series A, Biological Sciences and Medical Sciences, 57*, M155–M161.

Moos, R. H., Schutte, K. K., Brennan, P. L., & Moos, B. S. (2005). The interplay between life stressors and depressive symptoms among older adults. *Journals of Gerontology: Series B, Psychological Sciences and Social Sciences, 60*, P199–P206.

Moretti, R., Torre, P., Antonello, R. M., Cazzato, G., & Bava, A. (2002). Depression and Alzheimer's disease: Symptom or comorbidity? *American Journal of Alzheimer's Disease and Other Dementias, 17*, 338–344.

National Institute of Mental Health. (2001). *Depression research at the National Institute of Mental Health*. Available at www.nimh.gov.publicat/depresfact.cfm.

Norton, M. C., Skoog, I., Toone, L., Corcoran, C., & Tschanz, J. T. (2006). Three-year incidence of first-onset depressive syndrome in a population sample of older adults: The Cache County Study. *American Journal of Geriatric Psychiatry, 14*, 237–245.

Nygaard, I., Turvey, C., Burns, T. L., Crischilles, E., & Wallace, R. (2003). Urinary incontinence and depression in middle-aged United States women. *Obstetrics and Gynecology, 101*, 149–156.

Olin, J. T., Katz, I. R., Meyers, B. S., Schneider, L. S., & Lebowitz, B. D. (2002a). Provisional diagnostic criteria for depression of Alzheimer disease. *American Journal of Geriatric Psychiatry, 10*, 129–141.

Olin, J. T., Schneider, L. S., Katz, I. R., Meyers, B. S., Alexopoulos, G. S., Breitner, J. C., et al. (2002b). Provisional diagnostic criteria for depression of Alzheimer disease. *American Journal of Geriatric Psychiatry, 10*, 125–128.

Oxman, T. E., & Sengupta, A. (2002). Treatment of minor depression. *American Journal of Geriatric Psychiatry, 10*, 256–264.

Penninx, B. W. J. H., Rejeski, W. J., Pandya, J., Miller, M. E., Di Bari, M., Applegate, W. B., et al. (2002). Exercise and depressive symptoms: A comparison of aerobic and resistance exercise effects on emotional and physical function in older persons with high and low depressive symptomatology. *Journals of Gerontology: Series B, Psychological Sciences and Social Sciences, 57*, P124–P132.

Piven, M. L. (2001). Detection of depression in the cognitively intact older adult protocol. *Journal of Gerontological Nursing, 27*(6), 8–14.

Piven, M. L., & Buckwalter, K. C. (2001). Depression. In M. L. Maas, K. C. Buckwalter, M. D. Hardy, T. Tripp-Reimer, M. G. Titler, & J. P. Specht (Eds.), *Nursing care of older adults: Diagnoses, outcomes, & interventions* (pp. 521–542). St. Louis: Mosby.

Piven, M. L. S. (May 2005). Detection of depression in the cognitively intact older adult. Iowa City, IA: University of Iowa Gerontological Nursing Interventions Research Center, Research Dissemination Core.

Remick, R. A. (2002). Diagnosis and management of depression in primary care: A clinical update and review. *Canadian Medical Association Journal, 167*, 1253–1260.

Robison, J., Gruman, C., Gaztambide, S., & Blank, K. (2002). Screening for depression in middle aged and older Puerto Rican primary care patients. *Journals of Gerontology: Series A, Biological Sciences and Medical Sciences, 57*, M308–M314.

Roff, S. (2001). Suicide and the elderly. *Journal of Gerontological Social Work, 35*(2), 21–36.

Rozzini, R., Giovanni, B., Sabatini, T., & Trabucchi, M. (2002). The association of depression and mortality in elderly persons [comment]. *Journals of Gerontology: Series A, Biological Sciences and Medical Sciences, 57*, M144–M155.

Seligman, M. E. P. (1981). A learned helplessness point of view. In L. P. Rehm (Ed.), *Behavior therapy for depression* (pp. 123–141). New York: Academic Press.

Shanmugham, B., Karp, J., Drayer, R., Reynolds, C. F., & Alexopoulos, G. (2005). Evidenced-based interventions for geriatric depression. *Psychiatric Clinics of North America, 28*, 821–835.

Simpson, S., Baldwin, R. C., Jackson, A., Burns, A., & Thomas, P. (2000). Is the clinical expression of late-life depression influenced by brain changes? MRI subcortical neuroanatomical correlates of depressive symptoms. *International Psychogeriatrics, 12*, 425–434.

Singh, N. A., Clements, K. M., & Singh, M. A. F. (2001). The efficacy of exercise as a long term antidepressant in elderly subjects: A randomized, controlled trial. *Journals of Gerontology: Series A, Biological Sciences and Medical Sciences, 56*, M497–M504.

Snow, V., Lascher, S., & Mottur-Pilson, C. (2000). Pharmacologic treatment of acute major depression and dysthymia. *Annals of Internal Medicine, 132*, 738–742.

Strawbridge, W. J., Deleger, S., Roberts, R. E., & Kaplan, G. A. (2002). Physical activity reduces the risk of subsequent depression for older adults. *American Journal of Epidemiology, 156*, 328–334.

Sumaya, I. C., Rienzi, B. M., Deegan, J. F., & Moss, D. E. (2001). Bright light treatment decreases depression in institutionalized older adults: A placebo controlled crossover study. *Journals of Gerontology: Series A, Biological Sciences and Medical Sciences, 56*, M356–M360.

Sutcliffe, C., Cordingley, L., Burns, A., Mozley, C. G., Bagley, H., Challis, D., et al. (2000). A new version of the Geriatric Depression Scale for nursing and residential home populations: The Geriatric Depression Scale. *International Psychogeriatrics, 12*, 173–181.

Tateno, A., Kimura, M., & Robinson, R. G. (2002). Phenomenological characteristics of poststroke depression. *American Journal of Geriatric Psychiatry, 10*, 575–581.

Thobaben, M. (2002). Screening for depression: Ask clients two simple questions. *Home Health Care Management & Practice, 15*(1), 82–83.

Turvey, C. L., Conwell, Y., Jones, M. P., Phillips, C., Simonsick, E., & Pearson, J. L. (2002). Risk factors for late life suicide. *American Journal of Geriatric Psychiatry, 10*, 398–406.

Uncapher, H., & Arean, P. A. (2000). Physicians are less willing to treat suicidal ideation in older patients. *Journal of the American Geriatrics Society, 48*, 188–192.

Unutzer, K., Patrick, D. L., Marmon, T., Simon, G. E., & Katon, W. J. (2002). Depressive symptoms and mortality in a prospective study of 2,558 older adults. *American Journal of Geriatric Psychiatry, 10*, 521–530.

Waern, M., Rubenowitz, E., Runeson, B., Skoog, I., Wilhelmson, K., & Allebeck, P. (2002). Burden of illness and suicide in elderly people: A case-control study. *British Medical Journal, 324*, 1355.

Williams, J. W., Mulrow, C. D., Chiquette, E., Noel, P. H., Aguilar, C., Cornell, J., et al. (2000). A systematic review of newer pharmacotherapies for depression in adults. *Annals of Internal Medicine, 132*, 743–756.

Xavier, F. M. F., Farraza, M. P. T., Argimon, I., Trentini, C. M., Poyares, D., Bertollucci, P. H., et al. (2002). The DSM-IV "minor depression" disorder in the oldest-old: Prevalence rate, sleep patterns, memory function and quality of life in elderly people of Italian descent in Southern Brazil. *International Journal of Geriatric Psychiatry, 17*, 107–116.

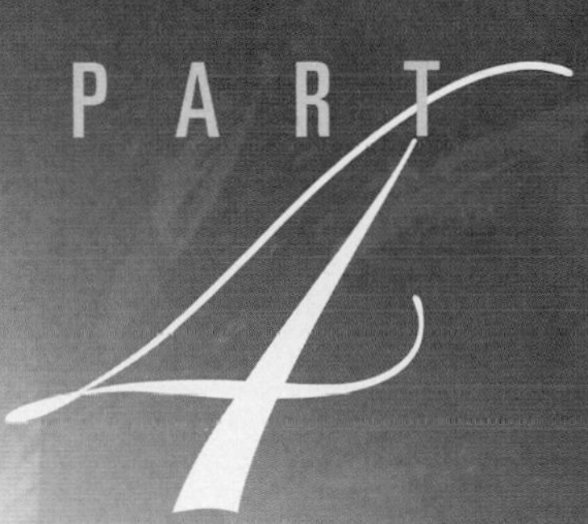

Promoting Wellness in Physical Function

CHAPTER 16

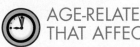

Hearing

Learning Objectives

After reading this chapter, you will be able to:

1. Describe age-related changes that affect hearing.
2. Identify risk factors that affect hearing wellness.
3. Discuss the functional consequences that affect hearing wellness.
4. Conduct a nursing assessment of hearing, with emphasis on identifying opportunities for health promotion.
5. Identify interventions to enhance the auditory abilities of older adults and address risk factors that interfere with hearing.

Key Terms

assistive listening device
cerumen
hearing aid
noise-induced hearing loss (NIHL)
otosclerosis
phonemes
presbycusis
tinnitus

Performance of many important daily activities—including communicating, protecting oneself from danger, and enjoying music, voices, and sounds—is highly dependent on good hearing. In older adults, age-related changes combine with risk factors to affect hearing wellness. Nurses enhance quality of life for older adults when they use health promotion interventions to improve hearing and communication. This chapter addresses the functional consequences associated with hearing in older adults and provides guides for nursing assessment and interventions.

AGE-RELATED CHANGES THAT AFFECT HEARING

Auditory function depends on a sequence of processes, beginning in the three compartments of the ear and ending with the processing of information in the auditory cortex of the brain. Sounds are coded according to intensity and frequency. Intensity, or amplitude, reflects the loudness or softness of the sound and is measured in decibels (dB). Frequency, which is measured in cycles per second (cps) or hertz (Hz), determines whether the pitch is high or low. Risk factors affect both sound intensity and frequency, and

Promoting Hearing Wellness in Older Adults

Nursing Assessment
- Risk factors
- Hearing Handicap Inventory
- Hearing impairment
- Effects of hearing loss

Age-Related Changes
- ↑ keratin
- Stiffer membrane, muscles
- Calcified ossicles
- ↓ neurons, blood, endolymph

Negative Functional Consequences
- ↓ ability to hear high-pitched sounds
- ↑ risk for impacted wax
- ↓ communication
- ↓ quality of life

Risk Factors
- Impacted wax
- Exposure to noise
- Ototoxic medications
- Smoking
- Diseases (diabetes, Ménière's)

Nursing Interventions
- Teaching about risk factors
- Removing and preventing impacted wax
- Referring for audiology
- Using hearing and listening aids
- Communication techniques

Wellness Outcomes
- Improved communication
- Increased social interaction
- Increased safety and functioning
- Better quality of life

even in the absence of risk factors, normal age-related changes affect frequency, causing hearing problems for many older adults.

External Ear

Hearing begins in the external or outer ear, which consists of the pinna and the external auditory canal (Fig. 16-1). These cartilaginous structures localize sounds so the person can identify the sources. The pinna undergoes changes in size, shape, flexibility, and hair growth with increasing age, but these changes do not affect the conduction of sound waves in healthy older adults. The auditory canal is covered by skin and lined with hair follicles and cerumen-producing glands. **Cerumen**, or wax, is a natural substance that is genetically determined to be either dry (flakey and gray) or wet (moist

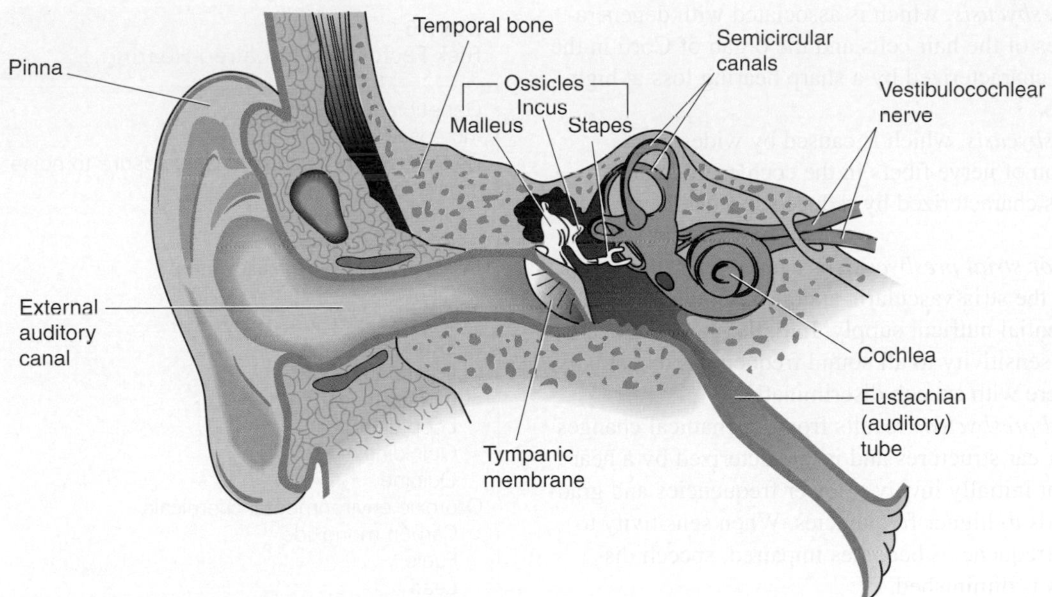

FIGURE 16-1 The ear. Age-related changes in structures of the ear can affect hearing in older adults.

and brown or tan). The function of cerumen is to cleanse, protect, and lubricate the ear canal. Cerumen is naturally expelled, but it can build up in older adults because of age-related changes such as an increased concentration of keratin, the growth of longer and thicker hair (especially in men), and thinning and drying of the skin lining the canal. An age-related diminution in sweat gland activity further increases the potential for cerumen accumulation by making the wax drier and more difficult to remove. A prolapsed or collapsed ear canal is another age-related change that can occur and affect localization and perception of high-frequency sounds.

Diversity Note

Whites and African Americans are likely to have wet cerumen, whereas Asians and Native Americans are likely to have dry cerumen.

Middle Ear

The tympanic membrane is a transparent, pearl-gray, slightly cone-shaped layer of flexible tissue separating the outer and middle ear. Its primary functions are to transmit sound energy and protect the middle and inner ear. With increased age, collagenous tissue replaces the elastic tissue, resulting in a thinner and stiffer eardrum. Sound vibrations pass through the tympanic membrane to the three auditory ossicles: the malleus, incus, and stapes. These bones are connected to each other but move independently, acting as a lever to amplify sound. Their primary function is to transmit vibrations across the air-filled middle ear, through the oval window, and to the fluid-filled inner ear. Transmission of sounds is influenced by the frequency of each sound and is most effective in the middle-frequency range of normal voices and least effective at the lowest and highest frequencies. Age-related calcification of the ossicular bones can interfere with the transfer of sound vibrations from the tympanic membrane to the oval window.

The middle ear muscles and ligaments contract in response to loud noises, stimulating the acoustic reflex, which protects the delicate inner ear and filters out auditory distractions originating from one's own voice and body movements. With increased age, the middle ear muscles and ligaments become weaker and stiffer and have a detrimental effect on the acoustic reflex. In addition, these degenerative changes diminish the resiliency of the tympanic membrane.

Inner Ear

In the inner ear, vibrations are transmitted to the cochlea, where they are converted to nerve impulses and coded for intensity and frequency. Nerve impulses stimulate fibers of the eighth cranial nerve and send the auditory message to the brain. This process transpires primarily in the sensory hair cells of the organ of Corti in the cochlea.

Age-related changes of the inner ear include loss of hair cells, reduction of blood supply, diminution of endolymph production, decreased basilar membrane flexibility, degeneration of spiral ganglion cells, and loss of neurons in the cochlear nuclei. These inner ear changes result in the degenerative hearing impairment termed **presbycusis**. One commonly used classification system for presbycusis is based on the specific structural source of the impairment, and can be categorized as follows:

- *Sensory presbycusis*, which is associated with degenerative changes of the hair cells and the organ of Corti in the cochlea, is characterized by a sharp hearing loss at high frequencies.
- *Neural presbycusis*, which is caused by widespread degeneration of nerve fibers in the cochlea and spiral ganglion, is characterized by reduced speech discrimination.
- *Metabolic or strial presbycusis* is caused by degenerative changes in the stria vascularis and a subsequent interruption in essential nutrient supply. Initially, these changes reduce the sensitivity to all sound frequencies; eventually, they interfere with speech discrimination.
- *Mechanical presbycusis* results from mechanical changes in the inner ear structures and is characterized by a hearing loss that initially involves lower frequencies and gradually spreads to higher frequencies. When sensitivity to the higher frequencies becomes impaired, speech discrimination is diminished.

Although useful for analyzing the physiologic basis for various types of presbycusis, this classification is limited because presbycusis usually involves not one, but several, age-related processes.

Auditory Nervous System

From the inner ear, the auditory nerve fibers pass through the internal auditory meatus and enter the brain. Functions of the auditory nerve pathway include localizing sound direction, fine-tuning auditory stimuli, and transferring information from the primary auditory cortex to the auditory association area.

With increased age, degenerative changes affect the entire auditory nerve pathway and related structures and cause hearing deficits in older adults. Hair cell atrophy in the organ of Corti, narrowing of the auditory meatus from bone apposition, and degeneration of the arteries that supply the auditory nerve are age-related changes that affect the auditory nervous system. Age-related changes in the central nervous system, such as those that affect speed of information processing, also can interfere with hearing abilities (Schneider et al., 2005).

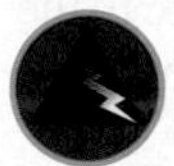

RISK FACTORS THAT AFFECT HEARING WELLNESS

In addition to the age-related changes that affect hearing, factors associated with lifestyle, heredity, environment, medications, impacted wax, and disease processes also can contribute to the development of hearing loss. Much research is being done on factors that threaten hearing wellness, with emphasis on modifiable risk factors, such as noise, that can be addressed through health promotion interventions. Research is also focusing on the interrelationship between risk factors, such as between noise and ototoxic substances and between heredity and ototoxic substances. Most likely, some hearing loss attributed to age-related changes actually results from risk factors such as exposure to noise or ototoxic substances. Thus, there is increasing emphasis on health education about preventive strategies. Box 16-1 summarizes some risk factors that interfere with hearing wellness.

Box 16-1
Risk Factors for Impaired Hearing

- Genetic predisposition
- Increased age
- Recreational or occupational exposure to noise
- Cigarette smoking
- Ototoxic medications
  - Aminoglycosides
  - Aspirin and other salicylates
  - Cisplatin
  - Erythromycin
  - Ibuprofen
  - Imipramine
  - Indomethacin
  - Loop diuretics
  - Quinidine
  - Quinine
- Ototoxic environmental chemicals
  - Carbon monoxide
  - Fuels
  - Lead
  - Mercury
  - Organophosphates
  - Styrene
  - Toluene

Lifestyle and Environmental Factors

The most prevalent risk factor for impaired hearing is exposure to noise, which can be viewed as both a lifestyle choice and an environmental factor. Prolonged or intermittent exposure to noise during occupational or leisure activities is a common and usually avoidable risk factor for damage to the auditory system. *Healthy People 2010* identifies **noise-induced hearing loss (NIHL)** as the most common occupational disease and one of the most modifiable risk factors (USDHHS, 2000). People who have an increased risk for NIHL because of their occupations include miners, farmers, plumbers, musicians, carpenters, firefighters, and armed services members. Common noise hazards that cause NIHL in farmers, for example, include tractors, animals, firearms, bulldozers, workshop tools, small motors, shearing sheds, cotton presses, and heavy machinery (Depczynski et al., 2005; Hass-Slavin et al., 2005). Intermittent noise exposure—such as that experienced by emergency medical service professionals—also has been identified as a factor in NIHL (McReynolds, 2005).

Older adults today are likely to have worked in noisy settings before noise level recommendations were enforced by the National Institute for Occupational Safety and Health. For instance, older people who were once employed as weavers or textile workers are likely to have been exposed to detrimentally noisy environments during their work years. Because the effects of NIHL and age-related changes are cumulative, the hearing loss may not be noticed until later adulthood. Some research suggests that exposure to noise during earlier years exacerbates the age-related changes in the cochlea and produces an age–noise interaction (Kujawa & Liberman, 2006). Thus, when hearing impairment is noticed during later adulthood, it may be falsely attributed to age-related changes alone.

Exposure to toxic chemicals in the workplace or the environment is another risk factor for hearing loss that has been under investigation since the 1990s, with current research focusing on metals, solvents, asphyxiants, and pesticides/herbicides. Hunting, woodworking, and other leisure-time activities also can contribute to NIHL, especially if people engaging in these activities do not use protective ear devices. Other activities that are likely to cause sensorineural damage unless protective mechanisms are used include listening to loud music; operating tractors, chain saws, or leaf blowers; and riding motorcycles, airplanes, snowmobiles, or motorboats. Figure 16-2 illustrates the noise levels of various activities. Sounds louder than 80 dB are considered potentially ototoxic.

Cigarette smoking, as well as living in a household with a smoker, is another lifestyle and environmental factor being investigated as a risk for hearing impairment. Cigarette smoking is both an independent risk factor for impaired hearing and a factor that potentiates the effects of noise to cause hearing loss (Burr et al., 2005; Wild et al., 2005). Thus, people who smoke are at even higher risk for NIHL.

Diversity Note

White men have higher rates of noise-induced hearing loss than African Americans or women (Helzner et al., 2005).

Impacted Cerumen

Impacted cerumen is common in older adults as a leading cause of hearing loss. Age-related changes can cause wax to accumulate and occlude the auditory canal, and the use of hearing aids increases the possibility of impacted wax. Cerumen accumulation is an easily preventable and treatable cause of hearing deficits; most important, it is readily amenable to nursing interventions, as discussed later in this chapter. A higher incidence of excessive or impacted cerumen is associated with increased levels of dependency, ranging from 9% of older adults in independent living settings to 82% of residents in nursing care facilities (Culbertson et al., 2004).

Medication Effects

Medications can cause or contribute to hearing impairments by damaging the cochlear and vestibular divisions of the auditory nerve. Despite the fact that quinine and salicylate ototoxicities were first observed more than a century ago, the ototoxic effects of medication have received little attention in clinical settings. Although age alone does not increase the risk for ototoxicity, older adults are more likely to be taking ototoxic medications, such as aspirin and furosemide. Other contributing factors that commonly occur in older adults and increase the risk for ototoxicity include renal failure, long-term use of ototoxic medications, and potentiation between two ototoxic medications, such as furosemide and aminoglycoside antibiotics. Medications that are likely to be ototoxic are listed in Box 16-1. Ototoxicity is often dose related, and hearing loss may be temporary if medications are discontinued or the dose is reduced. Although ototoxicity is potentially reversible, medications may be overlooked as a causative factor if the hearing loss is mistakenly ascribed to inevitable and irreversible degenerative changes.

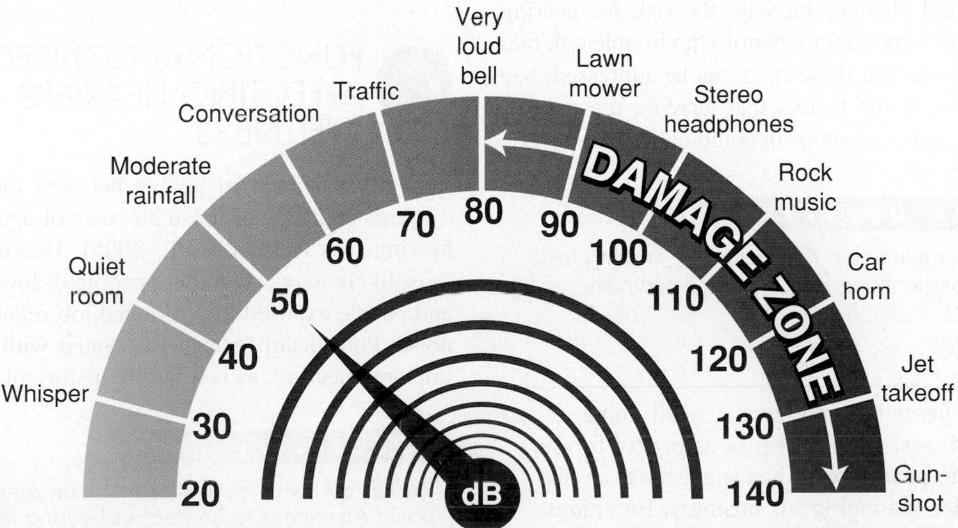

FIGURE 16-2 Noise levels associated with common activities are measured in decibels (dB). Sounds louder than 80 dB are potentially harmful to ears.

Disease Processes

Otosclerosis is a hereditary disease of the auditory ossicles that causes ankylosis of the footplate of the stapes to the oval window. Otosclerosis usually begins in youth or early adulthood, but the hearing loss may not be detected until middle or later adulthood, when age-related middle ear changes compound the disease-related changes. Otosclerosis primarily causes a conductive hearing loss, but some sensorineural loss also may occur. Initially, it is difficult to hear soft and low-pitched sounds; as the hearing loss worsens, the person is likely to experience dizziness, tinnitus, or balance problems.

Ménière's disease and acoustic neuromas are auditory system diseases that commonly cause hearing impairment. Diabetes and cerebrovascular disorders are examples of diseases that increase the risk of hearing loss, particularly in whites (Helzner et al., 2005). Other conditions and systemic diseases that cause or contribute to hearing impairment include syphilis, myxedema, hypertension, meningitis, hypothyroidism, head trauma, high fevers, Paget's disease, and viral infections (e.g., measles and mumps). Radiation for head and neck cancers has also been identified as a risk factor for high-frequency hearing loss (Pan et al., 2005).

Combinations of Risk Factors

Combinations of risk factors can be especially harmful. For example, people who take ototoxic medications or are genetically predisposed to hearing loss may be even more susceptible to the damaging effects of noise exposure. Similarly, people with a genetic predisposition to hearing loss may be more susceptible to hearing loss from ototoxic drugs. Researchers currently are focusing on synergistic effects of noise and chemicals. For example, ototoxicity from a combination of noise and hydrocarbons, as experienced by aircraft maintenance workers, is likely to cause more hearing impairment than either risk factor alone (Kaufman et al., 2005). Because age-related changes increase the risk for hearing loss, it is especially important to identify modifiable risk factors in older adults so that those risks can be addressed. See Box 16-1 for a list of the factors that increase the risk for impaired hearing, either alone or in combinations.

Wellness Opportunity

Modifiable and preventable risk factors for hearing loss include noise, medications, and impacted cerumen.

Mr. H. is 60 years old and owns a small home remodeling business. He has been a carpenter for 38 years, but in the past 9 years has spent most of his time in the office managing his business. He enjoys hunting and fishing on weekends. He smokes two packs of cigarettes a day and has smoked since he was 16 years old. His wife has been telling him she thinks he has "selective hearing" and hears only what he wants to hear. Mr. H. admits that he turns the television volume up louder than he used to, but denies having any "real hearing problem."

THINKING POINTS

- What age-related changes and risk factors contribute to Mr. H's hearing loss?
- Describe the hearing loss that Mr. H is likely to be experiencing.
- What environmental conditions will contribute to Mr. H's hearing difficulty?

PATHOLOGIC CONDITION AFFECTING HEARING: TINNITUS

Tinnitus is the persistent sensation of ringing, roaring, blowing, buzzing, or other types of noise that do not originate in the external environment. Tinnitus is a common pathologic condition in older adults that is highly associated with hearing loss, ototoxic medications, and Ménière's disease. It can be caused by impacted wax, especially if the wax is attached to the tympanic membrane. Caffeine, alcohol, or nicotine can exacerbate tinnitus. People with tinnitus should be evaluated for associated pathologic conditions or any of the contributing factors.

Wellness Opportunity

Nurses promote self-care by teaching people with tinnitus about the exacerbating effects of controllable factors, such as cigarette smoking and drinking alcoholic or caffeinated beverages.

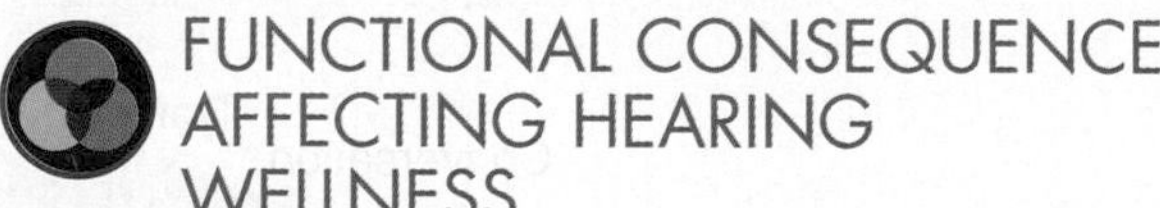

FUNCTIONAL CONSEQUENCES AFFECTING HEARING WELLNESS

Thirty-five percent of people between the ages of 65 and 79 years and 53% of those 80 years of age and older have a hearing loss (Caban et al., 2005). Hearing impairment is most likely to occur in men, people of low economic status, and people exposed to prolonged job-related or recreational noise. Poor health is also associated with a higher risk for impaired hearing, as is a family history of otosclerosis.

Diversity Note

Whites are twice as likely as African Americans or Hispanic Americans to be deaf or hearing impaired. Men are more likely than women to experience hearing loss.

Hearing losses are categorized according to the site of the impairment. Abnormalities of the external and middle ear impair the sound conduction mechanism and are classified as *conductive hearing losses*. Abnormalities of the inner ear interfere with the sensory and neural structures and are classified as *sensorineural hearing losses*. Sensorineural hearing loss often is age related or noise induced. Hearing losses that involve both conductive and sensorineural impairments are called *mixed hearing losses*.

Effects on Communication

Accurate comprehension of speech depends on speech pace, sound frequencies, environmental noise, and internal auditory function. Hearing acuity for high-frequency tones begins to decline in early adulthood, and by the age of 30 years for men and 50 years for women, there is some decline in hearing sensitivity at all frequencies. The rate of change in hearing level is more than twice as fast in men than in women, and the cumulative effects are usually noticed by men in their 50s and women in their 60s (Fozard & Gordan-Salant, 2001).

Speech comprehension is most directly influenced by the frequency of **phonemes**, the smallest units of sound. Each phoneme in a word has a different frequency; generally, vowels have lower frequencies and consonants have higher frequencies. Although most word phonemes have lower-range frequencies, sibilant consonants (those that have a whistling quality, such as *ch, f, g, s, sh, t, th,* and *z*) have higher-range frequencies. Because the earliest and most universal age-related changes affect one's ability to code higher-frequency sounds, words rich in sibilants will be most affected by age-related changes of the auditory system.

Presbycusis, as mentioned earlier, is the sensorineural hearing loss associated with an age-related degeneration of the auditory structures. Presbycusis usually occurs in both ears, but the degree of impairment in each ear can vary. An early functional consequence of presbycusis is the loss of ability to hear high-pitched sounds and sibilant consonants. When high-pitched sounds are filtered out, words become distorted and jumbled, and sentences become incoherent. For example, someone with presbycusis might interpret a sentence like "I think she should go to the store" as "I wish we could go to the show." This characteristic, known as diminished speech discrimination, is influenced by the speaker's rate of speech: rapid, slow, or slurred speech patterns make it increasingly difficult for the older person to discern words. As the hearing loss progresses, explosive consonants, such as *b, d, k, p* and *t,* also become distorted. Thus, by the ninth decade, older adults experience more difficulty understanding speech (Divenyi et al., 2005).

Background noise and environmental conditions, such as echoing or poor acoustics, compound the effects of sensorineural hearing loss, causing even greater difficulty with speech comprehension. Even older adults with little or no hearing loss have more difficulty than younger adults recognizing words in noisy environments (Thornton & Light, 2006). Thus, older adults in a hospital or long-term care facility, for example, may be particularly sensitive to background noises to which the staff may have become accustomed. People with sensorineural hearing loss are sometimes hypersensitive to high-frequency sounds, causing a very narrow range in which sound is heard adequately and comfortably. This condition makes it difficult to adjust hearing aids or assistive listening devices for optimal comfort and amplification (Palmer & Ortmann, 2005).

Diversity Note

Men report more difficulty with background noise than women, and a greater aversion to amplified sound (Fozard & Gordon-Salant, 2001).

A conductive hearing loss is characterized by a reduced intensity of sounds and difficulty hearing vowels and low-pitched tones. In contrast to presbycusis, all frequencies of sounds are heard equally once the sound threshold is reached, and background noise does not interfere as much with speech comprehension. Often there is a history of otosclerosis, perforated eardrum, or other ear disease. In older adults, impacted cerumen is a common contributing factor. Depending on the causative factor, conductive hearing loss occurs in one or both ears. Table 16-1 summarizes the functional consequences of age-related changes affecting hearing.

TABLE 16-1 Functional Consequences of Age-Related Changes Affecting Hearing

	Change	Consequence
External Ear	• Longer, thicker hair • Thinner, drier skin • Increased keratin	Potential for impacted cerumen and subsequent impaired sound conduction
Middle Ear	• Diminished resiliency of tympanic membrane • Calcified, hardened ossicles • Weakened and stiff muscles and ligaments	Impaired sound conduction
Inner Ear and Nervous System	• Diminished neurons, endolymph, hair cells, and blood supply • Degeneration of spiral ganglion and arterial blood vessels • Decreased flexibility of basilar membrane • Degeneration of central processing systems	*Presbycusis:* diminished ability to hear high-pitched sounds, especially in the presence of background noise

Effects on Quality of Life, Safety, and Functioning

Because it is a primary component of communication, hearing enables people to enjoy humor, appreciate music, obtain information, relate to others, and respond to threats. Thus, hearing deficits inevitably affect usual daily activities and have a variety of impacts on quality of life, safety, and functioning.

Hearing loss is associated with declines in cognitive function and many other negative psychosocial consequences (Scialfa & Fernie, 2006). For example, people who cannot discriminate words may be reluctant to respond to questions and may refrain from answering rather than risk feeling foolish. Performance on mental status examinations can be influenced negatively by a person's fear of not hearing the questions accurately as well as by the concomitant reduction of sensory stimuli. Poor performance on tests of cognitive abilities can mistakenly lead to a perception that the person has dementia when, in fact, the person simply has a hearing loss. Additional psychosocial consequences of hearing loss include fear, boredom, apathy, anxiety, depression, social isolation, and low self-esteem. When hearing loss interferes with one's ability to perceive reality accurately, it can lead to suspiciousness, paranoia, and loss of contact with reality. When only parts of a conversation are heard, a person is likely to believe that the conversation is about him or her, and persecutory delusions can develop.

The extent of psychosocial consequences of hearing impairment depends on the lifestyle of the person affected. For example, hearing impairments are relatively more detrimental for people whose occupations or interests are highly dependent on good hearing. By contrast, hearing loss is less likely to have detrimental effects for people who have few social relationships and who do not depend on hearing for occupational or leisure activities.

Diversity Note

Studies of gender differences in perceived hearing handicap suggest that hearing loss has a greater social impact on older men and a greater emotional impact on older women. Thus, men may withdraw from social interactions and women may continue to be active but worry about how well they can participate (Taylor & Jurma, 2003).

In addition to having a negative influence on quality of life, hearing deficits can affect the safety and functioning of older adults. For example, people with hearing impairments are likely to be less responsive when warning signals are sounded for fires, ambulances, and other emergencies. Besides creating actual safety hazards, the hearing deficit can lead to fear and anxiety about personal safety. Even mild hearing impairment in older adults is associated with functional decline and increased dependency in daily activities.

Negative societal attitudes about aging and hearing loss can result in a doubly negative effect on the person who is old as well as hard of hearing. The older person may be reluctant to acknowledge a hearing deficit, choosing to limit opportunities for communication rather than face the stigma associated with hearing impairments. These attitudes and accompanying behaviors can cause other psychosocial consequences such as loneliness, social isolation, and even a more rapid progression of the hearing loss. Geropsychologists who studied the relationship between age stereotypes and hearing loss found that negative perceptions of aging—particularly those related to physical appearance—were associated with a greater decline in hearing over a 3-year period (Levy et al., 2006). Moreover, Levy and colleagues found that age stereotypes had a greater influence on hearing loss than other risk factors such as age, sex, depression, or smoking history.

Wellness Opportunity

Nurses can initiate conversations that reflect positive and nonjudgmental attitudes about aging and hearing loss.

Mr. H. is now 69 years old and has been retired for several years. He spends several days a week hunting and fishing seasonally. He also spends time in his basement making small pieces of furniture and doing other woodworking. He continues to smoke, but has cut down to one pack per day. His wife and he attend the weekly "Lunch Bunch" group at the local senior center where you are the nurse. They make an appointment to talk with you because Mrs. H. is concerned about her husband's hearing. Mr. H., who blames his problem on "old age," refuses to have an evaluation for a hearing aid because he doesn't think an aid would do any good and "besides, it would stick out like a sore thumb."

THINKING POINTS

- What factors contribute to Mr. H's hearing loss?
- What environmental and other conditions might make the hearing loss worse?
- What myths or misunderstandings are likely to influence Mr. H's perception of his hearing problem and potential interventions for it?

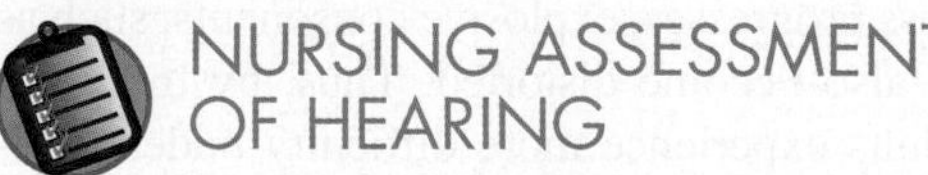

NURSING ASSESSMENT OF HEARING

Nursing assessment of hearing is aimed at identifying

- Factors that interfere with hearing wellness
- Actual hearing deficit
- The impact of any hearing deficits on the person's safety and quality of life

- Opportunities for health promotion
- Barriers to implementing interventions

Each of these factors is important in helping older adults and their caregivers compensate for hearing deficits. Assessment is accomplished through interviewing the person, observing behavioral cues, and administering hearing tests.

Interviewing About Hearing Changes

Interview questions are used to acquire information about (1) present and past risk factors, (2) the person's awareness and acknowledgment of a hearing impairment, (3) the psychosocial impact of any hearing deficit, and (4) attitudes that might influence health promotion interventions (Box 16-2). The hearing assessment interview begins with questions about family history of hearing impairments and a personal history of prolonged exposure to loud noises. Identification of ototoxic medications as a risk factor can be included as part of the hearing assessment or as part of the medication history. Nurses can use questions to prompt the person to acknowledge a hearing problem, particularly if they discuss these factors in relation to increasing the risk for hearing loss.

If the older adult does not initiate a discussion of hearing problems, the nurse asks direct questions about the person's discernment of any hearing deficit. If the older adult denies having a hearing problem but shows behavioral cues indicative of a hearing deficit, the nurse elicits further information by asking leading questions such as "I notice you turn your left ear toward me. Is your hearing better in that ear?"

Nurses ask questions about changes in the older adult's social activities to identify psychosocial consequences of hearing impairment that can be addressed through interventions. If no hearing impairment is present, questions about lifestyle do not necessarily have to be included as part of the hearing assessment. When a person acknowledges the existence of a hearing impairment, however, the nurse then asks about any associated changes in social and occupational activities.

Wellness Opportunity

Nurses address the whole person by including questions about the impact of a hearing loss on his or her quality of life.

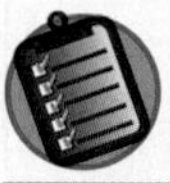

Box 16-2
Guidelines for Assessing Hearing

Questions to Identify Risk Factors for Hearing Loss

- Do you have a family history of hearing loss or deafness?
- Have you been exposed to loud noises in your job or leisure activities?
- Do you have a history of any of the following: diabetes, hypothyroidism, Ménière's disease, or Paget's disease?
- What medications do you take? (Refer to Box 16-1 to identify potentially ototoxic medications.)
- Have you ever had impacted wax in your ears?

Questions to Assess Awareness and Presence of Hearing Deficit

- Do you have any trouble with your hearing?
- Have you noticed any change in your ability to understand conversations or hear words?
- Are you bothered by any noises in your ears, such as ringing or buzzing?

Questions to Ask if Hearing Loss Is Acknowledged

- How long have you noticed a hearing loss?
- Do you notice differences in hearing in your left ear, versus your right ear?
- Has there been a progressive loss, or did the hearing problem begin suddenly?
- Describe your hearing difficulty.
- Are there any conditions, such as noisy environments or particular voices or sounds, that especially interfere with your hearing?
- Does your hearing loss interfere with your ability to communicate with others, either individually or in groups?
- Are there any activities that you would like to do, but feel you cannot because of hearing problems?
- Have you ever had, or thought about having, an evaluation for a hearing aid?
- Have you ever tried using a hearing aid?

Questions to Identify Opportunities for Education About Disease Prevention and Health Promotion

- Does the person engage in any activities that expose him or her to loud noises, such as woodworking or lawn mowing? If so, does he or she understand the importance of wearing ear protectors?
- If the person has a history of impacted wax, does he or she take preventive measures?
- Does the person smoke cigarettes or live in a household with a smoker? (If so, does the person realize that this is a risk factor for hearing loss?)
- What are the person's attitudes about hearing loss?
- Is hearing loss considered normal and untreatable?
- Is a hearing aid considered to be a stigma?
- If the person is resistant to an audiologic evaluation, what are the barriers? (For example, are there financial or transportation limitations that interfere with obtaining a hearing aid?)
- Does the hearing loss contribute to a sense of isolation, depression, paranoia, or low self-esteem?
- What are the person's usual communication opportunities, and how does the hearing loss influence these usual patterns? (For instance, does the person live in an environment where it is important to be able to use the phone?)
- Does the person live in a noisy environment and find relief in the hearing impairment?
- If the person lives in an environment where group activities are a large part of daily activities, does the person want to participate in these activities?

The nurse assesses the older person's attitudes toward hearing loss, hearing aids, and assistive listening devices because these attitudes influence his or her acceptance of interventions. Moreover, when nurses identify attitudinal barriers, they can plan health education interventions to address myths or misunderstandings. For example, older adults may believe that hearing aids are too costly or of little use, or they may be embarrassed to use a device that is visible to others. They also may not know how to go about arranging for an evaluation, and may distrust advertisements about hearing aids. Resistance toward hearing aids can also arise from lack of money, transportation, or motivation to communicate. Thus, the nurse focuses part of the assessment on barriers that are likely to interfere with interventions for hearing wellness.

The Hearing Handicap Inventory for the Elderly (HHIE-S) is a 10-item questionnaire that can be administered to older adults in about 5 minutes (Fig. 16-3). This tool was developed in the early 1980s for use with cognitively intact older adults in a variety of clinical and community settings. Both the Hartford Institute for Geriatric Nursing and the American Speech-Language-Hearing Association recommend this tool for assessing the effect of hearing impairment on an older person's daily function.

Wellness Opportunity

Nurses promote self-care by asking an older adult to use the HHIE-S and then reviewing the results of this assessment to identify goals.

Observing Behavioral Cues

Behavioral cues related to hearing loss provide important information about the presence of a hearing impairment, the psychosocial consequences of any such impairment, and

ITEM	YES (4 pts)	SOMETIMES (2 pts)	NO (0 pts)
Does a hearing problem cause you to feel embarrassed when you meet new people?	____	____	____
Does a hearing problem cause you to feel frustrated when talking to members of your family?	____	____	____
Do you have difficulty hearing when someone speaks in a whisper?	____	____	____
Do you feel handicapped by a hearing problem?	____	____	____
Does a hearing problem cause you difficulty when visiting friends, relatives, or neighbors?	____	____	____
Does a hearing problem cause you to attend religious services less often than you would like?	____	____	____
Does a hearing problem cause you to have arguments with family members?	____	____	____
Does a hearing problem cause you difficulty when listening to TV or radio?	____	____	____
Do you feel that any difficulty with your hearing limits or hampers your personal or social life?	____	____	____
Does a hearing problem cause you difficulty when in a restaurant with relatives or friends?	____	____	____

RAW SCORE_______ (sum of the points assigned each of the items)

INTERPRETING THE RAW SCORE

0 to 8 = 13% probability of hearing impairment (no handicap/no referral)
10 to 24 = 50% probability of hearing impairment (mild-moderate handicap/refer)
26 to 40 = 84% probability of hearing impairment (severe handicap/refer)

FIGURE 16-3 The screening version of the Hearing Handicap Inventory for the Elderly (HHIE-S). (Reprinted with permission from Ventry, I. & Weinstein, B. [1983, July]. *Identification of elderly people with hearing problems* [pp. 37–42]. Rockville, MD: American Speech-Language-Hearing Association. Copyright American Speech-Language-Hearing Association.)

the person's attitudes about assistive devices. If the older adult denies a hearing deficit that has been noticed by others, behavioral cues can be an important source of assessment information. Denial of a hearing deficit can be rooted in lack of awareness of the impairment because of gradual onset or, if the older person is socially isolated, can be caused by a paucity of opportunities for communication. Feelings of embarrassment or misconceptions that the hearing loss is an inevitable and untreatable consequence of aging can also contribute to denial. Box 16-3 lists behavioral cues that the nurse should observe as part of the hearing assessment.

Using an Otoscope and Tuning Fork

Nurses assess hearing by using an otoscope to examine the ear and a tuning fork to check hearing. The purpose of the otoscopic examination is to identify impacted wax and other factors that can interfere with hearing, whereas the purpose of the tuning fork test is to detect hearing impairments and to differentiate between conductive and sensorineural losses.

Box 16-4 describes the procedure for performing a nursing assessment of hearing using the otoscope and tuning fork. When a hearing deficit is identified, the nurse can recommend that further evaluation be conducted at a speech and hearing center or by a specialized physician, such as an otolaryngologist.

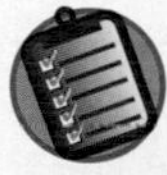

Box 16-3
Guidelines for Assessing Behavioral Cues Related to Hearing

Behavioral Cues to a Hearing Deficit

- Inappropriate or no response to questions, especially in the absence of opportunities for lip reading
- Inability to follow verbal directions without cues
- Short attention span, easy distractibility
- Frequent requests for repetition or clarification of verbal communication
- Intense observation of the speaker
- Mouthing of words spoken by the speaker
- Turning of one ear toward the speaker
- Unusual physical proximity to the speaker
- Lack of response to loud environmental noises
- Speech that is too loud or inarticulate
- Abnormal voice characteristics, such as monotony
- Misperception that others are talking about him or her

Behavioral Cues About Psychosocial Consequences

- Uncharacteristic avoidance of group settings
- Lack of interest in social activities, especially those requiring verbal communication or those that the person enjoyed in the past (e.g., bingo, card games)

Behavioral Cues About Assistive Devices

- Not using a hearing aid that has been purchased
- Failure to obtain batteries for a hearing aid
- Expression of embarrassment about using assistive devices

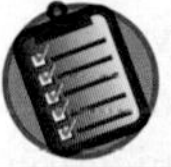

Box 16-4
Guidelines for Otoscopic and Tuning Fork Assessment

Using the Otoscope to Assess Factors That Could Interfere With Hearing

- Hold the otoscope upside down, resting your hand on the person's head to stabilize the instrument.
- Before inserting the speculum, pull the pinna upward and backward, while tilting the person's head slightly back and toward the opposite shoulder.
- If cerumen has accumulated to the point of interfering with the examination or occluding the canal, follow the cerumen removal procedure described in the section on Nursing Interventions.
- Normal otoscopic findings in older adults include the following:
  - Small amount of cerumen
  - Pinkish-white epithelial lining, no redness or lesions
  - Pearl-gray tympanic membrane, which is less translucent than in younger adults
  - Light reflex anteroinferiorly from the umbo
  - Visible landmarks

Using the Tuning Fork to Detect Hearing Impairment

- Use a tuning fork with frequencies of 512 to 1024 cps (Hz).
- Hold the tuning fork firmly at the stem.
- Strike the fork against the palm of your hand, or strike the fork with a rubber reflex hammer, to set it in motion.

Weber's Test

Procedure: Place the tip of a vibrating tuning fork at the center of the person's forehead. Ask where they hear the sound and whether it is louder in one ear than in the other.
Normal finding: The tuning fork is heard equally in both ears.
Abnormal finding: The tuning fork is heard better in one ear, indicating a possible hearing loss.

Rinne's Test

Procedure: Mask one ear, then place a vibrating tuning fork on the mastoid process of the opposite ear until the person indicates that it can no longer be heard. Then, quickly place the tuning fork in front of the ear canal with the top near the ear canal.
Normal finding: The length of time the tuning fork can be heard over the ear canal is about twice as long as the time it can be heard over the mastoid bone.
Abnormal finding: The length of time the tuning fork is heard in front of the ear is shorter than twice as long as the time it can be heard when placed on the mastoid process. In such a case, the person should undergo further tests for impaired hearing.

Recall that Mr. H. is a 69-year-old participant in activities at the local senior center where you are the nurse. You are meeting with Mr. and Mrs. H. to discuss Mrs. H.'s concerns about her husband's hearing problem.

THINKING POINTS

- Which of the questions and considerations in Boxes 16-2 and 16-3 would you use in assessing Mr. H.?
- Would you involve Mrs. H. in any part of the assessment? If so, how would you involve her?
- What health promotion advice would you give Mr. H. at this time?

NURSING DIAGNOSIS

Based on the nursing assessment, the nurse might identify an actual hearing deficit or risk factors for impaired hearing. An appropriate nursing diagnosis for an older adult with a hearing impairment would be Disturbed Sensory Perception: Auditory. This diagnosis is defined as the "state in which the individual/group experiences or is at risk of experiencing a change in the amount, pattern, or interpretation of incoming stimuli" (Carpenito-Moyet, 2006, p. 439). If the focus of care is on the person's responses to the hearing loss, then the nursing diagnosis of Impaired Communication might be applicable. Impaired Communication is "the state in which an individual experiences or is at high risk to experience difficulty exchanging thoughts, ideas, wants, or needs with others" (Carpenito-Moyet, 2006, p. 68). Related factors that are common in older adults are hearing loss, auditory nerve damage, ototoxic medications, and environmental conditions, such as background noise. If psychosocial consequences are identified, other pertinent nursing diagnoses might include Anxiety, Impaired Adjustment, Impaired Social Interaction, and Ineffective Individual Coping. When the hearing impairment is severe and uncompensated to the point that the person does not function safely, then Risk for Injury might be an applicable nursing diagnosis.

Wellness Opportunity

Nurses can use the wellness nursing diagnosis of Readiness for Enhanced Communication for older adults who are willing to explore possibilities for improving their hearing through health promotion interventions.

PLANNING FOR WELLNESS OUTCOMES

When older adults experience impaired hearing or when risk factors threaten hearing wellness, nurses identify wellness outcomes as an essential part of the planning process. The Nursing Outcomes Classification (NOC) that most directly relates to interventions to improve hearing for an older adult is Hearing Compensation Behavior, defined as "personal actions to identify, monitor, and compensate for hearing loss" (Johnson et al., 2006, p. 628). Another pertinent NOC is Sensory Function: Hearing, defined as the "extent to which sounds are correctly sensed" (Johnson et al., 2006, p. 636). In addition, any of the following nursing-sensitive outcomes are applicable to describe the effectiveness of interventions to improve hearing:

- Loneliness Severity
- Communication Ability
- Risk Control: Hearing Impairment
- Social Involvement
- Social Interaction Skills
- Personal Safety Behavior

Specific interventions to achieve these outcomes are discussed in the following section.

Wellness Opportunity

Quality of Life is a wellness outcome that is achieved through nursing interventions that improve communication for older adults with impaired hearing.

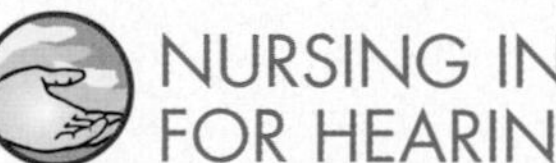

NURSING INTERVENTIONS FOR HEARING WELLNESS

Nursing interventions aim to promote hearing wellness through preventing hearing loss, assisting older adults to compensate for hearing deficits, and using communication methods that facilitate optimal communication. Specific interventions to achieve these goals are discussed in detail in the following sections. Nurses can use any of the following examples of pertinent Nursing Interventions Classification (NIC) terminology in care plans: Communication Enhancement: Hearing Deficit, Ear Care, Environmental Management, Environmental Management: Safety, Health Education, Health Screening, Health System Guidance, and Risk Identification.

Wellness Opportunity

Nurses can emphasize that even though interventions to prevent hearing loss ideally begin early in life, it is never too late to begin protecting ears from noise.

Promoting Health for Hearing Wellness

Nurses can challenge the perception that all hearing loss is an inevitable consequence of growing older by teaching about interventions to protect hearing, with emphasis on NIHL. Many older adults engage in recreational or occupational activities that can cause NIHL, and may not realize that age-

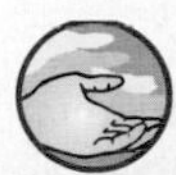

Box 16-5
Health Promotion Teaching About Hearing

Prevention and Early Detection of Hearing Loss

- Use ear protection devices when engaging in activities that omit loud noise.
- Have hearing screening done with questionnaire or audiometry when any change in hearing is noted.
- Have ears checked for impacted wax; use ceruminolytic agents if needed.

Interventions for Compensating for Hearing Loss

- Obtain evaluation at a Speech and Hearing Center for a hearing aid, assistive hearing device, or aural rehabilitation services.

Nutritional Considerations

- Adequate intake of zinc, magnesium, and vitamins A, D, and E

Commonly Used Complementary and Alternative Care Practices

- Herbs for tinnitus: ginkgo, sesame, goldenseal, black cohosh
- Herbs to improve circulation to the ear: ginger, ginkgo
- Homeopathic remedies for tinnitus: salicylic, carbonium sul, China sul, Kali iod, Kali carb, two drops of almond oil in each ear weekly
- Homeopathic remedies to reduce earwax: causticum
- Remedy for earwax removal: warm one drop of German camomile oil in five drops of olive oil and instill in the ear

related changes increase their susceptibility to development of hearing loss. Nurses can address the *Healthy People 2010* goal of reducing adult hearing loss in the noise-exposed public (USDHHS, 2000) by using information in Box 16-5. In addition, nurses can educate older adults about the potentiating effects of two or more risk factors, such as smoking and age-related changes, or medication effects and a genetic predisposition to ototoxicity. People who already experience a mild hearing impairment may be motivated to protect their hearing by avoiding hazardous noise and protecting their ears when they are exposed to noise. Similarly, if they are experiencing a hearing loss and recognize that nicotine can be ototoxic, they may be more motivated to quit smoking.

Another goal of *Healthy People 2010* is to "increase the proportion of persons who have had a hearing examination on schedule" (USDHHS, 2000, p. 28-14). Although guidelines for audiology screening are not specific, *Healthy People 2010* recommends screening once every 10 years between the ages of 18 and 50 years, "with more frequent monitoring after age 50 years" (USDHHS, 2000, p. 28-14). Whenever a nursing assessment identifies a hearing impairment, nursing interventions should include a referral for medical and audiology evaluations. Sometimes the nursing interventions also need to address barriers to obtaining a hearing aid, as discussed in the section on hearing aids. Nurses in community or residential settings for older adults may be able to find an audiologist who is willing to provide screening programs at little or no cost. As long as the sponsors of these programs do not have a vested interest in promoting a particular type of hearing aid, they may be effective resources for screening programs.

Wellness Opportunity

Nurses help meet the objectives of *Healthy People 2010* by teaching about NIHL and facilitating referrals to local speech and hearing centers.

Nurses promote hearing wellness by focusing their health education on modifiable risk factors such as smoking, exposure to noise, and use of ototoxic medication. For example, nurses can teach older adults and their caregivers about the potential ototoxicity of the medications listed in Box 16-1. This information is particularly important for older adults who have other risk factors for impaired hearing. When effective alternatives are available, or when the older adult is experiencing hearing difficulties, efforts should be made to avoid the use of these medications. As with other questions about medication, older adults and their caregivers should be advised to discuss their concerns about ototoxic medications with the prescribing health care practitioner. Nurses can use health education materials from resources listed at the end of this chapter to teach older adults how to protect themselves from NIHL. Similarly, nurses can use health education materials from resources listed at the end of Chapter 21 to teach about smoking cessation.

Nurses also promote hearing wellness through nursing interventions and health education aimed at alleviating or preventing hearing impairment caused by impacted wax. Over-the-counter emollient solutions containing ingredients such as glycerin, hydrogen peroxide, mineral oil, carbamide peroxide, and propylene glycol can prevent cerumen accumulation when periodically instilled in the ear canal (Saloranta & Westermarck, 2005). Liquid forms of docusate sodium (but not syrup forms) have been found to be an effective ceruminolytic (Singer et al., 2000). This solution is inexpensive and readily available in many settings where older adults receive care. The schedule for instillation of otic drops varies from semiweekly to monthly.

When an ear canal is impacted with cerumen, the nurse must determine whether there are any contraindications to irrigating, such as pain, swelling, a recent ear infection, or a history of ruptured tympanic membrane. If any of these conditions are identified, the nurse instructs the person to seek medical care from an otolaryngologist or other qualified professional.

If there are no contraindications, the following procedure should clear the canal of cerumen:

1. Soften the cerumen with a ceruminolytic agent.
2. Irrigate the canal with body-temperature tap water using a syringe and gentle pressure.
3. Aim water at the sides of the canal, and allow drainage from the ear to collect in a basin.

4. Drain excessive fluid from the ear by tilting the head toward the affected side.
5. If the cerumen is difficult to remove, instill a softening preparation twice daily for several days, and then attempt irrigation again.

After the wax build-up has been removed, teach the person to prevent the recurrence of impacted cerumen by using a ceruminolytic agent, as discussed earlier in this section.

Compensating for Hearing Deficits

Interventions for people who are hearing impaired should be considered only after a medical evaluation is done to identify treatable causes of the hearing loss. An audiologist can then evaluate more thoroughly to determine the best approach for facilitating communication. People with irreversible hearing deficits who are interested in corrective measures can be encouraged to participate in an aural rehabilitation program. One goal of *Healthy People 2010* is to "increase access by persons who have hearing impairments to hearing rehabilitation services and adaptive devices, including hearing aids, cochlear implants, or tactile or other assistive or augmentative devices" (USDHHS, 2000, p. 28-13). Individualized aural rehabilitation programs consist of counseling, together with any or all of the following services: amplification devices, auditory training, lip reading, and speech skills. These programs are available at speech and hearing centers, which are often affiliated with hospitals, medical centers, or universities. Internet resources, such as The National Association for Hearing and Speech Action website and others listed in the Educational Resources section of this chapter, can provide information about local resources for the evaluation and treatment of hearing disorders. Nurses play an important role in suggesting referrals for aural rehabilitation, discussing such programs with older adults and their caregivers, and facilitating or encouraging the use of recommended sound amplification devices.

Sound amplification generally is achieved by using hearing aids or assistive listening devices. Hearing aids are individually prescribed and require audiology services, whereas assistive listening devices are not individualized and are available without professional assistance or recommendation. These two types of sound amplification are discussed in the following sections.

Surgical implantation of an electronic device, such as a cochlear implant, may be indicated to compensate for damaged or nonfunctional parts of the inner ear. Adults who have lost all or most of their hearing later in life are candidates for this type of surgery, but extensive evaluation of the person is necessary to determine the appropriateness of the procedure. As this procedure becomes more common, nurses will be caring for more older adults who have had cochlear implants. One nursing implication is that the implanted devices are not compatible with magnetic resonance imaging (MRI), so nurses need to make sure that MRIs are not ordered for people with cochlear implants.

Assistive Listening Devices

Any device that amplifies or replaces sounds for individual or group communication without being individualized is categorized as an **assistive listening device**. These devices are sometimes called *personal listening systems*. A stethoscope is an assistive listening device commonly used by health care workers, and megaphones and microphones are examples of amplification devices used for group communication. Closed-captioned television is an assistive device that substitutes visual cues for auditory cues. Consumer information about assistive listening devices is widely available through catalogues and Internet sites such as Self Help for Hard of Hearing People (SHHH), listed in the Educational Resources section of this chapter. Local chapters of SHHH provide information about public buildings that are equipped with assistive listening devices.

Assistive listening devices, which consist of a small, battery-powered amplifier and headphones, can be used easily in any setting to improve communication temporarily. Advantages of assistive listening devices over hearing aids include lower cost and the fact that several people can share the device. In addition, most of these devices do not require as much manual dexterity as hearing aids, and some of them are more effective than hearing aids in filtering out background noise. Assistive listening devices can be used alone or in conjunction with hearing aids. Figure 16-4 shows one example of a very portable assistive listening device that enhances communication with someone who is hard of hearing.

Assistive listening devices are available for home use to amplify specific sounds, such as those from the radio, doorbell, television, or telephone. Telephone receivers with an amplifying device, called a *T-coil*, can be used in conjunc-

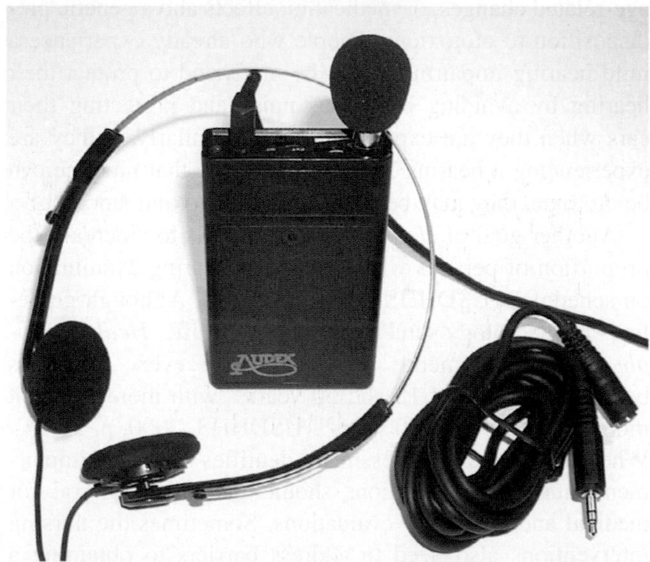

FIGURE 16-4 This assistive listening device (with extension cord) is very portable and can be used in a variety of settings to facilitate communication with hearing-impaired people. (Courtesy of Audex, Longview, TX.)

tion with the "T" position on a hearing aid. Other devices serve as substitutes for sound when amplification is impractical or ineffective: flashing lights for doorbells or doormats, and alarm clocks that vibrate the pillow or flash a light, for example. People with more serious hearing impairments but with adequate vision may benefit from closed captioned television, which provides subscripts for many programs. Since 1990, all televisions with screens 13 inches or larger are required to include a closed-captioned option.

Portable assistive listening devices are available for use in public places. Churches, theaters, and government buildings sometimes equip their facilities with assistive devices to amplify sound, and hearing-impaired people can ask about arrangements for using these devices. Small, hand-sized amplifiers can be attached temporarily to any telephone, and special devices are also available for mobile phones. In residential and institutional settings for older adults, having an assistive listening device available may be useful for nurses, especially when they are providing health education interventions.

Hearing Aids

A **hearing aid** is a battery-operated device that consists of an amplifier, a microphone, and a receiver. Hearing aids can be classified by size, location worn, and technology. The largest are about the size of a deck of cards and are worn on the body, whereas the new, smaller types fit completely in the ear canal. These smaller types can be seen only with close inspection of the ear and have a nylon string attached for insertion and removal. Preferred hearing aid locations include in-the-ear, in-the-canal, and completely-in-the-canal (Fig. 16-5). Body-worn and behind-the-ear hearing aids have become much less popular in recent years because of the availability of smaller, more powerful hearing aids made possible by newer technology.

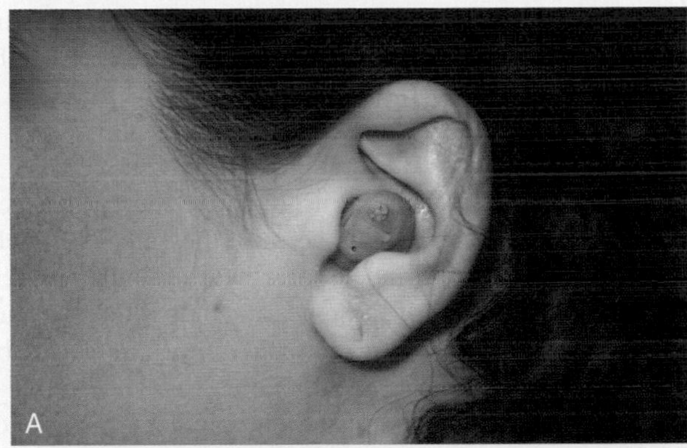

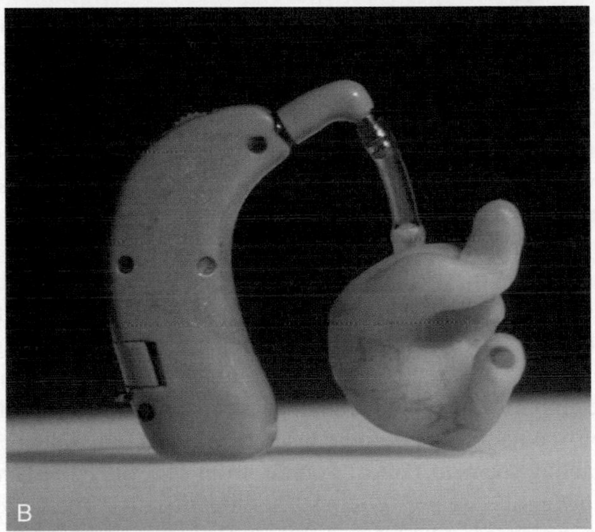

FIGURE 16-5 Sample hearing aids: in-the-ear **(A)**, behind-the-ear **(B)**. (From Craven, R. F., & Hirnle, C. J. [2007]. *Fundamentals of nursing: Human health and function* [5th ed.]. Philadelphia: Lippincott Williams & Wilkins.)

Until recently, the amplifying power of a hearing aid was strongly associated with its size because most hearing aids used the same type of technology, and severely impaired people needed larger, body-worn aids. New technology, however, has made available a variety of types of hearing aids that can be programmed and adjusted for individual differences. Currently, the effectiveness of a hearing aid is associated more with the type of technology used than with its size. Hearing aids are classified by whether they are analog or digital and according to the degree of individualized adjustments or programming possible. As discussed later, the cost of hearing aids increases as the programming becomes more adjustable and individualized.

Conventional, or traditional, hearing aids use analog technology to amplify sound but they do not correct distortions. These aids are the simplest type and are adjusted by the manufacturer based on an evaluation by an audiologist. Although the person wearing the aid can adjust its volume and the audiologist can make some minor adjustments, the aid becomes less effective as the person's hearing changes and may need to be replaced if the hearing loss progresses. Because analog aids amplify all sounds equally, they tend to be unsatisfactory for people who have only a mild high-frequency hearing loss and may be more beneficial to people with impairments at multiple frequencies. This characteristic also makes analog aids difficult to use in noisy environments, but older adults may find that they are satisfactory in quiet situations and one-on-one conversations. Nurses may need to encourage the selective use of analog aids in their appropriate environments. These aids are the least expensive type, with the cost beginning around $400. Cost is an important consideration because only the most comprehensive health insurance policies cover the cost of hearing aids and most people pay out-of-pocket for hearing aids. Until the cost of more sophisticated hearing aids decreases, these conventional hearing aids are likely to remain the most popular choice for older adults.

A variation of the conventional hearing aid is the recently developed disposable hearing aid, which lasts for about 30 to 40 days and costs about $40. They were developed for people with a mild to moderate hearing loss, and are about as effective as other analog hearing aids. Because they are not customized, they may not fit as well and are more likely to be associated with discomfort or feedback problems.

These aids were approved by the U.S. Food and Drug Administration (FDA) in 2000 and cannot be obtained without a prescription from a qualified hearing specialist. If these disposable hearing aids become more popular, it is likely that choices in size and amplification will increase.

Programmable analog hearing aids are more advanced than conventional hearing aids because they are selectively programmed to meet the needs of a hearing-impaired person. A major advantage of these hearing aids is that they are acoustically superior to conventional models and can be adjusted for different listening situations. Some programmable aids can automatically adjust their volume to the level of incoming sound by making soft sounds louder and loud sounds softer. Some programmable aids are equipped with a tiny remote control device, so the user can conveniently make adjustments for different environments. Remote devices are sometimes built into a wristwatch. Disadvantages include the need to train the wearer, the cost of up to several thousand dollars, and the need for frequent adjustments by the hearing health care professional.

Digital hearing aids use the most advanced technology and are the most flexible for individual needs because the audiologist uses a computer to program the aid to amplify specific frequencies for each person's hearing loss. The digital technology examines the incoming sounds and adapts the amplification without adding noise or distortion. In addition, some of these aids have directional microphones, enabling them to collect sounds from two directions and allowing the wearer to adjust the directionality. These aids can be programmed for different listening environments, and the wearer can use a remote control device to adjust the aid for various listening situations. The only disadvantage of these aids is their high cost, which is at least several thousand dollars.

Despite the major improvements in hearing aids in the last decade, only about 20% of people who could benefit from a hearing aid actually use one. Health education interventions can address negative attitudes and perceptions and have a positive effect on the use of hearing aids (Saunders et al., 2005). Nurses can play an important role in helping older adults to explore the many options for amplification by encouraging them to obtain accurate information from the organizations listed in the Educational Resources section. Nurses can encourage older adults and their families to obtain initial information about hearing aids from consumer and health care organizations, rather than primarily from a hearing aid dealer who sells only one kind of device. Many websites provide objective information about the various types of hearing aids. The International Hearing Society, for example, distributes a Hearing Aid Helpline consumer kit free of charge, and the Better Business Bureau provides information about local hearing aid dispensers. If financial or transportation limitations are problematic for an older person who is otherwise receptive to obtaining a hearing aid, nursing interventions can be aimed at identifying community resources to address these concerns.

In addition to the high cost of hearing aids, common barriers to obtaining and using them are the high levels of manual dexterity, fine motor movement, and good vision required to adjust the volume and other controls and to change batteries. Many of these barriers can be addressed by selecting the most appropriate hearing aid and through innovative techniques such as using a magnetic tool when changing the batteries and color coding battery doors (Saunders et al., 2005). Benefits of improved hearing include less paranoia and depression and higher levels of social support (Scialfa & Fernie, 2006).

Nurses who work with older adults in residential or other institutional settings can teach about the most effective use of hearing aids in different circumstances. For example, the older adult can be encouraged to use the aid for one-on-one conversations, but to remove it in the dining area or other large social areas where there is a lot of background noise. Nurses promote realistic expectations with regard to hearing aids by explaining that hearing aids do not restore normal hearing, but do improve communication and quality of life. Studies have found that the level of satisfaction with hearing aids increases gradually during the first year of use (Saunders et al., 2005).

Although it is impossible to know about all the available hearing aids, nurses need to keep up to date on various types and their implications for older adults. For example, it is important for nurses to know whether a person has an analog or a digital hearing aid, because the person with an analog aid may not be willing to use it in settings where background noise is problematic. It is also important for nurses to know if the person has a remote control device for the hearing aid, so the nurse can assist with adjusting the settings and give special attention to keeping track of the device.

Nurses must be familiar enough with hearing aids to assist older adults and their caregivers with their use and care. Although nurses can expect that hearing aid dispensers will provide initial instructions regarding use and care of the aid, these instructions may have to be reviewed or revamped as dependency needs and caregiver roles change. Older adults who normally depend on family members for assistance with their hearing aid may not be able to use and care for it properly when they are in a hospital or nursing home. Likewise, nurses in home settings may have to teach caregivers about hearing aids if the older adult needs assistance that was not previously provided by that caregiver. This situation is likely to arise if the caregiver changes, or if the older adult becomes more dependent because of increased functional impairment. Box 16-6 summarizes the teaching points related to the use and care of hearing aids.

Wellness Opportunity

Nurses promote self-care by providing educational brochures about the types and benefits of amplification devices and encouraging older adults to ask their primary care practitioners about an audiology referral.

Box 16-6
Use and Care of Hearing Aids

Guidelines for Insertion and Use

- With the volume of the device turned off and the canal portion pointing into the ear, insert the hearing aid.
- Make sure the aid fits snugly in the ear canal.
- The M, T, and O settings designate microphone, telephone, and off, respectively.
- Turn the M-T-O switch to M.
- Turn the volume up slowly, beginning at one third to one-half volume, until a comfortable level is reached.
- If whistling (feedback) is heard, check the position of the device in the ear and the volume. The aid may not fit snugly enough, or the volume may be too high.
- Begin wearing the aid for short periods, in a familiar and quiet environment, and in one-on-one conversations.
- Gradually increase the length of time the aid is worn, the variety of environments, and the number of people included in conversations.
- Allow several months before expecting to feel totally comfortable with the hearing aid.
- Avoid noisy environments and eliminate background noise when possible (e.g., turn off televisions and radios; close doors to rooms).
- Use the appropriate setting (T) for telephone calls.
- Understand that hearing aids do not restore hearing to normal, but rather amplify sound, including all environmental noises.

Guidelines for Care and Maintenance

- Keep a fresh battery available (batteries can be expected to last for 70 to 85 hours), but do not purchase batteries more than 1 month in advance.
- Turn off the hearing aid before changing the battery.
- Remove the battery or turn off the aid when not in use.
- Clean the aid weekly, using warm, soapy water for the earmold and a toothpick or pipe cleaner for the channel.
- Never use alcohol on the earmold because this will cause drying and cracking.
- Check the earmold for cracks or scratches.
- Avoid extreme heat, cold, or moisture (e.g., do not leave the hearing aid near the stove, do not wear it while using a hair dryer, and do not wear it outside in rainy or extremely cold weather unless it is protected well).
- Avoid exposure to chemicals, such as hairspray or permanent solutions.
- Avoid dropping the aid on a hard surface; when handling it, keep it over a soft or padded surface.

Communicating With Hearing-Impaired Older Adults

Good communication techniques are essential in assisting older adults to compensate for hearing deficits. The primary functional consequence of presbycusis is a diminished acuity for high-frequency sounds, which is exacerbated by fast speech pace and environmental noise. Therefore, communication interventions are directed toward improving the clarity of words, slowing the rate of speech, and eliminating environmental noise and distractions. Verbal techniques that enhance auditory communication should be augmented by nonverbal techniques such as body language and written communication, as described in Box 16-7. Nurses can apply these techniques and use this box for teaching caregivers how to improve communication with hearing-impaired people. In recent years, increased attention has been directed toward planning or modifying environments to diminish background noise and to improve the ability of people to hear. Although some noise control modifications, such as

Box 16-7
Techniques for Communicating With Hearing-Impaired People

- Stand or sit directly in front of, and close to, the person.
- Talk toward the better ear, but make sure your lips can be seen.
- Make sure the person pays attention and looks at your face.
- Address the person by name, pause, and then begin talking.
- Speak distinctly, slowly, and directly to the person.
- Do not exaggerate lip movements because this will interfere with lip reading.
- Avoid chewing gum, covering your mouth, or turning your head away.
- If the person does not understand, repeat the message using different words.
- Avoid or eliminate any background noise.
- Do not raise the volume of your voice; rather, try to lower the tone while still speaking in a moderately loud voice.
- Keep all instructions simple and ask for feedback to assess what the person heard.
- Avoid questions that elicit simple yes or no answers.
- Keep sentences short.
- Use body language that is congruent with what you are trying to communicate.
- Demonstrate what you are saying.
- Use large-print written communication and pictures to supplement verbal communication.
- Make sure only one person talks at a time; arrange for one-on-one communication whenever possible.
- If eyeglasses normally are worn to improve vision, make sure they are clean.
- Provide adequate lighting so that the person can see your lips; avoid settings in which there is glare behind or around you.

using window draperies, are relatively simple and can be applied to many settings, other measures, such as selection of building materials, need to be implemented while environments are being designed.

Mr. H. is now 83 years old and has been a widower for 1 year. He has given up hunting and woodworking because he developed Parkinson's disease 11 years ago and cannot manage the necessary fine motor movements. He continues to fish seasonally, play poker monthly, and smoke one pack per day of cigarettes. In addition to Parkinson's disease, he has hypertension and coronary artery disease. He still lives in his own home and attends the local senior center for meals and social activities three times a week. His hearing loss has progressed to the point that he has difficulty with phone conversations and has to turn the television up loud. He cannot hear the doorbell. At the senior center, participants avoid conversations with him because he has difficulty hearing.

You are the nurse at the senior center and you see him during your weekly "Wellness Clinic" for blood pressure checks. One week he tells you that his daughter is upset with him because he never answers his phone when she calls and she cannot have a decent phone conversation with him. She lives in another state and worries about him. She has offered to pay for a hearing aid evaluation for him, but he has told her "those things stick out like a sore thumb and they don't do any good anyway. I can hear anything I want to hear and there's a lot I don't care to hear so why should you spend a lot of money for something that I won't use." He asks your opinion about this and is wondering if he should at least get a checkup to pacify his daughter. He expects he will be told that nothing can be done, and that his daughter will have to be satisfied with the situation.

THINKING POINTS

- Which information in Box 16-2 would be most pertinent to obtain at this time?
- What myths and misunderstandings influence Mr. H.?
- What nursing diagnosis would you apply to Mr. H.?
- Which information in Box 16-5 would be pertinent to this situation?
- What health promotion teaching would you do to address Mr. H.'s resistance to having his hearing evaluated?
- What additional health promotion advice would you give?
- Because you usually see Mr. H. weekly, you can develop a long-term teaching plan. How would you establish priorities for immediate and long-term goals?

EVALUATING EFFECTIVENESS OF NURSING INTERVENTIONS

Nurses observe compensatory behaviors of hearing-impaired older adults to evaluate the effectiveness of interventions for the nursing diagnosis of Disturbed Sensory Perception: Auditory. The following are indicators of successful interventions:

- Improved ability to communicate
- Effective use of hearing aids and amplification devices
- Increased participation in social activities
- Environmental modifications to eliminate background noise
- Appropriate participation in aural rehabilitation programs

Evaluation of effectiveness of interventions varies in different health care settings. For example, nurses in short-term settings provide health education as part of a discharge plan that includes information about resources for hearing evaluations. Evaluation of the effectiveness of this intervention is based on the patient's positive response to the nurse's suggestions, but the nurse is not likely to know whether the person followed through with the referral and had beneficial outcomes. In home, community, and long-term care settings, nurses address long-term goals by facilitating referrals for audiology services. In these settings, the evaluation of interventions is based on the person's use of additional resources to improve communication abilities.

Mr. H. is an 89-year-old widower who has had Parkinson's disease for 17 years. Presbycusis is listed as an additional diagnosis on his medical record. He is being admitted to a nursing home because his condition has declined to the point that his daughter, Ms. D., can no longer manage his care in her home, where he has lived for several years. He is medically stable but needs assistance in all activities of daily living.

NURSING ASSESSMENT

During the admission interview, you notice that Mr. H. has difficulty hearing your questions and that he frequently asks his daughter to give the requested information. He

(case study continues on page 333)

shows no significant cognitive deficits, but he seems to have difficulty understanding verbal communication. When you ask about any hearing impairment, Ms. D. tells you that her father has used hearing aids for 5 years and has been reevaluated periodically at a speech and hearing center. Two months ago, he obtained new hearing aids, but wears them only for one-on-one conversations with her. Because of Mr. H.'s tremors and difficulty with fine motor movements, Ms. D. cares for his hearing aids and assists with their insertion and removal.

Ms. D. has encouraged her father to wear his hearing aids during family gatherings, but he says the noise from small children is too annoying. Except for family gatherings, Mr. H. has very few opportunities for social interaction, and he has become more and more withdrawn. He used to enjoy playing poker, but has not played in several years because all of his friends have died. Now he spends much of his time watching closed-captioned television programs. Ms. D. hopes that her father will respond to the opportunities for social interaction provided at the nursing home and that his quality of life will improve.

NURSING DIAGNOSIS

In addition to nursing diagnoses related to Mr. H.'s chronic illness and self-care deficits, you identify a nursing diagnosis of Impaired Social Interaction related to the effects of hearing loss. You select this, rather than Disturbed Sensory Perception: Auditory as a nursing diagnosis because Mr. H.'s hearing impairment has already been evaluated and sound amplification devices are available to him.

NURSING CARE PLAN FOR MR. H.

In your care plan, you address the psychosocial consequences of Mr. H.'s hearing impairment. Your nursing care is directed toward improving his social interaction through the use of available devices and through other communication techniques that will enhance his social interaction skills.

Expected Outcome	Nursing Interventions	Nursing Evaluation
Mr. H. will develop effective communication techniques for resident-staff interactions.	• During the initial interview, talk with Mr. H. and Ms. D. about the importance of good verbal communication with staff; emphasize the need for the staff to get to know Mr H so his needs can be addressed. • Ask Mr. H. to wear his hearing aids during all one-on-one interactions with staff. • Use good communication techniques when talking with Mr. H (as in Box 16-7). • Make sure all staff members provide appropriate assistance with insertion and removal of Mr. H.'s hearing aids. • Include hearing aid maintenance as part of the daily responsibilities of the nursing aide.	• Mr. H. will wear his hearing aids during all one-on-one conversations with staff. • Mr. H. will report satisfactory verbal interactions with the staff. • Mr. H.'s hearing aids will be maintained in good operating condition.
Mr. H. will engage in social interaction with one other resident.	• During the initial care plan conference, identify several other residents who might converse with Mr. H. • Ask the staff to encourage one-on-one conversations between Mr. H. and the selected resident (e.g., suggest that they watch closed-captioned television programs together).	• Mr. H. will wear his hearing aids at least once daily for a conversation with one other resident.

(case study continues on page 334)

Expected Outcome	Nursing Interventions	Nursing Evaluation
	• Ask Mr. H. to wear his hearing aids during one-on-one interactions with residents. • Provide assistance with inserting and removing hearing aids as needed. • Provide a quiet environment for one-on-one conversations with other residents.	
Mr. H. will engage in small group activities with other residents.	• During the first monthly care review conference, ask the activities staff to invite Mr. H. to a poker game with three other residents in the small-group room. • Make sure that environmental noise is controlled as much as possible.	• By the second month in this facility, Mr. H. will participate in weekly poker games with three other residents.

THINKING POINTS

- What nursing responsibilities would you have with regard to addressing Mr. H's hearing impairment? How would you work with other staff to implement the care plan described in the concluding case example?
- What are some of the advantages and disadvantages of hearing aids in a long-term care setting? How would you address the disadvantages?
- How would you involve Ms. D. in the care plan to address Mr. H.'s hearing impairment?
- If Mr. H. were in an acute care setting, how would you address his hearing problem?

CHAPTER HIGHLIGHTS

Age-Related Changes That Affect Hearing (Table 16-1)

- External ear: thicker hair, thinner skin, increased keratin
- Middle ear: less resilient tympanic membrane, calcified ossicles, stiffer muscles and ligaments
- Inner ear and auditory nervous system: fewer neurons and hair cells, diminished blood supply, degeneration of spiral ganglion and central processing systems

Risk Factors That Affect Hearing Wellness (Fig. 16-2, Box 16-1)

- Lifestyle and environmental factors: smoking, background noise, exposure to noise or toxic chemicals
- Genetic predisposition to otosclerosis
- Impacted cerumen
- Ototoxic medications: aminoglycosides, aspirin, loop diuretics, quinine
- Disease processes: diabetes, Paget's disease, Ménière's disease

Pathologic Condition Affecting Hearing

- Tinnitus: persistent sensation of noises that do not originate in the external environment

Functional Consequences Affecting Hearing Wellness (Table 16-1)

- Presbycusis: diminished ability to hear high-pitched sounds, especially in the presence of background noise
- Predisposition to impacted cerumen
- Psychosocial consequences: depression, social isolation, declines in cognitive function, diminished quality of life

Nursing Assessment of Hearing (Fig. 16-3, Boxes 16-2, 16-3, and 16-4)

- Screening tool: The Hearing Handicap Inventory for the Elderly
- Past and present risk factors (e.g., use of ototoxic medications, noise exposure, family history of otosclerosis)
- Attitudes about hearing aids if impairment is present
- Impact of hearing impairment on communication and quality of life
- Behavioral cues to impaired hearing
- Otoscopic examination for impacted cerumen
- Tuning fork tests for hearing

Nursing Diagnosis

- Readiness for Enhanced Communication
- Disturbed Sensory Perception: Auditory
- Additional diagnoses that address the functional consequences of impaired hearing: Impaired Communication, Anxiety, Impaired Adjustment, Impaired Social Interaction, and Ineffective Individual Coping, Risk for Injury

Planning for Wellness Outcomes

- Improved communication
- Increased social interactions
- Improved quality of life
- Increased safety and functioning

Nursing Interventions for Hearing Wellness (Fig. 16-4, Boxes 16-5, 16-6, and 16-7)

- Teaching about interventions to address modifiable risk factors: smoking, exposure to noise, use of ototoxic medications

- Removing and preventing impacted cerumen
- Promoting referrals for audiology services
- Using assistive listening devices
- Teaching about the use and care of a hearing aid
- Communicating with hearing-impaired older adults
- Compensating for hearing deficits by using hearing devices and hearing aids

Evaluating Effectiveness of Nursing Interventions

- Improved communication
- Use of appropriate amplification aids
- Appropriate environmental modifications
- Increased participation in social activities

Critical Thinking Exercises

1. Describe presbycusis and explain the functional consequences of this condition as it affects the everyday life of an older adult.
2. What risk factors would you consider in an 83-year-old person who complains of recent problems with hearing?
3. What advice would you give to someone who asks you about a brochure she received from a hearing aid company that offers free hearing screenings describing a new high-powered hearing aid? The person has trouble hearing, but has never had an evaluation.
4. Describe at least 10 ways in which you can adapt your communication for a hearing-impaired person.
5. Find at least one resource (*not* a hearing aid dealer) in your community that you could recommend to an older adult who needs a hearing evaluation.
6. Visit at least three Internet sites that provide educational materials about hearing impairment, and choose the one you think would be best for obtaining health information brochures.

Educational Resources

American Speech-Language-Hearing Association (ASHA)
www.asha.org

American Tinnitus Association (ATA)
www.ata.org

Better Hearing Institute (BHI)
www.betterhearing.org

Canadian Hard of Hearing Association
www.chha.ca

International Hearing Society (HIS)
www.ihsinfo.org

National Campaign for Hearing Health (NCHH)
www.hearinghealth.net

National Institute on Deafness and Other Communication Disorders (NIDCD)
www.nidcd.nih.gov/

Self Help for Hard of Hearing People, Inc. (SHHH)
www.shhh.org

References

Burr, H., Lund, S. P., Sperling, B. B., Kristensen, T. S., & Poulsen, O. M. (2005). Smoking and height as risk factors for prevalence and 5-year incidence of hearing loss: A questionnaire-based follow-up study of employees in Denmark aged 18–59 years and unexposed to noise. *International Journal of Audiology, 44*, 531–539.

Caban, A. J., Lee, D. J., Bomez-Marin, O., Lam, B. L., & Zheng, D. D. (2005). Prevalence of concurrent hearing and visual impairment in U.S. adults: The National Health Interview Survey, 1997–2002. *American Journal of Public Health, 95*, 1940–1942.

Carpenito-Moyet, L. J. (2006). *Handbook of nursing diagnosis* (11th ed.). Philadelphia: Lippincott Williams & Wilkins.

Culbertson, D. S., Griggs, M., & Hudson, S. (2004). Ear and hearing status in a multilevel retirement facility. *Geriatric Nursing, 25*, 93–98.

Depczynski, J., Franklin, R. C., Challinor, K., Williams, W., & Fragar, L. J. (2005). Farm noise emissions during common agricultural activities. *Journal of Agricultural Safety and Health, 121*, 325–334.

Divenyi, P. L., Stark, P. B., & Haupt, K. M. (2005). Decline of speech understanding and auditory thresholds in the elderly. *Journal of the Acoustical Society of America, 118*, 1089–1100.

Fozard, J., & Gordon-Salant, S. (2001). Changes in vision and hearing with age. In J. E. Birren & K. W. Schaie (Eds.), *The handbook of the psychology of aging* (5th ed., pp. 241–266). San Diego: Academic Press.

Hass-Slavin, L., McColl, M. A., & Pickett, W. (2005). Challenges and strategies related to hearing loss among dairy farmers. *Dairy Farmers, 21*, 329–326.

Helzner, E. P., Cauley, J. A., Pratt, S. R., Wisniewski, S. R., & Zmunda, J. M. (2005). Race and sex differences in age-related hearing loss: The health, aging and body composition study. *Journal of American Geriatrics Society, 53*, 2119–2127.

Johnson, M., Bulechek, G. M., Dochterman, J. M., Maas, M. L., Moorhead, S., Swanson, E., et al. (2006). *NANDA, NOC, and NIC linkages* (2nd ed.). St. Louis: Mosby Elsevier.

Kaufman, L. R., LeMasters, G. K., Olsen, D. M., & Succop, P. (2005). Effects of concurrent noise and jet fuel exposure on hearing loss. *Journal of Occupational and Environmental Medicine, 47*, 212–218.

Kujawa, S. M., & Liberman, M. C. (2006). Acceleration of age-related hearing loss by early noise exposure: Evidence of a misspent youth. *Journal of Neuroscience, 26*, 2115–2123.

Levy, B. R., Slade, M. D., & Gill, T. M. (2006). Hearing decline predicted by elders' stereotypes. *Journals of Gerontology: Series B, Psychological Sciences and Social Sciences, 61*, P82–P87.

McReynolds, M. C. (2005). Noise-induced hearing loss. *Air Medical Journal, 24*(2), 73-78.

Palmer, C. V., & Ortmann, A. (2005). Hearing loss and hearing aides. *Neurologic Clinics, 23*, 901–918.

Pan, C. C., Eisbruch, A., Lee, J. S., Snorrason, R. M., & Snorrason, R. M. (2005). Prospective study of inner ear radiation dose and hearing loss in head-and-neck cancer patients. *International Journal of Radiation Oncology, Biology and Physics, 61*, 1393–1402.

Saloranta, K., & Westermarck, T. (2005). Prevention of cerumen impaction by treatment of ear canal skin: A pilot randomized controlled study. *Clinical Otolaryngology, 30*, 112–114.

Saunders, G. H., Chisolm, T. H., & Abrams, H. B. (2005). Measuring hearing aid outcomes—not as easy as it seems. *Journal of Rehabilitation Research and Development, 42*, 157–168.

Schneider, B. A., Daneman, M., & Murphy, D. R. (2005). Speech comprehension difficulties in older adults: Cognitive slowing or age-related changes in hearing? *Psychology and Aging, 20*, 261–271.

Scialfa, C. T., & Fernie, G. R. (2006). Adaptive technology. In J. E. Birren & K. W. Schaie (Eds.), *The handbook of the psychology of aging* (6th ed., pp. 425–441). San Diego: Academic Press.

Singer, A. J., Sauris, E., & Viccellio, A. W. (2000). Ceruminolytic effects of docusate sodium: A randomized, controlled trial. *Annals of Emergency Medicine, 36*, 228–232.

Taylor, K. S., & Jurma, W. E. (2003, November 3). Gender-specific audiologic rehabilitation programs and self-perception of handicap in the elderly. *Audiology Online* (available at www.Audiologyonline.com/articles/article_detail.asp?article_id=509).

Thornton, R., & Light, L. L. (2006). Language comprehension and production in normal aging. In J. E. Birren & K. W. Schaie (Eds.), *The handbook of the psychology of aging* (6th ed., pp. 261–287). San Diego: Academic Press.

U.S. Department of Health and Human Services (USDHSS). (2000). *Healthy people 2010* (2nd ed.). Washington, DC: U.S. Government Printing Office.

Wild, D. C., Brewster, M. J., & Banerjee, A. R. (2005). Noise-induced hearing loss is exacerbated by long-term smoking. *Clinical Otolaryngology, 30*, 517–520.

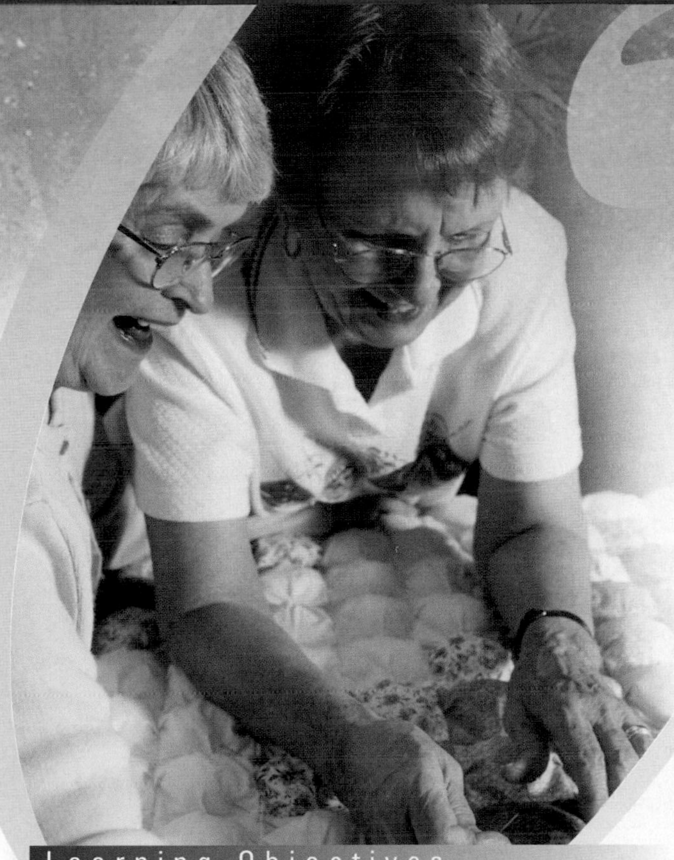

CHAPTER 17

Vision

Learning Objectives

After reading this chapter, you will be able to:

1. Describe age-related changes that affect vision.
2. Identify risk factors that can affect visual wellness.
3. Describe three pathologic conditions that cause vision impairments in older adults.
4. Discuss the functional consequences that affect visual wellness.
5. Conduct a nursing assessment of vision.
6. Identify environmental modifications and other interventions to facilitate visual wellness in older adults.

Key Terms

acuity
age-related macular degeneration (AMD)
arcus senilis
blepharochalasis
cataracts
color perception
critical flicker fusion
dark adaptation
depth perception
ectropion
enophthalmos
entropion
glare
glaucoma
low-vision aids
ophthalmologist
optician
optometrist
presbyopia
visual field

Because important daily activities—including communicating, enjoying visual images, and maneuvering in the environment—are highly dependent on eyesight, visual impairments can profoundly affect a person's safety, functioning, and quality of life. In older adults, age-related changes combine with risk factors to affect visual wellness. Fortunately, nurses have an array of interventions to assist older adults in maintaining optimal visual function. This chapter addresses functional consequences affecting vision in older adults and the impact of these changes on their vision. In addition, the chapter focuses on the role of the nurse in assessing vision and helping older adults to achieve visual wellness.

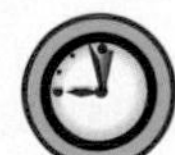 AGE-RELATED CHANGES THAT AFFECT VISION

Visual function depends on a sequence of processes, beginning with the perception of an external stimulus and ending with the processing of neural impulses in the cerebral cortex. Age-related changes affect all of the structures involved in visual function and alter visual perception for the older adult. In the absence of disease processes, these gradual changes have only a subtle impact on the daily activities of the older person. Unless compensatory actions are taken, however, age-related vision changes can interfere with the older person's quality of life and influence the enjoyment and safe performance of many activities.

Promoting Visual Wellness in Older Adults

Nursing Assessment
• Risk factors
• Environmental conditions (glare, lighting)
• Effects on daily activities
• Health behaviors (eye exams, protective measures)
Age-Related Changes
• ↓ elasticity in eyelids
• ↓ tear production
• ↑ corneal opacity
• Degenerative changes in all structures involved in visual function
Negative Functional Consequences
• ↓ ability to focus on near objects
• ↑ sensitivity to glare
• Need for ↑ illumination
• Dry eyes
• Difficulty driving at night
Risk Factors
• Glare, poor lighting
• Exposure to ultraviolet rays
• Smoking
• Nutrient deficiencies
• Adverse medication effects
• Diseases (diabetes, hypertension)
Nursing Interventions
• Addressing risk factors
• Modifying environments
• Suggesting aids to improve vision
• Referring for eye care
• Teaching about dry eyes
Wellness Outcomes
• Improved vision
• ↑ safety and functioning
• Better quality of life

Eye Appearance and Tear Ducts

Age-related changes in the tear ducts and the appearance of the eye and eyelids usually do not affect vision, but they are likely to affect visual wellness by causing anxiety and discomfort. Nurses can promote wellness by teaching older adults about comfort measures to relieve bothersome symptoms, as discussed later in this chapter.

As the eye ages, lipids accumulate in the outer part of the cornea, and a yellow or gray-white ring develops between the iris and the sclera. This phenomenon, termed **arcus senilis**, is the most common age-related corneal change and can be observed in most eyes by the age of 80 years in men and 90 in women (Yanoff, 2004). Other changes in the eye's appearance include diminished corneal translucency, yellowing of the sclera, and fading of the pigment in the iris.

Diversity Note

In whites and younger men, but not in African Americans, arcus senilis may be a sign of hyperlipidemia and increased risk for cardiovascular disease (Yanoff, 2004; Morrow et al., 2005).

Changes in the eyelids and surrounding skin include loss of orbital fat, development of wrinkles, decreased elasticity of the eyelid muscles, and accumulation of dark pigment around the eyes. These changes contribute to the overall appearance of sunken eyes, called **enophthalmos**. Loss of orbital fat and muscle elasticity can progress to the point of causing a lid fold and impairing vision. This condition, termed **blepharochalasis**, can be surgically treated. Relaxation of the lower lid muscles to an extreme degree results in the age-related conditions of ectropion or entropion. In **ectropion**, the lower lid falls away from the conjunctiva, blocking the flow of tears through the lower punctum and decreasing lubrication of the conjunctiva. In **entropion**, the lower lid becomes inverted and the eyelashes irritate the cornea, eventually leading to infection.

Age-related diminution in tear production leads to dry eye syndrome and complaints of dryness, burning, or photosensitivity. Subsequent irritation and rubbing of the cornea can lead to infections. Contrary to what might be expected, dry eye syndrome can cause excessive tearing because the lack of normal lubricating tears stimulates the production of reflex tears.

The Eye

Age-related changes in the eye itself also affect visual wellness. Specific structures of the eye that change with age include the cornea, lens, iris and pupil, ciliary body, vitreous, and retina (Fig. 17-1).

The *cornea* is a translucent covering over the eye that refracts light rays and provides 65% to 75% of the focusing power of the eye. As the eye ages, the cornea becomes opaque and yellow, interfering with the passage of light, especially ultraviolet rays, to the retina. Other corneal changes, such as the accumulation of lipid deposits, can cause an increased scattering of light rays and have a blurring effect on vision. In addition, age-related changes in the curvature of the cornea influence the refractive ability.

The *lens* consists of concentric and avascular layers of clear, crystalline protein. The lens has no blood supply, so it depends on the aqueous humor for metabolic and support functions. The transparent lens fibers are continually forming new layers without shedding old layers. As new layers form peripherally, the old layers are compressed inward toward the center, where they eventually become absorbed into the nucleus. This process gradually increases the size and density of the lens, causing a tripling of its mass by 70 years of age. Thus, the lens gradually becomes stiffer, denser, and more opaque.

Because of these age-related changes, the lens moves forward in the eye and is less responsive to the ciliary muscle. These changes also interfere with the transmission of light rays, diffusing the rays that pass through the lens and reducing the amount of light reaching the retina. These changes do not affect all wavelengths equally; rather, the most detrimental effect occurs with the shorter blue and violet wavelengths.

The *iris* is a pigmented sphincter muscle that dilates and contracts to control pupillary size and regulate the amount of light reaching the retina. With increasing age, the iris becomes more sclerotic and rigid, reducing the size of the *pupil* and interfering with its ability to respond to changes in light. The pupillary size begins to diminish during the third decade and levels off during the seventh decade. This condition, called *pupillary miosis*, significantly interferes with

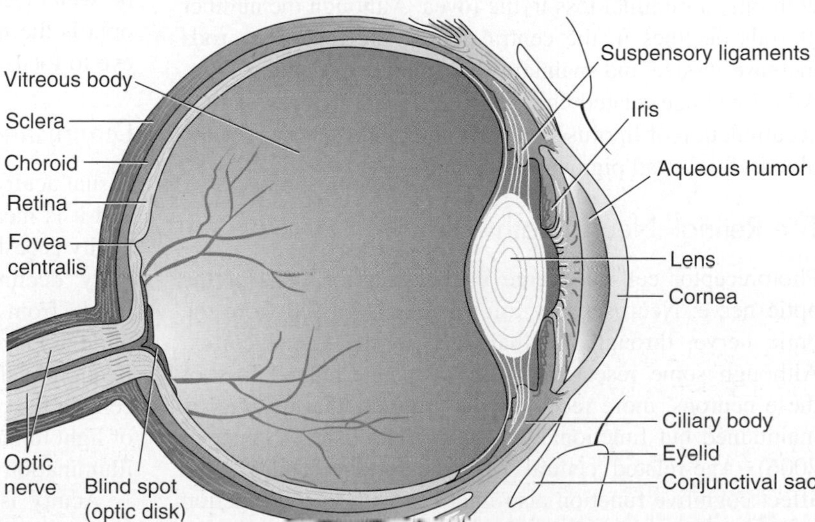

FIGURE 17-1 The eye. Age-related changes in structures of the eye can affect vision in older adults.

light reaching the retina, and is most pronounced in low levels of light (Schieber, 2006).

The *ciliary body* is a mass of muscles, connective tissue, and blood vessels surrounding the lens. These muscles regulate the passage of light rays through the lens by changing the shape of the lens. The ciliary body is responsible for accommodation, a process that controls one's ability to focus on near objects. In addition, the ciliary body produces aqueous fluid. Beginning in the fourth decade, the ciliary body gradually atrophies, and muscle cells are replaced with connective tissue. By the sixth decade, the ciliary body is smaller, stiffer, and less functional. With advanced age, diminished secretion of aqueous humor interferes with nourishment and cleansing of the lens and cornea.

The *vitreous* is a clear, gelatinous mass that forms the inner substance and maintains the spherical shape of the eye. During the fifth decade, this gelatinous substance begins to shrink and the proportion of liquid increases. These age-related changes can cause the vitreous body to pull away from the retina, resulting in symptoms such as floaters, blurred vision, distorted images, or light flashes. In addition, these changes can cause light to scatter more diffusely through the vitreous, reducing the amount of light reaching the retina.

The process of transforming visual stimuli into neural impulses begins in the rods and cones, which are pigment-producing photoreceptor cells in the *retina*. Rods do not perceive colors, but they are responsible for vision under low light. Cones require high levels of light to function effectively, and they are responsible for **color perception** and **acuity**, which is the ability to detect details and discern objects. Rods are distributed throughout the peripheral retina and cones are concentrated in the central and most sensitive part of the macula, called the *fovea*. Age-related changes affect the photoreceptor cells, with rod density beginning to diminish during the fourth decade and the loss of cones occurring at a slower pace (Schieber, 2006). The loss of cones occurs primarily in the periphery of the retina, with only a minimal loss in the fovea. Although the number of rods declines in the central retina, the remaining rods increase in size and maintain their ability to capture light. Additional age-related changes in retinal structures include accumulation of lipofuscin and thinning and sclerosis of the blood vessels and pigment epithelium.

The Retinal–Neural Pathway

Photoreceptor cells converge in the ganglion cells of the optic nerve. Neurosensory information is passed from the optic nerve, through the thalamus, to the visual cortex. Although some researchers report an age-related loss of these neurons, more recent studies suggest that quantity is maintained but functional efficiency diminishes (Schieber, 2006). Age-related central nervous system changes that affect cognitive function also interfere with visual function in older adults.

EFFECTS OF AGE-RELATED CHANGES ON VISION

All adults, regardless of race, sex, ethnicity, or socioeconomic status, notice some changes in their visual abilities by their fifth decade because age-related vision changes are an early biomarker of aging. Even the rare person who has 20/20 visual acuity at the age of 90 years experiences subtle changes in overall vision. However, despite the universal prevalence of age-related vision changes, most older adults can perform their usual activities by using low-vision aids and modifying their environment. Visual impairment, which is defined as vision loss that cannot be corrected by eyeglasses or contact lenses alone, ranges from mild impairment to blindness. Mild visual impairments are caused by normal age-related changes, but they are significantly exacerbated by environmental conditions such as glare and poor lighting. Compensatory interventions for the effects of age-related vision changes are quite effective for promoting visual wellness. For example, people who use reading glasses and bright but nonglaring light to improve their ability to read are compensating for mild visual impairment. These mild visual impairments are discussed in the following sections, and consequences of more significant visual impairments are discussed in the section that follows, Pathologic Conditions Affecting Vision.

Loss of Accommodation

Presbyopia is the loss of accommodation, which is the ability to focus clearly and quickly on objects at various distances. Presbyopia is an initial and universal age-related vision change, which begins in early adulthood and affects all humans to some degree by their mid-50s (Croft & Kaufman, 2006). This vision change is caused by degenerative changes in the lens and the ciliary body. Functionally, accommodative changes gradually extend the near point of vision, which is the closest point at which a small object can be seen clearly. A typical example of the effects of presbyopia is the need to hold reading materials farther from the eye to focus clearly on the print.

Diminished Acuity

Visual acuity is customarily assessed using a Snellen chart, and it is measured against a normal value of 20/20. Visual acuity is best around the age of 30 years, after which it gradually declines with increasing age. Diminished acuity results from age-related ocular changes, including decreased pupillary size, scatter of light in the cornea and lens, opacification of the lens and vitreous, and loss of photoreceptor cells in the retina. These changes interfere with the passage of light to the retina, causing a threefold reduction in retinal illumination between the ages of 20 and 60 years.

Acuity is also influenced by extraocular factors, such as the size and movement of an object and the amount of light reflected off an object. Low or poor illumination compounds the effects of age-related ocular changes, particularly on visual acuity. Visual acuity is more impaired for moving objects than for stationary objects, and it becomes more impaired with increasing speed of the object. This combination of age-related changes and external factors hinders the older person's ability to see moving objects and to perform tasks in low illumination. Consequently, older people require a relatively greater degree of illumination and may experience a marked decline in night driving competence.

Delayed Dark and Light Adaptation

The ability to respond to dim light, called **dark adaptation**, begins to decline around 20 years of age and diminishes more markedly after the age of 60 years. This decline is associated with decreased retinal illumination as well as age-related changes in the retina and retinal–neural pathways. The functional impact of these changes is that the older adult requires more time to adapt to dim lighting when moving from a brighter to a darker environment. For instance, when entering a darkened movie theater, an older person needs extra time to adapt to the changes in lighting before proceeding to a seat.

Age-related changes in the lens and pupil interfere with the response to bright lights because they reduce the amount of light reaching the retina. In practical terms, this means that an older person responds more slowly to lights such as car headlights and requires more time to recover from exposure to glare and bright lights.

Increased Glare Sensitivity

Glare occurs when scattered light in the optic media reduces the clarity of visual images. Glare is experienced when light is reflected from shiny surfaces, when the light is excessively bright or inappropriately focused, or when bright light originates from several sources at once. Glare is classified according to three types: veiling, dazzling, and scotomatic. *Veiling glare* is caused by the scattering of light over the retinal surface and results in diminished contrast of the viewed object. Veiling glare occurs, for example, when bright fluorescent lights in a grocery store reflect on the clear plastic covering over food products in a white case. *Dazzling glare*, which is caused by bright visual displays, interferes with the ability to discern details. Glass-covered directories in brightly lit shopping malls produces a dazzling glare that interferes with a person's ability to read the words in the directory, particularly if there is poor contrast between the letters and the background. *Scotomatic glare* is a blinding glare caused by loss of retinal sensitivity and overstimulation of retinal pigments during exposure to bright lights. For example, sunshine can create scotomatic glare, especially at sunrise or sunset.

Beginning in the fifth decade, age-related changes increase a person's sensitivity to glare and the time required to recover from glare. Glare sensitivity is influenced primarily by opacification of the lens; however, it also is affected by age-related changes in the pupil and vitreous. Functionally, these changes can significantly affect the person's ability to read signs, see objects, drive at night, and maneuver safely in bright environments. In many modern buildings and shopping malls, the bright lights, large windows, and highly reflective floors generate glare that can lead to accidents and inaccurate perceptions.

Reduced Visual Field

A **visual field** is an oval-shaped area encompassing the total view that people perceive while looking at a fixed point straight ahead. The scope of the visual field narrows slightly between the ages of 40 and 50 years and then declines steadily. Functionally, the visual field is important when people engage in tasks that require a broad perception of the environment and moving objects. Walking in crowded places and driving a vehicle are examples of activities that depend on the field of vision.

Diminished Depth Perception

Depth perception is the visual skill responsible for locating objects in three-dimensional space, judging differences in the depth of objects, and observing relationships among objects in space. Functionally, depth perception enables people to use objects effectively and to maneuver safely in the environment. As with many other visual skills, depth perception depends on interactions between ocular and extraocular factors. *Stereopsis*, or the disparity between retinal images that is caused by the separation of the two eyes, is the primary ocular characteristic that affects depth perception. Extraocular factors that influence depth perception include prior perceptual experiences of the observer; movement of the observer's head or body; and characteristics of the object, such as size, height, distance, texture, brightness, and shading. Depth perception declines with increasing age, and this can contribute to falls and tripping because of miscalculations about the distance and height of objects.

Altered Color Vision

Pigments in the retinal cones absorb light in the red, blue, or yellow ranges of the spectrum. As with many other visual functions, color perception is influenced by the type and quantity of light waves reaching the retina. Consequently, any age-related changes that interfere with retinal illumination—including lens opacification, pupillary miosis, retinal or retinal–neural changes—can interfere with accurate color perception. Opacification and yellowing of the lens interferes most directly with shorter wavelengths, causing an altered perception of blues, greens, and violets. Low levels of illumination and other environmental factors also interfere with color perception.

Functionally, altered color perception is manifested as a relative darkening of blue objects and a yellowed perception of white light. Accurate color perception is not essential in all daily activities, but it is important, for instance, in differentiating between medications that are similar in color or tone, especially those in the blue-green and yellow-white ranges. In addition, altered color perception can interfere with the detection of spoiled food.

Diminished Critical Flicker Fusion

Critical flicker fusion is the point at which an intermittent light source is perceived as a continuous, rather than flashing, light. The ability to perceive flashing lights accurately is a function of the retinal receptors and is influenced by extraocular factors, such as the size, color, and luminance of the object. Age-related changes in the retina and retinal–neural pathway, as well as changes that decrease retinal illumination, interfere with critical flicker fusion. Low levels of illumination further exacerbate the effects of these changes. Functionally, diminished critical flicker fusion distorts the perception of a flashing light, making it appear to be a continuous light. Thus, diminished critical flicker fusion can interfere with the discernment of emergency vehicles and road construction lights, especially at night.

Slower Visual Information Processing

Age-related changes of the retinal–neural pathway affect the accuracy and efficiency of visual information processing. Thus, older adults generally need more time to process visual information, but the effects are minimal or negligible when tasks are familiar. Table 17-1 summarizes age-related vision changes and their effects on vision.

TABLE 17-1 Age-Related Changes Affecting Vision

Change	Consequence
Appearance and Comfort	
• Decreased elasticity of the eyelid muscles	Potential for ectropion, entropion, blepharochalasis
• Enophthalmos	
• Decreased tears	Potential for dry eye syndrome
Structures	
• Yellowing and increased opacity of cornea	**Presbyopia:** diminished ability to focus on near objects
• Changes in the corneal curvature	
• Increase in lens size and density	Diminished accommodation
• Sclerosis and rigidity of the iris	Diminished acuity
• Decrease in pupillary size	Slower response to changes in illumination
• Atrophy of the ciliary muscle	Increased sensitivity to glare
• Shrinkage of gelatinous substance in the vitreous	Narrowing of the visual field
• Atrophy of photoreceptor cells	Diminished depth perception
• Thinning and sclerosis of retinal blood vessels	Altered color perception
• Degeneration of neurons in the visual cortex	Distorted perception of flashing lights Slower processing of visual information

RISK FACTORS THAT AFFECT VISUAL WELLNESS

Lifestyle and environmental factors—including both immediate and long-term conditions—exacerbate age-related vision changes and interfere with visual wellness. Forexample, long-term exposure to ultraviolet light (i.e., sunlight) is associated with the development of cataracts and loss of photoreceptor cells, particularly the cones. Furthermore, older adults are more vulnerable to eye damage from sunlight because age-related changes alter the protective response to harmful ultraviolet light. Warmer environmental temperatures are associated with an earlier age of onset for presbyopia (i.e., loss of near vision). Dry eyes can be caused by environmental conditions such as wind, sunlight, low humidity, and cigarette smoke. Other environmental influences on visual wellness include glare, dim lighting, and poor color contrast. Cigarette smoking is a lifestyle factor that increases the risk for cataracts and macular degeneration.

Wellness Opportunity

Poor lighting and exposure to sunlight are risk factors that can readily be addressed through simple self-care practices.

Chronic conditions can adversely affect visual function in a variety of ways. Vision impairments commonly occur in people with Alzheimer's or Parkinson's disease, even during the early stages. People with diabetes are at increased risk of development of cataracts, glaucoma, and diabetic retinopathy. People with hypertension or hypercholesterolemia are at higher risk for age-related macular degeneration (AMD). Malnutrition has been associated with cataract development, and vitamin A deficiency has been associated with dry eyes from reduced tear production.

Medications that are associated with adverse effects on vision include aspirin, haloperidol, nonsteroidal anti-inflammatory agents, tricyclic antidepressants, digitalis, anticholinergics, phenothiazines, isoniazid, tamoxifen, amiodarone, sildenafil, and oral or inhaled corticosteroids. Cataracts are common in people with glaucoma because of the anticholinesterase drugs used in glaucoma treatment. Medications that can cause or contribute to dry eyes include estrogen, diuretics, antihistamines, anticholinergics, phenothiazines, beta-blockers, and antiparkinson agents. Systemic anticoagulants can precipitate intraocular hemorrhage in people with preexisting macular degeneration.

Mrs. F. is 60 years old and has used "readers" (reading glasses) for 15 years, but has never needed glasses for anything other than reading and sewing. She recently noticed that she has trouble reading the glass-enclosed directory at the shopping mall. She works in an office building with an atrium that has skylights, and she has trouble reading the signs on the doors.

THINKING POINTS

- What age-related factors contribute to the vision changes that Mrs. F. notices?
- What environmental factors are likely to contribute to Mrs. F.'s difficulty when she is in the shopping mall or at work?
- When Mrs. F. is in her home environment, what tasks might be more difficult because of age-related vision changes?

PATHOLOGIC CONDITIONS AFFECTING VISION

Chronic conditions that interfere with visual wellness occur very commonly in older adults, so nurses have important roles in detecting and managing these conditions. Health promotion interventions are particularly important with conditions like glaucoma because interventions can prevent vision impairment. However, this condition is often undiagnosed so the interventions are not implemented in a timely manner. Among older adults, the three most common pathologic eye conditions are cataracts, AMD, and glaucoma (Fig. 17-2, Table 17-2).

Cataracts

Cataracts are the leading and most reversible cause of visual impairment in older adults. About one fourth of noninstitutionalized people 70 years of age and older reported that they

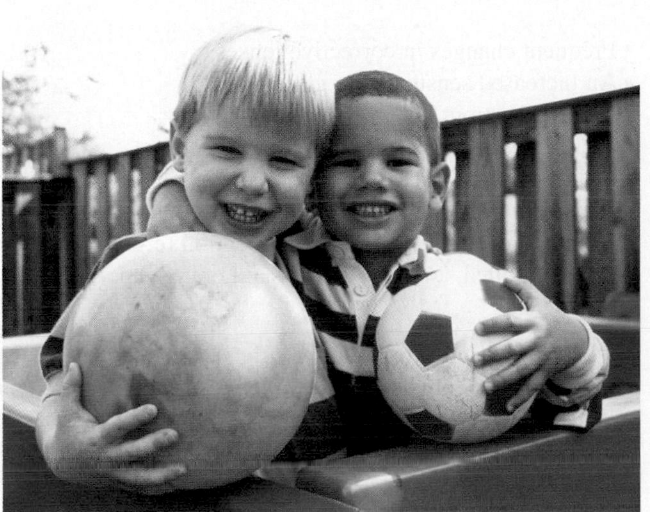

Normal vision

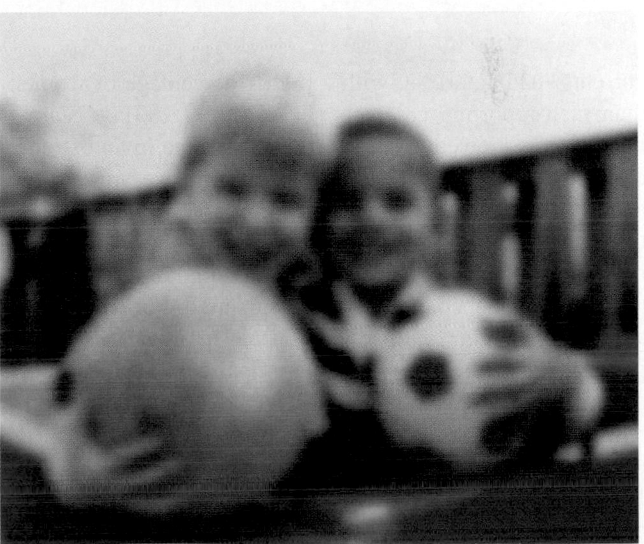

Cataracts

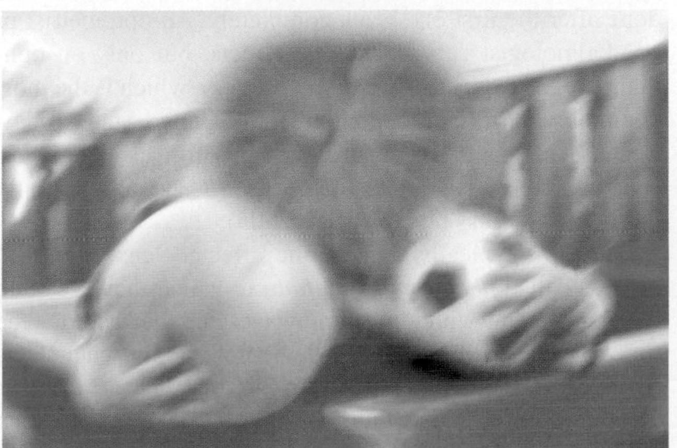

Macular degeneration

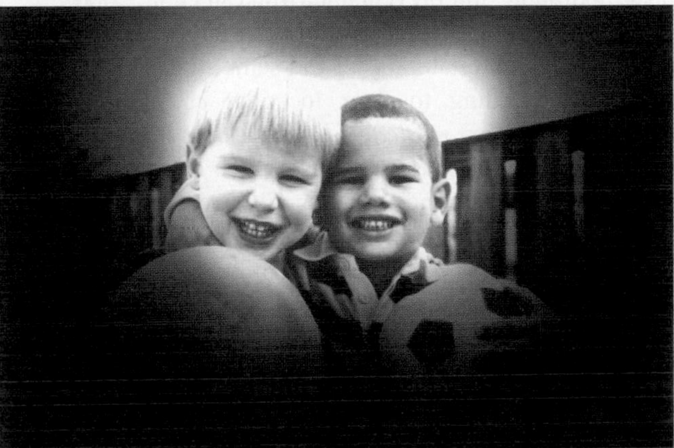

Glaucoma

FIGURE 17-2 Examples of normal vision, vision with cataracts, vision with age-related macular degeneration, and vision with glaucoma. (Courtesy of the National Eye Institute, National Institutes of Health.)

TABLE 17-2 Common Disease Conditions Affecting Vision

	Risk Factors	Symptoms	Management
Cataract	Advanced age, exposure to sunlight, smoking, diabetes, malnutrition, trauma or radiation to the eye or head, medications (corticosteroids, phenothiazines, amiodarone, benzodiazepines, anticholinesterases)	Increased sensitivity to glare, decreased contrast sensitivity, blurred vision, distorted images, double vision, diminished color perception, frequent eyeglass prescription changes	Surgical removal of lens followed by implantation of an intraocular lens
Age-Related Macular Degeneration (AMD)	Advanced age, non-Hispanic white ethnicity, family history of AMD, smoking, hypertension, hyperlipidemia, medications (tamoxifen, phenothiazines, chloroquine)	Gradual progressive loss of central vision, distorted straight lines, blurred vision	Visual rehabilitation programs, argon laser therapy for wet type, experimental treatments under investigation for both types
Glaucoma	Advanced age, African American race, family history of glaucoma, diabetes, medications (anticholinergics, corticosteroids)	**Chronic:** Slow onset, diminished vision in dim light, increased sensitivity to glare, decreased contrast sensitivity, diminished peripheral vision	**Chronic**: Medical therapy with miotics, adrenergic agonists, carbonic anhydrase inhibitors, beta-blockers, and prostaglandins (administered as eye drops)
		Acute: sudden onset, intense pain, blurred vision, halos around lights, nausea and vomiting	**Acute**: immediate treatment with medications to reduce pressure, followed by laser surgery

currently had cataracts, with a higher percentage of women than men reporting cataracts (Desai et al., 2001). Cataract formation is viewed as an age-related change in an extreme degree because changes in the lens begin in everyone by the age of 40 years and eventually can progress to the point of total opacification. As cataracts progress, the normally transparent lens becomes cloudy, transmission of light to the retina is diminished, and vision is impaired. For some older adults, the degree of opacification never progresses to the point of causing significant visual impairment, but for many older adults it does. In addition to being caused by age-related changes, risk factors include systemic disease, medications, and environmental factors, as summarized in Table 17-2. Also, cataracts are likely to occur more commonly after glaucoma surgery or other types of eye surgery. Among risk factors for cataracts, cigarette smoking is a factor that is the most modifiable and preventable (Mukesh et al., 2006).

Cataracts usually occur in both eyes, but they do not necessarily progress bilaterally at the same rate. Cataracts are classified according to their location: *cortical* cataracts occur in the cortex, *nuclear* cataracts occur in the nucleus, and *posterior subcapsular* cataracts occur on the back of the membrane that surrounds the lens. The location of cataracts significantly influences their impact, with nuclear cataracts interfering the most with vision.

In their early stages, cataracts do not necessarily affect visual acuity, but as they progress, they cause difficulty performing activities such as reading and night driving (see Fig. 17-2). People with cataracts are likely to experience any of the following vision changes:

- Dimmed or blurred vision
- Distorted or double images
- Frequent changes in corrective lenses
- An increased sensitivity to glare
- A need for more light when reading
- The perception of a "film" over the eye
- A diminished ability to discern contrast
- The perception of halos around bright lights
- Distorted or diminished color perception (e.g., blue appears dulled, and red, yellow, and orange appear brighter).

Cataracts cannot be treated with medication, but in the early stages they are managed by the prescription of stronger eyeglasses or contact lenses. When visual acuity declines to about 20/50 and cataracts affect the person's safety or quality of life, cataract surgery is usually recommended. When surgery is required for both eyes, the procedure is usually done on one eye at a time, with the second surgery being done after the first one heals completely. An optometrist or ophthalmologist can diagnose cataracts, but only an ophthalmologist can perform cataract surgery, which is the most commonly performed operation in the United States today. Because of many recent advances in surgical techniques, cataract surgery is simpler than it used to be and currently has a 99% success rate (Slusher, 2005).

Surgeons typically remove the affected lens through a process called *phacoemulsification*, in which they break up the clouded lens with ultrasound waves and then aspirate the tiny particles with a suction device. After the cataract is removed, the surgeon implants an intraocular lens. The surgical procedure is done with local anesthesia, takes less than 1 hour, and has a very low rate of complications. If the person needed corrective lenses before the surgery, the surgeon can insert an intraocular lens that mimics the natural focusing ability of the eye and results in improved vision with little or no need for additional correction. Although there is a high rate of satisfaction with this type of intraocular lens, patients commonly report continued difficulty with glare and halos (Slusher, 2005).

Nurses have an important role in dispelling myths that might interfere with older adults obtaining surgical treatment for cataracts. For example, older adults might think that cataract surgery is riskier or more complicated than it actually is because they are familiar with experiences of older friends or relatives who had cataract surgery many years ago. Nurses can emphasize that significant progress has been made in techniques for cataract surgery in recent years and that there are many benefits, especially when the vision impairment interferes with safety and quality of life. Wellness outcomes after cataract surgery include significant improvements in visual and cognitive function as well as emotional and general well-being (Gray et al., 2006).

Diversity Note

Among Medicare recipients, African Americans are only 60% as likely as whites to undergo cataract surgery (Wilson & Eezzuduemhoi, 2005).

Although nurses need not be thoroughly familiar with the surgical techniques, they can emphasize that the techniques used today are much simpler and have an extremely high success rate. Moreover, nurses can encourage older adults to seek reliable information and periodic evaluations from eye care professionals, rather than simply tolerating a loss of vision due to cataracts. Nurses also can emphasize that studies indicate that cataract surgery can significantly improve safety, functioning, and quality of life (Foss et al., 2006)

Wellness Opportunity

Nurses promote responsible decision making by encouraging older adults and their caregivers to explore risks and benefits of cataract surgery.

Age-Related Macular Degeneration

Age-related macular degeneration (AMD) is the leading cause of severe vision loss in older adults in the United States and other developed countries. AMD, in various stages, affects 18% of people between the ages of 70 and 74 years, and 47% of people 85 years of age and older. In younger adults, the prevalence of AMD does not differ significantly by sex or race, but in people 70 years and older, AMD affects women more than men and non-Hispanic whites more than African Americans. AMD is associated with the risk factors summarized in Table 17-2.

Early in the disease, deposits of yellow byproducts of retinal pigment, called *drusen*, build up in the macula, which is the area in the middle of the retina where visual acuity is best. As the disease progresses, it is classified either as *dry type*, which accounts for 80% to 90% of cases, or *wet (exudative) type*. In the dry type, damage is caused by death of the photoreceptors, which is seen on funduscopy as tiny areas of atrophy of the retinal pigment epithelium. The dry type of AMD usually progresses slowly and does not cause total blindness; however, if the wet type develops, visual loss can be rapid and severe. In the wet type, the damage is caused by the formation of new blood vessels in the choroid, a process called *choroidal neovascularization*, followed by hemorrhage into the subretinal space.

In the early stage of AMD, the person experiences blurred vision and has difficulty reading, especially in dim light. Like most other eye conditions, AMD occurs in both eyes, but it can appear initially in only one eye and its course may differ in each eye. As AMD progresses, it affects central vision and significantly interferes with activities such as reading, driving, watching television, recognizing people, and performing many other self-care activities (see Fig. 17-2). The primary treatment goal for patients with either type of AMD is to reduce the risk of further vision loss.

Laser photocoagulation and photodynamic therapy are two interventions that are effective in treating the choroidal neovascularization that occurs in the wet type of AMD. Not all people with the wet form meet the medical criteria for these two treatments, however. Another disadvantage of these treatments is that only a small percentage of patients experience significant long-term effects. Some progress is being made with regard to biologic or pharmacologic agents that halt the disease process, so nurses can encourage anyone with AMD to obtain information about clinical trials and new developments through reliable sources such as the National Eye Institute and other organizations listed in the Educational Resources section.

Nurses often serve in support roles by encouraging older adults to participate in vision rehabilitation programs so they can learn the most effective ways of compensating for declining vision. People with AMD are usually taught to test their eyes daily using the Amsler grid (Fig. 17-3) so they will be aware of sudden changes. In long-term care settings and for older adults with memory problems, nurses may have to provide daily reminders or assistance with carrying out this task. Nurses also need to encourage people with AMD to receive ongoing evaluation by eye care practitioners to detect treatable aspects of this disease.

Wellness Opportunity

Nurses holistically address needs of people with AMD by encouraging them to explore support groups and educational services associated with a Sight Center.

Glaucoma

The term **glaucoma** refers to a group of eye diseases in which the ganglion cells of the optic nerve are damaged by an abnormal build-up of aqueous humor in the eye. Aqueous

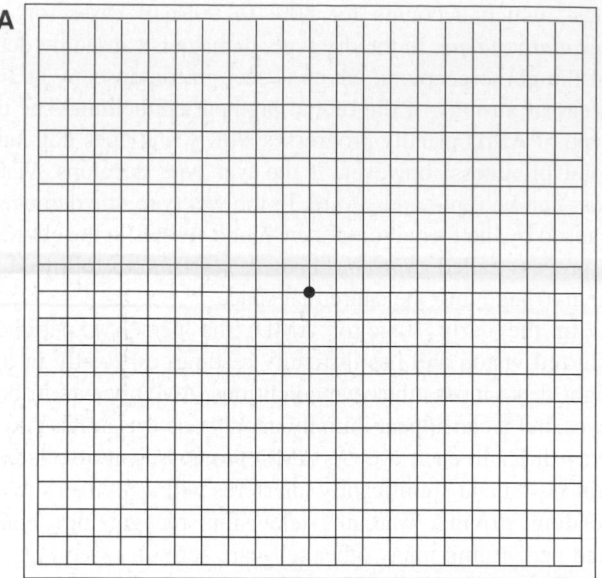

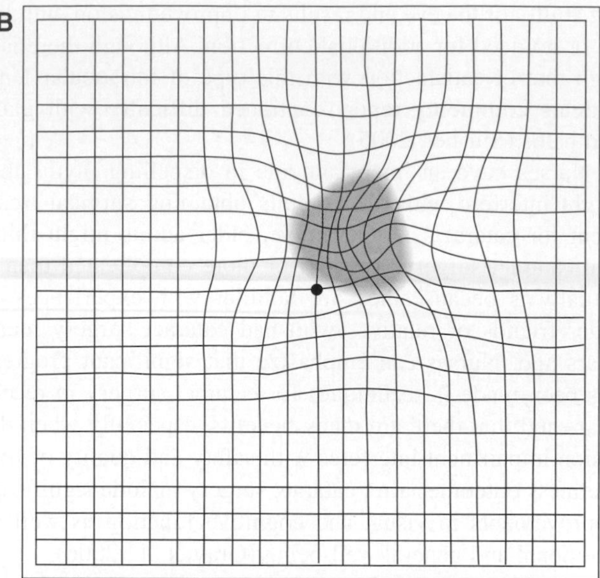

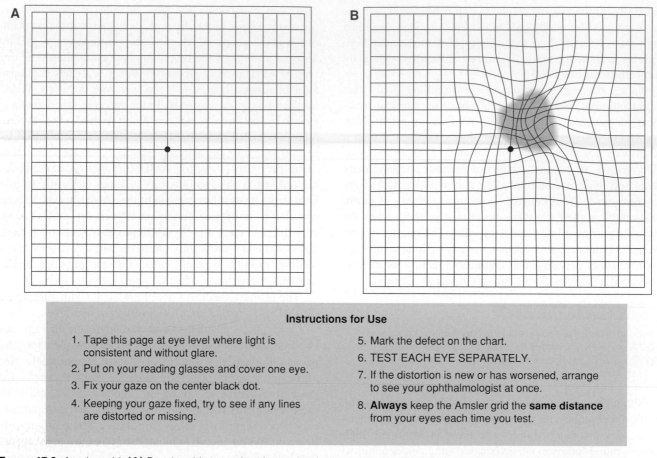

Instructions for Use

1. Tape this page at eye level where light is consistent and without glare.
2. Put on your reading glasses and cover one eye.
3. Fix your gaze on the center black dot.
4. Keeping your gaze fixed, try to see if any lines are distorted or missing.
5. Mark the defect on the chart.
6. TEST EACH EYE SEPARATELY.
7. If the distortion is new or has worsened, arrange to see your ophthalmologist at once.
8. **Always** keep the Amsler grid the **same distance** from your eyes each time you test.

FIGURE 17-3 Amsler grid. **(A)** People with age-related macular degeneration (AMD) use the Amsler grid to perform a simple daily test for sudden changes in their condition. **(B)** This is what the Amsler grid might look like to someone with AMD. (*Part A:* Reprinted with permission from American Macular Degeneration Foundation, 888-MACULAR, www.macular.org.)

humor is a clear fluid that is produced in the anterior chamber of the eye and normally maintains eye pressure between 10 and 20 mm Hg. If the fluid cannot flow out of the anterior chamber of the eye through the channel between the iris and the cornea, it accumulates and pushes the optic nerve into a cupped or concave shape. The resulting damage to the optic nerve causes a loss of peripheral vision. If left untreated, the damage can progress to blindness. About 8% of noninstitutionalized older adults have glaucoma, with a much higher prevalence among African Americans (15%) than whites (7%) (Desai et al., 2001). Glaucoma is the second leading cause of blindness in the United States, and the leading cause of irreversible blindness in African Americans.

Diversity Note

African Americans have an earlier age of onset of glaucoma than do whites.

Chronic (open-angle) glaucoma, which accounts for as much as 90% of cases of glaucoma in the United States, occurs when the drainage canals become clogged. This condition has an insidious onset and affects vision when the optic nerve becomes damaged. Early signs include increased intraocular pressure, poor vision in dim lighting, and increased sensitivity to glare. If the condition progresses, manifestations include headaches, "tired eyes," impaired peripheral vision, a fixed and dilated pupil, the perception of halos around lights, and frequent changes in the prescription for corrective lenses. Chronic glaucoma usually occurs in both eyes, but can begin in only one eye and does not necessarily progress at the same rate in both eyes. Because chronic glaucoma progresses slowly and causes little or no visual impairment in the early stage, annual assessments of intraocular pressure are necessary to detect the condition before visual impairments occur. Chronic glaucoma is most commonly managed with medications, but surgical treatment options include argon laser surgery and other types of eye surgery. Medication management commonly includes one or more of the following types of eye drops: miotics, prostaglandins, beta-blockers, adrenergic agonists, and carbonic anhydrase inhibitors.

Normal-tension glaucoma is another type of glaucoma that occurs in older adults. With this type of glaucoma, the intraocular pressure is within the normal range, but the optic nerve is damaged and the visual field is narrowed (see

Fig. 17-2). This condition is often managed with the same medications and surgical approaches that are used for chronic glaucoma.

Acute (closed-angle) glaucoma is caused by a sudden complete blockage of the flow of aqueous humor. This condition has an abrupt onset in one or both eyes and should be considered a medical emergency. People with acute glaucoma present with increased intraocular pressure, severe eye pain, clouded or blurred vision, dilation of the pupil, and nausea and vomiting. This condition can be precipitated by medications that cause pupil dilation, such as anticholinergics. Immediate treatment with medications is usually effective for acute attacks, but surgical intervention is often needed.

Health education for older adults with glaucoma focuses on the importance of adhering to ongoing medication routines and regularly being evaluated by their eye care practitioner. If older adults with glaucoma are admitted for institutional care, nurses need to ensure that prescribed eye drops are administered as ordered. In home care situations, nurses may need to develop a plan for administering eye drops on a daily or more frequent basis. If an older adult has memory problems, establishing a routine for administering eye drops can be quite challenging. Many times, complicated eye drop regimens can be simplified by working with the eye care practitioner to decrease the number of eye drops that are necessary or to prescribe a longer-acting medication that can be administered less frequently.

Wellness Opportunity

Nurses promote self-care by teaching people with glaucoma to be aware of prescription and over-the-counter medications that can exacerbate glaucoma.

Mrs. F. is now 72 years old and has been retired for several years. You are the nurse at her local senior center and she makes an appointment to see you. Mrs. F.'s medical history indicates that she has smoked a pack of cigarettes a day for 40 years and has been taking medications for hypertension and arthritis for 5 years. During a recent medical checkup, her doctor said he thought she had early cataracts, but he told Mrs. F. that he felt it was too early to do anything about them. She has never had an eye examination, other than what her regular doctor does periodically. When asked about her symptoms, Mrs. F. tells you that she sometimes feels like there is a film over her eyes and she has trouble seeing when she is outside on sunny days. Mrs. F. says that she never liked wearing sunglasses and hopes she won't have to start wearing them now. She has recently purchased stronger reading glasses, and these help a little with reading and sewing.

THINKING POINTS

- What factors likely contributed to the development of Mrs. F.'s cataracts?
- When Mrs. F. is driving during the day, what difficulties might she notice because of vision changes? Because of environmental conditions?
- When Mrs. F. is driving at night, what difficulties might she notice because of vision changes? Because of environmental conditions?
- When Mrs. F. is in her home, what changes in visual abilities might she notice because of cataracts?

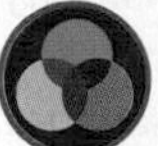

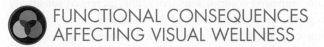

FUNCTIONAL CONSEQUENCES AFFECTING VISUAL WELLNESS

The most serious visual impairments that affect older adults are associated with pathologic conditions, such as cataracts, glaucoma, or AMD, all of which are increasingly likely to occur with advanced age. Visual impairments are categorized as "functional" when acuity is 20/50 or worse, as "low vision" when it is between 20/70 and 20/200, and as "blindness" when it is 20/400 or worse. People 65 years of age and older account for 30% of all visually impaired people in the United States, and for almost 37% of all visits to physicians' offices for eye care. Trouble seeing, even with corrective lenses, affects 14% of people between the ages of 70 and 74 years and 32% of those 85 years and older (Desai et al., 2001). The following sections describe the functional consequences that are associated with the types of visual impairments that are most likely to occur in older adults.

Diversity Note

African Americans and Hispanic Americans have a higher prevalence of blindness and visual impairment than do whites.

Effects on Safety and Function

Because visual impairments are associated with many aspects of safety and functioning, people who are visually impaired are likely to be more dependent in their activities of daily living. Age-related vision changes most directly influence the following activities:

- Getting outside
- Driving a vehicle
- Shopping for groceries
- Going up and down stairs
- Getting in and out of bed or a chair
- Maneuvering safely in dark or unfamiliar environments
- Seeing markings on clocks, radios, thermostats, appliances, and televisions
- Reading newspapers, directories, small-print signs and posters, and labels on food items and medication containers

Most of these activities are affected by alterations in several visual skills. In addition, the ability to perform these activities is influenced significantly by glare, lighting, and other environmental factors.

Visual impairments threaten safe functioning because they can affect gait, balance, and postural stability. They also increase the risk of falls, fractures, and other serious injury secondary to falling. Lord and Dayhew (2001), in a 1-year study of 156 community-living people between the ages of 63 and 90 years, found that impaired vision is an important and independent risk factor for falls. Age-related vision changes that increase the risk for falls include diminished acuity, reduced visual field, diminished depth perception, impaired contrast sensitivity, and increased sensitivity to glare. In addition, delayed processing of visual information can interfere with the quick responses necessary for avoiding falls.

The negative impact of visual impairments can exacerbate the effects of other functional impairments. For example, people who have Parkinson's or Alzheimer's disease are more likely to experience visual hallucinations if they also have decreased visual acuity (Matsui et al., 2006). Similarly, impaired vision is likely to exacerbate the effects of postural instability and increase the risk for falls.

Effects on Quality of Life

Age-related vision changes develop gradually and often go unnoticed for many years. As the changes progress and interfere with usual activities, older adults may withdraw from activities rather than acknowledge a vision problem or adjust to the changes. In a study of the impact of sensory impairment on older African-American men and women, visual impairments were associated with a lower level of psychological well-being even after other factors such as functional limitations were controlled for (Bazargan et al., 2001). Rovner and Casten (2002) found a high incidence of depression in older adults with AMD, with the level of depression increasing in relation to decreased participation in valued activities. In addition, depression contributed to excess disability by exacerbating visual limitations beyond what would be explained independently by the severity of visual loss (Rovner & Casten, 2002).

Of course, a person's usual lifestyle influences the extent of any psychosocial impact related to vision changes. If the preferred leisure activities require good visual skills, the older adult is likely to become bored and even depressed when vision changes interfere with endeavors such as reading, sewing, or needlework. Similarly, when artistic pursuits and entertainment events are important activities, diminished visual function can interfere with the person's quality of life. By contrast, the effect of vision impairment on lifestyle might be minimal for people who prefer music or other activities that are less dependent on visual skills.

One's living environment and support systems are other determinants of the psychosocial consequences of vision changes. Good visual skills are more important for people who live alone or who provide care for others than they are for people who live with, or have frequent contact with, others who have good vision. Also, if visually impaired people can modify their living environment to compensate for the impairments, the psychosocial consequences will be minimized. By contrast, people who live in institutional settings may experience relatively greater negative consequences because of their inability to alter environmental conditions.

Some older adults who notice declines in their vision develop fears that negatively affect their quality of life. For example, people may mistakenly fear going blind if they think they have a serious and progressive disease when, in reality, they have a treatable condition. Fear of blindness may be based on myths, inaccurate information, or the experiences of friends who have serious visual impairments. Negative or hopeless attitudes about vision changes can deter the older person from acknowledging the problem or seeking help. Fear of falling is another source of anxiety associated with impaired vision. Inaccurate depth perception can lead to frequent bumping into objects, and the older adult may feel insecure and unsafe, even in familiar environments. If the person has experienced falls or tripping, or knows someone who suffered a fracture as a result of falling, the fears may be magnified.

Wellness Opportunity

Nurses assess the impact of vision impairment on the whole person so they can address fears, anxieties, and other responses that affect quality of life.

Effects on Driving

Vision changes can significantly affect driving skills and exert a profound impact on older adults, their families, and society. Because driving is associated with considerable safety and independence concerns for drivers and their families—and because unsafe drivers place others at risk—there has been intense and increasing interest in the effects of vision changes on the driving skills of older adults. Visual dimensions that influence driving abilities are near vision, visual search, dynamic vision, light sensitivity, and visual processing speed. Consequences of visual impairment with regard to driving include the following:

- Slower dark and light adaptation creates problems when driving in and out of tunnels and when driving at night on streets with variable lighting.
- Decreased peripheral vision interferes with the wide visual field that is important for avoiding collisions.
- Decreased acuity interferes with the perception of moving objects, especially fast-moving vehicles.
- Diminished accommodation and acuity create problems when the older adult tries to read dashboard indicators after focusing on the road.

- Glare interferes with the perception of objects and is heightened by rainy, snowy, or sunny conditions.
- Bright sunlight shortly after sunrise or before sunset can significantly interfere with the perception of red and green traffic lights because of increased sensitivity to glare.
- If the car has tinted windows, the diminished illumination further interferes with visual skills.

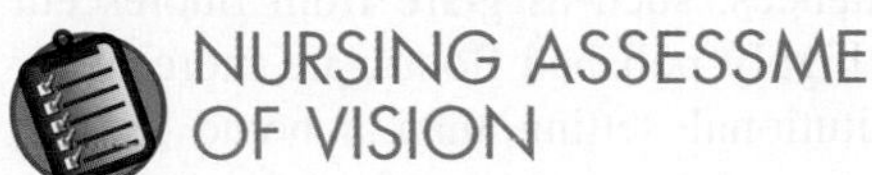

Nurses need to be aware of the far-reaching implications of the ability to drive not only on safety of the individual and others, but on independence and quality of life.

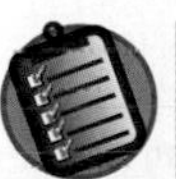

NURSING ASSESSMENT OF VISION

Nursing assessment of vision is aimed at identifying

- Factors that interfere with visual wellness
- Vision problems
- The impact of vision changes on safety, independence, or quality of life
- Opportunities for promoting visual wellness
- Barriers to implementing interventions

Nursing assessment of visual function is not a substitute for an examination by an eye care specialist. Whereas the purpose of an examination by an eye care specialist is to detect and initiate appropriate treatment of vision problems, the goal of the nursing assessment is to assist the older adult in minimizing the negative consequences of vision changes. Nursing assessment also aims at identifying modifiable risk factors that can be addressed through health promotion. Nurses assess visual abilities by interviewing the older adult (or caregivers of dependent older adults), by observing the older adult's ability to perform activities of daily living, and by testing the older adult's visual skills.

Interviewing About Vision Changes

Nurses use interview questions to elicit the following information: past and present risk factors for vision impairment, the person's awareness of any vision changes, the impact of these changes on daily activities and quality of life, and the person's attitudes about interventions (Box 17-1). The interview begins with direct questions about the person's awareness of any changes in vision. If the person acknowledges a visual impairment, the nurse elicits additional details about the onset and progression of vision changes. Nurses also ask about symptoms that cause discomfort or that indicate the possible presence of disease processes.

Nurses then ask about the impact of vision changes on the person's usual or desired activities. If the person has acknowledged vision changes, nurses can ask specific questions about how these changes have influenced usual activities. If the person is not aware of vision changes, the nurse inquires about any difficulties performing complex activities, such as driving, shopping, and meal preparation.

Box 17-1 Guidelines for Assessing Vision

Questions to Assess Awareness and Presence of Vision Impairment

- Have you noticed any changes in your vision during the past few years?
- Do you experience any uncomfortable symptoms, such as dry eyes?
- Do you have difficulty managing any of your usual activities because you have trouble seeing? (For instance, ask about the following: sewing, reading, driving, grooming, hobbies, preparing meals, watching television, managing money, writing letters, using the telephone, using dials on appliances, shopping for groceries, and going up and down stairs.)
- Have you ever tripped or fallen because you had trouble seeing?
- Have you stopped doing any activities because of vision problems? (For example, have you stopped driving at night because of difficulty seeing?)
- Are there things you would do if you could see better?

Questions to Ask if Vision Loss Is Acknowledged

- When did you first notice a loss of vision or a change in your ability to see?
- Have the changes been gradual, or did you notice sudden changes at any particular time?
- How would you describe the changes in your ability to see?
- Have you noticed pain, blurred vision, burning or itching, halos around lights, intolerance to bright light, a difference between day and night vision, or spots or flashing lights in front of your eyes?
- What kind of medical evaluation and care, if any, have you had for this problem?

Questions to Identify Opportunities for Education About Disease Prevention and Health Promotion

- When was the last time you had your eyes checked?
- Where do you go for eye care?
- Have you ever had your eyes checked for cataracts, glaucoma, and other eye conditions?
- What do you think about going for regular checkups for glaucoma and other eye problems?

Questions to Identify Risk Factors for Vision Loss

- When you spend time outdoors in the sun, do you use sunglasses or a hat to protect your eyes from bright light?
- Do you smoke cigarettes?
- Do you have a history of diabetes or hypertension?
- What medications do you take? (Refer to Table 17-2 to identify medications that may increase the risk for vision loss.)

Questions about leisure interests are incorporated into the interview to obtain information about the psychosocial consequences of vision impairments. Although the older adult may not associate lifestyle changes with vision impairments, questions about changes in hobbies and leisure activities can help the nurse identify the need for interventions to improve visual wellness. Because poor vision increases the risk for falls, especially tripping-related falls, nurses ask about a history of tripping, falling, and near-falling.

Wellness Opportunity

Nurses assess the impact of vision changes on the person's relationships with other people as one aspect of quality of life.

Identifying Opportunities for Health Promotion

Nurses identify opportunities for health promotion by asking about the person's usual eye care practices and about factors that can interfere with visual wellness. Information about the source, frequency, and dates of the person's eye examinations is particularly useful for planning health promotion interventions that address the early detection of eye disease. Nurses also listen for indicators of myths or misunderstandings that should be addressed through health education. If the person has cataracts, glaucoma, or another chronic condition affecting vision, the nurse asks questions to ascertain the person's self-care practices and attitude toward eye examinations and disease management. If a visual impairment has been denied, the nurse assesses attitudes about early detection of treatable conditions.

Last, identification of modifiable risk factors provides an opportunity for health education. For example, it is especially important to ask about cigarette smoking if the person has cataracts, AMD, or a family history of AMD. If the older person is likely to spend time outdoors in sunny climates, the nurse asks about exposure to sunlight. Placing this question toward the end of the interview sets the stage for health education about protective measures, such as the use of sunglasses.

Wellness Opportunity

Nurses pave the way for teaching about self-care by assessing attitudes about preventive and protective activities, such as obtaining eye examinations and wearing sunglasses.

Observing Cues to Visual Function

Reliable information about a person's visual function can be obtained simply by being observant. For example, nurses can observe for any abnormalities of the eyelids, such as serious lid lag, that might interfere with visual wellness. Nurses can detect other, more subtle, indications that visual function is impaired by observing the person's appearance and ability to perform daily activities. Finally, when possible, nurses observe older adults in their usual environments for a more accurate assessment of conditions that can affect visual wellness.

Nurses consider their observations in relation to the person's usual patterns of activities and personal care. For example, observation of spots and soiled marks on clothing would be interpreted differently for someone known to be meticulous about his or her appearance than for someone who had never showed much concern about this. When assessing older people who are not in their usual environment, the nurse should note any circumstances that might influence their visual performance, either positively or negatively. An example of a positive influence might be the presence of good lighting and color contrast. Some negative influences, such as glare from fluorescent lights reflecting on highly polished floors, are more likely to exist in an institutional setting than a home setting. Assessment of the person's visual performance outside the home setting also must take into account the influences of factors such as illness, medication effects, psychological stress, unfamiliar environments, and unavailability of corrective lenses. These influences are of particular concern in institutional settings and are likely to have a negative impact on the older person's performance of daily activities. In these settings, nurses can ask the older person and caregivers for information about the person's abilities in the home setting. Suggestions for observing behavioral and environmental cues related to visual function are listed in Box 17-2.

Using Standard Vision Tests

Nurses assess peripheral vision and acuity for near and distant objects by using both formal and informal tests. Some tests, such as checking distance vision with the Snellen chart, assessing visual fields with the confrontation test, and evaluating near vision by asking the person to read small-print text, require minimal equipment. Nursing assessment of these three parameters provides information about visual functions that often are affected by age-related changes and that influence the safe performance of daily activities. These tests are not a substitute for a complete eye examination, but they provide information that is useful for planning care and identifying the need for further evaluation.

For accurate assessment of visual skills, place a light source above the person's head to provide good lighting while avoiding shadows. If the person normally wears corrective lenses, make sure that they are clean and in place. Test each eye separately, using an appropriate eye cover; avoid using a hand as a cover.

Nurses can assess near acuity by asking the person to read a newspaper or other printed material of various type sizes. Another method is to ask the person to read a line or two of a form that needs to be signed and then observe the person's ability to find the signature line. Nurses can create additional opportunities for assessing acuity by providing

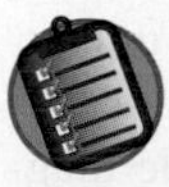

Box 17-2
Guidelines for Assessing Behavioral and Environmental Cues Related to Visual Performance

Behavioral Cues

- Is clothing spotted, soiled, or mismatched, in contrast to a former pattern of neatness and sense of style?
- Is makeup applied in heavy quantities, in contrast to the usual manner of application?
- Does the person rely heavily on nonvisual cues in performing usual activities, especially maneuvering in the environment (e.g., using the hands to find objects or to probe for obstacles)?

Environmental Cues

- What kind of lighting is used for various tasks? If the lighting is not adequate, can adjustments be made to improve the person's visual abilities?
- Does the person try to economize at home by using dim lights or no lights at all? If so, does this interfere with visual abilities or safe functioning?
- Where does the person usually sit in relation to light sources? Does glare from a window interfere with vision? Do shadows from lamps interfere with vision? Do overhead lights cause glare? Are light bulbs of sufficient wattage?
- What are the sources of light on stairways and hallways?
- Is there sufficient color contrast in the following areas: walls and floors; stairs and landings; furniture; eating utensils and place settings; cooking utensils and counter tops; markings and background on appliance dials?
- Are nightlights used in hallways and bathrooms?

written educational materials and asking the person to read a specific part, such as a phone number.

The Snellen chart, described in Box 17-3, is a standard test for measuring distance acuity. Nurses can informally assess distance acuity by asking the person to look out a window or down a hallway and to describe certain details, such as the words on a sign. This test is based on the assumption that the nurse's distance acuity is normal. When performing any distance vision tests in older adults, eliminate all sources of glare and make sure that color contrast for the viewed object is adequate.

A standard confrontation test provides a gross estimate of the peripheral visual fields of the examinee, as measured against the examiner's peripheral vision (Fig. 17-4). As with informal distance acuity tests, the results of the confrontation test are based on a comparison with the examiner's visual skill, which must be normal for an accurate comparison to be made. Instructions for performing the confrontation test are given in Box 17-3.

Recall that you are the nurse at the senior center in Mrs. F.'s neighborhood. During a recent visit, the 72-year-old Mrs. F. told you that she feels like there is a "film" over her eyes, and she has trouble seeing when she is outside on sunny days. Several months ago, Mrs. F's doctor told her that she has "early cataracts," but she has not had any further evaluation.

(case study continues on page 352)

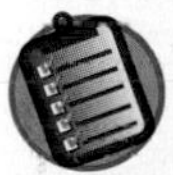

Box 17-3
Guidelines for Using Vision Screening Tests

Using the Snellen Chart to Assess Distance Acuity

- Position the chart 20 feet away from the person, at eye level.
- If space does not permit a 20-foot distance, the distance between the person and the chart should be either 15 or 10 feet, with final measurements adjusted for distance. Alternatively, a scaled-down Snellen card can be used, if available.
- If the person usually wears corrective lenses, test the corrected vision.
- Ask the person to start reciting the letters in the line that can be read most easily; then ask him or her to read as many letters as possible in the lines directly below that line.
- Document the findings for each eye by noting the figure at the end of the last line on which at least half of the letters were read correctly.
- The upper figure denotes the distance of the person from the chart, whereas the lower figure denotes the distance from the chart at which a person with normal vision would be able to read the line. (That is, a vision measurement of 20/50 indicates that the person being tested can see things at a distance of 20 feet that a person with normal vision would be able to see at a distance of 50 feet.)
- Normal Snellen chart test results for older adults are as follows:
  - A corrected vision of 20/20 is considered to be normal.
  - If a distance of 10 feet is used, the corrected vision should be 10/10.
  - The average corrected vision for older adults ranges from 20/20 to 20/50.

Performing the Confrontation Test to Assess Peripheral Vision

- Sit directly across from the older person, about 2 feet away.
- Cover your left eye and have the examinee cover his or her right eye.
- Instruct the examinee to focus on your right eye while you focus on the examinee's left eye.
- Fully extend your right arm midway between you and the examinee.
- Slowly move your right hand, with the fingers wiggling, from the outer periphery toward the center, testing visual fields from top to bottom.
- While maintaining continuous eye contact, ask the examinee to report the point at which your fingers are visualized.
- Repeat these steps, covering your right eye and the examinee's left eye and using your left arm.
- Normal confrontation test results for older adults: your wiggling fingers should be seen simultaneously by both you and the older person in all quadrants.

THINKING POINTS

- Which questions from Box 17-1 would you ask Mrs. F. at this time?
- What sort of information might you be able to glean from behavioral or environmental cues about Mrs. F.'s ability to see (see Box 17-2)?
- Would assessing Mrs. F.'s vision using vision screening tests be appropriate (see Box 17-3)? If so, which tests would you perform?
- What health promotion education would you give Mrs. F. at this time?

NURSING DIAGNOSIS

Based on the nursing assessment, the nurse might identify an actual vision impairment or risk factors for impaired vision. An appropriate nursing diagnosis for an older adult with impaired vision would be Disturbed Sensory Perception: Visual. This is defined as a "state in which the individual/group experiences or is at risk of experiencing a change in the amount, pattern, or interpretation of incoming stimuli" (Carpenito-Moyet, 2006, p. 439). Related factors that commonly affect older adults include age-related vision changes (e.g., presbyopia), sensory organ alterations (e.g., glaucoma), and environmental factors (e.g., glare, dim lighting, or poor color contrast). The care plan at the end of this chapter is based on a nursing diagnosis of Disturbed Sensory Perception: Visual related to age-related changes, sensory organ alterations, and environmental factors. Other nursing diagnoses might be addressed if the visual impairment interferes with the older adult's safety, quality of life, or performance of activities of daily living. Possible diagnoses to address these functional consequences include Anxiety, Ineffective Coping, Self-Care Deficit, Risk for Injury, Impaired Social Interaction, Readiness for Enhanced Coping, and Readiness for Enhanced Self-Care.

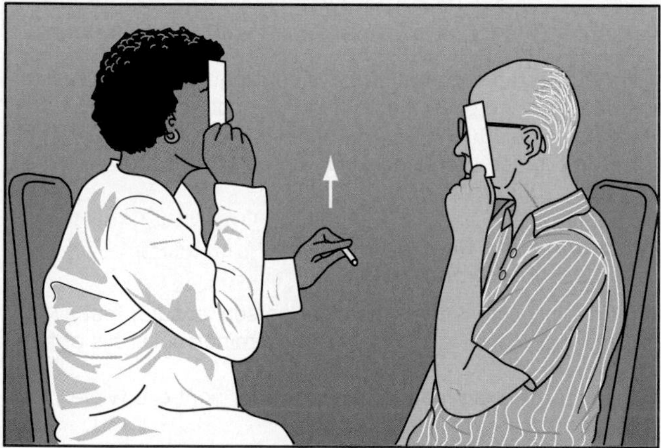

FIGURE 17-4 Performing the confrontation test to assess visual fields. The nurse and the patient sit approximately 2 feet apart. The patient covers his left eye, while the nurse covers her right eye. To test the inferior visual field, the nurse extends her left arm and slowly moves a pencil upward until the patient sees the pencil. The test is repeated for each of the remaining three visual fields (i.e., superior, temporal, and nasal), and then the four visual fields are tested for the other eye. With normal peripheral vision, the patient will see the pencil at the same time the nurse sees it.

Wellness Opportunity

The wellness nursing diagnosis of Readiness for Enhanced Knowledge: Improved Vision would be applicable for older adults who are willing to explore interventions that improve their visual abilities.

PLANNING FOR WELLNESS OUTCOMES

When older adults experience vision impairments or have risk factors that affect visual functioning, nurses identify wellness outcomes as an essential part of the planning process. The Nursing Outcomes Classification (NOC) that most directly relates to interventions to improve vision for older adults is Vision Compensation Behavior, defined as "personal actions to compensate for visual impairment" (Johnson et al., 2006, p. 638). Another pertinent NOC is Sensory Function: Vision, defined as "extent to which visual images are correctly sensed" (Johnson et al., 2006, p. 636). In addition, nurses can use any of the following NOCs to describe the effectiveness of interventions to improve vision: Coping, Adaptation to Physical Disability, Self-Care: Activities of Daily Living, Stress Level, Knowledge: Personal Safety, Fall Prevention Behavior, and Risk Control: Visual Impairment. Specific interventions to achieve these outcomes are discussed in the following section.

Wellness Opportunity

Quality of Life is a wellness outcome that is achieved through nursing interventions that improve visual function.

Health promotion goals are long term and focus on maintaining vision at an optimal level. For example, one goal might be for an older adult to obtain evaluation of vision problems. Nurses in institutional settings address these goals through a discharge plan that includes information about local resources for further evaluation. Also, the discharge plan might include suggestions for obtaining educational materials from a local sight center or the resources listed at the end of this chapter.

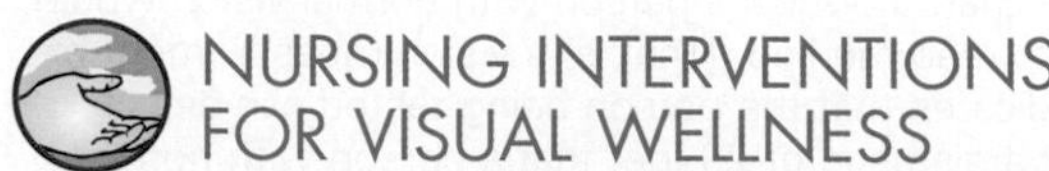

NURSING INTERVENTIONS FOR VISUAL WELLNESS

Nurses promote visual wellness through interventions directed toward preventing vision loss, promoting comfort measures for dry eyes, and implementing or teaching about methods to foster optimal visual function. Interventions to achieve these goals are discussed in detail in the following sections. The following pertinent Nursing Interventions Classification (NIC) terminology may be applicable to care plans: Communication Enhancement: Visual Deficit, Coping Enhancement, Eye Care, Environmental Management, Environmental Management: Safety, Health Education, Health Screening, Health System Guidance, Risk Identification, and Fall Prevention.

Health Promotion for Visual Wellness

Prevention strategies focus on health education about reducing or eliminating risk factors that can cause visual impairments (Box 17-4). Because prolonged exposure to ultraviolet light (especially UV-B) can lead to visual impairment, nurses should teach older adults about the importance of protecting their eyes from sunlight. Broad-brimmed hats and close-fitting sunglasses with UV-B–absorbing lenses have the long-range effect of protecting the eyes from harmful rays; they also have the immediate benefit of screening out sun glare that can interfere with visual function. Nurses can teach older adults, as well as their caregivers, about the benefits of these simple measures. Another modifiable risk factor for eye disease is smoking. People who have a diagnosis or family history of AMD should be taught about the relationship between smoking and AMD and encouraged to quit smoking. Strategies for encouraging older adults to quit smoking are discussed in Chapter 21. To reduce the risk for eye disease, people should be encouraged to include foods that are high in antioxidants in their daily diet. Box 17-4 provides additional details about nutritional considerations.

Because most eye diseases progress very slowly, disease prevention must also focus on regular vision examinations to detect the leading causes of visual impairment: cataracts, AMD, glaucoma, and diabetic retinopathy. Three objectives of *Healthy People 2010* are directed toward the early detection of cataracts, glaucoma, and diabetic eye disease; this is the first time vision objectives have been included in Healthy People initiatives (USDHHS, 2000). Nurses play an important role in achieving these objectives when they educate older adults and their caregivers about the importance of early detection of glaucoma and about treatments available for cataracts, glaucoma, and other eye disorders.

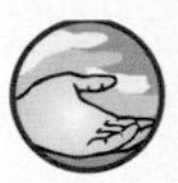

Box 17-4 Health Promotion Teaching About Vision

Nurses can educate the older adult in the following areas:

Prevention and Early Detection of Disease

- The damaging effects of UV light and how to minimize exposure (broad-brimmed hats, close-fitting sunglasses with UV-absorbing lenses)
- The importance of annual eye examinations, including screening for glaucoma, cataracts, and retinal disease
- Eye care practitioners and what they do (see Box 17-5)
- The importance of managing diabetes and hypertension
- Smoking cessation
- The importance of timely evaluation of any changes in vision

Nutritional Considerations

- Include foods high in antioxidants (fruits and vegetables) and B-complex vitamins daily.
- Vitamins A, C, and E may have a protective role in preventing cataracts.
- People who have AMD may benefit from a daily supplement containing the following antioxidants and minerals: 500 mg vitamin C, 400 IU vitamin E, 15 mg beta-carotene, 80 mg zinc oxide, and 2 mg cupric oxide (copper).

Compensating for Visual Impairments

- Referrals for vision rehabilitation if appropriate
- Bright, nonglare lighting and environmental modifications (see Boxes 17-6 and 17-7)
- Low-vision aids (see Boxes 17-8 and 17-9)

Diversity Note

About half of people with glaucoma do not know they have it, but Quigley and colleagues (2001) found that 62% of Hispanic Americans with glaucoma were undiagnosed.

It is recommended that people 35 years of age and older undergo biannual measurements of intraocular pressure to screen for glaucoma, and that people 65 years and older undergo such measurements annually. Annual dilated eye examinations are recommended for people with diabetes. Nurses can encourage older adults to take advantage of vision screening tests that might be available in the community through nonprofit organizations such as the Lions Club International. Even in the absence of disease conditions, annual eye examinations are important for identifying people who would benefit from changes in eyeglasses. Munoz and colleagues (2000) studied Americans between the ages of 65 and 84 years and found that one third of the subjects with impaired vision improved to an acuity of 20/40 with refraction. In this same study, more than half of the subjects with visual impairment or blindness had conditions that were treatable or potentially preventable with interventions.

In providing health education, it may be helpful to review the differences between opticians, optometrists, and ophthalmologists with the client (Box 17-5). Educational materials describing the scope of services of these eye care providers are distributed by some of the organizations listed in the Educational Resources section at the end of this chapter. The older adult may also benefit from the many educational brochures that are available on the subjects

Box 17-5
Eye Care Practitioners

Practitioners

Ophthalmologists are licensed doctors of medicine (M.D.) or osteopathy (D.O.) who are trained to diagnose and treat diseases and conditions of the eye. Ophthalmologic services include:

- Comprehensive eye examinations
- Diagnosis of eye diseases and disorders of the eye
- Prescription medications for eye problems (e.g., glaucoma)
- Eye surgery and postoperative care (e.g., cataracts)
- Laser treatments (e.g., retinopathy)
- Prescriptions for eyeglasses and contact lenses
- Prescriptions for low-vision aids
- Referrals for low-vision aids and training
- Medical referrals for diseases of the body that affect the eyes

Optometrists are licensed doctors of optometry (O.D.), not physicians, who are trained to examine eyes, screen for common eye problems, and prescribe eye exercises or corrective lenses. Optometrists use diagnostic medications, and in more than half the states in America, they can prescribe certain therapeutic drugs for eye diseases. Optometric services include:

- Comprehensive eye examinations
- Eye refractions to determine the need for corrective lenses
- Prescriptions for eyeglasses, contact lenses, and low-vision aids
- Vision therapy to improve certain skills, such as tracking and focusing the eyes
- Referrals for low-vision aids and training
- Referrals to physicians for surgery, medication, or further evaluation
- Diagnosis of eye disorders (in some states)
- Postoperative care (in some states)

Opticians are eye care practitioners who are trained to fit, adjust, and dispense eyeglasses and contact lenses that have been prescribed by an optometrist or ophthalmologist. In many states, opticians are licensed. They do not perform eye examinations or refractions, and they cannot prescribe corrective lenses or medications.

Health Insurance Coverage

Medicare and other health insurance programs cover many optometric and ophthalmologic services for the diagnosis and treatment of eye diseases. Routine eye examinations and corrective lenses usually are not covered, except by some supplemental or managed care plans. Beginning in 2002, Medicare covers annual dilated eye examinations for all people at high risk for glaucoma. After cataract surgery, eyeglasses and contact lenses are usually covered by health insurance if they are considered part of the cataract treatment. Optician services are not covered by Medicare.

of eye diseases, common vision problems, age-related eye changes, and low-vision aids. Nurses can use these publications to supplement and reinforce the health education components of their care plans. Local sight centers, or the organizations listed in the Educational Resources section at the end of this chapter, provide these materials at little or no cost, and some brochures are available in Spanish and other languages. In addition, much of the information can be obtained and printed directly from these organizations' websites. The National Association for the Visually Handicapped (NAVH) is an excellent resource for information about interventions for older adults with visual impairments. In contrast to publications from organizations that focus primarily on blindness, materials from the NAVH are written for people with gradual and partial visual losses. The American Academy of Ophthalmology and the American Optometric Association also are good sources of free pamphlets about eye problems that commonly affect older adults. Do-it-yourself eye test kits are available from Prevent Blindness America. This kit enables people to determine whether they are seeing as well as they should and provides guidelines for obtaining further evaluation.

Wellness Opportunity

Nurses promote self-care by encouraging older adults and their families to obtain information from resources listed at the end of this chapter.

Comfort Measures for Dry Eyes

If pertinent, simple measures to relieve dry eyes can be discussed. Use of over-the-counter artificial tears or ocular lubricants, especially before reading or engaging in other activities that require frequent eye movements, usually will afford symptomatic relief. People who use eye drops more frequently than every 3 hours should be advised to use preservative-free solutions to prevent any adverse effects from the preservatives. Other comfort measures, such as applying cold compresses or wearing wraparound glasses, are designed to prevent evaporation of tears. Maintenance of adequate environmental humidity, especially during the winter months or in dry climates, also decreases evaporation of eye moisture and adds to eye comfort. People who experience discomfort from dry eyes should avoid irritants, such as smoke and hairspray, as well as adverse environmental conditions, such as hot rooms and high wind. People who are bothered by dry eyes and are taking a medication that might exacerbate the discomfort should be encouraged to discuss the problem with their primary care practitioner.

Environmental Modifications

Simple environmental modifications can improve the older person's safe performance of activities of daily living, thereby reducing risks of falls and accidents. Because many functional consequences result from the age-related reduction in retinal illumination, proper lighting is the single most important intervention that improves an older adult's vision. Increased illumination is one of the easiest and least costly modifications that can be made in any setting (Box 17-6). Both the quality and quantity of light are important when providing illumination for optimal visual performance. For example, selection of broad-spectrum fluorescent lights and daylight-simulating lamps may be particularly beneficial in compensating for age-related vision changes.

Another important consideration in adapting the environment for optimal visual function is color contrast. Appliances and other items, such as ovens, irons, radios, thermostats, and televisions, may be difficult to use because of poor color contrast around the control mechanisms. Modifications can easily be made to improve the older person's ability to use these items safely and accurately. For example, two dots of red nail polish can be used to mark a designated and commonly used temperature setting, and the older adult can be instructed to turn the dial above or below the matching dots for higher or lower settings.

Architectural designs and institutional constraints may limit the extent of environmental adaptations that nurses can implement, especially in institutional settings. In most settings, however, nurses can improve the visual abilities of older adults by using appropriate colors to enhance contrast, by using curtains to control light and glare, and by placing chairs in positions that enhance illumination and avoid glare. Nurses have many opportunities to teach older adults and their caregivers about the environmental modifications that are most effective for optimal visual function. Box 17-7 summarizes some environmental adaptations that can be used to compensate for deficits in visual skills and improve safety. All older adults can benefit from these environmental modifications, even in the absence of diagnosed eye disorders, because they are effective ways of improving vision for all people.

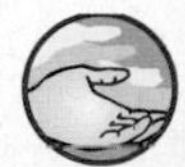

Box 17-6
Considerations for Optimal Illumination

- Older adults need at least three times as much light as younger people do.
- Older adults function best in environments with bright, broad-spectrum, nonglaring, indirect sources of light.
- Place sources of illumination 1 to 2 feet away from the object to be viewed.
- Flickering light, such as that generated by a single fluorescent tube, will cause fatigue and decreased visual performance.
- Light bulbs should be kept clean.
- Replace light bulbs when they become dim, rather than waiting for them to burn out.
- The amount of light decreases fourfold when the distance is doubled.
- Increased illumination has a greater positive effect on impaired vision than it does on normal vision.
- A gradual decrease in illumination from foreground to background is better than sharp contrasts in lighting.
- Moderate overhead lighting can be used to enhance brighter foreground lighting and prevent sharp contrasts.
- To reduce glare from reading material, place the light source to the left side of right-handed readers and to the right side of left-handed readers.
- Avoid glossy paper for reading materials.

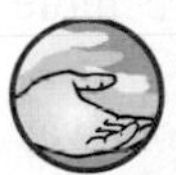

Box 17-7
Environmental Adaptations for Improving Visual Performance

Illumination, Glare Control, and Dark/Light Adaptation

- Position a 60- or 75-watt soft-white light bulb above and close to the head of the older person.
- Use a clear plastic shower curtain, rather than solid colors or printed curtains, for the tub or shower.
- Use light-colored, sheer curtains to eliminate glare from windows.
- Place nightlights in hallways and bathrooms, or keep a high-intensity flashlight at the bedside.
- Use illuminated light switches.
- Provide good lighting in stairways and hallways.
- Use illuminated or magnified mirrors.

Color Contrast

- Use brightly colored tape or paint on the edges of stairs, especially on the top and bottom steps.
- Use light-colored and dark-colored cutting boards to contrast with dark and light foods.
- Use contrasting, rather than matching, colors for china, placemats, and napkins.
- Use a toilet seat that contrasts with the bathroom walls and floor. Use colored bars of soap on white sinks and tubs.
- Use utensils with brightly colored handles.
- Place pillows of contrasting colors on stuffed furniture.
- Use decorative or lighted plates over light switches and wall sockets; avoid light switch plates that blend in with the wallpaper or paint.
- Place decorative items of contrasting colors, such as plants and ceramics, on tables to provide clues to depth, especially on light-colored furniture that is in a room with light-colored walls.
- Use brightly colored grooming utensils, such as combs, brushes, and razors.
- Use pens with black ink rather than blue ink.

General Adaptive Measures and Environmental Modifications

- Do not rearrange furniture without informing or showing the older person.
- Advise older adults to pause in doorways when going from light to dark rooms (or vice versa) to allow time for their eyes to adjust to the light change.
- Teach older people to use their feet and hands as probes to feel for curbs, steps, edges of chairs, and the like.
- When walking with an older person, stop when necessary to allow a change in focus from near to far and from light to dark.

Low-Vision Aids

People with visual impairments can improve their safety and quality of life through the use of **low-vision aids** that improve focus, contrast, magnification, or illumination (Box 17-8). Low-vision aids are most beneficial when used in conjunction with environmental modifications. For example, magnifiers are most effective when combined with measures that improve illumination and control glare. Reading glasses and other optical aids that magnify an image for visual tasks are available with or without a prescription. Nonoptical aids are devices that enhance contrast, reduce glare, improve lighting, or enlarge the image. Printed and Internet catalogues with illustrations of low-vision aids are available through many organizations (see the Educational Resources section). Also, local sight centers are good sources of low-vision aids, as well as training related to their use.

Although special low-vision aids must be ordered through catalogues or obtained at sight centers, everyday items, if used advantageously, can serve as low-vision aids. An example of a low-vision aid that may be available to nurses is a photocopy machine that can be used to convert regular-print materials into large-print materials. Likewise, household lamps, placed in the correct position and equipped with the right wattage bulb, can also serve as low-vision aids. Lighthouse International (listed in the Educational Resources section) provides educational materials that illustrate examples of effective color contrast and effective ways of making text legible. These free materials, which can be obtained through the mail or from the Internet, can be used as guides for developing more readable printed materials for signage, health education, and other purposes.

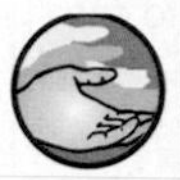

Box 17-8 Low-Vision Aids for Improving Visual Performance

Enlargement Aids

- Microscopic spectacles
- Hand-held or standing magnifiers
- Binoculars and hand-held or spectacle-mounted telescopes
- Magnifying sheets
- Field expanders for diminished peripheral vision
- Large-print books, magazines, and newspapers
- Photocopy machines or laser printers (used to enlarge print)
- Telephones with enlarged letters and numbers, or a pad with enlarged letters and numbers designed to fit over rotary-dial or push-button phones
- Large numbers on rulers, playing cards, and other items
- Thermometers with good color coding and enlarged numbers
- Large-eye needles

Illumination Aids

- High-intensity lights
- Gooseneck lamps
- Floor or table lamps with three-way light bulbs

Contrast Aids

- Use of broad-tipped felt markers in dark, yet bright, colors and colored construction paper for making signs
- Red print on a yellow background or white letters on a green background
- Reading and signature guides (typoscopes)
- Clip-on yellow lenses

Glare Control Aids

- Sunglasses with UV-absorbing lenses
- Sun visors and broad-brimmed hats
- Nonglare (antireflective) coating on eyeglasses
- Yellow and pink acetate sheets
- Pinhole occluders

Box 17-9 Guidelines for Using Magnifying Aids

Using a Hand-Held Magnifier

- Begin with the magnifier close to the reading material.
- Slowly move the magnifier toward the face until the image totally fills the lens.
- For optimal focus, move the magnifier back toward the print about a distance of 2 cm.

Using a Stand Magnifier

- Rest the stand flat against the reading material.
- Do not move the stand.

Using a Spectacle-Mounted Magnifier

- Begin with the reading material close to the nose.
- Slowly move the material away until it becomes clear.

Nurses can teach about the appropriate use of low-vision aids so the most effective outcomes are achieved. For example, if people understand that halving the distance of a light source increases illumination by fourfold, they are more likely to place lights in the most effective positions. As an illustration of this principle, a light bulb that is 1 foot away from someone will provide four times as much illumination as one that is 2 feet away. Nurses can use Boxes 17-6 and 17-9 to teach about effective use of lights and magnification. Local sight centers provide detailed training in the use of low-vision aids, and the NAVH publishes a helpful guide regarding their use. *Healthy People 2010* objective 28-10 is to "increase the use of vision rehabilitation services and adaptive devices by people with visual impairments" (USDHHS, 2000).

Wellness Opportunity

Nurses help meet objectives of *Healthy People 2010* by facilitating referrals to local vision rehabilitation services and encouraging older adults and their families to use these resources.

Maintaining and Improving Quality of Life

As discussed earlier, the psychosocial consequences of impaired vision can be quite significant for older adults.

Many of the interventions that help older adults compensate for visual deficits and function at their highest level also will improve their quality of life and address the psychosocial consequences of impaired vision. For example, the use of appropriate reading glasses and good environmental lighting may enable the older adult to read books, newspapers, and magazines. Subsequently, their quality of life may improve because they experience satisfying social interactions and increased intellectual stimulation. Nurses also encourage participation in support and educational groups because these interventions serve an important role in improving quality of life for people with significant or progressive vision loss.

Mrs. F. is now 81 years old. She had cataract surgery and an intraocular lens implant in her left eye when she was 76 years old, and in her right eye when she was 77. Her vision was good until a year ago, when she developed macular degeneration. She knows this condition will be progressive, but she continues to drive and live alone. Her current medical conditions are arthritis, hypertension, and coronary artery disease. She quit smoking several years ago after she was hospitalized for coronary artery disease. You are the nurse at the senior center where Mrs. F. comes for lunch several times a week. During an appointment with you, Mrs. F. confides that she is terrified of becoming totally blind and of losing her independence. Her grandmother went blind several years before she died and she had to go to a long-term care facility.

THINKING POINTS

- Which nursing diagnosis or diagnoses would you apply to Mrs. F. at this time?
- Which information in Boxes 17-4 through 17-9 might be appropriate for Mrs. F.?
- What health promotion advice would you give?
- Would you suggest any referrals for information or community resources?
- What interventions would address Mrs. F.'s fear of becoming blind and losing her independence?

EVALUATING EFFECTIVENESS OF NURSING INTERVENTIONS

Nurses observe compensatory behaviors of visually impaired older adults to evaluate the effectiveness of interventions for Disturbed Sensory Perception: Visual. The following are indicators of successful interventions:

- Use of corrective lenses and low-vision aids to achieve best possible visual function
- Adaptations of the environment for safety and improved visual function (e.g., bright, nonglare lighting, good color contrast)
- Expressed feelings of safety in relation to visual function
- Maximum independence in activities such as dressing, personal care, using appliances, and managing medications
- Expressed feelings of minimal negative impact on quality of life.

Nurses evaluate the effectiveness of interventions to improve independence by assessing and reassessing the older adult's abilities before and after interventions. When interventions address the psychosocial impact of visual impairment, nurses observe the extent to which the person's quality of life and ability to participate in enjoyable activities is improved. For example, better lighting and the use of a large-print *Reader's Digest* may enable someone to enjoy reading again.

Nurses evaluate the effectiveness of health education interventions according to the person's expressed intent to follow through with the recommended referral or course of action. In home, community, and long-term care settings, nurses may be able to facilitate referrals for vision screening or other vision care services. In these settings, nurses evaluate the effectiveness of interventions based on feedback from the older adults or their caregivers about the actual use of suggested resources.

Mrs. F. is now 86 years old and is recovering from a recent fractured hip, which occurred when she fell while getting out of bed to go to the bathroom at night. After a brief hospitalization for surgical repair of the fractured hip and a 2-week period of skilled rehabilitation, Mrs. F. was referred to a home care agency for therapy, assessment, monitoring of her medical status, and evaluation of her ability to manage at home.

In addition to AMD, Mrs. F.'s current medical diagnoses include arthritis, hypertension, coronary artery disease, and congestive heart failure. Mrs. F.'s medical conditions had been stable for several years, but during her hospitalization for the fractured hip she was started on oxygen and her medications were changed. Current medications are furosemide, 40 mg daily; digoxin, 0.125 mg daily; and enalapril, 10 mg twice daily. A 2-g sodium diet has been prescribed, and she has been discharged with an order for oxygen per nasal cannula at a rate of 2 L/minute as needed.

(case study continues on page 358)

Before her accident, despite the visual limitations from macular degeneration, Mrs. F. had lived alone in her own home, but her daughter has become increasingly concerned about her mother's safety. Now Mrs. F.'s daughter is convinced that her mother should not remain in her own home but should instead move to an assisted-living facility. Mrs. F. is adamant in her desire to stay in her own home and says the only reason she fell and broke her hip was because she was rushing to get to the bathroom. She says she has learned a lesson and will not hurry when she gets up at night. Furthermore, she says, she gave up driving to satisfy her daughter last year—now she's to give up her home, too? Mrs. F.'s daughter is staying with her mother for a couple of weeks until her mother regains her mobility to the point of independence. The daughter hopes that in the interim, she will be able to convince her mother to move to an assisted-living facility. You are the home care nurse working with Mrs. F. in her home.

NURSING ASSESSMENT

During your initial nursing assessment, you determine that Mrs. F. is motivated to regain her mobility and manage her medical conditions, but she has difficulty reading small-print instructions because of poor vision. When you review Mrs. F.'s medications with her, you observe that she cannot read the labels on the bottles. You also observe that Mrs. F. keeps her medications on the shelf above the kitchen counter, where the lighting is very dim. When you review the proper use of the oxygen, you note that she has difficulty seeing the markings on the flowmeter. Her daughter has been helping her with these regimens, but Mrs. F. hopes to perform these activities independently so she can remain in her own home.

Mrs. F. tells you that she is not concerned about falling because she walks slowly and carefully when she gets up during the night to go to the bathroom. She now uses a walker and says she feels safe. Her daughter expresses concern about her mother managing the oxygen and the walker when going to the bathroom. Mrs. F. uses the oxygen when she sleeps and her daughter is skeptical about her ability to get to the bathroom without rushing.

You observe that the hallway between the bedroom and bathroom is dark, and that the bedroom has an overhead light, but no bedside lamp. The bathroom has a narrow doorway and the toilet is at the other side of the sink. You assess the home for safety and determine that the pathways are clear and there is good lighting on the stairway and in the living areas. You identify no additional risks (e.g., throw rugs) to Mrs. F.'s safe mobility, but you do have concerns about Mrs. F.'s ability to navigate safely to the toilet with a walker.

When questioned about her vision problems, Mrs. F. gives her history of successful cataract surgery and a diagnosis of AMD at the age of 80 years. She sees her ophthalmologist every year, and he has told her that her vision will get worse and that nothing can be done about it. He had mentioned that the local sight center provides some rehabilitation services for people with low vision but he told her that those services are mostly for "younger blind people." Also, she is concerned that the sight center will suggest she purchase items that cost a lot of money, which she wouldn't be able to afford anyway. She says her daughter got her a subscription for the large-print *Reader's Digest*, which she enjoys, and that she's not interested in reading the newspaper because she watches the news on television. She has an appointment to see her eye doctor next month.

NURSING DIAGNOSIS

In addition to the nursing diagnoses related to Mrs. F.'s medical condition, you identify a nursing diagnosis of Disturbed Sensory Perception: Visual, related to age-related changes, sensory organ alterations, and environmental factors. Supporting evidence for this diagnosis can be found in Mrs. F.'s inability to read labels, instructions, or the flowmeter markings, and the environmental factors that contribute to unsafe mobility. The nursing

(case study continues on page 359)

diagnoses of Anxiety, Self-Care Deficit, and Risk for Injury might also be applicable. The diagnosis of Disturbed Sensory Perception: Visual, however, addresses the source of Mrs. F.'s anxiety, risk for injury, and inability to perform her instrumental activities of daily living, and therefore is probably the most comprehensive diagnosis. Also, this diagnosis prompts you to include a long-term goal of encouraging further evaluation and management of the visual impairments.

NURSING CARE PLAN FOR MRS. F.

Expected Outcome	Nursing Interventions	Nursing Evaluation
Mrs. F. will manage her medication regimen accurately and independently.	• Print simplified medication instructions on large index cards using black felt-tip marker. • Use colored dots to match pill bottles with instruction cards. • Establish a medication management system using pill organizer boxes with markings that are bold and have good color contrast. • Teach Mrs. F. how to fill the pill boxes weekly, using the index cards you prepared for her. • Suggest that Mrs. F. fill the pill boxes at the kitchen table during daylight hours while using overhead light.	• Mrs. F. will demonstrate that she can accurately fill the pill boxes. • Mrs. F. will take her medications correctly. • Mrs. F.'s daughter will observe that her mother follows the prescribed regimen.
Mrs. F. will self-administer oxygen as needed.	• Use a copy machine to enlarge the small-print instructions for the oxygen equipment. • Place a colored dot at the 2-L mark on the flowmeter. • Keep the oxygen tank in a well-lit location and suggest using a flashlight to help illuminate the flowmeter setting.	• Mrs. F. will demonstrate the safe and independent operation of the oxygen equipment. • Mrs. F.'s daughter will observe that her mother administers her oxygen correctly.
Mrs. F. will be able to use a commode safely and independently.	• Ask Mrs. F. to use a bedside commode during the night; emphasize the importance of preventing another fall. • Work with physical and occupational therapists to (1) evaluate the feasibility of installing grab bars or other devices that will assist Mrs. F. in safely using the toilet; (2) identify a safe way for Mrs. F. to use the bathroom during the daytime; (3) teach Mrs. F. to transfer between the bed and commode for nighttime use; (4) teach her to empty the bedside commode. • Place a lamp on the nightstand and make sure that Mrs. F. can turn it on easily while in bed. Teach Mrs. F. to turn the bedside lamp on and sit at the edge of the bed for a few minutes before getting up at night.	• Mrs. F. will demonstrate that she safely uses the bathroom during the day and a bedside commode at night. • Mrs. F. will be able to empty the commode independently. • Mrs. F. will have no further falls in the bathroom.
Mrs. F. will compensate as much as possible for her progressive visual loss.	• Educate Mrs. F. and her daughter about the services provided at the local sight center for people with low vision; emphasize that these services address the needs of older adults and people with recent and progressive visual loss. The services are for anyone with low vision, and there are many low-vision aids available to improve the visual function of people with macular degeneration. • Suggest that Mrs. F. ask her eye doctor for a referral to the sight center when she sees him next month. • Include Mrs. F.'s daughter in the discussion about these services, and ask her to assist with following through once a referral is obtained.	• Mrs. F. will make and keep an appointment for an initial evaluation at the sight center. • Mrs. F. will use low-vision aids to improve visual function.

(case study continues on page 360)

THINKING POINTS

- How would you address concerns about Mrs. F. living alone? What aspects of her safety and quality of life would you consider?
- How would you use any of the boxes in this chapter for health promotion teaching?
- What additional nursing diagnoses and outcomes would you identify for Mrs. F.?
- What additional interventions and referrals would you consider for Mrs. F.?
- Identify at least one resource in your community that might provide help or information for Mrs. F. Call that agency to obtain information about their services.

CHAPTER HIGHLIGHTS

Age-Related Changes That Affect Vision (Table 17-1)

- Changes in appearance include arcus senilis, loss of orbital fat, diminished elasticity of eyelid muscles
- Diminished tear production
- Degenerative changes affect all structures of the eye, the retinal–neural pathway, and the visual cortex of the brain

Effects of Age-Related Changes on Vision

- Diminished ability to focus clearly on objects at various distances
- Diminished ability to detect details and discern objects
- Slower adaptive response to changes in lighting
- Increased sensitivity to glare
- Narrowed visual field
- Diminished depth perception
- Altered color perception so objects look darker and whites appear more yellowed
- Diminished ability to perceive flashing lights
- Slower processing of visual information

Risks Factors That Affect Visual Wellness

- Environmental factors: glare, sunlight, poor lighting, low humidity
- Lifestyle factors: poor nutrition, cigarette smoking
- Chronic conditions: diabetes, hypertension, Alzheimer's or Parkinson's disease
- Adverse medication effects: estrogen, corticosteroids, anticholinergics, beta-blockers, antiparkinson agents

Pathologic Conditions Affecting Vision (Figs. 17-2 and 17-3, Table 17-2)

- Cataracts
- AMD
- Glaucoma

Functional Consequences Affecting Visual Wellness

- Presbyopia (diminished ability to focus on near objects)
- Need for three to five times more light than previously
- Difficulty with night driving
- Increased risk for unsafe mobility
- Increased difficulty in performing usual activities

Nursing Assessment of Vision (Fig. 17-4, Boxes 17-1 through 17-3)

- Vision screening tests
- Risk factors that affect vision
- Influence of vision changes on performance of activities of daily living
- Attitudes about eye examinations and preventive measures
- Attitudes regarding use of low-vision aids

Nursing Diagnosis

- Readiness for Enhanced Knowledge: Improved Vision
- Disturbed Sensory Perception: Visual
- Additional diagnoses that address the functional consequences of visual impairment include: Anxiety, Ineffective Coping, Self-Care Deficit, Risk for Injury, Impaired Social Interaction, Readiness for Enhanced Coping, and Readiness for Enhanced Self-Care

Planning for Wellness Outcomes

- Improved visual function
- Increased safety
- Improved independence in activities of daily living
- Improved quality of life

Nursing Interventions for Visual Wellness (Boxes 17-4 through 17-9)

- Prevention and detection of eye disease
- Comfort measures for dry eyes
- Environmental modifications (e.g., optimal illumination)
- Low-vision aids

Evaluating Effectiveness of Nursing Interventions

- Use of corrective lenses and other aids that improve vision
- Environmental adaptations for optimal safety and visual function
- Improved independence in daily activities
- Expressed feelings of improved quality of life in relation to visual function

CRITICAL THINKING EXERCISES

1. Describe presbyopia and explain the functional consequences of this condition in the everyday life of an older adult.
2. What environmental factors are likely to interfere with the visual function of older adults?
3. Describe the specific effects of glaucoma, cataracts, or AMD on one's ability to see a television program.

4. How would you assess the visual abilities of an older adult?
5. Explain the differences between opticians, optometrists, and ophthalmologists.
6. List at least 10 adaptations that might be implemented to improve the visual function of older adults.

Educational Resources

American Academy of Ophthalmology
www.eyenet.org

American Foundation for the Blind
www.afb.org

American Optometric Association
www.aoanet.org

Canadian National Institute for the Blind
www.cnib.ca

The Glaucoma Foundation
www.glaucoma-foundation.org

Lighthouse International
www.lighthouse.org

Lions Clubs International
www.lionsclubs.org

National Association for Visually Handicapped (NAVH)
www.navh.org

National Eye Institute (NEI)
www.nei.nih.gov

Prevent Blindness America
www.preventblindness.org

References

Bazargan, M., Baker, R. S., & Bazargan, S. H. (2001). Sensory impairments and subjective well-being among aged African American persons. *Journals of Gerontology: Series B, Psychological Sciences and Social Sciences, 56,* P268–P278.

Carpenito-Moyet, L. J. (2006). *Handbook of nursing diagnosis* (11th ed.). Philadelphia: Lippincott Williams & Wilkins.

Croft, M. A., & Kaufman, P. L. (2006). Accommodation and presbyopia: The ciliary neuromuscular view. *Ophthalmology Clinics of North America, 19,* 13–24.

Desai, M., Pratt, L. A., Lentzner, H., & Robinson, K. N. (2001). Trends in vision and hearing among older Americans. In *Aging trends, no. 2.* Hyattsville, MD: National Center for Health Statistics.

Foss, A. J., Harwood, R. H., Osborn, F., Gregson, R. M., Zaman, A., & Masud, T. (2006). Falls and health status in elderly women following second eye cataract surgery: A randomized controlled trial. *Age and Ageing, 35,* 66–71.

Gray, C. S., Karimova, G., Hildreth, A. J., Crabtree, L., Allen, D., & O'Connell, J. E. (2006). Recovery of visual and functional disability following cataract surgery in older people: Sunderland Cataract Study. *Journal of Cataract and Refractive Surgery, 32*(1), 60–66.

Johnson, M., Bulechek, G. M., Dochterman, J. M., Maas, M. L., Moorhead, S., Swanson, E., et al. (2006). *NANDA, NOC, and NIC linkages* (2nd ed.). St. Louis: Mosby Elsevier.

Lord, S. R., & Dayhew, J. (2001). Visual risk factors for falls in older people. *Journal of American Geriatrics Society, 49,* 508–515.

Matsui, H., Udaka, F., Tamura, A., Oda, M., Kubori, T., Nishinaka, K., et al. (2006). Impaired visual acuity as a risk factor for visual hallucinations in Parkinson's disease. *Journal of Geriatric Psychiatry Neurology, 19,* 36–40.

Morrow, D. A., Gersh, B. J., & Braunwald, E. (2005). Chronic coronary artery disease. In D. P. Zipes, P. Libby, R. O. Bonow, & E. Braunwald (Eds.), *Braunwald's heart disease* (7th ed.). Philadelphia: Elsevier Saunders.

Mukesh, B. N., Le, A., Ahmed, S., Taylor, H. R., & McCarty, C. A. (2006). Development of cataract and associated risk factors: The Visual Impairment Project. *Archives of Ophthalmology, 124,* 79–85.

Munoz, B. West, S. K., Rubin, G. S., Scheim, O. D., Quigley, H. A., Bressler, S. B., & Bandeen-Roche, K. (2000). Causes of blindness and visual impairment in a population of older Americans: The Salisbury Eye Evaluation Study. *Archives of Ophthalmology, 118,* 819–825.

Quigley, H. A., West, S. K., Rodriguez, J., Munoz, B., Klein, R., & Snyder, R. (2001). The prevalence of glaucoma in a population-based study of Hispanic subjects: VER. *Archives of Ophthalmology, 119,* 1819–1826.

Rovner, B. W., & Casten, R. J. (2002). Activity loss and depression in age-related macular degeneration. *American Journal of Geriatric Psychiatry, 10,* 305–310.

Schieber, F. (2006). Vision and aging: In J. E. Birren & K. W. Schaie (Eds.), *Handbook of the psychology of aging* (6th ed., pp. 129–161). San Diego: Academic Press.

Slusher, M. M. (2005). What's new in ophthalmic surgery? *Journal of the American College of Surgeons, 201,* 742–745.

U.S. Department of Health and Human Services (USDHSS). (2000). *Healthy people 2010* (2nd ed.). Washington, DC: U.S. Government Printing Office.

Wilson, M. R., & Eezzuduemhoi, D. R. (2005). Ophthalmologic disorders in minority populations. *Medical Clinics of North America, 89,* 795–804.

Yanoff, M. (2004). *Ophthalmology* (2nd ed.). St. Louis: Mosby Elsevier.

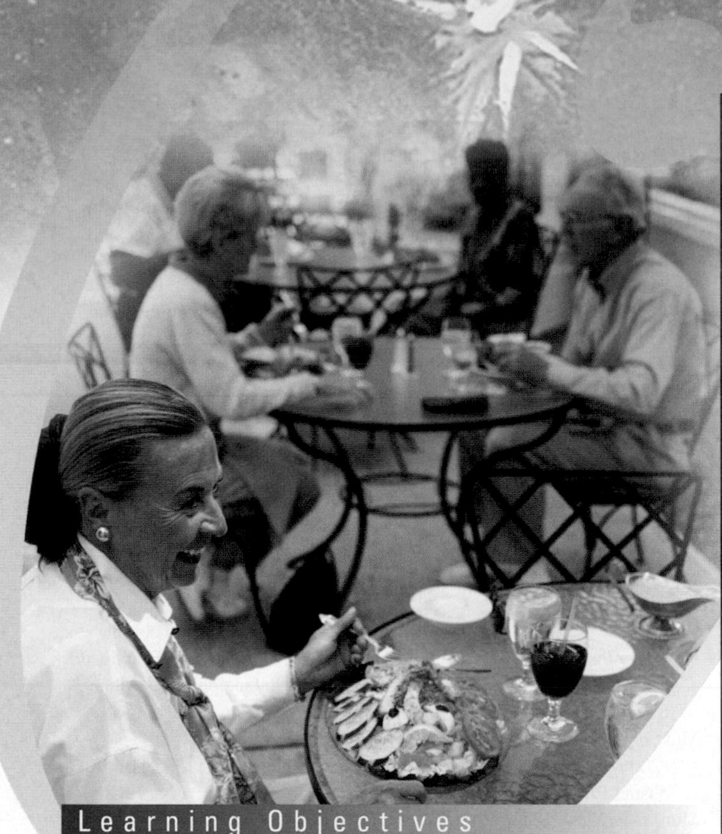

CHAPTER 18

Digestion and Nutrition

Learning Objectives

After reading this chapter, you will be able to:

1. Describe age-related changes that affect eating patterns and digestive processes.
2. List age-related changes in nutritional requirements.
3. Identify risk factors that affect the digestion and nutrition of older adults.
4. Explain the effects of age-related changes and risk factors on digestion and nutrition.
5. Assess aspects of nutrition, digestion, behaviors that affect eating and food preparation, and oral care pertinent to care of older adults.
6. Identify nursing interventions to promote optimal nutrition, digestion, and oral care.

Key Terms

achlorhydria
body mass index (BMI)
cholelithiasis
constipation
dietary fiber
dysphagia
early satiety
functional fiber
insoluble fibers
kwashiorkor
lipofuscin
marasmus
presbyesophagus
presbyphagia
protein-energy undernutrition
xerostomia

Digestion of food and maintenance of nutrition are influenced to a small degree by age-related gastrointestinal changes and to a large degree by risk factors that commonly occur in older adulthood. Older adults can easily adjust their eating habits to compensate for age-related changes in the digestive tract, but have more difficulty compensating for the consequences of the many factors that interfere with their ability to obtain, prepare, and enjoy food. This chapter discusses age-related changes and functional consequences in relation to digestion, eating patterns, and nutritional requirements.

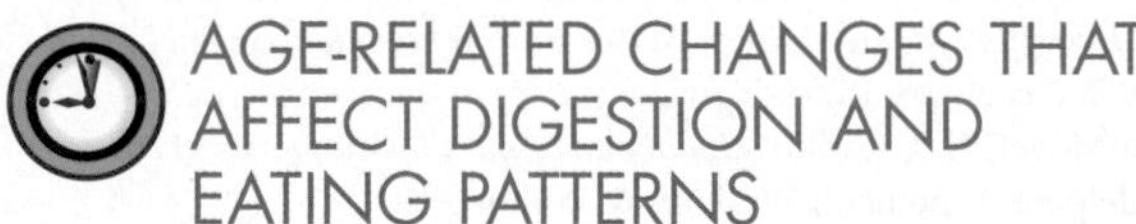

AGE-RELATED CHANGES THAT AFFECT DIGESTION AND EATING PATTERNS

Age-related changes affect the senses of smell and taste and all the organs of the digestive tract. These changes have very few functional consequences for healthy older adults, but they increase the vulnerability of older adults to risk factors.

Smell and Taste

Although the senses of both taste and smell affect food enjoyment, the sense of smell has a more significant influence and declines more than does the sense of taste in older adults. The ability to smell depends on the perception of odorants by the sensory cells in the olfactory mucosa and on central nervous system processing of that information. The ability to detect and identify odors is best around the age of 30 years, and then gradually declines. Age-related brain changes contribute to this decline, even in healthy older adults (Gilbert et al., 2006). Additional conditions that also

Promoting Digestive and Nutritional Wellness in Older Adults

Nursing Assessment
• Usual nutrient intake
• Usual eating patterns
• Risks that affect food preparation, intake, and enjoyment
• Measures of nutritional status
Age-Related Changes
• Less efficient chewing
• ↓ senses of smell and taste
• ↓ saliva secretion
• Slower motility
• Degenerative changes affecting digestion
• Daily intake: need fewer but higher quality calories
Negative Functional Consequences
• Difficulty procuring and preparing food
• ↓ enjoyment of food
• ↓ absorption of nutrients
• ↑ tendency to develop constipation
Risk Factors
• Conditions that affect ability to obtain, prepare, consume, or enjoy food
• Poor oral care
• Effects of medications
• Cultural and socioeconomic factors
• Environmental factors
Nursing Interventions
• Teaching about nutrition and digestion
• Preventing/addressing constipation
• Promoting oral and dental care
• Referring for home-delivered meals and group meal progams
Wellness Outcomes
• Improved nutritional status
• Improved oral hygiene
• Elimination of risk factors
• ↑ sense of well-being

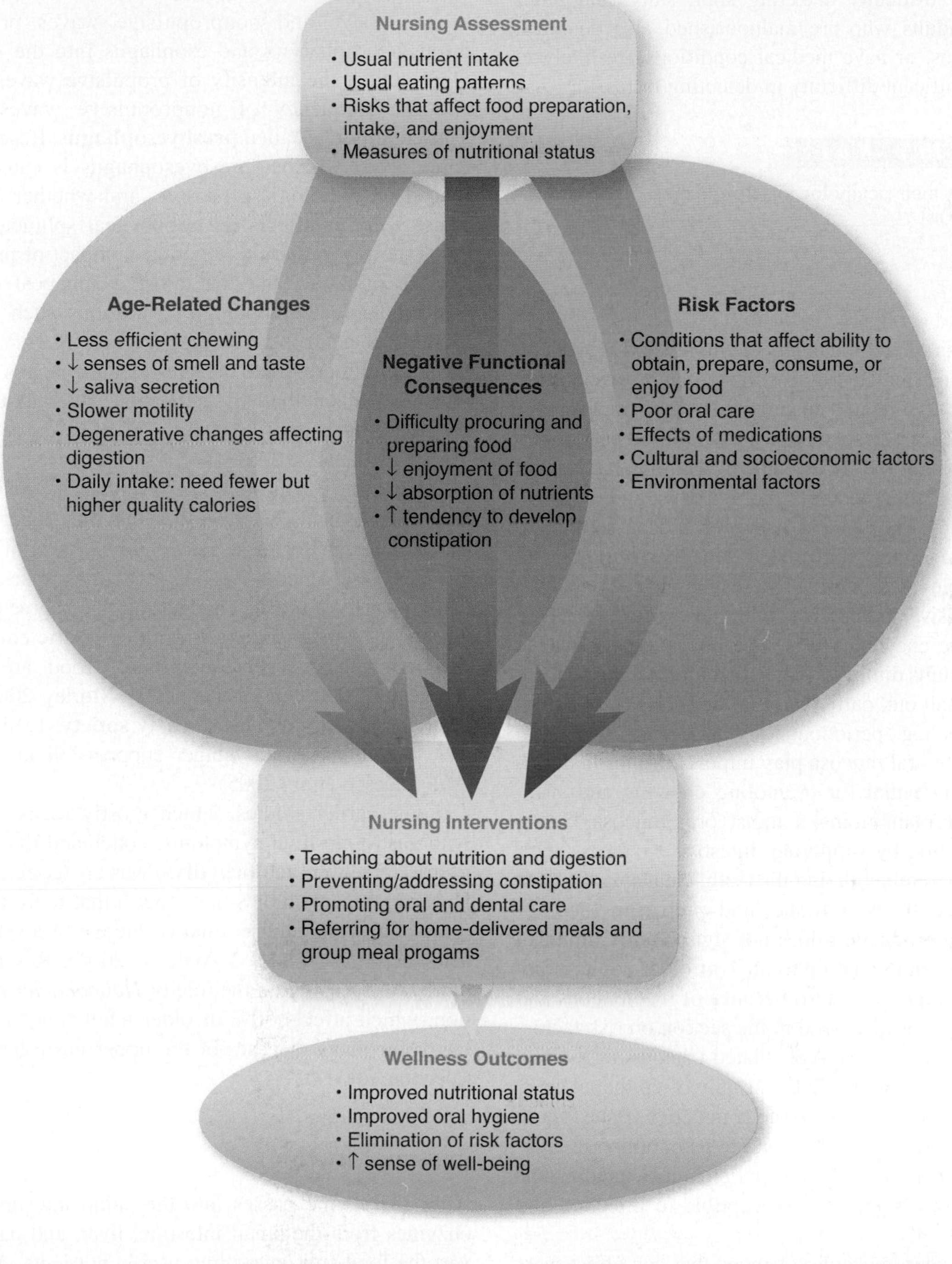

can contribute to this decline include smoking or chewing tobacco, vitamin B_{12} deficiency, radiation to the head or neck (beginning during the third week and lasting as long as 1 year), medications (e.g., anticoagulants, antihistamines, salicylates, hypoglycemics, antiparkinson drugs, psychoactive drugs), periodontal disease and oral infections, upper respiratory diseases (e.g., sinusitis), systemic diseases (e.g., dementia, diabetes, hypothyroidism), and occupational experiences (e.g., working in a factory) (Finkel et al., 2001; Morley, 2002; Dudek, 2007).

The ability to taste depends primarily on receptor cells in the taste buds, which are located on the tongue, palate, and tonsils. Characteristics of taste sensation are measured according to the ability to perceive intensity of taste, which diminishes with aging, and the ability to identify different tastes. Although some early studies suggested that the number of taste buds declined with aging, more recent studies have found that taste cells can regenerate but that the lag time of this turnover may account for diminished taste response in older adults (Fukunaga et al., 2005). Because age-related changes do not affect all taste sensations equally, healthy older adults maintain the ability to detect sweet taste but have more difficulty detecting sour, salty, and bitter tastes. Older adults who are malnourished, use dentures, take medications, or have medical conditions are likely to experience significant difficulty in detecting tastes.

Diversity Note

Women retain their acuity for taste and smell better than men (Yen, 2004).

Oral Cavity

Digestion begins when food enters the mouth and is acted on by the teeth, saliva, and neuromuscular structures responsible for mastication. Age-related changes in the teeth and support structures influence digestive processes and food enjoyment. With increased age, the tooth enamel becomes harder and more brittle, the dentin becomes more fibrous, and the nerve chambers become shorter and narrower. Because of these age-related changes, the teeth are less sensitive to stimuli and more susceptible to fractures. These changes, along with decades of abrasive and erosive action, also cause a gradual flattening of the chewing cusps. The bones supporting the teeth of older adults diminish in height and density, and teeth may loosen or fall out, particularly in the presence of pathologic conditions (e.g., periodontal disease).

Saliva and the oral mucosa play important roles in digestion. Saliva is essential for promoting chewing and swallowing and for maintaining a moist oral mucosa. Saliva facilitates digestion by supplying digestive enzymes, regulating oral flora, remineralizing the teeth, cleansing the taste buds, lubricating the soft tissue, and preparing food for chewing. Saliva production does not significantly diminish in healthy older adults, but up to 38% of older adults experience **xerostomia** (dry mouth) because of medications and disease processes, as discussed in the section on risk factors (Matear & Barbaro, 2005). Age-related changes of the oral mucosa include loss of elasticity, atrophy of epithelial cells, and diminished blood supply to the connective tissue. These changes can be exacerbated by conditions common in older adults (e.g., xerostomia, vitamin deficiencies), making the oral mucosa more friable and susceptible to infection and ulceration.

Age-related neuromuscular changes that can affect mastication and swallowing include diminished muscle strength and slower swallowing. Although these age-related changes do not have a major impact on healthy older adults, they may increase the probability that older adults will develop dysphagia and other swallowing problems (Nicosia et al., 2000). Problems with chewing and swallowing in older adults are generally attributable to risk factors, such as tooth loss or neurologic conditions, rather than to age-related changes alone.

Esophagus and Stomach

The second phase of digestion occurs when a combination of propulsive and nonpropulsive waves propels food through the pharynx and esophagus into the stomach. In older adults, the intensity of propulsive waves decreases, and the frequency of nonpropulsive waves increases. This condition is called **presbyesophagus**. Researchers disagree about whether presbyesophagus is caused by age-related or pathologic processes, and whether it slows the transit time or affects the esophageal sphincter. They do agree, however, that the functional impact of presbyesophagus is minimal, and that most esophageal dysfunction is attributable to pathologic conditions such as diabetes mellitus or neurologic disease (Achem & DeVault, 2005). **Presbyphagia** refers to the age-related changes in the swallow mechanism that affect healthy older adults and can increase the risk for aspiration (Leslie et al., 2005; Yoshikawa et al., 2006).

After passing through the esophageal sphincter, food enters the stomach, where gastric enzymes liquefy it and gastric action transforms it into chyme. As with esophageal changes, researchers disagree about the cause, extent, and consequences of gastric changes, but they agree that aging is associated with a modest slowing of gastric emptying, particularly when larger amounts of food are consumed (Horowitz, 2000; Jensen et al., 2001; Morley, 2002). Delayed gastric emptying may cause **early satiety** (feeling full with less food intake) and hunger suppression in older adults (DiFrancesco et al., 2005).

Some earlier studies, which mostly focused on people with gastrointestinal symptoms, concluded that diminished gastric secretion (**achlorhydria**) was an age-related change. However, recent studies have found that more than 80% of older adults maintain normal or increased levels of gastric acid secretion (Linder & Wilcox, 2001). Researchers currently are focusing on the role of *Helicobacter pylori* infection, which affects 50% of older adults and is a causative factor for many diseases of the upper gastrointestinal tract (Newton, 2004).

Intestinal Tract

After the chyme passes into the small intestine, digestive enzymes from the small intestine, liver, and pancreas convert the food substances into usable nutrients. A process of segmentation moves the chyme backward and forward, facilitating the digestion of food and the absorption of nutrients through the villi in the walls of the small intestine. Age-related changes that occur in the small intestine include atrophy of muscle fibers and mucosal surfaces; reduction in the number of lymphatic follicles; gradual reduction in the weight of the small intestine; and shortening and widening of the villi, which gradually form parallel ridges rather than finger-like projections. These structural changes do not significantly affect small intestinal motility, permeability, or transit time; however, they may affect immune function and absorption of some nutrients, such as calcium and vitamin D.

After nutrients are absorbed in the small intestine, the chyme passes into the large intestine, where water and electrolytes are absorbed and waste products are expelled. Age-related changes in the large intestine include reduced secretion of mucus, decreased elasticity of the rectal wall, and diminished perception of rectal wall distention. These age-related changes have little or no impact on motility of feces through the bowel, but they may predispose the older person to constipation because larger rectal volumes are needed before the urge to defecate is perceived (Prather, 2000).

Liver, Pancreas, and Gallbladder

The liver assists in digestion by producing and secreting bile, which is essential for the utilization of fats. It also plays an important role in the metabolism and storage of medications and nutrients, such as vitamins and carbohydrates. With increasing age, the liver becomes smaller and more fibrous, **lipofuscin** (a brown pigment) accumulates, and blood flow to the liver decreases by about one third. However, some of these changes may be pathologic, rather than age-related, in origin. Despite any age-related or pathologic changes, the liver has an enormous regenerative and reserve capacity, which allows it to compensate for such changes without significantly affecting digestive function.

A primary digestive function of the pancreas is the secretion of enzymes essential for neutralizing acids in the chyme and breaking down fats, proteins, and carbohydrates in the small intestine. The pancreas also functions as an endocrine gland and produces insulin and glycogen, which are essential for glucose metabolism. Age-related changes in the pancreas include decreased weight, hyperplasia of the duct, fibrosis of the lobe, and decreased responsiveness of pancreatic B cells to glucose. Although these changes have little or no direct impact on digestive functioning, diminished insulin secretion increases the susceptibility of older adults to the development of glucose intolerance and type 2 diabetes (Horowitz, 2000).

Age-related changes that affect the gallbladder and biliary tract include diminished bile acid synthesis, widening of the common bile duct, and increased secretion of cholecystokinin, a peptide hormone that contracts the gallbladder and relaxes the biliary sphincter. Effects of these age-related changes include biliary stasis, increased biliary bacterial flora, and increased incidence of **cholelithiasis** (gallstones) in older adults (Horowitz, 2000; Ross & Forsmark, 2001). In addition, the higher level of cholecystokinin that occurs in older adults may suppress the appetite and reduce food intake (Morley, 2002).

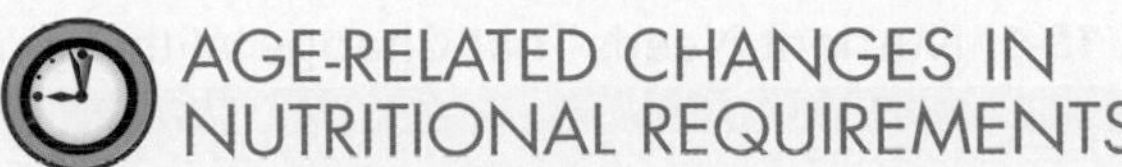

AGE-RELATED CHANGES IN NUTRITIONAL REQUIREMENTS

Until recently, little attention was focused on age-related changes in nutritional requirements for healthy older adults. A review of studies of nutrient intakes across the adult life span found some evidence that older adults require an increased intake of several nutrients because of diminished absorption and utilization, but "nutrition research is urgently needed to determine metabolic changes and nutrient needs of older people" (Wakimoto & Block, 2001, p. 79). Until the late 1990s, the Recommended Dietary Allowances (RDA) of the National Academy of Sciences (introduced in 1941) was the primary reference standard for measuring the intake levels of essential nutrients that were considered adequate for meeting the nutrient needs of healthy people. An important limitation of the RDA is that a single standard applied to all people age 51 years and older.

In January 2001, the Food and Nutrition Board, the Institute of Medicine, the National Academy of Sciences, and Health Canada jointly published a major revision of the RDA. This Dietary Reference Intakes (DRIs) set standards for meeting the basic nutrient needs of healthy adults and include indicators for preventing chronic disease and avoiding the harmful effects of consuming too much of a nutrient. In addition to focusing on the role of nutrients in health promotion, the DRIs address specific age groups (e.g., adults aged 51 to 70 years and those 70 years and older). Because these standards apply only to healthy older adults, they need to be adjusted to compensate for conditions such as nutrient deficiencies and medical conditions. In addition, adjustments for food and drug interactions may be necessary for people who take one or more medications. For example, people with gastroesophageal reflux disease are likely to need significantly increased intake or supplements of vitamin B_{12} because the condition and many medications used for it interfere with this vitamin's absorption. Table 18-1 summarizes some of the age-related changes in nutrient requirements.

Calories

The energy-producing potential of food is measured in units called *calories*. Caloric requirements are determined by a combination of factors, including height, weight, sex, body build, health–illness state, and usual level of physical activity. Because energy requirements gradually decrease throughout adulthood—owing to decreased physical activity and the decline in basal metabolic rate that is associated with diminished muscle mass—nutritional guidelines recommend a gradual reduction in calories beginning around the age of 40 to 50 years. Surveys of the nutritional status of older adults indicate that mean daily energy intake declines by 1000 to 1200 calories in men and by 600 to 800 calories in women between the ages of 20 and 80 years (Wakimoto & Block, 2001). Distribution of calories also changes, with

TABLE 18-1 Nutrient Needs That Change With Aging

Nutrient	Age (Years)			Rationale for Change
	31–50	51–70	>70	
Iron (mg)				
Men	**8**	**8**	**8**	
Women	**18**	**8**	**8**	Cessation of menses
Calcium (mg)				
Men	1000	1200	1200	Efficiency of Ca absorption decreases with age.
Women	1000	1200	1200	
Vitamin D (mcg)				
Men	5	10	15	Ability to synthesize vitamin D from sunlight decreases with age.
Women	5	10	15	
Vitamin B_{12} (mcg)				
Men	**2.4**	**2.4***	**2.4***	*The *amount* of vitamin B_{12} does not change, but the recommended source does. Because many older adults have impaired absorption of food-bound vitamin B_{12}, it is recommended that people older than 50 meet their RDA mainly from B_{12} fortified foods or vitamin supplements.
Women	**2.4**	**2.4***	**2.4***	
Vitamin B_6 (mcg)				
Men	**1.3**	**1.7**	**1.7**	Aging alters vitamin B_6 metabolism to increase need.
Women	**1.3**	**1.5**	**1.5**	

Bold items are Recommended Dietary Allowances (RDA), whereas Adequate Intakes (AI) appear in ordinary type.
From Dudek, S. G. (2007). *Nutrition essentials for nursing practice* (5th ed., rev. reprint, p. 354). Philadelphia: Lippincott Williams & Wilkins.

older adults needing to consume a higher percentage of calories in carbohydrates and a lower percentage in fats, while maintaining a relatively stable protein intake (Wakimoto & Block, 2001). Any decrease in caloric intake requires a proportionate increase in the quality of calories (nutritional density) to meet minimal nutritional requirements. Thus, nutritional deficiencies will occur unless a reduced caloric intake is accompanied by an increased intake of foods with a high nutritional value and a concomitant decrease in the intake of foods containing little or no nutrients.

Diversity Note

Mean caloric intake for groups in the United States is highest in whites, lower in Mexican Americans, and lowest in African Americans (Wakimoto & Block, 2001).

Protein

Protein provides the essential components for new tissue growth in the human body. Age-related changes, such as decreased lean body mass and muscle tissue and decreased plasma albumin and total body albumin levels, may influence protein requirements in older adults, but little is known about the specific effects of these changes in healthy older adults. A minimum daily protein intake of 1 g/kg of body weight is recommended for older adults, and this can be achieved if approximately 10% to 20% of the daily caloric intake is derived from protein. Older adults with acute medical conditions may need a daily protein intake of 1.5 g/kg of body weight (Jensen et al., 2001).

Carbohydrates and Fiber

Carbohydrates provide an essential source of energy and fiber. Without an adequate intake of carbohydrates, the body will derive energy from fat and protein, causing an increase in serum cholesterol and triglyceride levels and a depletion of water, electrolytes, and amino acids. Fiber has received much attention in recent years, primarily for its role in disease prevention, as an essential food component. *Soluble fibers*, found in oats and pectin, are beneficial in lowering serum cholesterol levels and improving glucose tolerance in people with diabetes. **Insoluble fibers**, found in most grains and many vegetables, are important for maintaining good bowel function and for preventing constipation. Definitions recently proposed by the National Academy of Sciences (2002) recommend that fiber be categorized as **dietary fiber** when it is an intrinsic component of food and as **functional fiber** when it is an isolated or extracted nondigestible carbohydrate that has beneficial physiologic effects in humans. Some fibers, such as cellulose, can be either dietary (when it occurs naturally in foods) or functional (when it is added to foods). The average daily intake of fiber for Americans is 10 to 15 g, which is significantly less than the 25 to 38 g/day recommended by the National Cancer Institute and other health authorities (DeBusk, 2002; National Academy of Sciences, 2002). Dietary guidelines suggest a daily intake of five to nine servings of fruits and vegetables, with at least 55% of the total calories consumed derived from complex carbohydrates.

Fats

The primary functions of fat are to assist in temperature regulation, provide a reserve source of energy, facilitate the absorption of fat-soluble vitamins, and reduce acid secretion and muscular activity of the stomach. Fats are also useful in providing a feeling of satiety and improving the taste of foods. Fats are categorized according to their source. Saturated fats are derived from animals, whereas unsaturated fats are found in vegetables. Although either type of fat can meet nutritional needs, only the saturated fats are associated with the detrimental accumulation of serum cholesterol. Adults in most industrialized societies consume far more calories in fats than is healthy or necessary. Because excessive fat intake is associated with harmful effects, such as hyperlipidemia, fat should constitute no more than 10% to 30% of a person's daily caloric intake. Those fats that are consumed should be polyunsaturated and monounsaturated fatty acids, rather than cholesterol and saturated fats (see Chapter 20 for further discussion of types of fat).

Water

Water is such a commonly available substance that it is often overlooked as a nutritional requirement. However, it is essential for all metabolic activities and must be consumed in adequate amounts for proper physiologic performance. The functions of water include regulating body temperature, maintaining a suitable metabolic environment, diluting water-soluble medications, and facilitating renal and bowel excretion. Potential consequences of reduced body water include decreased efficiency of thermoregulation, increased susceptibility to dehydration, and increased concentrations of water-soluble medications in the body.

Throughout life, the proportion of total body water as a percentage of body weight gradually decreases. Whereas water constitutes about 80% of a newborn infant's weight, it represents 60% of a younger adult's weight, and about 50% or less of an older adult's weight. This decrease in total body water is associated with a loss of lean body mass and is influenced by sex and degree of leanness, with women and obese people having a lower percentage of body water than men and lean, muscular people. In older adults, total body water may be further diminished by poor fluid intake secondary to age-related factors, such as diminished thirst sensation. It is recommended that older adults consume 1500 to 2000 mL (6 to 8 glasses) of noncaffeinated fluid daily to maintain adequate hydration.

RISK FACTORS THAT AFFECT DIGESTION AND NUTRITION

Certain behaviors and common disease processes are likely to interfere with nutrition and digestion in older adults. Behaviors that are detrimental to nutrition and digestion, such as limiting fluid intake and avoiding fresh fruit, may be based on myths and misconceptions. Although these conditions can create risks for people at any age, they occur more commonly in older adults, and the potential for harm is much greater than in other age groups because of the collective effects of risk factors and age-related changes. Risk factors affect every phase of digestion and nutrition and they can significantly influence eating patterns and nutritional intake. One study identified the following predictors of poor nutrition in newly admitted nursing home residents (Crogan & Corbett, 2002):

- Recent weight loss
- Psychiatric diagnosis
- Missing all or some teeth
- Living alone before admission
- Using a diuretic or antidepressant
- A decline in functional status from morning to evening

Risks that can cause specific nutrient deficiencies are listed in Table 18-2, along with the related functional consequences.

Inadequate Oral Care

Inadequate oral care practices have been cited as a factor that very commonly contributes to poor nutrition, particularly for older adults in institutional settings. Studies in Europe and North America have found widespread occurrence of poor oral health in nursing home residents, and one survey cited routine oral hygiene as the greatest single need among older nursing home residents (Coleman, 2002). Poor oral hygiene results in stomatitis, xerostomia, tooth loss, dental caries, and periodontal disease—all conditions that can interfere with nutrition and food selection and enjoyment. Although inadequate oral care is a common and serious risk factor for problems associated with nutrition and digestion, staff in long-term care facilities generally do not recognize it as a serious problem, nor do they consider it a priority for nursing care (Chung et al., 2000; Wardh et al., 2000). Thus, attitudes and behaviors of nurses related to provision of oral care for dependent older adults is a common risk factor that needs to be addressed through interventions (Ship, 2002).

Xerostomia and tooth loss are common among older adults, but both conditions are attributable to risk factors rather than to age-related changes. For example, more than 400 medications have been cited as the most common cause

TABLE 18-2 Causes and Consequences of Nutrient Deficiencies

Nutrient	Possible Causes of Deficiency	Functional Consequences of Deficiency
Calories	Anorexia, depression, mental or physical impairments	Weight loss, lethargy, edema, anemia
Protein	Lack of teeth or dentures, anorexia, depression, dementia, high alcohol or carbohydrate consumption	Poor tissue healing, hypoalbuminemia, reduced protein binding of drugs
Fat	Neomycin, phenytoin, laxatives, alcohol, colchicine, cholestyramine	Inability to absorb vitamins A, D, E, and K
Vitamin A	Mineral oil, neomycin, alcohol, cholestyramine, aluminum antacids, liver disease	Dry skin and eyes, photophobia, night blindness, hyperkeratoses
Thiamine (B_1)	High consumption of alcohol or caffeinated tea, pernicious anemia, diuretics	Neuropathy, muscle weakness, heart disease, dementia, anorexia
Riboflavin (B_2)	Malabsorption syndromes, chronic diarrhea laxative abuse, alcoholism, liver disease	Cheilitis, glossitis, photophobia, blepharitis, conjunctivitis
Niacin (B_3)	Poor dietary habits, diarrhea, cirrhosis, alcoholism	Dermatitis, stomatitis, diarrhea, dementia, depression
Pyridoxine (B_6)	Diuretics, hydralazine	Dermatitis, neuropathy
Folate (B_9)	Anticonvulsants, triamterene, sulfonamides, alcohol, smoking	Macrocytic anemia, elevated levels of homocysteine
Vitamin B_{12}	Malabsorption syndrome, H_2-receptor blockers, proton pump inhibitors, colchicine, oral hypoglycemics, potassium supplements, vegetarian diet	Pernicious anemia, weakness, dyspnea, glossitis, numbness, dementia, depression
Vitamin C	Aspirin, tetracycline, lack of fruits and vegetables in diet	Lassitude, irritability, anemia, ecchymosis, impaired wound healing
Vitamin D	Phenytoin, mineral oil, phenobarbital, sunlight deprivation	Muscle weakness and atrophy, osteoporosis, fractures
Vitamin E	Malabsorption syndromes	Peripheral neuropathy, gait disturbance, retinopathy
Vitamin K	Mineral oil, warfarin sodium (Coumadin), antibiotics, cholestyramine, phenytoin	Ecchymosis; hemorrhage involving the gastrointestinal, urinary, or central nervous system
Calcium	Phenytoin, aluminum-based antacids, laxatives, tetracycline, corticosteroids, furosemide, high intake of fiber or caffeine	Osteoporosis, fractures, low back pain
Iron	Achlorhydria; neomycin; aspirin; antacids; low intake of animal protein; high consumption of fiber, caffeine, or tannic acid (contained in some teas)	Anemia, weakness, lassitude, pallor
Magnesium	Alcohol, diuretics, diarrhea, bulk-forming laxatives	Cardiac arrhythmias, neuromuscular and central nervous system irritability, disorientation
Zinc	Penicillamine, aluminum-based antacids, bulk-forming laxatives, high consumption of fiber	Poor wound healing, hair loss
Potassium	Laxatives, furosemide, antibiotics, corticosteroids, diarrhea	Weakness, cardiac arrhythmias, digitalis toxicity
Water	Diuretics, laxatives, immobility, incontinence, diarrhea	Dry skin and mouth, dehydration, constipation
Fiber	Poor dietary habits	Constipation, hemorrhoids

of xerostomia in older people (Matear & Barbaro, 2005). A review of data concluded that 95% of older adults have dental caries, with the highest risk being associated with mental confusion, physical frailty, and dependency on others for oral care (Ettinger, 2001). Until recently, tooth loss was so common among older people that it has been inaccurately viewed as a normal consequence of aging; but the oral health of older people has improved in the past few decades so that older adults today are less likely to be edentulous (without any teeth). In the late 1990s, about half of all nursing home residents 75 years of age and older and one third of noninstitutionalized people 65 years of age or older were edentulous (Ritchie, 2002). Tooth loss in older adulthood is often attributable to inadequate dental care, xerostomia and periodontal disease, and other pathologic conditions that occur with increasing frequency in later years. Women and people who smoke have higher rates of tooth loss (Randolph et al., 2001). Some factors that contribute to inadequate dental care include

- Low income
- Less education
- Lack of transportation
- Lack of dental insurance
- High cost of dental services
- More urgent health concerns
- Inaccessibility of services as a result of distance or environmental barriers, such as stairs to dental offices

Diversity Note

African Americans, Native Americans, and Alaska Natives are more likely than white Americans to have fewer natural teeth (USDHHS, 2000).

Negative attitudes on the part of dentists or older adults also may interfere with the provision of dental services. For example, if a dentist or an older adult views tooth loss as an inevitable concomitant of old age, restorative and preventive dental services may not be offered by the dentist or not be requested by the patient. In addition, many older adults have been fully or partially edentulous since the 1930s and 1940s because of the dental practices of that era, which espoused the removal, rather than the preservation, of teeth. Because preventive dental care is a recent trend, older adults may believe that they should visit a dentist only when a toothache does not respond to home remedies.

Wellness Opportunity

Nurses promote wellness by exploring reasons that older adults do not obtain dental care so they can address these barriers.

Functional Impairments and Disease Processes

Functional impairments are strongly associated with poor nutrition and difficulty procuring food, particularly in community-living older adults (Sharkey, 2002). For example, mobility or visual impairments can interfere with the ability to procure and prepare food. In community settings, however, the extent to which functional impairments affect nutrition depends to a large degree on the availability of social supports, such as family, friends, or agencies who assist with provision of food. As many as 60% of nursing home residents have some degree of **dysphagia** (difficulty swallowing), a functional impairment that can significantly affect nutrition (Lewis, 2001). Dysphagia in older adults most commonly is caused by neurologic disorders, such as stroke and dementia.

Disease processes also increase the risk for nutritional and digestive consequences. Chronic gastritis (an inflammation of the gastric mucosa) is common in older adults and is a leading cause of vitamin B_{12} deficiency (Andres et al., 2002). Pernicious anemia, peptic ulcers, and stomach cancer occur more often in older adults, and these conditions may be associated with diminished capacity of the gastric mucosa to resist damage (Newton, 2004). Other pathologic conditions interfere with appetite and enjoyment of food in many ways. For example, infections, hyperthyroidism, hypoadrenalism, and congestive heart failure are associated with anorexia, and rheumatoid conditions and chronic obstructive pulmonary disease (COPD) are associated with both decreased appetite and increased energy expenditure. Alzheimer's disease and other dementias often have serious negative effects on eating and nutrition related to procuring and preparing food, remembering to eat, and chewing and swallowing food. Risk factors associated with unintentional weight loss include dementia, depression, malignancies, gastrointestinal disease, and endocrine and cardiovascular disorders (Alibhai et al., 2005).

Medication Effects

Medications can create risk factors for impaired digestion and inadequate nutrition through their effects on digestion, eating patterns, and utilization of nutrients (Table 18-3). Although these medication effects are not uniquely age related, they are more likely to occur in older adults because of their increased use of prescription and over-the-counter medications. Moreover, because medication effects can exacerbate and interact with age-related changes and other risk factors, they are likely to be more detrimental in older adults.

Medications can interfere with digestion and eating through adverse effects such as anorexia, xerostomia, early satiety, and impaired smell and taste perception. In addition to being a common cause of xerostomia, medications are a common cause of eating or chewing discomfort. For example, gum hyperplasia is associated with phenytoin, nifedipine, diltiazem, and cyclosporine. Medications can alter chemosensory perceptions through their action at peripheral receptors, neural pathways, and the brain. More than 250 medications are associated with abnormal or dulled taste sensation (Staveren et al., 2002).

Constipation is another common adverse effect of many medications, especially agents that act on the central nervous system. Paralytic ileus, which has a serious impact on digestive function, may arise from anticholinergic medications or from hypokalemia caused by potassium-wasting diuretics. Medications also cause adverse effects that interfere with the ability to procure, prepare, eat, and enjoy food. For example, medications that cause confusion, depression, and other mental changes can indirectly but significantly affect the older person's eating patterns.

Medications can affect nutrition by interfering with the absorption and excretion of nutrients, as in the following examples:

- Broad-spectrum antibiotics can alter intestinal flora and impair nutrient synthesis.
- Medications and vitamins that are similar in chemical structure may compete at sites of action, altering their excretion pattern.
- Some medications bind to particular ions and form compounds that cannot be absorbed (e.g., tetracycline can bind to iron and calcium).
- Diuretics can interfere with the transport of water, sodium, glucose, and amino acids.
- Nutritional supplements and herbal preparations also can affect nutrients (e.g., long-term use of beta-carotene supplements can cause a vitamin E deficiency).

Additional food, herb, and medication interactions are discussed in Chapter 8.

Lifestyle Factors

Alcohol and smoking can alter an older person's nutritional status in several ways. Alcohol has a high caloric content but low nutrient value, so it provides empty calories. In addition, it interferes with the absorption of the B-complex vitamins and vitamin C. Alcoholism is often unrecognized and under-

TABLE 18-3 Potential Effects of Medications on Digestion and Nutrition

Medications	Potential Effect on Digestion and Nutrition
Digoxin, theophylline, fluoxetine, antihistamines (including over-the-counter cold or sleep preparations)	Anorexia
Anticholinergics, narcotics, iron sulfate, antidepressants, antipsychotics, aluminum- and calcium-based antacids	Constipation
Cimetidine, laxatives, antibiotics, iron sulfate, cardiovascular drugs, antidementia drugs	Diarrhea, nausea, vomiting
Diuretics, ibuprofen, hypnotics, antipsychotics, antidepressants, antihistamines, decongestants, antiadrenergic agents (e.g., clonidine), any medication that has anticholinergic effects	Dry mouth
Ibuprofen, phenylbutazone, indomethacin, aspirin, phenobarbital, corticosteroids	Gastric irritation
Anticholinergics, potassium-depleting medications (e.g., furosemide)	Paralytic ileus
Bulk-forming agents (e.g., psyllium, methylcellulose), when taken before meals	Early satiety
Diuretics, vasodilators, antihistamines, antimicrobials, antihypertensives, hypoglycemic agents, psychotropic medications	Diminished smell and taste sensations
Mineral oil, cholestyramine	Diminished absorption of vitamins A, D, E, and K
Anticonvulsants	Diminished storage of vitamin K, decreased absorption of calcium
Aluminum- or magnesium-based antacids	Diarrhea; decreased levels of calcium, fluoride, and phosphorus
Products containing sodium bicarbonate	Sodium overload, water retention
Gentamicin and penicillin	Hypokalemia
Tetracyclines	Diminished absorption of zinc, iron, calcium, and magnesium
Neomycin	Diminished absorption of fat, iron, lactose, nitrogen, calcium, potassium, and vitamin B_{12}
Aspirin	Gastrointestinal bleeding; decreased levels of iron, folate, and vitamin C
Corticosteroids	Increased need for calcium, phosphorus, B vitamins, and vitamins C and D
Cimetidine, potassium supplements	Diminished absorption of vitamin B_{12}
Nonsteroidal anti-inflammatory drugs (NSAIDs)	Nausea, vomiting, gastrointestinal ulcers and bleeding, diminished absorption of iron

treated in older adults and may be a common contributing factor to nutritional disorders (Meyyazhagan & Palmer, 2002). Smoking diminishes the ability to smell and taste food and interferes with absorption of vitamin C and folic acid.

Psychosocial Factors

Psychosocial factors are likely to affect an older person's appetite and eating patterns. Any changes in mealtime companionship, as may occur through loss or disability of a spouse, are likely to have a negative impact on eating patterns. Eating alone has been associated with a 30% decline in caloric intake compared with caloric intake of people who eat in the company of others, and loneliness has been identified as a risk factor for anorexia in older adults (de Castro, 2002; Staveren et al., 2002). When older adults have established a long-term pattern of preparing meals for family and spouse, it may be especially difficult for the older adult to adjust to purchasing, preparing, and eating food for just one person. Similarly, older adults who have never participated in the purchase or preparation of foods may have great difficulty assuming these tasks after the loss of a spouse or other person who performed these tasks. If the older adult depends on others for assistance in procuring food, any factors that limit the availability of support resources may affect the older adult's ability to obtain food.

Wellness Opportunity

Nurses can work with older adults to identify ways of promoting positive social interaction during mealtimes.

Stress and anxiety affect digestive processes through their influence on the autonomic nervous system. Although stress-related effects on digestion are not unique to older adults, any alteration of the autonomic nervous system may compound age-related effects that otherwise would not have much effect. Older adults who are depressed are likely to experience anorexia and loss of interest in food. Confusion, memory problems, and other cognitive deficits may significantly interfere with eating patterns and the ability to prepare food.

Cultural and Socioeconomic Factors

Ethnic background, religious beliefs, and other cultural factors strongly influence the way people define, select, prepare, and eat food and beverages. Cultural factors also can influence eating patterns and selection of food in relation to health status. For example, some Asian and Hispanic people may classify foods, beverages, and medicines as hot or cold, and they may select a particular food based on their belief that their illness would respond to warm, hot, cool, or cold types of remedies. According to this health belief model, illnesses are caused by an imbalance between hot and cold, and so must be treated with substances that have the opposite characteristics.

Cultural dietary customs usually are not detrimental for healthy older adults, as long as the diet includes essential nutrients and avoids extremes. However, for the older adult with a medical condition that requires diet modification (e.g., diabetes or hypertension), cultural food patterns may aggravate the condition and create barriers to nutritional therapy. For example, the use of large amounts of high-sodium sauces may contribute to hypertension. Cultural Considerations 18-1 summarizes some of the food habits that are associated with major cultural and religious groups in the United States. Nurses should remember, though, that individual older adults vary in their eating patterns and may not adhere to the patterns of their cultural group. It is usually not necessary to try to change culturally influenced eating patterns, but it is important to recognize any cultural factors that may affect an older adult's nutritional status.

Wellness Opportunity

Nurses address cultural needs by identifying food preferences and finding ways to provide these foods.

A person's past and present economic status also influences food choices. If nutrient intake has been inadequate because of long-standing financial limitations, the progressive effects of poor nutrition may precipitate new problems in older adults, especially in combination with age-related changes in nutrient intake and utilization. People of low socioeconomic status usually have a narrower selection of foods than do people of higher socioeconomic status. Edentulism is almost twice as common in people with incomes below the poverty line than in those with incomes at or above the poverty line (Vargas et al., 2001). Education also may affect nutritional status, with limited education being associated with poor nutrition and less use of dental services. For example, people who have more than a high school education are twice as likely to have visited a dentist in the past year as those with less education (Vargas et al., 2001).

Diversity Note

Lack of access to adequate nutrition affects 18.9% of black, 15.4% of Hispanic, and 3.7% of white older adults in the United States (American Dietetic Association, 2005).

Cultural Considerations 18-1

Cultural Influences on Eating Patterns

African Americans

- "Soul food" is common, particularly in the southern United States.
- Common main courses: wild game, fried fish and poultry, pork and all parts of the pig
- Common vegetables and side dishes: corn, rice, okra, greens, legumes, tomatoes, hot breads, sweet potatoes
- Methods of food preparation: stewing, barbecuing, and frying with lard or saltpork
- Low consumption of milk (possibly owing to lactose intolerance)
- Low calcium dietary intake

Asian Americans

- Common foods: rice, wheat, pork, eggs, chicken, soybean products, and a variety of vegetables
- Methods of food preparation: stir-frying with lard, peanut oil, or sesame oil; seasoning with ginger, soy sauce, sesame seeds, and monosodium glutamate
- Beverages: green tea; rare use of milk products because lactose intolerance is common

Hispanic Americans

- Common main courses: eggs, tacos, chicken, corn tortillas, pinto or calico beans
- Common vegetables and side dishes: rice, corn, squash, bread, tomatoes
- Methods of food preparation: frying with lard; seasoning with garlic, onions, and chili powder
- Beverages: herbal teas, carbonated soda, milk in hot beverages

Native Americans

- May obtain foods from their natural environment (e.g., fish, roots, fruits, berries, wild greens, and wild game)
- May rely on nonperishable foods because of lack of refrigeration
- May depend on commodity foods provided by the U.S. Department of Agriculture
- May be influenced by tribal culture
- May have limited use of dairy products because of lactose intolerance

Religious Influences

- Some groups of Jews follow prescribed rules for preparing and serving foods (e.g., they eat only kosher meat and poultry and do not eat shellfish or any pork products).
- Mormons do not drink tea, coffee, or alcohol.
- Hindus are vegetarians.
- Seventh Day Adventists are lacto-ovovegetarians.
- Roman Catholics do not eat meat on Ash Wednesday or Good Friday.

Environmental Factors

Environmental factors affect the enjoyment of food as well as the ability to obtain and prepare it. Many barriers to food enjoyment have been identified in the dining environments of long-term care facilities and other institutional settings. Limited food selection and low staffing levels are two of the most commonly identified barriers to nutrition care in nursing homes (Crogan et al., 2001; Simmons et al., 2001). Older adults in congregate housing and long-term care facilities may find it difficult to adjust to unfamiliar environments. Moreover, they many not desire the mealtime social interaction that is part of the institutional environment. A noisy or crowded dining room may have a negative impact on food enjoyment and consumption. Such an environment may be particularly stressful for an older adult who uses a hearing aid or who is accustomed to eating alone. The potential outcomes of a move to a new environment include poor nutrition and loss of interest in eating, particularly during the initial adjustment period.

Environmental influences, such as inclement weather conditions, particularly affect functionally impaired older adults who live in their own homes. For example, an older person who walks to the store or depends on public transportation may be unable or unwilling to obtain groceries in snowy or rainy weather. Likewise, the older adult may not be able to tolerate hot or sultry conditions, especially if car transportation is not readily available. People who depend on others for transportation or who have difficulty maneuvering in adverse weather conditions are likely to shop for groceries less frequently and to purchase their groceries at smaller convenience stores, where prices are higher and selection is limited. The additional cost and limited selection may interfere with food intake and lead to nutrient deficiencies. Finally, environmental conditions and packaging trends in the grocery store may create additional difficulties for older people, especially those who are functionally impaired. For example, the combined glare of fluorescent lights, highly polished floors, cellophane wrappers, and white freezer cases often make it extremely difficult, if not impossible, for the older adult with vision changes to read labels, especially when the print is small and contrasts poorly against the background.

Behaviors Based on Myths and Misunderstandings

Myths and misunderstandings may be detrimental to a person's food intake and behaviors related to bowel function. For example, during the 1950s and 1960s, a widely held belief was that roughage and raw fruits or vegetables were harmful to the older person. It is now known that lack of roughage in the diet and consumption of only cooked fruits and vegetables are eating patterns that contribute to constipation by slowing the transit time of feces through the large intestine. Another commonly held belief is that a daily bowel movement is the norm for good digestive function. Rigid adherence to this standard may, in fact, lead to the unnecessary and detrimental use of laxatives. Advertisements have further reinforced this false belief by implying that daily bowel movements should be attained through medication. Although recent advertising trends emphasize the achievement of healthy bowel patterns through the ingestion of high-fiber food items, the negative impact of long-term beliefs may be difficult to overcome.

Misunderstandings about fluid intake also may interfere with digestion and nutrition. Many older adults reduce the amount of liquids they consume in an attempt to decrease the incidence of urinary incontinence. Fluid intake also may be restricted if functional limitations, such as impaired mobility or manual dexterity, interfere with either the ability to obtain liquids or the ease of urinary elimination. Reduced fluid intake can have a number of detrimental consequences, such as constipation, xerostomia, and diminished food enjoyment.

Wellness Opportunity

Nurses identify myths and misunderstandings about constipation and teach older adults about habits that promote healthy elimination patterns.

PATHOLOGIC CONDITION AFFECTING DIGESTIVE WELLNESS: CONSTIPATION

Constipation—defined as "stasis of the large intestine, resulting in infrequent (two or less weekly) elimination and/or hard, dry feces" (Carpenito-Moyet, 2006, p. 88)— is one of the most common pathologic conditions associated with digestion. Up to 80% of institutionalized older adults and 45% of community-living older adults report constipation problems (Frank et al., 2001). Prevalence of constipation is highest among women, African Americans, people older than 60 years, and people who have low incomes, less education, and lower levels of physical activity (Hinrichs, et al., 2001).

Definitions of constipation usually are based on characteristics of bowel movements, including frequency and difficulty passing the stool. The normal frequency for bowel movements, which shows significant individual variation but does not necessarily change with aging, ranges from three times daily to once or twice weekly. Constipation is characterized by all of the following conditions:

- The stool is excessively hard.
- There is a decrease in the person's normal frequency pattern.
- The stool is difficult to pass (i.e., straining with bowel movements).
- The person experiences a feeling of incomplete evacuation after a bowel movement.

Although constipation is a common complaint of older adults, it is caused by risk factors rather than age-related changes. It is often associated with functional impairments (e.g., diminished mobility), pathologic conditions (e.g., hypothyroidism), adverse medication effects (including long-term laxative abuse), and poor dietary habits (e.g., inadequate intake of bulk, fiber, and fluid). Because constipation occurs so commonly in older adults, nurses assess for risk factors and initiate health promotion interventions, as discussed in the sections on Nursing Assessment and Nursing Interventions.

Mr. and Mrs. D., who are 71 and 72 years old, respectively, attend the senior center where you provide monthly group health education sessions and weekly one-on-one "Counseling for Wellness" sessions. Mrs. D. makes an appointment to see you because her bowels get "bound up" and she always feels "bloated." When you ask about her bowel patterns she reports that she has a bowel movement "about every other day" and has to "sit on the commode for a good half-hour before anything happens." She has taken Milk of Magnesia every night for about 20 years, but "it doesn't seem to be any help anymore." She avoids fresh fruits and vegetables because her mother always told her that canned fruits and vegetables were easier to digest. She rarely eats cereal and uses white bread. Her weight is about 125% of her ideal body weight, and she does not walk often because of trouble with arthritis. She takes levothyroxine (Synthroid), 100 mcg once daily, and an over-the-counter generic calcium supplement that contains 500 mg calcium carbonate twice daily.

THINKING POINTS

- Identify at least five risk factors that are likely to contribute to Mrs. D.'s constipation.
- Describe how you would begin addressing one of these risk factors in health education.

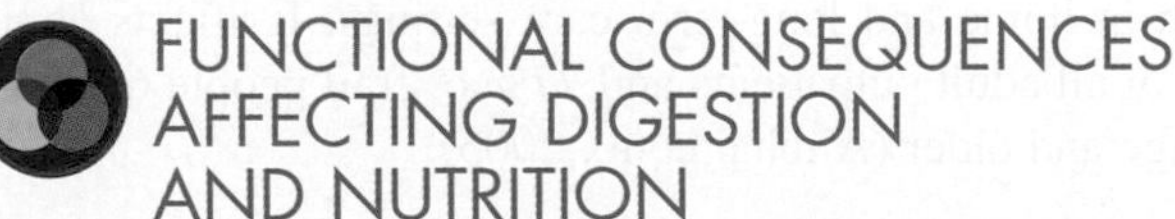

FUNCTIONAL CONSEQUENCES AFFECTING DIGESTION AND NUTRITION

Functional consequences affect the following aspects of digestion and nutrition of older adults:

- Procurement, preparation, and enjoyment of food
- Mastication and digestion of food
- Nutritional status
- Psychosocial function

Negative functional consequences occur primarily because of the many risk factors that affect older adults, rather than because of age-related changes alone.

Ability to Procure, Prepare, and Enjoy Food

Activities involved in procuring, preparing, consuming, and enjoying food depend on the skills of cognition, balance, mobility, and manual dexterity, as well as on the five senses. Food procurement depends on getting to the grocery store, pushing a shopping cart, reaching for food items on high shelves, reading the small print on shelves and food packages for cost and nutrition information, and coping with the glare of bright lights, especially in the frozen food sections. Age-related changes and conditions that may interfere with these activities include vision impairments and any illness, such as arthritis, that limits mobility, balance, or manual dexterity.

Food preparation activities that are likely to be more difficult for older adults include cutting food items, measuring ingredients accurately, carrying food and liquid without spilling, standing for long periods in the kitchen, reaching for items on high shelves and in cupboards, safely using the oven or stove, and reading the temperature controls correctly. Impairments of vision, balance, cognition, mobility, or manual dexterity are likely to cause difficulties in the performance of these tasks.

Diminished sensory function can affect food enjoyment in all the following ways:

- Inaccurate perception of color, taste, or smell can interfere with appetite and food appeal.
- Diminished gustatory and olfactory sensitivity may lead to excessive use of condiments and seasonings, such as salt and sugar.
- Visual and olfactory impairments may make it difficult to detect spoiled food.

Moreover, food choices are influenced by the condition of the oral cavity and teeth, as well as by the quantity and quality of natural or replacement teeth.

Wellness Opportunity

Nurses promote wellness through interventions that improve the older adult's independence in procuring and preparing satisfying meals.

Oral Function and Digestion of Food

Digestive processes in healthy older adults are not significantly affected by age-related changes, but older adults often have digestive complaints (e.g., "heartburn," constipation) caused by commonly occurring risk factors. For example, many negative functional consequences are associated with medications (see Table 18-3). Xerostomia causes negative functional consequences because it can interfere with oral comfort, food enjoyment, and taste sensitivity. It also interferes with digestion because diminished saliva production makes it more difficult to chew food and increases the susceptibility of the teeth and tongue to bacterial action. Studies have identified the following consequences of impaired salivary function (Ghezzi et al., 2000; Ship et al., 2002):

- Gingivitis
- Dry lips
- Dental caries
- Excessive plaque
- Periodontal disease
- Difficulty swallowing
- Speech dysfunction
- Poorly fitting dentures
- Decreased nutritional intake
- Inflammation of the mucous membrane
- Oral mucosal infections (e.g., candidiasis)
- Traumatic oral lesions

The functional consequences of being edentulous or using dentures include avoidance of certain foods, decreased chewing efficiency, and increased susceptibility to accidental choking from ineffective mastication. Because edentulous people tend to avoid meats, salads, fresh fruits, and raw vegetables they may be at risk for nutritional deficiencies (Hutton, 2002; Vargas et al., 2001).

Nutritional Status and Weight Changes

Because older adults need fewer calories, a deficiency of essential minerals or vitamins is likely to occur if the quantity of calories is reduced without a corresponding increase in the quality of the food consumed. In addition, risk factors (e.g., medications and pathologic processes) that commonly occur in older adults often cause nutrient deficiencies. For example, iron deficiency is associated with chronic diseases and low socioeconomic status. Other minerals and vitamins that commonly are deficient in older adults are zinc, calcium, most B vitamins, and vitamins D and E. See Table 18-2 for examples of nutrient deficiencies and associated risk factors and functional consequences that are likely to affect older adults.

Some researchers have identified the prevalence of specific nutritional deficits among older adults, but conclusions of the studies are clouded by a lack of common definitions. The following findings are indicative of significant concerns about nutritional intake among older adults (Johnson et al., 2002; Meyyazhagan & Palmer, 2002; Milne et al., 2006):

- Fifty percent of older adults have a vitamin and mineral intake less than the recommended dietary allowance.
- Undernutrition occurs in 5% to 12% of community-living older adults, in up to 55% of hospitalized elderly, and in 52% to 85% of older adults in long-term care facilities.
- Ten to 30% of older adults have abnormally low serum levels of vitamins and minerals.
- Vitamin D deficiency occurs in 5% to 25% of community-living older adults and in 48% to 80% of older adults in long-term care facilities.
- Vitamin B_{12} deficiency occurs in 12% to 14% of community-living older adults and in up to 25% of older adults in long-term care facilities.
- Malnutrition is associated with poorer recovery across many conditions.

A type of malnutrition that is common in frail older adults is **protein-energy undernutrition** (also called *protein-calorie undernutrition*), which occurs when the intake of calories and protein is less than the amount required to meet daily needs. This condition is associated with a high-carbohydrate, low-protein diet, which often results from one or several of the risk factors already discussed (e.g., depression, loss of appetite, pathologic conditions). Characteristics of mild or moderate protein-energy undernutrition (called **marasmus**) include weakness, lethargy, unintentional weight loss, diminished muscle mass, marked decrease in subcutaneous fat, and impaired ability to respond to physiologic stresses (e.g., surgery, infection). If the condition progresses and becomes severe (a state called **kwashiorkor**), it is characterized by edema and loss of visceral protein. In a study of patients between the ages of 65 and 99 years, Liu and colleagues (2002) found that protein-energy undernutrition is a significant independent factor for increased risk of mortality in the year following hospitalization. Additional consequences of undernutrition in older adults that have been identified in studies are anemia, weakness, fatigue, infections, electrolyte imbalance, functional disability, altered skin integrity, and increased morbidity, mortality, and admissions to long-term care facilities (Furman, 2006).

Older adults are susceptible to unintentional weight gains and losses. Age-related changes in body composition and carbohydrate metabolism contribute to gradual weight gains. The proportion of body fat to lean tissue begins to increase around 30 years of age and leads to disproportionately increased abdominal fat during later adulthood. This pattern of fat distribution is associated with increased risk for insulin resistance, diabetes mellitus, and cardiovascular disease (Rincon et al., 2006). Obesity is a major public health concern for all population groups, but it is most prevalent among people in their sixth and seventh decades, which is attributable in part to retirement and decreased work hours (Chung, 2006). Unintentional weight loss is a common problem for medically compromised older adults, both in home and long-term care settings. It affects about 8% of all adult outpatients and 27% of frail people 65 years of age and older (Alibhai et al., 2005).

Diversity Note

Men generally reach peak weight between 55 years and the early 60s; for women it is between 65 and 70 years (Noel & Reddy, 2005).

Quality of Life

Good food and nutrition are essential components of health-related quality of life, particularly for older adults (Amarantos et al., 2001). In day-to-day life, many food-related activities are associated with pleasurable events, and mealtime activities often are associated with caring, comfort, nurturing, and social interaction. For example, in certain circumstances, food is a focal point of celebrations, religious rituals, or gatherings to share significant events. Thus, when mealtime enjoyment is affected in any way, the psychosocial aspects of eating are also affected. Older adults who enjoyed participating in family meals or eating in restaurants may withdraw from these activities if food is no longer enjoyable. Consequently, they may lose the social interaction that occurs in these settings.

Perhaps even more detrimental than the psychosocial consequences of diminished food enjoyment are the psychosocial effects of inadequate nutrition. When fluid or nutrient intake is inadequate, older adults are likely to develop malnutrition and dehydration because of impaired homeostatic mechanisms. Changes in mental status, including memory impairment, are among the early signs of malnutrition, dehydration, and electrolyte imbalance in older adults. Sometimes these mental changes are attributed incorrectly to irreversible conditions (e.g., dementia) rather than to a treatable and reversible metabolic imbalance. For example, folate and vitamin B_{12} deficiencies are two of the most common nutritional causes of mental changes.

Last, negative psychosocial consequences are associated with loss of teeth and poor oral health. Edentulism, dental caries, and periodontal disease are factors that contribute to diminished self-esteem (Vargas et al., 2001).

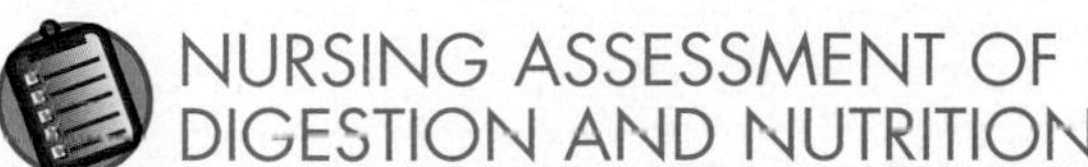

NURSING ASSESSMENT OF DIGESTION AND NUTRITION

Nurses assess digestion and nutrition to identify (1) effects of age-related changes on digestion, nutrition, and eating patterns; (2) risk factors that interfere with optimal nutrition; (3) cultural factors that influence eating patterns; (4) nutritional status and usual eating patterns; and (5) negative functional consequences of altered digestion or inadequate nutrition. Based on this assessment information, nurses identify opportunities for health promotion interventions.

Interviewing About Digestion and Nutrition

Nurses use an assessment interview to identify opportunities for health promotion by asking about the following information:

- Usual eating patterns and nutrient intake
- Health behaviors associated with oral care
- Age-related changes and risk factors that affect nutritional needs or digestive processes
- Environmental or social support factors that affect the procurement, preparation, and enjoyment of food
- Symptoms of gastrointestinal dysfunction

A dietary history is important in assessing the adequacy of nutrient intake. For example, nurses can ask older adults to describe foods and beverages consumed during an average day or during the past 24-hour period. If the older person is unable to convey this information accurately, the nurse can obtain the information from caregivers. A logical sequence for assessment questions is to begin with information about the oral cavity and end with information about bowel elimination. A major goal for assessing patterns of bowel elimination is to identify opportunities for health education about constipation. Hinrichs and colleagues (2001) developed an excellent research-based protocol for nursing assessment and management of constipation. Box 18-1 summarizes interview questions for a nursing assessment of nutrition and digestion in older adults.

Wellness Opportunity

Nurses promote personal responsibility by asking older adults to keep a 7-day diary of food and beverage intake and eating patterns and reviewing this to identify strengths and weaknesses.

Observing Cues to Digestion and Nutrition

Nurses observe eating patterns and environments and also assess social and cultural factors that influence eating and nutrition. Nurses in institutional settings can assess behavioral cues to digestion and nutrition by observing older adults during meals. Nursing assessment of chewing and swallowing is especially important for older adults at risk for dysphagia, which often develops gradually and eventually causes serious complications such as aspiration pneumonia. If dysphagia is suspected, a bedside or mealtime swallowing evaluation can be performed by a speech therapist. Shanley and O'Loughlin (2000) provide a comprehensive protocol for assessment and management of dysphagia in nursing home residents.

Nurses also observe all the following aspects of oral health:

- Condition of lips, teeth, gums, tongue, and oral mucous membrane
- Number of teeth and use of full or partial dentures and bridges
- Fit of dentures
- Oral care items (i.e., condition of toothbrush, type of toothbrush or denture cleaning supplies)

Box 18-2 summarizes behavioral cues to nutrition and digestion, including cultural considerations, observations related to eating patterns and the eating environment, and indicators of dysphagia.

Wellness Opportunity

Nurses observe environmental conditions to identify positive or negative effects on eating patterns.

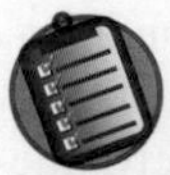

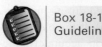

Box 18-1
Guidelines for Assessing Digestion and Nutrition

Assessing Oral Comfort and Chewing Ability

- Do you have any difficulty with soreness or bleeding in your mouth?
- Do you have any teeth that hurt, are loose, or are sensitive to hot or cold temperatures?
- Do your gums bleed?
- Do you have any problems chewing or swallowing food or liquids? *If yes, ask about particular types of food or liquids that are problematic.*
- Are there foods you avoid because of problems with chewing or swallowing?
- Does your mouth or tongue ever feel dry?

Assessing Dental Habits and Attitudes Toward Dental Care

- How often do you see a dentist?
- When is the last time you had dental care?
- Where do you go for dental care?
- *If the person does not seek dental care at least once per year:* What prevents you from seeing the dentist?
- How do you care for your teeth?
- Do you use dental floss? *If yes:* How often? *If no:* Have you ever been taught to use dental floss?

Assessing Nutritional Needs

- Do you have diabetes, heart disease, or any condition that requires dietary modifications?
- Do you have any food allergies?
- What medications do you take?
- What is your usual daily activity pattern?

Identifying Patterns of Food Procurement

- How do you get your grocery shopping done?
- Do you have any help getting to the store?
- Where and how often do you do your grocery shopping?
- What is your usual food budget?
- Do you have any difficulty getting food because of problems with vision, walking, or transportation?

Identifying Patterns of Food Preparation and Consumption

- Where do you eat your meals?
- With whom do you eat?
- Does anyone help you prepare your meals?
- Do you have any trouble fixing your meals (e.g., difficulty opening containers)?
- Do you have any difficulties getting around your kitchen, using appliances, or reaching the cupboards?
- Have there been recent changes in your eating or food preparation patterns (e.g., loss of eating companion or change in caregiver situation)?

Assessing Patterns of Bowel Elimination

- How often do you have a bowel movement?
- Have you noticed any recent changes in your pattern of bowel movements?
- Do you have any difficulty with your bowel movements? (e.g., Do you strain with bowel movements? or Is the stool hard, dry, or difficult to pass?)
- Do you ever have problems with loose stools or diarrhea?
- Do you take laxatives or any other products to help you move your bowels?
- Do you ever have pain or bleeding when you move your bowels?

Using Physical Assessment and Laboratory Information

Physical assessment and laboratory data provide important additional information for assessing the older adult's nutritional and hydration status. Height, weight, and **body mass index (BMI)** provide important clues to nutritional status. The BMI—a measure of body composition related to body fat—is commonly used as an indicator of malnutrition. Healthy BMI (weight [lb]/height [in]^2 $\times$ 705) is between 18.5 and 24.9 for adults. Although there is no benefit to severe obesity, some studies suggest that a higher BMI—30 to 35 for women and 27 to 30 for men—is helpful for withstanding metabolic demands of illness and is associated with lower risk of mortality after the age of 70 years (Dudek, 2007).

Nurses need to consider individual circumstances in relation to ideal body weight because standardized tables do not necessarily provide the most realistic or appropriate goal for older adults. Rather, for many older adults, maintenance of a stable weight may be more important because patterns of weight loss and gain are important indicators of overall health condition. Weight loss is considered in relation to percentage of loss, which is calculated by subtracting current weight from usual weight and dividing that by the usual weight—for example, (160 lb – 120 lb)/160 lb = 40 lb, or a 25% weight loss. An unintentional weight loss of more than 5% of body weight in 1 month, more than 7.5% in 3 months, or more than 10% in 6 months is considered a significant indicator of poor nutrition (Omran & Salem, 2002).

Physical assessment of hydration in older adults is particularly challenging because effects of age-related changes or pathologic conditions often mimic the typical manifestations of dehydration. For example, dry mucous membranes is a common indicator of dehydration in younger adults, but it also is likely to occur in older adults as an adverse medication effect. Assessment of skin turgor in older adults may be more accurate on the forehead and over the anterior chest wall because these areas are less affected by age-related skin changes. Orthostatic hypotension, oliguria or anuria, changes in mental status, and dry tongue and mucous membranes are common manifestations of dehydration in older

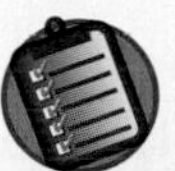

Box 18-2
Behavioral Cues to Nutrition and Digestion

Cultural Considerations That May Influence Nutrition and Eating Patterns

- What are the usual patterns of meals eaten (e.g., content, frequency, timing)? What is the usual social context of meals?
- Are there any culturally influenced food taboos or preferences? (Refer to Cultural Considerations 18-1.)
- Are there any special foods that are important because of religious or cultural factors? (If yes, are they accessible to the older adult?)
- Are certain foods or beverages avoided or preferred in relation to an illness or chronic condition (e.g., foods or beverages that are considered yin and yang foods)?
- Is there a preference for the temperature of beverages (e.g., use of iced or heated beverages)?
- Is the person's ethnic background likely to increase his or her chance of being lactose intolerant? (Prevalence is highest among Asians, American Indians, and African and American blacks; high among Hispanics; and lowest among whites of northern European descent.)

Observations To Assess Eating Patterns

- Does the person seem to enjoy eating meals with others, or does the presence of other people seem to interfere with mealtime enjoyment?
- If the person has dentures, are they worn at meals? If not, why not?
- What are the person's between-meal food and fluid consumption patterns?
- Are enjoyable noncaffeinated liquids readily available for between-meal fluid intake?
- What cultural influences affect the person's food preferences and preparation?

Observations To Assess the Eating Environment

- Do environmental or social influences negatively affect mealtime enjoyment (e.g., a noisy dining room or disruptive mealtime companions)?
- If the person eats alone, is this the best arrangement, or should consideration be given to providing mealtime social interaction?

Indicators of Dysphagia

- Drooling
- Slurred speech
- Incomplete lip closure
- Nasal regurgitation of food
- Pocketing of food in cheeks
- Refusing or resisting food or drink
- Increased congestion or secretions after eating
- Wet, hoarse, or gurgly voice after swallowing
- Slow chewing or slow or delayed swallowing
- Coughing or choking (while or soon after drinking thin liquids or chewing and swallowing food)

adults. Urinalysis provides clues to a person's hydration status, with highly concentrated urine being an indicator of dehydration. Blood values that may be altered in dehydration include sodium, hematocrit, creatinine, osmolality, and blood urea nitrogen, all of which may be elevated. In addition, a sudden loss of body weight might be an indicator of dehydration.

Laboratory data can provide clues to nutritional deficiencies, even before any clinical signs are evident; however, test results must be evaluated in relation to the person's overall health status. For instance, dehydration falsely elevates hemoglobin, hematocrit, and serum albumin. Low serum albumin levels are associated with poor nutrition; however, they also occur under the following conditions: trauma, edema, infection, neoplasm, overhydration, nephrotic syndrome, and malabsorption syndromes (Lewis, 2001). Box 18-3 summarizes information about physical assessment indicators and laboratory values that are especially important in assessing the nutritional status of older adults. Additional indicators of nutrient deficiencies are listed in Table 18-2 in the column describing functional consequences.

Using Assessment Tools

Recently, nutrition assessment tools have been promoted for identifying people at risk for dehydration and nutritional problems so that preventive and therapeutic interventions can be implemented (Patterson, 2002; Thomas et al., 2000; Vellas et al., 2006; Zembrzuski, 2000). The parameters most frequently included in nutrition assessment tools are diet history, clinical presentation, anthropometric measurements, and laboratory and immunologic assessments (Wakefield, 2001). The Mini Nutritional Assessment and the Nutritional Form for the Elderly are widely used in a variety of settings as reliable and validated assessment tools for identifying older adults who are malnourished or at risk for poor nutrition (Bleda et al., 2002; Delahunt, 2002; Salva & Pera, 2001; Soderhamn, 2002; Vellas et al., 2006). A short six-item form, which can be administered in 5 minutes, has also been found to be reliable as a first-step screening process for identifying older adults who should be assessed further for poor nutrition (Fig. 18-1).

Recall that you are the nurse at the senior center attended by Mr. and Mrs. D., who now are 75 and 76 years old, respectively. During a "Counseling for Health" session, Mrs. D. asks your advice about her gradual unintended weight loss over the past few months. Although Mrs. D. continues to cook meals because her husband enjoys eating, she states that food no longer appeals to her. You notice that her

(case study continues on page 378)

mouth is very dry and her teeth are in poor condition. She had a stroke 2 years ago and recovered well except for some dysphagia and right-sided weakness. She takes an antidepressant and two blood pressure medications, but does not know the names of the pills. She asks what she can do about the weight loss.

THINKING POINTS

- What risk factors are likely to be contributing to Mrs. D.'s weight loss?
- Make a list of assessment questions you would use with Mrs. D. Select applicable questions from Box 18-1 and list any additional questions that you would use for further assessment.
- What would you ask Mrs. D. to do to provide additional assessment information so that you can plan some teaching interventions?

NURSING DIAGNOSIS

The nursing assessment may identify problems related to nutrition, digestion, or oral health. If nutritional deficits are identified, a pertinent nursing diagnosis is Imbalanced Nutrition: Less than Body Requirements. This diagnosis is defined as "the state in which an individual, who is not NPO, experiences or is at risk for inadequate intake or metabolism of nutrients for metabolic needs with or without weight loss" (Carpenito-Moyet, 2006, p. 293). Related factors that may affect older adults include medications, anorexia, depression, chewing or swallowing difficulties, social isolation, and inability to procure or prepare food.

If the nursing assessment identifies constipation or risks for constipation, the applicable nursing diagnosis is Constipation. The nursing assessment may also identify certain oral health problems that are common in older adults. These include xerostomia, medication effects, chewing difficulties, periodontal disease, diminished taste sensation, ill-fitting

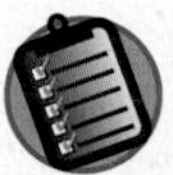

Box 18-3
Physical Assessment and Laboratory Data

Examination of the Oral Cavity

- Inspect the oral cavity using a tongue depressor and a light.
- Observe for evidence of oral disease, including pain, lumps, soreness, bleeding, swelling, loose teeth, and abraded areas.
- Note the presence or absence of teeth, dentures, and partial bridges.

Normal Findings

- Lips: pink, moist, symmetrical
- Teeth: intact, without cavities or tartar
- Gums: pink, no bleeding
- Mucous membranes: pink, moist
- Tongue: pink, moist; presence of numerous varicosities on undersurface
- Pharynx: soft palate rises slightly when "ahh" is vocalized

Indicators of Nutritional Deficiency

- Lips: dry, fissured, cracked at corners
- Teeth: decayed or missing
- Gums: red, swollen, recessed, spongy or prone to bleeding
- Mucous membranes: dry, ulcerated, inflamed, bleeding, white patches
- Tongue: dry, swollen, reddened, or very smooth

Examination of the Abdomen and Rectum

- Examine the abdomen with the person lying comfortably in the supine position.
- Perform a rectal examination with the person in the side-lying position.

Normal Findings

- Symmetrical, soft abdomen that moves with respirations
- Audible bowel sounds (heard through the diaphragm of a stethoscope) occurring at irregular intervals (5 to 15 seconds apart)
- Smooth skin around anus; no evidence of hemorrhoids, fissures, inflammation, or rectal prolapse
- Soft, brown stool that tests negative for occult blood

Indicators of Nutritional Deficiency

- Swollen abdomen
- Stool that tests positive for occult blood

General Physical Assessment Indicators of Malnutrition

- Weight loss
- Lack of subcutaneous fat
- Diminished size and strength of muscles
- Skin that is dry, rough, or tissue thin
- Abnormal pulse or blood pressure
- Edema, especially in the face or lower extremities
- Hair that is dry, dull, thin, brittle, or sparse
- Dry or dull-looking eyes
- Listless, apathetic, or depressed mood
- Difficulty with walking or maintaining balance

Laboratory Data

- Biochemical data that will provide information about nutritional status: serum ferritin; serum or red blood cell folate and vitamin B_{12}; complete lipid profile; and serum albumin, glucose, sodium, and potassium levels
- Urinalysis results should be within the normal adult range, except for a slight decrease in the upper limit for specific gravity

Indicators of Nutritional Deficiency

- Anemia
- Lymphocytopenia
- Serum albumin level of less than 3.5 g/dL
- Cholesterol levels of less than 160 mg/dL
- Total iron-binding capacity less than 250 mcg/dL

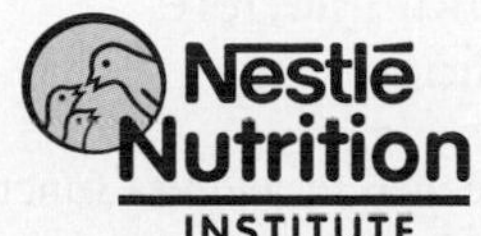

Mini Nutritional Assessment MNA®

Last name: First name: Sex: Date:

Age: Weight, kg: Height, cm: I.D. Number:

Complete the screen by filling in the boxes with the appropriate numbers.
Add the numbers for the screen. If score is 11 or less, continue with the assessment to gain a Malnutrition Indicator Score.

Screening

A Has food intake declined over the past 3 months due to loss of appetite, digestive problems, chewing or swallowing difficulties?
0 = severe loss of appetite
1 = moderate loss of appetite
2 = no loss of appetite ☐

B Weight loss during the last 3 months
0 = weight loss greater than 3 kg (6.6 lbs)
1 = does not know
2 = weight loss between 1 and 3 kg (2.2 and 6.6 lbs)
3 = no weight loss ☐

C Mobility
0 = bed or chair bound
1 = able to get out of bed/chair but does not go out
2 = goes out ☐

D Has suffered psychological stress or acute disease in the past 3 months
0 = yes 2 = no ☐

E Neuropsychological problems
0 = severe dementia or depression
1 = mild dementia
2 = no psychological problems ☐

F Body Mass Index (BMI) (weight in kg) / (height in m)²
0 = BMI less than 19
1 = BMI 19 to less than 21
2 = BMI 21 to less than 23
3 = BMI 23 or greater ☐

Screening score (subtotal max. 14 points) ☐☐
12 points or greater Normal – not at risk – no need to complete assessment
11 points or below Possible malnutrition – continue assessment

Assessment

G Lives independently (not in a nursing home or hospital)
0 = no 1 = yes ☐

H Takes more than 3 prescription drugs per day
0 = yes 1 = no ☐

I Pressure sores or skin ulcers
0 = yes 1 = no ☐

Ref. Vellas B, Villars H, Abellan G, et al. Overview of the MNA® - Its History and Challenges. J Nutr Health Aging 2006;10:456-465.
Rubenstein LZ, Harker JO, Salva A, Guigoz Y, Vellas B. Screening for Undernutrition in Geriatric Practice: Developing the Short-Fom Mini Nutritional Assessment (MNA-SF). J. Geront 2001;56A: M366-377.
Guigoz Y. The Mini-Nutritional Assessment (MNA®) Review of the Literature - What does it tell us? J Nutr Health Aging 2006; 10:466-487.

For more information : www.mna-elderly.com

J How many full meals does the patient eat daily?
0 = 1 meal
1 = 2 meals
2 = 3 meals ☐

K Selected consumption markers for protein intake
- At least one serving of dairy products (milk, cheese, yogurt) per day yes ☐ no ☐
- Two or more servings of legumes or eggs per week yes☐ no☐
- Meat, fish or poultry every day yes ☐ no ☐

0.0 = if 0 or 1 yes
0.5 = if 2 yes
1.0 = if 3 yes ☐.☐

L Consumes two or more servings of fruits or vegetables per day?
0 = no 1 = yes ☐

M How much fluid (water, juice, coffee, tea, milk…) is consumed per day?
0.0 = less than 3 cups
0.5 = 3 to 5 cups
1.0 = more than 5 cups ☐.☐

N Mode of feeding
0 = unable to eat without assistance
1 = self-fed with some difficulty
2 = self-fed without any problem ☐

O Self view of nutritional status
0 = views self as being malnourished
1 = is uncertain of nutritional state
2 = views self as having no nutritional problem ☐

P In comparison with other people of the same age, how does the patient consider his/her health status?
0.0 = not as good
0.5 = does not know
1.0 = as good
2.0 = better ☐.☐

Q Mid-arm circumference (MAC) in cm
0.0 = MAC less than 21
0.5 = MAC 21 to 22
1.0 = MAC 22 or greater ☐.☐

R Calf circumference (CC) in cm
0 = CC less than 31 1 = CC 31 or greater ☐

Assessment (max. 16 points) ☐☐.☐

Screening score ☐☐.☐

Total Assessment (max. 30 points) ☐☐.☐

Malnutrition Indicator Score
17 to 23.5 points at risk of malnutrition ☐
Less than 17 points malnourished ☐

FIGURE 18-1 The Mini Nutritional Assessment (MNA). (From Nestlé Nutrition Services. © Nestlé, 1994, Revision 2006. Available at www.mna-elderly.com.)

dentures, inadequate oral hygiene, and broken or missing teeth. A relevant nursing diagnosis to address these problems would be Impaired Oral Mucous Membrane.

Wellness Opportunity

Nurses can use the wellness diagnosis of Readiness for Enhanced Nutrition for older adults who express an interest in improving nutritional patterns.

PLANNING FOR WELLNESS OUTCOMES

Nurses can apply the following Nursing Outcomes Classification (NOC) terms to address risk factors and promote improved nutrition in older adults:

- Appetite
- Bowel Elimination
- Health Beliefs
- Knowledge: Diet
- Loneliness Severity
- Nutritional Status
- Oral Hygiene
- Self-Care: Eating
- Sensory Function: Taste and Smell
- Swallowing Status
- Weight: Body Mass
- Weight Control

NOCs related to Constipation include Hydration, Bowel Elimination, Medication Response, and Symptom Control.

Wellness Opportunity

Knowledge: Health Promotion would be an NOC for older adults who are ready to improve their nutrition to protect themselves from illness.

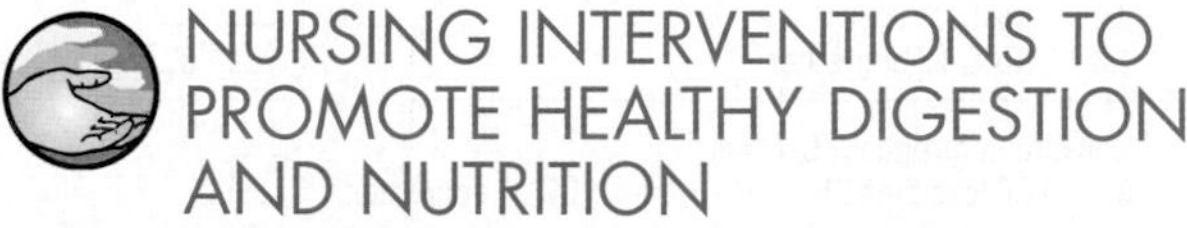

NURSING INTERVENTIONS TO PROMOTE HEALTHY DIGESTION AND NUTRITION

Nurses can apply the following Nursing Interventions Classification (NIC) terminology in care plans: Bowel Management, Environmental Management, Health Education, Nutrition Management, Nutritional Counseling, Oral Health Maintenance/Promotion, Referral, Self-Care Assistance, and Weight Management. Nursing interventions to promote healthy digestion and nutrition in older adults include health education about optimal nutrition and disease prevention and direct interventions to eliminate risk factors that interfere with digestion, nutrition, and oral health.

Addressing Risk Factors That Interfere With Digestion and Nutrition

Nursing interventions may be needed to address functional consequences of age-related changes even in healthy older adults. For example, if older adults experience early satiety during meals, they may benefit from eating five smaller meals a day, rather than the customary three meals a day. Similarly, nurses can encourage older adults to maintain a sitting or upright position during eating and for $^1/_2$ to 1 hour after eating to compensate for any effects of presbyesophagus.

When functional limitations interfere with the activities involved in procuring, preparing, and enjoying food, interventions focus on improving the person's access to palatable and nutritious meals. For the community-living older adult, this may involve identifying resources that offer assistance in obtaining food. Home-delivered meal programs may be available to older adults at minimal cost, and group meal programs are available in almost every community through the federally funded National Nutrition Program for the Elderly, established under the Older Americans Act. Studies have found that formal meal programs are effective in reducing nutritional risk for community-living older adults (Keller, 2006). In addition to providing inexpensive and nutritionally balanced meals, these programs provide opportunities for social interaction. Local offices on aging may provide assistance with transportation or grocery shopping and are an excellent source of information about group and home-delivered meal programs. When environmental barriers, such as high cupboards, interfere with the older adult's ability to prepare meals safely, environmental modifications can be made. Nurses can apply many of the environmental adaptations suggested in the chapters on vision (see Chapter 17) and mobility (see Chapter 22) to improve the ability of the older person to prepare meals.

In institutional settings, environmental factors may interfere with food enjoyment. Although modifying large institutional environments is often difficult or impossible, nurses may be able to identify simple interventions that will increase food enjoyment, particularly in long-term care facilities. For example, the seating arrangement in a dining room might be planned to improve social interaction and to minimize the negative effects of disruptive people. In some long-term care settings, two mealtimes are scheduled for each meal to allow increased flexibility in seating arrangements. Additional examples of environmental modifications that nurses can implement to improve nutrition and eating in long-term care facilities are described in gerontological journals (e.g., Brush et al., 2002; Roberts & Durnbaugh, 2002).

In long-term care settings, inadequate access to enjoyable beverages is a common barrier to optimal fluid intake that nurses can address through interventions. For example, one nursing home used a colorful beverage cart and colorful pitchers and glasses to serve a variety of hot and cold beverages twice daily to the residents. This intervention was cost-effective because outcomes of improved hydration for the residents included reduction in laxative use, increased frequency of bowel movements, and a decline in the number of falls and other negative outcomes of dehydration (Robinson & Rosher, 2002).

Food additives can be used to enhance food flavors for people with diminished smell and taste sensations. Although the use of monosodium glutamate as a flavor enhancer has been discouraged because it contains sodium, the use of very small amounts of flavor enhancers containing monosodium glutamate can improve food palatability and increase nursing home residents' dietary intake without significantly increasing their sodium intake (Mathey et al., 2001). Nurses can encourage the use of low- or no-sodium food additives and flavor enhancers, such as herbs and lemon.

Nursing interventions also address smoking and poor oral care when these are risk factors that interfere with food enjoyment. Good oral hygiene, especially before meals, can be effective in enhancing food flavors. If older adults smoke, encourage them to abstain from smoking for 1 hour before meals.

When the older adult is misinformed about constipation, or when other risk factors (e.g., a low-fiber diet) interfere with good bowel function, nursing interventions are directed toward education. Examples of effective programs for the prevention and management of constipation are found in nursing and medical literature (e.g., Hinrichs et al., 2001). Daily use of bran cereals or bran mixed with other foods is a common and effective strategy for preventing constipation. Howard and colleagues (2000) found that daily use of a mixture of applesauce, wheat bran, and unsweetened prune juice resulted in decreased use of medications for constipation and improved predictability of bowel movements so that patients could be toileted more accurately. Box 18-4 identifies some of the foods and other interventions that aid in preventing constipation.

Wellness Opportunity

Nurses try to find "teachable moments" so they can correct any myths or misconceptions associated with unhealthy eating patterns.

When medications affect nutrition and digestion, the nurse, caregiver, or older adults can discuss this problem with the prescribing health care practitioner to identify ways of alleviating this risk or addressing the consequences. If over-the-counter medications have a detrimental effect on nutrition or digestion, the nurse educates the older adult about medication–nutrient interactions and discusses ways of addressing the negative effects. Pharmacists may be helpful in suggesting interventions that will compensate for, or minimize, the effects of both prescription and over-the-counter medications on nutrition and digestion.

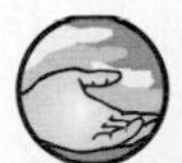

Box 18-4
Health Education Regarding Constipation

- A bowel movement every day is not necessarily the norm for every adult.
- Each adult has an individual pattern of bowel regularity, with the normal range varying from 3 times a day to 2 times a week.
- Include several portions of the following high-fiber foods in your daily diet: fresh, uncooked fruits and vegetables; bran and other cereal products made from whole grains.
- Drink 8 to 10 glasses of noncaffeinated liquid, including fruit juices, every day.
- Avoid laxatives and enemas.
- If medication is needed to promote bowel regularity, a bulk-forming agent (e.g., psyllium or methylcellulose) is least likely to have detrimental effects, especially if fluid intake is adequate.
- Do not ignore the urge to defecate; try to respond as soon as you feel the urge.
- Exercise regularly.

When consumption of alcohol interferes with nutrition, interventions might address the potential problem of alcoholism, or they may be aimed at compensating for the detrimental effects on nutrition. Nurses can recommend vitamin supplementation for people with a history of alcoholism after a medical evaluation has been performed to identify any underlying conditions, such as pernicious anemia.

Promoting Oral and Dental Health

In its goals related to oral health conditions, *Healthy People 2010* includes the objective of improving access to dental care for older adults, particularly for residents of long-term care facilities (USDHHS, 2000). This goal is addressed through dental services and good daily oral care; nurses have important responsibilities in implementing interventions to achieve this goal. If the older adult has avoided dental care because of resignation to poor oral health or a poor understanding of the need for preventive dental care, the nurse attempts to change these attitudes through education. Nurses also emphasize the importance of obtaining dental care every 6 months and, if appropriate, facilitate referrals for dental care. For homebound older adults, home dental services are often available, especially in large urban communities. In addition, low-cost dental services and dentures may be available through schools of dentistry. Nurses need to be familiar with local resources so that they can teach older adults and their caregivers about the dental services that are available in their community. In long-term care settings, nurses are usually responsible for facilitating referrals for dental care every 6 months. For older adults in any setting, if xerostomia interferes with digestion or nutrition, the nurse may suggest or facilitate a referral for a medical evaluation to identify disease processes or medication effects that may be contributing factors.

Good oral care is an essential, but often overlooked, component of daily nursing care for dependent older adults. An important initial intervention in institutional settings may be educational strategies to develop a culture "that promotes, values, and communicates oral health caregiving as fundamental to geriatric nursing practice as are restraint reduction and skin care practices" (Coleman, 2002, p. 193). An intervention that has been found to be effective in long-term care facilities is the use of specially trained aides whose only responsibility is to provide oral care to residents. Because the cost of implementing this model is offset by reducing the cost of care related to consequences of poor oral hygiene (e.g., aspiration pneumonia), this model may be associated with measurable cost savings (Terpenning & Shay, 2002). Excellent oral hygiene protocols for older adults in institutional settings can be found in nursing journals (e.g., Gil-Montoya et al., 2006) and at www.geronurseonline.org.

Nurses and researchers also are trying to identify cost-effective oral care products that improve oral hygiene and are easy to use. For example, Simons and colleagues (2002) found that older residents of residential homes who had some natural teeth and chewed sugar-free gum containing xylitol alone or xylitol and chlorhexidine for 15 minutes after the morning and evening meals had significant increases in saliva flow rates and reductions in denture stomatitis, angular cheilitis, and denture debris scores compared with a control group that did not chew gum. A recent nursing review of oral care products suggested that ultrasonic oral care devices or specially designed manual brushes (e.g., the Collis-curve brush, available at www.colliscurve.com) are more effective and convenient than traditional manual brushes for use with dependent older adults (Coleman, 2002). Nurses can adapt handles of toothbrushes, or obtain specially designed brushes, to increase the self-care abilities of people with functional limitations that interfere with normal use of a toothbrush. Battery-operated brushes are effective, easy to use, and relatively inexpensive. Child-size toothbrushes (manual or automatic) may be easier to use for dependent older adults, especially if access to all their teeth is limited. Although foam swabs have been commonly used in institutional settings for several decades, they are not effective for cleaning teeth or removing plaque. Similarly, lemon and glycerin swabs, which have been available since the 1940s, are no longer recommended because they reduce the oral pH and dehydrate oral mucous membranes. Prescription mouth rinses containing chlorhexidine (e.g., Peridex) are effective in inhibiting plaque and treating periodontal disease and have been used as an alternative to mechanical plaque removal for frail or dependent older adults (MacEntee, 2000). Over-the-counter products (e.g., Listerine and generic equivalents) also help control plaque, but many of these have a high alcohol content (Momeyer & Luggen, 2005). Box 18-5 can be used as a

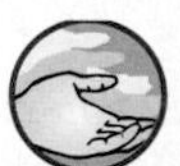

Box 18-5
Health Education Regarding Oral and Dental Care

Health Education Regarding Care of the Teeth and Gums

- Oral care should include daily use of dental floss as well as twice daily brushing of all tooth surfaces.
- Use a soft-bristled toothbrush and fluoridated toothpaste.
- If you have any limitations that interfere with your ability to use a regular toothbrush, you may benefit from using an electric or battery-powered brush or a brush with a specially designed handle (available where medical supplies are sold).
- Easy-to-use floss aids are inexpensive and widely available for facilitating dental flossing; they are especially helpful for people with any limitations in manual strength or dexterity or limited range of motion in the upper extremities.
- Some mouth rinses have cleansing, antimicrobial, and moisturizing effect, but they are used in conjunction with, not instead of, brushing.
- Avoid the use of alcohol-containing mouthwashes because of their drying effect.
- Because sugar is a major contributing factor to tooth decay, it is important to limit the intake of sugary substances, especially substances that are kept in the mouth for long periods (e.g., gum, hard candy).
- After eating sugar-containing foods, rinse your mouth or brush your teeth.
- Visit a dentist every 6 months for regular oral care.
- If partial or complete dentures are worn, remove them at night, keep them in water, and clean them before placing them back in your mouth.

Health Education Regarding Dry Mouth

- Excessive dry mouth may be caused by medical conditions or medication effects and should be evaluated before symptomatic treatment is initiated.
- Drink at least 10 to 12 glasses of noncaffeinated fluid during the day, and drink sips of water at frequent intervals.
- Suck on xylitol-flavored fluoride tablets or sugar-free hard candies to stimulate saliva flow.
- Chew sugar-free gum with xylitol for 15 minutes after meals to stimulate saliva flow and promote oral hygiene.
- Try using one of the many brands of saliva substitutes available at drugstores, but avoid those that contain sorbitol because this can worsen the condition.
- Avoid sucking lozenges containing citric acid because of their detrimental effects on tooth enamel.
- Avoid alcohol, alcohol-containing mouthwashes, and highly acidic drinks (e.g., orange or grapefruit juice) because these tend to exacerbate the condition.
- Avoid smoking because this exacerbates the symptoms and further irritates the oral mucous membranes.
- Pay particular attention to oral hygiene because a dry mouth increases the risk for gum and dental diseases.
- Maintain optimal room humidity, especially at night.

guide to health education about interventions for oral care and alleviation of xerostomia.

Wellness Opportunity

Nurses promote independence and self-care in oral hygiene by facilitating referrals for occupational therapists for older adults with functional impairments.

Promoting Optimal Nutrition and Preventing Disease

Therapeutic diets have long been recognized as essential interventions for some diseases (e.g. diabetes, renal or liver failure), and in recent years the role of nutrients is increasingly being supported as an important health promotion and disease prevention intervention for people of all ages. For example, a goal of *Healthy People 2010* is to "promote health and reduce chronic disease associated with diet and weight" (USDHHS, 2000, p. 19-9). Specific objectives address food and nutrient consumption of fruit, grains, sodium, calcium, vegetables, and total and saturated fats. Gerontologists and gerontological health care practitioners currently emphasize the role of nutrition as secondary prevention interventions that can contribute to improved health and longer life expectancy for older adults (Chernoff, 2001). Nutritional interventions for older adults are directed specifically toward conditions such as diabetes, obesity, hypertension, osteoporosis, cardiovascular disease, and age-related macular degeneration.

Recent attention also is focused on nutritional interventions for healthy aging, with many recommendations emphasizing the inclusion of foods containing antioxidants and other nutrients that may play a protective and preventive role. Researchers are exploring the role of nutrients as primary prevention interventions for age-associated conditions such as dementia, cataracts, cardiovascular disease, and age-related macular degeneration (Smeeding, 2001), but results of studies are not likely to be available in the near future. In analyzing information about potential benefits of nutrients as preventive interventions, distinctions must be made between nutrients obtained from foods and those that are found in supplements. For example, a high dietary intake of a particular nutrient (e.g., carotenoids) may be beneficial in health promotion or disease prevention, but a dietary supplement product with the same nutrient may not necessarily have the same beneficial effects. Thus, nurses need to educate older adults about the importance of obtaining nutrients from food sources rather than relying primarily on dietary supplements.

Nurses teach older adults about basic nutritional requirements, using easy-to-understand educational materials. Healthy older adults generally maintain optimal nutritional status through the daily intake of the foods listed in Box 18-6 and illustrated in Figure 18-2. If the older adult has any illness or takes any medications or chemicals that interfere with homeostasis, digestion, or nutrition, the daily diet will have to be modified to compensate for these effects. If, for any reason, the food intake is inadequate to meet daily nutritional requirements, the older adult can be encouraged to use a broad-spectrum vitamin and mineral supplement. Box 18-7 summarizes health education guidelines regarding nutritional supplements and complementary and alternative practices related to digestion and nutrition.

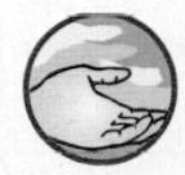

Box 18-6
Guidelines for Daily Food Intake for Older Adults

- Nutrient requirements do not diminish with age, but caloric needs decrease gradually in older adulthood. Therefore, it is important to select a variety of high-quality foods.
- Use salt, sugar, and sodium only in moderation.
- The amount of each type of food will vary according to the caloric needs of each older person, with men generally needing a greater number of servings than women.
- Basic nutritional requirements will be met if the daily diet includes at least the minimum number of servings from each food group listed below and if it includes complex carbohydrates and high-fiber foods. Basic nutritional requirements are as follows:

Servings	***Food Group***
6–9	Bread, rice, pasta, and cereal
3–4	Vegetables
2–3	Fruits
2–3	Meat, fish, poultry, or legumes (dried peas and beans, lentils, nut butters, soy products)
2–3	Milk, cheese, yogurt, and dairy desserts
8 or more	8-ounce glasses of noncaffeinated liquid

Wellness Opportunity

Nurses promote personal responsibility by suggesting that older adults use the modified food guide pyramid shown in Figure 18-2 to identify beneficial and detrimental eating patterns.

Nutrition education can be provided on an individual basis or in group settings, perhaps in conjunction with registered dietitians. In acute care settings, registered dietitians are usually available, but their services are often limited to people who have special dietary needs or an identified nutritional problem. In long-term care settings, a registered dietitian generally assesses the nutritional needs and usual eating patterns of older adults and establishes a plan of care aimed at attaining and maintaining optimal nutrition. In community settings, nurses sometimes provide nutrition education to groups of older adults. Nurses making home visits include nutrition education in their health teaching, make referrals for registered dietitian assessment and recommendations, and use available community resources to

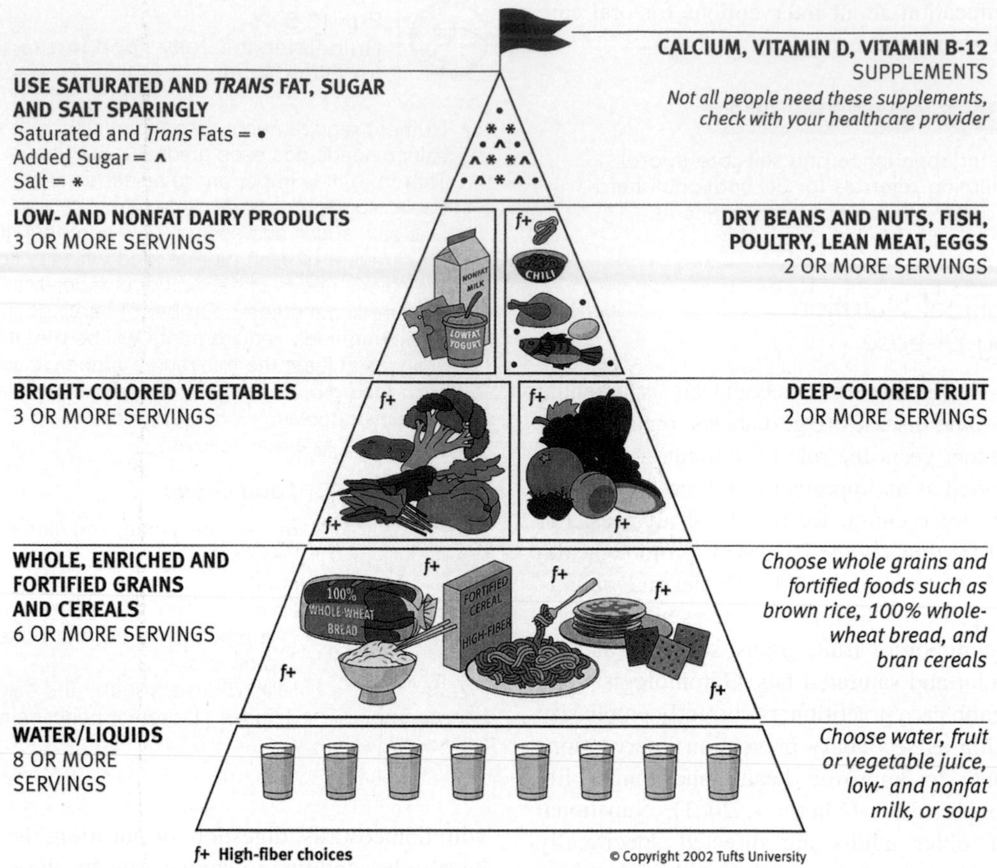

FIGURE 18-2 The modified food guide pyramid for people older than 70 years. (Available at http://nutrition.tufts.edu. Courtesy of Tufts University.)

supplement these interventions. Nurses can use the Transtheoretical Model (discussed in Chapter 5) as an effective approach to working with older adults toward improved nutrition and changes in eating patterns (Burkholder & Evers, 2002).

Determining the appropriate role of nutritional supplements is becoming increasingly difficult, despite their burgeoning availability and variety, because much of the information about them is provided by groups that benefit from their sale. Thus, nurses need to keep abreast of scien-

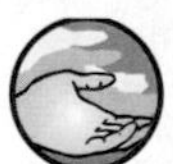

Box 18-7
Health Education About Nutritional Supplements and Complementary and Alternative Practices

Guidelines for Vitamin Supplementation in Older Adults

The following daily vitamin supplements are recommended for older adults:

- One multivitamin
- A total of 600 IU vitamin D for people with osteoporosis or risks for osteoporosis or vitamin D deficiency (e.g., sunlight deprivation)
- A total of 1 mg folate for people with cardiovascular risk factors (especially smoking) and for people with alcoholism
- Up to a total of 10 mg thiamine for people with alcoholism
- Up to a total of 2000 IU vitamin E for people with dementia (but observe for signs of toxicity—e.g., malaise, headache, gastrointestinal disturbances—in doses of 1000 IU or higher)

Guidelines Regarding Complementary and Alternative Practices

- Moderate amounts of the following herbs may be effective for constipation: flax, aloe, senna, fennel, rhubarb, buckthorn, cascara, psyllium, fenugreek, and licorice.
- Avoid large amounts of herbal laxatives (including teas) because these may adversely affect the gastrointestinal tract.
- Homeopathic remedies that may be helpful for constipation include graphites, bryonia, alumina, nux vomica, and natrum muriaticum.
- Complementary and alternative practices that may be helpful for treating constipation include yoga, acupuncture, acupressure, reflexology, gentle massage of the abdomen, and hot compresses to the abdomen.

tifically based research and resources relating to this topic by using the Educational Resources section at the end of this chapter. In acute and long-term care settings, inexpensive oral nutritional supplements can be used to increase weight and improve nutritional status (Levinson, et al., 2005; Milne et al., 2006).

Mrs. D. returns for a "Counseling for Health" follow-up session with a 7-day diet history and a list of her medications, as you requested. You review the diet history and find that in response to your previous health education about constipation Mrs. D. now uses whole-wheat bread instead of white and eats more fresh fruits and vegetables. You assess that her daily intake is only about 800 calories, of which pastries account for a high percentage. She rarely eats meat, perhaps because of the poor condition of her teeth. Her medications include citalopram (Celexa) 20 mg daily; clonidine (Catapres) 0.2 mg daily; and triamterene 37.5 mg/hydrochlorothiazide 25 mg (Dyazide) daily.

THINKING POINTS

- What specific risk factors do you address in your health teaching interventions?
- What health teaching would you give about alleviating risk factors?
- What interventions would you suggest to improve Mrs. D.'s nutrition?
- What interventions would you suggest to address Mrs. D.'s dry mouth (which you noticed during Mrs. D.'s last visit)?
- What health teaching would you provide about oral and dental care?

EVALUATING EFFECTIVENESS OF NURSING INTERVENTIONS

Nursing care for older adults with Imbalanced Nutrition: Less than Body Requirements is evaluated by determining whether the older adult has a daily nutrient intake that corresponds with metabolic needs and by the older adult's achieving a body weight within 110% of the ideal body weight for that individual. For older adults with Constipation, or risks for constipation, evaluation criteria would depend on the older adult's verbalizing accurate information about constipation, identifying the factors that contribute to constipation, and reporting that he or she passes soft stools on a regular basis without any straining or discomfort.

Mr. D. is an 85-year-old widower who was referred for home care after a hospitalization in the Acute Care for the Elderly (ACE) unit for congestive heart failure. During the hospitalization, the geriatric assessment team diagnosed protein-energy undernutrition because Mr. D.'s weight (116 pounds) is only 75% of his ideal body weight (155 pounds). In addition, laboratory work revealed the following abnormal values: hemoglobin, 11%; hematocrit, 35%; and serum albumin, 3.2 g/dL. Mr. D.'s congestive heart failure is stable and he ambulates with a walker but is very weak. In addition to orders pertaining to assessment and management of the newly diagnosed congestive heart failure, home care orders include nursing assessment of his home situation, nutrition education, and monitoring of weight. The geriatric assessment team in the ACE unit, which included a registered dietitian, recommended that Mr. D. have a daily intake of 1600 calories, including a minimum of 60 g of protein (240 calories). Mr. D. could meet this goal if his daily intake included the minimum number of servings from each food group as listed in Box 18-6.

NURSING ASSESSMENT

Mr. D. lives alone in a senior high-rise apartment and, until recently, participated in social activities and took advantage of van transportation to get to medical appointments and the grocery store. He used to prepare his own meals and shop for his groceries once a week, but has not been out of his apartment in the past month because of gradually increasing weakness, shortness of breath, and swelling in his legs. After his health began declining, a neighbor began doing his grocery shopping. Typical meals are toast and coffee for breakfast; canned soup, a lunchmeat sandwich, and cookies for lunch; and a "Budget Gourmet" entree for supper. Mr. D. says that he never really learned to cook very well, but

(case study continues on page 386)

that he got along "well enough for a man my age." He says that he does not particularly enjoy the convenience foods that he eats, but states, "They sure are easy to fix, even if they are boring." Mr. D. acknowledges that he has thought about going to the daily noon meal offered at a nearby church, but has not followed through because "the senior van doesn't go there, but it does go to the grocery store. Besides, I'm never very hungry because food just doesn't interest me the way it used to when I had Magda's good Hungarian cooking." Mr. D. reports a gradual weight loss of about 50 pounds since his wife died 2 years ago. He says that he was too heavy when his wife used to do the cooking, so he is not concerned about his weight loss. He has full dentures but has not used them for the past year because they do not fit well anymore. He has not done anything about his dentures because he manages to chew the kinds of food he buys. In addition, his dentist retired 2 years ago and he has not considered going to a new one.

NURSING DIAGNOSIS

One of the nursing diagnoses that you address in your home care plan is Altered Nutrition: Less than Body Requirements, related to social isolation, declining health, ill-fitting dentures, and lack of enjoyment of food. You also question whether depression may be a contributing factor. Evidence comes from his low body weight, laboratory data consistent with poor nutritional status, and his descriptions of his eating and food preparation patterns.

NURSING CARE PLAN FOR MR. D.

Expected Outcome	Nursing Interventions	Nursing Evaluation
Mr. D. will state what his daily needs are for each food group.	• Give Mr. D. a copy of Box 18-6 and use it as a basis for teaching about daily nutrient requirements.	• Mr. D. will describe an eating pattern that meets his daily nutritional needs.
Mr. D. will identify a method for meeting his nutrient needs.	• Gain Mr. D.'s permission to arrange for home health aide assistance three times weekly for meal preparation and grocery shopping. • Explore with Mr. D. various options for broadening his food selection to improve his nutritional intake (e.g., including dairy products and more fruits and vegetables). • Develop a meal plan with Mr. D. that includes foods that he enjoys but are not currently part of his diet. Discuss the nutritional value of these foods and suggest that he add new food items in each of the food group categories in which he is deficient.	• Mr. D. will describe an acceptable plan for meeting his nutritional needs. • Mr. D. will gain between 1 and 2 pounds weekly until he reaches the goal of 150 to 155 pounds.
Mr. D. will have his dentures evaluated and modified or replaced.	• Discuss with Mr. D. the importance of dentures in chewing efficiency and food enjoyment. • Discuss the long-term detrimental effects of lack of dentures. • Explore ways of obtaining a dental evaluation.	• Mr. D. will chew his food with dentures that fit properly.

THINKING POINTS

- What risk factors are likely to be contributing to Mr. D.'s gradual weight loss during the past 2 years?
- What further assessment information would you want to have?

Chapter Highlights

Age-Related Changes That Affect Digestion and Eating Patterns
- Diminished senses of smell and taste
- Less efficient chewing
- Decreased saliva secretion
- Slower propulsive waves in esophagus
- Degenerative changes in the intestinal tract, liver, pancreas, and biliary tract

Age-Related Changes in Nutritional Requirements (Table 18-1)
- Calories: need less quantity, better quality
- Fiber: 25 to 38 g/day
- Protein: minimum daily intake of 1 g/kg of body weight (1.5 g/kg for older adults with acute medical conditions)
- Fat: no more than 10% to 30% of daily caloric intake

Risk Factors That Affect Digestion and Nutrition
- Poor oral care
- Conditions that can lead to nutritional deficiencies (Table 18-2)
- Pathologic process or functional impairment that interferes with ability to obtain, prepare, consume, or enjoy food
- Effects of medications (Table 18-3)
- Psychosocial factors (e.g., dementia, depression, loneliness)
- Cultural and socioeconomic factors (Cultural Considerations Box 18-1)
- Environmental factors (e.g., noisy or unpleasant environment in institutional setting)
- Behaviors based on myths and misunderstandings (e.g., overuse of laxatives because of poor understanding of normal bowel function)

Pathologic Condition Affecting Digestive Wellness
- Constipation: two or fewer bowel movements weekly, or hard, dry feces

Functional Consequences Affecting Digestion and Nutrition
- Difficulty with procuring food and preparing meals
- Diminished enjoyment of food
- Impaired digestion
- Decreased absorption of nutrients
- Tendency to develop constipation as a result of risk factors

Nursing Assessment of Digestion and Nutrition (Fig. 18-1, Boxes 18-1 through 18-3)
- Usual nutrient intake and eating patterns
- Risks that interfere with any aspect of obtaining, preparing, eating, and enjoying food
- Physical examination and laboratory data regarding nutritional status

Nursing Diagnosis
- Readiness for Enhanced Nutrition
- Altered Nutrition: Less than Body Requirements
- Constipation
- Impaired Oral Mucous Membrane

Planning for Wellness Outcomes
- Improved: appetite, nutritional status, oral hygiene, depression level
- Self-care: eating, oral hygiene
- Increased knowledge about diet, improved health beliefs about constipation

Nursing Interventions to Promote Healthy Digestion and Nutrition (Fig. 18-2, Boxes 18-4 through 18-7)
- Teaching older adults about nutrition and digestion
- Applying daily food guide to older adults
- Promoting oral and dental health
- Referring for community resources (e.g., home-delivered meals, group meal programs)

Evaluating Effectiveness of Nursing Interventions
- Daily nutrient intake that corresponds to metabolic needs
- Achieving/maintaining body weight within 110% of ideal body weight for the individual
- Achieving/maintaining regular bowel elimination

Critical Thinking Exercises

1. Discuss specific ways in which each of the following conditions might influence the eating patterns of older adults: depression, medications, sensory changes, cognitive impairments, functional impairments, economic factors, social circumstances, and oral health factors.
2. Describe at least three characteristics of eating patterns for each of the following cultural groups: Native Americans, Hispanic Americans, African Americans, and Asian Americans.
3. How would you assess digestion and nutrition for an older adult in each of the following settings: home, long-term care facility, and acute care facility?
4. Outline a health education plan for teaching older adults about constipation. Include the following points: definition of constipation, risk factors for constipation, and interventions to prevent and address constipation.
5. Outline a health education plan for teaching older adults about oral and dental care.

Clinical Tool Resources

Hartford Institute for Geriatric Nursing
Try This: Best Practices in Nursing Care to Older Adults
Issue Number 9 (Revised Summer 2004), Assessing Nutrition in Older Adults
www.hartfordign.org/resources/education/tryThis.html

Educational Resources

American Dietetic Association
www.eatright.org

Canadian Council of Food and Nutrition
www.nin.ca

Food and Drug Administration
www.fda.gov

Food and Nutrition Information Center
www.nal.usda.gov/fnic

Mini Nutritional Assessment
www.mna-elderly.com

National Dairy Council
www.dairyinfo.com

National Oral Health Information Clearinghouse
www.nohic.nidcr.nih.gov/

Nutrition Screening Initiative
http://www.aafp.org/nsi.xml

References

Achem, S. R., & DeVault, K. R. (2005). Dysphagia in aging. *Journal of Clinical Gastroenterology, 39*, 357–371.

Alibhai, S. M. H., Greenwood, C., & Payette, H. (2005). An approach to the management of unintentional weight loss in elderly people. *Canadian Medical Association Journal, 172*, 773–780.

Amarantos, E., Martinez, A., & Dwyer, J. (2001). Nutrition and quality of life in older adults. *Journals of Gerontology: Series A, Biological Sciences and Medical Sciences, 56* (Special Issue II), 54–64.

American Dietetic Association. (2005). Position paper of the American Dietetic Association: Nutrition across the spectrum of aging. *Journal of the American Dietetic Association, 105*, 616–633.

Andres, E., Kaltenbach, G., Perrin, A. E., Kurtz, J. E., & Schlienger, J. L. (2002). Food-cobalamin malabsorption in the elderly. *American Journal of Medicine, 13* (4), 351–352.

Bleda, M. J., Bolibar, I., Pares, R., & Alava, A. (2002). Reliability of the Mini Nutritional Assessment (MNA) in institutional elderly people. *The Journal of Nutrition, Health and Aging, 6*, 134–137.

Brush, J. A., Meehan, R. A., & Calkins, M. P. (2002). Using the environment to improve intake for people with dementia. *Alzheimer's Care Quarterly, 3*, 330–338.

Burkholder, G. J., & Evers, K. A. (2002). Application of the Transtheoretical Model to several problem behaviors. In P. M. Burbank & D. Riebe (Eds.), *Promoting exercise and behavior change in older adults: Interventions with the transtheoretical model* (pp. 85–145). New York: Springer.

Carpenito-Moyet, L. J. (2006). *Handbook of nursing diagnosis* (11th ed.). Philadelphia: Lippincott Williams & Wilkins.

Chernoff, R. (2001). Nutrition and health promotion in older adults. *Journals of Gerontology: Series A, Biological Sciences and Medical Sciences, 56* (Special Issue II), 47–53.

Chung, J.-P., Mojon, P., & Budtz-Jorgensen, E. (2000). Dental care of elderly in nursing homes: Perceptions of managers, nurses, and physicians. *Special Care Dentistry, 20*, 12–17.

Chung, S. (2006). *Retirement and obesity among the near elderly*. PhD Thesis. Chapel Hill, NC: The University of North Carolina at Chapel Hill.

Coleman, P. (2002). Improving oral health care for the frail elderly: A review of widespread problems and best practices. *Geriatric Nursing, 23*, 189–197.

Crogan, N. L., & Corbett, C. F. (2002). Predicting malnutrition in nursing home residents using the minimum data set. *Geriatric Nursing, 23*, 224–226.

Crogan, N. L., Shultz, J. A., Adams, C. E., & Massey, L. K. (2001). Barriers to nutrition care for nursing home residents. *Journal of Gerontological Nursing, 27* (12), 25–31.

DeBusk, R. M. (2002). Oats vs. wheat for heart health. *The Integrative Medicine Consult, 108*, 117–118.

De Castro, J. M. (2002). Age-related changes in the social, psychological and temporal influences on food intake in free living, healthy, adult humans. *Journals of Gerontology: Series A, Biological Sciences and Medical Sciences, 57*, M368–M377.

Delahunt, A. (2002). The use of the Mini Nutritional Assessment tool for older people attending a day hospital. *Irish Journal of Medical Science, 170*(3), 106–126.

DiFrancesco, V., Zamboni, M., Dioli, A., Zoico, E., Mazzali, G., Omizzolo, F., et al. (2005). Delayed postprandial gastric emptying and impaired gallbladder contraction together with elevated cholecystokinin and peptide YY serum levels sustain satiety and inhibit hunger in healthy elderly persons. *Journals of Gerontology: Series A, Biological Sciences and Medical Sciences, 60*, 1581–1585.

Dudek, S. G. (2007). *Nutrition essentials for nursing practice* (5th ed., rev. reprint). Philadelphia: Lippincott Williams & Wilkins.

Ettinger, R. (2001). Oral health. In E. A. Swanson, T. Tripp-Reimer, & K. Buckwalter (Eds.), *Health promotion and disease prevention in the older adult* (pp. 81–101). New York: Springer.

Finkel, D., Pedersen, N. L., & Larsson, M. (2001). *Journals of Gerontology: Series B, Psychological Sciences and Social Sciences, 56*, P226–P233.

Frank, L., Flynn, J., & Rothman, M. (2001). Use of a self-report constipation questionnaire with older adults in long-term care. *The Gerontologist, 41*, 778–786.

Fukunaga, A., Uematsu, H., & Sugimoto, K. (2005). Influences of aging on taste perception and oral somatic sensation. *Journals of Gerontology: Series A, Biological Sciences and Medical Sciences, 60*, 109–113.

Furman, E. F. (2006). Undernutrition in older adults across the continuum of care: Nutritional assessment, barriers, and interventions. *Journal of Gerontological Nursing, 32*(1), 22–27.

Ghezzi, E. M., Wagner-Lange, L. A., Schork, M. A., Meter, E. J., Baum, B. J., Streckfus, C. F., et al. (2000). Longitudinal influence of age, menopause, hormone replacement therapy, and other medications on parotid flow rates in healthy women. *Journals of Gerontology: Series A, Biological Sciences and Medical Sciences, 55*, M34–M42.

Gilbert, P. E., Pirogovsky, E., Ferdon, S., & Murphy, C. (2006). The effects of normal aging on source memory for odors. *Journals of Gerontology: Series B, Psychological Sciences and Social Sciences, 61*, P58–P60.

Gil-Montoya, J. A., DeMello, A. L. F., Cardenas, C. B., & Lopez, I. G. (2006). Oral health protocol for the dependent institutionalized elderly. *Geriatric Nursing, 27*, 95–101.

Hinrichs, M., Huseboe, J., Tang, J., & Titler, M. G. (2001). Research-based protocol: Management of constipation. *Journal of Gerontological Nursing, 27*(2), 17–28.

Horowitz, M. (2000). Aging and the gastrointestinal tract. In M. H. Beers & R. Berkow (Eds.), *The Merck manual of geriatrics* (3rd ed., pp. 1000–1006). Whitehouse Station, NJ: Merck Research Laboratories.

Howard, L. V., West, D., & Ossip-Klein, D. J. (2000). Chronic constipation management for institutionalized older adults. *Geriatric Nursing, 21*, 78–81.

Hutton, B. (2002). Is there an association between edentulism and nutritional state? *Journal of the Canadian Dental Association, 68*, 182–187.

Jensen, G. L., McGee, M., & Brinkley, J. B. (2001). Gastrointestinal disorders in the elderly: Nutrition in the elderly. *Gastroenterology Clinics, 30*, 313–334.

Johnson, K. A., Bernard, M. A., & Funderburg, K. (2002). Vitamin nutrition in older adults. *Clinics in Geriatric Medicine, 18*, 773–801.

Keller, H. H. (2006). Meal programs improve nutritional risk: A longitudinal analysis of community-living seniors. *Journal of the American Dietetic Association, 106*, 1042–1048.

Leslie, P., Drinnan, M. J., Ford, G. A., & Wilson, J. A. (2005). Swallow respiratory patterns and aging: Presbyphagia or dysphagia? *Journals of Gerontology: Series A, Biological Sciences and Medical Sciences, 60*, 391–395.

Lewis, M. M. (2001). Long-term care in geriatrics: Nutrition in long term care. *Clinics in Family Practice, 3*, 627–651.

Levinson, Y., Dwolatzky, T., Epstein, A., Adler, B., & Epstein, L. (2005). Is it possible to increase weight and maintain the protein status of debilitated elderly residents of nursing homes? *Journals of Gerontology: Series A, Biological Sciences and Medical Sciences, 60*, 878–881.

Linder, J. D., & Wilcox, C. M. (2001). Gastrointestinal disorders in the elderly: Acid peptic disease in the elderly. *Gastroenterology Clinics, 30*, 363–376.

Liu, L., Bopp, M. M., Roberson, P. K., & Sullivan, D. H. (2002). Undernutrition and risk of mortality in elderly patients within 1 year of hospital discharge. *Journals of Gerontology: Series A, Biological Sciences and Medical Sciences, 57*, M741–M746.

MacEntee, M. (2000). Oral care for successful aging in long-term care. *Journal of Public Health Dentistry, 60*, 326–329.

Matear, D. W., & Barbaro, J. (2005). Effectiveness of saliva substitute in the treatment of dry mouth in the elderly: A pilot study. *Journal of the Royal Society for the Promotion of Health, 125*, 35–41.

Mathey, M.-F., Siebelink, E., de Graaf, C., & Van Staveren, W. A. (2001). Flavor enhancement of food improves dietary intake and nutritional status of elderly nursing home residents. *Journals of Gerontology: Series A, Biological Sciences and Medical Sciences, 56*, M200–M205.

Meyyazhagan, S., & Palmer, R. M. (2002). Nutritional requirements with aging. *Clinics in Geriatric Medicine, 18*, 557–576.

Milne, A. C., Avenell, A., & Potter, J. (2006). Meta-analysis: Protein and energy supplementation in older people. *Annals of Internal Medicine, 144*, 37–48.

Momeyer, M. A., & Luggen, A. S. (2005). Geriatric nurse practitioner guideline: Periodontal disease in older adults. *Geriatric Nursing, 26*, 197–200.

Morley, J. E. (2002). Pathophysiology of anorexia. *Clinics in Geriatric Medicine, 18*, 661–674.

National Academy of Sciences. (2002). Dietary, functional, and total fiber. In *Dietary reference intakes for energy, carbohydrates, fiber, fat, protein and amino acids (macronutrients)* (pp. 265–334). Washington, DC: National Academy of Sciences.

Newton, J. L. (2004). Changes in upper gastrointestinal physiology with age. *Mechanisms of Ageing and Development, 125*, 867–870.

Nicosia, M. A., Hind, J. A., Roecker, E. B., Carnes, M., Doyle, J., Dengel, G. A., et al. (2000). Age effects on the temporal evolution of isometric and swallowing pressure. *Journals of Gerontology: Series A, Biological Sciences and Medical Sciences, 55*, M634–M640.

Noel, M., & Reddy, M. (2005). Nutrition and aging. *Primary Care Clinics in Office Practice, 32*, 659–669.

Omran, M. L., & Salem, P. (2002). Diagnosing undernutrition. *Clinics in Geriatric Medicine, 18*, 719–737.

Patterson, A. J. (2002). Relationship between nutrition screening checklist and the health and well-being of older Australian women. *Public Health Nutrition, 5*(1), 65–71.

Prather, C. M. (2000). Constipation, diarrhea, and fecal incontinence. In M. H. Beers & R. Berkow (Eds.), *The Merck manual of geriatrics* (3rd ed., pp. 1080–1095). Whitehouse Station, NJ: Merck Research Laboratories.

Randolph, W. M., Ostir, G. V., & Markides, K. S. (2001). Prevalence of tooth loss and dental service use in older Mexican Americans. *Journal of the American Geriatrics Society, 49*, 585–589.

Rincon, M., Muzumdar, R., & Barzilai, N. (2006). Aging, body fat, and carbohydrate metabolism. In E. J. Masoro & S. N. Austad (Eds.), *Handbook of the biology of aging* (6th ed., pp. 498–511). San Diego: Academic Press.

Ritchie, C. S. (2002). Oral health, taste, and olfaction. *Clinics in Geriatric Medicine, 18*, 709–718.

Roberts, S., & Durnbaugh, T. (2002). Enhancing nutrition and eating skills in long-term care. *Alzheimer's Care Quarterly, 3*, 316–329.

Robinson, S. B., & Rosher, R. B. (2002). Can a beverage cart improve hydration? *Geriatric Nursing, 23*, 208–211.

Ross, S. O., & Forsmark, C. E. (2001). Gastrointestinal disorders in the elderly. *Gastroenterology Clinics, 30*, 531–545.

Salva, A., & Pera, G. (2001). Nutrition and ageing: Screening for malnutrition in community-dwelling elderly. *Public Health and Nutrition, 4*, 1375–1378.

Shanley, C., & O'Loughlin, G. (2000). Dysphagia among nursing home residents: An assessment and management protocol. *Journal of Gerontological Nursing, 26*(8), 35–48.

Sharkey, J. R. (2002). The interrelationship of nutritional risk factors, indicators of nutritional risk, and severity of disability among home-delivered meal participants. *The Gerontologist, 42*, 373–380.

Ship, J. A. (2002). Improving oral health in older people. *Journal of the American Geriatric Society, 50*, 1454–1455.

Ship, J. A., Pillemer, S. R., & Baum, B. J. (2002). Xerostomia and the geriatric patient. *Journal of the American Geriatrics Society, 50*, 535–543.

Simons, D., Brailsford, S. R., Kidd, E. A. M., & Beighton, D. (2002). The effects of medicated chewing gums on oral health in frail older people: A 1-year clinical trial. *Journal of the American Geriatrics Society, 50*, 1348–1353.

Simmons, S. F., Osterseil, D., & Schnelle, J. F. (2001). Improving food intake in nursing home residents with feeding assistance: A staffing analysis. *Journals of Gerontology: Series A, Biological Sciences and Medical Sciences, 56*, M790–M794.

Smeeding, S. J. W. (2001). Nutrition, supplements, and aging. *Geriatric Nursing, 22*, 219–224.

Soderhamn, U. (2002). Reliability and validity of the nutritional form for the elderly (NUFFE). *Journal of Advanced Nursing, 37*(1), 28–34.

Staveren, W. A., de Graaf, C., & de Groot, L. C. P. G. M. (2002). Regulation of appetite in frail persons. *Clinics in Geriatric Medicine, 18*, 675–685.

Terpenning, M., & Shay, K. (2002). Oral health is cost-effective to maintain but costly to ignore. *Journal of the American Geriatrics Society, 50*, 584–585.

Thomas, D. R., Ashmen, W., Morley, J. E., Council for Nutritional Strategies in Long-Term Care. (2000). Nutritional management in long term care: Development of a clinical guideline. *Journals of Gerontology: Series A, Biological Sciences and Medical Sciences, 55*, M725–M734.

U.S. Department of Health and Human Services (USDHHS). (2000). *Healthy people 2010* (2nd ed.). Washington, DC: U.S. Government Printing Office.

Vargas, C. M., Kramarow, E. A., & Yellowitz, J. A. (2001). The oral health of older Americans. *Aging trends, no. 3*. Hyattsville, MD: National Center for Health Statistics.

Vellas, B. C., Villars, H., Abellan, G., Soto, M. E., Rolland, Y., Guigoz, Y., et al. (2006). Overview of MNA: Its history and challenges. *Journal of Nutrition, Health, and Aging, 10*, 456–465.

Wakefield, B. (2001). Altered nutrition: Less than body requirements. In M. L. Maas, K. C. Buckwalter, M. D. Hardy, T. Tripp-Reimer, M. G. Titler, & J. P. Specht (Eds.), *Nursing care of older adults: Diagnoses, outcomes, and interventions* (pp. 145–157). St. Louis: Mosby.

Wakimoto, P., & Block, G. (2001). Dietary intake, dietary patterns, and changes with age: An epidemiological perspective. *Journals of Gerontology: Series A, Biological Sciences and Medical Sciences, 56* (Special Issue II), 65–80.

Wardh, I., Hallberg, L., Beggren, U., Andersson, L., & Sorensen, S. (2000). Oral health care: Low priority in nursing. *Scandinavian Journal of Caring Sciences, 14*, 137–142.

Yen, P. K. (2004). Nutrition and sensory loss. *Geriatric Nursing, 25*, 118-119.

Yoshikawa, M., Yoshida, M., Nagasaki, T., Tanimoto, K., Tsuga, K., & Akagawa, Y. (2006). Influence of aging and denture use on liquid swallowing in healthy dentulous and edentulous older people. *Journal of the American Geriatrics Society*, 54, 444–449.

Zembrzuski, C. (2000). Nutrition and hydration. *Journal of Gerontological Nursing, 26*(12), 6–7.

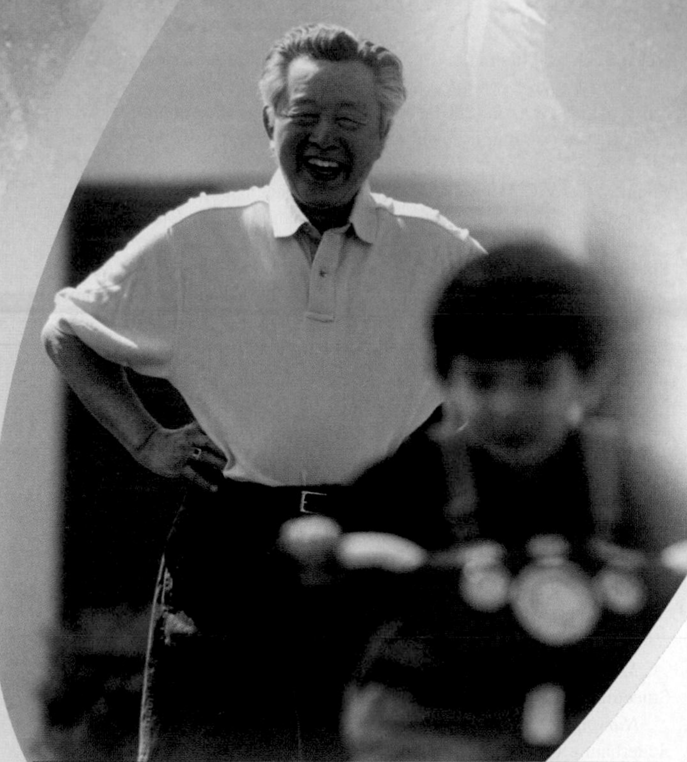

CHAPTER 19

Urinary Function

Learning Objectives

After reading this chapter, you will be able to:

1. List age-related changes that affect the complex processes involved in urinary elimination.
2. Describe risk factors that influence kidney function and urinary elimination.
3. Define urge, stress, mixed, and functional incontinence.
4. Describe functional consequences of age-related changes and risk factors related to each of the following aspects of urinary function: elimination of medications and metabolic wastes, patterns of urinary elimination, and consequences of incontinence for older adults and their caregivers.
5. Describe interview questions, observations, and laboratory data that are used in the nursing assessment of urinary function in older adults.
6. Identify interventions for addressing risk factors that influence urinary elimination and for alleviating and managing incontinence.

Key Terms

detrusor overactivity incontinence
mixed urinary incontinence
nocturia
overactive bladder
postural sway
stress urinary incontinence
urethral relaxation incontinence
urge syndrome *or* urgency-frequency syndrome
urge urinary incontinence
urinary incontinence

The primary function of urinary elimination is the excretion of water and chemical wastes, such as metabolic and pharmacologic byproducts, that would become toxic if allowed to accumulate. Efficient urinary excretion depends on renal blood flow, filtering activities within the kidneys, good functioning of the urinary tract muscles, and nervous system control over voluntary and involuntary mechanisms of elimination. Control of urinary elimination also depends on ambulatory and sensory abilities and on social, emotional, cognitive, and environmental factors.

In the absence of risk factors, healthy older adults experience very few functional consequences affecting urinary elimination. In the presence of risk factors, however, negative functional consequences, such as urinary incontinence, are common. **Urinary incontinence** is defined as "the complaint of any involuntary leakage of urine" (Abrams et al., 2002, p. 118). An important risk factor—and one that can be alleviated through health education interventions—is the false belief that urinary incontinence is an inevitable part of aging. Nurses have many opportunities to improve quality of life for older adults by addressing the risk factors that contribute to urinary incontinence.

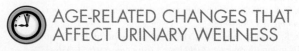

 AGE-RELATED CHANGES THAT AFFECT URINARY WELLNESS

Age-related changes in the kidneys, bladder, urethra, and control mechanisms in the nervous and other body systems

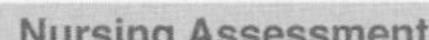
Promoting Urinary Wellness in Older Adults
Nursing Assessment
• Attitudes and knowledge
• Usual patterns of fluid intake and voiding
• Risk factors (drugs, diseases, functional limitations)
• Environmental barriers
• Signs and symptoms of urinary dysfunction
Age-Related Changes
• ↓ functioning nephrons
• ↓ renal blood flow
• ↓ elasticity in urinary tract muscles
• Degenerative changes in cerebral cortex
Negative Functional Consequences
• ↓ ability to maintain homeostasis
• ↓ clearance of some drugs
• ↓ bladder capacity
• Urgency
• Chronic residual urine
• Predisposition to urinary incontinence
Risk Factors
• Myths and misperceptions
• Functional impairments
• Environmental barriers
• Diseases (vaginitis, BPH, UTI)
• Medication effects (diuretics)
Nursing Interventions
• Teaching about normal urinary function
• Teaching about preventing and alleviating incontinence
• Managing incontinence
Wellness Outcomes
• Longer intervals of continence
• Self-care practices
• ↑ self-esteem
• Improved quality of life

affect the physiologic processes that control urinary elimination. In addition, any age-related change that interferes with the skills involved in socially appropriate urinary elimination can interfere with urinary control. Age-related changes that directly or indirectly affect urinary function and control are discussed in the next two sections.

Changes in the Kidneys

The complex process of urinary excretion begins in the kidneys with the filtering and removal of chemical wastes from the blood. Blood circulates through glomeruli, where liquid wastes, called *glomerular filtrate*, pass through Bowman's capsule and the renal tubules to the collecting ducts. During this process, substances needed by the body (such as water, glucose, and sodium) are retained, and waste products are excreted in the urine. These functions are important for maintaining homeostasis and excreting many medications. Excretory function, which is measured by the glomerular filtration rate (GFR), depends on the number and efficiency of nephrons and on the amount and rate of renal blood flow.

The kidney increases in weight and mass from birth until early adulthood, when the number of functioning nephrons begins to decline, particularly in the cortex, where the glomeruli are located. This decline continues throughout life, resulting in approximately a 25% decrease in kidney mass by the age of 80 years. The remaining glomeruli undergo various age-related changes, such as increased size, diminished lobulation, and thickened basement membrane. In addition, the proportion of sclerotic glomeruli increases from fewer than 5% at the age of 40 years to 35% by the age of 80 years. Beginning in the fourth decade, renal blood flow gradually diminishes, particularly in the cortex, at a rate of 10% per decade.

An average decline in renal function of 1% per year has been widely accepted since the 1970s as a hallmark of aging that begins between the ages of 30 and 40 years. However, longitudinal studies indicate that there is a great deal of individual variation in renal function among healthy older adults, and about one third of older people show no decrease in renal function (Masoro, 2006). Any substantial decline in renal function is more likely associated with common pathologic conditions, such as hypertension, rather than age-related changes alone.

Renal tubules regulate the dilution and concentration of urine, and subsequent excretion of water from the body, in a diurnal rhythm. The physiologic processes responsible for urine concentration and water excretion are influenced by the following factors:

- The amount of fluid in the body
- Resorption of water through, and transport of substances across, the tubular membrane
- Osmoreceptors in the hypothalamus, which regulate the level of circulating antidiuretic hormone (ADH) according to plasma water concentration
- Substances and activities that influence ADH secretion, such as caffeine, medications, alcohol, pain, stress, and exercise
- The concentration of sodium in the glomerular filtrate

Normally, production of ADH is stimulated by hemorrhage, dehydration, and other conditions that affect plasma volume or osmolality. This physiologic protective mechanism helps to maintain plasma volume and conserve fluid and sodium under conditions of water or sodium deprivation.

Many age-related changes affect the renal tubules, and thereby affect dilution and concentration of urine. These changes include fatty degeneration, the presence of diverticula, a loss of convoluted cells, and alterations in the composition of the basement membranes. Functionally, the renal tubules in older adults are less efficient in the exchange of substances, the conservation of water, and the suppression of ADH secretion in the presence of hypo-osmolality. Age-related changes also decrease the ability of the older kidney to conserve sodium in response to salt restriction. These age-related changes predispose healthy older adults to hyponatremia and other fluid and electrolyte imbalances, especially in the presence of any condition that alters renal circulation, water or sodium balance, or plasma volume or osmolality.

Changes in the Bladder and Urinary Tract

After being filtered by the kidneys, liquid wastes pass through the ureters into the bladder for temporary storage. The bladder is a balloon-like structure composed of collagen, smooth muscle (called *detrusor*), and elastic tissue. Liquid wastes are eliminated from the bladder through a complex physiologic process involving the following mechanisms:

- The ability of the bladder to expand for adequate storage and to contract for complete expulsion of liquid wastes
- The maintenance of higher urethral pressure relative to intravesicular pressure
- Regulation of the lower urinary tract through autonomic and somatic nerves
- Voluntary control of urination (micturition) through the cerebral centers

Age-related changes alter each of these mechanisms and affect urinary function in older adults.

In younger adults, the bladder stores 350 to 450 mL of urine before the person experiences sensations of fullness and discomfort. With increasing age, hypertrophy of the bladder muscle and thickening of the bladder wall interfere with its ability to expand, limiting the amount of urine that can be stored comfortably to about 200 to 300 mL.

As urine flows into the bladder, the smooth muscle expands without increasing intravesical pressure, and the urethral pressure increases, to the point that it is slightly higher than the intravesical pressure. As long as the volume of urine does not rise above 500 to 600 mL, this balance can be maintained, and urination can be controlled voluntarily. If the volume rises above this level, or if the detrusor muscle contracts involuntarily, the intravesical pressure will exceed the urethral pressure, and leakage of urine is likely to occur. In addition to the amount of urine in the bladder, the following factors influence the balance between intravesical and urethral pressure:

- Abdominal pressure
- Thickness of the urethral mucosa
- Tone of the pelvic, detrusor, urethral, and bladder neck muscles
- Replacement of smooth muscle tissue in the bladder and urethra with less elastic connective tissue

Internal and external sphincters regulate urine storage and bladder emptying. The internal sphincter is part of the base of the bladder and is controlled by autonomic nerves. The external sphincter is part of the pelvic floor musculature and is controlled by the pudendal nerve. When urination takes place, the detrusor and abdominal muscles contract, and the perineal and external sphincter muscles relax. When necessary, the external sphincter contracts to inhibit or interrupt voiding and to compensate for sudden surges in abdominal pressure. Age-related changes involving loss of smooth muscle in the urethra and relaxation of the pelvic floor muscles reduce the urethral resistance and diminish the tone of the sphincters.

Changes in Control Mechanisms

Changes in the nervous system and other regulatory systems affect urinary function. For example, motor impulses in the spinal cord control urination, but higher centers in the brain are responsible for detecting the sensation of bladder fullness, for inhibiting bladder emptying when necessary, and for stimulating bladder contractions for complete emptying. As the bladder fills, sensory receptors in the bladder wall send a signal to the sacral spinal cord. In healthy older adults, degenerative changes in the cerebral cortex may alter both the sensation of bladder fullness and the ability to empty the bladder completely. In younger adults, a sensation of fullness begins when the bladder is about half full. This sensation occurs at a later point for older adults, so the interval between the initial perception of the urge to void and the actual need to empty the bladder is shortened, which may trigger an episode of incontinence.

Many structures involved in urination contain estrogen receptors and are affected by hormonal changes, especially those that occur in menopausal women. For example, diminished estrogen causes a loss of tone, strength, and collagen support in the urogenital tissues and can contribute to a decrease in urethral closure pressure, which predisposes to urinary leakage problems. Also, because nerve endings depend on estrogen, diminished estrogen increases sensitivity to irritating stimuli, which leads to an increased urge to void. The decline in estrogen associated with menopause may partially account for the increased prevalence and earlier onset of incontinence in women.

Diminished thirst perception is another age-related change that can affect homeostasis and urinary function. Healthy older adults who are deprived of fluid do not sense thirst, experience discomfort from dry mouth, or drink enough water to rehydrate themselves. In the presence of conditions that place additional demands on fluid and electrolyte balance, such as fever or infection, diminished thirst sensation can interfere with the mechanisms that normally compensate for these physiologic stresses. Consequently, older people are likely to be at increased risk of dehydration because of inadequate fluid intake.

Changes Affecting Control Over Socially Appropriate Urinary Elimination

Control over urination depends not only on satisfactory functioning of the urinary tract and nervous system, but also on other functional aspects, such as adequate cognition and mobility, that significantly affect the skills needed for socially appropriate urinary elimination. The following factors affect a person's capacity for socially appropriate urinary elimination:

- Identification of a designated receptacle in a private area
- Accessibility and acceptability of toilet facilities
- Ability to get to and use a suitable receptacle
- The interval between the perception of the urge to void and the actual need to empty the bladder
- Voluntary control over the urge to void from the time of its perception until the person is able to use an appropriate receptacle

These factors are influenced by age-related changes that directly affect urinary elimination, as well as by those changes that affect the ability to identify and reach appropriate toileting facilities. Thus, balance, mobility, visual impairments, manual dexterity, and age-related vision changes are some of the factors that may influence urinary control. Older adults often experience an increase in **postural sway**, an age-related change that can interfere with one's ability to stand still. With increasing postural sway, older men may find it more difficult to maintain a standing position for urination. If urinary incontinence does occur, a diminished ability to smell may interfere with the older adult's perception of offensive odors. Although this does not have a functional impact on urinary elimination, the presence of urinary odors is viewed as socially inappropriate and may lead to isolation and rejection of the older adult.

Standards for socially appropriate urinary elimination may vary according to different social environments. For example, an independent, community-living older adult is expected to remain free of urinary odors or wetness and to urinate in private, designated places; however, a dependent or institutionalized older adult may not be expected to adhere so strictly to these standards. In any setting, attitudes and behaviors of caregivers can significantly influence patterns of urinary elimination, as discussed in the following section on Risk Factors.

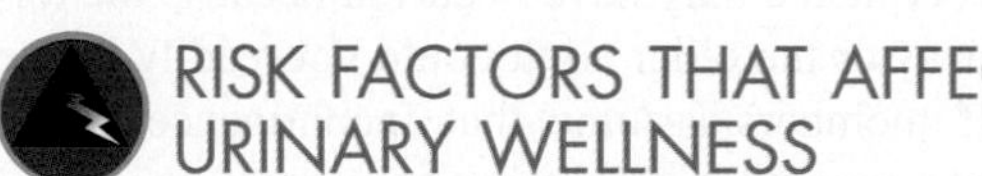

RISK FACTORS THAT AFFECT URINARY WELLNESS

As with many other areas of functioning, risk factors play a more significant role than age-related changes in causing negative functional consequences for urinary function. Epidemiologic studies have shown a strong association between urinary incontinence and all of the following risk factors: obesity, increasing age, childbirth, white race, and medical comorbidity (Melville et al., 2005). Other studies have shown conflicting results regarding an association between urinary incontinence and menopause, depression, smoking, diabetes, and a history of hysterectomy or cesarean section (Melville et al., 2005). Types of risk factors that can significantly affect urinary function include behaviors based on myths and misunderstandings, functional impairments, disease processes, medications, and environmental and lifestyle influences.

Behaviors Based on Myths and Misunderstandings

Attitudes based on myths or lack of knowledge about urinary function can have a detrimental effect on the behavior of older adults and their caregivers. For example, the perception of urinary incontinence as an inevitable consequence of aging deters older adults from seeking help from health care professionals. Physicians and nurses often reinforce these misperceptions and fail to ask about incontinence, even though most older adults are willing to discuss this sensitive topic if the health care provider is receptive (Palmer & Newman, 2006). Nurses in care facilities are likely to view incontinence as inevitable, with fewer than 3% of nurses addressing this in their care plans despite high rates of urinary incontinence among residents (Mangnall et al., 2006).

Because of such attitudes of resignation, early signs and symptoms of urinary dysfunction may be managed inappropriately, and the problem may progress. For example, older adults often underestimate the interval between the perception of the urge to void and the actual need to empty the bladder. When incontinence results, they may compensate by decreasing their fluid intake or urinating at more frequent intervals. However, these compensatory actions can lead to further urgency and incontinence, which, in turn, may reinforce the myth that incontinence is an inevitable problem of aging.

Attitudes, behaviors, and expectations of caregivers also interfere with the older adult's urinary continence. For example, when episodes of incontinence are noted soon after admission of an older adult to a long-term care facility, nursing staff members are likely to view the resident as having chronic incontinence, and their subsequent behaviors may reinforce the expectation of incontinence. In reality, the episode of incontinence may have occurred because the toilet is too far away or the older adult could not readily locate it. When staff members assume that incontinence is the norm for that person, they might initiate use of absorbent products by the resident, giving the older adult the message that voluntary control over urination is not expected.

In acute and long-term care settings, staff attitudes and nursing procedures strongly influence the standards for urinary elimination. In acute care facilities, indwelling catheters are commonly used because of patient illness, surgical procedures, or staff convenience. Once an indwelling catheter is inserted, it frequently remains in place until the person is discharged, allowing little or no time to reestablish normal voiding patterns during the hospitalization. In long-term care facilities, heavy workloads, poor communication, lack of teamwork, or inadequate knowledge about appropriated interventions are barriers to continence care (Mather & Bakas, 2002). In any setting, caregivers may believe that the use of pads or other incontinence products for the management of incontinence is easier and more convenient than preventing incontinence by assisting with toileting activities at the necessary intervals. For example, if an older adult needs a great deal of assistance with mobility, caregivers encourage the use of incontinence products because this is less time consuming than assisting the person to the bathroom. In these situations, dependent older adults are likely to behave according to the expectations of the caregivers, and incontinence will be the inevitable consequence. Medicare policies also may influence the caregiver's approach to urinary management because reimbursement for skilled care services is provided for people with indwelling catheters, but not for those who manage incontinence by other methods.

Limited fluid intake in response to the fear or onset of incontinence—or for any reason—is another behavior that can unintentionally exacerbate incontinence. Johnson and colleagues (2000) found that almost 37% of incontinent older adults limited their fluid intake as a self-care practice. If bladder fullness is not adequately achieved, as in states of dehydration or limited fluid intake, the neurologic mechanism that controls bladder emptying will not function effectively, and incontinence can occur because the person does not perceive the urge to void. Dehydration and inadequate hydration also cause increased bladder irritability, with subsequent uninhibited contractions and incontinence.

Wellness Opportunity

Nurses should examine their own attitudes and behaviors about incontinence to be sure they are based on accurate information rather than on misperceptions or ageist perspectives that could blind them to opportunities to promote urinary wellness.

Functional Impairments

Functional impairments are a major risk factor for the development of incontinence in older adults because they can interfere with the ability to recognize and respond to the urge to void in a timely manner. In the presence of age-related changes that shorten the interval between the perception of the urge to void and the actual need to empty the bladder, any delay in reaching an appropriate receptacle can result in incontinence. Thus, dependency in performing activities of daily living (ADLs) for any reason is strongly associated with incontinence. For example, conditions such as arthritis or Parkinson's disease may slow the ambulation of older adults as well as their ability to manipulate clothing. Likewise, dementia and other conditions that impair cognitive abilities can interfere with the timely processing of information that is necessary for maintaining voluntary control over urination. Finally, restraints can cause significant functional limitations and increase the risk of development of incontinence. Nurses should keep in mind that when older adults are dependent on family caregivers for assistance, the needs of the family are likely to influence the toileting practices.

Disease Processes

Disease processes that commonly increase the risk of urinary incontinence in older adults include those that directly involve the urinary tract and those that affect other systems and indirectly cause incontinence. Most of the conditions that affect the urinary tract are gender-specific, whereas those that affect other systems can affect all older adults.

Conditions of the Genitourinary Tract

Weakening of pelvic floor muscles in women, which may be secondary to postmenopausal estrogen depletion or to pregnancy, increases the risk of development of incontinence. With weakening of the pelvic muscles, any sudden increase in abdominal pressure may cause the involuntary expulsion of small amounts of urine. A cystocele, rectocele, or urethrocele may develop because of extreme pelvic muscle stretching or relaxation. These disorders, which frequently coexist with uterovaginal prolapse, are frequently associated with urinary incontinence. Pelvic muscle weakness also interferes with complete emptying of the bladder, resulting in residual urine and increased risk of bacteriuria. In addition to causing degenerative changes in the pelvic floor muscles, decreased estrogen levels cause atrophy of the vaginal and trigonal tissue with subsequent diminished resistance to pathogens. Vaginitis and trigonitis may develop and cause urinary urgency, frequency, and incontinence.

Benign prostatic hyperplasia is a common cause of voiding problems in older men, and prostatic carcinoma is a less common cause. In its early stage, prostatic hyperplasia obstructs the vesical neck and compresses the urethra, causing a compensatory hypertrophy of the detrusor muscle and subsequent outlet obstruction. With progressive hypertrophy, the bladder wall loses its elasticity and becomes thinner. Subsequently, urinary retention occurs, increasing the risk of bacteriuria and infection. Eventually, the ureter and kidney are affected, and hydroureter, hydronephrosis, diminished GFR, and uremia may develop. Men with prostatic hyperplasia may experience **nocturia** (excessive urination at night), decreased urine flow, incomplete bladder emptying, and urinary urgency and frequency. Another cause of decreased urethral resistance in men is the residual effect of transurethral surgery or radical prostatectomy.

Urinary tract infections are a common cause of incontinence in older adults, with an annual incidence of 10%. Manifestations of urinary tract infections in older adults may be very subtle; urinary incontinence may be the initial or primary sign. A change in behavior or level of functioning may be the presenting sign, especially in people with dementia. Older adults also are likely to have chronic bacteriuria, a condition characterized as 10^5 or more colony-forming units without symptoms of urinary tract infection. Of residents who reside in a nursing home, 25% to 50% of women and 15% to 40% of men are chronically bacteriuric (Juthani-Mehta et al., 2005).

Diversity Note

Women are twice as likely as men to have a urinary tract infection.

Other Conditions That Cause Urinary Incontinence

Many pathologic conditions affecting either the central or peripheral nervous system increase the risk of development of incontinence. Dementia is strongly associated with urinary incontinence, but the relationship between these two conditions is complex; incontinence should not be viewed as an inevitable and untreatable component of dementia (Ostbye et al., 2002). For example, older adults with dementia may lack the perceptual abilities that are necessary for finding and using appropriate facilities, but they may be able to maintain continence when given appropriate cues and reminders. Similarly, behavioral interventions can effectively resolve urinary incontinence in people with dementia when it is associated with functional declines such as impaired mobility (Holroyd-Leduc et al., 2006).

Conditions of the gastrointestinal tract that can cause incontinence include gastroenteritis, constipation, and fecal impaction. The mass of stool that is present with constipation or fecal impaction places pressure on the bladder and diminishes its storage capacity. In turn, this causes urinary frequency, urgency, and incontinence. Fecal impaction also can obstruct the bladder outlet, causing bladder distention and urinary retention or incontinence.

Other conditions that are highly associated with incontinence are obesity, diabetes, alcoholism, multiple sclerosis, Parkinson's disease, cerebrovascular accident, and chronic obstructive pulmonary disease (COPD). A longitudinal study found an independent association between diabetes mellitus and nocturia, and also found an association between hypertension and nocturnal polyuria and nocturia (Johnson et al., 2005b).

Metabolic disturbances that induce diuresis, such as diabetes and hypercalcemia, can lead to incontinence. Conditions that affect mental status, such as delirium, may be manifested or accompanied by urinary incontinence. Likewise, many conditions that affect physiologic processes, such as acute illness, can cause or exacerbate incontinence. Any acute illness or surgical intervention that temporarily limits mobility or compromises mental abilities also represents a risk factor for urinary incontinence. Hip fracture is a common cause of hospital-acquired incontinence, and the risk is exacerbated in older adults who are cognitively impaired and those with prior mobility limitations (Palmer et al., 2002).

Wellness Opportunity

Nurses holistically assess older adults by recognizing that urinary incontinence can be an indicator of physiologic disturbances (e.g., urinary tract infection), psychosocial conditions (e.g., dementia or depression), or a combination of functional limitations and environmental barriers.

Medication Effects

Medications influence urinary function in a number of ways and are common risk factors in the development of urinary incontinence. For example, loop diuretics increase urinary output, placing additional demands on the urinary system and compounding the effects of an age-related decrease in bladder capacity. Many medications, especially those that act on the central or autonomic nervous system, directly affect the urinary tract and cause incontinence. Older adults with other urinary tract conditions may be particularly susceptible to adverse medication effects. For example, men with prostatic hyperplasia may be especially prone to development of urinary retention when they take an adrenergic or anticholinergic agent (even those in over-the-counter decongestants and antihistamines). Similarly, alpha-adrenergic blocking agents (commonly used for hypertension) may contribute to stress incontinence (explained in the section on Pathologic Condition Affecting Urinary Function) in women with estrogen depletion. Some medications that are used to treat incontinence also can cause incontinence. For example, terazosin is used for benign prostatic hyperplasia but it can cause urethral relaxation and stress incontinence. Thus, it is imperative that causes of incontinence be identified accurately before treatment is initiated.

In addition to causing incontinence through their direct effects on the urinary tract, medications can cause incontinence through their effects on functional abilities. For example, anticholinergics (including those in over-the-counter agents) are commonly associated with cognitive and other functional impairments, which can interfere with the older adult's voluntary control over urination. Anticholinergics also cause dry mouth, and the subsequent increased fluid intake and diuresis can precipitate incontinence. Many medications cause constipation, which is a causative factor for incontinence. This adverse effect may be especially detrimental in the presence of prostatic hyperplasia or weakened pelvic floor muscles.

In addition to creating risk factors for incontinence, medications can compromise kidney function through the overstimulation of ADH secretion, which may compound age-related effects that predispose older adults to hyponatremia. Medications that stimulate ADH secretion include aspirin, narcotics, acetaminophen, antidepressants, barbiturates, chlorpropamide, clofibrate, fluphenazine, and haloperidol. Table 19-1 summarizes some types and examples of medications that can cause incontinence in older adults.

Dietary and Lifestyle Factors

Smoking of cigarettes and other nicotine-containing products increases the risk of urinary urgency, frequency, and urge incontinence. Certain foods (e.g., chocolate and spicy or acidic foods), food additives (e.g., aspartame and other artificial sweeteners), and caffeinated or carbonated beverages can cause incontinence. These substances can cause urinary urgency, frequency, and incontinence through the following mechanisms: increased diuresis, irritation of the bladder mucosa, and involuntary bladder contractions (Bottomley, 2000).

Specific nutrients also can affect urinary incontinence. A 1-year study of almost 6000 women aged 40 years and older

TABLE 19-1 Medications That Can Cause Urinary Incontinence

Medication Type	Examples	Mechanism of Action
Diuretics	Furosemide, bumetanide	Increased diuresis can cause urinary urgency, frequency, and polyuria
Anticholinergic agents	Antihistamines, antipsychotics, antidepressants, antispasmodics, anti-parkinsonian agents	Decreased bladder contractility and relaxed bladder muscle can cause urinary retention, frequency, and incontinence
Adrenergics (alpha-adrenergic agonists)	Decongestants	Decreased bladder contractility and increased sphincter tone can cause urinary retention, frequency, and incontinence
Alpha-adrenergic blockers	Prazosin, terazosin, doxazosin	Decreased urethral and internal sphincter tone can cause leakage and stress incontinence
Calcium channel blockers	Nifedipine, nicardipine, isradipine, felodipine, nimodipine	Decreased bladder contractility can cause urinary retention, frequency, nocturia, and incontinence
Angiotensin-converting enzyme inhibitors	Captopril, enalapril, lisinopril	Can cause chronic cough, which precipitates or exacerbates stress incontinence
Hypnotics and antianxiety agents	Benzodiazepines	Can interfere with voluntary control over urination by causing sedation, delirium, and cognitive impairments
Alcohol	Wine, beer, hard liquor	Can interfere with voluntary control over urination by causing sedation, delirium, increased diuresis, and cognitive impairments

found an association between increased risk for stress urinary incontinence and diets high in fat, particularly saturated fat and, to a lesser degree, monounsaturated fatty acids (Dallosso et al., 2004). This same study analyzed micronutrient intake and found that zinc and vitamin B_{12} were positively associated with onset of stress urinary incontinence. Dallosso and colleagues suggested that either an excess or a deficiency of zinc can contribute to stress urinary incontinence.

Environmental Factors

Environmental factors may impede or prevent older adults—especially those with mobility limitations—from reaching and using the toilet in home, public, and institutional settings. Examples of environmental obstacles include stairs, an absence of grab bars and railings, and toilet seats that are not the appropriate height. Box 19-1 summarizes some environmental risk factors that may contribute to the incidence of incontinence in older adults.

PATHOLOGIC CONDITION AFFECTING URINARY FUNCTION: URINARY INCONTINENCE

Although age-related changes alone do not cause urinary incontinence, they predispose older adults to it, making it the most commonly occurring pathologic condition associated with the urinary tract in older adults. Prevalence of incontinence in various groups of older adults is as follows (Anger et al., 2006; Jewart et al., 2005):

- 33% to 38% of older women
- 15% to 20% of older men
- 50% of all frail elderly persons
- 60% to 80% of nursing home residents

Box 19-1
Environmental Factors That Can Contribute to Urinary Incontinence

- Stairways between the bathroom level and the living or sleeping areas
- A distance to the bathroom that is more than 40 feet
- Living arrangements where several or many people share a bathroom
- Small bathrooms and narrow doors and halls that do not accommodate walkers or wheelchairs
- Chair designs and bed heights that hinder mobility
- Poor color contrast, as between a white toilet and seat and light-colored floor or walls
- Public settings with poorly visible or poorly color-contrasted signs designating gender-specific bathroom facilities
- Public settings with dim lighting and out-of-the-way bathroom facilities
- Very bright environments, where glare interferes with the perception of signs for bathrooms
- Mirrored walls, which reflect bright lights and create glare

Diversity Note

Prevalence rates for urinary incontinence in community-based women in the National Health and Nutrition Examination Survey for 2000 were as follows: non-Hispanic white, 41%; Mexican American, 36%; and non-Hispanic black, 20% (Anger et al., 2006).

Urinary incontinence is a focus of much attention among health care consumers and practitioners. Although the condition is physiologic, it has many psychosocial effects, and researchers and clinicians are identifying and addressing the impact of incontinence on quality of life (Abrams et al., 2002). The International Continence Society promotes the use of standardized terms related to urinary and pelvic floor function and dysfunction. Box 19-2 summarizes some definitions that are pertinent to nursing care of older adults. Full recommendations, which are periodically updated, are available at www.icsoffice.org.

Urinary incontinence is categorized according to the signs and symptoms. **Urge urinary incontinence** is characterized by involuntary urinary leakage due to the inability to hold urine long enough to reach a toilet after perceiving the urge to void. **Stress urinary incontinence** is characterized by an involuntary leakage of urine as a result of an activity that increases abdominal pressure (e.g., lifting, coughing, sneezing, laughing, or exercise). **Detrusor overactivity incontinence** is urinary leakage due to an involuntary detrusor contraction, and **urethral relaxation incontinence** is due to relaxation of the urethra that occurs concurrently with increased abdominal pressure or detrusor overactivity. **Mixed urinary incontinence** is characterized by leakage of urine with both the sensation of urgency and activities such as coughing, sneezing, or exertion.

In recent years, **overactive bladder** has become a common term for a syndrome characterized by bothersome urgency, usually accompanied by nocturia and daytime frequency, and sometimes accompanied by urge urinary incontinence (Gray, 2005). This term, which is equated with the **urge syndrome** or **urgency-frequency syndrome,** refers to a constellation of symptoms that are difficult to define and quantify (Sand & Dmochowski, 2002). When any type of urinary incontinence develops, a comprehensive assessment is warranted to identify causes and risk factors that can be addressed through interventions, as discussed later in this chapter.

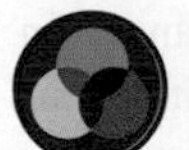

FUNCTIONAL CONSEQUENCES AFFECTING URINARY WELLNESS

Despite the many age-related changes in the urinary tract, the elimination of wastes is not significantly affected in healthy, nonmedicated, older adults. However, in the presence of any unusual physiologic demands, such as those that occur with medications or disease conditions, older adults are likely to experience functional consequences affecting

Box 19-2
Standardized Terminology for Lower Urinary Tract Function

Terms Related to the Control of Urination (Micturition)

Urinary incontinence—the complaint of any involuntary leakage of urine

Overactive bladder syndrome—a symptom syndrome characterized by bothersome urgency, usually accompanied by daytime voiding frequency and nocturia, and sometimes accompanied by urinary incontinence

Urgency—the complaint of a sudden compelling desire to pass urine, which is difficult to defer

Urge urinary incontinence—involuntary leakage accompanied by or immediately preceded by urgency

Stress urinary incontinence—involuntary leakage on effort or exertion, or on sneezing or coughing

Detrusor overactivity incontinence—leakage due to an involuntary detrusor contraction

Urethral relaxation incontinence—leakage due to urethral relaxation in the presence of raised abdominal pressure or detrusor overactivity

Mixed urinary incontinence—involuntary leakage associated with urgency and also with exertion, effort, sneezing, or coughing

Enuresis—any involuntary loss of urine

Continuous urinary incontinence—continuous leakage

Terms Related to Urinary Bladder Physiology and Function

Urinary bladder—the entire vesica urinaria organ

Detrusor—the smooth muscle structure that controls micturition

- *Normal detrusor function*—allows bladder filling with little or no change in pressure
- *Detrusor overactivity*—involuntary detrusor contractions during the filling phase
- *Detrusor underactivity*—a contraction of reduced strength or duration, resulting in prolonged bladder emptying or failure to achieve complete bladder emptying within a normal time span

Bladder sensation

- *Normal*—awareness of bladder filling and increasing sensation up to a strong urge to void
- *Increased*—sensation of an early and persistent desire to void
- *Reduced*—awareness of bladder filling but no sensation of a definite desire to void
- *Absent*—no sensation of bladder filling or desire to void
- *Nonspecific*—no specific bladder sensation, but perception of bladder filling as abdominal fullness, vegetative symptoms, or spasticity

Urinary flow pressures

- *Urethral*—fluid pressure needed to just open a closed urethra
- *Intravesical*—pressure within the bladder
- *Abdominal*—pressure surrounding the bladder

Postvoid residual (PVR)—the volume of urine left in the bladder at the end of micturition

Terms That Should No Longer Be Used

Dysuria
Detrusor instability
Reflex incontinence
Overflow incontinence

Adapted from Abrams, P., Cardozo, L., Fall, M., Griffiths, D., Rosier, P., Ulmsten U., et al. (2002). The standardisation of terminology of lower urinary tract function: Report from the Standardisation Sub-committee of the International Continence Society. *American Journal of Obstetrics and Gynecology, 187*, 116–126; and Sand, P. K., & Dmochowski, R. (2002). Analysis of the standardization of terminology of lower urinary tract dysfunction. *Neurourology and Urodynamics, 21*, 167–178.

homeostatic mechanisms and urinary control. Age-related changes and risk factors also cause functional consequences in patterns of urinary elimination and predispose older adults to incontinence. When incontinence occurs, additional functional consequences, especially psychosocial effects, can be quite serious.

Effects on Homeostasis

Age-related changes have only a limited effect on renal function in healthy older adults, but functional consequences include impaired absorption of calcium and a predisposition to hyponatremia and hyperkalemia. Age-related changes in the kidney and in aldosterone secretion interfere with compensatory mechanisms that maintain fluid and electrolyte balance, so older adults have a delayed and less effective response to variations in sodium intake. Similarly, diminished renal function lengthens the time needed for pH imbalances to be corrected in older adults. Even with normal states of hydration, a decrease in GFR delays water excretion and may lead to hyponatremia in healthy older adults. Likewise, even routine daily activities can challenge the renal function of older adults because of diminished renal efficiency. For example, when older adults perspire during exercise, they may tire easily because of age-related delays in the mechanisms controlling water and sodium conservation.

With increasing age, the kidneys become less responsive to ADH and are less able to concentrate urine, causing a decrease in the maximal urinary concentration. Age-related changes also cause a doubling of urine production at night in older adults compared with younger adults, even in the absence of pathologic factors (Miller, 2000).

Older adults who take medications or have medical conditions are likely to experience functional consequences such as the following:

- Diuretics are more likely to cause hypovolemia and dehydration in older adults than in younger people.
- Under conditions of physiologic stress (e.g., surgery, infection, or excessive fluid loss), older adults are likely to develop dehydration, volume depletion, and other fluid and electrolyte imbalances.

- Volume depletion may occur soon after the onset of fever-producing illnesses because of the inability to compensate for insensible fluid losses.
- Any condition or medication that stimulates ADH secretion, such as pneumonia or chlorpropamide, is likely to cause water intoxication and hyponatremia in older adults because of their diminished ability to compensate for excessive levels of ADH.

Diminished renal function contributes to the increased incidence of drug interactions and adverse medication reactions in older adults. These age-related changes are most likely to affect water-soluble medications that are highly dependent on GFR (e.g., digoxin, cimetidine, and aminoglycoside antibiotics) or renal tubular function (e.g., penicillin and procainamide). Unless medication doses are adjusted to account for age-related changes in GFR and renal tubular function, excretion may be delayed and toxic substances are likely to accumulate. As a rule, older adults require a 50% higher urine volume to excrete the same solute load as their younger counterparts. These adverse medication effects can significantly impair physical and mental abilities and have profound functional consequences, as discussed in Chapter 8.

Effects on Voiding Patterns

Because of age-related changes, the bladder of the older adult has a smaller capacity, empties incompletely, and contracts during filling. Thus, older adults experience shorter intervals between voiding, and they have less time between the perception of the urge to void and the actual need to empty the bladder. Older adults often describe this by saying, "When you gotta go, you gotta go." Another consequence is that the bladder retains up to 50 mL of residual urine after voiding, causing symptomatic or asymptomatic bacteriuria and predisposing older adults to urinary tract infections.

Age-related changes in the diurnal production of urine in the kidneys cause a shift in voiding pattern to more urinary output at night than during the day. By later adulthood, the average day and night urine volumes for older adults are 50 mL/hour and 70 mL/hour, respectively, compared with 75 mL/hour and 35 mL/hour in young adults (Miller, 2000). In addition, an overactive bladder and smaller bladder capacity contribute to nocturia in older adults. Functional consequences of nocturia include disrupted sleep and increased risk for nighttime falls (Johnson et al., 2005a).

Consequences of Urinary Incontinence

Urinary incontinence can negatively affect an older adult's quality of life through both physical and psychosocial consequences. Physical consequences of incontinence include a predisposition to falls, fractures, urosepsis, perineal rashes, pressure ulcers, and urinary tract infections (Resnick & Yalla, 2002). Consequences of limited fluid intake, a commonly used compensatory action, include increased risk of dehydration, bacteriuria, incontinence, constipation, adverse drug effects, and impaired homeostatic mechanisms. Additional serious psychosocial consequences associated with urinary incontinence include shame or embarrassment, anxiety, depression, social isolation, and loss of self-confidence. Another consequence is that people who have experienced episodes of incontinence may become preoccupied with covering up any evidence of wetness or urinary odors so they can avoid social stigma. Studies indicate that older adults are likely to conceal urinary incontinence because loss of control over bodily functions is strongly associated with the inability to live independently (Horrocks et al., 2004).

A Student's Perspective

One morning, I was caring for a client with a Foley catheter. While preparing her to go to breakfast, I noticed there was not a cover on her catheter bag and asked her if she had one. My client explained she once had a cover, but the nurses did not know where it went. I decided to do some searching, which only required my asking the laundry lady, and discovered several covers were stored in the linen closet. When I came back to her room with the cover, my client was so grateful. She said she had been asking for a long time if she could get another one, but the nurses and aides never cared to search for one. She explained that she doesn't like everyone to be able to see her catheter bag as she rides around the nursing home in her wheelchair. My finding the cover for her catheter bag was a very simple act requiring very little effort, but it showed me the importance of putting a little extra time into the client's care. Although this seemed like a miniscule problem to the nurses, it was a real concern to my client. I hope that as we continue in our nursing careers we remember to do these simple acts, because a seemingly insignificant thing to us can mean the world to a client.

Katrina D.

Psychosocial consequences also arise if caregivers have infantilizing attitudes and behaviors (e.g., unnecessarily using incontinence products rather than providing assistance with toileting) toward the older person who is incontinent. These attitudes and behaviors can have a devastating effect on the older adult's dignity and self-esteem. In addition, older adults who do not understand age-related changes may have exaggerated fears of progressive incontinence, triggered by the onset of urgency or frequency. Even in older adults who are not incontinent, the experience of urinary urgency and frequency can cause psychosocial consequences, such as anxiety, restricted activity, feelings of insecurity and powerlessness, and embarrassment about frequent trips to the bathroom.

For caregivers of dependent older adults in home settings, the onset of urinary incontinence may create additional stress, especially if urinary incontinence is compounded by environmental barriers or functional limitations. Caregivers report that tasks related to incontinence are some of the most difficult and stressful aspects of providing care. Langa and colleagues (2002) found that caregivers of community-living older adults spent an additional 1 hour daily for care specifically related to incontinence. Because urinary incontinence adds to the burden of caregiving stress, it is a major factor influencing the decision to seek institutional care for the dependent person, as indicated by studies that identify urinary incontinence as a major factor that precipitates nursing home placement for people with dementia (Jewart et al., 2005).

Caregivers in home settings are likely to feel angry, guilty, frustrated, or inadequate when dealing with incontinence on a daily basis. Lifelong attitudes about control over urination may contribute to feelings of disgust about the care demands, which may be further compounded by feelings of guilt about this initial reaction to caregiving tasks. If the caregiver perceives intentionality on the part of the dependent person in his or her failure to control urination, these feelings will likely be intensified. In institutional settings, nursing staff and other caregivers may experience these same feelings to a lesser degree.

Wellness Opportunity

Nurses address the person's relationships with others by being sensitive to the psychosocial responses of family caregivers who are dealing with incontinence.

Mr. and Mrs. U., who are 69 and 68 years old, respectively, attend the senior center where you provide monthly group health education sessions, weekly blood pressure checks, and one-on-one "Counseling for Wellness" sessions. During a recent health counseling session, Mrs. U. confided that she does not know what to do about her husband's "smelly dribbling" and that she worries that he has prostate problems. She has perceived a strong odor of urine and has noticed yellow stains on his clothing when she does the laundry. Even their children have mentioned the odor to her, but when she tries to discuss it with her husband, he changes the subject. She says that he will not talk with his doctor about it because he "hears so much about prostate cancer and he's afraid that he has an untreatable condition." She asks your advice about this and asks if you would talk with him when he comes to see you next week. Your next group health education session is entitled "Control of Urine: What's Normal With Aging?" and you plan to have separate group discussions for the men and women. Since Mr. and Mrs. U. usually attend these sessions, you see this as an opportunity to initiate health education about this sensitive topic.

THINKING POINTS

Decide what information you would include in the group session about each of the following topics:

- What can older men (women) expect of their urinary tract?
- What factors increase the risk of having problems with urinary control in older men (women)?

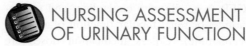

NURSING ASSESSMENT OF URINARY FUNCTION

Nurses can identify opportunities for health promotion interventions by assessing all of the following aspects of urinary function:

- Risk factors that influence overall urinary function
- Risk factors that increase the potential for incontinence
- Signs and symptoms of any dysfunction involving urinary elimination
- Fears and attitudes about urinary dysfunction
- Psychosocial consequences of incontinence

In long-term care settings, nurses also perform a comprehensive "bladder assessment" of all residents who have urinary incontinence or an indwelling catheter on admission, as well as residents who experience any changes in mental status, urinary function, or physical abilities (Newman et al., 2005). Nurses obtain most of this information by interviewing older adults and caregivers of dependent older adults. In addition, the nurse obtains objective data from laboratory tests and by observing behaviors, behavioral cues, and environmental influences.

Talking With Older Adults About Urinary Function

Because urinary elimination is associated with certain social expectations, discussion of this topic may especially be influenced by a person's attitudes and feelings. Although nurses usually learn to discuss urinary elimination with relative ease, older adults may feel uncomfortable with the topic, especially if there are gender or age differences between the older person and the nurse, or if a communication barrier, such as a hearing impairment, exists. In addition, older adults may be reluctant to discuss urinary problems because they tend to accept urinary leakage as an inevitable consequence of aging and gradually increase their tolerance threshold (Horrocks et al., 2004).

Terminology related to urinary elimination presents further difficulties in interviewing older adults. In social settings, people commonly use euphemisms to avoid directly discussing urination (e.g., "I'm going to the powder room,"

"I'm going to take a leak," "I have to use the john"). Even the sounds associated with urinary elimination may be viewed as embarrassing, so people may run the faucet or flush the toilet to disguise the sound of urination when others are present. Because of this social context, successful interviewing about urinary elimination and incontinence depends on identifying the terms that are least embarrassing and most understandable to the older adult. If any hearing impairment is present, a term such as "urinate," which is not used in everyday social language, or a one-syllable word like "pee" may be difficult to understand or may be misinterpreted. Although phrases like "use the toilet" and "go to the bathroom" are not specific to urinary elimination, they may prove to be acceptable, especially if additional questions are asked in order to distinguish between urinary and bowel elimination. Similarly, the term "incontinence" may be problematic for people who may not be familiar with this term. Hearing impairments, if present, may further interfere with comprehension of this word. Rather than referring to incontinence, it may be more acceptable to older adults to discuss "trouble holding their water." Older adults may tend to use phrases, such as "accidents," "leaking," "weak kidneys," or "bladder trouble," to describe incontinent episodes.

The nurse can set the stage for direct questions about urinary elimination by focusing initial questions on risk factors. Nurses can indirectly assess perception of and attitudes about urinary incontinence and its psychosocial consequences by observing responses to the interview questions. If the older adult acknowledges incontinence, asking about what actions the person has taken may help to identify fears and attitudes that contribute to psychosocial consequences or interfere with interventions. If depression and social withdrawal preceded the onset of incontinence, this can be a clue that the condition is affecting the person's self-esteem and usual activities. If older adults are willing to discuss their incontinence, the nurse asks direct questions about its impact on their daily activities and social life.

Wellness Opportunity

Nurses need to be cautious about using the term "diapers" because older adults may view this as an indicator of disrespect.

Identifying Opportunities for Health Promotion

Box 19-3 summarizes interview questions related to urinary elimination. If information is already available from other parts of an assessment (e.g., medication use and medical history), the nurse incorporates it into the assessment of urinary elimination rather than repeating questions. Nurses supplement their assessment interview by obtaining information about the person's patterns of urinary elimination and by assessing environmental factors that may interfere with control over urinary elimination.

A bladder diary—also called a bladder record, incontinence chart, or voiding or urinary diary—is one method of obtaining information about patterns of urinary elimination (Fig. 19-1). This widely recommended assessment tool is used to document information about pad usage, fluid intake, the degree of urgency, the times and volumes of urinations, and times and degree of incontinence episodes (Dowling-Castronovo, 2001; Locher et al., 2002). Although the length of time for keeping a bladder diary varies between 3 and 14 days, a 1-week period of data collection provides stable and reliable assessment information (Locher et al., 2002). Nurses use information from the bladder diary to identify potential causes of and interventions for incontinence, particularly with regard to identifying opportunities for health education.

Wellness Opportunity

Nurses promote self-care by encouraging older adults to assess their patterns of urinary elimination in relation to factors such as food and fluid intake.

Older adults who are cognitively impaired or dependent on others for their care may not be able to keep a bladder diary. In these situations, or when incontinence is an unacknowledged problem, observations about patterns of urinary elimination are particularly important. In long-term care facilities and other institutional settings, nurses have many opportunities to observe behavioral cues to incontinence. In home settings, caregivers of dependent older adults may observe behavioral cues and provide valuable information about urinary elimination patterns. Box 19-4 summarizes specific observations that may yield important assessment information.

Home environments are assessed for barriers that might interfere with the quick performance of urinary elimination (refer to Box 19-1). Stairways, long hallways, poor lighting, and cluttered surroundings can lengthen the time needed to get to the toilet, especially for people who have any functional impairment or use assistive devices, such as a walker. Also, it is important to assess the environment for the presence of safety and assistive devices or their potential benefit to the individual. For instance, an elevated toilet seat, grab bars near the toilet, and grab bars on the walls leading to the toilet may improve the person's ability to urinate safely. See Box 19-4 for specific environmental factors that can influence socially appropriate urinary elimination.

Using Laboratory Information

Data from urinalysis and blood chemistry tests contribute important information to the assessment of urinary elimination. A midstream or second-void specimen is the best type

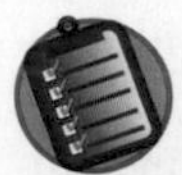

Box 19-3
Guidelines for Assessing Urinary Elimination

Interview Questions to Assess Risk Factors Influencing Urinary Elimination

- *(Men)* Have you had any surgery for prostate or bladder problems?
- *(Men)* Have you ever been told you had prostate problems? (or, Do you think you have prostate problems?)
- *(Women)* Have you had any children? (If yes, ask about the number of pregnancies and any problems with childbirth.)
- *(Women)* Have you had any surgery for pelvic, bladder, or uterine disorders?
- *(Women)* Have you had any infections in your vaginal area?
- Do you have any pain, burning, or discomfort when you urinate (pass water)?
- Have you had any urinary tract infections?
- Do you have any chronic illnesses?
- What medications do you take?
- Do you have any problems with your bowels?
- How much water and other liquids do you drink during the day? (Ask for details about timing and the amount of alcoholic, carbonated, and caffeinated beverages consumed.)

Interview Questions to Assess Risk Factors for Socially Appropriate Urinary Elimination

- Do you have any trouble walking or any difficulty with balance?
- Do you have any trouble reading signs or finding restrooms when you're in public places?

Interview Questions to Assess Signs and Symptoms of Urinary Dysfunction

- Do you ever leak urine?
- Do you ever wear pads or protective garments to protect your clothing from wetness?
- Do you ever have difficulty holding your urine (water) long enough to get to the toilet? (or, How long can you hold your urine after you first feel the need to go to the bathroom?)
- Do you have trouble holding your urine (water) when you cough, laugh, or make sudden movements?
- Do you wake up at night because you have to go to the bathroom to urinate (pass water)? (If the response is affirmative, try to differentiate between this symptom and the habit of going to the bathroom after waking up for some other reason.)
- Immediately after urinating (passing your water), does it feel like you haven't emptied your bladder completely?
- Do you have to exert pressure during urination to feel like your bladder is being completely emptied?
- *(Men)* When you urinate (pass water), do you have any difficulty starting the stream or keeping the stream going?

Interview Questions if Incontinence Has Been Acknowledged

- When did your incontinence begin?
- What have you done to manage the problem? (Have you cut down on the amount of liquids you drink? Do you empty your bladder at frequent intervals as a precautionary measure?)
- Are there certain things that make the problem worse or better?
- Does it happen all the time, or just at certain times?
- Do you have any pain when you urinate (pass water)?
- *(Women)* Do you feel any pressure in your pelvic area?

Interview Questions to Assess Fears, Attitudes, and Psychosocial Consequences of Incontinence

- Have you ever sought help or talked to a primary care provider or other health care professional about this problem?
- Have you changed any of your activities because you need to stay near a toilet?
- Do you avoid going to certain places because of difficulty holding your urine (water)?

of sample for a urinalysis. At the age of 80 years, the normal upper limit for specific gravity is 1.024, and slight proteinuria is normal in older adults. Other than these two variations, the urinalysis results should be within the normal range for healthy older adults.

Blood chemistry values that may be helpful in assessing renal function include the following: electrolyte level, creatinine level, creatinine clearance, nonprotein nitrogen level, and blood urea nitrogen level. In older adults, the serum creatinine may not be an accurate indicator of the GFR, but a 24-hour urine collection for creatinine clearance may have greater value as an indicator of renal functioning. Renal function in older adults is best assessed according to the Cockcroft-Gault formula for predicting creatinine clearances from serum creatinine concentrations. This formula, which uses a person's age and weight to calculate creatinine clearance, is as follows (for men):

$$\text{Creatinine clearance} = \frac{(140 - \text{age}) \times \text{weight [kg]}}{72 \times \text{serum creatinine [mg/100 mL]}}$$

The same calculation applies to women, except that the resulting value must be multiplied by 0.85.

Recall that you are the nurse at the senior center attended by Mr. and Mrs. U. After your class ("Control of Urine: What's Normal With Aging?"), Mr. U. schedules an appointment for a Counseling for Wellness session. He tells you that he has a "little dribbling" problem but has ignored it because it did not bother him very much. He has not talked with any doctor about this because he thought it was "to be expected," but now that he attended your session, he thinks that maybe he should have the problem evaluated and wants further information from you. During other health counseling sessions with Mr. U., he has told you that he is taking medications for hypertension and Parkinson's disease.

THINKING POINTS

- What risk factors are likely to be contributing to Mr. U.'s problems with urinary control?

(case study continues on page 403)

Bladder Diary ("Uro-Log")

Complete one form for each day for four days before your appointment with a healthcare provider. In order to keep the most accurate diary possible, you'll want to keep it with you at all times and write down the events as they happen. Take the completed forms with you to your appointment.

Your Name: ____________

Date: ____________

Time	Fluids		Foods		Did you urinate?		ACCIDENTS			
							Leakage	Did you feel an urge to urinate?		What were you doing at the time?
	What kind?	How much?	What kind?	How much?	How many times?	How much? (sm, med, lg)	How much? (sm, med, lg)			Sneezing, exercising, etc.
Sample	Coffee	1 cup	Toast	1 slice	✓✓	med	sm	Yes	(No)	Running
6-7 a.m.								Yes	No	
7-8 a.m.								Yes	No	
8-9 a.m.								Yes	No	
9-10 a.m.								Yes	No	
10-11 a.m.								Yes	No	
11-12 noon								Yes	No	
12-1 p.m.								Yes	No	
1-2 p.m.								Yes	No	
2-3 p.m.								Yes	No	
3-4 p.m.								Yes	No	
4-5 p.m.								Yes	No	
5-6 p.m.								Yes	No	
6-7 p.m.								Yes	No	
7-8 p.m.								Yes	No	
8-9 p.m.								Yes	No	

Provided by the National Association For Continence; (800)BLADDER; www.nafc.org

FIGURE 19-1 Example of a bladder diary. (Courtesy of the National Association for Continence [NAFC]. Available at www.nafc.org/Uploads/OnlineUroLog.pdf.)

- Make a list of assessment questions that you would use with Mr. U. (Use applicable questions from Box 19-3 and any additional questions that might be appropriate.)
- What observations would you make as part of your assessment?
- What would you teach Mr. U. about filling out the voiding diary (see Fig. 19-1)?

NURSING DIAGNOSIS

When the nursing assessment identifies any risk factors for incontinence or any complaints about or evidence of incontinence, an applicable nursing diagnosis would be Impaired Urinary Elimination, defined as the "state in which an individual experiences, or is at risk for experiencing, urinary elimination dysfunction" (Carpenito-Moyet, 2006, p. 503). Major defining characteristics commonly found in older adults include urgency, frequency, dribbling, nocturia, hesitancy, and incontinence.

When nurses identify negative functional consequences related to urinary problems, the following nursing diagnoses might be applicable: Anxiety, Social Isolation, Disturbed Body Image, Disturbed Sleep Pattern, Impaired Skin Integrity, or Caregiver Role Strain (or Risk for).

Wellness Opportunity

Nurses can use the wellness nursing diagnosis of Readiness for Enhanced Urinary Elimination for older adults who are interested in learning self-care practices, such as pelvic floor muscle training.

PLANNING FOR WELLNESS OUTCOMES

Nursing care plans are directed toward preventing, minimizing, or compensating for the negative functional consequences that affect urinary elimination. Specific outcomes

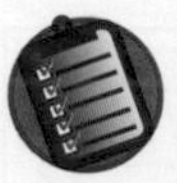

Box 19-4
Guidelines for Assessing Behavioral Cues to and Environmental Influences on Incontinence

Behavioral Cues

- Does the older adult use disposable or washable pads or products?
- Is there an odor of urine on clothing, floor coverings, or furniture (especially couches and stuffed chairs)?
- Has the older adult withdrawn from social activities, especially those held away from home?

Environmental Influences

- Where are the bathroom facilities located in relation to the older adult's usual daytime and nighttime activities?
- Does the person have to go up or down stairs to use the toilet at night or during the day?
- Are there any grab bars or other aids in, near, or on the way to the bathroom?
- Would the person benefit from using an elevated toilet seat?
- Does the person use a urinal or other aid to cut down on the number of trips to the bathroom?
- How many people share the same bathroom facilities?
- Is privacy ensured?

related to urinary elimination include Fluid Balance or Kidney Function (maintenance of homeostasis) and Risk Detection or Medication Response (prevention of adverse medication effects). Outcomes for older adults who have urinary incontinence include achieving continence and preventing negative consequences; initial outcomes focus on controlling and alleviating, rather than simply managing, incontinence.

The following Nursing Outcomes Classification (NOC) terminology is pertinent to older adults who experience urinary incontinence and related consequences: Urinary Continence, Urinary Elimination, Self-Care: Toileting, Depression Self-Control, Fear Level, Health Beliefs: Perceived Control, Immobility Consequences: Physiological, and Tissue Integrity: Skin.

In addition, any of the following NOCs may be pertinent to caregivers, especially family members, who are caring for someone with urinary incontinence: Caregiver Stressors, Caregiver Well-Being, Caregiver Performance: Direct Care, Caregiver Lifestyle Disruption, Caregiver Emotional Health, and Caregiver Endurance Potential.

Wellness Opportunity

Quality of Life is an outcome that can be achieved for older adults and their caregivers through nursing interventions that are effective in alleviating or managing urinary incontinence.

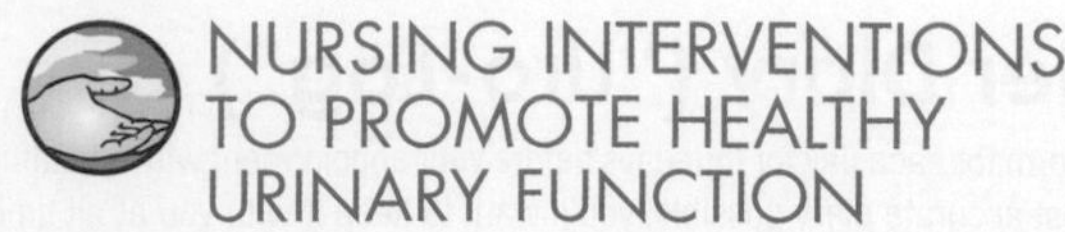

NURSING INTERVENTIONS TO PROMOTE HEALTHY URINARY FUNCTION

Nurses have numerous opportunities to promote wellness in relation to urinary function, particularly for older adults who have difficulty maintaining urinary control. For example, nurses can challenge myths about urinary incontinence, address attitudes of resignation, and teach self-care interventions. The following Nursing Interventions Classification (NIC) terminology is pertinent to promoting urinary continence and addressing the associated psychosocial consequences: Biofeedback, Emotional Support, Environmental Management, Exercise Promotion, Fluid Management, Health Education, Pelvic Muscle Exercise, Perineal Care, Prompted Voiding, Referral, Self-Esteem Enhancement, Teaching: Individual, Urinary Bladder Training, Urinary Elimination Management, and Urinary Habit Training.

Teaching About Urinary Wellness

Healthy older adults are not significantly affected by age-related kidney changes during normal activities; however, under conditions of physiologic stress, such as exercise, homeostasis can be affected unless the older adult initiates compensatory actions. Thus, nurses teach older adults about functional consequences affecting homeostasis and self-care actions to prevent problems. For example, nurses can explain that exercising in a cool (rather than hot) environment and increasing one's fluid intake before exercise may compensate for the age-related diminished ability to conserve water and sodium. Nurses also can suggest that older adults can take protective measures when they are in very hot and humid environments. Examples of appropriate protective measures are using fans and air conditioners; increasing fluid intake; and avoiding alcoholic, carbonated, and caffeinated beverages.

Older adults taking normal doses of water-soluble medications are likely to experience adverse medication effects because of diminished renal function. Therefore, when water-soluble medications are prescribed for older adults, dose adjustments should be based on an accurate assessment of kidney function and serum drug levels. Nurses need to be aware of and teach older adults about the increased potential for adverse medication effects, especially when the older adult is taking more than one medication. Further information about adverse medication effects and interventions for medication management is discussed in Chapter 8.

Perhaps the risk factor most amenable to nursing interventions is the false perception of incontinence as an inevitable effect of aging for which nothing can be done. Because this attitude is based on myths or a lack of information, it can be changed through education. Nurses can emphasize the need for a comprehensive evaluation of urinary incontinence so risk factors can be alleviated. For example, teaching older adults the rationale for maintaining adequate fluid intake as a means of preventing incontinence and maintaining good urinary function is a simple but important intervention. Older adults may be more willing to increase their fluid intake if they understand that concentrated urine due to fluid restriction can cause incontinence by stimulating bladder contractions. Nurses also can explain that because older adults often do not experience a sensation of thirst, even in the presence of dehydration, their intake of liquids may be inadequate if they drink fluids only when thirsty. Interventions to promote adequate fluid intake include identifying nonalcoholic, noncaffeinated, and noncarbonated beverages that the older adult will accept and consume readily, even in the absence of thirst sensation. Teaching about normal age-related changes, such as decreased sensation of thirst, can help to challenge ageist beliefs that negative functional consequences are inevitable.

When a risk factor contributes to incontinence or otherwise interferes with normal urinary elimination, interventions focus on optimal management of the precipitating factor. For example, if postmenopausal estrogen depletion leads to vaginitis and trigonitis, health education is directed toward encouraging the older woman to seek medical treatment for the underlying condition. When fecal impaction or chronic constipation are risk factors for urinary incontinence, interventions are aimed at attaining and maintaining good bowel function, as discussed in Chapter 18. Pelvic floor muscle training (PFMT), as discussed in the next section, is another health promotion intervention that can be performed by men and women who are at increased risk of developing, or already are experiencing, urinary incontinence.

Nurses also can teach about appropriate fluid intake as a factor that can significantly affect control over urination. As discussed in the section on risk factors, inadequate fluid intake can contribute to incontinence. Nurses can talk with older adults about drinking adequate amounts of noncaffeinated beverages at suitable intervals during the day. Also, nurses need to recognize that no studies have found that evening fluid restriction reduces nocturia, except for patients who clearly and intentionally drink large quantities before retiring to bed (Johnson et al., 2005b). Thus, it is imperative that nurses discuss fluid intake in relation to all aspects of urinary control and based on the needs and habits of each individual. Box 19-5 summarizes teaching points about self-care activities that promote optimal overall urinary function and help older adults maintain continence.

Wellness Opportunity

Nurses promote personal responsibility by encouraging older adults to talk with their primary care practitioner about identifying risk factors for urinary incontinence that can be addressed through self-care measures.

Promoting Continence and Alleviating Incontinence

If self-care interventions cannot alleviate urinary incontinence, a comprehensive evaluation must be done to determine the underlying cause of the incontinence. Nurses can facilitate referrals to specialty clinics, primary care practitioners, or a geriatric assessment program for an evaluation. Interventions also address contributing factors such as environmental conditions, resources and abilities of caregivers, functional and cognitive abilities of the older adult, and

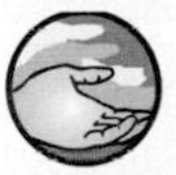

Box 19-5
Health Education to Promote Urinary Wellness

Health Promotion Activities for Good Urinary Function

- Drink 8 to 10 glasses of noncaffeinated liquid every day.
- Do not depend on thirst sensation as an accurate indicator for adequate fluid intake—drink liquids even if you do not feel thirsty.
- Avoid excessive use of alcoholic, caffeinated, or carbonated beverages, especially before bedtime.
- Avoid foods and beverages that can irritate the bladder (e.g., sugar, caffeine, alcohol, chocolate, artificial sweeteners, and spicy and acidic foods).
- Drink 1 or 2 glasses of fluid before, and every 15 minutes during, periods of sweat-producing exercise or activity.
- Avoid smoking.
- Maintain ideal body weight and good physical fitness.
- Take steps to prevent constipation (refer to Chapter 18, Box 18-4).
- Practice pelvic muscle exercises (refer to Box 19-6).

Correction of Myths About Incontinence

- Incontinence is not an inevitable age-related change.
- Normal age-related changes affecting urination include a shortened interval between the perception of the urge to void and the actual need to empty the bladder, an increased frequency of voiding, and the need to get up to urinate several times during the night.
- Nocturia, urgency, and frequency do not necessarily lead to total incontinence.
- If incontinence occurs, a pathologic condition or other influencing factor can usually be identified through a comprehensive evaluation.
- One of the requirements for voluntary control over urination is the signal of the need to void because of a full bladder. Restricting fluid intake interferes with this signal.
- Highly concentrated urine, from inadequate fluid intake, will stimulate involuntary bladder contractions and may lead to incontinence.
- Consistently emptying the bladder at intervals of less than 1 or 2 hours may contribute to problems with incontinence.
- Seek medical advice from a knowledgeable practitioner about any difficulties with urinary continence.

negative effects and social acceptability of the intervention. Evidence-based guidelines are available on evaluation and management of urinary incontinence, but the scope of the guidelines varies, with some focusing on a specific target group, clinical setting, or professional group (e.g., women, acute care, nurses). The National Guideline Clearinghouse provides an excellent and periodically updated comparison of the guidelines, available at www.guideline.gov.

The following types of interventions are used, often in combination, for control of incontinence: PFMT, biofeedback and stimulation devices, urinary control devices, continence training, environmental modifications, medications, and surgical and minimally invasive procedures. Health education provided by nurses is an important component of behavioral interventions (Borrie et al., 2002; Dougherty et al., 2002). If incontinence cannot be alleviated, aids and equipment can be used to minimize the functional consequences.

Pelvic Floor Muscle Training

When weakening of the pelvic floor musculature contributes to incontinence, exercises to strengthen these muscles can cure or improve incontinence. PFMT was first advocated in the late 1940s by A. H. Kegel, an American gynecologist, for postpartum therapy. Since then, many variations of these exercises have been promoted, both for control of incontinence and for enhancement of sexual pleasure. Other terms used interchangeably with PFMT include Kegels, Kegel exercises, pelvic muscle exercises, pelvic floor training, and pelvic muscle rehabilitation. This intervention is sometimes used in combination with biofeedback, behavioral training, or pelvic floor electrical stimulation for improved effectiveness. Studies support the effectiveness of PFMT, either alone or in combination with other interventions, for incontinent people, including those older than 75 years of age, who are motivated and cognitively intact (Perrin et al., 2005).

The goal of PFMT is improvement of urethral resistance through active exercise of the pubococcygeal muscle. There are no contraindications to or negative effects of these exercises, which can be initiated by any motivated person who is able to learn the technique. They are recommended for women with stress incontinence and for men and women as adjuncts to bladder training and other interventions for urge and mixed incontinence (Holroyd-Leduc et al., 2006; Schnelle & Smith, 2001). A very important aspect of teaching about PFMT is to help the person accurately identify the pubococcygeal muscle. Once the pubococcygeal muscle is identified, the person must practice contracting and relaxing this muscle, gradually increasing the ability to hold the contraction. It is important to emphasize that improvement is very gradual, and full effects are not noticed until 3 to 6 months of regular exercise have been completed. Even after full effects are achieved, daily maintenance exercises must be continued. Box 19-6 summarizes the points to cover when teaching adults to do these exercises.

In recent years, devices and equipment have become available as PFMT training aids, many of which are available without prescription. For example, weighted vaginal cones can be used gradually to improve the strength of contractions. A pelvic floor muscle exerciser, consisting of a vaginal

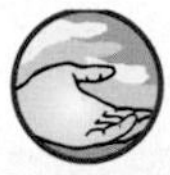

Box 19-6
Instructions for Performing Pelvic Muscle Exercises

Purpose: To prevent the involuntary loss of urine by strengthening the pelvic floor muscles

Frequency: Minimum of 60 times daily for at least 6 weeks; ideally working up to 150 contractions daily in several sessions of at least 15 exercises per session (e.g., 3 to 10 sets of 15 exercises, or 4 to 6 sets of 20 exercises), continued indefinitely

Position: Lying, sitting, or standing

Identifying the Pubococcygeal Muscle

- Identify the pubococcygeal muscle by contracting the muscle that stops the flow of urine. Do NOT do this regularly when urinating
- *(Women)* Lie down and insert a finger about three quarters of the way up your vagina. Squeeze the vaginal wall so you feel pressure on your finger and a sensation in your vagina.
- *(Men)* Stand in front of a mirror and try to make your penis move up and down without moving the rest of your body.
- Biofeedback, weighted vaginal cones, or a perineometer (a balloon-like device that is placed in the vagina) can be used to assist in identifying the pubococcygeal muscle and in measuring the strength of the contraction.

Method

- Tighten your pubococcygeal muscle and hold for a period of 3 seconds.
- Relax this muscle for an equal period.
- Repeat the contraction—relaxation cycle (one exercise) for your scheduled number of times.
- Breathe normally during these exercises and do NOT tighten other muscles at the same time. Be careful not to contract your legs, buttocks, or abdominal muscles while you are contracting your pubococcygeal muscle.
- Repeat this exercise daily in several sessions for a total of 60 to 150 exercises.
- For each of the daily sessions, vary your position (e.g., perform the exercise while lying down in the morning, standing in the afternoon, and sitting in the evening).
- Gradually increase the duration of each exercise up to a count of 10 for a contraction and 10 for a relaxation.

Additional information: The National Association for Continence, (800) 252-3337, has audiotapes and written materials available about pelvic muscle exercises.

probe connected to a hand-held indicator, can be used to monitor the strength of contractions. Referrals can be made to physical therapists for patient education about PFMT. Educational materials are available from the organizations listed in the Educational Resources section of this chapter.

Biofeedback and Stimulation Devices

Biofeedback and various methods of nerve stimulation are sometimes used as interventions for stress, urge, or mixed incontinence, either alone or in conjunction with other treatments such as PFMT or bladder training. Most nurses are not directly involved with administering these therapies, but they need to be familiar with the range of treatment options for incontinence so they can facilitate appropriate referrals. Nurses can emphasize that many effective and noninvasive therapies are available and they can encourage incontinent older adults to obtain information about these therapies from knowledgeable health care practitioners.

Biofeedback involves the use of monitoring devices to provide information about the physiologic activity involved in urination. Typically, a sensor is placed in the vagina of women, or in or around the anus of men, and connected to a computer that feeds back information about how the pelvic floor muscles are relaxing and contracting. The person uses this information to monitor the strength of muscle contractions to improve the effectiveness of PFMT.

Pelvic floor electrical stimulation, which can be done in office and home settings, uses an electrode to deliver small amounts of electrical stimulation to the nerves and muscles of the bladder and pelvic floor. This stimulation improves continence by increasing the sphincter tone and strengthening the levator and periurethral muscles. Devices that deliver pulsed magnetic fields to the pelvic floor muscles also are used as noninvasive methods of treating incontinence. Pulsed magnetic therapy is a passive treatment that does not depend on the person's ability to perform PFMT. Sacral nerve stimulation therapy is effective for urge incontinence and involves the surgical implantation of a neurostimulator under the abdominal skin. The neurostimulator, which is about the size of a stopwatch and can be adjusted nonsurgically, sends mild electrical pulses to the sacral nerves that control bladder function. This improves continence by inhibiting involuntary bladder contraction and promoting an increase in bladder volume.

Wellness Opportunity

Using biofeedback and other devices acknowledges the connection between the person's body and mind and may enhance self-care abilities.

Urinary Control Devices

A variety of intravaginal or intraurethral devices are available for resolving stress incontinence. Pessaries have been used for many decades to treat cystocele in women. These pelvic organ support devices are placed in the vagina to support the bladder, compress the urethra, or both. They are available in many sizes and shapes and are individually fitted by a primary care practitioner (Fig. 19-2). Pessaries need to be removed and reinserted at intervals ranging from nightly to once every few months, depending on the type that is used.

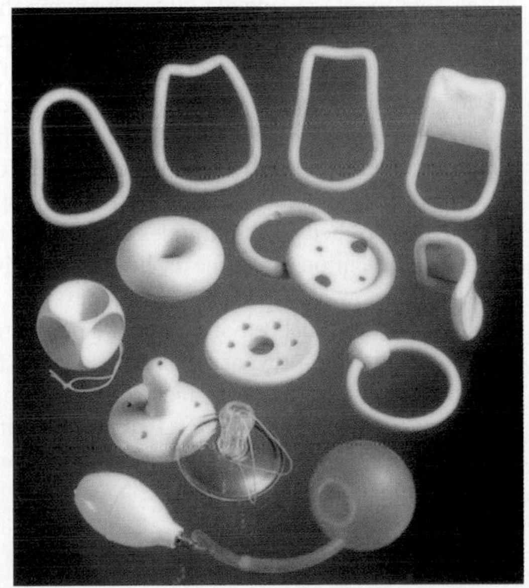

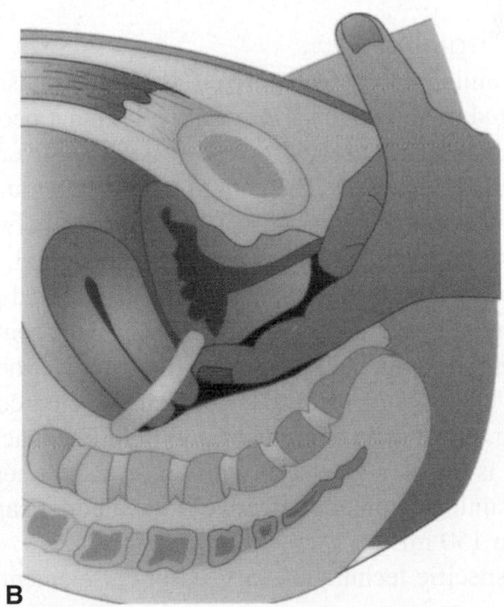

FIGURE 19-2 Examples of pessaries. (**A**) Various shapes and sizes of pessaries available. (**B**) Insertion of one type of pessary. (From Smeltzer, S. C., Bare, B. G., Hinkle, J. E., & Cheever, K. [2008]. *Brunner and Suddarth's textbook of medical-surgical nursing* [11th ed.]. Philadelphia: Lippincott Williams & Wilkins.)

In recent years, many urinary control devices have become available or are in clinical trials for self-insertion into the urethra. For example, one type of device controls urination through the inflation and deflation of a small balloon that rests at the bladder neck. Other currently available devices for women include urethral plugs; intraurethral catheters with unidirectional valves; and external occlusive devices, which cover the external urinary meatus and provide a watertight seal to prevent leakage. For men, foam-cushioned penile clamps with compression mechanisms are available. Because the options of urinary control devices for both men and women are rapidly evolving, nurses should encourage people with urinary incontinence to obtain current information from a qualified health care provider or from the National Association for Continence, listed in the Educational Resources section at the end of this chapter.

Indwelling catheters have been widely used for decades as a urinary control device for incontinence. However, in recent years, their use has been questioned because of the high rate of associated urinary tract infections and other complications. Their use in long-term care facilities has come under particular scrutiny, and the number of residents who have indwelling catheters is viewed as an indictor of quality of care in long-term care facilities (with lower numbers of indwelling catheters being associated with better quality of care). The only acceptable indications for the use of internal catheters, according to the Centers for Medicare and Medicaid Services (CMS), are stage III or IV pressure sores when urine impedes healing, urinary retention that cannot be treated medically or surgically, or terminal illnesses with which position changes are painful (Holroyd-Leduc et al., 2006). Intermittent clean catheterization is sometimes used as a self-care or caregiver-administered intervention for some types of incontinence.

Continence Training

Continence training can be categorized as (1) methods that are self-directed by motivated and cognitively intact people; or (2) methods that are directed by motivated caregivers of cognitively impaired people. The goal of continence training is to achieve a continent interval of 2 to 4 hours between voiding. These intervals will not necessarily be equal, and will usually be longer during the night. In self-directed programs, the person hopes to regain voluntary urinary control, whereas in caregiver-directed programs, the caregiver hopes to reduce the episodes of incontinence. Self-directed continence training, alone or in combination with biofeedback or medications, is most successful with urge incontinence. Continence training cannot be effective if the bladder capacity is less than 150 mL.

Although specific techniques vary, essential elements of any continence training program include motivation, an assessment of voiding patterns, an individualized and carefully timed intake of about 2000 mL of fluid per day, timed voiding in the most appropriate place, methods of reinforcing expected behaviors, and ongoing monitoring. During the initial assessment, diaries are used to record times and circumstances of toileting, as well as times of and reasons for any episode of incontinence. After the usual voiding pattern is identified, the older adult is encouraged to resist the sensation of urgency and to postpone voiding rather than responding immediately to an urge.

With caregiver-directed methods—often referred to as prompted voiding programs—the caregiver uses the initial assessment of voiding patterns to establish a schedule for assisting with voiding. The caregiver gradually increases the interval between voidings until the person can maintain continence for 2 to 4 hours. These methods are most successful when the timed intervals are flexible and are based on a good assessment of the person's needs and voiding patterns. For example, caregivers need to adjust schedules for diurnal variations and during the night. Prompted voiding has successfully decreased incontinent episodes by increasing self-initiated voiding in patients with dementia who recognize their name and objects (Holroyd-Leduc et al., 2006). Combining anticholinergics with prompted voiding may be helpful for individuals who do not respond to prompted voiding alone (Holroyd-Leduc et al., 2006). Caregiver-directed programs may include the use of electronic alarm devices or behavior modification techniques. These programs also incorporate social feedback (e.g., praising the person for behaviors such as staying dry between scheduled trips to the bathroom and self-initiating requests to toilet) (Lyons et al., 2000). Box 19-7 identifies some of the terms used for and the general principles of continence training programs.

Environmental Modifications

When incontinence is associated with the inability to reach an appropriate receptacle after perceiving the need to void, interventions are directed toward modifying the environment and improving functional abilities. If environmental adaptations cannot be made, as in public places, older adults are encouraged to become familiar with the location and arrangement of the bathroom facilities before the need to urinate is imminent. In home and institutional settings, the provision of bedside commodes and privacy can be an effective intervention. If space is limited or privacy cannot be assured, however, bedside commodes may not be acceptable. Box 19-8 lists environmental modifications that can be implemented to prevent incontinence when functional limitations are a contributing factor. Interventions discussed in chapters on vision (Chapter 17) and mobility (Chapter 22) can address functional limitations that can contribute to incontinence.

Wellness Opportunity

Nurses promote self-care by helping older adults identify ways of improving their functional abilities that can affect urinary control.

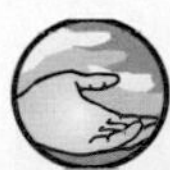

Box 19-7
Continence Training Programs

Goal of Programs: To achieve voluntary control over urination at intervals of 2 to 4 hours

Terminology

Terms used for self-directed programs: bladder drill, bladder training, bladder retraining, bladder exercise, bladder retention exercise

Terms used for caregiver-directed programs: scheduled toileting, routine toileting, prompted voiding, timed voiding, habit training

Method

Step 1: Identify the usual voiding pattern, noting the times of incontinence and information about fluid intake. During the first few days, keep a diary to record the following information at hourly intervals: dry or wet, amount voided, place of voiding, fluid intake, and sensation and awareness of need to void.

Step 2: Using information from the voiding diary, establish a schedule that allows for emptying of the bladder before incontinence is likely to occur.

Step 3: Provide the equipment and assistance necessary for optimal voiding at scheduled times.

Step 4: Provide 2000 mL of noncaffeinated liquids per day for liquid intake. Consume the largest amounts during the early part of the day, and limit fluid intake about 2 to 4 hours before bedtime.

Step 5: Gradually increase the length of time between voidings until the interval is 2 to 4 hours long.

Box 19-8
Environmental Modifications for Preventing Incontinence

Modifications to Enhance Visibility of Facilities

- Use contrasting colors for the toilet seat and surroundings.
- Provide adequate lighting in and near toilet areas, but avoid creating glare.
- Use nightlights in the pathway between the bedroom and bathroom.

Modifications to Improve the Ability to Use the Toilet in Time

- Encourage the use of chairs or beds that are designed to help the person arise unaided after sitting or lying.
- Install handrails in the hallway(s) leading to the bathroom.
- Make sure the pathway to the bathroom is safe and uncluttered.

Modifications to Improve the Ability to Use the Toilet

- Place grab bars at appropriate places to facilitate getting on and off the toilet and to assist men in maintaining their balance when standing at the toilet.
- Use elevated toilet seats or an over-the-toilet chair to compensate for any functional limitations of the lower extremities.
- If the person has functional limitations involving the upper extremities, clothing for the lower body should feature easy-open closures, such as Velcro or elastic waistbands.

Medications

Medications have varying degrees of success for treatment of incontinence, but their effectiveness depends greatly on identifying and addressing the specific type of incontinence. Medications also can effectively treat an underlying condition that contributes to incontinence (e.g., vaginitis and benign prostatic hyperplasia). If medications are prescribed, nurses are responsible for knowing their expected positive effects, as well as their potential adverse effects.

Medications that act on the autonomic nervous system are most often used for control of incontinence. Alpha-adrenergic agents control stress incontinence by increasing bladder outlet resistance through stimulating receptors at the trigone and internal sphincter. Alpha-adrenergic blocking agents, used either alone or in combination with cholinergic agents, can treat incontinence by decreasing bladder outlet resistance. Anticholinergic medications (e.g., antimuscarinic agents) can control the uninhibited or unstable bladder by blocking the transmission of nerve impulses, and cholinergic medications can prevent urinary retention by stimulating bladder contractions or increasing intravesical pressure. In recent years, geriatricians have expressed concern about adverse effects of antimuscarinic agents, which are used increasingly for treatment of overactive bladder. In particular, these medications are likely to cause cognitive dysfunction (including memory problems), especially in older adults who have dementia or mild cognitive impairment (Kay et al., 2005). Thus, nurses need to raise questions about a potential relationship between the onset or worsening of mental changes in anyone taking medications, such as oxybutynin or darifenacin, with antimuscarinic action. Table 19-2 summarizes the specific types and modes of actions for medications used in the treatment of incontinence.

Surgical and Minimally Invasive Procedures

Surgical procedures have been used for many decades to control incontinence when structural abnormalities, such as a cystocele, are identified as the underlying cause. For example, several types of bladder suspension surgery or "sling" procedures are used for stress incontinence. The goal of bladder suspension surgery is to reposition the urethra so that the pelvic floor muscles can squeeze it more effectively. When urinary incontinence is caused by loss of sphincter control, it may be treated successfully by surgical implantation of an artificial urinary sphincter, a device with an inflatable cuff that is placed around the urethra to hold it closed. To operate the artificial urinary sphincter, men squeeze a pump in the scrotum, whereas women press a valve in the labia to deflate the cuff, which automatically reinflates after

TABLE 19-2 Medications for Treating Urinary Incontinence

Type of Urinary Incontinence	Type of Medication	Examples
Urge incontinence and overactive bladder syndrome	Anticholinergic action to relax the bladder and inhibit uncontrolled contractions	oxybutynin (Ditropan) tolterodine (Detrol) darifenacin (Enablex) solifenacin (VESIcare) tricyclic antidepressants
Stress incontinence	Alpha-adrenergic stimulation to increase the strength of bladder muscle contractions	phenylpropanolamine (Entex LA) pseudoephedrine (Sudafed)
Incontinence and retention associated with prostatic hyperplasia	Antiadrenergic action to relax smooth muscle of the urethra and prostatic capsule	doxazosin (Cardura) terazosin (Hytrin) tamsulosin (Flomax) finasteride (Proscar) dutasteride (Avodart)
Urinary retention with incontinence	Cholinergic action stimulates bladder contractions	bethanechol (Urecholine)

voiding is completed. About 70% of men who have intrinsic sphincter deficiency after prostatectomy regain continence with this procedure (Resnick, 2002).

In recent years, several minimally invasive surgical procedures have been developed for the treatment of incontinence. For example, periurethral injections of a bulking agent (e.g., collagen) may be effective in treating stress incontinence in men and women with intrinsic sphincter deficiency; however, several injections may be required, especially in men. A recently developed treatment for stress incontinence in women is the tension-free vaginal tape system. This procedure involves the surgical insertion of a meshlike tape through the vagina to support the bladder neck and mid-section of the urethra. Minimally invasive surgical procedures for men, such as visual laser ablation and transurethral needle ablation, are being used to treat benign prostatic hyperplasia. In addition, a wire mesh stent can be placed in the man's urethra to maintain the flow of urine through an enlarged prostate.

Wellness Opportunity

Nurses promote self-care by encouraging older adults to seek further evaluation from qualified physicians, rather than relying solely on the reported experiences of friends.

Managing Incontinence

When incontinence cannot be alleviated, it can be managed with the use of various aids and equipment, including disposable and washable incontinence products; and collecting devices, such as urinals and commodes. When used in conjunction with environmental modifications to increase accessibility of toilet facilities, such equipment usually has beneficial effects; however, when aids and equipment are used by caregivers as substitutes for other methods of promoting continence, they are beneficial only to the caregiver and are detrimental to the older adult. For example, if protective products are used to manage incontinence, the positive effect for the caregiver may be the ease of care; however, the negative effects for the older adult include the likelihood of skin breakdown and decreased self-esteem. Because continence aids can be beneficial as well as detrimental, they should be used only after careful evaluation of all contributing factors.

When an older adult depends on a caregiver for assistance with urinary elimination, the nurse must consider the needs, limitations, and abilities of the caregiver when planning interventions. In institutional settings, staff is expected and trained to care for incontinent patients or residents using the most appropriate interventions. In home settings, the nurse must consider the total caregiving situation, and the needs of the caregiver may take precedence over the needs of the older adult, especially if the caregiver has functional limitations.

Numerous products are available for managing incontinence, and selection of a product depends on factors such as cost, convenience, and effectiveness. Economic considerations are particularly important because disposable incontinence products can be quite expensive, especially if used daily. Initial and periodic cost of reusable products also needs to be considered, as does the time and expense of laundering. Many types of products are designed specifically for either male or female incontinence. Products are also available according to degrees of absorbency, ranging from light to heavy protection. Absorbency of some disposable products is enhanced by the addition of gel or fiber materials. Often different products will be needed to address incontinence under particular circumstances. For example, a person may need a product with light protection during the day and heavy protection during the night. Ease of use is a major consideration, especially for people who are able to manage incontinence with little or no supervision. "Pull-ups" now provide a convenient alternative to the products with tabs that cannot be easily removed before and reapplied after toileting. Box 19-9 lists factors to be considered in selecting and using various types of aids and equipment for

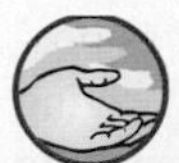

Box 19-9
Considerations Regarding Continence Aids and Equipment

Assessment Considerations

- What are the costs of various disposable and washable products, both initially and over a period of time? (Include the time and expense of laundry when considering costs of washable products.)
- What are the preferences of the incontinent person? (e.g., Is a "brief" or "pull-up" style garment more acceptable than a "diaper" style product? Also, how much noise a product makes when the person is walking or moving around in social settings may influence acceptability of a product.)
- What level of absorbency is appropriate for different circumstances?
- What are the needs and abilities of the caregivers of dependent older adults in home settings? (Can the caregiver manage the tasks involved in toileting?)
- What are the secondary benefits of various aids? (For example, in home settings, if the care of an individual with an indwelling catheter is covered by Medicare as skilled care, will additional services, such as home health aide assistance, also be covered?)
- What are the consequences if the incontinence cannot be managed in the home setting? (For example, will the older adult be institutionalized?)

Teaching Related to Aids and Equipment

- Many types of external collecting devices are available for men and women (e.g., male or female urinals, condom catheters, retracted penis pouches, and bedside urinals with attached drainage bags).
- An elevated toilet seat with rails can be used to increase safety and transfer mobility.
- Commodes are useful in diminishing the distance between the place of usual activities and toilet facilities.
- A variety of commodes are available and can be selected according to needs and preferences of the dependent person.
- If commodes are viewed as socially unacceptable, measures can be taken to ensure privacy and increase their social acceptability. Privacy can be ensured by placing an attractive screen around the commode.
- Commodes are now available that are attractively designed to resemble normal furniture items.
- A bedpan can be placed on a regular chair, especially in the bedroom, and removed when not in use.

managing urinary incontinence. Nurses can keep up to date on new developments in incontinence products by visiting the Internet sites listed in the Educational Resources section of this chapter.

Mr. and Mrs. U. are now 73 and 72 years old, respectively, and continue to attend the senior center where you are the nurse. Mr. U. has been under the care of a urologist for 3 years and has been taking terazosin for prostatic hyperplasia. Until recently, he had been able to maintain urinary continence, but lately his Parkinson's has worsened and 1 month ago he started taking furosemide 80 mg daily for congestive heart failure. He makes an appointment to ask your advice about incontinence products that would be best for him because "it's just hopeless to get to the toilet on time because our only bathroom is upstairs and I like to be downstairs during the day." He reports that he limits his fluid intake to 4 cups of liquid daily, which includes 2 cups of black coffee. Because of his Parkinson's disease, he has trouble standing at the toilet and usually sits down; however, he is "slow and clumsy" in managing his clothing. His son bought him some "jogging" outfits with elastic waists, but he does not wear them because he prefers to "dress up" when he goes to the senior center, so he wears trousers with belts.

THINKING POINTS WITH REGARD TO MR. U.

- What risk factors are likely to be contributing to Mr. U.'s incontinence, and which factors might be alleviated with interventions?
- What environmental modifications might be helpful in addressing the incontinence?
- What health education would you give about alleviating risk factors?
- What health education would you give about incontinence products?

Mrs. U. also makes an appointment to see you to discuss her recent problem with incontinence. She tells you that for several years she has been wearing "light-days pads" because "I have trouble holding my water whenever I sneeze or cough." In the past few months, she notices that she has to go to the bathroom every hour or two and is reluctant to be away from her house for more than an hour at a time. Her health has been good overall, but her arthritis has been getting worse and she is very slow in her mobility, especially when she needs to go up and down stairs. She drinks about 6 cups of liquid daily, consisting mostly of tea and coffee. She's heard some of her friends talking about "those Kegel exercises we

(case study continues on page 412)

had to do when we had our babies." One friend even talked about having some "cones she puts in to help her with exercises."

THINKING POINTS WITH REGARD TO MRS. U.

- What risk factors are likely to be contributing to Mrs. U.'s incontinence?
- What environmental modifications might be helpful in addressing the incontinence?
- What health education would you give about alleviating risk factors?
- What health education would you give about Kegel exercises?
- What health education would you give about incontinence products?

EVALUATING EFFECTIVENESS OF NURSING INTERVENTIONS

Nursing care for older adults with urinary incontinence is evaluated by measuring the extent to which the person is able to achieve periods of continence that are as long as possible. When older adults attribute incontinence to aging processes, nurses evaluate the effectiveness of their teaching by the degree to which the person verbalizes accurate information and understands the importance of identifying treatable causes. Another measure of the effectiveness of nursing interventions in such cases would be that the person seeks evaluation for his or her incontinence, rather than accepting this condition as inevitable.

If incontinence cannot be resolved, nursing care is directed toward managing urinary elimination in such a way as to maintain the dignity of the older adult and prevent negative consequences. In these situations, effectiveness of nursing interventions might be measured by the extent to which the person maintains their daily activities. For example, if older adults restrict their social activities because of incontinence, a measure of the success of nursing interventions might be that they begin using incontinence products to permit them to be away from their home for 4 hours at a time. For people with total incontinence, a measure of the effectiveness of nursing interventions would be the absence of skin irritation and breakdown.

Mrs. U., who is now 79 years old, is being transferred to a long-term care facility for rehabilitation after sustaining a hip fracture. An indwelling catheter was inserted before her hip surgery 7 days ago, and it was removed yesterday. She is ambulating with a walker but needs one-person assistance. The discharge summary describes her as incontinent of urine. Mrs. U. hopes to regain her independence in performing ADLs so that she can return to her own home, where she lives with her husband.

NURSING ASSESSMENT

During your functional assessment, Mrs. U. tells you she has had "trouble holding her water" since they removed the catheter yesterday. She is quite embarrassed about this and has not discussed it with any other health care practitioner. She says that she had too many other questions to discuss with her orthopedic surgeon, and states that the nurses kept a large absorbent pad on her bed so that she wouldn't have to walk to the bathroom. When she went to physical therapy, she used sanitary napkins, which her friend brought to her. She limited her fluid intake to a cup of coffee with each meal and a few sips of water with her pills.

Further assessment of Mrs. U's incontinence reveals that, for many years, she has had difficulty with "leaking," particularly when she coughs, sneezes, or exercises. Also, she gets up to urinate about four to five times nightly. It was during one of these trips to the bathroom that she tripped and fractured her hip. She says that she wakes up a lot during the night and goes to the bathroom because she's afraid of wetting the bed. She does not feel the need to urinate every time she wakes up, but goes to the bathroom to prevent any leakage. She limits her fluid intake to 6 glasses per day and does not drink anything after 5 PM. A few years ago, a nurse taught her how to do "Kegels and they helped for a couple years, but I don't bother to do them anymore." She tearfully confides that she thinks that the orthopedic surgeon damaged a nerve in her bladder, which she believes is the reason she has such little control over urination since the surgery. She thinks that the hospital staff inserted the catheter because she has "weak kidneys." She states, "Before I had this

(case study continues on page 413)

fractured hip, I just had the usual problems holding water like all my friends have but now it's really bad and I'll probably never be able to hold my water again. I wish you'd just put that tube back in me so I can go home again and not worry about accidents."

NURSING DIAGNOSIS

In addition to the nursing diagnoses related to Mrs. U.'s impaired mobility, you address her problem with urinary incontinence. In deciding which type of urinary incontinence to include in your nursing diagnosis, you conclude that both Stress Incontinence and Functional Incontinence are appropriate because of the combination of long-term and recent factors that contribute to her incontinence. Your nursing diagnosis is Stress/Functional Incontinence related to limited mobility, recent indwelling catheter, and insufficient knowledge of normal urinary function and pelvic muscle exercises. Evidence for this diagnosis can be found in Mrs. U.'s statements reflecting misconceptions and lack of information and in her description of current and past problems with incontinence. Evidence also is derived from your observations that she needs one-person assistance for walking and that she uses sanitary napkins and bedpads for urinary incontinence.

NURSING CARE PLAN FOR MRS. U.

Expected Outcome	Nursing Interventions	Nursing Evaluation
Mrs. U.'s knowledge of normal urinary function will increase.	• Discuss normal urinary function, using a balloon partially filled with water and a simple illustration of the female urinary tract. • Emphasize the relationship between adequate fluid intake and continence.	• Mrs. U. will be able to describe normal urinary function and the mechanisms involved in maintaining continence.
Mrs. U.'s knowledge about causative factors for incontinence will increase.	• Describe age-related changes that contribute to incontinence, using the information in Box 19-5. • Discuss the effects of frequent bladder emptying and limited fluid intake on the maintenance of continence. • Discuss the relationship between limited mobility and urinary incontinence.	• Mrs. U. will describe age-related changes that influence urinary elimination. • Mrs. U. will identify risk factors that contribute to her incontinence.
Mrs. U.'s misconceptions about her urinary incontinence will be corrected.	• Emphasize that as Mrs. U. regains her mobility, she will regain continence. • Emphasize that urinary incontinence is not an inevitable consequence of aging. • Explain that the orthopedic surgeon was not operating on or near her bladder or urinary tract. • Explain that the Foley catheter probably contributed to her current incontinence, but that this is a temporary situation that will resolve with proper interventions. • Emphasize that the nursing home staff will work with her to improve or alleviate her incontinence.	• Mrs. U. will state correct information about the relationship between her hip surgery and her incontinence. • Mrs. U. will express confidence in regaining urinary control.
The factors that contribute to Mrs. U.'s functional incontinence will be eliminated.	• Provide a bedside commode for Mrs. U.'s use until she is able to walk to the bathroom without assistance. • Work with the physical therapy staff to teach Mrs. U. a proper technique for independent transfer to the commode. • The nursing and dietary staff will provide 2000 mL of fluids/day, taking into consideration Mrs. U.'s preferences.	• Mrs. U. will be continent of urine, except for stress incontinence.

(case study continues on page 414)

Expected Outcome	Nursing Interventions	Nursing Evaluation
	• The nursing and dietary staff will work with Mrs. U. to schedule her fluid intake at acceptable times of the day, with minimal intake in the evening. • Talk with Mrs. U. about eliminating the bedpads as soon as she feels confident about maintaining continence.	
Mrs. U. will regain full control over urination.	• Suggest that Mrs. U. seek a comprehensive assessment of her urinary incontinence. • Give Mrs. U. a copy of Box 19-6 as a guide for performing PFMT. • Emphasize the need to perform PFMT on an ongoing basis for alleviation of stress incontinence. • Give Mrs. U. information about educational resources that might be helpful for her.	• Mrs. U. will report a reduction in or elimination of her stress incontinence.

THINKING POINTS

- What myths and misunderstandings affect Mrs. U's attitude about urinary incontinence?
- What risk factors are contributing to Mrs. U's urinary incontinence?
- What additional assessment information would you want to obtain?

Chapter Highlights

Age-Related Changes That Affect Urinary Wellness

- Kidney: diminished blood flow, decreased number of functioning nephrons, degenerative changes in tubules
- Urinary muscles: hypertrophy of bladder muscle, replacement of smooth muscle with connective tissue, relaxation of pelvic floor
- Neurologic control: degenerative changes in cerebral cortex
- Postural sway

Risk Factors That Affect Urinary Wellness

- Misperceptions and attitudes (e.g., resignation, viewing urinary incontinence as "normal," staff and caregiver attitudes that interfere with maintaining continence)
- Functional impairments that affect control over socially appropriate urinary elimination (dependency in ADLs)
- Conditions of the genitourinary tract (e.g., vaginitis, benign prostatic hyperplasia, urinary tract infections)
- Other pathologic conditions (e.g., dementia, Parkinson's, metabolic disturbances)
- Medication effects (Table 19-1)
- Dietary and lifestyle factors (e.g., obesity, tobacco smoking, intake of caffeinated beverages)
- Environmental factors (Box 19-1)

Pathologic Condition Affecting Urinary Function

- Urinary incontinence

Functional Consequences Affecting Urinary Wellness

- Effects on homeostasis: diminished ability to maintain electrolyte balance (especially sodium), changes in diurnal pattern of urine production (shift to increased nighttime output)
- Delayed excretion of water-soluble medications and increased risk of drug interactions and adverse effects
- Diminished bladder capacity; urinary urgency and frequency
- Decrease in interval between the signal of the need to void and the actual need to empty the bladder
- Chronic residual urine and consequent predisposition to bacteriuria
- Predisposition to urinary incontinence
- Diminished quality of life due to urinary incontinence
- Practical and psychosocial effects of urinary incontinence on the older adult and caregivers

Nursing Assessment of Urinary Function (Fig. 19-1, Boxes 19-2, 19-3, and 19-4)

- Talking with older adults about urinary function (finding appropriate terminology)
- Identifying usual voiding patterns and influencing factors (Fig. 19-1)
- Identifying risk factors for urinary incontinence
- Identifying risk factors that influence renal function and homeostasis
- Identifying symptoms of impaired urinary elimination
- Being alert to misunderstandings about urinary elimination
- Psychosocial consequences of incontinence (e.g., anxiety, depression, social isolation)

Nursing Diagnosis

- Readiness for Enhanced Urinary Elimination

- Impaired Urinary Elimination
- Social Isolation
- Caregiver Role Strain (or Risk for)

Planning for Wellness Outcomes
- Urinary Continence
- Urinary Elimination
- Health Beliefs: Perceived Control
- Caregiver Stressors
- Caregiver Endurance Potential

Nursing Interventions to Promote Healthy Urinary Function (Table 19-2, Boxes 19-5 through 19-9)
- Teaching older adults about age-related changes and preventing urinary incontinence
- Promoting continence and alleviating incontinence (pelvic floor muscle training, biofeedback and stimulation devices, urinary control devices, continence training, environmental modifications, medications, and surgical or minimally invasive procedures)
- Managing urinary incontinence

Evaluating Effectiveness of Nursing Interventions
- Longer intervals of continence
- Accurate understanding of normal urinary function and risks for incontinence
- Self-care practices to promote continence and urinary wellness
- Use of resources for further evaluation of incontinence when appropriate

Critical Thinking Exercises

1. Describe how each of the following age-related changes or risk factors might influence urinary function in older adults: medications, renal function, functional abilities, environmental conditions, altered thirst perception, changes in the urinary tract and nervous system, and myths and misunderstandings on the part of older adults, their caregivers, and health care professionals.
2. What are the psychosocial consequences of urinary incontinence for older adults and their caregivers?
3. Describe how you would address the following statement made by a 74-year-old woman: "Of course I have to wear pads all the time, just like when I was a teenager. I haven't talked to the doctor because I figured this was pretty normal at my age."
4. Describe the nursing assessment, with regard to urinary elimination, for a 75-year-old man and a 75-year old woman.

Clinical Tool Resources

Hartford Institute for Geriatric Nursing
Try This: Best Practices in Nursing Care to Older Adults
Issue Number 11 (March 2001), Urinary Incontinence Assessment
www.hartfordign.org/resources/education/tryThis.html

Educational Resources

The Canadian Continence Foundation
www.continence-fdn.ca

The American Geriatrics Society (AGS) Foundation for Health in Aging
www.healthinaging.org

International Continence Society
www.icsoffice.org

National Association for Continence (NAFC)
www.nafc.org

The Simon Foundation for Continence
www.simonfoundation.org

United States Department of Health and Human Services Agency for Healthcare Research and Quality, AHRQ Publications Clearinghouse
www.ahrq.gov

References

Abrams, P., Cardozo, L., Fall, M., Griffiths, D., Rosier, P., Ulmsten U., et al. (2002). The standardisation of terminology of lower urinary tract function: Report from the Standardisation Sub-committee of the International Continence Society. *American Journal of Obstetrics and Gynecology, 187*, 116–126.

Anger, J. T., Saigal, C. S., Litwin, M. S., & The Urologic Diseases of America Project. (2006). The prevalence of urinary incontinence among community dwelling adult women: Results from the National Health and Nutrition Examination Survey. *Journal of Urology, 175*, 601–604.

Borrie, M. J., Bawden, M., Speechly, M., & Kloseck, M. (2002). Interventions led by nurse continence advisers in the management of urinary incontinence: A randomized controlled trial. *Canadian Medical Association Journal, 166*, 1267–1273.

Bottomley, J. M. (2000). Complementary nutrition in treating urinary incontinence. *Topics in Geriatric Rehabilitation, 16*(1), 61–77.

Carpenito-Moyet, L. J. (2006). *Handbook of nursing diagnosis* (11th ed.). Philadelphia: Lippincott Williams & Wilkins.

Dallosso, H., Matthews, R., McGrother, C., Donaldson, M., & The Leicestershire MRC Incontinence Study Group. (2004). Diet as a risk factor for the development of stress urinary incontinence: A longitudinal study in women. *European Journal of Clinical Nutrition, 58*, 920–926.

Dougherty, M. C., Dwyer, J. W., Pendergrast, J. F., et al. (2002). A randomized trial of behavioral management for continence with older rural women. *Research in Nursing and Health, 25*, 3–13.

Dowling-Castronovo, A. (2001). Urinary incontinence assessment. *Journal of Gerontological Nursing, 27*(5), 5–8.

Gray, M. (2005). Overactive bladder: An overview. *Journal of Wound, Ostomy and Continence Nursing*, 32(3), S1–S5.

Holroyd-Leduc, J. M., Lynder, C. H., & Tannenbaum, C. (2006). Practical management of urinary incontinence. *Annals of Long-Term Care, 14*(2), 30–37.

Horrocks, S., Somerset, M., Stoddart, H., & Peters, T. (2004). What prevents older people from seeking treatment for urinary incontinence? A qualitative exploration of barriers to the use of community continence services. *Family Practice, 21*, 689–696.

Jewart, R. A., Green, J., Lu, C., Cellar, J., & Tune, L. E. (2005). Cognitive, behavioral, and physiological changes in Alzheimer disease patients as a function of incontinence medications. *American Journal of Geriatric Psychiatry, 13*, 324–328.

Johnson, T. M., Burgio, K. L., Redden, D. T., Wright, K. C., & Goode, P. S. (2005a). Effects of behavioral drug therapy on nocturia in older incontinent women. *Journal of the American Geriatrics Society, 53*, 846–850.

Johnson, T. M., Kincade, J. E., Bernard, S. L., Busby-Whitehead, J., & Defriese, G. H. (2000). Self-care used by older men and women to manage urinary incontinence: Results for the national follow-up survey on self-care and aging. *Journal of the American Geriatrics Society, 48*, 894–902.

Johnson, T. M., Sattin, R. W., Parmelee, P., Fultz, N. H., & Ouslander, J. G. (2005b). Evaluating potentially modifiable risk factors for prevalent and incident nocturia in older adults. *Journal of the American Geriatrics Society, 53*, 1011–1016.

Juthani-Mehta, M., Drickamer, M. A., Towle, V., Zhang, Y., Tinetti, M. E., & Quagliarello, V. J. (2005). Nursing home practitioner survey of diagnostic criteria for urinary tract infections. *Journal of the American Geriatrics Society, 53*, 1986–1990.

Kay, G. G., Abou-Donia, M. B., Messer, W. S., Murphy, D. G., Tsao, J. W., & Ouslander, J. G. (2005). Antimuscarinic drugs for overactive bladder and their potential effects on cognitive function in older patients. *Journal of the American Geriatrics Society, 53*, 2195–2201.

Langa, K. M., Fultz, N. H., Saint, S., Kabeto, M. U., & Herzog, R. (2002). Informal caregiving time and cost for urinary incontinence in older individuals in the United States. *Journal of the American Geriatrics Society, 50*, 733–737.

Locher, J. L., Burgio, K. L., Goode, P. S., Roth, D. L., & Rodriguez, E. (2002). Effects of age and causal attribution to aging on health related behaviors associated with urinary incontinence in older women. *The Gerontologist, 42*, 515–521.

Lyons, S. S., Specht, P., Mentes, J. C., & Titler, M. G. (2000). Prompted voiding protocol for individuals with urinary incontinence. *Journal of Gerontological Nursing, 12*(6), 5–13.

Masoro, E. J. (2006). Are age-associated diseases an integral part of aging? In E. J. Masoro & S. N. Austad (Eds.), *Handbook of the biology of aging* (6th ed., pp. 43–62). San Diego: Academic Press.

Mangnall, J., Taylor, P., Thomas, S., & Watterson, L. (2006). Continence problems in care homes: Auditing assessment and treatment. *Nursing Older People, 18*(2), 20–22.

Mather, K. F., & Bakas, T. (2002). Nursing assistants' perceptions of their ability to provide continence care. *Geriatric Nursing, 23*, 76–82.

Melville, J. L., Katon, W., Delaney, K., & Newton, K. (2005). Urinary incontinence in US women. *Archives of Internal Medicine, 165*, 537–542.

Miller, M. (2000). Nocturnal polyuria in older people: Pathophysiology and clinical implications. *Journal of the American Geriatrics Society, 48*, 1321–1329.

Newman, D., Gaines, T., & Snare, E. (2005). Innovation in bladder assessment: Uses of technology in extended care. *Journal of Gerontological Nursing, 12*, 33–41.

Ostbye, T., Hunskaar, S., & Sykes, E. (2002). Predictors and incidence of urinary incontinence in elderly Canadians with and without dementia. *Canadian Journal on Aging (La Revue Canadienne du Vieillissement), 2*(1), 95–102.

Palmer, M. H., Baumgarten, M., Langengerg, P., & Carson, J. L. (2002). Risk factors for hospital-acquired incontinence in elderly female hip fracture patients. *Journals of Gerontology: Series A, Biological Sciences and Medical Sciences, 57*, 672–678.

Palmer, M. H., & Newman, D. K. (2006). Bladder control: Educational needs of older adults. *Journal of Gerontological Nursing, 1*, 28–32.

Perrin, L., Dauphinee, S. W., Corcos, J., Hanley, J. A., & Kuchel, G. A. (2005). Pelvic floor muscle training with biofeedback and bladder training in elderly women. *Journal of Wound, Ostomy and Continence Care, 32*(3), 186–199.

Resnick, N. M., & Yalla, S. V. (2002). Geriatric incontinence and voiding dysfunction. In W. C. Walsh (Ed.), *Campbell's urology* (pp. 1218–1223). Philadelphia: W. B. Saunders.

Sand, P. K., & Dmochowski, R. (2002). Analysis of the standardization of terminology of lower urinary tract dysfunction. *Neurourology and Urodynamics, 21*, 167–178.

Schnelle, J. C., & Smith, R. L. (2001). Quality indicators for the management of urinary incontinence in vulnerable community-dwelling elders. *Annals of Internal Medicine, 135*, 752–758.

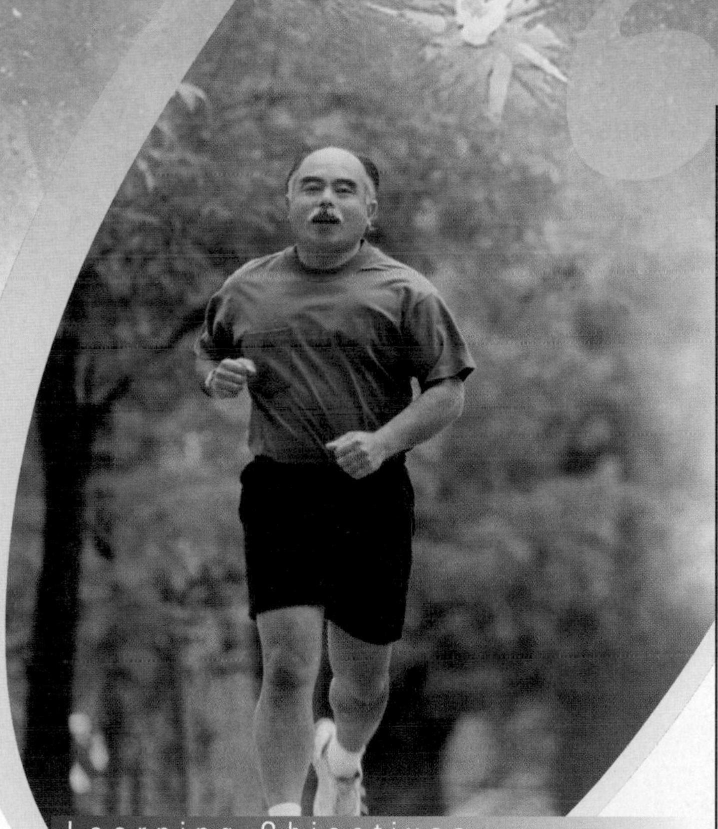

CHAPTER 20

Cardiovascular Function

Learning Objectives

After reading this chapter, you will be able to:

1. Describe age-related changes that affect cardiovascular function.
2. List risk factors for cardiovascular disease and orthostatic and postprandial hypotension.
3. Identify the functional consequences of age-related changes and risk factors that affect cardiovascular function.
4. Describe the assessment of cardiovascular function and risks for cardiovascular disease in older adults.
5. Identify interventions directed toward achieving optimal cardiovascular performance, reducing risk factors for cardiovascular disease, and preventing and managing hypertension, dyslipidemia, and orthostatic and postprandial hypotension in older adults.

Key Terms

adaptive response
atherosclerosis
baroreflex mechanisms
dyslipidemia
hypertension
orthostatic hypotension
physical deconditioning
postprandial hypotension
postural hypotension

A primary function of the cardiovascular system is to maintain homeostasis by circulating blood cells containing oxygen and nutrients to organs and tissues and by transporting carbon dioxide and other waste products for removal by other body systems. Like many other physiologic systems, the cardiovascular system has a tremendous adaptive capacity to compensate for age-related changes. Healthy older adults, therefore, will not notice any significant change in cardiovascular performance because of age-related changes. In the presence of risk factors, however, the cardiovascular system is less efficient in performing life-sustaining activities, and serious negative functional consequences can occur.

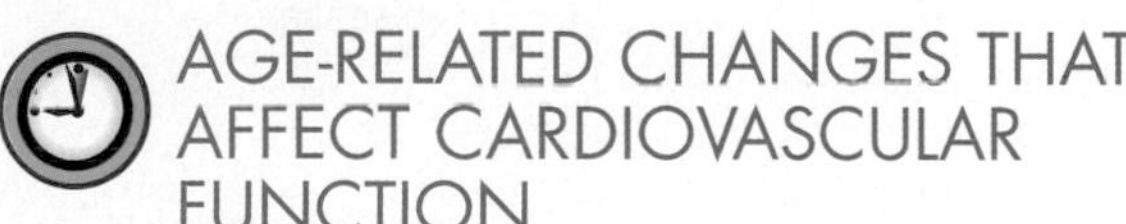

AGE-RELATED CHANGES THAT AFFECT CARDIOVASCULAR FUNCTION

As with many other aspects of physiologic function, it is difficult to determine whether changes in cardiovascular function are attributable to normal aging or pathologic processes. Knowledge about distinct age- or disease-related changes in cardiovascular function is confounded by the fact that, until recently, no medical technology existed to detect asymptomatic pathologic cardiovascular processes (e.g., occlusion of a major coronary artery). Thus, early studies provided more information about common cardiovascular changes that affect older people and less information about age-related changes. Currently, researchers focus on subjects who have been carefully screened for cardiovascular disease.

In addition to differentiating between age- and disease-related changes in cardiovascular function, researchers are trying to distinguish between changes that are age related

Promoting Cardiovascular Wellness in Older Adults

Nursing Assessment
• Usual heart rate, sounds, rhythm
• Blood pressure, including hypotension
• Risks for cardiovascular disease
• Signs and symptoms of cardiovascular disease
• Knowledge about cardiovascular disease
Age-Related Changes
• Myocardial degenerative changes
• Arterial stiffening
• ↑ peripheral resistance
• Altered baroreflex mechanisms
Negative Functional Consequences
• ↓ adaptive response to exercise
• ↑ susceptibility to hypertension, hypotension
• ↑ susceptibility to arrhythmias
• ↓ cerebral blood flow
Risk Factors
• Hypertension, hyperlipidemia
• Inactivity
• Obesity
• Dietary habits
• Tobacco smoking
• Stress, depression
• ↓ social supports
Nursing Interventions
• Teaching about diet, exercise, optimal weight
• If applicable, teaching about smoking cessation
• Teaching about hypertension and dyslipidemia
• Teaching about signs and symptoms of heart disease
Wellness Outcomes
• Improved cardiovascular function
• Prevention of cardiovascular disease
• Normal blood pressure and serum lipids
• Improved longevity and quality of life

and those that can be linked to risk factors. For example, perhaps more than any other aspect of physiologic function, lifestyle factors significantly influence cardiovascular performance. Smoking, dietary habits, some medical conditions, and physical exercise are all known to have long-term effects on cardiovascular function. It is particularly difficult to identify specific effects of lifestyle factors when entire societies are affected by these factors. Blood pressure, for example, has been found to increase gradually in adulthood in people who live in Western societies but not in people from less industrialized societies. Therefore, changes that are thought to be age related because they occur consistently in large population samples may be found to be related to lifestyle when cross-cultural studies are done. Lifestyle and environmental influences are important factors in explaining the wide range of variability in cardiovascular function among older adults, even for changes that are not disease-related.

Myocardium and Neuroconduction Mechanisms

Age-related changes of the myocardium include amyloid deposits, lipofuscin accumulation, basophilic degeneration, myocardial atrophy or hypertrophy, valvular thickening and stiffening, and increased amounts of connective tissue. Researchers currently are investigating the extent to which these changes are age related or disease related, but they agree that myocardial atrophy is disease related and that a slight, but not marked, increase in left ventricular wall thickness is the primary age-related change (Lakatta, 2000). In addition, the left atrium enlarges, even in healthy older adults. Other age-related changes include thickening of the atrial endocardium, thickening of the atrioventricular valves, and calcification of at least part of the mitral annulus of the aortic valve. These changes interfere with the ability of the heart to contract completely. With less effective contractility, more time is required to complete the cycle of diastolic filling and systolic emptying. In addition, the myocardium becomes increasingly irritable and less responsive to the impulses from the sympathetic nervous system.

Age-related changes in cardiac physiology are minimal, and the changes that do occur affect cardiac performance only under conditions of physiologic stress. Even under stressful conditions, the heart in healthy older adults is able to adapt, but the adaptive mechanisms may differ from those of younger adults or be slightly less efficient. The age-related changes that cause functional consequences primarily involve the electrophysiology of the heart (i.e., the neuroconduction system). Age-related changes in the neuroconduction system include a decrease in the number of pacemaker cells; increased irregularity in the shape of pacemaker cells; and increased deposits of fat, collagen, and elastic fibers around the sinoatrial node.

Vasculature

Age-related changes affect two of the three vascular layers, and functional consequences vary, depending on which layer is affected. For example, changes in the tunica intima, the innermost layer, have the most serious functional consequences in the development of atherosclerosis, whereas changes in the tunica media, the middle layer, are associated with hypertension. The outermost layer (the tunica externa) does not seem to be affected by age-related changes. This layer, composed of loosely meshed adipose and connective tissue, supports nerve fibers and the vasa vasorum, the blood supply for the tunica media.

The tunica intima consists of a single layer of endothelial cells on a thin layer of connective tissue. It controls the entry of lipids and other substances from the blood into the artery wall. Intact endothelial cells allow blood to flow freely without clotting; however, when the endothelial cells are damaged, they function in the clotting process. With increasing age, the tunica intima thickens because of fibrosis, cellular proliferation, and lipid and calcium accumulation. In addition, the endothelial cells become irregular in size and shape. These changes cause the arteries to become dilated and elongated and, as a result, the arterial walls are more vulnerable to atherosclerosis (discussed in the section on Pathologic Condition Affecting Cardiovascular Wellness).

The tunica media is composed of single or multiple layers of smooth muscle cells surrounded by elastin and collagen. The smooth muscle cells are involved in the tissue-forming functions of producing collagen, proteoglycans, and elastic fibers. Because it provides structural support, this layer controls arterial expansion and contraction. Age-related changes that affect the tunica media include an increase in collagen and a thinning and calcification of elastin fibers, resulting in stiffened blood vessels. These changes are particularly pronounced in the aorta, where the diameter of the lumen increases to compensate for the age-related arterial stiffening. Although these changes are viewed as age related, longitudinal and cross-cultural studies are beginning to raise questions about the impact of lifestyle variables on arterial stiffness.

Age-related changes in the tunica media cause increased peripheral resistance, impaired baroreceptor function, and diminished ability to increase blood flow to vital organs. Although these changes do not cause serious consequences in healthy older adults, they increase the resistance to blood flow from the heart so the left ventricle is forced to work harder. Moreover, the baroreceptors in the large arteries become less effective in controlling blood pressure, especially during postural changes. Overall, the increased vascular stiffness causes a slight increase in the systolic blood pressure.

Veins undergo changes similar to those affecting the arteries, but to a lesser degree. Veins become thicker, more dilated, and less elastic with increasing age. Valves of the large leg veins become less efficient in returning blood to the heart. Peripheral circulation is further influenced by an age-related reduction in muscle mass and a concurrent reduction in the demand for oxygen.

Baroreflex Mechanisms

Baroreflex mechanisms are physiologic processes that regulate blood pressure by increasing or decreasing the heart rate and peripheral vascular resistance to compensate for transient decreases or increases in arterial pressure. Age-related changes that alter baroreflex mechanisms include arterial stiffening and reduced cardiovascular responsiveness to adrenergic stimulation. These changes cause a blunting of the compensatory response to both hypertensive and hypotensive stimuli in older adults, so the heart rate does not increase or decrease as efficiently as in younger adults.

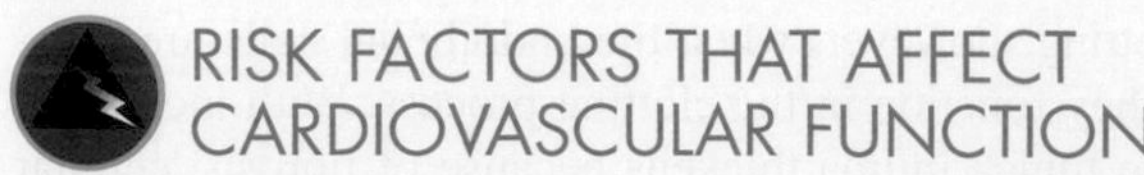

RISK FACTORS THAT AFFECT CARDIOVASCULAR FUNCTION

Physical Deconditioning

Physical deconditioning (i.e., lack of exercise) is a risk factor for diminished cardiovascular function, even in healthy older adults, because it "influences every known heart disease risk factor except family history" (Gibbons & Clark, 2001, p. 348). Gerontologists and exercise physiologists have suggested that physical deconditioning, rather than age-related changes, is the major causative factor for many of the cardiovascular changes that affect older adults (Lakatta, 2000). A particular focus of current research is to identify the extent to which physical deconditioning affects cardiovascular response to exercise. There is increasing and irrefutable evidence that physical conditioning can improve the aerobic capacity of older adults by increasing cardiac output and oxygen utilization (Lakatta, 2000). Thus, a sedentary lifestyle may be the major contributing, and potentially reversible, risk factor that affects the cardiovascular response to exercise in older adults. Factors that contribute to physical deconditioning include acute illness, a sedentary lifestyle, mobility limitations, cardiac disease or other diseases that interfere with physical activity, and psychosocial influences, such as depression or lack of motivation.

Risks for Cardiovascular Disease

Atherosclerosis and other cardiovascular diseases are associated with physical inactivity, race, sex, increased age, obesity, diabetes, heredity, socioeconomic and psychosocial factors, tobacco smoke, chemical and nutritional factors, hypertension, and dyslipidemia. In addition, subclinical conditions (i.e., those that are not symptomatic but can be identified by diagnostic tests) are a focus of recent studies as factors that increase the risk for coronary heart disease. For example, researchers are trying to identify clinical measurements (e.g., C-reactive protein, hypertension, diabetes mellitus) that are present in older adults whose risk of coronary heart disease could be reduced with pharmacologic measures (Kuller et al., 2006). Similarly, studies are focusing on whether treatment of subclinical hypothyroidism would reduce the risk for congestive heart failure among older adults (Rodondi et al., 2005).

Diversity Note

Prevalence of having two or more risk factors for cardiovascular disease is highest among blacks (48.7%) and Native Americans/Alaska Natives (46.7%) and lowest among Asians (25.9%) (American Heart Association, 2006).

Socioeconomic and Psychosocial Factors

Low socioeconomic status is widely recognized as a risk factor for cardiovascular disease. For example, being a college graduate and having a household income of $50,000 or more is associated with a prevalence of multiple risk factors that is about half the rate of people with less than a high school diploma and income of $10,000 or less (American Heart Association, 2006).

Psychosocial risk factors that studies have identified as being associated with an increased risk for cardiovascular disease include anxiety, depression, job strain, social isolation, poor social supports, high anger and hostility indices, stressful family relationships, and physical or emotional stress reaction (Arthur, 2006; Eaton & Anthony, 2002; Williams et al., 2002). For several decades, studies have shown an association between hostility and cardiovascular disease, with one review panel indicating that hostility is comparable with smoking as a risk factor (Bono & McCullough, 2004). Recent studies indicate that people who are high in hostility measures respond to social stressors (e.g., criticism) with higher blood pressures and increased triglycerides and low-density lipoprotein (LDL) cholesterol levels (Aldwin et al., 2006).

Wellness Opportunity

Nurses promote cardiovascular wellness by encouraging older adults to develop the habit of forgiveness, which is associated with lower levels of anger and hostility (Krause, 2006).

Tobacco Smoking

Tobacco smoking is a major avoidable cause of cardiovascular disease, and there is indisputable evidence that all forms of tobacco (smoking and smokeless or exposure to secondhand smoke) increase the risk for cardiovascular disease (Teo et al., 2006). Substantial evidence links nicotine to all the following cardiovascular effects in people who smoke (American Heart Association, 2006):

- Acceleration of atherosclerotic processes
- Increase in systolic blood pressure
- Increase in LDL cholesterol
- Decrease in high-density lipoprotein (HDL) cholesterol

Studies have also identified cardiovascular effects of exposure to secondhand smoke. Even brief exposure to secondhand smoke increases the risk of a heart attack because of immediate adverse effects on the heart, blood, and vascular systems (USDHHS, 2006). In addition, the risk of development of heart diseases is 25% to 30% greater in nonsmokers who are exposed to secondhand smoke at home or work (USDHHS, 2006). It should be emphasized that these cardiovascular effects are in addition to the effects of nicotine on respiratory function (see Chapter 21) and other aspects of health (e.g., increased risk for development of many cancers).

Chemical and Nutritional Factors

Researchers also are investigating the potential roles of antioxidants, alcohol intake, diet and nutrition, and nonsteroidal anti-inflammatory drugs (NSAIDs) as factors that can increase or decrease the risk for development of cardiovascular disease. For example, there is increasing attention to the role of nonaspirin NSAIDs because studies have found an increased risk of hypertension and other cardiovascular effects in people taking these agents. As a result of these studies, in 2005 the U.S. Food and Drug Administration requested that pharmaceutical companies include a warning box highlighting potential cardiovascular effects of all prescription and over-the-counter NSAIDs (National Clearinghouse Guidelines, 2005). In addition, researchers are investigating the role of dietary sodium and potassium in increasing or reducing the risk for stroke, hypertension, and other cardiovascular diseases (Aviv, 2001; Hajjar et al., 2001).

Hypertension

In the United States, about 60% of people between the ages of 65 and 75 years and 70% of those 75 years of age and older have hypertension (Aronow, 2002b). **Hypertension** is defined as blood pressure of 140/90 mm Hg or higher, or a blood pressure that requires treatment with an antihypertensive medication. Researchers have found that blood pressure even at the high end of normal (i.e., 130 to 139/85 to 89 mg Hg) is a risk factor for stroke, myocardial infarction, sudden cardiac death, coronary heart disease, heart failure, renal disease, and all-cause mortality (Deaton et al., 2004; Prospective Studies Collaboration, 2002; Vasan et al., 2001). Until recently, elevated diastolic blood pressure was considered a stronger risk factor for cardiovascular disease than elevated systolic blood pressure, and some questions were raised about the value of treating isolated systolic hypertension, especially in older adults. Recent studies, however, have confirmed the importance of both diastolic blood pressure and systolic blood pressure (Benetos et al., 2002; Mancia et al., 2002). Risk factors for hypertension include obesity, physical inactivity, and high-sodium diets. Older adults and African Americans may have a heightened salt sensitivity and therefore may be more likely than other groups to develop hypertension in response to sodium intake (Vollmer et al., 2001).

The Joint National Committee on Detection, Evaluation, and Treatment of High Blood Pressure (JNC) has published seven reports, most recently in 2003. Because each of these reports revised the classification of hypertension, a blood pressure measurement that was considered "normal" in 1980 could be deemed pathologic in the 1990s. Similarly, until recently parameters for judging the significance of elevated blood pressure were determined at least in part by age. For example, "100 plus your age" was the "normal upper range" for systolic blood pressure, so an 84-year-old person could have a systolic blood pressure of 184 and not be diagnosed as having hypertension. This perspective has gradually changed so the same standards for determining hypertension apply to adults of all ages.

The JNC recommends a classification of hypertension by stages to emphasize the risk of any degree of high blood pressure as a factor in cardiovascular disease (JNC, 2003). To clarify various terms, Table 20-1 defines some of the criteria used regarding blood pressure in older adults.

TABLE 20-1 Criteria for Normal Blood Pressure and Stages of Hypertension

Adult BP	Systolic (mm Hg)		Diastolic (mm Hg)
Normal	<120	and	<80
Prehypertension	120–139	or	80–89
Hypertension, Stage I	140–159	or	90–99
Hypertension, Stage II	≥160	or	≥100

(JNC. [2003]. The seventh report of the Joint National Committee on Prevention, Detection, Evaluation, and Treatment of High Blood Pressure. *Journal of the American Medical Association, 289,* 2560–2577.)

Diversity Note

Prevalence of hypertension increases with age and is greater in women than men and in African Americans than in whites or Mexican Americans (Laucka & Trotter, 2001).

Dyslipidemia

Dyslipidemia (i.e., abnormal serum lipoprotein levels) is a risk factor for cardiovascular disease when LDL cholesterol levels are high or HDL cholesterol levels are low. In contrast, high levels of HDL are considered protective against atherosclerosis and are associated with a lower risk for cardiovascular disease.

Public awareness of the importance of addressing dyslipidemia as a risk factor for cardiovascular disease has been gradually increasing since the early 1980s, when *saturated fat* and *polyunsaturated fat* became household words. By the late 1980s, mass screening programs for serum cholesterol levels were as popular as the mass blood pressure screenings of the 1970s. During the 1990s, there was much debate about the value of cholesterol screening for older adults and little consensus about treatment of dyslipidemia in older adults, particularly those older than 75 years. During the early 2000s, observational studies supported the value of identifying and treating dyslipidemia in older adults, even in nonagenarians (Aronow, 2002a). In 2001, the National Cholesterol Education Program published *Adult Treatment Panel (ATP) III*, which provides updated guidelines for identifying and treating dyslipidemia, with particular emphasis on people aged 50 years and older (Expert Panel, 2001). This report emphasizes the importance of considering all of the following risk factors in assessing the additional risk posed by dyslipidemia:

- Cardiovascular disease (e.g., angina, angioplasty, bypass surgery)
- Cerebrovascular conditions (e.g., ischemic stroke, transient ischemic attacks, symptomatic carotid artery stenosis)

- Peripheral vascular conditions
- Diabetes mellitus

The report categorizes three levels of risk and recommends acceptable lipoprotein ranges according to the person's number of risk factors. For example, treatment is recommended for people with cardiovascular disease if their LDL cholesterol is higher than 130 mg/dL, but is recommended for healthy people without any risk factors only if their LDL cholesterol is higher than 160 mg/dL (Expert Panel, 2001). The Expert Panel recommends that at least once every 5 years healthy older adults have their triglyceride, total cholesterol, HDL cholesterol, and LDL cholesterol levels checked. In contrast to previous reports that determined risk based partially on the ratio between LDL and HDL cholesterol, the updated report recognizes that HDL cholesterol should be maintained above 60 mg/dL and LDL cholesterol should be low regardless of any ratio (Eidelman et al., 2002).

Diversity Note

African Americans and Mexican Americans are less likely than whites to be screened for dyslipidemia (Nelson et al., 2002).

Gender-Specific Risks

Because cardiovascular disease has long been viewed as a disease of middle-aged men, early research focused primarily, or exclusively, on men. In the early 1990s, researchers began recognizing that the prevalence of cardiovascular disease in women increases dramatically after the age of 50 years and continued to increase until it surpasses that of men by the eighth decade. In early and middle adulthood, however, male sex is a risk factor because women tend to get cardiovascular disease about 10 years later than men with similar risk factor profiles (Keevil et al., 2002).

Several major research initiatives address questions about gender-specific risk factors for cardiovascular disease, with particular emphasis on estrogen as an influencing factor. Many of the longitudinal studies are ongoing and several of the studies address the influence of hormonal therapy for postmenopausal women. A review of research by Eaton and Anthony (2002) identified the following characteristics that contribute to the increased risk of cardiovascular disease in postmenopausal women:

- An atherogenic lipid profile (i.e., low HDL cholesterol, high LDL cholesterol, and elevated triglycerides)
- Increased abdominal fat
- Increased incidence of obesity
- Increased incidence of hypertension, including isolated systolic hypertension
- Increased incidence of diabetes and insulin resistance

Hormonal therapy for menopausal women has been the focus of many studies since the 1960s. Initial studies with mostly observational data suggested that hormonal therapy reduced the risk of cardiovascular disease in postmenopausal women, but many of these studies did not adjust for confounding variables such as socioeconomic status (Humphrey et al., 2002; Laine, 2002). More recent randomized trials have shown no benefit of hormonal therapy for either primary or secondary prevention of cardiovascular disease in older women, and there is some indication that hormonal therapy may actually increase the risk for ischemic stroke (Hsia et al., 2006; Lemaitre et al., 2006; Women's Health Initiative Investigators, 2002).

Diversity Note

In the United States alone, more than a half million women die of cardiovascular disease each year, exceeding the number of deaths in men and the next seven causes of death in women combined (Mosca et al., 2004).

Risks for Orthostatic and Postprandial Hypotension

The prevalence of both orthostatic and postprandial hypotension rises significantly after the age of 75 years, and it is usually due to a combination of age-related changes (e.g., decreased baroreflex sensitivity) and risk factors (Iwanczyk et al., 2006). Pathologic conditions and medications that affect the autonomic or central nervous systems increase the risk for orthostatic and postprandial hypotension (Box 20-1). For example, Parkinson's disease increases the risk for orthostatic hypotension through its effects on the nervous system and through the effects of medications (e.g., levodopa) used to treat this condition. Additional risk factors that can cause orthostatic hypotension include prolonged immobility, surgical sympathectomy, and the Valsalva maneuver during voiding.

PATHOLOGIC CONDITION AFFECTING CARDIOVASCULAR WELLNESS: ATHEROSCLEROSIS

Atherosclerosis is a disorder of the medium and small arteries in which patchy deposits of lipids and connective tissue (atherosclerotic plaques) reduce or obstruct blood flow. Several theories about the pathophysiology of atherosclerosis have been proposed since the first "reaction to injury" theory was proposed by Ross and Glomset (1976). Recent studies emphasize that the early stages of atherosclerosis are attributed to either abnormal cholesterol and saturated fat intake or abnormal lipid metabolism related to a genetic predisposition. Atherosclerosis develops because of the following processes (Tierney et al., 2005):

1. An accumulation of lipids and lipid-laden monocytes (macrophages) first appears as a "fatty streak" in the subendothelial layer of the artery.

Box 20-1
Risk Factors for Hypotension

Risks for Orthostatic Hypotension

Pathologic Processes

- Hypertension, including isolated systolic hypertension
- Parkinson's disease
- Cerebral infarct
- Diabetes
- Anemia
- Peripheral neuropathy
- Arrhythmias
- Volume depletion (e.g., dehydration)
- Electrolyte imbalances (e.g., hyponatremia, hypokalemia)

Medications

- Antihypertensives
- Anticholinergics
- Phenothiazines
- Antidepressants
- Levodopa
- Vasodilators
- Diuretics
- Alcohol

Risks for Postprandial Hypotension

Pathologic Processes

- Systolic hypertension
- Diabetes mellitus
- Parkinson's disease
- Multisystem atrophy

Medications

- Diuretics
- Antihypertensive medications ingested before meals

2. Macrophages migrate into the subendothelial space and take up lipids, giving the appearance of "foam" cells (i.e., plaque).
3. This process continues and smooth cells also migrate to the site; at this point the endothelial function is compromised and the ability to protect against further invasion of lipoproteins is limited.
4. If the plaque remains stable, a fibrous cap forms over the lesion, the lesion becomes calcified, the vessel wall remodels, and eventually the lumen becomes narrowed.
5. If the plaque does not remain stable, it progresses gradually or ruptures.
6. When the plaque ruptures through the vessel wall, a cascade of physiologic processes culminates in intravascular thrombosis.
7. The result is either partial or complete occlusion of the artery or a restabilization of the plaque, which can lead to more severe stenosis.
8. Damage to the myocardial cells by lack of oxygenated blood flow results in an elevation of troponin levels, which is an indicator of the degree of myocardial cellular damage.

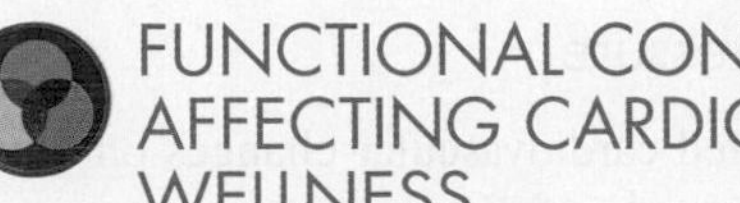

FUNCTIONAL CONSEQUENCES AFFECTING CARDIOVASCULAR WELLNESS

Older adults who have no pathologic conditions experience no significant cardiovascular effects in the resting state, but their cardiovascular performance is less efficient during exercise. In addition, they are likely to experience orthostatic or postprandial hypotension because of a combination of age-related changes and risk factors. However, older adults who have hypertension, atherosclerosis, or other pathologic cardiovascular conditions are likely to experience negative functional consequences.

Effects on Cardiac Function

Cardiac output, the amount of blood pumped by the heart per minute, is an important measure of cardiac performance because it represents the heart's ability to meet the oxygen requirements of the body. Although reduced cardiac output is common in older adults, it is associated primarily with pathologic, rather than age-related, conditions. With the exception of a slight decrease in cardiac output at rest in older women, healthy older adults do not experience any decline in cardiac output.

The heart rates of healthy older people decrease gradually, from an average intrinsic sinus rate of 104 beats/minute at the age of 20 years to 92 beats/minute between the ages of 45 and 55 years (Lakatta, 2000). Age-related changes in cardiac conduction mechanisms are likely to cause harmless ventricular and supraventricular arrhythmias, even in healthy older adults. Atrial fibrillation—a more serious arrhythmia—commonly occurs in older adults, but this is more likely to be caused by pathologic conditions (e.g., hypertension, coronary artery disease) than by age-related changes alone.

Effects on the Response to Exercise

A negative functional consequence that affects cardiovascular performance in healthy older adults is a blunted adaptive response to physical exercise. Physiologic stress, such as that associated with exercise, increases the demands on the cardiovascular system by four to five times the basal level. The **adaptive response** involves many aspects of physiologic function, including the respiratory, cardiovascular, musculoskeletal, and autonomic nervous systems. The maximum heart rate achieved during exercise is markedly decreased, and the peak exercise capacity and oxygen consumption decline in older adults; however, physical deconditioning and other risk factors account for some of this decline. Whereas a younger adult's heart rate speeds up to 180 to 200 beats per minute under stress (e.g., physical exercise), the heart rate of an 80-year-old person accelerates to only 135 to 150 beats per minute. Likewise, oxygen consumption during exercise diminishes by 50% between the ages of 20 and 80 years (Lakatta, 2000).

Effects on Blood Pressure

The effects of age-related cardiovascular changes on blood pressure can be summarized as follows:

- In men, diastolic blood pressure increases steadily at a rate of 1 mm Hg per decade without any plateau or decline.
- In women, diastolic blood pressure increases significantly between the ages of 40 and 60, then stabilizes, and may decline slightly after the age of 70 years.
- Systolic blood pressure gradually increases by 5 to 8 mm Hg per decade beginning around the age of 50 years in men and 40 years in women.
- Beginning around the age of 30 years, systolic blood pressure increases to a greater degree than diastolic blood pressure, so the pulse pressure gradually widens.
- In older adults, the increase in systolic blood pressure that occurs in response to aerobic exercise is sustained for a longer period of time than in younger adults.

Age-related changes predispose older adults to orthostatic hypotension and postprandial hypotension. These two distinct conditions are both associated with dysregulation of the autonomic nervous system and other risk factors; they tend to occur in older people who have hypertension, but do not necessarily occur together (O'Mara & Lyons, 2002; Vloet et al., 2005). Geriatricians are emphasizing the importance of assessing for and treating both conditions because they are associated with falls, syncope, and cerebrovascular damage (Fisher et al., 2005; Vloet & Jansen, 2005).

Orthostatic hypotension (also called **postural hypotension**) is defined as a reduction in systolic blood pressure and diastolic blood pressure of at least 20 mm Hg or 10 mm Hg, respectively, that occurs within 1 to 4 minutes of standing after being recumbent for at least 5 minutes. An additional criterion in some definitions is assessing blood pressure at two time periods of 1 and 3 minutes after standing (Irvin & White, 2004). Orthostatic hypotension occurs in about 10% to 15% of community-dwelling adults older than 65 years and in one third to one half of older adults in nursing homes (Iwanczyk et al., 2006; Mukai & Lipsitz, 2002). Orthostatic hypotension can occur in healthy older adults as a result of age-related changes, but, as noted earlier, is more likely to occur in older adults who have additional risk factors.

Although many people with orthostatic hypotension report no symptoms, studies have found the following signs and symptoms were most common: lightheadedness (88%), weakness or tiredness (72%), cognitive difficulties (47%), blurred vision (47%), tremulousness (38%), and pallor (31%) (Iwanczyk et al., 2006). Orthostatic hypotension might seem to be relatively harmless; however, it can affect the safety and quality of life of older adults and lead to serious negative functional consequences. Studies have found that it is associated with increased mortality and it is an independent risk for falling among older nursing home residents (Iwanczyk et al., 2006). Moreover, people with orthostatic hypotension are at increased risk for strokes, coronary events, and transient ischemic attacks (Weiss et al., 2002).

Postprandial hypotension, a blood pressure reduction of 20 mm Hg within 75 minutes of eating a meal (particularly breakfast), occurs in 20% to 40% of healthy older adults, 36% of nursing home residents, and 82% of older adults with parkinsonism (Mehagnoul-Schipper et al., 2001; O'Mara & Lyons, 2002; Puisieux et al., 2000). Physiologic changes that are likely to cause postprandial hypotension include impaired baroreflex mechanisms, quicker rate of gastric emptying, the release of vasoactive gastrointestinal hormones, and impaired autonomic regulation of gastrointestinal perfusion. Some studies indicate that postprandial hypotension is associated with the consumption of carbohydrates, particularly glucose, and is more likely to occur after a consumption of warmer foods that are high in carbohydrate content (Jansen, 2005; Maurer et al., 2000). Postprandial hypotension is now considered an important geriatric condition because it contributes to falls, syncope, hip fractures, myocardial infarction, stroke-related dizziness, and frailty and malnutrition (Morley, 2001; Puisieux et al., 2000). Geriatricians recommend that any older adult who falls, has syncope, or loses consciousness be evaluated for postprandial hypotension (O'Mara & Lyons, 2002).

Effects on Circulation

Functional consequences also can affect circulation to the brain and the lower extremities. For example, age-related changes in cardiovascular and baroreflex mechanisms can reduce cerebral blood flow to some extent in healthy older adults and to a greater extent in older adults who have diabetes, hypertension, dyslipidemia, and heart disease. In addition, increased tortuosity and dilation of the veins, along with decreased efficiency of the valves, lead to impaired venous return from the lower extremities. Consequently, the older adult may have stasis edema of the feet and ankles and an increased susceptibility to certain diseases or conditions, such as venous stasis ulcers.

Mr. C. is a 64-year-old African American who frequently comes to your Senior Wellness Clinic for a blood pressure check. He has been taking hydrochlorothiazide, 25 mg, and verapamil, 120 mg, every morning, and his blood pressures range between 126/80 mm Hg and 130/84 mm Hg. Mr. C. sees his primary care provider once a year and obtains additional health care through community resources, such as health fairs. Mr. C.'s 86-year-old mother recently died from a cerebrovascular accident, and his father died in his early fifties from a heart attack. Mr. C. has had hypertension since the age of 24 years, and both of his daughters have high blood pressure as well. Neither Mr. C. nor anyone in the household smokes tobacco. He gets very little exercise and weighs 210 pounds, about 30 pounds more than

(case study continues on page 425)

his ideal weight. He reports that he "gets winded easily" when walking up or down a flight of steps or when he has to walk "a long distance" (which he defines as the distance across the parking lot to the senior center). He attributes this to "getting old."

THINKING POINTS

- What age-related changes in cardiovascular function is Mr. C. likely to be experiencing?
- What risk factors are likely to be contributing to Mr. C.'s experience of "getting winded?"
- What risk factors does Mr. C. have for cardiovascular disease?
- What further information would you want to obtain for assessing his risk for cardiovascular disease?

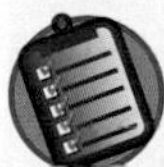

NURSING ASSESSMENT OF CARDIOVASCULAR FUNCTION

Identification of risks for cardiovascular disease is one of the most important aspects of the nursing assessment of cardiovascular function because many risks can be addressed through health promotion interventions. From a wellness perspective, it is especially important to assess the older adult's knowledge about risks for cardiovascular disease. Moreover, when older adults would benefit from improving their health-related behaviors (e.g., diet, exercise), nurses need to assess their readiness for changing behaviors, as discussed in Chapter 5. Assessment of physical aspects of cardiovascular function (e.g., heart rate, blood pressure) is similar in older and younger adults, but nurses also need to assess for hypotension. In addition, nurses need to consider that older adults are more likely than younger adults to have asymptomatic myocardial ischemia or atypical manifestations of a heart attack. Nurses can use the assessment guidelines reviewed in this text along with the usual methods of assessing cardiovascular function in any adult.

Wellness Opportunity

Nurses address body-mind-spirit interconnectedness by identifying stress-related factors that increase the risk for cardiovascular disease (refer to Chapters 12 and 13).

Assessing Baseline Cardiovascular Function

With the exception of a slightly lower range for heart rate for older adults, physical assessment indicators of cardiovascular function (e.g., peripheral pulses, heart rhythm and sounds) are the same for all healthy adults. Nurses must keep in mind, however, that older adults are more likely to have chronic conditions that affect cardiovascular function. The following findings are common in older adults, but in the absence of symptoms or other abnormal findings, they are usually not indicative of any serious pathologic process:

- Auscultation of a fourth heart sound
- Auscultation of short systolic ejection murmurs
- Difficulty percussing heart borders
- Diminished or distant-sounding heart sounds
- Electrocardiographic changes such as arrhythmias, left axis deviation, bundle branch blocks, ST-T wave changes, and prolongation of the P-R interval

If a murmur, arrhythmia, or any other unusual finding is detected, it is important to determine whether it reflects a new development, a preexisting but previously unidentified condition, or a preexisting condition that has already been evaluated. The nurse asks questions to determine the person's awareness of such abnormal findings. Any of the following terms might be used by older adults to describe arrhythmias: fluttering, palpitations, skipped beats, extra beats, or flip-flops. It is advisable to ask the older person about a history of arrhythmias before auscultation, because asking immediately after auscultation could cause undue concern. Arrhythmias may be caused by cardiac diseases, electrolyte imbalances, physiologic disturbances, or adverse medication effects; alternatively, they may be harmless manifestations of age-related changes. Likewise, murmurs may be caused by age- or disease-related conditions. Therefore, when murmurs or arrhythmias are detected, their significance is assessed in relation to the person's history, as well as in relation to the potential underlying causes. It is also important to find out the date of the person's last electrocardiogram because this may provide baseline information regarding the duration of asymptomatic or unrecognized changes.

Assessing Blood Pressure

Although only a few nurses have primary responsibility for medical management of blood pressure, all nurses are responsible for accurate assessment of blood pressure and for decisions regarding the implications of these findings. Thus, all nurses need to be familiar with the most current guidelines for detection of hypertension so that health promotion efforts can be directed toward interventions. Despite mounting medical evidence that the identification and management of hypertension has important health benefits for people of any age—including the "oldest old"—only about one fourth of community-living older adults with hypertension have adequately controlled blood pressure (Hajjar et al., 2002). Nurses are in a key position to detect hypertension, provide health education, and refer older adults for further medical evaluation and treatment.

Accurately assessing blood pressure in older adults may be more difficult than in younger adults for several reasons. First, blood pressure in older adults is more variable and has an increased tendency to fluctuate in response to postural changes and other factors. In addition, assessment of older adults commonly finds "pseudohypertension," which is the phenomenon of elevated systolic blood pressure readings that result from the inability of the external cuff to compress the arteries in older people with arteriosclerosis. This phenomenon explains the finding of extremely elevated systolic blood pressure readings in people without any evidence of end-organ damage and with normal diastolic blood pressure readings. Another assessment consideration is the common occurrence of "white coat hypertension" (also called "isolated office hypertension"), which is the phenomenon of blood pressure readings being high during office visits to a primary care practitioner but normal when self-assessed at home.

The practice of self-measurement of blood pressure, called *home blood pressure monitoring*, has become increasingly more accepted, and even encouraged, by primary care practitioners. Because older adults and people with hypertension are particularly susceptible to white coat hypertension, self-measurement of blood pressure in the home environment can provide additional assessment information that is important in management of hypertension. Self-monitoring also makes it easier to obtain an increased number of measurements, which is particularly important for older adults because they are likely to have fluctuating blood pressures. Moreover, patients who are being treated for hypertension can monitor their blood pressure before taking medications to assess effectiveness at the end of the dosing interval (Artinian, 2004).

Assessment of blood pressure in older adults is aimed at detecting not only hypertension but orthostatic or postprandial hypotension, because an older adult may have two or more of these conditions concomitantly. Box 20-2 summa-

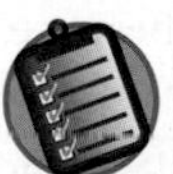

Box 20-2 Guidelines for Assessing Blood Pressure

For Accurate Blood Pressure Measurement in Older Adults

- Recognize that blood pressure readings are likely to vary, particularly in response to external factors (e.g., meals or postural changes).
- Blood pressure measurements may be lower in hot weather or at very warm indoor temperatures.
- Blood pressure measurements are likely to have a diurnal variation, with lowest levels during the night and highest levels after rising in the morning.
- The person should wait 1 hour after eating to have his or her blood pressure checked.
- The person should not have ingested caffeine or smoked a cigarette within $^1/_2$ hour before having his or her blood pressure checked.
- The person should be seated and resting for 5 minutes before having his or her blood pressure checked.

For Assessment of Orthostatic Hypotension

- Obtain initial blood pressure reading after the person has been in a sitting or lying position for at least 5 minutes.
- Obtain second blood pressure reading after the person has been standing for 1 to 3 minutes.

For Assessment of Postprandial Hypotension

- Obtain initial blood pressure reading before a meal.
- Obtain second and third reading at 15-minute intervals after the meal is completed.

Method of Assessing Blood Pressure

- The person should be seated with arm bared and feet flat on the floor.
- Support the person's arm as near to the heart level as possible.
- Ask the person to refrain from talking while you check his or her blood pressure.
- Use a sphygmomanometer that has been checked for accuracy.
- Use an appropriate-sized cuff (i.e., the length of the cuff bladder should be at least 80% of the circumference of the arm, and the width should be 20% wider than the diameter of the arm).
- Record the cuff size that is used. (Cuffs that are too small will yield falsely high readings, whereas cuffs that are too large will yield falsely low readings.)
- Fit the deflated cuff firmly around the upper arm, with the center of the cuff bladder over the brachial artery and the bottom of the cuff about 1 to 1$^1/_2$ inches above the bend of the arm.
- Inflate the cuff to 20 or 30 mm Hg above the palpated systolic blood pressure.
- Deflate the cuff at a rate of 2 to 3 mm Hg per second.
- Measure systolic blood pressure at the first sound and diastolic blood pressure at the onset of silence.
- If auscultatory gaps are heard, estimate the systolic blood pressure by applying the cuff, palpating the radial pulse, and inflating the cuff until the pulse is no longer felt.
- Record the magnitude and range of the gap (e.g., 184/82 mm Hg, auscultatory gap 176–148).
- If a very low diastolic blood pressure is heard, record the onset of Korotkoff phases IV and V (e.g., 138/72/10 mm Hg). Also, be sure not to press too hard on the stethoscope.
- Measure blood pressure in both arms the first time it is assessed, then measure it in the arm with the higher reading on subsequent determinations.
- If sounds are difficult to auscultate, support the person's arm above his or her head for 30 seconds. Then inflate the cuff, have the person lower the arm, and measure the blood pressure.
- If it is necessary to recheck the blood pressure in the same arm, deflate the cuff fully before reinflating it and wait at least 2 minutes before taking another measurement.

Normal Findings

- Normal blood pressure is less than 120 mm Hg systolic blood pressure, and less than 80 mm Hg diastolic blood pressure.
- The normal difference between lying/sitting and standing systolic blood pressure is 20 mm Hg or less after standing for 1 minute.
- The normal difference between lying/sitting and standing diastolic blood pressure is 10 mm Hg or less after standing for 1 minute.

rizes guidelines for accurate assessment of blood pressure in older adults, including the technique for assessing for orthostatic and postprandial hypotension.

Identifying Risks for Cardiovascular Disease

The assessment of risks for cardiovascular disease, with emphasis on identification of modifiable risk factors, provides a basis for health promotion interventions directed toward preventing negative functional consequences. Hypertension, dyslipidemia, and smoking cessation (discussed in Chapter 21) have been identified as the most important remediable factors for older adults who have these risks. Obesity, physical inactivity, and dietary habits are important lifestyle factors that can significantly affect the risk for development of cardiovascular disease. Figure 20-1 is an example of one of the many easy-to-use assessment tools that are available to identify risk factors. Nurses can use Box 20-3 as a guide for nursing assessment of risks.

Wellness Opportunity

Nurses promote personal responsibility and self-awareness by teaching older adults to use self-assessment tools (e.g., Fig. 20-1) to identify their risks for heart disease.

Assessing Signs and Symptoms of Heart Disease

Assessment of older adults for cardiac disease is complicated by the fact that the primary symptom often differs from the expected manifestations of cardiac disease. Congestive heart failure, for example, often begins very subtly, and the early manifestations may be mental changes secondary to the physiologic stress. Thus, older adults are likely to be in more advanced stages of heart failure before an accurate diagnosis is made. Likewise, older people with angina and acute myocardial infarctions are likely to have subtle and unusual manifestations, rather than the classic symptom of chest pain. Studies have found that between 25% and 68% of all myocardial infarctions are not clinically recognized as such, and the incidence of these unrecognized episodes is higher in women and older adults (Aronow, 2003; Sheifer et al., 2001). Compared with younger adults, older adults are more likely to have dyspnea or neurologic symptoms, rather than chest discomfort, as a primary sign of myocardial ischemia or acute myocardial infarction (Aronow, 2003; Williams et al., 2002). Canto and colleagues (2002) found that only 48% of people with unstable angina have typical manifestations, such as chest pain, and that factors associated with atypical manifestations included older age and a history of dementia. In this study, the predominant presenting atypical symptoms included nausea; shortness of breath; sharp, burning, or pleuritic chest discomfort; and pain or discomfort localized to an area of the upper body. Rather than complaining of chest pain, older adults are likely to have vague symptoms, such as fatigue, dyspnea, syncope, indigestion, and mental or behavioral changes. In addition, older adults who have mobility impairments or other functional limitations may not be active enough to experience exertion-related symptoms.

Diversity Note

Myocardial infarction is more likely to be unrecognized in African Americans (23%) than in whites (19%) (Boland et al., 2002).

Because manifestations of myocardial ischemia or other cardiac disturbances are often subtle or different from what is expected, patients as well as health care professionals may falsely attribute complaints to a noncardiac cause such as indigestion or arthritis in the shoulder. Therefore, nurses need to keep in mind that complaints about digestion, respiration, or pain or discomfort in the arms, shoulders, or upper trunk can be indicators of cardiac disease. Assessment of these complaints is complicated by the fact that older adults often have more than one underlying condition that could be responsible for these symptoms. It is not unusual, for example, for an older person to have an esophageal reflux disorder as well as a history of ischemic heart disease. Therefore, in addition to asking questions specifically related to cardiovascular function, the nurse must consider assessment information regarding other functional areas in relation to cardiovascular function. In addition, a baseline electrocardiogram is helpful in establishing the possibility of silent or atypical myocardial ischemia.

Assessing Knowledge About Heart Disease

In addition to assessing signs and symptoms, nurses need to assess the older adult's knowledge about manifestations of heart disease. This is particularly important because immediate medical attention is a major factor in determining outcomes of heart attacks and all people need to be aware of the warning signs so they can initiate appropriate help-seeking actions. Thus, nurses ask at least one question to determine the older adult's knowledge about the signs and symptoms of a heart attack. Nurses also can include a question about what the person would do and whom they would call if they thought they were experiencing a heart attack. Box 20-4 summarizes the guidelines for assessing cardiovascular function and detecting cardiovascular disease in older adults, emphasizes the assessment components that are unique to older adults, and refers to additional assessment components that apply to adults in general.

Diversity Note

Studies have found that women delay seeking treatment for symptoms of acute myocardial infarction longer than men (Rosenfeld et al., 2005).

What Is Your Risk of Developing Heart Disease or Having a Heart Attack?

In general, the higher your LDL level and the more risk factors you have (other than LDL), the greater your chances of developing heart disease or having a heart attack. Some people are at high risk for a heart attack because they already have heart disease. Other people are at high risk for developing heart disease because they have diabetes (which is a strong risk factor) or a combination of risk factors for heart disease. Follow these steps to find out your risk for developing heart disease.

Step 1 **Check the table below to see how many of the listed risk factors you have; these are the risk factors that affect your LDL goal.**

Major Risk Factors That Affect Your LDL Goal

- ❍ Cigarette smoking
- ❍ High blood pressure (140/90 mmHg or higher or on blood pressure medication)
- ❍ Low HDL cholesterol (less than 40 mg/dL)*
- ❍ Family history of early heart disease (heart disease in father or brother before age 55; heart disease in mother or sister before age 65)
- ❍ Age (men 45 years or older; women 55 years or older)

**If your HDL cholesterol is 60 mg/dL or higher, subtract 1 from your total count.*

Even though obesity and physical inactivity are not counted in this list, they are conditions that need to be corrected.

Step 2 **How many major risk factors do you have? If you have 2 or more risk factors in the table above, use the risk scoring tables on the opposite page (which include your cholesterol levels) to find your risk score. Risk score refers to the chance of having a heart attack in the next 10 years, given as a percentage.**

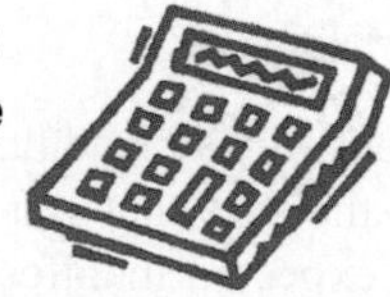

(Use the Framingham Point Scores on the opposite page.)

My 10-year risk score is _______%.

Step 3 **Use your medical history, number of risk factors, and risk score to find your risk of developing heart disease or having a heart attack in the table below.**

If You Have	You Are in Category
Heart disease, diabetes, or risk score more than 20%*	I. Highest Risk
2 or more risk factors and risk score 10-20%	II. Next Highest Risk
2 or more risk factors and risk score less than 10%	III. Moderate Risk
0 or 1 risk factor	IV. Low-to-Moderate Risk

**Means that more than 20 of 100 people in this category will have a heart attack within 10 years.*

My risk category is _______.

FIGURE 20-1 Example of an easy-to-use assessment tool for identifying risk factors for cardiovascular disease. An interactive tool for assessing risk factors is available at http://hp2010.nhlbihin.net/atpiii/calculator.asp. (From U.S. Department of Health and Human Services, Public Health Service, National Institutes of Health, National Heart, Lung, and Blood Institute. [May 2001]. *What is your risk of developing heart disease or having a heart attack?* NIH publication no. 01-3290. Rockville, MD: Author.)

Men

Estimate of 10-Year Risk for Men

(Framingham Point Scores)

Age	Points
20-34	-9
35-39	-4
40-44	0
45-49	3
50-54	6
55-59	8
60-64	10
65-69	11
70-74	12
75-79	13

Total Cholesterol	Points				
	Age 20-39	Age 40-49	Age 50-59	Age 60-69	Age 70-79
<160	0	0	0	0	0
160-199	4	3	2	1	0
200-239	7	5	3	1	0
240-279	9	6	4	2	1
≥280	11	8	5	3	1

	Points				
	Age 20-39	Age 40-49	Age 50-59	Age 60-69	Age 70-79
Nonsmoker	0	0	0	0	0
Smoker	8	5	3	1	1

HDL (mg/dL)	Points
≥60	-1
50-59	0
40-49	1
<40	2

Systolic BP (mmHg)	If Untreated	If Treated
<120	0	0
120-129	0	1
130-139	1	2
140-159	1	2
≥160	2	3

Point Total	10-Year Risk %
<0	< 1
0	1
1	1
2	1
3	1
4	1
5	2
6	2
7	3
8	4
9	5
10	6
11	8
12	10
13	12
14	16
15	20
16	25
≥17	≥ 30

10-Year risk _____%

Women

Estimate of 10-Year Risk for Women

(Framingham Point Scores)

Age	Points
20-34	-7
35-39	-3
40-44	0
45-49	3
50-54	6
55-59	8
60-64	10
65-69	12
70-74	14
75-79	16

Total Cholesterol	Points				
	Age 20-39	Age 40-49	Age 50-59	Age 60-69	Age 70-79
<160	0	0	0	0	0
160-199	4	3	2	1	1
200-239	8	6	4	2	1
240-279	11	8	5	3	2
≥280	13	10	7	4	2

	Points				
	Age 20-39	Age 40-49	Age 50-59	Age 60-69	Age 70-79
Nonsmoker	0	0	0	0	0
Smoker	9	7	4	2	1

HDL (mg/dL)	Points
≥60	-1
50-59	0
40-49	1
<40	2

Systolic BP (mmHg)	If Untreated	If Treated
<120	0	0
120-129	1	3
130-139	2	4
140-159	3	5
≥160	4	6

Point Total	10-Year Risk %
< 9	< 1
9	1
10	1
11	1
12	1
13	2
14	2
15	3
16	4
17	5
18	6
19	8
20	11
21	14
22	17
23	22
24	27
≥25	≥ 30

10-Year risk _____%

U.S. DEPARTMENT OF HEALTH AND HUMAN SERVICES
Public Health Service
National Institutes of Health
National Heart, Lung, and Blood Institute

NIH Publication No. 01-3290
May 2001

FIGURE 20-1 (continued)

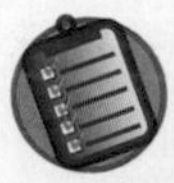

Box 20-3
Guidelines for Assessing Risks for Cardiovascular Disease in Older Adults

Questions to Identify Risk Factors for Cardiovascular Disease

- Do you have, or have you ever had, any heart or circulation problems (e.g., stroke, angina, heart attack, blood clots, or peripheral vascular disease)? *If yes, ask the usual questions about type of therapy, and so on.*
- When was the last time you had an electrocardiogram done?
- What is your normal blood pressure? Have you ever been told that you have high blood pressure, or borderline high blood pressure?
- Do you take, or have you ever taken, medications for heart problems or blood pressure? *If yes, ask the usual questions about type, dose, duration of therapy, and the like.*
- Do you smoke, or have you ever smoked? *If yes, ask additional questions, such as those appropriate for assessing respiratory function, Chapter 21.*
- Do you know what your cholesterol levels are? When was the last time you had your cholesterol checked?
- Do you have diabetes? When was the last time you had your blood sugar (glucose) level checked?
- What is your usual pattern of exercise?

Additional Considerations Regarding Risk Factors

- Compare the person's ideal weight to his or her present weight.
- Determine usual dietary habits, paying particular attention to the person's intake of sodium, fiber, and types of fat. (This information is usually obtained during the nutritional assessment.)

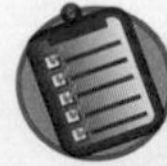

Box 20-4
Guidelines for Assessing Cardiovascular Function in Older Adults

Questions to Assess for the Presence of Cardiovascular Disease

- Do you ever have chest pain or tightness in your chest? *If yes, ask the usual questions to explore the type, onset, duration, and other characteristics.*
- Do you ever have difficulty breathing? *If yes, ask the usual questions regarding onset and other characteristics.*
- Do you ever feel lightheaded or dizzy? *If yes, ask about specific circumstances, medical evaluation, and methods of dealing with symptoms and ensuring safety.*
- Do you ever feel like your heart is racing, is irregular, or has extra or skipped beats? *If yes, ask about any prior medical evaluation.*
- Have you ever been told that you had a heart murmur? *If yes, ask about any prior medical evaluation.*

Information Obtained During Other Portions of an Assessment That May Be Useful in Assessing Cardiovascular Function

- Do you tire easily or feel that you need more rest than is ordinarily required?
- Do you have any problems with indigestion?
- Do your feet or ankles ever get swollen?
- Do you wake up at night because of difficulty breathing or because of any other discomfort? Have you made any adjustments in your sleeping habits because of difficulty breathing (e.g., do you use more than one pillow or sleep in a chair)?
- Do you have any pain in your upper back or shoulders?

Interview Questions to Assess for Postural Hypotension

- Do you ever feel lightheaded or dizzy, especially when you get up in the morning or after you've been lying down?
- *If yes:* Is this feeling accompanied by any additional symptoms, such as sweating, nausea, or confusion?
- *If yes:* Do any of the risks listed in Box 20-1 apply to you? *If yes, ask about any prior medical evaluation.*

NURSING DIAGNOSIS

If the nursing assessment identifies risks for impaired cardiovascular function in a healthy older adult, a nursing diagnosis of Ineffective Health Maintenance may be applicable. This diagnosis is defined as "the state in which an individual or group experiences or is at risk of experiencing a disruption in health because of an unhealthy lifestyle or lack of knowledge about managing a condition" (Carpenito-Moyet, 2006, p. 197). Related factors common in older adults include lack of regular exercise; cultural influences on patterns of food intake and preparation; and insufficient knowledge about low-sodium diets, dietary measures to control cholesterol levels, and the effects of tobacco use.

For older adults with impaired cardiovascular function, applicable nursing diagnoses may include Activity Intolerance, Decreased Cardiac Output, and Ineffective Tissue Perfusion (Cardiopulmonary). The nursing diagnosis of Risk for Injury may be appropriate for older adults with orthostatic or postprandial hypotension, particularly in the presence of additional risk factors for falls and fractures (e.g., osteoporosis, neurologic disorders, and medication side effects).

Wellness Opportunity

Nurses can use the wellness nursing diagnoses Readiness for Enhanced Nutrition or Readiness for Enhanced Knowledge for older adults who are interested in developing heart-healthy dietary habits or learning about health-promoting behaviors to prevent heart disease.

PLANNING FOR WELLNESS OUTCOMES

When older adults have risks for cardiovascular disease, nurses can apply any of the following Nursing Outcomes Classification (NOC) terminology to identify wellness outcomes in their care plans: Health Orientation, Health Promoting Behavior, Knowledge: Diet, Knowledge: Health

Behavior, Risk Control: Cardiovascular Health, Risk Control: Tobacco Use, and Weight Control. Wellness outcomes for older adults with cardiovascular disease include Cardiac Disease Self-Management, Circulation Status, Health Seeking Behavior, Knowledge: Cardiac Disease Management, Tissue Perfusion: Cardiac, and Tissue Perfusion: Peripheral. Additional outcomes include maintaining blood pressure within the normal range and preventing negative consequences of orthostatic or postprandial hypotension (e.g., falls and fractures).

Wellness Opportunity

Nurses address body-mind-spirit interconnectedness by including Stress Level as an outcome directed toward reducing the risk for cardiovascular disease.

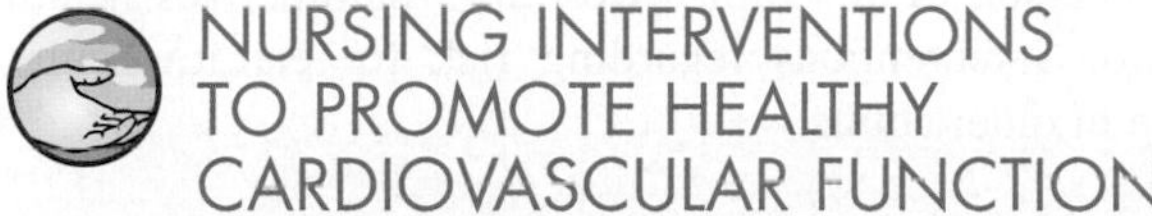

NURSING INTERVENTIONS TO PROMOTE HEALTHY CARDIOVASCULAR FUNCTION

Nursing interventions to promote healthy cardiovascular function focus on primary and secondary prevention of cardiovascular disease. These nursing interventions address *Healthy People 2010*'s goal of improving cardiovascular health and quality of life through the "prevention, detection, and treatment of risk factors; early identification and treatment of heart attacks and strokes; and prevention of recurrent cardiovascular events" (USDHHS, 2000, p. 12-15). Health promotion interventions for older adults who have risk factors focus on smoking, hypertension, obesity, dyslipidemia, and sedentary lifestyle. For all older adults, health promotion focuses on optimal exercise, a heart-healthy diet, and stress-reduction actions. Although pharmacologic and medical interventions are often used to reduce risk factors, teaching about health promotion actions is a nursing intervention that is appropriate in almost all situations. In addition to addressing risks for cardiovascular disease, nurses can address orthostatic or postprandial hypotension and the related functional consequences, such as falls and fractures.

Nurses can use the following Nursing Interventions Classification (NIC) terminology in care plans to promote cardiovascular wellness: Cardiac Care, Coping Enhancement, Counseling, Exercise Promotion, Health Education, Meditation Facilitation, Nutritional Counseling, Self-Responsibility Enhancement, Simple Guided Imagery, Simple Relaxation Therapy, and Teaching: Individual.

Addressing Risks Through Nutrition and Lifestyle Interventions

Nutrition interventions can be effective in reducing the risk of cardiovascular disease in all adults and are particularly important for prevention or management of hypertension and dyslipidemia. There is increasing recognition of the importance of fiber, folic acid, and vitamins B_6, B_{12}, C, D, and E in prevention of cardiovascular disease. For example, consuming more than eight servings a day of fruits and vegetables, particularly green leafy vegetables and vitamin C–rich fruits and vegetables, may diminish the risk for cardiovascular disease (Joshipura et al., 2001). Other nutrients that are helpful in preventing cardiovascular disease include calcium, potassium, magnesium, fiber, and soy protein (e.g., legumes) (Bazzano et al., 2001). Longitudinal data from the Women's Health Study indicate that a higher intake of magnesium-rich foods can prevent hypertension in women (Song et al., 2006).

Studies also have addressed the effects of beverages on cardiovascular function and have found light to moderate cardiovascular effects (DiCastelnuovo, 2002; Hirano et al., 2002; Hodgson et al., 2001). A large longitudinal study in Japan found that consumption of five or more cups of green tea daily was associated with a reduction in all-cause mortality of 12% for men and 23% for women, with a 31% reduction in the cardiovascular mortality rate for women (Kuriyama et al., 2006).

Nutritional interventions also are important in helping older adults to achieve and maintain their ideal body weight; nurses can encourage any person who is 20% or more heavier than the ideal body weight or has a body mass index (BMI) of 27 or more to lose weight. Nurses also can encourage older adults to ask their primary care practitioners about taking dietary supplements to reduce the risk of cardiovascular diseases. For example, current evidence suggests that omega-3 fatty acid supplements are safe and can be effective in reducing triglycerides (Fletcher et al., 2005).

Lifestyle interventions that are effective for prevention of cardiovascular disease in healthy older adults include remaining physically active, refraining from smoking, and maintaining ideal body weight. In recent years, there is increasing evidence supporting the importance of physical exercise as an intervention for improving cardiovascular performance in healthy older adults and in those with cardiovascular disease (Fig. 20-2) (Fleg, 2007; Klieman et al., 2006; Resnick et al., 2006). Specific cardiovascular benefits include lower body fat ratios, lower blood pressure measurements, lower resting heart rates, improved physical working capacity, and lower rates of myocardial infarction. Fahlman and colleagues (2002) found that a regular program of resistance or endurance exercise significantly improved the serum lipoprotein profiles of healthy women between the ages of 70 and 87 years. Similarly, researchers have concluded that aerobic exercise is an important component of lifestyle modification for primary and secondary prevention of hypertension (Whelton et al., 2002). Additional positive effects of exercise in other functional areas are noted throughout this text, and this information can be used in educating older adults about the many positive functional consequences of regular physical exercise. Studies have found that older adults who have experienced acute cardiac events may be fearful of engaging in exercise programs and may benefit from participation in cardiac rehabilitation pro-

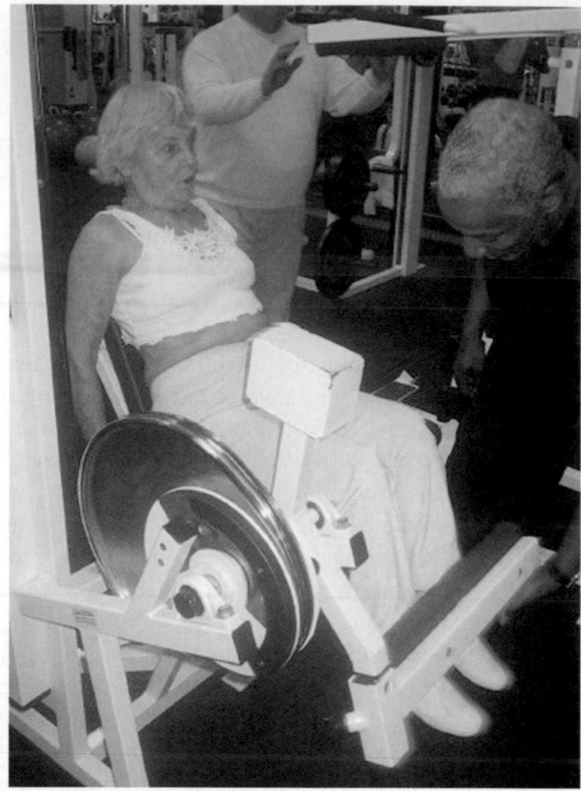

FIGURE 20-2 Exercise is an important preventive intervention. (Courtesy of Monte Unetic.)

grams which are widely available but underused by older adults (Dolansky et al., 2006).

Smoking is a major risk factor for cardiovascular disease, and quitting smoking has cumulative beneficial effects for people at any age. Williams and colleagues (2002) found that the benefits of smoking cessation as a secondary prevention intervention begin during the first year after myocardial infarction, and they are as effective in people older than 70 years of age as they are in younger people. People who cease smoking for 3 years after a myocardial infarction decrease their risk of recurrent coronary events to the equivalent of a nonsmoker's risk (Rea et al., 2002). An important nursing responsibility is to provide health education regarding smoking cessation, as discussed in Chapter 21.

Wellness Opportunity

Nurses communicate positive attitudes about aging by talking with older adults about personal responsibility for addressing risks for cardiovascular disease and communicating that it's never too late to incorporate healthy behaviors into daily life.

Addressing Risks Through Pharmacologic Interventions

Recently, some attention has been focused on the use of hormonal therapy for menopausal women and low-dose aspirin therapy as measures for preventing cardiovascular disease. In the 1990s, hormonal therapy was recommended for menopausal women as primary and secondary prevention of cardiovascular disease, but this recommendation was reversed in 2002 because of longitudinal and large-scale investigations showing that risks outweighed the benefits as a preventive intervention (U.S. Preventive Services Task Force, 2002). The use of low-dose aspirin to reduce the risk of coronary events also has been somewhat controversial because aspirin therapy, even when administered in low doses, is accompanied by increased risks for gastrointestinal bleeding and hemorrhagic stroke. Since the early 2000s, studies have concluded that the balance of benefit and harm is most favorable in people with a high risk for, or a history of, cardiovascular disease and that recommended doses of 75 to 162 mg aspirin daily are appropriate for people who are at high risk and can tolerate this dose (Mosca et al., 2004; Pearson et al., 2002). Box 20-5 summarizes health education interventions regarding risk for cardiovascular disease in older adults.

Preventing and Managing Hypertension

Although relatively few nurses prescribe medications for hypertension, all nurses have a great deal of decision-making responsibility regarding the management of hypertension because they are responsible for taking appropriate steps when they assess blood pressure. Thus, nurses need to understand current guidelines and recommendations for management of hypertension so they can make appropriate

Box 20-5
Health Promotion Activities to Reduce the Risks for Cardiovascular Disease

Detection of Risks

- Have blood pressure checked annually.
- If the total serum cholesterol level is less than 200 mg/dL, have it rechecked every 5 years. If the total serum cholesterol level is between 200 and 239 mg/dL, follow dietary measures to reduce it and have it rechecked annually. If the total serum cholesterol level is 240 mg/dL or more, obtain a further medical evaluation.

Reduction of Risks

- Give high priority to smoking cessation, if you smoke.
- Avoid passive smoking (i.e., inhaling smoke from other people's cigarettes).
- Maintain weight at a level less than 110% of ideal weight.
- Exercise daily, and engage in aerobic exercise (i.e., exercise that increases the pulse rate) several times weekly for 30 to 45 minutes each time.
- Avoid foods that are high in sodium, and follow dietary measures to reduce serum cholesterol levels.
- Discuss with your primary care provider the use of low-dose aspirin therapy as a preventive measure, particularly if there is any history of coronary artery disease or cerebrovascular events.

decisions about discussing blood pressure findings with primary care providers. Nurses also are responsible for evaluating the response of an older person to prescribed medications and for educating older adults and their caregivers about interventions for hypertension.

The stepped-care approach to management of hypertension was introduced in the first JNC report, published in the 1970s, and it has been consistently recommended in subsequent reports. This approach recommends that lifestyle modifications might be tried initially, followed by pharmacologic interventions to achieve ideal blood pressure. Weight reduction and regular physical exercise can be effective first-line interventions for hypertension in people who are overweight or sedentary (Hinderliter et al., 2002). Studies have found that reducing sodium intake can effectively reduce blood pressure in older adults (Appel et al., 2001). The National Institutes of Health have encouraged people to follow a nutrition plan called the Dietary Approaches to Stop Hypertension (DASH), health promotion materials for which are available at www.nih.gov. The recently updated dietary guidelines of the U.S. Department of Agriculture recommend that daily sodium intake be less than 2300 mg.

Many types of medications are used for treating hypertension, and selection of the best medication is based on a consideration of variables such as therapeutic effectiveness and the presence of concomitant conditions. Diuretics, either alone or in combination with beta-blockers or angiotensin-converting enzyme (ACE) inhibitors, are commonly used as initial therapy for hypertension, and calcium channel blockers are used as adjunct therapy when needed (Moser, 2001). There is increasing emphasis on selecting a medication that is effective not only in treating hypertension but in addressing coexisting cardiovascular disease. For example, beta-blockers are indicated for people with hypertension and a history of myocardial infarction, and ACE inhibitors are recommended for treatment of hypertension in people with diabetes or heart failure (Kudzma, 2001). Another consideration is the potential for preventing cardiovascular events. Studies indicate that treatment of hypertension with a thiazide diuretic reduces the risk for ischemic stroke (Klungel et al., 2001). In addition, selection of medication is based on consideration of potential adverse effects, which is particularly important for older adults with functional impairments because the degree of risk from adverse effects is at least partially related to the type of functional impairment that exists. For example, if orthostatic hypotension is an adverse effect of a medication, this is potentially more detrimental to a frail but ambulatory 85-year-old woman than to a nonambulatory older adult.

Increasing attention also is focused on the influence of genetic factors and variations in response to drugs of different ethnic and cultural groups. For example, current research is attempting to identify variations in response to antihypertensive agents in whites, Asians, Hispanics, and African Americans (Kudzma, 2001). Sareli and colleagues (2001) found that calcium channel blockers are more effective than thiazides in African Americans for initial treatment of hypertension. Researchers also are addressing questions about age and sex differences in response to hypertensive medications. For example, women and older people experience greater antihypertensive effects from the extended-release form of the calcium channel blocker verapamil compared with men and younger people (White, 2001). Some cultural aspects of hypertension prevalence and treatment are summarized in Cultural Considerations 20-1. Box 20-6 summarizes guidelines for interventions for hypertension and includes health education information about nutrition and lifestyle interventions.

Cultural Considerations 20-1

Cultural Considerations in Medication Management of Hypertension

- African Americans tend to respond best to thiazide diuretics or calcium channel blockers.
- Whites may respond best to beta-blockers and angiotensin-converting enzyme (ACE) inhibitors.
- Asian Americans tend to respond best to calcium channel blockers, diuretics, and beta-blockers.
- Asian Americans may need lower doses of beta-blockers.
- Arab Americans may respond to lower doses of anti-hypertensive agents.
- Chinese Americans and some other cultural groups are likely to use herbal medicines for hypertension.

Wellness Opportunity

Nurses promote personal responsibility for managing hypertension by talking with older adults about self-monitoring of blood pressure.

Mr. C. is now 70 years old and his blood pressure fluctuates between 130/88 mm Hg and 146/94 mm Hg. He continues to take hydrochlorothiazide, 25 mg, and verapamil, 120 mg, every morning. Mr. C. and his wife live with their daughter and her teenage children. Mr. and Mrs. C. usually do the family grocery shopping, and his wife and daughter prepare the family meals. A diet history reveals that the family usually eats fried fish or chicken about four times a week and pig's feet or ham hocks for the other main meals. Common side dishes are corn, okra, grits, cornbread, sweet potatoes, black-eyed peas, and fried greens. For cooking, the family uses lard, salt pork, or bacon drippings. Their usual beverage is decaffeinated coffee with sugar and cream. The family

(case study continues on page 434)

generally has cereal and toast for breakfast, but they have bacon and eggs on Saturdays and Sundays. Mr. and Mrs. C. eat their noon meal at the senior center 5 days a week. Mr. C.'s weight is still about 30 pounds over his ideal weight. For the past several years he has participated in the exercise program at the senior center, but gets little additional exercise and continues to complain of "getting winded" when he walks across the parking lot.

THINKING POINTS

- What additional information would you obtain for further assessment of Mr. C.'s cardiovascular status?
- What nutritional and lifestyle interventions would you discuss with Mr. C. regarding his hypertension?
- What teaching materials would you use for health education with Mr. C.?

Preventing and Managing Dyslipidemia

Nurses do not usually prescribe medications for treatment of dyslipidemia, but do frequently have responsibility for collecting information about serum lipid levels of their patients and for providing health education about prevention and management of dyslipidemia. Thus, nurses need to be familiar with dyslipidemia treatment guidelines, such as the *Adult Treatment Panel (ATP) III*. This revised report focuses on people aged 50 years and older and encourages health care providers to consider a number of risk factors for people of any age when evaluating the need for interventions. Thus, goals for lipid profiles vary depending on the number of risk factors. For example, the LDL goal for healthy people with no risk factors is less than 160 mg/dL, but the LDL goal for someone with multiple risks is less than 100 mg/dL. The Expert Panel (2001) identifies the following conditions as risk factors:

- Cardiovascular disease (e.g., angina, angioplasty, bypass surgery)
- Cerebrovascular conditions (e.g., ischemic stroke, transient ischemic attacks, symptomatic carotid artery stenosis)
- Peripheral vascular conditions
- Diabetes mellitus

As with treatment of hypertension, nutrition and lifestyle interventions are the first-line approaches, and medications (e.g., statins) are used as necessary if goals are not achieved with nonpharmacologic interventions (Zarowitz et al., 2006). Essential nutrition and lifestyle interventions for dyslipidemia include dietary modifications, maintenance of ideal body weight, and incorporation of regular exercise in one's daily routine. One study found that a 6-month program of aerobic and resistance training lowered diastolic, but not systolic, blood pressure in older adults with mild hypertension (Stewart et al., 2005). Nutrition interventions focus on

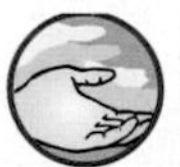

Box 20-6
Guidelines for Nursing Management of Hypertension

Health Promotion Interventions

The following lifestyle modifications are recommended for all people with hypertension:

- Avoidance of tobacco
- Weight reduction when appropriate (i.e., when the person weighs more than 110% of his or her ideal weight)
- 30 to 45 minutes of exercise, such as brisk walking, at least 5 times weekly
- Limitation of alcohol intake to 1 drink per day (e.g., 2 ounces of 100-proof whiskey, 8 ounces of wine, or 24 ounces of beer)

The following nutritional interventions are recommended for all people with hypertension:

- Intake of no more than 2.4 g sodium daily
- Avoidance of processed foods
- Daily intake of 7 to 8 servings of grains and grain products and 8 to 10 servings of fruits and vegetables

Considerations Regarding the Treatment of Hypertension

- Risks from and definitions of hypertension apply to all age categories (refer to Table 20-1 for criteria).
- A person's blood pressure should be measured at least three times before making any decisions about treatment.
- The safety of antihypertensive agents is improved by carefully selecting the medication, starting with low doses, and changing the medication regimen gradually, in small increments, if necessary.

Treatment Goals

- The goals of hypertensive treatment are to control blood pressure by the least intrusive means and to prevent cardiovascular morbidity and mortality.
- Treatment is directed toward achieving and maintaining a systolic blood pressure of less than 140 mm Hg and a diastolic blood pressure of less than 90 mm Hg (< 130/80 mm Hg in people with diabetes or chronic kidney disease).
- Blood pressure reduction to 130/85 mm Hg is recommended if this can be achieved without compromising cardiovascular function.
- For older adults with isolated systolic hypertension or systolic blood pressure levels of 140 to 160 mm Hg, lifestyle modifications should be the first treatment step.
- The initial goal of therapy for those with a systolic blood pressure of greater than 180 mm Hg is to reduce the systolic blood pressure to less than 160 mm Hg.
- For older adults with systolic blood pressure measurements of between 160 and 179 mm Hg, the initial goal is to reduce the systolic blood pressure by 20 mm Hg. If initial treatment is well tolerated, further reduction of the systolic blood pressure should be considered.

dietary fat intake, with emphasis on limiting foods containing saturated fats and trans fatty acids and increasing foods that are high in polyunsaturated and monounsaturated fats. Recent large-scale epidemiologic studies support the intake of foods containing omega-3 fatty acids (e.g., fish, seafood), which are also called *polyunsaturated fatty acids*, and food and oils containing alpha-linoleic acids (e.g., walnuts, soybeans, flaxseeds, and canola oil) (Harper & Jacobson, 2001; Kris-Etherton et al., 2002). Daily supplementation with 1 g of elemental calcium is another nonpharmacologic intervention that may increase serum HDL cholesterol and reduce serum LDL cholesterol (Reid et al., 2002). Box 20-7 summarizes health education interventions for prevention and management of dyslipidemia in older adults.

Diversity Note

Nutrition and exercise interventions may be particularly effective in Native American populations (Kudzma, 2001).

Preventing and Managing Orthostatic or Postprandial Hypotension

Interventions aimed at preventing orthostatic and postprandial hypotension can be initiated as health measures for older adults who have any of the risk factors listed in Box 20-1. For older adults with symptomatic orthostatic hypotension, interventions to alleviate the problem are important for maintaining quality of life and preventing serious consequences. When symptomatic orthostatic hypotension cannot be alleviated, interventions must be directed toward ensuring the individual's safety, particularly by preventing falls and fractures.

For older adults with postprandial hypotension, interventions can be implemented around mealtimes. In institutional or home care settings, registered dietitians may be helpful in developing a plan for addressing postprandial hypotension, but in any setting nurses assume responsibility for health education about interventions. In older adults with postprandial hypotension, low-carbohydrate meals are associated with significantly shorter periods of hypotension, significantly smaller declines in systolic blood pressure, and less frequent and less severe symptoms compared with normal and high-carbohydrate meals (Jansen, 2005). Xylose (found in gum) and guar gum (a natural food supplement) may slow the rate of gastric emptying and be effective in alleviating postprandial hypotension (Jones et al., 2001). Additional interventions are summarized in Box 20-8, which can be used as a tool for health education about orthostatic and postprandial hypotension.

Box 20-7
Nutritional Interventions for People With High Cholesterol

Dietary Measures to Promote a Healthy Lipid Profile

- Include foods that are high in fiber content in your daily diet (e.g., whole grains).
- Include soy proteins in your daily diet (e.g., tofu, soy milk).
- Eat a minimum of two servings of fatty fish weekly.
- Limit total fat intake to less than 30% of your total daily calorie intake.
- Limit total daily cholesterol intake to between 250 and 350 mg.
- Use nonfat or low-fat dairy desserts.
- Limit consumption of butter or margarine.
- Limit consumption of egg yolks, including those in food, to two or three per week.
- Use egg whites or egg substitutes instead of whole eggs.
- Limit consumption of lean meats to five or fewer 3- to 5-ounce servings per week. Trim fat off meats and the skin off poultry.
- Avoid eating processed meats (e.g., bacon, bologna, sausage, hot dogs).
- Avoid gravies, fried foods, and organ meats.

Guide to Types of Fats

Type of Fat	Sources	Examples	Effect on Lipid Profile
Saturated fatty acids	Animal fats and some vegetable oils (usually solid at room temperatures)	Meat, poultry, butter, lauric and palm oils	Negative: increases LDL and total cholesterol
Trans fatty acids	Vegetable oils that are processed into margarine or shortening	Dairy products, baked goods, snack foods	Negative: increases LDL cholesterol and lowers HDL cholesterol
Monounsaturated fatty acids	Vegetable oils (usually liquid at room temperatures)	Olive, peanut, and canola oils	Positive: decreases LDL
Polyunsaturated fatty acids	Seafood and vegetable oils (soft or liquid at room temperatures)	Corn, sunflower, safflower, canola, and linoleic oils	Positive: decreases LDL
Omega-3 fatty acids	Fatty fish	Tuna, salmon, herring, mackerel	Positive: decreases LDL cholesterol and triglycerides

LDL, low-density lipoprotein; HDL, high-density lipoprotein.

Box 20-8
Education Regarding Orthostatic and Postprandial Hypotension

Prevention and Management of Both Orthostatic and Postprandial Hypotension

- Maintain adequate fluid intake (i.e., eight glasses of noncaffeinated beverages daily).
- Eat five or six smaller meals daily, rather than large meals.
- Avoid excessive alcohol consumption.
- Avoid sitting or standing still for prolonged periods, especially after meals.

Health Promotion Measures Specific to Orthostatic Hypotension

- Change your position slowly, especially when moving from a sitting or lying position to a standing position.
- Before standing up, sit at the side of the bed for several minutes after rising from a lying position.
- Maintain good physical fitness, especially good muscle tone, and engage in regular, but not excessive, exercise. (Swimming is an excellent form of exercise because the hydrostatic pressure prevents blood from pooling in the legs.)
- Wear a waist-high elastic support garment or thigh-high elastic stockings during the day, and put them on before getting out of bed in the morning.
- Sleep with the head of the bed elevated on blocks.
- During the day, rest in a recliner chair with your legs elevated.
- Take measures to prevent constipation and avoid straining during bowel movements.
- Avoid medications that increase the risk for orthostatic hypotension, particularly if additional risk factors are present (refer to Box 20-1).
- Avoid sources of intense heat (e.g., direct sun, electric blankets, and hot baths and showers) because these cause peripheral vasodilation.
- If taking nitroglycerin, do not take it while standing.

Health Promotion Measures Specific to Postprandial Hypotension

- Minimize the risk for postprandial hypotension by taking antihypertensive medications 1 hour after meals rather than before meals.
- Eat small, low-carbohydrate meals.
- Avoid alcohol consumption.
- Avoid strenuous exercise, especially for 2 hours after meals.

Safety Precautions if Hypotension Cannot Be Prevented

- Reduce the potential for falls and other negative functional consequences of postprandial hypotension by remaining seated (or by lying down) after meals.
- Call for assistance if help is needed with walking.
- Adapt the environment to minimize the risk and consequences of falling (e.g., ensure good lighting, install grab bars, keep pathways clear).

EVALUATING EFFECTIVENESS OF NURSING INTERVENTIONS

One measure of the effectiveness of health promotion interventions is the extent to which the older adult verbalizes correct information about the risks. Also, the older adult may verbalize intent to change or eliminate the lifestyle factors that increase the risk of impaired cardiovascular function. For example, the older adult may agree to join an exercise program and follow dietary measures to reduce serum cholesterol levels. Effectiveness of interventions also can be measured by determining the actual reduction in risk factors. For example, the person's serum cholesterol level may decrease from 238 to 198 mg/dL after 6 months of regular exercise and dietary modifications. For older adults with impaired cardiovascular function, nurses evaluate the extent to which the signs and symptoms are alleviated and the extent to which older adults verbalize correct information about managing their condition.

Mr. C. is now 74 years old and continues to come to the Senior Wellness Clinic for monthly blood pressure checks. He reports that his doctor recently started him on a medication for high cholesterol and told him to "watch my diet," but gave no further information or educational materials about what to do about his cholesterol.

NURSING ASSESSMENT

Mr. C. has no knowledge about dietary sources of cholesterol, and is unaware that his diet, which he terms "soul food," is high in cholesterol. Although he says that he has heard a lot about "good and bad cholesterol" in the news, he does not know which foods are good or bad. He tries to buy foods that say "no cholesterol" on the label, but says that the labels are too confusing about the different kinds of fats.

(case study continues on page 437)

NURSING DIAGNOSIS

Your nursing diagnosis is Altered Health Maintenance related to lack of regular exercise, dietary habits that contribute to hyperlipidemia, and insufficient information about lifestyle factors that increase the risk of cardiovascular disease. Evidence of these risk factors comes from Mr. C.'s inactivity, eating patterns, history of hypertension, and family history of cardiovascular disease. Also, Mr. C. has verbalized insufficient information about the relationship between exercise and cardiovascular function and about dietary measures to control cholesterol.

NURSING CARE PLAN FOR MR. C.

Expected Outcome	Nursing Interventions	Nursing Evaluation
Mr. C.'s knowledge of risk factors for cardiovascular impairment will increase.	• Discuss the risk factors for impaired cardiovascular function, using Figure 20-1 and information from Box 20-3. • Emphasize the risk factors that can be addressed through lifestyle modifications (e.g., exercise, weight loss, and dietary measures to control cholesterol levels).	• Mr. C. will be able to describe his risk factors for cardiovascular disease. • Mr. C. will identify those risk factors that he can address through lifestyle changes.
Mr. C.'s knowledge of the relationship between diet and serum cholesterol levels will increase.	• Use teaching materials obtained from the American Heart Association to illustrate the relationship between diet and serum cholesterol levels. Provide a copy of these pamphlets for Mr. C. to take home. • Suggest that Mr. C. discuss the information in the pamphlets with his wife and daughter. • Ask Mr. C. to bring his wife to the nursing clinic next month so that you can talk with both of them about dietary measures to control cholesterol.	• Mr. C. will accurately describe the relationship between food intake and cholesterol levels. • Mr. C. will identify family eating habits that contribute to his elevated serum cholesterol level.
Mr. C. will modify one dietary habit that contributes to his high cholesterol level.	• Work with Mr. C. to make a list of the foods associated with high cholesterol levels (e.g., fried foods, ham hocks, lard, bacon, and eggs). • Give Mr. C. a copy of Box 20-7 and use it to discuss dietary measures to reduce cholesterol. • Ask Mr. C. to select one change in dietary habits that will have a positive effect on his cholesterol level (e.g., switching from lard to vegetable oil for frying foods).	• Mr. C. will state that he is willing to change one eating habit that contributes to his high cholesterol level. • Next month, Mr. C. will report that he has changed one eating pattern that contributes to high cholesterol levels.
Mr. C. will increase his knowledge about the relationship between exercise and cardiovascular function.	• Use pamphlets from the American Heart Association to teach about the effects of aerobic exercise on cardiovascular function. • Review information about the relationship between exercise and weight.	• Mr. C. will describe the beneficial effects of regular aerobic exercise.
Mr. C. will begin exercising on a regular basis.	• Discuss ways in which Mr. C. can incorporate regular exercise into his daily activities • Invite Mr. C. and his wife to participate in the daily Eldercise program that is offered following the noon meal at the senior center.	• Mr. C. will verbalize a commitment to perform 30 minutes of exercise 3 days a week.

(case study continues on page 438)

Expected Outcome	Nursing Interventions	Nursing Evaluation
Mr. C. will eliminate lifestyle factors that increase the risk for cardiovascular disease.	• Ask Mr. C. to invite his wife to your monthly appointments so that she can also receive important health education. • Identify a plan that will enable Mr. and Mrs. C. to incorporate additional dietary measures aimed at reducing cholesterol gradually into the family meal plans. • Identify a plan that will enable Mr. and Mrs. C. to include 30 minutes of exercise 5 times a week. • Discuss weight reduction with Mr. C. and emphasize that dietary modifications and regular exercise are interventions that should facilitate weight loss.	• Mr. C.'s total cholesterol level will be ≤200 mg/dL at the end of 6 months. • Mr. C.'s serum cholesterol level will remain below 200 mg/dL. • Mr. C. will report that he engages in 30 minutes of exercise 5 times weekly. • Mr. C. will report that he follows the dietary measures presented in Box 20-7. • Mr. C.'s weight will be reduced to between 180 and 198 pounds, and he will maintain that weight.

THINKING POINTS

- What factors affect Mr. C.'s ability to manage his cardiovascular condition and address his risk factors, and how would you address these factors in your interventions?
- Explore some of the educational resources listed at the end of this chapter to find teaching tools that would be appropriate for Mr. C.

CHAPTER HIGHLIGHTS

Age-Related Changes That Affect Cardiovascular Function

- Degenerative changes of myocardium
- Arterial stiffening
- Thicker, less elastic, more dilated veins
- Increased peripheral resistance
- Altered baroreflex mechanisms

Risk Factors That Affect Cardiovascular Function

- Inactivity, obesity, tobacco smoking, dietary habits
- Low socioeconomic status
- Psychosocial factors (e.g., stress, depression, anxiety, poor social support)
- Hypertension, dyslipidemia
- Gender-specific risks (e.g., menopausal status)
- Conditions that predispose the person to orthostatic or postprandial hypotension (Box 20-1)

Pathologic Condition Affecting Cardiovascular Function

- Atherosclerosis

Functional Consequences Affecting Cardiovascular Wellness

- Slight decrease in normal pulse rate
- Diminished adaptive response to exercise
- Increased susceptibility to cardiac arrhythmias
- Increased susceptibility to orthostatic and postprandial hypotension
- Decreased cerebral blood flow
- Varicosities, increased susceptibility to venous stasis

Nursing Assessment of Cardiovascular Function (Fig. 20-1; Table 20-1; Boxes 20-2 through 20-4)

- Baseline cardiovascular function (heart rate, sounds, and rhythm)
- Blood pressure, including hypertension and orthostatic or postprandial hypotension
- Risks for cardiovascular disease
- Signs and symptoms of heart disease
- Knowledge about manifestations of heart disease

Nursing Diagnosis

- Readiness for Enhanced Knowledge
- Decreased Cardiac Output
- Health Maintenance

Planning for Wellness Outcomes

- Health Promoting Behaviors
- Risk Control: Cardiovascular Health
- Risk Control: Tobacco Use
- Cardiac Disease Self-Management

Nursing Interventions to Promote Healthy Cardiovascular Function (Boxes 20-5 through 20-8)

- Teaching about interventions to promote optimal cardiovascular function (exercise, heart-healthy diet, optimal body weight, cessation of smoking if applicable)
- Teaching about medications for primary and secondary prevention of cardiovascular disease
- Medication, nutrition, and lifestyle interventions for hypertension
- Medication, nutrition, and lifestyle interventions for dyslipidemia
- Prevention and management of orthostatic and postprandial hypotension

Evaluating Effectiveness of Nursing Interventions

- Verbalization of correct information about risks
- Reported participation in health promotion interventions

(e.g., heart-healthy diet, regular exercise, weight reduction and smoking cessation when applicable)
- Indicators of cardiovascular function within normal range (e.g., blood pressure, serum lipids)
- If applicable, alleviation of signs and symptoms of cardiovascular disease

Critical Thinking Exercises

1. Discuss how each of the following factors influences cardiovascular function, including orthostatic hypotension: lifestyle, medications, age-related changes, and pathologic conditions.
2. Demonstrate how you would teach a home health aide to assess blood pressure and orthostatic hypotension correctly.
3. Describe the questions and considerations that you would include in an assessment of cardiovascular function in an older adult who has no complaints of heart problems, but who has a history of falling twice in the past month and who has not been evaluated by a primary care provider in the past year.
4. You are asked to give a health education talk entitled "Keeping Your Heart Healthy" at a senior center. What information would you include in the presentation? What local resources (i.e., specific contact information for agencies or organizations in your area) would you suggest your audience contact for further information? What audiovisual aids would you use? How would you involve the participants in the discussion?
5. You are working in an assisted-living facility in which several of the residents have orthostatic hypotension. What would you include in your health education regarding management of orthostatic hypotension?

Educational Resources

American Heart Association
www.americanheart.org

American Stroke Association
www.strokeassociation.org

Heart and Stroke Foundation of Canada
www.heartandstroke.ca

National Heart, Lung, and Blood Institute Information Center
www.nhlbi.nih.gov

National Stroke Association
www.stroke.org

References

Aldwin, C. M., Spiro III, A., & Park, C. L. (2006). Health, behavior, and optimal aging: Life span developmental perspective. In J. E. Birren & K. W. Schaie (Eds.), *Handbook of the psychology of aging* (6th ed., pp. 85–125). San Diego: Elsevier Academic Press.

American Heart Association. (2006). *Heart disease and stroke statistics: 2006 Update.* Dallas: Author.

Artinian, N. T. (2004). Can NPs rely on self-blood pressure measurements? *The Nurse Practitioner, 29*(5), 46–52.

Appel, L. J. Espeland, M. A., Easter, L., Wilson, A. C., Folmar, S., & Lacy, C. R. (2001). Effects of reduced sodium intake on hypertension control in older individuals: Results for the trial of nonpharmacologic interventions in the elderly (TONE). *Archives of Internal Medicine, 161,* 685–693.

Aronow, W. S. (2002a). Should hypercholesterolemia in older persons be treated to reduce cardiovascular events? *Journals of Gerontology: Series A, Biological Sciences and Medical Sciences, 57,* M411–M413.

Aronow, W. S. (2002b). What is the appropriate treatment of hypertension in elders? *Journals of Gerontology: Series A, Biological Sciences and Medical Sciences, 57,* M483–M486.

Aronow, W. S. (2003). Silent MI: Prevalence and prognosis in older patients diagnosed by routine electrocardiograms. *Geriatrics, 58*(1), 24–40.

Arthur, H. M. (2006). Depression, isolation, social support, and cardiovascular disease in older adults. *Journal of Cardiovascular Nursing, 21,* S2–S7.

Aviv, A. (2001). Salt and hypertension: The debate that begs the bigger question. *Archives of Internal Medicine, 161,* 507–510.

Bazzano, L. A., He, J., Ogden, L. G., Loria, C., Vupputuri, S., Myers, L., & Whelton, P. K. (2001). Legume consumption and risk of coronary heart disease in US men and women. *Archives of Internal Medicine, 161,* 2573–2578.

Benetos, A., Thomas, F., Bean, K., Gautier, S., Smulyan, H., & Guize, L. (2002). Prognostic value of systolic and diastolic pressure in treated hypertensive men. *Archives of Internal Medicine, 162,* 577–581.

Boland, L. L., Folsom, A. R., Sorlie, P. D., Taylor, H. A., Rosamond, W. D., Chambless, L. E., et al. (2002). Occurrence of unrecognized myocardial infarction in subjects aged 45 to 65 years (the ARIC study). *American Journal of Cardiology, 90,* 927–931.

Bono, G., & McCullough, M. E. (2004). Religion, forgiveness, and adjustment in older adulthood. In K. W. Schaie, N. Krause, & A. Booth (Eds.), *Religious influences on health and well-being in the elderly* (pp. 163–186). New York: Springer.

Canto, J. G., Fincher, C., Kiefe, C. L., Allison, J. J., Li, Q., Funkhouser, E., et al. (2002). Atypical presentation among Medicare beneficiaries with unstable angina pectoris. *American Journal of Cardiology, 90,* 248–253.

Carpenito-Moyet, L. J. (2006). *Handbook of nursing diagnosis* (11th ed.). Philadelphia: Lippincott Williams & Wilkins.

Deaton, C., Bennett, J. A., & Riegel, B. (2004). State of the science for care of older adults with heart disease. *Nursing Clinics of North America, 39,* 495–528.

DiCastelnuovo, A. (2002). Meta-analysis of wine and beer consumption in relation to vascular risk. *Circulation, 105,* 2836–2844.

Dolanksy, M. A., Moore, S. M., & Visovsky, C. (2006). Older adults' views of cardiac rehabilitation programs: Is it time to reinvent? *Journal of Gerontological Nursing, 32*(2), 37–44.

Eaton, C. B., & Anthony, D. (2002). Cardiovascular disease and the maturing woman. *Clinics in Family Practice, 4*(1), 71–88.

Eidelman, R. S., Lamas, G. A., & Hennekens, C. H. (2002). The new National Cholesterol Education Program guidelines. *Archives of Internal Medicine, 162,* 2033–2036.

Expert Panel on Detection, Evaluation, and Treatment of High Blood Cholesterol in Adults. (2001). Executive summary of the Third Report of the National Cholesterol Education Program (NCEP) Expert Panel on Detection, Evaluation, and Treatment of High Blood Cholesterol in Adults (ATP III). *Journal of the American Medical Association, 285,* 2486–2497.

Fahlman, M. M., Boardley, D., Lambert, C. P., & Flynn, M. G. (2002). Effects of endurance training and resistance training on plasma lipoprotein profiles in elderly women. *Journals of Gerontology: Series A, Biological Sciences and Medical Sciences, 57,* B54–B60.

Fisher, A. A., Davis, M. W., & Le Couteur, D. G. (2005). The effect of meals at different mealtimes on blood pressure and symptoms in geriatric patients with postprandial hypotension: Letter to the editor. *Jour-*

nals of Gerontology: Series A, Biological Sciences and Medical Sciences, 60, 184–186.

Fleg, J. L. (2007). Exercise therapy for elderly heart failure patients. *Clinics in Geriatric Medicine, 23*, 221–234.

Fletcher, B., Berra, K., Ades, P., Braun, L. T., Burke, L. E., Durstine, J. L., et al. (2005). Managing abnormal blood lipids: A collaborative approach. *Circulation, 112*, 3184–3209.

Gibbons, L. W., & Clark, S. M. (2001). Exercise in the reduction of cardiovascular events: Lessons for epidemiologic trails. *Cardiology Clinics, 19*, 347–355.

Hajjar, I., Miller, K., & Hirth, V. (2002). Age-related bias in the management of hypertension: A national survey of physicians' opinions on hypertension in elderly adults. *Journals of Gerontology: Series A, Biological Sciences and Medical Sciences, 57*, M487–M491.

Hajjar, I. M., Grim, C. E., George, V., & Kotchen, T. A. (2001). Impact of diet on blood pressure and age-related changes in blood pressure in the US population. *Archives of Internal Medicine, 161*, 589–593.

Harper, C. R., & Jacobson, T. A. (2001). The fats of life: The role of omega-3 fatty acids in prevention of coronary heart disease. *Archives of Internal Medicine, 161*, 2185–2192.

Hinderliter, A., Sherwood, A., Gullette, E. C. D., Babyak, M., Waugh, R., Georgiades, A., et al. (2002). Reduction of left ventricular hypertrophy after exercise and weight loss in overweight patients with mild hypertension. *Archives of Internal Medicine, 162*, 1333–1339.

Hirano, R., Momiyama, Y., Takahashi, R., Taniguchi, H., Kondo, K., Nakamura, H., et al. (2002). Comparison of green tea intake in Japanese patients with and without angiographic coronary artery disease. *American Journal of Cardiology, 90*, 1150–1153.

Hodgson, J. M., Puddey, I. B., Mori, T. A., Baker, R. I., & Beilin, L. J. (2001). Effects of regular ingestion of black tea on haemostasis and cell adhesion molecules in humans. *European Journal of Clinical Nutrition, 55*, 881–886.

Hsia, J., Langer, R. D., Manson, J. E., Kuller, L., Johnson, K. C., Hendrix, S. L., et al. (2006). Conjugated equine estrogens and coronary heart disease. *Archives of Internal Medicine, 166*, 357–365.

Humphrey, L. L., Chan, B. K. S., & Sox, H. C. (2002). Postmenopausal hormone replacement therapy and the primary prevention of cardiovascular disease. *Annals of Internal Medicine, 137*, 273–284.

Irvin, D. J., & White, M. (2004). The importance of accurately assessing orthostatic hypotension. *Geriatric Nursing, 25*(2), 99–101.

Iwanczyk, L., Weintraub, N. T., & Rubenstein, L. Z. (2006). Orthostatic hypotension in the nursing home setting. *Journal of American Medical Directors Association, 7*, 163–167.

Jansen, R. W. M. M. (2005). Postprandial hypotension: Simple treatment but difficulties with the diagnosis. *Journals of Gerontology: Series A, Biological Sciences and Medical Sciences, 60*, 1268–1270.

Joint National Committee on Prevention, Detection, Evaluation, and Treatment of High Blood Pressure (JNC). (2003). The seventh report of the Joint National Committee on Prevention, Detection, Evaluation, and Treatment of High Blood Pressure (JNC IV). *Journal of the American Medical Association, 289*, 2560–2577.

Jones, K. L., MacIntosh, C., Su, Y. C., Wells, F., Chapman, I. M., Tonkin, A., et al. (2001). Guar gum reduces postprandial hypotension in older people. *Journal of the American Geriatrics Society, 49*, 162–167.

Joshipura, K. J., Hu, F. B., Manson, J. E., Stampfer, M. J., Rimm, E. B., Speizer, F. E., et al. (2001). The effect of fruit and vegetable intake on risk for coronary heart disease. *Annals of Internal Medicine, 134*, 1106–1114.

Keevil, J. G., Stein, J. H., & McBride, P. E. (2002). Cardiovascular disease prevention. *Primary Care: Clinics in Office Practice, 29*, 667–777.

Klieman, L., Hyde, S., & Berra, K. (2006). Cardiovascular disease risk reduction in older adults. *Journal of Cardiovascular Nursing, 55*, S27–S39.

Klungel, O. H., Heckbert, S. R., Longstreth, W. T., Furberg, C. D., Kaplan, R. C., Smith, N. L., et al. (2001). Antihypertensive drug therapies and the risk of ischemic stroke. *Archives of Internal Medicine, 161*, 37–43.

Krause, N. (2006). Religion and health in later life. In J. E. Birren & K. W. Schaie (Eds.), *Handbook of the psychology of aging* (6th ed., pp. 500–518). San Diego: Elsevier Academic Press.

Kris-Etherton, P. M., Harris, W. S., & Appel, L. J. (2002). Fish consumption, fish oil, omega-3 fatty acids, and cardiovascular disease. *Circulation, 106*, 2747–2757.

Kudzma, E. C. (2001). Cultural competence: Cardiovascular medicine. *Progress in Cardiovascular Nursing, 16*, 152–160, 169.

Kuller, L. H., Arnold, A. M., Psaty, B. M., Robbins, J. A., O'Leary, D. H., Tracy, R. P., et al. (2006). 10-Year follow-up of subclinical cardiovascular disease and risk of coronary heart disease in the Cardiovascular Health Study. *Archives of Internal Medicine, 166*, 71–78.

Kuriyama, S., Shimazu, T., Ohmori, N., Kikuchi, N., Nakaya, N., Nishino, Y., et al. (2006). Green tea consumption and mortality due to cardiovascular disease, cancer, and all causes in Japan: The Oshaki Study. *Journal of the American Medical Association, 296*, 1255–1265.

Laine, C. (2002). Postmenopausal hormone replacement therapy: How could we have been so wrong? *Annals of Internal Medicine, 137*, 290.

Lakatta, E. G. (2000). Cardiovascular aging in health. *Clinics in Geriatric Medicine, 16*, 419–444.

Laucka, P. V., & Trotter, J. M. (2001). Medication management of hypertension. *Topics in Geriatric Rehabilitation, 17*(2), 61–82.

Lemaitre, R. N., Weiss, N. S., Smith, N. L., Psaty, B. M., Lumley, T., Larson, E. B., et al. (2006). Esterified estrogen and conjugated equine estrogen and the risk of incident myocardial infarction and stroke. *Archives of Internal Medicine, 166*, 399–404.

Mancia, G., Bombelli, M., Lanzarotti, A., Grassi, G., Ceasana, G., Zanchetti, A., et al. (2002). Systolic vs diastolic blood pressure control in the hypertensive patients of the PAMELA population. *Archives of Internal Medicine, 162*, 582–586.

Maurer, M. S., Karmally, W., Rivadeneira, H., Parides, M. K., & Bloomfield, D. M. (2000). Upright posture and postprandial hypotension in elderly. *Annals of Internal Medicine, 133*, 533–536.

Mehagnoul-Schipper, D. J., Boerman, R. H., Hoefnagels, W. H. L., & Jansen, R. W. M. M. (2001). Effects of levodopa on orthostatic and postprandial hypotension in elderly parkinsonian patients. *Journals of Gerontology: Series A, Biological Sciences and Medical Sciences, 56*, M749–M755.

Morley, J. E. (2001). Postprandial hypotension: The ultimate Big Mac attack. *Journals of Gerontology: Series A, Biological Sciences and Medical Sciences, 56*, M741–M743.

Mosca, L., Appel, L. J., Benjamin, E. J., Berra, K., Chandra-Strobos, N., Fabunmi, R. P., et al. (2004). Evidence-based guidelines for cardiovascular disease prevention in women. *Circulation, 109*, 672–693.

Moser, M. (2001). Is it time for a new approach to the initial treatment of hypertension? *Archives of Internal Medicine, 161*, 1140–1144.

Mukai, S., & Lipsitz, L. A. (2002). Orthostatic hypotension. *Clinics in Geriatric Medicine, 18*, 253–268.

National Clearinghouse Guidelines. (2005). Seventh Report of the Joint National Committee on Prevention, Detection, Evaluation, and Treatment of High Blood Pressure, Summary updated on July 15, 2005. Available at http://www.guideline.gov/summary. Accessed on 6/24/07.

Nelson, K., Norris, K., & Mangione, C. M. (2002). Disparities in the diagnosis and pharmacologic treatment of high serum cholesterol by race and ethnicity. *Archives of Internal Medicine, 162*, 929–935.

O'Mara, G. O., & Lyons, D. (2002). Postprandial hypotension. *Clinics in Geriatric Medicine, 18*, 307–321.

Pearson, T. A., Blair, S. N., Daniels, S. R., Eckel, R. H., Fair, J. M., Fortmann, S. P., et al. (2002). AHA Guidelines for primary prevention of cardiovascular disease and stroke: 2002 update. *Circulation, 106*, 388–391.

Prospective Studies Collaboration. (2002). Age-specific relevance of usual blood pressure to vascular mortality: A meta-analysis of individual data for one million adults in 61 prospective studies. *Lancet, 360*, 1903–1913.

Puisieux, F., Bulckaen, H., Fauchais, A. L., Drumez, S., Salomez-Granier, F., & Dewailly, P. (2000). Ambulatory blood pressure monitoring and postprandial hypotension in elderly persons with falls or syncopes. *Journals of Gerontology: Series A, Biological Sciences and Medical Sciences, 55*, M535–M540.

Rea, T. D., Heckbert, S. R. Kaplan, R. C., Smith, N. L., Lemaitre, R. N., & Psaty, B. M. (2002). Smoking status and risk for recurrent coronary events after myocardial infarction. *Annals of Internal Medicine, 137*, 494–500.

Reid, I. R., Mason, B., Horne, A., Ames, R., Clearwater, J., Bava, U., et al. (2002). Effects of calcium supplementation on serum lipid concentrations in normal older women: A randomized controlled trial. *American Journal of Medicine, 112*, 343–347.

Resnick, B., Ory, M. G., Rogers, M. E., Page, P., Lyle, R. M., Sipe, C., et al. (2006). Screening for and prescribing exercise for older adults. *Geriatrics and Aging, 9*(3), 174–182.

Rodondi, N., Newman, A. B., Vittinghoff, E., de Rekeneire, N., Satterfield, S., Harris, T. B., et al. (2005). Subclinical hypothyroidism and the risk of heart failure, other cardiovascular events, and death. *Archives of Internal Medicine, 165*, 2460–2466.

Rosenfeld, A. G., Lindauer, A., & Darney, B. G. (2005). Understanding treatment-seeking delay in women with acute myocardial infarction: Descriptions of decision-making patterns. *American Journal of Critical Care, 14*, 285–292.

Ross, R., & Glomset, J. (1976). The pathogenesis of atherosclerosis. *New England Journal of Medicine, 295*, 369–377, 420–425.

Sareli, P., Radecski, I. V., Valtchanova, Z. P., Lighaber, E., Candy, G. P., Hond, E. D., et al. (2001). Efficacy of different drug classes used to initiate antihypertensive treatment in black subjects. *Archives of Internal Medicine, 161*, 965–971.

Sheifer, S. E., Manolio, T. A., & Gersh, B. J. (2001). Unrecognized myocardial infarction. *Annals of Internal Medicine, 135*, 801–811.

Song, Y., Sesso, H. D., Manson, J. E., Cook, N. R., Buring, J. E., & Liu, S. (2006). Dietary magnesium intake and risk of incident hypertension among middle-aged and older US women in a 10-year follow-up study. *American Journal of Cardiology,* 98, 1616–1621.

Stewart, K. J., Bacher, A. C., Turner, K. L., Fleg, J. L., Hees, P. S., Shapiro, E. P., et al. (2005). Effect of exercise on blood pressure in older persons: A randomized controlled trial. *Archives of Internal Medicine, 165*, 756–762.

Teo, K. K., Ounpuu, S., Hawken, S., Pandey, M. R., Valentin, V., Hunt, D., et al. (2006). Tobacco use and risk of myocardial infarction in 52 countries in the INTERHEART study: A case-control study. *Lancet, 368*, 647–658.

Tierney, L. M., McPhee, S. J., & Papadakis, M. A. (Eds.). (2005). *2006 Current medical diagnosis & treatment*. New York: McGraw-Hill.

U.S. Department of Health and Human Services (USDHHS). (2000). *Healthy people 2010* (2nd ed.). Washington, DC: U.S. Government Printing Office.

U.S. Department of Health and Human Services (USDHHS). (2006). *The health consequences of involuntary exposure to tobacco smoke. A report of the surgeon general*. Rockville, MD: Office of the Surgeon General.

U.S. Preventive Services Task Force. (October 2002). *Hormone replacement therapy for primary prevention of chronic conditions: Recommendations and rationale*. Rockville, MD: Agency for Healthcare Research and Quality. Available at www.ahrq.gov/clinic/3rduspstf/hrt/hrtr.htm.

Vasan, R. S., Larson, M. G., Leip, E. P., Evans, J. C., O'Donnell, C. J., Kannel, W. B., et al. (2001). Impact of high-normal blood pressure on the risk of cardiovascular disease. *New England Journal of Medicine, 345*, 1291–1297.

Vloet, L., & Jansen, R. W. M. M. (2005). The effect of meals at different mealtimes on blood pressure and symptoms in geriatric patients with postprandial hypotension: Authors' response. *Journals of Gerontology: Series A, Biological Sciences and Medical Sciences, 60*, 184–186.

Vloet, L. C. M., Pel-Little, R. E., Jansen, P. A. F., & Jansen, R. W. M. M. (2005). High prevalence of postprandial and orthostatic hypotension among geriatric patients admitted to Dutch hospitals. *Journals of Gerontology: Series A, Biological Sciences and Medical Sciences, 60*, 1271–1277.

Vollmer, W. M., Sacks, F. M., Ard, J., Appel, L. J., Bray, G. A., Simons-Morton, D. G., et al. (2001). Effects of diet and sodium intake on blood pressure: Subgroup analysis of the DASH-sodium trial. *Annals of Internal Medicine, 135*, 1019–1028.

Weiss, A., Grossman, E., Beloosesky, Y., & Grinblat, J. (2002). Orthostatic hypotension in acute geriatric ward: Is it a consistent finding? *Archives of Internal Medicine, 162*, 2369–2374.

Whelton, S. P., Chin, A., Xin, X., & He, J. (2002). Effect of aerobic exercise on blood pressure: A meta-analysis of randomized, controlled trials. *Annals of Internal Medicine, 136*, 493–503.

White, W. B. (2001). Gender and age effects on the ambulatory blood pressure and heart rate responses to antihypertensive therapy. *American Journal of Hypertension, 14*, 1239–1247.

Williams, M. A., Fleg, J. L., Ades, P. A., Chaitman, B. R., Millee, N. H., Mohiuddin, S. M., et al. (2002). Secondary prevention of coronary heart disease in the elderly (with emphasis on patients ≥75 years of age). *Circulation, 105*, 1735–1743.

Women's Health Initiative Investigators. (2002). Risks and benefits of estrogen plus progestin in healthy postmenopausal women: Principal results from the Women's Health Initiative randomized controlled trial. *Journal of the American Medical Association, 288*, 321–333.

Zarowitz, B. J., Aronow, W. S., Hollenack, K., & O'Shea, T. (2006). The application of evidence-based principles of care in older persons (issue 2): Management of lipid disorders. *Journal of American Medical Directors Association, 12*, 173–179.

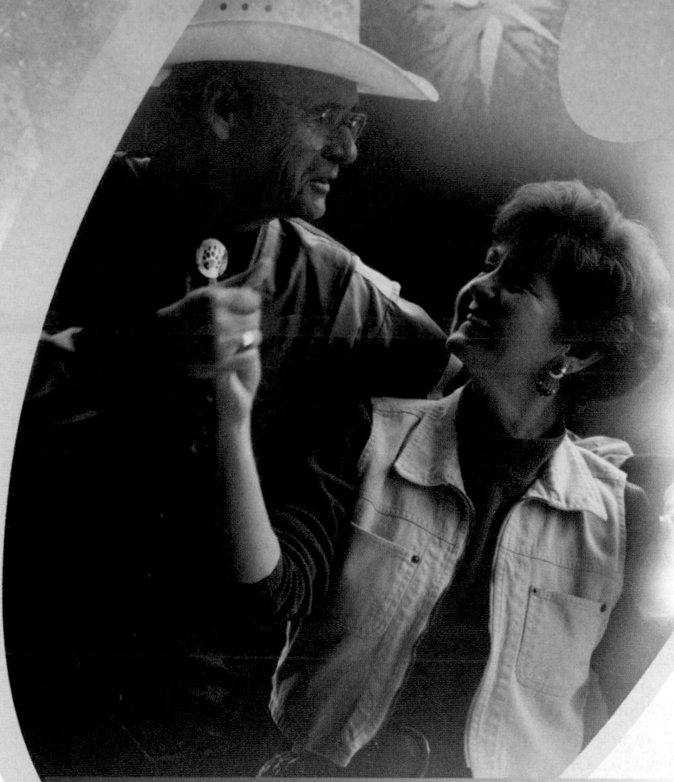

CHAPTER 21

Respiratory Function

Learning Objectives

After reading this chapter, you will be able to:

1. Describe age-related changes that affect respiratory function.
2. Identify risk factors that interfere with optimal respiratory function.
3. Discuss the functional consequences that affect respiratory wellness in older adults.
4. Assess respiratory function, with emphasis on identifying opportunities for health promotion.
5. Identify nursing interventions to improve respiratory function and reduce risk factors that interfere with respiratory wellness.

Key Terms

chronic obstructive pulmonary disease (COPD)
ductectasia
elastic recoil
kyphosis
lung parenchyma
secondhand smoke
smokeless tobacco

The primary functions of respiration are to supply oxygen to and remove carbon dioxide from the blood. Adequate respiratory performance is essential to life because all body organs and tissues need oxygen. Thus, it is noteworthy that the respiratory system shows less age-related decline than other body systems in healthy, nonsmoking, older adults. Because of genetic factors, respiratory function in older adults shows great individual variations. The age-related changes that do affect respiratory performance are subtle and gradual and healthy older adults are able to compensate for these changes. However, when illness, anesthesia, or another complicating factor places extraordinary demands for oxygen on the body, age-related respiratory changes can influence the overall function of the older adult.

AGE-RELATED CHANGES THAT AFFECT RESPIRATORY FUNCTION

As with other physiologic functions, it is difficult to distinguish the effects of age-related changes from those caused by disease processes and external influences, such as tobacco smoking. Although these influences occur throughout the life span, their cumulative effects become more pronounced in older adults. In addition, the cumulative effects are likely to have a greater effect when they interact with age-related changes, such as diminished immune response, or with risk factors, such as diminished mobility.

Upper Respiratory Structures

The nose is often overlooked in discussions of respiratory function, but age-related changes of the upper respiratory

Promoting Respiratory Wellness in Older Adults

Nursing Assessment
- Overall respiratory function
- Signs and symptoms of infection
- Tobacco use and attitudes about quitting
- Immunization status

Age-Related Changes
- ↑ stiffness of chest wall
- ↑ anteroposterior diameter
- Enlarged alveoli
- Weaker respiratory muscles
- ↓ response to hypercapnia or hypoxia

Negative Functional Consequences
- ↑ use of accessory muscles
- ↓ cough and gag reflexes
- ↑ energy expenditure for breathing
- ↓ efficiency of gas exchange
- ↑ susceptibility to respiratory infections

Risk Factors
- Tobacco smoking
- Environmental pollutants
- Occupational exposure to respiratory toxins

Nursing Interventions
- Teaching about smoking cessation
- Teaching about flu and pneumonia immunizations
- Teaching about preventing respiratory infections

Wellness Outcomes
- Improved respiratory function
- Decreased risk of respiratory infection
- Improved health from quitting smoking

structures can influence both comfort and function. For example, age-related connective tissue changes cause the nose to have a retracted columella (the lower edge of the septum) and a poorly supported, downwardly rotated tip. Although these changes are often viewed as having cosmetic, but not functional, effects, they can also cause septal deviations that interfere with the flow of air through the nasal cavity. These changes also can contribute to mouth breathing during sleep, causing snoring and obstructive apnea.

With increasing age, blood flow to the nose diminishes, causing the nasal turbinates to become smaller. Age-related changes also affect the submucosal glands, causing diminished secretions, even in healthy older adults. Because the secretions from the submucosal glands are thin and watery, their function is to dilute the thicker mucus secretions from the goblet cells. With diminished submucosal gland secretions, the mucus in the nasopharynx is thicker and more difficult to remove. This combination of age-related changes in turbinates, blood flow, and submucosal glands results in the presence of thicker and dryer secretions and a perception of nasal stuffiness. It also can cause stimulation of the cough reflex and a persistent tickle in the throat.

The epiglottis and upper airway structures expel mucus and unwanted material from the lungs and protect the lower airway from harmful substances, ranging in size from microorganisms to large pieces of food. An age-related change that affects these structures is calcification of the cartilage, which causes the trachea to stiffen. Another is blunting of the cough and laryngeal reflexes, with a concomitant decrease in coughing in older adults. Age-related reductions in the number of laryngeal nerve endings also have been noted, and these may contribute to diminished efficiency of the gag reflex.

Chest Wall and Musculoskeletal Structures

The chest wall and lungs function as one like a bellows, with the chest expanding outward in relation to lung expansion. The rib cage and the vertebral musculoskeletal structures are affected by the same kind of age-related changes that affect other musculoskeletal tissue: the ribs and vertebrae become osteoporotic, the costal cartilage becomes calcified, and the respiratory muscles become weaker. Because of these age-related processes, the following structural changes, which can affect respiratory performance, occur: **kyphosis** (i.e., an increased curvature of the spine), shortened thorax, chest wall stiffness, and increased anteroposterior diameter of the chest. As a result of these changes, older adults experience diminished respiratory efficiency and reduced maximal inspiratory and expiratory force. To compensate for age-related changes, older adults depend increasingly on accessory muscles, particularly the diaphragm, so they are increasingly sensitive to any changes in intra-abdominal pressure. In summary, older adults expend more energy to achieve the same respiratory efficiency as younger adults, but the overall effects on healthy older people are minimal.

Lung Structure and Function

Even in healthy older adults, lungs become smaller and flabbier, and their weight diminishes by approximately 20%. The age-related changes that have the most significant functional consequences are those that occur in the **lung parenchyma**, which is the part of the respiratory system where gas exchange takes place. The affected structures include the terminal bronchioles, alveolar ducts, alveoli, and capillaries. Beginning at around the age of 20 or 30 years, the alveoli progressively enlarge and their walls become thinner. This process of **ductectasia** continues throughout adulthood, causing approximately a 4% loss of alveolar surface area per decade. Because of this loss of alveolar surface, the amount of anatomic dead space increases. Age-related changes also affect the pulmonary vasculature. The trunk of the pulmonary artery becomes thickened and less extensible, and its diameter widens. The number of capillaries also diminishes, and pulmonary capillary blood volume decreases. Finally, the mucosal bed, where diffusion takes place, thickens.

Elastic recoil is the characteristic that keeps the airway open during inspiration by resisting expansion and maintaining a positive pressure across the lung surface. During expiration, elastic recoil keeps the airways open until the pressure placed on them by the respiratory muscles forces them to collapse. If the airways close prematurely, air is trapped and the lungs cannot expire to their maximum capacity. In healthy older adults, elastic recoil diminishes by a small degree, owing to a combination of age-related changes in the parenchyma and alterations in the elastic fibers. The end result is early airway closure, the mechanism that is responsible for age-related changes in lung volumes and air flow rates.

Specific aspects of lung function, such as air volumes and airflow rates, are measured by pulmonary function tests. In older adults, air volumes are altered because of the age-related changes in the chest wall and in lung elastic recoil. Because various air volumes are interrelated, however, the total lung capacity remains essentially the same due to compensatory mechanisms. Airflow rates are affected to a small degree by age-related changes and to a greater degree by additional variables, such as height, sex, and air volumes. Overall, there is an age-related decline in all airflow rates, but because of the many additional factors, there is a wide range of normal levels. Table 21-1 summarizes the age-related changes of some lung function parameters.

Because gas exchange is the primary function of the respiratory system, it is the most important functional aspect to consider. Oxygen–carbon dioxide exchange depends on a close match between ventilation (i.e., the amount of air in the lungs) and perfusion (i.e., the amount of blood flowing into the lungs). Because of age-related changes, particularly early airway closure, gas exchange is more likely to be compromised in the lower, rather than upper, lung regions. Consequently, inspired air is preferentially distributed in the upper regions, and a ventilation-to-perfusion mismatch results. The result of this mismatch is a gradual decrease in arterial oxygen pressure (PaO_2) of approximately 4 mm Hg per decade.

Compensatory changes in respiratory rate are made under conditions of hypercapnia (too much carbon dioxide) or hypoxia (too little oxygen). The response mechanism varies, depending on the stimulus. The response to hypercapnia is initiated by the central chemoreceptor, located in the medulla, whereas the response to hypoxia is initiated by peripheral chemoreceptors, located in the carotid and aortic bodies. When these mechanisms operate efficiently, the respiratory rate and depth increase in response to either low levels of oxygen or high levels of carbon dioxide. Age-related changes cause a 40% to 50% reduction in the ventilatory response to both hypoxia and hypercapnia between the third and eighth decades. Thus, instead of experiencing breathlessness or other respiratory symptoms when blood gases are abnormal, older adults are likely to develop mental changes.

TABLE 21-1 Age-Related Changes in Indicators of Lung Function

Indicator	Definition	Age-Related Change
Tidal volume	Amount of air moved in and out during a normal breath	Slight decrease
Residual volume	Amount of air left in the lungs after a forced expiration	Increases by 5%–10% per decade
Forced expiratory volume	Amount of air expelled within 1 second after a maximum inspiration	Decreases 23–32 mL/yr in men, 19–26 mL/yr in women
Forced inspiratory volume	Maximum volume of air that can be inhaled in addition to tidal volume	Decreases
Forced vital capacity	Maximum volume of air that can be expelled following a maximum inspiration	Decreases 14–30 mL/yr in men, 14–24 mL/yr in women
Total lung capacity	Amount of air that can be held in the lungs after a maximum inspiratory effort	Unchanged, as a result of compensatory mechanisms
Diffusing capacity	Ability of lungs to transfer gases between the lungs and blood	Declines 2.03 mL/min/mm Hg per decade in men, and 1.47 mL/min/mm Hg in women
Arterial oxygen pressure (PaO_2)	Amount of oxygen in arteries	Declines 0.3% per year or 4 mm Hg per decade, but remains stable after age 75 years

RISK FACTORS THAT AFFECT RESPIRATORY WELLNESS

For people of any age, tobacco smoking is the single most important risk factor for lung disease and impaired respiratory function; these risks are both immediate and cumulative. Other risks are mentioned because, particularly for nonsmokers, they can be addressed through health promotion interventions to improve respiratory function. For smokers, however, these other risks are of minimal importance, and attention must be focused on the serious negative consequences of smoking.

Tobacco Smoking

Tobacco smoking causes detrimental effects through heat and chemical actions on the respiratory system. Burning cigarettes release toxic gases, including carbon monoxide, hydrogen cyanide, and nitrogen dioxide. In addition, burning cigarettes release tobacco tar, which contains nicotine and many other harmful chemicals. Harmful physiologic effects on the respiratory system include, but are not limited to the following:

- Bronchoconstriction
- Inflammation of the mucosa throughout the respiratory tract
- Early airway closure (which is also an age-related change)
- Inhibited ciliary action, leading to increased coughing and mucous secretions and diminished protection from harmful organisms

Age-related changes and the cumulative effects of cigarette smoking compound the risks for older adults. Even in otherwise healthy people, smokers have a doubled or tripled rate of decline, compared with nonsmokers, in the forced expiratory volume at 1 second (FEV_1). This reduced FEV_1 is an accelerated and exacerbated age-related change that increases the risk for diseases, such as chronic obstructive pulmonary disease (COPD). In addition to being associated with detrimental effects on lung functioning, tobacco smoking is strongly associated with increased risk for serious diseases of the lungs, cardiovascular system, and many other systems. Smoking is strongly correlated with a number of cancers, including acute myelogenous leukemia and cancer of the lung, lip, oral cavity, pharynx, larynx, esophagus, stomach, liver, pancreas, cervix, uterus, kidney, and bladder (Vollset et al., 2006).

Diversity Note

Smoking prevalence ranking among various groups in the United States, from highest to lowest, is Native Americans/Alaska Natives, African Americans, whites, Hispanics, Asians/Pacific Islanders (USDHHS, 2000).

Although pipes and cigars are often viewed as safer than cigarettes, pipe and cigar smoking still carries risks for cancer, cardiovascular disease, and increased mortality. A large prospective study showed that pipe smoking was associating with an increased risk of death from COPD, cerebrovascular disease, coronary artery disease, and cancers of the lung, larynx, oropharynx, esophagus, colorectum, and pancreas (Henley et al., 2004). Research also challenges the perception that cigar smoking is a safe alternative to cigarettes, particularly with regard to the risk for cardiovascular disease (Vlachopoulos et al., 2004) and cancer of the pancreas (Alguacil & Silverman, 2004). Regardless of whether the person inhales when smoking pipes or cigars, the effects of the environmental tobacco smoke can be harmful to everyone who is exposed to **secondhand smoke** (also called sidestream, passive, or environmental tobacco smoke).

Smokeless tobacco (also called nonsmoking tobacco) also has been falsely viewed as harmless, but its use is highly associated with increased risk of gingivitis, tooth loss, and cancers of the mouth; its only advantage is that it does not contribute to environmental tobacco smoke. Because the use of smokeless tobacco is increasing and is the most common type of tobacco used in some countries, studies are just beginning to focus on health effects of these products (Teo et al., 2006). For example, studies of oral snuff (chewing tobacco) users suggest that it is carcinogenic to the pancreas (Boffetta et al., 2005) and that it increases the risk for stroke and cardiovascular disease (Henley et al., 2005; Rohani & Agewall, 2004). Another potentially detrimental health effect of smokeless tobacco that nurses need to be aware of is potential drug interactions. For example, smokeless tobacco can significantly interfere with warfarin by increasing levels of vitamin K (Kuykendall et al., 2004). Additional examples of drug–nicotine interactions are discussed in Chapter 8.

Wellness Opportunity

Older adults need to be aware of potential interactions between medications and nicotine products so they can avoid negative functional consequences that can affect their health.

Environmental Factors

Along with the skin, the physiologic function of the respiratory system is the one most directly influenced by air quality and other environmental factors. The negative effects of secondhand smoke were first reported to the public in the 1972 Surgeon General's Report. Although this report was initially viewed with some skepticism, the National Institutes of Health is very clear about the cause-and-effect relationship between exposure to smoke and human cancer incidence. For instance, environmental tobacco smoke causes approximately 3400 lung cancer deaths annually and as many as 69,000 deaths from coronary heart disease among adult nonsmokers in the United States (CDC, 2006). A study of adults with asthma showed that exposure to secondhand smoke was associated with poorer health outcomes (Eisner et al., 2005). Environmental smoke contains the same chemical compounds as mainstream smoke, but the particles are smaller and can be inhaled more deeply in the lungs. In fact, some of the harmful chemical compounds are in greater concentrations than in mainstream smoke (Nurminen & Jaakkola, 2001).

Respiratory function also is affected by environmental humidity and other characteristics. For example, dry air can affect the upper airway by further drying the nasal secretions, causing them to be thicker and more difficult to remove. Another environmental risk factor that can lead to negative functional consequences is the inhalation of air pollutants. Like the effects of cigarette smoking, the effects of air pollution are cumulative over many years and, therefore, have an increased impact on older adults who have been exposed to it over much of their lifetime. For example, older adults who have lived their entire lives in urban environments may have been exposed to air pollutants for as many as 7 or 8 decades.

In addition to being exposed to general air pollutants, older adults who worked in occupations such as mining and firefighting might experience the cumulative and long-term effects of occupational exposure to toxic substances. Because hazards in the workplace were largely unregulated before the 1970s, many older people never benefited from the protections enforced under the Occupational Safety and Health Act. In addition, much of the information now available on the harmful effects of certain chemicals was not widely available when these older adults were working. Even though the exposure to harmful substances may have occurred long ago, occupational lung disease may not be identified until later adulthood, when the cumulative effects lead to signs and symptoms. Some of the job categories associated with an increased risk of respiratory disease are listed in Box 21-1.

Additional Risk Factors

A unique characteristic of respiratory performance is that the maximum level of function in middle and later adulthood is significantly influenced by the maximum level reached during the third decade of life, which is largely determined by factors that affected respiratory development in early life. Because respiratory complaints develop when pulmonary function is reduced to half of the maximally attained level, older adults whose peak level was higher during early adulthood can tolerate a greater degree of age-related changes and exposure to risk factors before experiencing respiratory dysfunction. Conversely, older adults who did not attain a high peak level during their twenties will experience the effects of age-related changes and risk factors at an earlier age.

In addition to the age-related changes that involve the respiratory system, age-related changes affecting other aspects of functioning can also affect respiratory performance. For example, both kyphosis, which is caused by age-related skeletal changes, and poor posture can interfere with maximum respiratory performance. A decline in immune response and host defense mechanisms is an age-related change that contributes to the increased morbidity and mor-

Box 21-1
Workforces With an Increased Risk for Harmful Respiratory Effects

Firefighters
Miners
Traffic controllers
Shipyard workers
Rubber workers
Aluminum workers
Iron and steel foundry workers
Tunnel and street repair workers
Asbestos workers
Quarry workers
Farmers, agricultural workers, grain handlers
Construction workers
Paper mill workers
Workers exposed to the following: dust, fumes, gases, nickel, arsenic, beryllium, chromium, or radiation

tality when older adults acquire pneumonia and other lower respiratory infections.

Any condition or chronic illness that interferes with chest wall expansion, which is already compromised by age-related changes, increases the risk for impaired respiratory function. For example, restricted activity, a recumbent position, and conditions that cause shallow breathing exacerbate the effects of age-related changes and result in compromised respiratory performance. Therefore, any older adult who is on bed rest, even for short periods, is at increased risk for impaired respiratory function.

Obesity is another health-related risk factor that can interfere with respiratory function through its effects on an individual's overall activity level. Obesity also affects the ability to take deep breaths and to ventilate the lower lobes of the lung. Even minor changes in body weight can affect ventilatory capacity, with weight gain and loss being associated with a decline or improvement in lung function (Aaron et al., 2004).

Medications increase the risk for impaired respiratory function in several ways. For example, sedatives and anticholinergic medications can affect upper airway function by drying the mucus. Medications also may influence cough reflexes. Angiotensin-converting enzyme inhibitors, for example, can cause persistent dry cough.

Although healthy older adults are not likely to develop aspiration pneumonia, this is a common and serious respiratory condition in long-term care residents and in older adults with compromised functional status. Factors that increase the risk for aspiration pneumonia include neoplasm, dysphagia, general debility, tube feeding, malnutrition and dehydration, poor oral hygiene, decreased cough reflex, diminished salivary flow, compromised immune function, altered levels of consciousness, and use of broad-spectrum antibiotics (Coleman, 2004).

PATHOLOGIC CONDITION AFFECTING RESPIRATORY FUNCTION: COPD

Chronic obstructive pulmonary disease (COPD) is a group of diseases, including emphysema, chronic bronchitis, and a subset of asthma, characterized by chronic airflow obstruction. Age and smoking are the two major risk factors for COPD that act synergistically. The prevalence of COPD among smokers between the ages of 76 and 77 years is reported to be approximately 50%, but the prevalence and severity of COPD is underdiagnosed in both the middle-aged and the older adult population groups (Lindberg et al., 2006). Risk factors for COPD include genetic predisposition, tobacco smoking, increased age, low socioeconomic status, exposure to environmental smoke and other toxins, and history of significant childhood respiratory disease. Although tobacco smoking increases the risk for COPD, nonsmokers account for 22% to 25% of the cases in the United States, the United Kingdom, and Spain (Behrendt, 2005).

A Student's Perspective

I was glad to interact with someone who has emphysema and to learn about her struggles and about how care needs to be specialized for her because of her condition. Listening to E.A.'s breath sounds was frightening to me. I knew she was unable to breathe well, but I had no idea it was that obstructed. The struggle and stress her condition puts on her body to breathe is saddening. I really am amazed she is able to function as well as she does with her decreased level of oxygen.

I really enjoyed how talkative E.A. was. I had no problem getting information from her to complete her functional health assessment. It really hit me after I walked out of the nursing home on Friday that she literally talked to me for 3 hours. She was absolutely beside herself just to have someone there to listen and to interact with. I was glad I was able to give that to her. I believe this experience with E.A. will help me in the future to remember to give the emotional care as well as the physical.

In the next week, the things I would like to improve include supporting and promoting E.A. to get up and get dressed. I would like to help her with performing ADLs and help make her morning more worthwhile. I think helping E.A. become a little more productive could also help improve her social interactions. This is an area she needs a lot of help with, and I hope this week I will be able to give her support in doing so.

Jenna W.

The most common manifestations of COPD are cough, dyspnea, wheezing, and increased sputum production. The condition is progressive and its cumulative effects become more disabling as the person ages. Older adults with COPD are likely to have longer hospitalizations and an increased risk for being discharged to nursing facilities. Another negative consequence of COPD is impaired health-related quality of life (Miravitlles et al., 2005).

Diversity Note

Although COPD is thought to be more prevalent among men than women, some of this disparity may be due to significant underdiagnosis of COPD, particularly in women (Chapman et al., 2001).

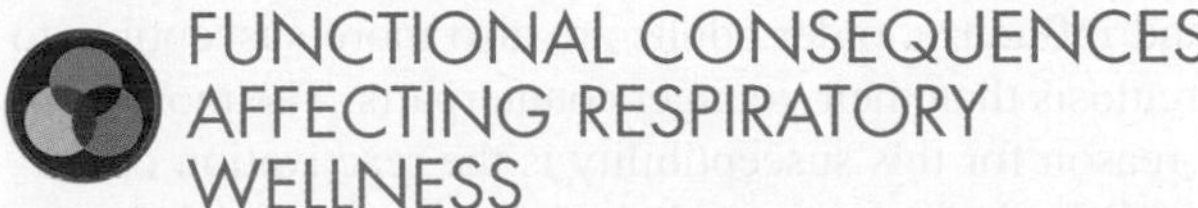

FUNCTIONAL CONSEQUENCES AFFECTING RESPIRATORY WELLNESS

In the absence of smoking and other risk factors, healthy older adults do not experience any significant functional consequences related to respiratory function when perform-

TABLE 21-2 Functional Consequences of Age-Related Changes Affecting Respiratory Function

Change	Consequence
Upper airway changes: calcification of cartilage, altered neuromuscular function and reflexes	Snoring, mouth breathing, diminished cough reflex, decreased efficiency of gag reflex
Increased anteroposterior diameter, chest wall stiffness, weakened muscles and diaphragm	Increased use of accessory muscles, increased energy expended for respiratory efficiency
Enlargement of alveoli, thinning of alveolar walls, diminished number of capillaries	Diminished efficiency of gas exchange, decreased arterial oxygen pressure (PaO_2)
Decreased elastic recoil and early airway closure	Changes in lung volumes, slight decrease in overall efficiency
Tidal volume unchanged or slightly diminished, increased residual volume, decreased vital capacity	Total lung capacity unchanged

ing ordinary activities. Under conditions of physical stress, however, older adults may become dyspneic and fatigued because their respiratory system is less efficient in gas exchange. Similarly, age-related changes in the respiratory system do not affect exercise capacity, but deconditioning and risk factors can compromise it. Table 21-2 summarizes the functional consequences of age-related changes that affect respiratory wellness.

For nonsmoking older adults, the most significant negative functional consequence of age-related changes and risk factors is an increased susceptibility to lower respiratory infections. The combination of age-related changes in respiratory function and age-related changes in immunity contributes to an increased risk of acquiring pneumonia and influenza in older adulthood. People older than 65 years of age are four times more likely to acquire pneumonia then their younger counterparts. Another functional consequence is that lower respiratory infections are likely to lead to death or cause a decline in functional status in older adults. For example, mortality rates for hospitalized older patients with community-acquired pneumonia are as high as 30%, and the rate for those with nursing home–acquired pneumonia is as high as 57% (Janssens & Krause, 2004). The higher morbidity and mortality is due in part to the difficulty of diagnosing pneumonia during early stages because the manifestations are subtle and nonspecific.

In addition to being increasingly susceptible to pneumonia and influenza, older adults are also more susceptible to tuberculosis than their younger counterparts. The most common reason for this susceptibility is the reactivation of dormant tuberculosis, particularly in the presence of risk factors such as smoking, diabetes, malnutrition, debilitating conditions, or long-term use of corticosteroids. The incidence of tuberculosis in community-living older adults is twice that of the general population; however, for older adults in long-term care facilities, the incidence is four times higher than that in the general population. Some of the cases of tuberculosis that affect long-term care residents are attributable to the ease with which this disease can spread among residents. Moreover, altered and more subtle disease manifestations interfere with identification and treatment of tuberculosis in older adults (as discussed in the section on Nursing Assessment of Respiratory Function). As with pneumonia, mortality rates for older adults with tuberculosis are higher than those for younger populations.

Older adults who smoke or have other risk factors experience the same negative consequences as younger adults, but the effects are cumulative. That is, they will have higher rates of cancer, cardiovascular disease, COPD, and other diseases than those without risk factors. For example, smokers age 65 and older have twice the cancer and cardiovascular mortality than their nonsmoking peers (Whitson et al., 2006).

Diversity Note

Tuberculosis is more prevalent in African Americans, Hispanics, Native Americans, and Asian Americans than in whites.

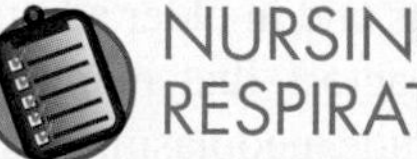

NURSING ASSESSMENT OF RESPIRATORY FUNCTION

Nursing assessment of respiratory function is similar for older and younger adults, but nurses must assess the different life experiences of older adults—particularly with regard to exposure to environmental toxins and attitudes about tobacco use—when identifying opportunities for health promotion. Nurses also must consider variations in the manifestations of lower respiratory infections and minor differences in the physical assessment of the respiratory system in older adults. Nursing assessment of respiratory function involves identifying opportunities for health promotion, detecting lower respiratory infections, assessing smoking behaviors, and identifying other risk factors.

Identifying Opportunities for Health Promotion

Nurses interview older adults, or their caregivers, to identify the risk factors that can be addressed through health promotion activities. Because tobacco smoking is the risk factor that contributes most to impaired respiratory function and lung diseases, nurses assess the potential for influencing all smokers, even older adults, to quit. Information obtained through assessment questions about smoking provides the base for health education approaches. Assessment questions also provide information about other preventive aspects, such as influenza and pneumonia vaccinations. Nurses iden-

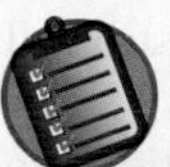

Box 21-2
Guidelines for Assessing Respiratory Function

Questions to Identify Risk Factors for Respiratory Problems

- Have you had any respiratory problems, such as asthma, chronic lung disease, pneumonia, or other infections?
- Do you have a family history of chronic lung disease?
- Have you ever had tuberculosis?
- Have you ever worked in a job where you were exposed to dust, fumes, smoke, or other air pollutants (e.g., in mining, farming, or any of the occupations listed in Box 21-1)?
- Have you lived in neighborhoods where there was a lot of pollution from traffic or factories?
- Do you smoke now, or have you ever smoked? (If yes, continue with the questions in Box 21-3.)
- Have you been exposed to passive smoke in home, work, or social environments?

Questions to Identify Opportunities for Education About Disease Prevention and Health Promotion

- Have you ever had a pneumonia vaccination? (If yes, ask about when the vaccination was administered and whether a booster was ever given.)
- Do you get annual influenza vaccinations?

Questions to Assess Overall Respiratory Function

- Do you have any problems with breathing?
- Do you have any wheezing?
- Do you have spells of coughing? *If yes:* When do they occur? How long do they last? What brings them on? Are they dry or productive? Does the phlegm come from your throat or lungs? What does the phlegm look like?
- Do you ever have trouble getting enough air during any particular activities or when you lie down at night?
- Have you stopped doing any particular activities because of problems breathing? For example, have you stopped going up or down stairs, or have you limited the amount of walking you do? (For people with mobility limitations, this question might not be relevant.)
- Do you ever have any chest pain, or feelings of heaviness or tightness in your chest?
- Do you use more than one pillow at night, or make any other adjustments, because of trouble with breathing?
- Do you wake up at night because of coughing or difficulty with breathing?
- Do you ever feel as though you can't catch your breath?
- Do you have trouble breathing when the weather is hot, cold, or humid?
- Do you tire easily?

tify attitudes of older adults about these preventive interventions, so they can plan appropriate health promotion approaches. Last, nurses ask older adults about their overall respiratory function to identify respiratory problems that can be addressed in the nursing care plan. Box 21-2 presents an interview format that nurses can use to assess risk factors, overall respiratory function, and opportunities for health education.

Wellness Opportunity

Nurses ask at least one question to identify the person's health-promoting behaviors, such as "What do you do to avoid environmental tobacco smoke?"

Detecting Lower Respiratory Infections

The term *detection* is more accurate than *assessment* with regard to lower respiratory infections because when older adults have pneumonia, they do not always meet the typical assessment criteria. Rather than presenting with a cough, chills, dyspnea, elevated temperature, and elevated white blood cell count, older adults are more likely to have subtler and nonspecific disease manifestations. Even an initial chest radiograph may not provide accurate diagnostic information. Rather, older adults are likely to present with an altered mental status (delirium) or other changes in functioning, such as incontinence, unexplained falls, sudden aggravation, or failure to thrive (Janssens & Krause, 2004). Other clinical manifestations of pneumonia most commonly seen in older adults, particularly during the early stages of the disease, are headache, weakness, anorexia, lethargy, dehydration, and a decline in overall function.

In respiratory infections such as pneumonia, the clinical symptoms of tachypnea and tachycardia are present in only about two thirds of older patients (Janssens & Krause, 2004). Temperature elevations may occur later in the disease process rather than earlier. The changes in lung sounds that are commonly associated with pneumonia may not be present; in fact, the only respiratory sign may be tachypnea. Dyspnea or breathlessness is likely to have a later onset, or it may be absent if the older adult restricts his or her activities to avoid dyspnea on exertion. In older adults with pneumonia, the most significant finding on physical assessment of the lungs may be a diminished intensity of lung sounds or the presence of rales and rhonchi, which are very nonspecific findings.

Nurses must keep in mind that although older adults may exhibit the typical manifestations of pneumonia, the absence of these manifestations is not as significant in older adults as it is in younger adults. In older adults, a change in mental status or another alteration in functional status, such as falls or incontinence, may be the major clue to the presence of pneumonia. Thus, an important nursing responsibility is to detect nonspecific manifestations of pneumonia and collect additional information. Astute nursing observations about nonspecific manifestations are essential for ensuring a timely diagnosis and preventing the progression of pneumonia.

In addition to being aware of the different manifestations of pneumonia in older adults, nurses also must be aware of the increased rates and varied manifestations of tuberculosis in this population. As with pneumonia, diagnosis and treatment of tuberculosis in older adults are often delayed because of nonspecific clinical and radiologic findings; at times, the disease is discovered only on autopsy (Van den Brande, 2005). Another reason that tuberculosis is more difficult to detect in older adults is that about one third of older adults have false-negative tuberculin skin test reactions. Because tuberculosis often occurs as a reactivation of dormant disease, nurses must be particularly alert for manifestations of this disease in older adults who have a history of tuberculosis. Older adults have a high rate of false-negative tuberculin skin test reactions, but the two-step Mantoux test with tuberculin purified protein derivative (PPD) is the recommended method of assessing for previous exposure to tuberculosis.

Assessing Smoking Behaviors

Although smoking affects all people, regardless of age, some aspects of smoking behaviors differ according to age cohorts. Therefore, an assessment of smoking as a risk factor must address the age-related factors that affect these behaviors. The cohort of people born between 1910 and 1930, for example, is the first age group to be exposed to the social pressures that encouraged smoking without knowing about its detrimental effects. As a result, people who began smoking in the early 1920s, when it became a popular habit for men in the United States, may have smoked for 4 or 5 decades before finding out that smoking is harmful. For women in the United States, smoking was not socially acceptable until the mid-1940s. Thus, the cohort of smoking women who are now in their sixties is the first group of women who have smoked throughout their adulthood. Not until 1964 did the U.S. Surgeon General issue the first report on the detrimental effects of cigarette smoking, *Smoking and Health*. By this time, men had been smoking for 4 decades and women had been smoking for 2 decades. Thus, older adults who have a long history of smoking may have an outlook reflected in statements such as, "If I've smoked this long and am still alive, why should I quit now?"

In addition to assessing attitudes about smoking, nurses should assess past and present smoking patterns. Frequency of smoking and type of tobacco smoked are important determinants of the relative risk of smoking. Smokeless tobacco, for example, is not as detrimental to respiratory and cardiovascular function as cigarette smoking, but it does increase the risk of oral cancer. Cigarettes vary in the amount of nicotine they contain, and this variable influences the degree of risk associated with a particular type of cigarette. In contrast to younger adults, who began smoking when cigarettes had filters and were lower in nicotine, older adults began smoking when cigarettes had no filters and contained greater amounts of tar and nicotine. Older adults, therefore, are likely to smoke cigarettes that have higher and more harmful nicotine levels. Some older adults, in fact, may still roll their own cigarettes using loose tobacco.

For older adults who smoke, nurses ask questions to determine their readiness to consider quitting smoking as well as their knowledge about the health effects of smoking. Nurses also assess the older adult's perception of smoking as a manifestation of his or her rights and autonomy. As with other health care decisions, adults are entitled to make decisions about their health-related behaviors, but these decisions should be based on full knowledge of the benefits and risks of their choices. Many beliefs and attitudes about smoking may arise primarily from lack of information. Wolfsen and colleagues (2001) found that elderly nursing home residents do not hold strong antismoking views and lack information about the relationships between smoking and health. Residents viewed smoking as "the singular remaining vestige of their former life as competent independent adults" (p. 10). The authors of this study suggested that educational interventions for nursing home residents might be a step toward reducing the prevalence of smoking in this population.

Nurses may need to examine their own attitudes about smoking, especially in relation to older adults. For example, it is important to identify ageist influences that can lead to the view that smoking cessation would not be beneficial for older adults. Similarly, although it is important to respect the rights of older adults who choose to smoke, health care professionals should not exclude older adults from health promotion interventions about smoking simply because they are old. Assessment questions designed to help determine smoking habits and attitudes about smoking are included in Box 21-3.

Wellness Opportunity

To assess smoking behaviors from a whole-person perspective, nurses need to ask questions about the older adult's knowledge about the detrimental effects of smoking as well as their perception of smoking as an expression of autonomy.

Identifying Other Risk Factors

In addition to assessing tobacco use as a risk factor, nurses identify other factors that affect respiratory function in less significant ways. Because maximum respiratory function is attained by early adulthood, nurses assess factors that may have influenced respiratory development in early life. For example, questions about nutrition, respiratory infections, and exposure to cigarette smoke may be helpful in assessing the older adult's maximum respiratory function and in providing information about the person's vulnerability to the effects of age-related changes and risk factors. For this reason, nurses incorporate questions about exposure to environmental tobacco smoke and harmful air pollutants in their assessments.

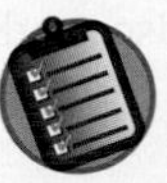

Box 21-3
Guidelines for Nursing Assessment of Older Adults Who Smoke

Questions to Assess Smoking Behaviors

- How long have you smoked?
- How much do you smoke?
- What do you smoke?
- Have you smoked other types of tobacco in the past?

Questions to Assess Knowledge of the Risk From Smoking

- Do you think there are any harmful effects of smoking for people in general?
- Do you think you are at risk for any harmful effects from smoking?
- Do you think there are any benefits to quitting smoking?

Questions to Assess Attitudes Toward Smoking

- Have you ever thought about quitting smoking?
- Has any health professional ever talked to you about quitting smoking?
- What do you think about the idea of quitting smoking?
- Have you ever tried to quit? *If yes:* What was your experience with the attempt?
- Would you be interested in finding out information about quitting smoking now?

Occupational exposure to certain harmful substances is particularly important for smokers because the risk of either one of these factors is compounded when the other factor is present. Nurses also assess the person's level of activity and identify factors that interfere with mobility or routine activities because these conditions can influence the degree to which the person can improve his or her level of activity. If, for example, people have limited mobility because of arthritis, they may not be able to engage in vigorous physical exercise, but they might benefit greatly from water exercises. Box 21-2 summarizes guidelines for assessing respiratory function in older adults.

Wellness Opportunity

To set the stage for health education about preventive measures, nurses asses the older adult's understanding of influenza and pneumonia vaccinations.

Physical Assessment Findings

Nurses use the usual methods of inspection, palpation, percussion, and auscultation to evaluate respiratory performance in both younger and older adults. Minor differences in assessment findings for healthy older adults include:

- Slight increase in the normal respiratory rate, which ranges from 16 to 24 respirations per minute
- Increased anteroposterior diameter
- Forward leaning posture because of kyphosis
- Increased resonance on percussion
- Diminished intensity of lung sounds
- Increased presence of adventitious sounds in the lower lungs

Nurses begin the assessment of respiratory function by observing the person's breathing pattern when he or she is walking, changing position, or even sitting. Asking the older adult to sit upright, cough before auscultation, and breathe as deeply as possible with his or her mouth open will facilitate auscultation of breath sounds. When nurses have an opportunity to observe respirations in a sleeping older adult, they may see frequent but brief periods of apnea. This phenomenon is common in older adults and is highly associated with sleep problems, as discussed in Chapter 24, Sleep and Rest. With the exceptions of pneumonia and tuberculosis, the manifestations of most respiratory diseases, such as influenza and COPD, do not differ in older and younger adults.

Mr. R. is 70 years old and comes with his wife to the senior center where you provide weekly nursing services. Both Mr. and Mrs. R. smoke one to two packs of cigarettes a day. Mr. R. has mild COPD and Mrs. R. has hypertension and coronary artery disease. Every October, the senior center offers flu shots for anyone over the age of 65 years. As you are preparing to give flu shots, Mr. and Mrs. R. come to you and ask, "Is this the shot that takes care of pneumonia? Our daughter said we should get a pneumonia shot every year, but we don't want a flu shot because our friend says she got the flu from one of those shots and she'll never get a shot again. Can you just give us the pneumonia shot today? We got one from the doctor last year but it's too expensive to get it from him."

THINKING POINTS

- What myths and misunderstandings do Mr. and Mrs. R. express?
- What further assessment questions would you ask?
- What health promotion teaching would you do?

NURSING DIAGNOSIS

The nursing diagnosis of Ineffective Breathing Pattern would be applicable when the nursing assessment identifies factors that may impair the older adult's respiratory function. This diagnosis is defined as "the state in which the individual experiences an actual or potential loss of adequate ventilation related to an altered breathing pattern" (Carpenito-Moyet, 2006, p. 376). Defining characteristics include cough, dyspnea, shortness of breath, and changes in respiratory rate or pattern from baseline. If impaired respiratory function interferes with activities of daily living, a nursing diagnosis of Activity Intolerance might be appropriate. Debilitated or chronically ill older adults who live in group settings may be at risk for infections, particularly pneumonia, influenza, and tuberculosis. For example, if a long-term care resident has active tuberculosis, the nursing staff might address the nursing diagnosis of Risk for Infection Transmission for the affected resident and the nursing diagnosis of Risk for Infection for all other residents. Likewise, when influenza affects one or more residents or staff of a long-term care or group living facility, the same nursing diagnoses may be applicable. Ineffective Health Maintenance is a nursing diagnosis that may be used for older adults who have insufficient knowledge about the detrimental effects of active or passive smoking.

Wellness Opportunity

When nurses provide pneumonia or influenza immunizations for older adults, they can use the wellness nursing diagnosis of Readiness for Enhanced Immunization Status.

PLANNING FOR WELLNESS OUTCOMES

When caring for older adults with respiratory problems, nurses identify wellness outcomes as an essential part of the planning process. Nurses can use the following Nursing Outcomes Classification (NOC) terminology in care plans that address the nursing diagnosis of Ineffective Breathing Pattern: Vital Signs, Respiratory Status: Airway Patency, and Respiratory Status: Ventilation.

For the majority of older adults who have adequate respiratory function, nurses plan for wellness outcomes by addressing their increased vulnerability to pneumonia, influenza, and tuberculosis. NOC terminology pertinent to the nursing diagnosis of Risk for Infection include Immune Status, Immunization Behavior, and Community Risk Control: Communicable Disease.

An appropriate wellness outcome for older adults who lack knowledge about preventing respiratory infections would be Knowledge: Health Behaviors. A specific and easily measured outcome of successful health education might be that older adults obtain immunizations against pneumonia and influenza.

Wellness Opportunity

Nurses promote wellness when their care plans address the immunization status of older adults.

Because tobacco smoking is the most important factor that influences respiratory function, nurses working with older adults who smoke should always consider the possibility of identifying and working toward a goal of reducing or eliminating tobacco use. Thus, for older adults who smoke, NOCs include Risk Control: Tobacco Use and Knowledge: Substance Use Control.

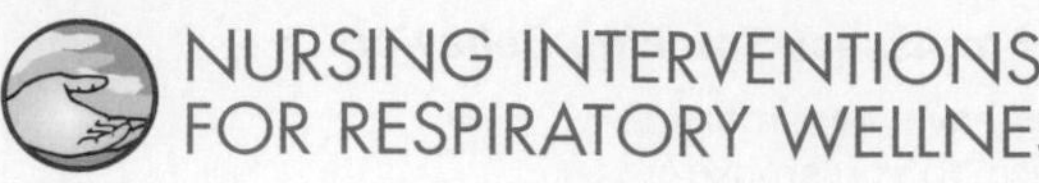

NURSING INTERVENTIONS FOR RESPIRATORY WELLNESS

For all older adults, nursing interventions to promote respiratory wellness focus on protection from secondhand smoke and prevention of respiratory infections. For those who smoke, teaching about smoking cessation is the most important intervention for respiratory wellness. The following Nursing Interventions Classification (NIC) terminology might be applicable in care plans to promote respiratory wellness: Environmental Risk Protection, Health Education, Immunization/Vaccination Management, Infection Control, Infection Protection, Referral, and Smoking Cessation Assistance.

Promoting Health for Respiratory Wellness

It is widely acknowledged that smoking is the single most important preventable cause of disease and death in the United States and therefore should be a major target of disease prevention activities. Because most older smokers already have at least minor smoking-related conditions affecting respiratory function and other systems, smoking cessation will address secondary or tertiary prevention rather than primary prevention. Smoking cessation is more cost-effective as a health promotion activity than other common preventive services, including mammography, Pap tests, colon cancer screening, and treatment of hypercholesterolemia or mild to moderate hypertension (CDC, 2000).

Healthy People 2010 addresses 21 national health objectives related to tobacco smoking and several additional objectives related to tuberculosis, pneumonia, occupational lung disease, and COPD (USDHHS, 2000). Disease prevention and health promotion interventions related to respiratory function that are particularly applicable to older adults include pneumonia and influenza vaccinations and education about the importance of stopping smoking and avoiding environmental tobacco smoke. These interventions are discussed in the following sections and summarized in Boxes 21-4 and 21-5. In addition, numerous educational materials are available for use in disease prevention and health promotion interventions, and many of these are available in languages other than English.

Since the early 1990s, the Centers for Disease Control and Prevention (CDC), the National Institutes of Health, and other governmental health agencies have emphasized the importance of diminishing environmental tobacco smoke. An objective of *Healthy People 2010* is to eliminate exposure to environmental tobacco smoke through laws, policies, and regulations requiring smoke-free environments in schools, work sites, and public places (USDHHS, 2000). Nurses address the influence of the environment on health

Box 21-4
Health Promotion Teaching About Respiratory Problems

Factors That Increase the Risk for Pneumonia and Influenza

- Diabetes or any chronic lung, heart, or kidney disease
- Hospitalization within the past year for heart or lung diseases
- Severe anemia or a debilitating condition
- Confinement to bed or very limited mobility
- Residence in a nursing home or other group living setting
- Immunosuppressive medications

Preventing Respiratory Infection

- Wash your hands frequently with an antibacterial soap or hand sanitizer.
- Avoid hand-to-mouth and hand-to-eye contact.
- Avoid inhaling air that has been contaminated with particles from the cough or sneeze of someone with an infection.
- Avoid crowds during the flu season.
- Be sure that influenza and pneumonia vaccinations are up to date.

Information About Influenza Vaccinations

- New vaccinations are developed every year, based on information about the strains of viruses that are most likely to affect people during the influenza season.
- Vaccines are made from inactivated viruses and, therefore, should have few or no side effects.
- People who are allergic to eggs and egg products should NOT receive influenza immunizations.
- Immunizations do not offer immediate protection because there is a 2- to 3-week delay in developing an antibody response.
- Every year, the manufacturers of the influenza vaccination provide recommendations as to the best time for administering the immunizations for optimal effectiveness. The best time is during the late fall, but the exact time period will vary slightly from year to year.
- Vaccines are not 100% effective, but they are helpful for most older people.
- Influenza immunizations provide protection against the most serious viruses but not against all types of respiratory infections.
- The duration of effectiveness of vaccinations may be shorter than 6 months in some older people; therefore, one vaccination might not protect the person through the entire season.
- In 1993, Medicare began paying for flu shots.

Information About Pneumonia Vaccinations

- Pneumonia vaccinations are recommended for people older than 65 years of age.
- Pneumonia vaccinations were considered one-time-only immunizations, but boosters are now being recommended for older adults who received their initial immunization 5 or more years ago.
- Side effects, if they occur, are not serious and will subside within a few days.
- Common side effects include a slight fever accompanied by pain, redness, or tenderness at the injection site.
- Pneumonia vaccinations are covered by Medicare and other health insurance.

Nutritional Considerations

- Include foods high in zinc and vitamins A, B-complex, C, and E.

Complementary and Alternative Care Practices

- Humidifier, vaporizer, air filter, mustard poultice, steam therapy
- Herbs for colds or coughs: thyme, yarrow, garlic, hyssop, coltsfoot, licorice, peppermint, Echinacea, marsh mallow, slippery elm, red sage
- Aromatherapy: thyme, lemon, menthol, camphor, eucalyptus, lavender, tea tree
- Acupuncture may be used for coughs, influenza, upper respiratory infections, nasal allergic conditions, and chronic respiratory conditions

by teaching about the importance of avoiding environmental tobacco smoke.

Wellness Opportunity

Nurses promote self-care behaviors by encouraging older adults to use patient teaching materials from the agencies listed in the educational resources list at the end of this chapter.

Preventing Lower Respiratory Infections

Interventions to prevent pneumonia and influenza are particularly important because these two conditions collectively constitute the fourth leading cause of death in people older than 65 years of age. Moreover, of all the leading causes of death in older adults, pneumonia and influenza are the only ones that can be prevented without the considerable investment of time, money, and motivation. Nurses also have important roles in addressing tuberculosis, particularly for medically compromised older adults in long-term and residential care facilities. The following sections discuss the role of the nurse in preventing these types of lower respiratory infections, with emphasis on health education interventions.

The influenza vaccine is safe and well tolerated in older adults and has been shown to reduce mortality and morbidity as well as decrease hospitalization admission rates for respiratory infection (Janssens & Krause, 2004). Despite the efficacy of influenza vaccinations, fewer than half of all older adults in the United States receive them each year. Many institutional settings have standing orders for influenza and pneumonia vaccinations, and nurses play a primary role in implementing this health promotion intervention in community, residential, and institutional settings. In addition, any health care worker who cares for older adults should receive annual influenza vaccinations to prevent transmission and thus indirectly reduce mortality from influenza in the older population.

Box 21-5
Health Promotion Teaching About Cigarette Smoking

Attitudes About Smoking

Stopping smoking at any age is more beneficial than continuing to smoke.

- Many of the harmful effects of smoking are reversed once the smoker quits.
- Although some of the effects of past smoking are irreversible, all of the harmful effects of future smoking can be avoided by quitting now.
- Smoking is a major risk factor for many cancers, including those of the lung, head, stomach, kidney, and pancreas.
- Smoking is a major risk factor for lung and heart disease, including high blood pressure and heart attacks.
- Passive smoking (inhaling smoke from the air) is associated with an increased risk for many diseases.

Type of Tobacco

- The lower the tar and nicotine content of cigarettes, the less harmful the effects. Many cigarettes with lower tar and nicotine levels, however, have additional chemical additives that can be harmful.
- Pipe and cigar smokers are at a higher risk for chronic lung disease than nonsmokers, just as cigarette smokers are.
- The harmful effects of tobacco use on the mouth and upper respiratory tract are equal for all types of tobacco, including smokeless tobacco. All smokers have the same risk for developing cancer of the mouth and upper respiratory tract. Snuff, chewing tobacco, and smokeless tobacco contain nicotine and many other harmful chemicals. The only advantage of smokeless tobacco is that it does not affect other people nearby.

Approaches to Quitting

- Any reduction in present tobacco use is better than maintaining the current level. The negative effects of smoking are directly proportional to the number of cigarettes inhaled.
- Various forms of prescription and over-the-counter nicotine substitutes (e.g., gum, skin patches, and nasal sprays) are available and may be helpful, especially when used in conjunction with counseling and self-help techniques.
- Besides nicotine substitutes, some non-nicotine prescription medications and over-the-counter products may be effective as a component of a smoking cessation program.
- People who are trying to quit smoking should discuss their goals with a health care professional to identify the methods that might be most effective.
- Many self-help programs are available for support and education regarding quitting smoking.
- Information about group programs can be obtained on the Internet or by calling the local office of any of the following organizations: American Lung Association, American Heart Association, or American Cancer Society.

Complementary and Alternative Care Practices to Help Quit Smoking

- Herbs: combination of coltsfoot and plantain
- Homeopathic remedies: plantain, nox vomica
- Citric acid throat spray
- Exercise, music, imagery, massage, meditation, affirmations, deep breathing, stress reduction, social support, individual or group counseling

Although the benefits of annual influenza immunizations are well accepted and well publicized, pneumonia vaccinations have received less attention. In immunocompetent older adults, efficacy of the pneumococcal vaccine is estimated to be 50% to 70% for the 23 organisms that most commonly cause pneumonia (Adis Data Group, 2005). The CDC recommends pneumonia vaccinations for all people aged 65 years and older. Since 1997, the CDC has recommended a one-time booster dose for all people aged 65 years or older if they received an initial pneumonia vaccination 5 or more years earlier and if they were younger than 65 years at the time of initial vaccination. Pneumonia vaccinations are also recommended for older adults who are uncertain about their vaccination status. Box 21-4 summarizes current information about influenza and pneumonia immunizations, along with information about risk factors for these illnesses.

In addition to promoting pneumonia and influenza immunizations, nurses need to promote adequate nutrition and hydration as preventive measures for all older adults. Nurses who care for long-term care residents and older adults with compromised functioning need to implement direct nursing interventions to prevent pneumonia, including aspiration pneumonia. Provision of good oral hygiene—including measures to prevent the accumulation of plaque on teeth and dentures—is important for reducing the growth of pathogens that lead to aspiration pneumonia. Additional nursing interventions for preventing lower respiratory infections include meticulous attention to handwashing and optimal positioning and turning of patients who have limited mobility.

Nurses working in long-term care or other group living facilities are responsible for implementing programs to detect and address tuberculosis. The CDC website (www.CDC.gov) provides up-to-date guidelines for screening and diagnostic methods, such as skin testing. It also provides information about interventions for residents with tuberculosis and prevention of the spread of infection among staff and residents. Any nurse or direct-care staff member working with older adults should undergo periodic skin testing to screen for exposure to tuberculosis.

Eliminating the Risk From Smoking

Nurses begin implementing educational interventions to help older smokers eliminate this risk factor by addressing attitudes that influence self-care behaviors. For example, if an older person expresses an "I'm-too-old-to-change" attitude, the initial intervention might be to explore the older adult's understanding of his or her ability to change behavioral patterns. Studies have shown that older smokers can successfully quit smoking at rates comparable with their younger counterparts, even though they are often viewed as chronic smokers who do not want to quit (Abdullah & Simon, 2006). Using information about psychosocial development in older adulthood, nursing interventions would be directed toward encouraging the older person to consider the possibility of a behavioral change. Nurses also can apply a health promotion model for behavior change, such as the transtheoretic model (discussed in Chapter 5), which has been widely studied as a model for smoking cessation programs for older adults (Burbank & Riebe, 2002).

Wellness Opportunity

Nurses support wellness in older adults by communicating that old age is not an inevitable barrier to changing health-related behaviors: It's never too late to quit.

Another commonly expressed belief that nurses can address through health education is "It's too late to do any good." When nurses encounter this type of attitude, they can challenge the underlying assumptions with the goal of improving the older adult's motivation to quit smoking. For example, nurses can emphasize that the substantial health benefits derived from quitting smoking include improved respiratory function and reduced risk for heart disease and lung cancer. Specific benefits from smoking cessation that have been identified in studies include improved quality of life, decreased susceptibility to smoking-related illnesses, and a more rapid recovery from illnesses that usually are exacerbated by smoking (Abdullah & Simon, 2006). Although health benefits of quitting smoking occur at any age, they vary according to the age at which people quit. Smokers who quit before 50 years of age reduce their risk of dying by half over the next 15 years (Mahon, 2005). Similarly, men and women who quite smoking at age 35 increase their life expectancy by 4.5 and 6.1 years, respectively, and those who quit at age 65 can expect an increase in life expectancy of 2.0 and 3.7 years, respectively.

Clinical practice guidelines emphasize the importance of nurses and other health care providers initiating the topic of smoking cessation and routinely identifying and intervening with all tobacco users at every opportunity (AHRQ, 2005). Guidelines for nursing interventions for smoking cessation can be found in nursing literature (e.g., O'Connell, 2001; Wynd & Dossey, 2005).

Health education includes information about the variety of approaches to smoking cessation, including various prescription or over-the-counter pharmacologic therapies that can help treat nicotine addiction. Methods for delivering nicotine substitutes include gum, patches, inhalants, lozenges, and nasal sprays. These products have all been found to be effective in significantly increasing the cessation rate, and some people may benefit from combining different types of products (Kenford & Fiore, 2004). In addition to nicotine substitution products, a sustained-release form of bupropion has been available since 1997 as the first non-nicotine medicinal aid to smoking cessation. A citric acid aerosol product is available as a smoking cessation aid. Nonpharmacologic interventions include the use of guided imagery, which has been has shown to be effective in long-term smoking cessation for abstinence in adult smokers (Wynd & Dossey, 2005). Regardless of the methods that are used, it is widely agreed that counseling from a health professional is an important component of any smoking cessation efforts. Educational materials about group and individual self-help programs are available through the organizations listed in the Educational Resources section. Nurses can use Box 21-5 as a guide for health education about helping older adults quit smoking.

Mr. R. is now 77 years old and attends the senior center with his wife three times a week for meal and social programs. During your weekly Senior Wellness Clinic, he comes to have his blood pressure checked and says that he is thinking about quitting smoking, but that his son just quit and gained a lot of weight and had a lot of trouble sleeping. He's not sure if quitting smoking is worth the effort, especially because his son has been so miserable since he quit. Also, at his age, it probably won't do any good to quit now, he says.

THINKING POINTS

- What further questions would you ask to assess Mr. R.'s readiness to discuss quitting smoking?
- What health promotion teaching would you do?
- What would your response be if you determine that Mr. R. is not ready to consider quitting smoking?

EVALUATING EFFECTIVENESS OF NURSING INTERVENTIONS

Measuring the effectiveness of interventions for the nursing diagnosis of Ineffective Breathing Pattern is based on a reassessment of subjective indicators such as ease of breathing and objective indicators such as lung sounds and respiratory rate and rhythm. An indicator of successful health education interventions for older adults with Ineffective Breathing Pattern is that they can accurately identify factors that can be addressed to improve their respiratory function. Disease prevention interventions for the nursing diagnosis of Risk for Infection could be documented on a record of the person's history of immunizations for pneumonia and influenza. For older adults who smoke and are willing to address this risk factor, effectiveness of interventions would be measured by the person's increased knowledge about the detrimental effects of smoking and by his or her willingness to develop a plan to stop smoking. Long-term effectiveness would be evaluated by the person's successful participation in the smoking cessation program.

Mr. R. is now 83 years old and recently moved into an assisted living complex where you are employed as the nurse. When he comes in for his flu shot, he asks you how he can get some nicotine gum because he has heard that this is a good way to cut down on cigarettes. Now that he lives in the assisted living complex, he can't smoke in the dining room, and he'd like to chew nicotine gum before and after he eats. He admits that he smokes a pack of cigarettes every day, but denies having experienced any bad effects from smoking. Mr. R. sees his doctor for COPD and takes Flovent, 2 puffs b.i.d. and Serevent, 2 puffs b.i.d.

NURSING ASSESSMENT

You begin your nursing assessment by exploring Mr. R.'s attitudes about smoking and ascertaining his knowledge about the harmful effects of cigarette smoking. Mr. R. says he thought about quitting smoking many times but never actually tried to quit because his wife smoked even more than he did until she died a few months ago. He felt it would be too hard to quit as long as she was smoking two packs per day. He also states that he's heard a lot about passive smoking and he figured it wasn't worth trying to quit as long as he was around his wife's cigarette smoke. He states that he's been smoking for 40 years, and if he hasn't gotten lung cancer by now, he's not going to get it at his age. To comply with the rules in the assisted living facility, Mr. R. says he plans to chew nicotine gum when he can't smoke cigarettes, but he sees no reason to quit.

In assessing Mr. R.'s knowledge about the effects of cigarette smoking, you determine that he is aware of some of the harmful effects of passive smoking but has very little information about the detrimental effects of cigarette smoking. He relates that his wife died of lung cancer, but he attributes her death to a history of breast cancer, which she had 10 years before the lung cancer. Mr. R. has no knowledge about cigarette smoking as a risk factor for cardiovascular disease, nor does he realize that his hypertension poses an additional risk. Mr. R. reports that he has experienced no ill effects from cigarette smoking, but when you ask about his history of respiratory infections, he admits he had pneumonia 3 years ago. He says that he received a pneumonia shot 2 years ago, so he doesn't have to worry about getting pneumonia again, and that he has had bronchitis several times, but now that he won't be out shoveling snow, he doesn't worry about getting any lung infections either.

NURSING DIAGNOSIS

Based on the assessment findings, an appropriate nursing diagnosis would be Ineffective Health Maintenance, related to insufficient knowledge about the effects of tobacco use and self-help resources. Some of Mr. R.'s statements reflect a lack of accurate information about the harmful effects of cigarette smoking, particularly regarding risks for respiratory infections and impaired cardiovascular function. Other statements probably reflect an intellectualization of his continued smoking. You intuit that, with some education and support, he may be willing to quit smoking.

NURSING CARE PLAN FOR MR. R.

Expected Outcome	Nursing Interventions	Nursing Evaluation
Mr. R. will increase his knowledge about the harmful effects of cigarette smoking.	• Give Mr. R. brochures and illustrations provided by the Office on Smoking and Health and use them to discuss the effects of cigarette smoking. • Use brochures from the American Heart Association to discuss the risk factors for cardiovascular disease.	• Mr. R. will verbalize correct information about the risks of cigarette smoking. • Mr. R. will describe the benefits derived from quitting smoking.

(case study continues on page 457)

Expected Outcome	Nursing Interventions	Nursing Evaluation
	• Discuss cigarette smoking as a risk factor for respiratory infections. • Give Mr. R. a copy of Box 21-5 and discuss the immediate and long-term benefits of quitting smoking.	
Mr. R. will be knowledgeable about techniques for quitting smoking.	• Using information from the American Lung Association, discuss some of the strategies for quitting smoking (e.g., quitting cold turkey, using nicotine substitutes, participating in self-help groups).	• Mr. R. will describe the advantages and disadvantages of the various methods of quitting smoking.
Mr. R. will quit smoking.	• Identify the method Mr. R. prefers for quitting smoking. • Emphasize the importance of nutrition, exercise, and adequate fluid intake. • Agree on realistic goals for smoking cessation. • Discuss supportive resources. Set up weekly appointments at the Senior Wellness Clinic for support and further discussions.	• Mr. R. will report that he has stopped or significantly reduced his smoking.

THINKING POINTS

- How would you assess Mr. R.'s readiness and motivation to quit smoking?
- What health education approach would you take with Mr. R.?
- What additional interventions or health education points would you use for Mr. R.?

CHAPTER HIGHLIGHTS

Age-Related Changes That Affect Respiratory Wellness (Tables 21-1 and 21-2)

- Upper airway changes (e.g., calcification of cartilage)
- Increased anteroposterior diameter
- Chest wall stiffness, weakened muscles
- Alveoli enlarged and have thinner walls
- Alterations in lung volumes and airflow
- Decreased compensatory response to hypercapnia and hypoxia

Risks Factors That Affect Respiratory Wellness (Box 21-1)

- Tobacco smoking
- Environmental factors (e.g., pollution, dry air, secondhand smoke)
- Occupational hazards

Pathologic Condition Affecting Respiratory Wellness: COPD

- Chronic obstructive pulmonary disease (COPD): a group of diseases, including emphysema, chronic bronchitis, and a subset of asthma, characterized by chronic airflow obstruction

Functional Consequences Affecting Respiratory Wellness

- Mouth breathing, diminished cough reflex, less efficient gag reflex
- Increased use of accessory muscles, increased energy expended for breathing
- Diminished efficiency of gas exchange, decreased PaO_2 levels
- Decreased vital capacity, slight decrease in overall efficiency
- Increased susceptibility to lower respiratory infections

Nursing Assessment of Respiratory Function (Boxes 21-2 and 21-3)

- Overall respiratory function
- Detection of lower respiratory infections
- Tobacco use and attitudes regarding smoking

Nursing Diagnosis

- Health-Seeking Behaviors
- Ineffective Breathing Pattern
- Risk for Infection

Planning for Wellness Outcomes

- Vital Signs, Respiratory Status: Airway Patency, and Respiratory Status: Ventilation
- Immune Status, Immunization Behavior, and Community Risk Control
- Knowledge: Health Behaviors
- Risk Control: Tobacco Use and Knowledge: Substance Use Control

Nursing Interventions for Respiratory Wellness (Boxes 21-4 and 21-5)

- Prevention and detection of pneumonia and influenza
- Health education about smoking cessation

Evaluating Effectiveness of Nursing Interventions

- Ease of breathing
- Up-to-date status for pneumonia immunization

- Influenza immunization every year
- For older adults who smoke: active participation in smoking cessation behaviors

Critical Thinking Exercises

1. What will a healthy, nonsmoking, 83-year-old person experience in his or her daily life with regard to respiratory function?
2. What would you include in a health education program, designed for older adults, on the prevention of pneumonia and influenza?
3. How would you address the following statement made by a 71-year-old person: "I've lived this long and don't have lung cancer; why should I start worrying now?"
4. Find the names, addresses, and phone numbers of local agencies that would be appropriate resources for someone interested in quitting smoking. Contact at least one of these organizations to find out specific information about support groups, written materials, and other resources.

Clinical Tool Resources

Hartford Institute for Geriatric Nursing
Try This: Best Practices in Nursing Care to Older Adults
Issue Number 21 (Revised 2007), Immunizations for the Older Adult
www.hartfordign.org/resources/education/tryThis.html

Educational Resources

Agency for Healthcare Research and Quality, U.S. Department of Health and Human Services
AHRQ National Guidelines Clearinghouse
www.ahrq.gov

American Cancer Society
www.cancer.org

American Heart Association
www.americanheart.org

American Lung Association
www.lungusa.org

Lung Association of Canada
www.lung.ca

National Heart, Lung, and Blood Institute Information Center
www.nhlbi.nih.gov/health/index.htm

Office on Smoking and Health, Centers for Disease Control and Prevention
www.cdc.gov/tobacco

References

Aaron, S. D., Fergusson, D., Dent, R., Chen, Y., & Vandemhee, K. L. (2004). Effects of weight reduction on respiratory function and airway reactive obese women. *Chest, 125*, 2046–2052.

Abdullah, A. S., & Simon, J. L. (2006). Health promotion in older adults: Evidence-based smoking cessation programs for use in primary care settings. *Geriatrics, 61*(3), 30–34.

Adis Data Group. (2005). Community-acquired pneumonia (CAP) remains a serious threat to the elderly and should be treated empirically based on disease severity. *Drugs & Therapy Perspectives, 21* (11), 10–13.

Agency for Healthcare Research and Quality (AHRQ). (2005). *Helping smokers quit: A guide for nurses*. Rockville, MD: Author.

Alguacil, J., & Silverman, D. T. (2004). Smokeless and other noncigarette tobacco use and pancreatic cancer: A case-control study based on direct interviews. *Cancer Epidemiology, Biomarkers and Prevention, 13*, 55–58.

Behrendt, C. E. (2005). Mild and moderate-to-severe COPD in nonsmokers. *Epidemiology, 128*, 1239–1244.

Boffetta, P., Aagnes, B., Weiderpass, E., & Anderson, A. (2005). Smokeless tobacco use and risk of cancer of the pancreas and other organs. *International Journal of Cancer, 114*, 992–995.

Burbank, P. M., & Riebe, D. (2002). *Promoting exercise and behavior change in older adults: Interventions with the transtheoretical model*. New York: Springer.

Carpenito-Moyet, L. J. (2006). *Handbook of nursing diagnosis* (11th ed.). Philadelphia: Lippincott Williams & Wilkins.

Centers for Disease Control and Prevention (CDC). (2000). Reducing tobacco use: A report of the Surgeon General. *Morbidity and Mortality Weekly Report, 16*(RR-16), 1–27.

Centers for Disease Control and Prevention (CDC). (2006). Fact sheet: Secondhand smoke (updated September 2006). CDC National Tobacco Control Program. Available at www.cdc.gov/tobacco/data_statistics/Factsheets/SecondhandSmoke.htm.

Chapman, K. R., Tashkin, D. P., & Pye, D. J. (2001). Gender bias in the diagnosis of COPD. *Chest, 199*, 1691–1695.

Coleman, P. R. (2004). Pneumonia in the long-term care setting: Etiology, management, and prevention. *Journal of Gerontological Nursing,* 30, 14–23.

Eisner, M. D., Klein, J., Hammond, S. K., Koren, G., & Lactao, G. (2005). Directly measured second-hand smoke exposure and asthma health outcomes. *Thorax, 60*, 794–795.

Henley, S. J., Thun, M. J., Chao, W., & Calle, E. E. (2004). Association between exclusive pipe smoking and mortality from cancer and other diseases. *Journal of the National Cancer Institute, 96*, 853–861.

Henley, S. J., Thun, M. J., Connell, C., & Calle, E. E. (2005). Two large prospective studies of mortality among men who use snuff or chewing tobacco (United States). *Cancer Causes and Control, 16*, 347–358.

Janssens, J., & Krause, K. (2004). Pneumonia in the very old. *The Lancet Infectious Diseases, 4*, 112–124.

Kenford, S. L., & Fiore, M. C. (2004). Promoting tobacco cessation and relapse prevention. *Medical Clinics of North America, 88*, 1553–1574.

Kuykendall, J. R., Houle, M. D., & Rhodes, R. S. (2004). Possible warfarin failure due to interaction with smokeless tobacco. *Annals of Pharmacotherapy, 38*, 595–597.

Lindberg, A., Bjerg-Backlund, A., Ronmark, E., Larrson, L., & Lundback, B. (2006). Prevalence and under-diagnosis of COPD by disease severity and the attributable fraction of smoking: Report from the Obstructive Lung Disease in Northern Sweden studies. *Respiratory Medicine, 100*, 264–272.

Mahon, S. M. (2005). Review of selected approaches in smoking cessation. *Clinical Journal of Oncology Nursing, 9*, 745–747.

Miravitlles, M., Ferrer, M., Pont, A., Viejo, J. L., & Fernando, M. (2005). Characteristics of population of COPD patients identified from a population-based study: Focus on previous diagnosis and never smokers. *Respiratory Medicine, 99*, 985–995.

Nurminen, M. M., & Jaakkola, M. S. (2001). Mortality from occupational exposure to environmental tobacco smoke in Finland. *Journal of Occupational and Environmental Medicine, 43*, 687–693.

O'Connell, K. A. (2001). Smoking cessation among older clients. In E. A. Swanson, T. Tripp-Reimer, & K. Buckwalter (Eds.), *Health promotion and disease prevention in the older adult* (pp. 102–118). New York: Springer.

Rohani, M., & Agewall, S. (2004). Oral snuff impairs endothelial function in healthy snuff users. *Journal of Internal Medicine, 255*, 379–383.

Teo, K. K., Ounpuu, S., Hawken, S., Pandey, M. R., Valentin, V., Hunt, D., et al. (2006). Tobacco use and risk of myocardial infarction in 52 countries in the INTERHEART study: A case-control study. *Lancet, 368*, 647–658.

U.S. Department of Health and Human Services (USDHHS). (2000). *Healthy people 2010* (2nd ed.). Washington, DC: U.S. Government Printing Office.

Van den Brande, P. (2005). Revised guidelines for the diagnosis and control of tuberculosis. *Drugs & Aging, 22*, 663–686.

Vlachopoulos, C., Alexopoulos, N., Panagiotakos, D., O'Rourke, M. F., & Stefanadis, C. (2004). Cigar smoking has an acute detrimental effect on arterial stiffness. *American Journal of Hypertension, 17*, 299–303.

Vollset, S. E., Tverdal, A., & Gjessing, H. K. (2006). Smoking and deaths between 40 and 70 years of age in women and men. *Annals of Internal Medicine, 144*, 381–389.

Whitson, H. E., Heflin, M. T., & Burchett, B. M. (2006). Patterns and predictors of smoking cessation in elderly cohort. *Journal of the American Geriatrics Society, 54*, 446–471.

Wolfsen, C., Barker, J. C., & Mitteness, L. S. (2001). Smoking and health: Views of elderly nursing home residents. *Journal of Gerontological Nursing, 27*(8), 6–12.

Wynd, C. A., & Dossey, B. M. (2005). Smoking cessation: Freedom from risk. In B. M. Dossey, L. Keegan, & C. E. Guzzetta (Eds.), *Holistic nursing: A handbook for practice* (4th ed., pp. 759–780). Boston: Jones and Bartlett.

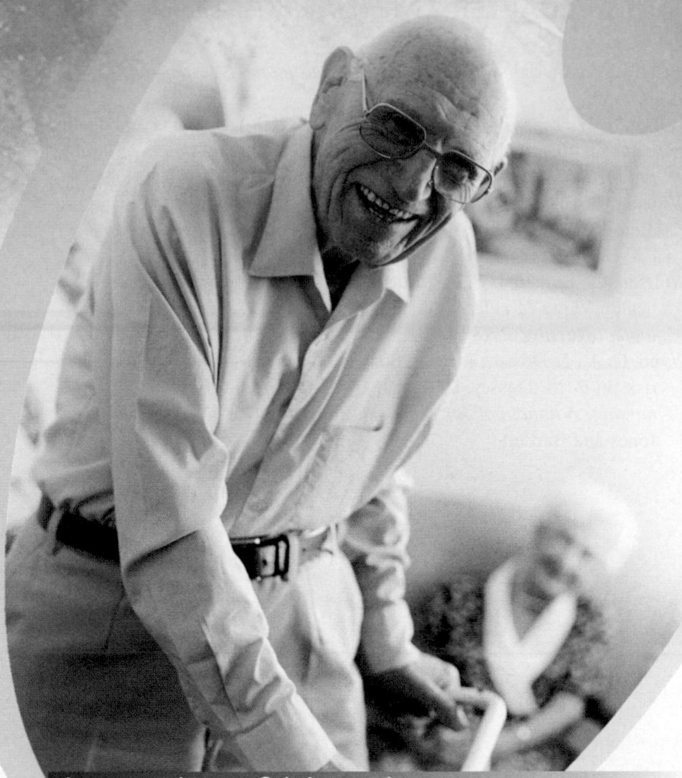

CHAPTER 22

Mobility and Safety

Learning Objectives

After reading this chapter, you will be able to:

1. Delineate age-related changes that affect mobility and safety.
2. Identify risk factors that increase the risk of osteoporosis and influence the safety and mobility of older adults.
3. Discuss the following functional consequences: diminished musculoskeletal function, increased susceptibility to fractures, and increased susceptibility to falls.
4. Discuss the psychosocial and long-term consequences of falls, fractures, and osteoporosis.
5. Conduct a nursing assessment of musculoskeletal performance and risks for falls and osteoporosis.
6. Identify interventions directed toward safe mobility and the elimination of risks for falls and osteoporosis.

Key Terms

body sway
fallaphobia
osteoarthritis
osteoporosis
post-fall syndrome

Mobility is one of the most important aspects of physiologic function because it is essential for maintaining independence and because serious consequences occur when independence is lost. For older adults, mobility is influenced by age-related changes to some extent, but risk factors play a much larger role. Because of the many risks that threaten mobility, falls are an unfortunately common occurrence in old age. Older adults, then, have the dual challenge of maintaining mobility skills and avoiding falls. For these reasons, safety is considered to be an integral aspect of mobility.

 AGE-RELATED CHANGES THAT AFFECT MOBILITY AND SAFETY

The bones, joints, and muscles are the body structures most closely associated with mobility, but many additional functional aspects are involved in safe mobility. Neurologic function, for example, influences all facets of musculoskeletal performance, and visual function influences the ability to interact safely with the environment. In the musculoskeletal system, osteoporosis is the age-related change that has the most significant overall impact, has been studied the most, and is most amenable to interventions aimed at prevention and management. For these reasons, osteoporosis is discussed separately from age-related changes in bones.

Bones

Bones provide the framework for the entire musculoskeletal system and work in conjunction with the muscular system to facilitate movement. Additional functions of bone in the

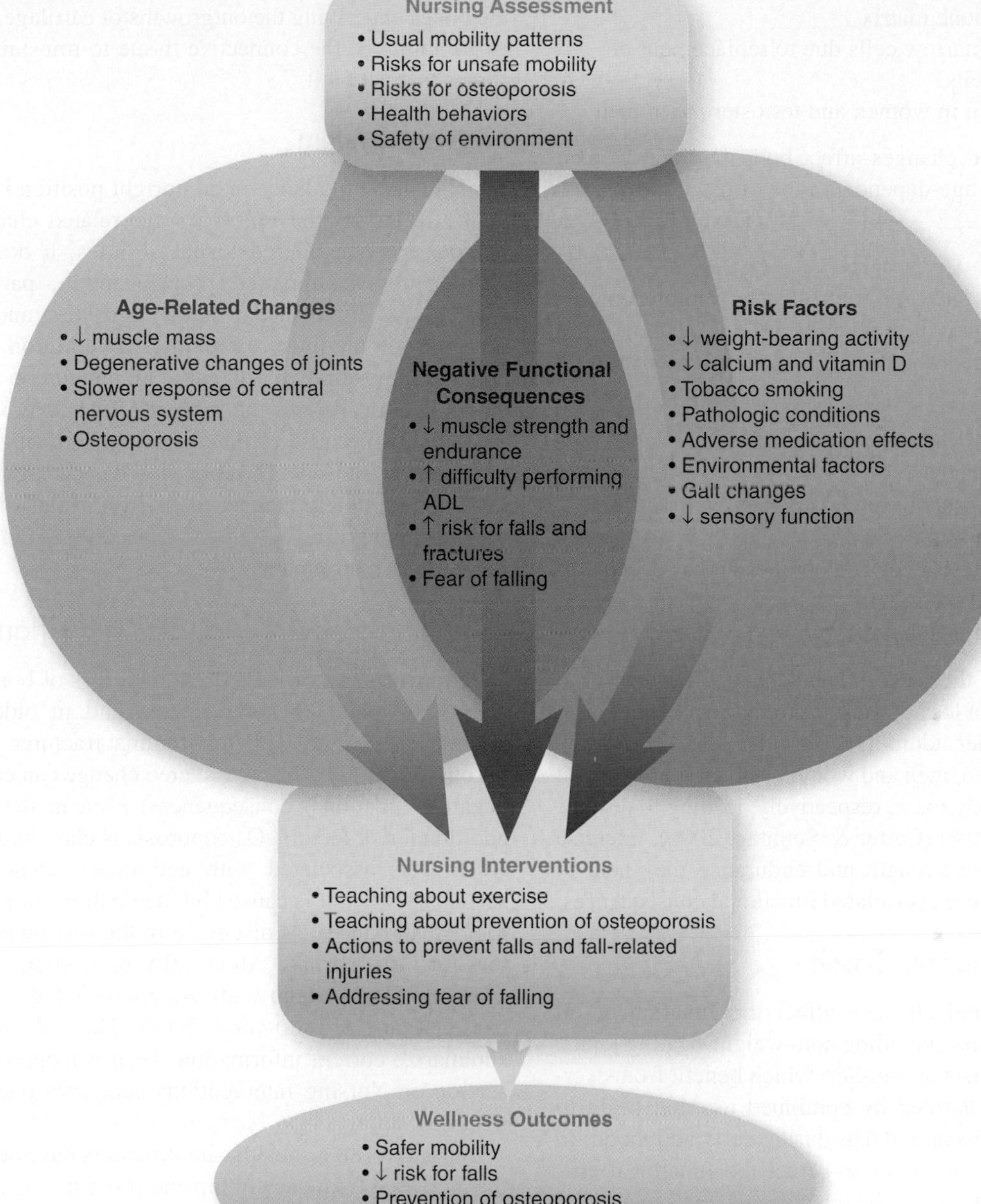
Promoting Musculoskeletal Wellness in Older Adults
Nursing Assessment
• Usual mobility patterns
• Risks for unsafe mobility
• Risks for osteoporosis
• Health behaviors
• Safety of environment
Age-Related Changes
• ↓ muscle mass
• Degenerative changes of joints
• Slower response of central nervous system
• Osteoporosis
Negative Functional Consequences
• ↓ muscle strength and endurance
• ↑ difficulty performing ADL
• ↑ risk for falls and fractures
• Fear of falling
Risk Factors
• ↓ weight-bearing activity
• ↓ calcium and vitamin D
• Tobacco smoking
• Pathologic conditions
• Adverse medication effects
• Environmental factors
• Gait changes
• ↓ sensory function
Nursing Interventions
• Teaching about exercise
• Teaching about prevention of osteoporosis
• Actions to prevent falls and fall-related injuries
• Addressing fear of falling
Wellness Outcomes
• Safer mobility
• ↓ risk for falls
• Prevention of osteoporosis
• ↓ risk for fractures
• Improved quality of life

human body include storing calcium, producing blood cells, and supporting and protecting body organs and tissues. Bone is composed of a hard outer layer, called cortical or compact bone, and an inner, spongy meshwork, called trabecular or cancellous bone. The proportion of cortical to trabecular components varies according to bone type. Long bones, such as the radius and femur, are composed of as much as 90% cortical cells, whereas flat and vertebral bones are composed primarily of trabecular cells. Both cortical and trabecular bone components are affected by age-related changes, but the rate and impact of age-related changes differ in the two types of bone.

Bone growth reaches maturity in early adulthood, but bone remodeling continues throughout one's lifetime. The following age-related changes affect this remodeling process:

- Increased bone resorption (i.e., breakdown of bone that is necessary for remodeling)
- Diminished calcium absorption

- Increased serum parathyroid hormone
- Impaired regulation of osteoblast activity
- Impaired bone formation secondary to reduced osteoblastic production of bone matrix
- Fewer functional marrow cells due to replacement of marrow with fat cells
- Decreased estrogen in women and testosterone in men

These age-related changes affect both men and women and account for the age-dependent type of osteoporosis.

Muscles

Skeletal muscles, which are controlled by motor neurons, directly affect all activities of daily living (ADLs). Age-related changes that have the greatest impact on muscle function include

- Decreased size and number of muscle fibers
- Loss of motor neurons
- Replacement of muscle tissue by connective tissue and, eventually, by fat tissue
- Deterioration of muscle cell membranes and a subsequent escape of fluid and potassium
- Diminished protein synthesis

The end result of these age-related changes is a decline in motor function and a loss of muscle strength and endurance, even in healthy older adults (McCarter, 2006). During the normal adult life span, men and women lose an average of 12 kg and 5 kg lean body mass, respectively, leading to disability and loss of function (Carter & Sonntag, 2006). Exercise programs to increase strength and endurance may help to delay the onset of these age-related functional consequences.

Joints and Connective Tissue

Numerous age-related changes affect the function of all musculoskeletal joints, including non–weight-bearing joints. In contrast to the bones or muscles, which benefit from exercise, the joints are harmed by continued use and begin to show the effects of wear and tear during early adulthood. In fact, degenerative processes that affect the functional efficiency of the joints begin in the third decade, before skeletal maturity is reached, and affect the tendons, ligaments, and synovial fluid.

Some of the most significant age-related joint changes include the following:

- Diminished viscosity of synovial fluid
- Degeneration of collagen and elastin cells
- Fragmentation of fibrous structures in connective tissue
- Outgrowths of cartilaginous clusters because of continuous wear and tear
- Formation of scar tissue and areas of calcification in the joint capsules and connective tissue
- Degenerative changes in the articular cartilage resulting in extensive fraying, cracking, and shredding, in addition to a pitted and thinned surface

Consequences of these changes include impaired flexion and extension, decreased flexibility of the fibrous structures, diminished protection from forces of movement, erosion of the bones underlying the outgrowths of cartilage, and diminished ability of the connective tissue to transmit the tensile forces that act on it.

Nervous System

Maintenance of balance in an upright position is a complex skill affected by the following age-related changes of the nervous system: altered visual abilities; a decline in the righting reflex; impaired proprioception, particularly in women; and diminished vibratory sensation and joint position sense in the lower extremities. In addition, age-related changes in postural control cause an increase in **body sway**, which is a measure of the motion of the body while standing. Finally, because of the age-related slowing in reaction time, older adults walk more slowly and are less able to respond in a timely manner to environmental stimuli. Thus, they are more at risk for falls, especially when they are in unfamiliar environments.

Osteoporosis as an Age-Related Change

Osteoporosis is a process of gradual loss of bone mass that affects all adults to some degree and in older adults is strongly associated with low-trauma fractures (i.e., osteoporotic fractures). This age-related change can cause serious negative functional consequences, even in the absence of additional risk factors. Osteoporosis is classified as primary when it is associated with age-related changes, and as secondary when it is caused by medications or pathophysiologic disturbances, as discussed in the section on Risk Factors for Osteoporosis. About 20% of women and between 40% and 50% of men with osteoporosis have a secondary cause (Kenny & Prestwood, 2000). The following sections summarize current information about osteoporosis, and the section on Nursing Interventions addresses prevention and treatment approaches.

Since the 1880s, health care providers have been aware of the increased frequency of hip and forearm fractures in older women. However, it was not until the 1940s that estrogen deficiency was recognized as a major risk factor for osteoporosis and fractures in older women. By the 1960s, primary care providers suspected that many fractures in older women were associated with moderate or no trauma. During the 1970s and 1980s, the use of noninvasive methods for measuring bone mineral density (BMD) led to much progress in the understanding of osteoporosis. During the 1990s, pharmaceutical companies focused on developing safe and effective treatments for both the prevention and treatment of osteoporosis. By the early 2000s, the widespread availability and low cost of noninvasive measurements of BMD and the development and availability of several pharmaceutical interventions for osteoporosis focused attention on the diagnosis, prevention, and treatment of osteoporosis in men as well as women. Until the mid-1990s, most research focused on women, but current research and recommendations are attempting to address osteoporosis in older men and high-risk groups such as residents of long-term care facilities and people who use certain medications for long periods.

Gender differences account for the relatively higher rate of osteoporosis among women compared to men. Both men and women reach peak bone mass in their mid-thirties, but there are significant differences in patterns of bone loss between men and women. Women have a period of bone mass stability between peak level and the onset of menopause, when declining estrogen levels significantly affect bone mass. During the first decade after the onset of menopause, the annual rate of bone loss may be as great as 7%, but after menopause it is between 1% and 2%. By contrast, the annual rate of bone loss in men is only about 1% after peak bone mass has been reached. Another gender difference is that men have more cortical bone than women, and gain cortical bone through periosteal bone deposition until the age of 75 years (Kenny & Prestwood, 2000). Consequently, bone diameter increases in men and confers a mechanical advantage in protecting from fractures (Shreyasee & Felson, 2001). In summary, primary osteoporosis occurs in both men and women, but women have a much greater percentage of bone loss over their lifetime and experience greater bone loss at an earlier age.

Diversity Note

Lifetime bone loss in women and men, respectively, is 35% and 23% of cortical bone and 50% and 33% of trabecular bone.

RISK FACTORS THAT AFFECT MOBILITY AND SAFETY

The risk factors for safe mobility that are of greatest concern are those that contribute to osteoporosis, fractures, and falls. These risks are of particular importance to nurses because health promotion interventions are appropriate for addressing many of the risk factors. In addition, eliminating or minimizing the risks is likely to prevent the serious functional consequences.

Risk Factors for Impaired Musculoskeletal Function

Although it is difficult to differentiate between factors that increase the risk for osteoporosis, fractures, and falls and those that affect overall musculoskeletal function, some nutritional and lifestyle factors have been identified that have a detrimental effect on general musculoskeletal function. Lack of exercise is a well-known risk factor for diminished musculoskeletal performance, and there is increasing evidence of the beneficial effects of physical activity for preventing age-induced declines in mobility. Nutritional factors also are associated with overall musculoskeletal function; Campbell and colleagues (2001) concluded that the Recommended Dietary Allowance of 0.8 g/kg/day for protein may not be adequate for maintaining optimal skeletal muscle function in older adults. Another analysis suggests that low levels of vitamin D contribute to diminished muscle strength, impaired muscular function, and increased disability in community-living older women (Zamboni et al., 2002).

Wellness Opportunity

Many lifestyle and environmental factors can be addressed for preventing falls and fractures. Prevention of falls is an important, but often overlooked, aspect of care.

Risk Factors for Osteoporosis and Fractures

Hormonal variations account for most gender differences in the development of primary osteoporosis. Researchers have focused on the role of estrogen in relation to osteoporosis in women for several decades; however, they are just beginning to address the role of testosterone, estrogen, and other hormones in men. In women, late menarche, early menopause, and low endogenous estrogen levels increase the risk for osteoporosis. In older men, low BMD is associated with low estradiol levels, rather than with low testosterone or adrenal androgens (Kamel, 2005; Shreyasee & Felson, 2001).

Lifestyle factors, such as cigarette smoking and inadequate amounts of weight-bearing activity, also can increase the risk for osteoporosis. Additional risk factors associated with low BMD include ethnicity, advanced age, low weight and body mass index, and maternal family history of hip fracture or falls. Nutritional factors that increase the risk of osteoporosis include daily intake of less than 1000 to 1500 mg of calcium and 400 to 600 International Units of vitamin D. In addition, for people with inadequate calcium intake, high intakes of dietary protein, caffeine, sodium, and phosphorus can negatively affect calcium balance and increase the risk of osteoporosis (NIH, 2001). Excessive alcohol consumption is another risk factor for osteoporosis, particularly in men.

Diversity Note

Varying rates of osteoporosis are found in the following groups (ranging from highest to lowest):

- Asians, Alaska Natives, Native Americans
- White non-Hispanic women
- Hispanic groups
- White men and African American women
- African American men

Pathologic conditions that are associated with secondary osteoporosis include hypogonadism, osteomalacia, hyperthyroidism, hyperparathyroidism, multiple myeloma, and malabsorption syndrome. Certain medications also affect bone remodeling and increase the risk for secondary osteoporosis. For example, one study found that anticlotting agents such as warfarin can interfere with the activation of bone matrix proteins (Gage et al., 2006). With long-term use, oral or inhaled corticosteroids—a common treatment for asthma, rheumatoid arthritis, and chronic obstructive pulmonary disease—are the medications most frequently associated with secondary osteoporosis. Antiseizure agents, such as phenytoin and valproic acid, also are associated with osteoporosis (Sato et al., 2001). The most widely acknowledged risks for development of osteoporosis are summarized in Box 22-1.

In recent years, researchers have tried to differentiate between the risks for osteoporosis and the risks for fractures, with particular emphasis on hip fractures. Factors that consistently have been associated with increased fracture risk include

- Impaired vision
- Impaired cognition
- History of falls
- History of fractures
- Environmental hazards
- Diminished physical function, such as slow gait
- Cigarette smoking, with increased risk for women after menopause (but no increase in risk after 15 years of cessation)

Screening for osteoporosis, by contrast, is a factor that has been associated with lowered fracture risk. A study of community dwellers 65 years of age and older reported that those patients who had received osteoporosis screening with hip dual-energy x-ray absorptiometry (DEXA) were 36% less likely to have a hip fracture over the next 6 years than those community dwellers who did not have this type of screening (Kern et al., 2005).

Researchers have tried to identify gender and racial differences in risks for fractures. Two gender differences relating to hip fractures are that men tend to be older than women when fractures occur, and they have more protection conferred by greater bone mass at maturity. Investigations of risk factors in older Mexican Americans found that hip fractures in women, but not in men, were associated independently with advanced age, history of a stroke, and living alone or being unmarried (Espino et al., 2000). Ottenbacher and colleagues (2002) found that diabetes was associated with an increased risk for hip fracture in older Mexican Americans.

Box 22-1
Risk Factors for Osteoporosis

Factors That Increase the Risk for Osteoporosis

- Female sex
- Increased age
- Small bones
- Thinness, less-than-normal weight
- White or Asian race
- Genetic predisposition
- Low calcium intake, both past and current
- Inadequate vitamin D intake
- Prolonged immobility
- Lack of weight-bearing activity
- Estrogen deficiency (women)
- Decreased testosterone levels (men)
- Cigarette smoking
- Excessive alcohol intake
- Long-term use of certain medications (e.g., corticosteroids, anticonvulsants, thyroid hormones, warfarin)
- Excessive use of antacids, particularly those that contain aluminum

Ms. M. is 55 years old and works as the secretary in the Senior Circle of Care program where you do health screening and educational programs. This program is a "senior wellness program" sponsored by one of the nonprofit hospitals in Minneapolis, Minnesota. Ms. M.'s responsibilities include finding and organizing health education materials under the direction of the nurses. You often go to lunch with her and discuss social and health-related topics. Ms. M. has always been inquisitive about health-related concerns, and one day she asks your advice about osteoporosis. She says that both she and her mother, who is 83 years old, have been receiving flyers about getting a bone density test, and that her mother asked if she would go with her so they could both be tested. You know from past conversations that Ms. M.'s mother fractured her wrist a long time ago, but otherwise is relatively healthy. Ms. M. is fairly healthy, although she admits that she "could stand to lose a little weight." You also know from previous discussions that Ms. M. has been taking hormonal replacement therapy for 5 years, because you have had more than one lunchtime conversation with her about the pros and cons of estrogen. In your work as the senior wellness nurse, you have developed and presented several health education programs about osteoporosis and are fairly familiar with recent literature on osteoporosis.

THINKING POINTS

- Based on what you know about Ms. M., what would you tell her about her risk factors for osteoporosis?
- Based on what you know about Ms. M.'s mother, what additional information would you want to know before advising her about a test for her mother?
- How would you answer Ms. M.'s inquiry?
- What suggestions would you make to help Ms. M. become more knowledgeable about osteoporosis?

Risk Factors for Falls

Falling is an age-related functional consequence that has been the focus of a great number of studies in Great Britain and the United States and continues to be a major concern today. A half century ago, an article titled "On the Natural History of Falls in Old Age" began with the following declaration: "The liability of old people to tumble and often to injure themselves is such a commonplace of experience that it has been tacitly accepted as an inevitable aspect of ageing, and thereby deprived of the exercise of curiosity" (Sheldon, 1960, p. 1685). In the last decade, geriatricians and gerontologists have challenged this view that falls are a normal consequence of aging or are accidental or random events. It is now widely agreed that falls and mobility problems result from multiple, diverse, and interacting factors. The current clinical approach is to identify the most likely causes and contributing conditions and to plan interventions that address these factors (Morley, 2002).

Risk factors for falls are categorized according to their origin as follows: age-related changes, common pathologic conditions and functional impairments, medication effects, and environmental factors (Box 22-2). Falls are the result of a combination of these factors, rather than one isolated risk factor, and the risk of falls increases in proportion to the number of fall risk factors. The many studies of reasons for falling in older adults have identified different underlying causes in different age groups. Falls in older adults younger than 75 years of age are often associated with trips and slips that are predominantly attributable to a combination of age-related changes, such as vision changes, and unfavorable environmental conditions, such as poor lighting. A study of falls after a trip in healthy older adults found that walking quickly may be the greatest cause of this type of fall (Pavol et al., 2001). By contrast, falls in people older than 75 years of age are usually associated with a combination of disease- and medication-related factors.

Risks for falls also vary according to the environment in which the older person lives. For example, falls in institutionalized older people are most often associated with weakness, dizziness, and gait and balance disorders, whereas falls in community-living populations tend to be associated with environmental factors (Rubenstein & Josephson, 2002). Basante and colleagues (2001) reviewed 21 studies of fall risks for older adults in long-term care facilities and identified medications (e.g., psychotropics), deconditioning (e.g., lower extremity weakness and gait and balance disorders), and physical restraints (e.g., vests, pelvic restraints, lap trays), or any combination of these factors, as the major contributing factors.

Age-Related Changes and Common Conditions

Nocturia, osteoporosis, gait changes, orthostatic hypotension, decreased muscle strength, hearing and vision changes, and central nervous system changes, such as decreased reaction time, are common age-related changes that can increase the risk of falls in older adults. Other age-related changes that are risk factors for falls were discussed earlier in this chapter.

In addition to these age-related changes, common pathologic conditions can also increase the risk of falls. For example, anemia is associated with twice the incidence of falls and with fall-related symptoms such as vertigo, orthostatic

Box 22-2
Risk Factors for Falls

Age-Related Changes

- Vision and hearing changes
- Osteoporosis
- Slowed reaction time
- Altered gait, increased sway
- Postural hypotension
- Nocturia

Pathologic Conditions and Functional Impairments

- Cardiovascular diseases (e.g., arrhythmias or myocardial infarction)
- Respiratory diseases (e.g., chronic obstructive pulmonary disease [COPD])
- Neurologic disorders (e.g., parkinsonism, cerebrovascular accident [CVA])
- Metabolic disturbances (e.g., dehydration, electrolyte imbalances)
- Musculoskeletal problems (e.g., osteoarthritis)
- Transient ischemic attack (TIA)
- Vision impairments (e.g., cataracts, glaucoma, macular degeneration)
- Cognitive impairments (e.g., dementia, confusion)
- Psychosocial factors (e.g., depression, anxiety, agitation)

Medication Effects and Interactions

- Anticholinergics, including ingredients in over-the-counter products (e.g., diphenhydramine)
- Diuretics
- Benzodiazepines and other hypnotics
- Antipsychotics
- Antidepressants
- Antihypertensives
- Nonsteroidal anti-inflammatory agents (NSAIDs)
- Alcohol

Environmental Factors

- Physical restraints, including bedrails
- Glare
- Inadequate lighting
- Lack of handrails on stairs
- Slippery floors
- Throw rugs
- Cords or clutter
- Unfamiliar environments
- Highly polished floors
- Improper height of beds, chairs, or toilets

hypotension, diminished muscle strength, and poor physical performance (Penninx et al., 2005). Another study found that a primary diagnosis of cerebrovascular accident was the only variable that increased the risk of falling (Patrick & Blodgett, 2001). Sleep problems also have been found to be an independent risk factor for falls in community-living older adults (Brassington et al., 2000). In general, pathologic conditions are associated with falls in older adults in all of the following ways:

1. Pathologic conditions may be treated with medications that create risks for falling.
2. Illnesses can cause functional impairments, such as vision or mobility limitations.
3. Illnesses may cause metabolic or other physiologic disturbances that create risks for falls.
4. Falls may be one manifestation of an acute illness or a change in a chronic illness.
5. Chronic illnesses interfere with optimal exercise and other health practices that are important in promoting safe mobility.

Functional impairments, regardless of cause, also increase the risk for falls, especially in combination with other risk factors. For example, nursing home residents with impaired visual-spatial abilities were three times more likely to fall than those who did not have impairments (Olsson et al., 2005). Similarly, Harrison and colleagues (2001) found that the number of falls increased during a 3-month period as the level of cognition declined in nursing home residents with dementia. Both dementia and depression diminish one's awareness of the environment and can interfere with the ability to process information about environmental stimuli. The following combination of factors is likely to increase the risk for falls in people with dementia: medications, concurrent conditions, decreased level of awareness, diminished ability to cope with environmental surroundings, and the severity of associated functional disabilities, such as mobility impairments (Shaw, 2002). Older adults who are depressed are at increased risk for falls secondary to gait changes, medication effects, and a diminished ability to concentrate on and respond to environmental factors. Considering all of these possible associations, it is not surprising that most falls resulting in injuries occur in people who have functional impairments and multiple, chronic medical problems.

Medication Effects

Numerous studies have identified hundreds of medications that can contribute to falls, and some studies have looked at the relationship between falls, medications, and diagnoses. Not all conclusions are consistent with regard to specific medications or diagnoses, but the key to identifying an association between medications and falls is to consider the underlying mechanism of the medication action, as well as the pathologic condition and the potential interactions between various factors. For example, orthostatic hypotension can result from pathologic conditions, age-related changes, or adverse medication effects, and can increase the risk for falls. If an 80-year-old person has a pathologic condition (e.g., hypertension) that may cause orthostatic hypotension, and if the person is taking a medication (e.g., a vasodilator) that causes orthostatic hypotension, the risk for falls is significantly increased. Therefore, rather than memorizing all of the medications that have been found to increase the risk for falls, nurses can focus their attention on the underlying mechanisms that increase the risk for falls.

The following medication effects can increase the risk for falls: confusion, depression, sedation, arrhythmias, hypovolemia, orthostatic hypotension, delayed reaction time, diminished cognitive function, and changes in gait and balance (e.g., ataxia, decreased proprioception, and increased body sway). Thus, any medication that has one or more of these adverse effects may increase the risk for falls. Benzodiazepines have been widely studied in relation to an increased risk for falls, and evidence suggests that their effect on psychomotor function may contribute to falls. This is just one of the adverse effects of benzodiazepines; others include sedation and impaired cognitive function. Even low doses of benzodiazepines can increase the risk for falls in community-living older adults (Gray et al., 2006).

Although atypical antipsychotics have a lower incidence of extrapyramidal side effects, they are still associated with an increased risk for falling (Hein et al., 2005). Also, selective serotonin reuptake inhibitors (SSRIs) have the same potential to cause falls and fractures as the older antidepressants; therefore, all psychotropics need to be used with caution in older people (Hein et al., 2005).

Other considerations that influence the risk of falls include medication–disease interactions, medication–medication interactions, and medication–alcohol interactions. Also, the dose, half-life, and administration time of the medication can affect the risk for falls. For example, benzodiazepines with long half-lives (e.g., flurazepam) have been associated with an increased risk for falls and fall-related injuries. Ray and colleagues (2000) found that the rate of falls among nursing home residents who were current users of benzodiazepines was increased 44% and that the risk of falls increased with higher doses, recent onset of use, and longer elimination half-life. In recent years, zolpidem has become a widely used nonbenzodiazepine sedative-hypnotic for older people because of the high association between benzodiazepines and falls. Wang and colleagues (2001), however, found that the use of zolpidem was associated with a 90% increased risk of hip fracture in a sample of older nursing home residents (mean age, 82 years), even after controlling for potential confounding effects.

Studies have focused primarily on prescription medications, but over-the-counter medications also can create risks for falls through their adverse effects on psychomotor function. For example, many over-the-counter preparations for pain, colds, and insomnia contain alcohol or anticholinergics. These ingredients may themselves pose risks, or may interact with other medications to increase the risk for falls. Recently, the adverse effects of diphenhydramine, a widely used ingredient in over-the-counter products for sleep, colds, and allergies, have received much attention in the media and medical literature. Diphenhydramine has been associated with significant adverse effects on the psychomotor skills necessary for safe driving, and many states include this and other over-the-counter agents in laws pertaining to driving while impaired. Studies have shown diphenhydramine to have adverse effects on mood, reaction time, attention, vigilance, working memory, and level of activity. These effects may persist through the next day after an evening dose (Kay, 2000). The effects of even these over-the-counter medications on frail older adults can be a risk factor for falls and fall-related injuries. Some of the types of medications that are likely to increase the risk for falls are listed in Box 22-2.

Environmental Factors

Some environmental hazards were discussed in Chapter 7, but additional environmental influences must be considered specifically in relation to falls. In hospitals and long-term care settings, for example, the first and second most common sites of falls are the bedroom and bathroom. In the bedroom, most falls occur while the person is getting in or out of bed, although some are related to climbing over side rails or footboards. In the bathroom, falls generally occur while transferring on or off of toilet seats or while hurrying to urinate or defecate. In community settings, most falls occur in the home, particularly in stairways, bedrooms, and living rooms. Activities that have been associated with falling in home settings include slipping on wet surfaces, slipping while descending stairs, getting in and out of beds and chairs, and tripping over floor coverings or objects on the floor.

Physical Restraints

Since the mid-1960s, physical restraints have commonly been used in institutional settings with the intent of protecting impaired people from injury and reducing staff work load. Historically, the belief that the use of physical restraints protects vulnerable people from falls and shields the institution from liability was widespread. Starting in the mid-1980s, however, the validity of this belief began to be questioned. Since the 1990s, there has been growing evidence that restraints not only do not reduce the risk of falls, but are more likely to lead to serious injury from falls when used for older adults (Twersky, 2001). Dunn (2001) found no significant difference in the number of falls, but a decrease in severity of fall-related injuries, after a restraint-free environment was established in a long-term care facility. In addition to being associated with fall-related injuries, restraints have been found to cause agitation, strangulation, deconditioning, and pressure ulcers (Shorr et al., 2002).

Since the late 1980s, bedrails have been considered a form of restraint, except when they are used to facilitate bed mobility. In recent years, many questions have been raised about their safety and effectiveness, particularly for people who are cognitively impaired and unable to understand the intent of bedrails. As with other restraints, evidence does not support their use, and studies have found that reducing the use of bedrails can decrease the risk of falls and serious fall-related injuries (Hoffman et al., 2003).

Since the 1990s, agencies such as the American Nurses Association, the U.S. Food and Drug Administration (FDA), the Centers for Medicare and Medicaid Services (CMS; previously known as the Health Care Financing Administration), and the Joint Commission (previously known as the Joint Commission on Accreditation of Healthcare Organizations) have challenged the use of restraints in hospitals and long-term care settings and urged the use of less restrictive safety measures. In 2001, the American Geriatrics Society, the British Geriatrics Society, and the American Academy of Orthopaedic Surgeons Panel on Fall Prevention in Older Persons concluded that there is no evidence to support the use of restraints for fall prevention and, in fact, restraints can contribute to serious injuries (American Geriatrics Society et al., 2001). These efforts have resulted in a 50% to 75% decrease in use of restraints in nursing homes since the late 1980s (Weintraub & Spurlock, 2002).

In summary, falls must be viewed as complex events that occur more commonly in older adults, with the risk increasing as the number of contributing factors increases. Contributing factors can be intrinsic or extrinsic, and the risk can often be reduced through interventions, as discussed later in this chapter.

Ms. M. is now 67 years old and has retired from her secretarial job. She attends weekly social and lunch gatherings at the local senior center, where you are the wellness nurse. One day she comes to the center with a cast on her left wrist and reports that she fractured her wrist when she slipped and fell on ice in her driveway. You know from prior conversations with her that she stopped taking hormonal therapy several years ago because she had been on it for over 10 years and was concerned about long-term effects. You also know that she takes medications for arthritis, hypertension, and depression and that she self-monitors her blood pressure. In the past 10 years, she has gradually gained "a little weight every year" and her current height/weight is 5′3″/172 pounds. She participates in the weekly "mall walkers" exercise program, but does not often exercise independently. She says that "my housework is enough exercise" and that the weekly group exercise activity is "as much as my arthritis will tolerate." She lives in a small one-floor house. Although Ms. M. says she is not really concerned about sustaining any more fractures because she views the recent fall as a "fluke of bad winter luck," she makes an appointment to talk with you. During the appointment, she reports that she is a "little concerned about osteoporosis."

(case study continues on page 468)

THINKING POINTS

- What risk factors for osteoporosis can you identify from what you already know about Ms. M.?
- What risk factors for falls and fall-related injuries can you identify from what you already know about Ms. M.?
- Can you identify any factors that diminish her risk for falls or fractures?
- What additional information about Ms. M. would be helpful in identifying additional risks for osteoporosis?
- What additional information would be helpful in identifying additional risks for falls and fractures?

PATHOLOGIC CONDITION AFFECTING MUSCULOSKELETAL FUNCTION: OSTEOARTHRITIS

Osteoarthritis is a degenerative inflammatory disease affecting joints and attached muscles, tendons, and ligaments that is characterized by pain, swelling, and limited movement in joints. Osteoarthritis is a leading cause of disability in the United States that affects women disproportionately (Burks, 2005). Because it occurs almost universally in older adults, osteoarthritis is often viewed as an extreme progression of age-related changes; however, not all older adults have symptoms of osteoarthritis (Loeser, 2000). Osteoarthritis is now considered a very complex disease process that results from the interplay of risk factors such as trauma, genetics, obesity, and age-related changes. Diminished estrogen also may be a contributing factor in postmenopausal women.

Diversity Note

Whites and African Americans have similar rates of arthritis, but African Americans have a higher rate of arthritis-related activity limitation.

Because self-care is an important aspect of managing osteoarthritis, nurses focus on health education interventions. Nurses can teach people with osteoarthritis about the following activities for prevention and treatment:

- Participating in a supervised, low-impact exercise program that focuses on improving musculoskeletal strength, balance, and endurance
- Avoiding high-impact activities
- Wearing good shock-absorbing shoes
- Balancing weight-bearing activities with rest periods
- Losing weight if appropriate
- Getting adequate intake of vitamins C and D
- Using walkers and other assistive devices as appropriate to relieve weight-bearing joints, improve balance, or achieve independent functioning
- Using moist heat and analgesics for pain

Care plans for managing osteoarthritis are most effective when they take an interdisciplinary approach that includes medicine, nursing, and physical and occupational therapy. Because there are many medical and surgical interventions for osteoarthritis, nurses emphasize the importance of obtaining regular medical care for ongoing evaluation and treatment as this condition changes. Complementary and alternative care practices commonly used for osteoarthritis include acupuncture; magnetic therapy; therapeutic touch; glucosamine and chondroitin; and vitamins C, D, and E. Nurses can encourage older adults to find reliable information about these approaches from sources such as the National Institutes of Health.

Wellness Opportunity

Older adults with osteoarthritis need to engage in self-care activities, including making responsible decisions about promoting optimal comfort and functioning.

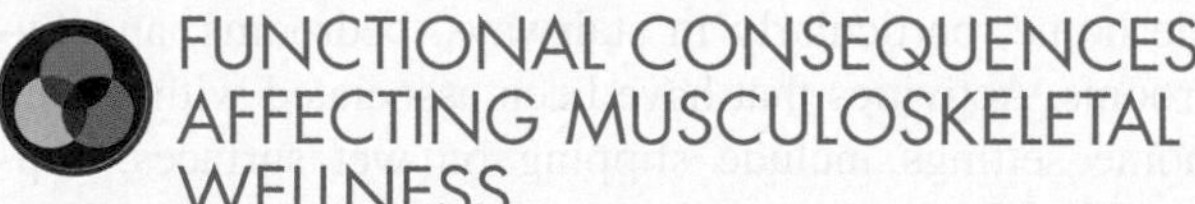

FUNCTIONAL CONSEQUENCES AFFECTING MUSCULOSKELETAL WELLNESS

Age-related changes affect musculoskeletal function to some degree, but older adults can compensate for functional consequences, at least in part, through exercise. Age-related changes in joint function have a slight impact on mobility and range of motion, but in the absence of osteoarthritis and other disease-related processes, the functional consequences are not serious. The functional consequences of osteoporosis, however, are quite serious, as are the functional consequences that result from the combination of age-related changes and the hundreds of risk factors that contribute to falls in older adults. As with many other aspects of function in older adulthood, cumulative and interacting effects of risk factors rather than age-related changes most significantly affect function and quality of life.

Effects on Musculoskeletal Function

Muscle strength, endurance, and coordination are affected to some extent by age-related changes, even in the absence of risk factors. Beginning around the age of 40 years, muscle strength declines gradually, resulting in an overall decrease of 30% to 50% by the age of 80 years, with a greater decline in muscle strength in the lower extremities than in the upper extremities. Diminished muscle strength is attributed primarily to age-related loss of muscle mass. In addition, a person's current level of activity and lifelong patterns of exercise can influence muscle strength at any age. Muscle endurance and coordination diminish as a result of age-related changes in the muscles and central nervous system. Because of these changes, older adults experience muscle fatigue after shorter periods of exercise compared with their younger counterparts.

Joint function begins to decline during early adulthood and progresses gradually to cause the following changes in range of motion:

- Decreased range of motion in the upper arms
- Decreased lower back flexion
- Decreased external rotation of the hip
- Decreased hip and knee flexion
- Decreased dorsiflexion of the foot

These changes result in slowed performance of daily activities such as writing, eating, grooming, and putting shoes and socks on; difficulty climbing stairs and curbs; and an overall diminished ability to respond to environmental stimuli.

Gait changes, which differ in men and women, are one of the more noticeable functional consequences that occur after the age of 75 years. Women have less muscular control, develop a narrower standing and walking gait, and develop bowlegged-type changes that affect the lower extremities and alter the angle of the hip. Older men develop a wider walking and standing gait, characterized by less arm swing, a shorter stride, decreased steppage height, and a more flexed position of the head and trunk than when they were younger. The overall impact of these changes is that older men and women have a slower walking speed and spend more time in the support phase of gait than in the swing phase. These changes can increase the risk for falls. Although many older adults have gait disorders, significant gait changes should not be considered an inevitable result of aging.

Susceptibility to Falls and Fractures

The combination of age-related changes and multiple interacting risk factors doubly jeopardizes older adults by increasing the probability of both falls and fractures. Fractures are not unique to older adults, but they do differ in many respects from those that occur in younger populations. First, bones of older adults can be fractured with little or no trauma, whereas bones of healthy children and younger adults are usually fractured in response to a forceful impact. Fractures are classified as osteoporotic, or fragility fractures, when they occur as the result of even minimal trauma—that is, trauma that is no more severe than that resulting from falling to the floor from a standing position. Second, the risk of fractures increases in direct relation to age (in older women the number of years since menopause may be a more accurate risk indicator than chronologic age). Third, it is more likely that fractures in older adults, particularly hip fractures, will have serious consequences affecting independence and quality of life, as discussed later in this section.

During childhood and young adulthood, boys and men sustain fractures more often than their female counterparts do, but after the age of 35 years, this begins to change. By the sixth decade, fracture rates for women become twice those in men (Walker-Bone et al., 2001).

> **Diversity Note**
>
> Whites and Asians have a much higher rate of osteoporotic fractures than do African Americans, but the reasons for this are not clear. Factors that may contribute to this discrepancy include the higher bone mass of African Americans at skeletal maturity, the greater bone density and thicker bone cortex of African Americans, and the slower rate of age- or menopause-related bone loss in the African American population.

One of the reasons that falls, fractures, and osteoporosis are the focus of attention is that these events have a tremendous impact on health care expenditures for older adults. Fall injuries account for 6% of all medical expenditures for adults older than 65 years of age (Komara, 2005). Even more important than the financial consequences are the quality-of-life consequences associated with falls and fractures.

To appreciate the serious implications of falls and fractures for older adults, consider these statistics (Aschkenasy & Rothenhaus, 2006; Ellis & Trent, 2001; Gass & Dawson-Hughes, 2006; Magaziner et al., 2000):

- Fall-related complications are the leading cause of death from injury in people age 65 years and older.
- Approximately 30% to 40% of community-living older adults will sustain a significant fall during the remainder of their lives.
- At least half of residents in long-term care facilities will experience a fall.
- Approximately 40% of white women who are 50 years and older will experience a hip, spine, or wrist fracture during the remainder of their lives.
- Hip fractures are associated with a substantial increase in the risk of dying; 18% to 33% of older people who fracture a hip die within a year.
- Both men and women who fracture a hip have an increased risk of dying within 2 years, but this outcome is significantly greater for men (Fransen et al., 2002).
- Vertebral fractures are associated with functional limitations, chronic back pain, and increased risk of dying or being in a hospital.
- Nearly 67% of people age 85 years or older admitted to a hospital for fall-related injuries are transferred to a long-term care facility.
- Almost half of older adults who live at home at the time of their fracture are admitted to long-term care, and 15% to 25% remain in a long-term care setting for a year after the fracture.

- As much as 75% of older adults who are independent before a hip fracture can neither walk independently nor achieve their previous level of independent living within 1 year of the fracture.

These statistics underscore the importance of nursing interventions to minimize the risk for osteoporosis, falls, and fall-related injuries in older adults.

Psychosocial Consequences

In the early 1980s, the phrase **post-fall syndrome** was used to describe a distinct gait pattern adopted by older people who have fallen and been admitted to the hospital for post-fall injuries (Murphy & Isaacs, 1982). People who have this syndrome do not have any neurologic or orthopedic problems that could account for the gait, and they did not display the syndrome's characteristic gait pattern before the fall. Post-fall syndrome comprises the following characteristics: an expressed fear of falling when standing erect, a tendency to grab and clutch at objects within view, and marked hesitancy and irregularity in walking attempts (Murphy & Isaacs, 1982).

Since the 1980s, the term **fallaphobia** has been used to describe the experience of the following sequence of events: (1) older people fall, lose their balance, or feel at risk for falling; (2) they lose confidence in their ability to perform the activity that led to or created a risk for falling; (3) they stop performing the activity; and (4) they eventually become homebound or chair bound (Tideiksaar & Kay, 1986). Fear of falling has been identified as "the most commonly reported anxiety among older people, exceeding even fear of robbery or financial difficulties" (Yardley & Smith, 2002, p. 17). Fear of falling is sometimes associated with a specific activity, such as bathing, toileting, climbing stairs, or walking outside. In these situations, people usually avoid the associated activity or become quite anxious when forced to participate in the feared activity. Sometimes the fear and avoidance eventually extends to other activities.

Fear of falling is often associated with the occurrence and severity of previous falls, but some studies have found that even nonfallers can develop a fear of falling (Murphy et al., 2002). Additional variables associated with a fear of falling include pain, frailty, anxiety, depression, poor health and balance, lower levels of mobility and activity, poorer quality of life, and use of prescription medications (Drozdick & Edelstein, 2001; Yardley & Smith, 2002). Cumming and colleagues (2000) found that fear of falling was a serious health problem even for nonfallers and that being afraid of falling was predictive of being admitted to a long-term care facility among fallers, but not among nonfallers. These researchers also found a strong relationship in both fallers and nonfallers between low fall-related self-efficacy and a decline in functional abilities.

One potentially positive effect of the fear of falling is that it can lead to gait changes that can prevent falls, such as slower gait, shorter and wider stride, and prolonged double-limb support time (Chamberlin et al., 2005). Although fear of falling can have a protective effect, it primarily causes detrimental effects such as shame, anxiety, depression, deconditioning, social isolation, excess disability, loss of confidence, and diminished quality of life. Moreover, fear of falling kindles additional fears about physical harm, long-term functional disability, loss of independence, social embarrassment and indignity, fear of becoming a burden, and damage to personal confidence and identity (Tischler & Hobson, 2005). Also, it often causes older people—especially those who are frail and have had an injurious fall—to excessively restrict their activities and avoid public settings (Murphy et al., 2002; Yardley & Smith, 2002).

Family caregivers of older adults also may be quite anxious about potential falls, and they may experience excessive worry about the possibility that the older person might fall. This fear can lead to decisions that restrict an older adult's activities unnecessarily or that result in a move to a setting that provides a greater level of assistance or supervision than the older person desires. Although a move to an unfamiliar environment will not necessarily protect the person from falls and may even increase the risk of falls, the caregivers who encourage or make such a decision may derive some peace of mind because they perceive that the older person is safer. It is now widely recognized that restraints do not prevent falls and are likely to contribute to more serious fall-related injuries; however, some people may falsely believe that restraints and restricted activity are safe and effective fall prevention interventions.

Wellness Opportunity

Nurses respect older adults' autonomy and involve them in decisions by creatively finding ways to ensure safety while also allowing as much freedom of movement as possible.

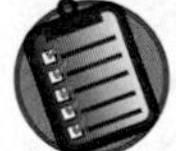

NURSING ASSESSMENT OF MUSCULOSKELETAL FUNCTION

Nursing assessment of musculoskeletal function focuses on identifying risk factors for falls and osteoporosis, as well as identifying the functional consequences of age-related musculoskeletal changes that affect ADLs. Assessment of risks for falls and osteoporosis should pay particular attention to those factors that can be modified or alleviated through health promotion and other nursing interventions. Also, it is important to identify the degree of risk for either osteoporosis or falls so that appropriate preventive interventions can be planned and implemented based on the degree of risk. Although even a low risk for falls or osteoporosis creates numerous opportunities for health promotion interventions, a higher risk is associated with greater nursing responsibility for health education and preventive interventions.

Assessing Musculoskeletal Performance

For healthy older adults, the primary effects of age-related changes on musculoskeletal performance are a change in gait and slower performance of some ADLs. Older adults who have osteoarthritis, neurologic conditions, dementia, or other conditions that can affect gait, balance, or joint function are likely to have additional functional consequences that affect their musculoskeletal function. In assessing overall musculoskeletal performance, it is important to identify whether the changes are due to age-related changes or a pathologic condition because interventions vary depending on the underlying cause. For example, interventions for older adults who have dementia must address the effects of cognitive impairment. One study found that 89% of residential care and assisted-living residents with dementia had some degree of impaired mobility, but 38% to 63% of these residents were not assessed or treated for these limitations (Williams et al., 2005). Considering the strong association between dementia and fall risk, a nursing assessment of musculoskeletal function is particularly important for older adults who are cognitively impaired.

Assessment of overall musculoskeletal performance begins with observation of the person's mobility and activities. In addition to watching the person walk, it is especially important to observe the person getting up from a hard-back chair without arms. Nurses obtain additional assessment information by asking questions about the person's ability to perform ADLs. When any limitations are identified, it is important to find out whether the older adult is using assistive devices to improve mobility, balance, or overall function; safety; and independence. If the person is not using such devices and may benefit from them, the nurse assesses both the person's knowledge about the availability of such devices as well as his or her attitude about using them because attitudes are likely to influence the acceptability of using recommended aids. Nurses can use the criteria for the functional assessment of all ADLs provided in Chapter 7 together with the assessment information in this chapter.

In addition to experiencing minor changes in performance of ADLs, older adults experience changes in posture and diminished height. Older adults may or may not be concerned about or aware of a loss of height; however, a loss of about 2 to 4 cm per decade is normal, owing to osteoporosis and other age-related changes. Including a question about the person's usual height and any noticeable loss of height will give the nurse an opportunity to assess the older adult's awareness of this change. Although the functional consequences of decreased height are minimal, older people who never were very tall may experience increased difficulty performing activities that depend on height. In these situations, they may find that it is safer and more effective to use assistive devices, such as long-handled reachers. They also may need encouragement to rearrange cupboards so the most frequently used items are accessible. Another assessment implication of decreased height is that the pants legs of older adults may be too long, especially if the person also has lost weight. Therefore, nurses observe whether the length of clothing increases the risk for falls. Box 22-3 summarizes guidelines for assessing overall musculoskeletal performance in older adults.

Identifying Risks for Osteoporosis

Because some health promotion interventions for osteoporosis—such as adequate intake of calcium and vitamin D and participation in regular weight-bearing exercise—are universally applicable, nurses assess risks in all older adults. Nurses also identify modifiable risk factors—such as smoking and drinking excessive amounts of alcohol—that can be alleviated through lifestyle interventions. If the nursing assessment identifies risk factors that cannot be modified (e.g., small bones), this information may be used to motivate the person to take action to eliminate the risks that can be. Nurses obtain much of the information regarding risks for osteoporosis during an overall assessment or health history, and they consider this information in relation to mobility and safety.

A diagnostic evaluation for osteoporosis is generally based on tests of BMD. Frequently used methods of measuring BMD include radiographic absorptiometry (RA), quantitative ultrasonography, dual-photon absorptiometry (DPA), single-photon absorptiometry (SPA), quantitative computed tomography (QCT), and dual-energy x-ray absorptiometry (DXA or DEXA). Sites that are evaluated include the hip, hand, wrist, heel, tibia, forearm, and lumbar spine. Although there are many ways to assess BMD, DXA of the spine and hip is the preferred method and is recommended for all women older than 64 years (Zarowitz et al., 2006). Medicare covers the cost of BMD testing every 2 years for the following groups: people with vertebral abnormalities or primary hyperparathyroidism, women who are estrogen deficient or at clinical risk for osteoporosis, and patients taking long-term corticosteroid therapy or being monitored for response to treatment with an FDA-approved osteoporosis medication.

Because these tests are widely available and community-based screening programs are becoming more common, nurses need to be knowledgeable about them so they can teach older adults about their value and the implications of their results. The operational definition of osteoporosis—which applies only to white women—is bone density that is at least 2.5 standard deviations below the mean for young adult white women (NIH, 2001). Similarly, a definition for osteoporosis in men is under consideration but currently specifies bone density that is more than 2.5 standard deviations below the mean for normal young men. Results of BMD tests can guide decisions about initiating medical treatment because some medical interventions involve risks (e.g., hormonal therapy) and can be quite expensive. Nurses should assess the older adult's awareness of BMD tests and ask whether the person has discussed them with his or her primary care practitioner. See Box 22-3 for assessment questions and considerations relating to osteoporosis.

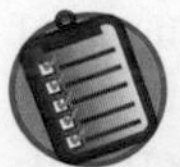

Box 22-3
Guidelines for Assessing Overall Musculoskeletal Function and Risks for Falls and Osteoporosis

Questions to Assess Overall Musculoskeletal Performance

- Do you have any trouble performing your usual activities because of joint limitations?
- Do you have any pain or discomfort in your joints?
- Do you ever feel like you are losing your balance?
- Do you have any trouble walking or getting around?
- Do you use any assistive devices (e.g., a walker, quad cane, or reaching devices) to help you do things?

Questions to Assess Risks for Osteoporosis

Questions to Ask All Older Adults

- Do you know of any blood relatives who have had osteoporosis or who have sustained fractures late in life?
- Have you sustained any fractures during your adult years? (If yes, ask additional questions regarding age at the time, type, location, circumstances, treatment, and so on.)
- Do you take any calcium or vitamin D supplements?
- Have you ever had your bone density measured?
- Have you ever talked with your primary care practitioner about prevention of osteoporosis?
- Do you take any medications for osteoporosis?

Questions to Ask Women

- When did you begin menopause?
- Do you take, or have you ever taken, estrogen or other hormonal therapy? (If yes, ask additional questions regarding type, dose, duration, and so on.)

Questions to Assess Risk for Falls and Fear of Falling

- Have you had any falls in the past few years? (If yes, ask additional questions about the circumstances and ask about pertinent risk factors as summarized in Box 22-2.)
- Are you afraid of falling? (If yes, ask additional questions about specific fears, such as, *What do you think might happen if you were to fall?*)
- Are there any activities you would like to do, but do not do, because of any difficulty moving or getting around? (If yes, ask about specific activities, such as shopping, using public transportation, and so on).
- Are there any activities you would like to do, but do not do, because you are afraid of falling? (If yes, ask about specific activities, such as going up or down stairs, taking a bath or shower, and so on).

Observations Regarding Overall Musculoskeletal Performance

- Measure and record the person's present height and stated peak height.
- Observe the individual's walking and gait pattern.
- Observe the person rising from a chair.

Information From the Overall Assessment That Is Also Useful in Assessing Musculoskeletal Function

- Observe and document a functional assessment, as described in Chapter 7.
- How much exercise does the person get on a regular basis? In particular, how much weight-bearing exercise?
- Does the person smoke cigarettes?
- How much alcohol does the person consume?
- What is the person's usual daily intake of calcium and vitamin D?
- Does the person have any medical conditions that are associated with falls or osteoporosis (as summarized in Boxes 22-1 and 22-2)?
- Is the person taking any medications that might create risks for falls (including over-the-counter medications)?
- Does the person have postural hypotension?
- Is the person moderately or seriously visually impaired?
- Does the person have any cognitive impairments or other psychosocial impairments that diminish his or her attention to the environment or interfere with the ability to respond to environmental stimuli?

Wellness Opportunity

From a holistic perspective, nurses ask older adults to identify enjoyable ways of engaging in weight-bearing activities.

Identifying Risks for Falls and Injury

Identifying fall risk is an essential part of health care for older adults because it is imperative to initiate preventive interventions for people at risk for falls. Standards for the management and prevention of falls in vulnerable older adults recommend that health care professionals ask an older person at least one screening question per year about the occurrence of falls (Rubenstein et al., 2001). This guideline is based on evidence that falls are common, often preventable, frequently unreported, and often the cause of injury and unnecessary restriction of activity, which results in a reduction of overall health and quality of life. In addition, a recent history of falls is a strong predictor of future falls (Rubenstein et al., 2001). Guidelines also recommend further assessment for all older people who report even a single fall and for those who are observed to be unsteady (American Geriatrics Society, 2001). Because prevention of falls and fall-related injuries is an important aspect of health promotion for older adults, all nurses working with older adults are responsible for assessing and documenting fall risk factors, particularly in institutional settings. Even in home and community settings where older adults are relatively independent, nurses can follow the guidelines of the American Geriatrics Society by observing for apparent risk factors and asking each person one question about the occurrence of falls annually. For any person with a history of falls or several other risk factors for falls, nurses must assess and document further fall risk so that any modifiable factors can be addressed. See Box 22-3 for guidelines for assessment questions that are applicable to older adults who are independent or relatively independent.

Fall risk assessment is multidimensional and ideally includes observing the person in his or her usual environment. Nurses in institutional settings focus their assessment on the immediate environment; however, they also need to be concerned about the person's home environment as part of their discharge planning. Although the same assessment criteria are used for environmental safety, regardless of the setting, specific fall risks will vary according to the environment. For example, poor lighting and throw rugs are common fall risks in home environments, whereas assistive devices are common fall risks in institutional settings. The best assessment information is obtained by observing the person in the environment and paying particular attention to the person's awareness of and attention to the environment. Observations are especially helpful in identifying discrepancies between the person's perception of his or her abilities and his or her actual performance. Observations also provide information about adaptive behaviors that otherwise might not be acknowledged. For example, a person might state that he or she has no difficulty with stair climbing, but observations might reveal that the person performs this activity in a highly unsafe manner. Nurses in institutional settings generally do not have opportunities to observe home environments directly, but they can observe the person in the immediate environment and ask the person or caregivers questions about the home setting and their ability to function safely in that setting. They can also consider referrals to home care agencies for home assessment as part of the discharge plan.

Another important aspect of assessing the environment in any setting is identifying the factors that are likely to cause serious injury if a fall does occur. For example, night stands or any heavy furniture can cause serious injuries, especially if someone hits his or her head while falling. Likewise, furniture with hard or sharp edges can cause serious injuries and bleeding, especially for people taking anticoagulants. The guidelines summarized in Chapter 7 can be used to assess the safety of any environment, and can be applied to all older adults, particularly those who have intrinsic risk factors for falls.

Wellness Opportunity

Whenever possible, nurses actively involve the older adult and family members in identifying environmental factors that either support or create risks for safe mobility.

In the past few decades, many fall risk assessment tools have been developed and are now readily available for use in different settings. The purpose of these tools is to identify people who are at risk for falls so that comprehensive assessment can be done and interventions can be planned. The two general types of fall risk assessment tools are functional assessment scales and nursing fall risk tools. Functional assessment scales, which focus on the person's mobility, are usually used by physical therapists or primary care practitioners. These tools specifically identify gait and balance problems that increase the risk for falls. Nurses can informally assess gait and balance by asking the person to sit in a firm, straight-backed chair with armrests, stand up from the chair and walk a few steps, then turn around and return to the chair. Nurses also can observe the usual walking pattern of the person, paying particular attention to any gait or balance unsteadiness or unusual patterns. If any abnormalities are noted, nurses can suggest that the patient receive further evaluation by a primary care provider. Nurses also can suggest referral to a physical therapist for further assessment and recommendations about a therapy program.

Nursing fall risk assessment tools are widely used in institutional settings as well as home and community-based settings. The Hartford Foundation for Geriatric Nursing recommends the use of the Hendrich II Fall Risk Model (Fig. 22-1) as a tool that has been validated with skilled nursing and rehabilitation populations (Gray-Miceli, 2006).

Fall risk assessment tools are useful in identifying people who are at high risk for falls, but they do not provide a base for comprehensive assessment of causative factors. If several risk factors are identified or if an older adult has already fallen, a more extensive assessment is required. Comprehensive fall assessments can be done by primary care practitioners, but they are often done in settings such as geriatric assessment or rehabilitation programs. Specialized fall assessment programs use a multidisciplinary approach to assess the following aspects of functioning: cognition, nutrition, medications, pathologic conditions, and gait and balance. Evaluation of previous falls and contributing factors also is included for people with a fall history. Be aware that any change in functioning, even an improvement in functioning, indicates the need for a reassessment of fall risk.

Because fear of falling has negative functional consequences in addition to those associated with actual falls, nurses include at least one question about fear of falling in any assessment of falls and fall risk. If the older person expresses a fear of falling, nurses ask additional questions in relation to specific activities that may be associated with fears or falls. Assessment questions aimed at identifying fear of falling and related negative functional consequences are included in Box 22-3.

Ms. M. is now 75 years old and goes to the senior center three or four times weekly for lunch. You have been the wellness nurse at the center for several years and are quite familiar with Ms. M. because she frequently attends your weekly "Healthy Aging" classes. After your recent class on "Keeping Your Bones Healthy and Moving Well," she made an appointment to see you. She tells you she has significantly cut down on her exercise because she experienced pain in one knee about a month ago after she took a long walk in the park with her dog. She talked with her doctor about this and was told to start taking ibuprofen, but she has not started taking it because she is not sure how much to take and her knee does not bother her except when she takes a long walk. She

(case study continues on page 474)

used to take her dog for daily walks, but now ties him out so she does not have to go out. Current prescription medications are enalapril, 5 mg twice daily and hydrochlorothiazide, 25 mg daily. She also takes a multiple vitamin daily and acetaminophen 1000 mg every 6 hours as needed. She continues to live in her one-floor house and is independent in doing all of her household chores. She also is responsible for all year-round outdoor maintenance activities, including mowing the lawn, raking leaves, and shoveling snow.

THINKING POINTS

- What assessment questions from Box 22-3 would you ask Ms. M. at this time?
- Would you use any information from Box 22-1 or 22-2 at this time?
- What myths or misunderstandings related to mobility and exercise might be influencing Ms. M.?
- Would you take any steps to assess her home environment for fall risks?

Hendrich II Fall Risk Model © 2006

Risk Factor	Risk Points	
Confusion/Disorientation/Impulsivity	4	
Symptomatic Depression	2	
Altered Elimination	1	
Dizziness/Vertigo	1	
Gender (Male)	1	
Any Administered Antiepileptics (anticonvulsants): *(Carbamazepine, Divalproex Sodium, Ethotoin, Ethosuximide, Felbamate, Fosphenytoin, Gabapentin, Lamotrigine, Mephenytoin, Methsuximide, Phenobarbital, Phenytoin, Primidone, Topiramate, Trimethadione, Valproic Acid)*	2	
Any Administered Benzodiazepines: *(Alprazolam, Chlordiazepoxide, Clonazepam, Clorazepate Dipotassium, Diazepam, Flurazepam, Halazepam, Lorazepam, Midazolam, Oxazepam, Temazepam, Triazolam)*	1	
Get-up-and-go Test: "Rising from a Chair" **If unable to assess, monitor for change in activity level, assess other risk factors, document both on patient chart with date and time.*		
Ability to rise in single movement-No loss of balance with steps	0	
Pushes up, successful in one attempt	1	
Multiple attempts but successful	3	
Unable to rise without assistance during test *(OR if a medical order states the same and/or complete bed rest is ordered)* **If unable to assess, document this on the patient chart with the date and time*	4	
(A score of 5 or greater = High Risk) **TOTAL SCORE**		

AHI
A VITAL SIGN FOR SAFETY™
Fall Prevention and Risk Management

FIGURE 22-1 The Hendrich II Fall Risk Model, a fall risk assessment tool recommended by the Hartford Institute for Geriatric Nursing. (©Ann Hendrich, Inc.) Used with permission.

NURSING DIAGNOSIS

Nurses working with older adults in any setting may identify risks for osteoporosis that they can address through health education. In community settings, postmenopausal women may express an interest in preventing osteoporosis because they are aware of the association between decreased estrogen and an increased likelihood of fractures. In these situations, Health-Seeking Behaviors may be an applicable nursing diagnosis, especially when there is a need for additional information about nutrition, exercise, and other interventions to prevent osteoporosis. This diagnosis is defined as "the state in which an individual in stable health actively seeks ways to alter personal health habits and/or the environment in order to move toward a higher level of wellness" (Carpenito-Moyet, 2006, p. 208). In long-term care and rehabilitation settings, nurses frequently address the needs of older adults who have a diagnosis of osteoporosis or a history of fractures. In these situations, as well as in any situation where someone has several risk factors for osteoporosis, a nursing diagnosis of Ineffective Health Maintenance can be used because the focus is on secondary prevention. This diagnosis is defined as "the state in which an individual or group experiences or is at risk of experiencing a disruption in health because of an unhealthy lifestyle or lack of knowledge about managing a condition" (Carpenito-Moyet, 2006, p. 197).

Impaired Physical Mobility is a nursing diagnosis that is applicable when the assessment identifies limitations in mobility of an older adult, and is particularly applicable in rehabilitation settings. This diagnosis is defined as "the state in which an individual experiences or is at risk of experiencing limitation of physical movement but is not immobile" (Carpenito-Moyet, 2006, p. 279). Related factors common in older adults include arthritis, depression, chronic pain, fractured hip and neurologic disorders (e.g., dementia or Parkinson's disease). If the nursing assessment identifies a history of falls or any risks for falls, the nursing diagnosis of Risk for Falls would be applicable. This diagnosis is defined as "the state in which an individual has increased susceptibility to falling" (Carpenito-Moyet, 2006, p. 250). Related factors common in older adults include all those factors listed in Box 22-2. When older adults express feelings associated with fallaphobia, the nurse may address this concern by applying a nursing diagnosis of Fear. Related factors would be postural instability, gait or balance disorders, or history of falls. This diagnosis is applicable when the nursing assessment reveals that the older adult limits his or her activities because of fallaphobia to the point that quality of life or level of functioning is affected.

Wellness Opportunity

Nurses can use the wellness nursing diagnosis Readiness for Enhanced Activity-Exercise Pattern for older adults who are willing to explore opportunities for improving musculoskeletal function and preventing falls and fractures.

PLANNING FOR WELLNESS OUTCOMES

When planning care for older adults who are at risk for osteoporosis, nurses identify wellness outcomes that focus on primary and secondary prevention. In these situations, any of the following Nursing Outcomes Classification (NOC) terms might be pertinent: Health Promoting Behavior, Knowledge: Health Behavior, Risk Control, or Risk Detection.

Nursing goals for an older adult with a nursing diagnosis of Impaired Physical Mobility focus on restoring functional abilities, preventing further loss of function, and preventing falls and injuries. NOC terminology applicable to an older adult with this nursing diagnosis include Balance, Endurance, Mobility, Pain Level, or Activity Tolerance.

Care of older adults with a nursing diagnosis of Risk for Falls focuses on preventing the occurrence of falls and fall-related injuries by implementing fall prevention programs. The following NOC terminology would be applicable with regard to safety and fall prevention: Risk Control, Risk Detection, Safety Behavior: Fall Prevention, Safety Behavior: Home Physical Environment, Safety Behavior: Personal, Safety Status: Physical Injury, or Safety Status: Falls.

Wellness Opportunity

Wellness outcomes that address the body–mind–spirit interrelatedness for people who are afraid of falling include Coping, Fear Control, Comfort Level, Anxiety Control, and Quality of Life.

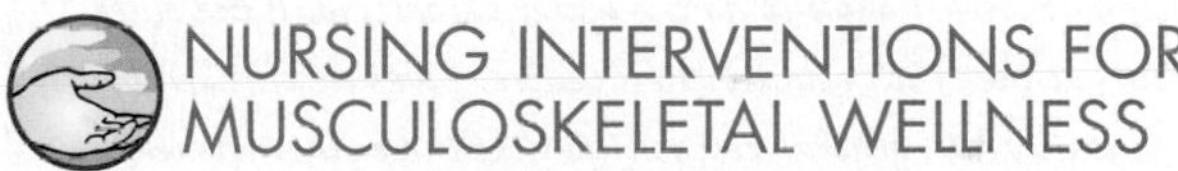

NURSING INTERVENTIONS FOR MUSCULOSKELETAL WELLNESS

Nurses have numerous opportunities to promote musculoskeletal wellness because most older adults would benefit from learning about health promotion interventions for overall physical fitness, preventing osteoporosis, and preventing falls. Thus, many of the interventions focus on teaching about eliminating or addressing risks. When nurses care for older adults in institutional settings, interventions also include direct actions to prevent falls and promote safe mobility. Some Nursing Interventions Classification (NIC) terminology that would be applicable to the interventions discussed in the following sections include Environmental Management, Exercise Promotion, Fall Prevention, Health Education, Risk Identification, and Teaching: Individual.

Promoting Healthy Musculoskeletal Function

Healthy older adults experience only a slight decline in overall musculoskeletal function, but they can compensate for these minor functional consequences by maintaining an active lifestyle. Various types of exercise are beneficial in promoting healthy musculoskeletal function and nurses can encourage older adults to incorporate several exercise strategies into their regular health behavior routines. Weight-bearing exercise is most helpful for osteoporosis, and a single set of seven resistance training exercises has been found to increase muscle size, strength, power, and endurance in older adults (Galvao & Taaffe, 2005). Flexibility exercises can improve range of motion, and balance training programs can improve safe mobility. Strength training has several positive effects, including improved balance. T'ai chi improves lower extremity strength, balance, flexibility, and coordination (Wallsten et al., 2006) and is becoming more widely available in community and long-term care settings. Maintaining an active lifestyle can be enjoyable as well as physically beneficial. Walking, dancing, swimming, t'ai chi, and bicycle riding are a few examples of recreational and relaxation activities that can have very positive health benefits for musculoskeletal function. The Gerontological Nursing Interventions Research Center at the University of Iowa developed an excellent evidence-based nursing protocol for promoting exercise in older adults. The purpose of this protocol is to "help health care providers in all settings enhance or maintain exercise behavior, particularly walking, in older adults" (Jitramontree, 2001, p. 7).

Wellness Opportunity

T'ai chi is an example of a wellness intervention that has positive effects on one's body, mind, and spirit.

A Student's Perspective

This past week I chose to do the water aerobics with the older adults at the Health and Fitness Centre. I was encouraged by the vitality and general zest for life that these older women showed. I was enlightened by their sense of pride in their health and level of activity. I left with the impression that this group activity was something that each of them attributed her good health to. I also noted that they got more out of this activity than just physical exercise. The social connection that these women had was truly admirable. They were constantly encouraging each other and me during the class. They also used the time just to connect with each other and discuss normal life events.

My take-away lesson from this experience was the importance of having opportunities like this for older adults to exercise their muscles as well as their social personalities. Older adults are often portrayed as socially inferior in today's popular culture, but I felt these older women were living truly balanced lives, maybe more so than me in some respects. I think that often I find myself so busy that I do not take time to invest myself in more meaningful relationships—something that these people are obviously benefiting from.

Clint H.

Preventing and Treating Osteoporosis

Health care providers are advised to incorporate interventions for prevention and treatment of osteoporosis as an integral part of fracture prevention regimens for older adults (Delaney, 2006; Gass & Dawson-Hughes, 2006). A recent report from the U.S. Surgeon General recommended a pyramidal treatment approach to osteoporosis that includes physical activity, fall prevention, and supplementation with calcium and vitamin D as the foundation of fracture prevention. Second and third levels of the pyramid include treatment of secondary causes of osteoporosis and pharmacotherapy for osteoporosis (USDHHS, 2004).

Goals of *Healthy People 2010* include reducing the proportion of adults with osteoporosis and reducing the proportion of adults who are hospitalized for vertebral fractures, which are the most common fractures due to osteoporosis (USDHHS, 2000). *Healthy People 2010* emphasizes that all older people, even those who have had a fracture, can benefit from treatment to prevent further bone loss or restore some lost bone to decrease the risk of further fractures. Osteoporosis is prevented and treated by using lifestyle, pharmacologic, and nutritional interventions. Lifestyle and nutritional interventions are applicable to all adults, and medical interventions are commonly used for people who have or are at risk for osteoporosis. Pharmacologic interventions are likely to be accompanied by at least a minimal risk of adverse effects, but for anyone with osteoporosis, the benefits and preventive effects are likely to far outweigh the risks. Because nutritional and lifestyle interventions have been found to be very safe as well as effective in both preventing and treating osteoporosis, there is much current emphasis on health education for all adults about them.

Although most studies on interventions for osteoporosis have focused on postmenopausal women, there is growing attention to osteoporosis interventions for men and residents of long-term care facilities. This attention is warranted because nursing home residents are more frail, vulnerable, and susceptible to the adverse effects of the failure to treat osteoporosis (Zarowitz et al., 2006). Up to 86% of white female nursing home residents have bone densities that meet the criteria for osteoporosis (Lee, 2001). Interventions for osteoporosis should be viewed as an important part of fracture prevention programs in long-term care facilities.

Despite the existence of research-based evidence that osteoporosis interventions are effective, studies have found that many older adults with risk factors for osteoporosis are untreated or undertreated (Bellantonio et al., 2001; Cuddihy et al., 2002; Gallagher et al., 2002; Khan et al., 2001). Some of this lack of treatment can be attributed to ageist perceptions that signs and symptoms of osteoporosis such as loss of height, dowager's hump, back pain, and fragility fractures are a normal part of aging (Zarowitz, et al., 2006). Nurses in any setting have numerous opportunities for teaching older adults about lifestyle, nutritional, and pharmacologic interventions for osteoporosis, as discussed in the following sections.

Health Education About Lifestyle and Nutritional Interventions

Because there is increasing attention to osteoporosis as a health concern that affects the majority of older adults in the United States, nurses have almost limitless opportunities for educating older adults about preventing osteoporosis and fractures. Public awareness about osteoporosis in women is high, but awareness about osteoporosis in men is just beginning to develop. Thus, nurses have a particular responsibility for raising the level of awareness about osteoporosis in men and educating older men about risk factors for osteoporosis and fractures. Nurses also focus health education on older adults who already have had fractures and on people who have other risk factors, because people who are more vulnerable to the serious consequences of osteoporosis may be more motivated to use preventive interventions.

Wellness Opportunity

Self-care practices to prevent osteoporosis are particularly important for older adults who have a history of falls or fractures.

Health education begins with providing information about risk factors for osteoporosis, as summarized in Box 22-1. Nurses can incorporate information about BMD tests in their health education about risk factors and advise older adults to discuss the appropriateness of this test with their primary care practitioner. Once risk factors are identified, nurses can help older adults develop a plan to address the modifiable risk factors. Nurses can encourage older adults with risk factors to discuss pharmacologic interventions with their primary care practitioner. Even in the absence of major risk factors, lifestyle and nutritional interventions should be encouraged for all older adults. Box 22-4 summarizes health promotion information that can be used as a guide for teaching older adults about osteoporosis.

Nurses can encourage all older adults to incorporate lifestyle interventions aimed at preventing osteoporosis because of their many overall benefits. For example, quitting smoking, limiting alcohol intake, and engaging in regular weight-bearing exercise are health-promoting behaviors that are likely to reduce the risk for fractures and osteoporosis, as well as being highly beneficial for other aspects of health and function. Successful implementation of lifestyle interventions depends to a large degree on motivation, but moti-

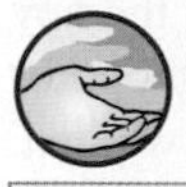

Box 22-4
Health Promotion Teaching About Osteoporosis

Health Promotion Interventions for Early Detection and Treatment

- Review risk factors for osteoporosis as summarized in Box 22-1.
- Plan interventions for modifiable risk factors using Box 22-1 as a guide.
- Encourage discussion with primary care provider about bone mineral density (BMD) tests.
- Encourage discussion with primary care provider about medical interventions for osteoporosis if risk factors are present.
- Encourage discussion with primary care provider about prevention of fractures if osteoporosis is diagnosed.

Lifestyle Interventions

- Implement weight-bearing exercise regimen for 1/2 hour daily.
- Wear good support shoes.
- Discontinue cigarette smoking.
- Maintain ideal body weight.
- Avoid excessive alcohol intake.

Nutritional Interventions

- Calcium supplements often are recommended so that the total intake is 1500 mg per day (average daily calcium intake of older adults is less than 800 mg).
- Foods that are high in calcium include milk, cheese, yogurt, custard, ice cream, raisins, tofu, canned salmon or sardines, and broccoli and other dark green vegetables.
- Provide adequate dietary intake of vitamin D and use 400 to 800 IU of vitamin D supplement daily.
- Calcium carbonate, which is found in some antacids, is an effective and inexpensive source of elemental calcium.
- Limit consumption of beverages containing alcohol, caffeine, or phosphorus.
- Avoid phosphate food additives.
- Increase intake of foods high in plant estrogen (e.g., tofu, soy foods).
- Herbal sources of calcium include nettle, parsley, horsetail, and dandelion leaf.
- Sources of natural estrogen include sage, ginseng, licorice, motherwort, dong quai, black cohosh, and chaste tree.

Special Precautions

- Vitamin D in amounts greater than 400 to 600 IU per day, and vitamin A in amounts exceeding 5000 IU per day, can have detrimental effects.
- Calcium supplements are not recommended for people with poor kidney function or a predisposition for kidney stones.
- Because calcium may contribute to constipation, measures should be taken to promote bowel function (e.g., regular exercise and adequate fiber and fluid intake).
- Calcium supplements can interact with some medications (e.g., calcium decreases absorption of tetracycline).

Complementary and Alternative Care Practices

- Engage in activities such as yoga, swimming, massage, acupressure, and t'ai chi.
- Acupuncture is helpful for arthritis and joint and muscle disorders.

vation for change is based at least in part on knowledge about risk factors. Therefore, nurses have an important responsibility to provide health information not only about risk for osteoporosis and fractures, but also about exercise and other lifestyle interventions that reduce this risk.

Nurses can also teach older adults and their caregivers about the importance of adequate intake of calcium and vitamin D. A registered dietician, if available, can evaluate a 3-day food history to determine the usual intake of calcium and vitamin D. If intake does not provide 1200 mg of calcium and 600 International Units of vitamin D, then health teaching focuses either on increasing dietary intake to the recommended amount or on taking a daily supplement. In long-term care facilities, nurses should include a review of nutritional interventions for osteoporosis in care plans, especially in relation to preventing fractures. Nurses can take the lead in initiating such a discussion and involving dieticians and primary care providers in developing and implementing appropriate preventive interventions. An article on management of osteoporosis in nursing homes stated that "unless there is clear contraindication, all residents should be taking recommended doses of calcium and vitamin D" (Lee, 2001, p. 34).

Adequate calcium is essential to maintaining musculoskeletal health, and there is widespread agreement that all adults age 51 years or older should have a daily calcium intake of 1200 to 1500 mg. Because the average American adult diet provides only between 500 and 800 mg of calcium daily, calcium supplements are usually necessary. Two reviews of studies concluded that calcium supplementation reduces bone loss, increases BMD, lowers the fracture rate in older adults, and may be particularly helpful for postmenopausal women (Grossman & MacLean, 2001; Morgan, 2001). Calcium supplements, however, may have detrimental effects in older adults who take medications or in those who have physiologic disturbances such as renal impairments. The supplements can interfere with absorption of zinc, iron, and other nutrients and medications such as atenolol, salicylates, propranolol, tetracyclines, and bisphosphonates. Absorption of calcium supplements is optimal at dosages of no more than 600 mg per dose (Morgan, 2001). The most common adverse effects of daily calcium supplements of 1500 mg or less are constipation, flatulence, and rebound gastric acidity.

An adequate intake of vitamin D also is essential for maintaining musculoskeletal health because it is necessary for the absorption of calcium. Most older adults do not have an adequate dietary intake of vitamin D. In addition, older adults who are not exposed to sunlight will not be able to synthesize vitamin D. Evidence supports the musculoskeletal benefits of 400 to 800 International Units of vitamin D supplement daily. Caution should be used, however, because vitamin D is fat soluble and excess amounts are not excreted. Adverse effects of vitamin D include hypercalciuria, hypercalcemia, and formation of kidney stones.

Pharmacologic Interventions

Effectiveness of pharmacologic interventions for osteoporosis is determined by their efficacy in both increasing BMD and reducing fracture risk. As new medications have become available, there has been more demand for randomized clinical trials that compare the effectiveness of various pharmacologic approaches for both treatment of osteoporosis and prevention of osteoporosis and fractures. Currently, major efforts focus on developing medications that will reduce the occurrence of fractures, especially hip fractures. Medications that were initially approved only for treating osteoporosis may undergo further clinical trials and become approved for the additional indications of preventing osteoporosis or fractures. Because clinical trials have only recently started to address osteoporosis in men, recommendations about pharmacologic interventions for osteoporosis in men are limited. However, this is a rapidly evolving area of medicine, and nurses need to keep up to date with new developments so they can provide appropriate health education. This section summarizes current information regarding medications for osteoporosis prevention and treatment in men and women.

Since the early 1980s, studies have consistently found that oral or transdermal estrogen is effective in preventing bone loss and reducing the incidence of fractures in postmenopausal women. Thus, for 2 decades hormonal therapy has been the most well-established approach for osteoporosis treatment and prevention in postmenopausal women. Although estrogen is most effective when administered early in the postmenopausal period, it is also effective in preventing further bone loss even when treatment begins at a late age. Many questions about the safety of estrogen replacement therapy arose during the 1970s, but at least some of the risk of the regimens initially prescribed has been reduced by using low doses and administering estrogen in combination with progesterone. In 2002, however, results of long-term studies identified additional serious risks from hormonal therapy, especially when it is used for more than a few years (see Chapter 26). Because of these findings, and because recent developments in pharmaceutical approaches to osteoporosis (discussed later in this section) have increased the number of medications available for prevention and treatment of osteoporosis, hormonal therapy is being used less commonly as a medical intervention for osteoporosis.

In 1984, the FDA approved calcitonin, a natural hormone that affects bone resorption, as the first nonestrogen medical intervention for treatment of osteoporosis. Initial limitations of calcitonin therapy included its high cost, the need for subcutaneous injections, and questions about its long-term effectiveness. In 1995, a nasal spray form of calcitonin was approved as an option for the treatment of low BMD. One therapeutic advantage of calcitonin over estrogen is that it has analgesic effects and can reduce the pain associated with vertebral fractures. Nasal calcitonin is approved for osteoporosis in women who have been postmenopausal for

5 years or more, but a disadvantage is that it may not be effective in preventing hip and other nonvertebral fractures (Gass & Dawson-Hughes, 2006).

The development of selective estrogen receptor modulators (SERMs) in the last decade created new hormonal treatment options for women with osteoporosis. SERMs, sometimes called *designer estrogens*, have estrogenic effects on bones and lipids but behave like estrogen blockers in the breast and uterus (Delaney, 2006). The goal of these agents is to provide the beneficial effects of estrogen without other unwanted effects. Tamoxifen is a SERM that has been used since 1994 to treat breast cancer, and in recent years there has been some evidence that it also maintains bone mass and may prevent fractures. Raloxifene is the most commonly used SERM for treating osteoporosis and reducing the risk of vertebral fracture; however, it has not been found to prevent nonvertebral fractures (Delaney, 2006). Raloxifene also improves serum lipids and may reduce the risk of breast cancer, but it increases the risk of deep vein thrombosis and pulmonary embolism (Gass & Dawson-Hughes, 2006). Adverse effects of SERMs include hot flashes, leg cramps, and deep vein thrombosis.

In the mid-1990s, the bisphosphonates became the first nonhormonal medications approved by the FDA for the prevention of fractures and bone loss. Currently, they are the most commonly used drugs for osteoporosis and are considered the gold standard against which other therapies are judged (Binkley & Krueger, 2005). Because bisphosphonates reduce bone resorption, they not only prevent bone loss but increase bone mass. Multiple randomized, controlled studies have found two bisphosphonates (alendronate and risedronate) to be effective in increasing BMD and reducing vertebral and nonvertebral fractures by 30% to 50% (Binkley & Krueger, 2005; NIH, 2001). Because of their effects on the gastrointestinal tract, bisphosphonates need to be taken in the morning with a full glass of water (not mineral water) at least a half hour before any food. In addition, the person must be in an upright position when taking this medication and avoid lying down for a half hour after the dose. Medically frail older adults may have difficulty meeting this requirement; this difficulty may be one of the factors that accounts for low use of bisphosphonates in nursing home residents (Jachna et al., 2005). Dosing frequency of bisphosphonates ranges from once daily to once monthly. Adverse effects of bisphosphonates include indigestion, diarrhea, flatulence, and abdominal pain.

The newest medical approach to treating osteoporosis is the use of parathyroid hormone (PTH), an anabolic agent that has been found to be effective in stimulating new bone growth. Teriparatide, the first drug in this class, is approved for the treatment of osteoporosis in women who are at high risk for fracture and in men with primary or hypogonadal osteoporosis who are at high risk for fracture. This drug is administered once daily as a subcutaneous injection; adverse effects include nausea, headache, and mild and transient hypercalcemia. The current recommendation is that teriparatide not be used for longer than 2 years because studies have not confirmed its long-term safety or efficacy.

Because most clinical trials of medical interventions for osteoporosis have focused primarily on women, much less evidence is available about safe and effective pharmacologic treatments for men with the disease. Bisphosphonates are the most widely studied pharmacologic interventions in men, and by 2002 the FDA had approved alendronate and risedronate for osteoporosis in men. It is likely that when additional bisphosphonates are approved for treatment of osteoporosis they will be approved for use in both men and women. Calcitonin is another medical intervention that can be used for men with osteoporosis, but its effectiveness in men is still being investigated. Testosterone therapy has been shown to improve BMD and it may, in turn, decrease the risk for fracture in men, but it has been shown to be effective only in men with secondary osteoporosis associated with hypogonadism. One study of healthy older men with low serum testosterone levels found that transdermal testosterone prevented bone loss at the femoral neck, decreased body fat, and increased lean body mass (Kenny et al., 2001). Although it has not been found to be beneficial for older men who have normal testosterone levels, the administration of testosterone, alone or in combination with growth hormone, is under investigation for its effects in increasing BMD in men with primary osteoporosis (Christmas et al., 2002).

In summary, there is sound evidence for pharmacologic treatment of osteoporosis because this intervention can improve BMD, reduce the rate of bone loss, and decrease the risk for fracture. Evidence is less clear about pharmacologic interventions for older adults who do not have osteoporosis but have risks for it. Decisions about preventive pharmacologic interventions for people at risk for osteoporosis and fractures must be based on an appraisal of the relative risks and benefits of any particular intervention. Pharmacologic treatment is just one component of a comprehensive management plan that also must include nutritional intake of calcium and vitamin D, physical activity to maintain musculoskeletal function and reduce the risk of falls, and patient education regarding osteoporosis and fall prevention (Binkley & Krueger, 2005).

Recall that you are the nurse at the wellness program where Ms. M., who is 75 years old, regularly attends your health education programs. Based on additional assessment information, you know that Ms. M. does not take any calcium or vitamin D supplements because she drinks milk twice daily and believes that this should be sufficient. She stopped having menstrual periods when she was 50 years old and began hormonal therapy at that time. She stopped taking estrogen when she was 63 because

(case study continues on page 480)

she began "hearing too many bad things about estrogen." When she fractured her wrist 8 years ago, the orthopedic surgeon said that her x-rays showed that her "bones were pretty good for her age." She has not had any further x-rays or any BMD tests and says her doctor has never brought up the subject of osteoporosis because "I guess he's too worried about my heart problems to be concerned about my bones." Although she fell once when she was raking leaves last fall and tripped over a small tree stump, she has had no serious fall-related injuries since she fractured her wrist. She does not smoke and drinks alcohol only on major social occasions. When you assessed her blood pressure, you found her blood pressure while standing was 146/86 mm Hg and while lying was 128/78 mm Hg. Her record of self-monitored blood pressure readings indicates that her usual blood pressure is around 134/82 mm Hg. Her vision is adequate, but she has stopped driving at night and is being monitored by her ophthalmologist for progression of bilateral cataracts. Her eye doctor told her she is likely to need cataract surgery sometime during the next 2 to 3 years.

THINKING POINTS

- What further assessment information would you want to have?
- What health promotion interventions would you advise for Ms. M.? Specifically, what health teaching would you do with regard to further assessment, lifestyle interventions, nutrition and nutritional supplements, and pharmacologic interventions?
- What educational materials would you use for Ms. M.?
- What follow-up health promotion would you consider for Ms. M.? Specifically, how would you work with Ms. M. to develop long-term health promotion interventions?

Preventing Falls and Fall-Related Injuries

Nurses intervene to prevent falls and fall-related injuries, but because falls are multifaceted in their causes, falls and fall-related injuries are best prevented through efforts of multidisciplinary teams. Multidisciplinary interventions focus on actions that nurses and other members of the health care team can take to eliminate and address all identified risk factors. Some of these interventions involve health education of older adults and their families. Formal fall prevention programs are now widely implemented in institutional as well as home care settings, and many guidelines have been developed based on nursing research (e.g., Lyons, 2004; O'Connell & Mion, 2003; Resnick, 2003; Theodos, 2004).

Implementing Fall Prevention Programs

Fall prevention programs may be designed to address a single risk factor or to address multiple risk factors. Examples of interventions addressing single risk factors include exercise to promote strength and balance; vision examinations with provision of corrective lenses and appropriate treatments; and education about ways of compensating for specific mobility problems and underlying causative factors (Lord et al., 2005). When impaired musculoskeletal function is combined with cognitive impairment, fall prevention programs should include treatment of psychiatric and behavioral symptoms (Kallin et al., 2005).

Fall prevention programs are more effective when an initial baseline assessment is done to estimate the person's overall risk for falls and to establish their basic performance level. Risk factors must be assessed (as discussed in the Assessment section) not only initially but at timely intervals, so the information can be incorporated as an integral part of the comprehensive fall prevention plan.

Each fall prevention program addresses risk factors that are common in that particular setting and those factors that are unique to each at-risk person. Attention must be paid to intrinsic and extrinsic risk factors for falls, to factors that reduce the risk of falls, and to factors that reduce the risk of fall-related injuries. Key aspects of fall prevention programs are the identification of people who are at risk for falls and the consistent implementation of preventive actions by all staff. Thus, an important part of these programs is the education of all professional and nonprofessional staff members who have contact with the person who is at risk for falls. Education may involve strategies to heighten staff awareness of the importance of reducing the risks of falls. For example, posters and brochures may be used initially and periodically as reminders. Also, some form of patient/resident or chart identification can be used to draw attention to those people who have an increased risk for falls. Box 22-5 describes a fall prevention program that could be adapted for use in institutional settings.

Because the prevalence of falls for residents in dementia care units is twice that in other institutional settings, staff in these units need to take special precautions (Detweiler et al., 2005). For example, studies have found that placing residents in a small group with intense, focused supervision by specially trained staff is effective in reducing falls and fall-related injuries. Staff responsibilities include observing to anticipate falls, keeping residents occupied, and intervening quickly to catch a falling resident (Detweiler et al., 2005).

Addressing Intrinsic Risk Factors. Because any gait and balance impairment increases the risk for falls, interventions that improve mobility are likely to be beneficial in preventing falls. Interventions for improving mobility are implemented primarily by therapists, nurses, and nursing staff, often through an interdisciplinary approach. Teaching about the proper use of mobility aids and other assistive devices is an important part of fall prevention programs (Fig. 22-2).

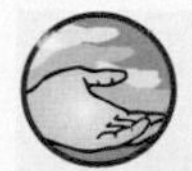

Box 22-5
A Fall Prevention Program for Older Adults Being Cared for in Hospitals or Nursing Homes

Identification of Patients/Residents Who Are at Risk for Falling

- During the initial nursing or multidisciplinary assessment, identify any risks for falling and fall-related injuries (e.g., medications, osteoporosis, medical conditions, history of falls, impaired cognition, diminished alertness, impaired mobility, age 75 years or older).
- Document the risk factors on the designated fall assessment guide.
- Address any risk factors for falls, osteoporosis, or fall-related injuries that can be modified; this often requires a multidisciplinary approach.
- Reassess the risks for falls and fall-related injuries at predetermined times (e.g., every shift, every day, whenever there is a change in the patient's/resident's functional status).
- Use color-coded items (e.g., brightly colored stickers for the chart, a brightly colored identification band for the person's wrist, and signs near the person's bed and outside the room) to identify those who are included in the fall prevention program.

Education of the Staff, Patient/Resident, and Family

- Instruct the patient or resident and family about the fall prevention program using brochures that provide information about preventing falls and obtaining help if falls occur.
- Provide staff education about the fall prevention program and the risk factors for falls, especially those factors that the staff influences (e.g., use of restraints, selection of footwear).
- Use posters and fliers to heighten staff awareness of the fall prevention program.

Interventions to Be Implemented for All High-Risk Patients/Residents

- Keep the call light within reach at all times.
- Make sure that ambulatory patients wear sturdy, nonslip footwear when out of bed.
- Offer assistance with activities of daily living (ADLs) and try to anticipate the person's needs before help is needed.
- Encourage the person to call for help when needed.
- Frequently check all people who cannot be relied on to call for help.
- Make sure the bed is in the lowest position possible and the wheels are locked.
- Carefully and frequently assess the environment for factors that increase the risk for either falls or fall-related injuries; address all modifiable risk factors.
- Consider the use of a movement detection device.
- Carefully evaluate the potential consequences of physical restraints, including bedrails.
- If restraints are used, reevaluate their use every shift.
- If appropriate, orient the person to person, place, and time every shift and as needed.
- Document fall prevention interventions on the person's chart.

Nurses are responsible for raising questions about whether an older adult may benefit from the use of mobility aids or assistive devices and facilitating a referral to a physical therapist for evaluation and teaching regarding their use. In community settings, nurses can teach older adults and their caregivers about the availability of various mobility aids, transfer assistance devices, and other aids that might improve safety. Nurses can suggest that older adults seek professional help with selecting appropriate mobility aids and assistive devices. Some suppliers of home health care equipment have therapists on staff who can provide advice and assist with processing claims if the aids are covered by insurance. When mobility aids are prescribed, nurses are responsible for encouraging the person to use the aids and making sure that the aids are accessible. Nurses are responsible for facilitating referrals for reassessment if questions arise about the safety or effectiveness of mobility aids that are being used.

Because proper footwear is essential to prevent slips and falls, nurses can advise older adults about wearing nonslip footwear for safety. Walking outdoors can be particularly hazardous, especially when winter conditions create a very dangerous environment for older people who have a predisposition for falls. Nurses can emphasize the importance of removing ice and snow from walkways and help older adults explore resources for assistance with this. In addition, a simple gait-stabilizing device, such as the Yaktrax Walker (Fig. 22-3), can be used for preventing outdoor falls when applied and worn properly (McKiernan, 2005).

In recent years, fall prevention literature has emphasized the effectiveness of various exercise routines as an intervention for reducing intrinsic fall risk. An important role for nurses is to identify those older adults who may benefit from gait and balance training programs and to facilitate referrals for physical therapy when appropriate. Nurses also are responsible for encouraging adequate and consistent follow-through with recommended exercise programs. In long-term care settings, nurses generally oversee restorative nursing programs in which nursing assistants help residents with walking and other exercise regimens established by physical therapists. These restorative nursing routines are essential aspects of fall prevention programs. Group exercise programs also are widely used as fall prevention interventions that are beneficial to all at-risk people. Many programs incorporate exercises aimed specifically at improving gait, balance, ankle strength, or other aspects of fall prevention. T'ai chi, for example, reduces the risk of falls and has been effective for addressing fear of falling in frail older adults (McKenna, 2001). Nurses can include information about the benefits of tai chi and other exercise routines into their health promotion education about fall prevention.

Fall prevention programs also include multidisciplinary interventions to address polypharmaceutic and pathologic

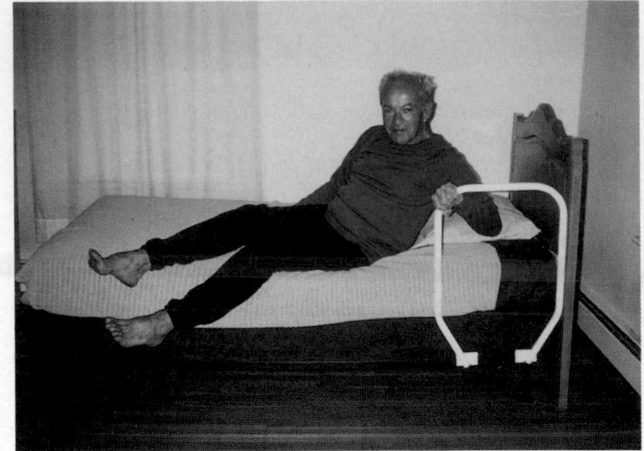

A

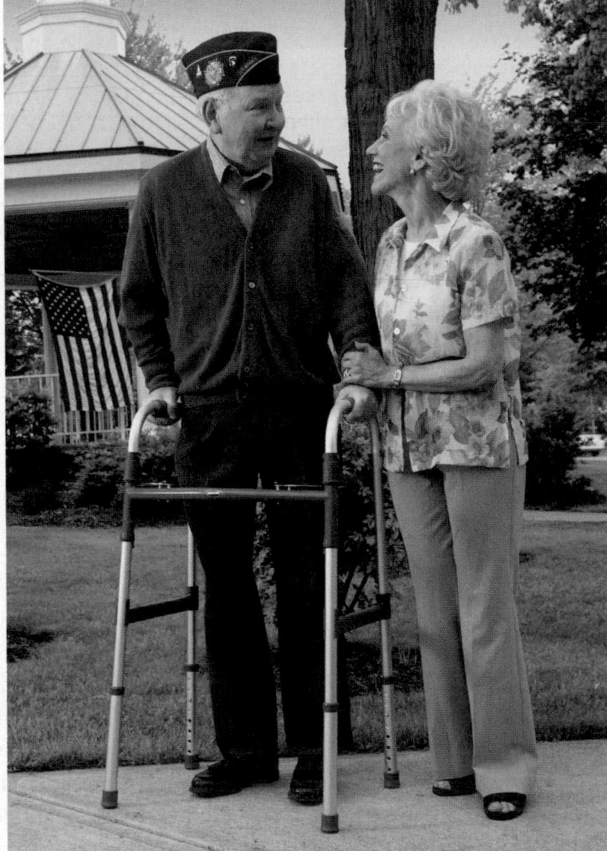

B

FIGURE 22-2 The use of assistive devices can help reduce the risk of falls. **(A)** Transfer assistive devices are used to facilitate safer transfer in and out of beds. (BED-BAR courtesy of Brown Engineering Corporation.) **(B)** Walkers are available in various styles with wheels, brakes, baskets, seats, and other features to improve safety and mobility. (Invacare Blue Release Walker. Photography ©2000 Invacare Corporation. Invacare is a registered trademark of Invacare Corporation.)

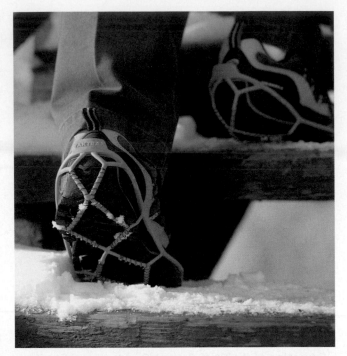

FIGURE 22-3 The Yaktrax Walker is an example of a gait-stabilizing device that can be used to prevent falls on slippery outdoor surfaces. (Photograph courtesy of Yaktrax, LLC.)

conditions that increase the risk for falls. Nurses are responsible for knowing the common adverse effects of medications and raising questions about these effects, particularly in relation to fall risk. Nurses should assess for postural hypotension, for example, as a potential adverse medication effect and as a risk factor for falls. Medication regimens should be reviewed periodically, and nurses can take the lead in suggesting that pharmacists and prescribing practitioners evaluate medications in relation to fall risks.

Addressing Extrinsic Risk Factors. Interventions for addressing extrinsic risk factors, such as environmental conditions and use of restraints, are applicable for older adults in any setting. Educational interventions and modifications to reduce risks based on a home hazard assessment have been found to be successful interventions in reducing fall hazards in homes (Stevens et al., 2001). Even an educational intervention as simple as raising awareness about the importance of modifying home environments for safety can be an effective fall prevention strategy (Gerson et al., 2005). Guidelines recommend that patients who are at risk for falls should receive referrals for environmental home assessments when they are discharged from hospitals (American Geriatrics Society, 2001). Environmental assessment guidelines provided in Chapter 7 can help with planning interventions that may eliminate or reduce environmental risks. In addition, environmental modifications to improve a person's vision, as discussed in Chapter 17, are applicable to fall prevention.

Wellness Opportunity

Fall-prevention interventions that address the person–environment relationship can be as simple and effective as involving older adults in decisions about removing or replacing slippery throw rugs.

Using Monitoring Devices. Monitoring devices can be very useful in alerting staff to potentially dangerous patient/resident activity, such as getting out of bed or a chair without assistance. Many types of devices are available, but they all transmit a signal to a remote location (e.g., a nursing station) when activated by certain levels of patient/resident movement. Some devices, such as a pad, are applied to the bed, whereas others are attached to the person's clothing. Other devices are programmed specifically for the person's movement in a confined environment such as his or her room. Most movement detection devices were originally designed for institutional use, but simplified monitoring and signal systems have now been developed for home use by family caregivers. In home settings, an auditory room monitoring device may be useful when caregivers need to detect the sound of someone moving around in another room. These devices are widely available in stores where infant care supplies are sold. A major limitation of any movement detection device is that its effectiveness depends on the timely response of someone who is able to prevent the fall. These devices are not useful for people living alone or for people without responsible and responsive caregivers.

Preventing Fall-Related Injuries and Death

In the United States, trauma is the fifth leading cause of death in people older than 65 years of age, and falls are responsible for 70% of the deaths due to trauma in people older than 75 years (Colon-Emeric, 2002; Fuller, 2000). When falls cannot be prevented, interventions are directed toward reducing the risk of fractures and other serious fall-related injuries. Because falls are the most common cause of injuries and trauma-related hospitalizations among older adults—with hip fractures being the most serious fall-related injury—one goal of *Healthy People 2010* is to reduce hip fractures in this population (USDHHS, 2000). Perhaps the most universally applicable intervention for prevention of fall-related injuries is to ensure that the measures for preventing and treating osteoporosis discussed earlier are taken. Environmental adaptations can also be considered universally as interventions to reduce the risk of fall-related injuries. For example, heavy furniture that is in a pathway where a fall is likely to occur can be moved out of the way, and sharp edges of furniture can be padded. Using a bed that can be adjusted to a low position can reduce risk of injury from falling out of bed. Soft mats can be placed near beds and in other locations where people are likely to fall, but caution must be used so these pads do not become fall risks. External hip protectors have been available since the 1990s, and at least ten types of hip protectors are now in use in both Europe and North America (Fig. 22-4). Hip protectors, which are designed to decrease the impact of a fall, consist of pads with or without hard shells that are placed over the hips and worn under garments. Some studies indicate that wearing these protectors can significantly reduce the risk of hip fracture in nursing home residents who are at high risk for falls. However, questions about effectiveness and concerns about cost, comfort, and appearance often limit their use (Lin & Lane, 2006).

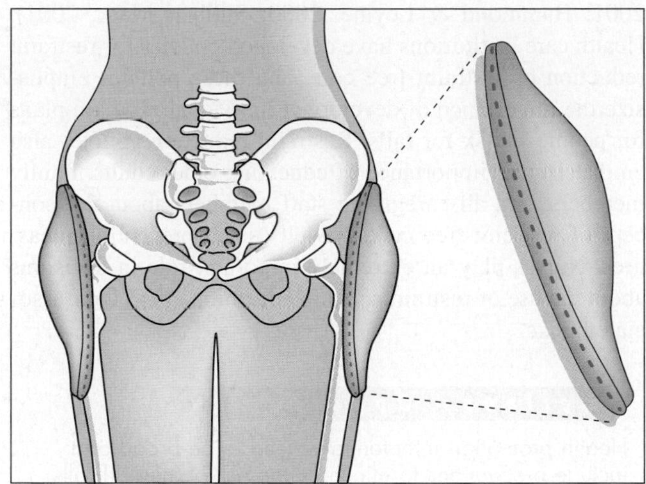

FIGURE 22-4 Hip protectors come in a variety of styles. This hip protector system consists of two padded shells that fit in pockets inside an undergarment.

For people living alone, interventions also are directed toward providing assistance in a timely manner. A personal emergency response system (PERS) can be useful in summoning help when falls cannot be prevented. These devices involve the use of a small portable transmitter that is worn on the person's body or clothing. Examples of such devices are beeper-type devices worn on the belt or pendants worn as necklaces or bracelets. When the person falls, he or she can summon help by using the transmitter to signal a receiver unit attached to the phone. In turn, a call is automatically made to the PERS provider, who then checks in with the person and calls the local emergency response team or a contact person, such as a neighbor or family member. Some of these devices are set up so that a check-up call is made to the person during any 24 hour period in which the person does not push a reset button or otherwise notify the company that he or she is well. The effectiveness of PERS depends on the ability of the fallen person to signal for help and on the availability of a helping person. A major limitation of such devices is that cognitively impaired people may not be able to learn to use them. Hospitals and home care agencies can provide information about local PERS programs, and information about national programs is available on the Internet. Cordless phones, especially if preprogrammed for emergency help and placed within reach where someone might fall, can also be used for obtaining help.

Finally, decisions regarding use of bedrails and other types of restraints should take into consideration that restraints do not necessarily reduce the risk of falls and are associated with more serious fall-related injuries. Numerous nursing references can be found in professional journals, and organizations such as the American Nurses Association, the CMS, and the Joint Commission have challenged the routine use of restraints (e.g., American Geriatrics Society,

2001; Hammond & Levine, 2000; Sullivan-Marx, 2001). Health care institutions have developed policies for restraint reduction or restraint-free care, and these policies emphasize the importance of developing individualized care plans for people at risk for falls. Restraint reduction policies also emphasize the importance of educating older adults, family members, and all caregiving staff members about the concept of restraint-free care as well as fall prevention measures. Nurses play an extremely important role in decisions about the use of restraints and in education about their associated risks.

Wellness Opportunity

Health promotion interventions need to be broad and include precautions to minimize the risk of injury if falls do occur.

Addressing Fear of Falling

Any interventions that reduce the risk of falls are likely also to reduce a person's fear of falling, but some people may need additional interventions to address this problem. Several models of group interventions have been published describing educational and psychosocial interventions to address fear of falling (Gentleman & Malozemoff, 2001; Tennstedt et al., 2001). The "Falls and Feelings" discussion group is a nursing model that was designed to facilitate discussion of feelings related to falling experiences. The goal for group members was "to enhance self-confidence and life satisfaction, resulting in empowerment of the individual to handle fear of falling" (Gentleman & Malozemoff, 2001, 36). Themes of the sessions included risks for falls, prevention of falls, falls and feelings, and fear as a consequence of falls (Gentleman & Malozemoff, 2001). Nurses can address fear of falling in the same way they address other fears: encourage the expression of feelings and provide education and reassurance about interventions that are being implemented as part of an individualized fall prevention care plan. Family members and caregivers should be included in nursing interventions and health education to address fear of falling. For people living alone, a PERS may be very reassuring and at least alleviate the fear of being helpless if a fall occurs.

Wellness Opportunity

Nurses address body–mind–spirit interrelatedness by talking with older adults about ways of diminishing their fear of falling and identifying ways of improving their safety.

EVALUATING EFFECTIVENESS OF NURSING INTERVENTIONS

Nursing care for older adults with impaired musculoskeletal function is evaluated by the degree to which the person achieves and maintains the highest possible level of independence and safe mobility. Nursing care of older adults who are at high risk for osteoporosis is evaluated according to the degree to which the older adult incorporates preventive measures in his or her daily life. For example, older adults might begin a regimen of three half-hour periods of weight-bearing exercise weekly. The nursing care of older adults who are at high risk for falls and fall-related injuries is evaluated according to the extent to which falls and serious injuries are prevented. Nurses cannot, of course, measure the number of falls that do not occur, but they can measure the risk factors that have been addressed in the care plan. Evaluation of these risk factors is facilitated by careful documentation of interventions, such as environmental modifications and fall prevention programs.

Ms. M. is now 89 years old and has been admitted to the hospital for heart failure. Additional medical problems include arthritis, osteoporosis, recurrent depression, early-stage dementia, and history of fractured hip. Current medications include furosemide, 40 mg twice daily; enalapril, 10 mg twice daily; digoxin, 0.125 mg daily; calcitonin nasal spray daily; OS-cal with D; and sertraline (Zoloft), 50 mg at bedtime. Ms. M. lives alone in an assisted-living facility, where she receives help with her medications and goes to the dining room for meals. You are the nurse on the acute care floor assigned to her care on the day of admission.

NURSING ASSESSMENT

During your initial nursing assessment, Ms. M. is quiet and withdrawn. When you ask about her living situation, she says she moved to the assisted-living facility 2 years ago, after she was hospitalized for treatment of a fractured hip. At the time of the injury, she had been living alone. She had fallen while making her way to the bathroom at night, and remained lying on the floor until her daughter came to visit her the next morning. During

(case study continues on page 485)

the past year, Ms. M. reports that she has fallen twice in her room, but that she has been able to call for help and has not had any serious injuries. You determine that Ms. M. will need help in ambulating to the bathroom and that she should be supervised whenever she gets out of bed.

Ms. M. confides that she is worried that she will have to move to the nursing home section of her facility if she falls again. She is very depressed about her lack of energy and her hospitalization for congestive heart failure. A mental status assessment indicates that Ms. M. is alert and oriented but that her short-term memory is impaired. She has a great deal of difficulty with abstract ideas, such as learning to use the call button. You check her vital signs, which are within normal range, with no evidence of postural hypotension.

NURSING DIAGNOSIS

In addition to the nursing diagnoses related to Ms. M.'s medical condition, you identify a nursing diagnosis of Risk for Falls. Related factors include weakness, diuretic and cardiovascular medications, a history of falls, depression, and impaired cognition. You are concerned about preventing falls during her hospitalization.

NURSING CARE PLAN FOR MS. M.

Expected Outcome	Nursing Interventions	Nursing Evaluation
Ms. M. will ambulate safely and avoid falls during her hospitalization.	• Identify Ms. M. as a participant in the fall prevention program by using an orange wrist bracelet, posting a Fall Alert sign near her bed, and placing an orange Fall Alert sticker on her chart. • Provide Ms. M. with a brochure that explains the fall prevention program. • Reassess fall risks every shift and document these on the Fall Assessment form included in Ms. M.'s chart. • Talk with Ms. M.'s physician about a referral for physical therapy. • Keep the call light button within her reach and review instructions for its use every shift. • Assess benefits and risks of using bedrails, and discuss with Ms. M. and her family. • Make sure that the bed is in the lowest possible position with the wheels locked. • Use a movement detection bed pad and explain to Ms. M. that the purpose of the pad is to ensure that the staff knows when she needs to get out of bed. • Every 2 hours, when Ms. M. is awake, the nursing staff will ask her if she needs to go to the bathroom.	• Ms. M. will receive assistance with ambulation every time she is out of bed. • Ms. M. will not fall during her hospitalization.

THINKING POINTS

- If you were the nurse on the acute care floor where Ms. M. was a patient, what concerns would you address in a discharge plan? Would you identify any additional nursing diagnoses related to safe mobility and musculoskeletal function? What additional nursing interventions would you plan to supplement the care plan described in this chapter?
- If you were a nurse in the assisted-living facility where Ms. M. lives, what concerns would you have about her care? How would you address these concerns in a care plan?

Chapter Highlights

Age-Related Changes That Affect Mobility and Safety

- Diminished muscle mass
- Degenerative changes in joints
- Slower response of central nervous system
- Osteoporosis

Risk Factors That Affect Mobility and Safety

- Risk factors for impaired musculoskeletal function: inactivity, inadequate protein and vitamin D intake
- Risk factors for osteoporosis and fractures: inadequate calcium and vitamin D intake, lack of weight-bearing activity, female gender, small bones, increased age, tobacco smoking, excessive alcohol drinking, certain medications (e.g., corticosteroids) (Box 22-1)
- Risk factors for falls: age-related changes in gait, sensory function, and central nervous system; pathologic conditions and functional impairments; medication effects and interactions; environmental factors (e.g., obstacles, throw rugs, physical restraints) (Box 22-2)

Pathologic Condition Affecting Musculoskeletal Wellness

- Osteoarthritis

Functional Consequences Affecting Musculoskeletal Wellness

- Diminished muscle strength, endurance, and coordination
- Increased difficulty performing ADLs
- Increased susceptibility to falls
- Increased susceptibility to fall-related injuries, including death
- Fear of falls

Nursing Assessment of Musculoskeletal Function (Box 22-3)

- Ability to walk safely and perform all ADLs
- Risks for osteoporosis (e.g., intake of calcium and vitamin D, history of fractures)
- Identifying risks for falls (Fig. 22-1)
- Assessing for safety of the environment

Nursing Diagnosis

- Wellness nursing diagnosis: Readiness for Enhanced Activity-Exercise Pattern
- Related to osteoporosis: Health-Seeking Behaviors, Ineffective Health Maintenance
- Related to fall risks: Impaired Physical Mobility, Risk for Falls
- Additional diagnoses that addresses fear of falling: Fear

Planning for Wellness Outcomes

- Balance, Endurance, Mobility, Activity Tolerance
- Risk Control, Risk Detection
- Safety Behavior: Fall Prevention, Home Physical Environment
- Coping, Fear Control, Comfort Level

Nursing Interventions for Musculoskeletal Wellness

- Teaching about exercise
- Teaching about osteoporosis (e.g., early detection and treatment, lifestyle interventions, nutritional interventions, medications) (Box 22-4)
- Implementing fall prevention programs (e.g., eliminating risks, using monitoring devices, addressing contributing factors) (Box 22-5)
- Preventing fall-related injuries and death (e.g., hip protectors, environmental interventions)
- Addressing fear of falling

Evaluating Effectiveness of Nursing Interventions

- Maintenance of highest level of safe mobility
- Incorporation of preventive measures in daily life to ensure safety and prevent osteoporosis
- Expressed feelings of safety and improved quality of life

Critical Thinking Exercises

1. Identify factors that increase or reduce the risk for osteoporosis.
2. Describe how each of the following age-related changes or risk factors might increase an older person's risk for falls and fractures: nocturia, osteoporosis, medications, altered gait, pathologic conditions, sensory impairments, cognitive impairments, functional impairments, slowed reaction time.
3. Describe the environmental factors that you would assess, in both home and institutional settings, to identify potential risks for falls.
4. Describe how you would design and implement a fall prevention program in a long-term care facility.
5. How would you deal with a daughter who demanded that restraints be used whenever her 84-year-old mother, who is a patient on your acute care floor, is sitting in a chair?
6. What information would you include in health education about osteoporosis?
7. Use the Internet to find information about fall prevention products that you might use in clinical practice.

Clinical Tool Resources

Hartford Institute for Geriatric Nursing
Try This: Best Practices in Nursing Care to Older Adults
Issue Number 8 (Revised 2007), Fall Risk Assessment for Older Adults: The Hendrich II Model
www.hartfordign.org/resources/education/tryThis.html

Educational Resources

American Menopause Foundation, Inc.
www.americanmenopause.org

Arthritis Foundation
www.arthritis.org

National Arthritis and Musculoskeletal and Skin Diseases Information Clearinghouse
National Institutes of Health
www.nih.gov/niams

National Center for Injury Prevention and Control
www.cdc.gov/ncipc

National Osteoporosis Foundation
www.nof.org

North American Menopause Society
www.menopause.org

Watch Your Step
Falls Prevention Initiative
www.chpna.ca/falls

REFERENCES

American Geriatrics Society, British Geriatrics Society, & American Academy of Orthopaedic Surgeons Panel on Falls Prevention. (2001). Guideline for the prevention of falls in older persons. *Journal of the American Geriatrics Society, 49*, 664–672.

Aschkenasy, M. T., & Rothenhaus, T.C. (2006). Trauma and falls in the elderly. *Emergency Medicine Clinics of North America, 24*, 413–432.

Basante, J., Bentz, E., Heck-Hakley, J., Kenion, B., Young, D., & Holm, M. B. (2001). Fall risks among older adults in long-term care facilities: A focused literature review. *Physical & Occupational Therapy in Geriatrics, 19*(2), 63–85.

Bellantonio, S., Fortinsky, R., & Prestwood, K. (2001). How well are community-living women treated for osteoporosis after hip fracture? *Journal of the American Geriatrics Society, 49*, 1197–1204.

Binkley, N., & Krueger, D. (2005). Current osteoporosis prevention and management. *Topics in Geriatric Rehabilitation, 21*(1), 17–29.

Brassington, G. S., King, A. C., & Bliwise, D. L. (2000). Sleep problems as a risk factor for falls in a sample of community-dwelling adults aged 64–99 years. *Journal of the American Geriatrics Society, 48*, 1234–1240.

Burks, K. (2005). Osteoarthritis in older adults: Current treatments. *Journal of Gerontological Nursing, 31*(5), 14–19.

Campbell, W. W., Trappe, T. A., Wolfe, R. R., & Evans. W. J. (2001). The recommended dietary allowance for protein may not be adequate for older people to maintain skeletal muscle. *Journals of Gerontology: Series A, Biological Sciences and Medical Sciences, 56*, M373–M380.

Carpenito-Moyet, L. J. (2006). *Handbook of nursing diagnosis* (11th ed.). Philadelphia: Lippincott Williams & Wilkins.

Carter, C. S., & Sonntag, W. E. (2006). Growth hormone, insulin-like growth factor-1, and the biology of aging. In E. J. Masoro & S. N. Austad (Eds.), *Handbook of the biology of aging* (6th ed., pp. 534–569). San Diego: Academic Press.

Chamberlin, M. E., Fulwider, B. D., Sanders, S. L., & Medeiros, X. (2005). Does fear of falling influence spatial and temporal gait parameters in elderly persons beyond changes associated with normal aging? *Journals of Gerontology: Series A, Biological Sciences and Medical Sciences, 60*, 1163–1167.

Christmas, C., O'Connor, K. G., Harman, S. M., Tobin, J. D., Münzer, T., Bellantoni, M. F., et al. (2002). Growth hormone and sex steroid effects on bone metabolism and bone mineral density in healthy aged women and men. *Journals of Gerontology: Series A, Biological Sciences and Medical Sciences, 57*, M12–M18.

Colon-Emeric, C. S. (2002). Falls in older adults: Assessment and intervention in primary care. *Hospital Physician, 4*, 55–65.

Cuddihy, M. T., Gabriel, S. E., Crowson, C. S., Atkinson, E. J., Tabini, C., O'Fallon, W. M., et al. (2002). Osteoporosis intervention following distal forearm fractures. *Archives of Internal Medicine, 162*, 421–426.

Cumming, R. G., Salkeld, G., Thomas, M., & Szonyi, G. (2000). Prospective study of the impact of fear of falling on activities of daily living, SF-36 scores, and nursing home admission. *Journals of Gerontology: Series A, Biological Sciences and Medical Sciences, 55*, M299–M305.

Delaney, M. F. (2006). Strategies for the prevention and treatment of osteoporosis during early postmenopause. *American Journal of Obstetrics and Gynecology, 194*, 12–23.

Detweiler, M. B., Kim, K. Y., & Taylor, B. Y. (2005). Focused supervision of high-risk fall dementia patients: A simple method to reduce fall incidence and severity. *American Journal of Alzheimer's Disease and Other Dementias, 20*(2), 97–104.

Drozdick, L. W., & Edelstein, B. A. (2001). Correlates of fear of falling in older adults who have experienced a fall. *Journal of Clinical Geropsychology, 7*(1), 1–13.

Dunn, K. S. (2001). The effect of physical restraints on fall rates in older adults who are institutionalized. *Journal of Gerontological Nursing, 27*(10), 40–48.

Ellis, A. A., & Trent, R. B. (2001). Do the risks and consequences of hospitalized fall injuries among older adults in California vary by type of fall? *Journals of Gerontology: Series A, Biological Sciences and Medical Sciences, 56*, M686–M692.

Espino, D. V., Palmer, R. F., Miles, T. P., Mouton, C. P., Wood, R. C., Bayne, N. S., et al. (2000). Prevalence, incidence, and risk factors associated with hip fractures in community-dwelling older Mexican Americans: Results of the Hispanic EPESE study. *Journal of the American Geriatrics Society, 48*, 1252–1260.

Fransen, M., Woodward, M., Norton, R., Robinson, E., Butler, M., & Campbell, A. J. (2002). Excess mortality or institutionalization after hip fracture: Men are at greater risk than women. *Journal of the American Geriatrics Society, 50*, 685–690.

Fuller, G. F. (2000). Falls and the elderly. *American Family Physician, 61*, 2159–2168, 2173–2174.

Gage, B. F., Birman-Deych, E., Radford, M. J., Nilasena, D. S., & Binder, E. F. (2006). Risk of osteoporotic fracture in elderly patients taking warfarin. *Archives of Internal Medicine, 166*, 241–246.

Gallagher, T. C., Geling, O., & Comite, F. (2002). Missed opportunities for prevention of osteoporotic fracture. *Archives of Internal Medicine, 162*, 450–456.

Galvao, D. A., & Taaffe, D. R. (2005). Resistance exercise dosage in older adults: Single- versus multi-set effects on physical performance and body composition. *Journal of the American Geriatrics Society, 53*, 2090–2097.

Gass, M., & Dawson-Hughes, B. (2006). Prevention osteoporosis-related fractures: An overview. *American Journal of Medicine, 119*(4, Suppl. 1), 3S–11S.

Gentleman, B., & Malozemoff, W. (2001). Falls and feelings: Description of a psychosocial group nursing intervention. *Journal of Gerontological Nursing, 27*(10), 35–39.

Gerson, L. W., Camargo, C. A., & Wilber, S. T. (2005). Home modification to prevent falls by older ED patients. *American Journal of Emergency Medicine, 23*, 295–298.

Gray, S. L., LaCroix, A. Z., Hanlon, J. T., Penninx, B. W., & Blough, D. K. (2006). Benzodiazepine use and physical disability in community-dwelling older adults. *Journal of the American Geriatrics Society, 54*, 224–230.

Gray-Miceli, D. (Winter 2006). Fall Risk Assessment for Older Adults: The Hendrich II Model. *Try this: Best practices in nursing care to older adults*, Issue 8. New York University, Hartford Institute for Geriatric Nursing. Available at www.hartfordign.org/resources/education/tryThis.html.

Grossman, J. M., & MacLean, C. H. (2001). Quality indicators for the management of osteoporosis in vulnerable elders. *Annals of Internal Medicine, 135*, 722–730.

Hammond, M., & Levine, J. M. (2000). Bedrails: Choosing the best alternative. *Geriatric Nursing, 20*, 297–300.

Harrison, B., Booth, D., & Algase, D. (2001). Studying fall risk factors among nursing home residents who fell. *Journal of Gerontological Nursing, 27*(10), 26–34.

Hein, L. T., Cumming, R. G., Cameron, I. D., Chen, J. S., & Lord, S. R. (2005). Atypical antipsychotic medications and risk of falls in residents of aged care facilities. *Journal of the American Geriatrics Society, 53*, 1290–1265.

Hoffman, S., Powell-Cope, G., MacClellan, L., & Bero, K. (2003). Bedsafe: A bed safety project for frail older adults. *Journal of Gerontological Nursing, 29*(11), 34–42.

Jachna, C. M., Shireman, T. I., Whittle, J., Ellerbeck, E. F., & Rigler, S. K. (2005). Differing patterns of antiresorptive pharmacotherapy in nursing facility residents and community dwellers. *Journal of the American Geriatrics Society, 53*, 1275–1281.

Jitramontree, N. (2001). Evidence-based protocol: Exercise promotion—encouraging older adults to walk. *Journal of Gerontological Nursing, 27*(10), 7–18.

Kallin, K., Gustafso, Y., Sandman, P., & Karlsson, S. (2005). Factors associated with falls among older cognitively impaired people in geriatric care settings. *American Journal of Geriatric Psychiatry, 13*, 501–509.

Kamel, H. K. (2005). Male osteoporosis: New trends in diagnosis and therapy. *Drugs & Aging, 22*, 741–748.

Kay, G. G. (2000). The effects of antihistamines on cognition and performance. *Journal of Allergy and Clinical Immunology, 105*, 622–627.

Kenny, A. M., & Prestwood, K. M. (2000). Osteoporosis: Pathogenesis, diagnosis, and treatment in older adults. *Rheumatic Disease Clinics of North America, 26*, 569–591.

Kenny, A. M., Prestwood, K. M., Gruman, C. A., Marcello, K. M., & Raisz, L. G. (2001). Effects of transdermal testosterone on bone and muscle in older men with low bioavailable testosterone levels. *Journals of Gerontology: Series A, Biological Sciences and Medical Sciences, 56*, M266–M272.

Kern, L. M., Powe, N. R., Levine, M. A., Fitzpatrick, A. L., & Harris, T. B. (2005). Association between screening for osteoporosis and the incidence of hip fracture. *Annals of Internal Medicine, 142*, 173–181.

Khan, S. A., de Geus, C., Holroyd, B., & Russell, A. S. (2001). Osteoporosis follow-up after wrist fractures following minor trauma. *Archives of Internal Medicine, 161*, 1309–1312.

Komara, F. A. (2005). The slippery slope: Reducing fall risk in older adults. *Primary Care Clinics in Office Practice, 32*, 683–697.

Lee, V. K. (2001). Management of osteoporosis in the nursing home setting. *Annals of Long-Term Care: Clinical Care and Aging, 9*(9), 32–42.

Lin, J. T., & Lane, J. M. (2006). Rehabilitation of the older adult with an osteoporosis-related fracture. *Clinics in Geriatric Medicine, 22*, 435–447.

Loeser, R. F., Jr. (2000). Aging and the etiopathogenesis and treatment of osteoarthritis. *Rheumatic Disease Clinics of North America, 26*, 547–567.

Lord, S. R., Tiedemann, A., Chapman, K., Munro, B., & Murray, S. M. (2005). The effect of an individualized fall prevention program on fall risk and falls in older people: A randomized, controlled trial. *Journal of the American Geriatrics Society, 53*, 1296–1304.

Lyons, S. S. (2004). *Fall prevention for older adults*. Iowa City, IA: University of Iowa Gerontological Nursing Interventions Research Center, Research Dissemination Core. Available at www.nursing.uiowa.edu.

Magaziner, J., Hawkes, W., Hebel, J. R., Zimmerman, S. I., Fox, K. M., Dolan, M., et al. (2000). Recovery from hip fracture in eight areas of function. *Journals of Gerontology: Series A, Biological Sciences and Medical Sciences, 55*, M498–M507.

McCarter, R. J. M. (2006). Differential aging among skeletal muscles. In E. J. Masoro & S. N. Austad (Eds.), *Handbook of the biology of aging* (6th ed., pp. 470–497). San Diego: Academic Press.

McKenna, M. (2001). The application of tai chi chuan in rehabilitation and preventive care of the geriatric population. *Physical and Occupational Therapy in Geriatrics, 18*(4), 23–34.

McKiernan, F. E. (2005). A simple gait-stabilizing device reduces outdoor falls and nonserious injurious falls in fall-prone older people during the winter. *Journal of the American Geriatrics Society, 53*, 943–947.

Morgan, S. L. (2001). Calcium and vitamin D in osteoporosis. *Rheumatic Disease Clinics of North America, 27*, 101–130.

Morley, J. E. (2002). A fall is a major event in the life of an older person. *Journals of Gerontology: Series A, Biological Sciences and Medical Sciences, 57*, M492–M495.

Murphy, J., & Isaacs, B. (1982). The post-fall syndrome. *Gerontology, 28*, 265–270.

Murphy, S. L., Williams, C. S., & Gill, T. M. (2002). Characteristics associated with fear of falling and activity restriction in community-living older persons. *Journal of the American Geriatrics Society, 50*, 516–520.

National Institutes of Health (NIH). (2001). *National Institutes of Health consensus development conference statement (March 27–29, 2000)*. Washington, DC: U. S. Department of Health and Human Services.

O'Connell, A. M., & Mion, L. C. (2003). Use of physical restraints in acute care setting. In M. Mezey, T. Fulmer, I. Abraham, & D. A. Zwicker (Eds.), *Geriatric nursing protocols for best practice* (2nd ed., pp. 251–264). New York: Springer.

Olsson, R. H., Wambold, S., Brock, B., Waugh, D., & Sprague, H. (2005). Visual spatial abilities and fall risk: An assessment tool for individuals with dementia. *Journal of Gerontological Nursing, 31*(9), 45–51.

Ottenbacher, K. O., Ostir, G. V., Peek, M. K., Goodwin, J. S., & Markides, K. S. (2002). Diabetes mellitus as a risk factor for hip fracture in Mexican American older adults. *Journals of Gerontology: Series A, Biological Sciences and Medical Sciences, 57*, M648–M653.

Patrick, L., & Blodgett, A. (2001). Selecting patients for falls-prevention protocols: An evidence-based approach on a geriatric rehabilitation unit. *Journal of Gerontological Nursing, 27*(10), 19–25.

Pavol, M. J., Owings, T. M., Foley, K. T., & Grabiner, M. D. (2001). Mechanisms leading to a fall from an induced trip in healthy older adults. *Journals of Gerontology: Series A, Biological Sciences and Medical Sciences, 56*, M428–M437.

Penninx, B. W., Pluijm, S. M., Lips, P., Woodman, R., & Miedema, K. (2005). Late-life anemia is associated with increased risk of recurrent falls. *Journal of the American Geriatrics Society, 53*, 2106–2111.

Ray, W. A., Thapa, P. B., & Gideon, P. (2000). Benzodiazepines and the risk of falls in nursing home residents. *Journal of the American Geriatrics Society, 48*, 682–685.

Resnick, B. (2003). Preventing falls in acute care. In M. Mezey, T. Fulmer, I. Abraham, & D. A. Zwicker (Eds.), *Geriatric nursing protocols for best practice* (2nd ed., pp. 141–164). New York: Springer.

Rubenstein, L. Z., & Josephson, K. R. (2002). The epidemiology of falls and syncope. *Clinics in Geriatric Medicine, 18*, 141–158.

Rubenstein, L. Z., Powers, C. M., & MacLean, C. H. (2001). Quality indicators for the management and prevention of falls and mobility problems in vulnerable elders. *Annals of Internal Medicine, 135*, 686–693.

Sato, Y., Kondo, I., Ishida, S., Motooka, H., Takayama, K., Tomita, Y., et al. (2001). Decreased bone mass and increased bone turnover with valproate therapy in adults with epilepsy. *Neurology, 57*, 445–449.

Shaw, F. E. (2002). Falls in cognitive impairment and dementia. *Clinics in Geriatric Medicine, 18*, 159–173.

Sheldon, J. H. (1960). On the natural history of falls in old age. *British Medical Journal, 2*, 1685–1690.

Shorr, R. I., Guillen, M., K., Rosenblatt, L. C., Walker, K., Caudle, C. E., & Kritchevsky, S. B. (2002). Restraint use, restraint orders, and the risk of falls in hospitalized patients. *Journal of the American Geriatrics Society, 50*, 526–529.

Shreyasee, A., & Felson, D. T. (2001). Osteoporosis in men. *Rheumatic Disease Clinics of North America, 27*, 19–47.

Stevens, M., Holman, C. D. J., & Bennett, N. (2001). Preventing falls in older people: Impact of an intervention to reduce environmental hazards in the home. *Journal of the American Geriatrics Society, 49*, 1442–1447.

Sullivan-Marx, E. M. (2001). Achieving restraint-free care of acutely confused older adults. *Journal of Gerontological Nursing, 27*(4), 56–61.

Tennstedt, S. L., Lawrence, R. H., & Kasten, L. (2001). An intervention to reduce fear of falling and enhance activity: Who is most likely to benefit? *Educational Gerontology, 27*, 227–240.

Theodos, P. (2004). Fall prevention in frail elderly nursing home residents: A challenge to case management, part II. *Lippincott's Case Management, 9*(1), 32–44.

Tideiksaar, R., & Kay, A. D. (1986). What causes falls? A logical diagnostic procedure. *Geriatrics, 41*(12), 32–50.

Tischler, L., & Hobson, S. (2005). Fear of falling: A qualitative study among community-dwelling older adults. *Physical and Occupational Therapy in Geriatrics, 23*(4), 37–53.

Twersky, J. I. (2001). Long-term care in geriatrics: Falls in the nursing home. *Clinics in Family Practice, 3*, 653–666.

U.S. Department of Health and Human Services (USDHSS). (2000). *Healthy People 2010* (2nd ed.). Washington, DC: U. S. Government Printing Office.

U.S. Department of Health and Human Services (USDHSS). (2004). Bone health and osteoporosis: A report of the Surgeon General. Rockville, MD: Public Health Service, Office of the Surgeon General.

Walker-Bone, K., Dennison, E., & Cooper, C. (2001). Epidemiology of osteoporosis. *Rheumatic Disease Clinics of North America, 27*, 1–18.

Wallsten, S. M., Bintrim, K., Denman, D. W., Parrish, J. M., & Hughes, G. (2006). The effect of Tai Chi Chuan on confidence and lower extremity strength and balance in residents living independently at a continuing care retirement community. *Journal of Applied Gerontology, 25*(1), 82–95.

Wang, P. S., Bohn, R. L., Glynn, R. J., Mogun, H., & Avorn, J. (2001). Zolpidem use and hip fractures in older people. *Journal of the American Geriatrics Society, 49*, 1685–1690.

Weintraub, D., & Spurlock, M. (2002). Change in the rate of restraint use and falls on psychogeriatric inpatient unit: Impact of the health care financing administration's new restraint and seclusions standards for hospitals. *Journal of Geriatric Psychiatry and Neurology, 15*, 91–94.

Williams, S. W., Williams, C. S., Zimmerman, S., Sloane, P. D., & Preisser, J. S. (2005). Characteristics associated with mobility limitation in long-term care residents with dementia. *The Gerontologist, 45*, 62–67.

Yardley, L., & Smith, H. (2002). A prospective study of the relationship between feared consequences of falling and avoidance of activity in community-living older people. *The Gerontologist, 42*, 17–23.

Zamboni, M., Zoico, E., Tosoni, P., Zivelonghi, A., Bortolani, A., Maggi, S., et al. (2002). Relation between vitamin D, Physical performance, and disability in elderly persons. *Journals of Gerontology: Series A, Biological Sciences and Medical Sciences, 57*, M7–M11.

Zarowitz, B. J., Stefanacci, R., Hollenack, K., & O'Shea, T. (2006). The application of evidence-based principles of care in older persons: Management of osteoporosis. *American Medical Directors Association, 7*, 102–108.

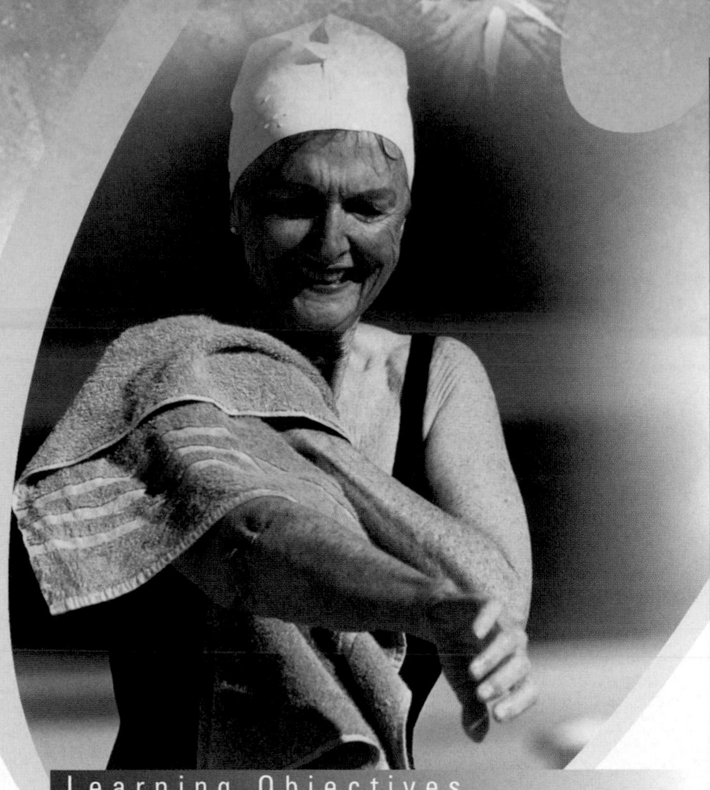

CHAPTER 23

Integument

Learning Objectives

After reading this chapter, you will be able to:

1. Delineate age-related changes that affect the skin, hair, nails, and glands.
2. Describe risk factors that can affect skin wellness for older adults.
3. Discuss the functional consequences of age-related changes and risk factors that affect the skin, hair, nails, and glands.
4. Assess skin in older adults and recognize normal and pathologic skin changes.
5. Describe assessment, prevention, and management of pressure ulcers.
6. Implement nursing interventions to address the following aspects of skin care: maintenance of healthy skin, prevention of xerosis, and referrals for treatment of pathologic skin lesions.

Key Terms

Mongolian spots
photoaging
photosensitivity
pressure ulcer
xerosis

For many people, and particularly for older adults, skin is an accurate and very visible indicator of the combined effects of biologic aging, lifestyle, and environment. Thus, the skin, hair, and nails not only have physiologic functions, but have many social functions. Physiologically, the skin directly affects all the following processes:

- Thermoregulation
- Excretion of metabolic wastes
- Protection of underlying structures
- Synthesis of vitamin D
- Maintenance of fluid and electrolyte balance
- Sensation of pain, touch, pressure, temperature, and vibration

The social functions of the skin include facilitating communication and serving as an indicator of race, gender, work status, and other personal characteristics.

Hair serves to protect underlying organs, primarily the skin, from injury and adverse temperatures. In addition, in social contexts the length and style of one's hair can reflect certain characteristics such as age, gender, and personality. Hair is one of the most visible manifestations of aging, and gray hair is an age-related characteristic that a person can easily alter if gray is viewed as an undesirable indicator of age. Like the skin and hair, nails also have both a physiologic and social capacity. Physiologically, nails protect the underlying tissue from injury. In social contexts, nails can reflect personal characteristics, such as grooming and occupational activities.

Promoting Skin Wellness in Older Adults

Nursing Assessment
- Usual activities that affect skin and risk for skin cancer
- Abnormal skin conditions
- Knowledge about risks and protective behaviors
- Risks for pressure ulcers

Age-Related Changes
- ↓ epidermal proliferation
- Thinner dermis, flattened dermal-epidermal junction
- ↓ moisture content
- ↓ sweat and sebaceous glands

Negative Functional Consequences
- Wrinkles, dry skin
- Slower wound healing
- ↓ sweating, shivering, tactile sensitivity
- ↑ susceptibility to skin cancer
- ↑ susceptibility to burns, bruises, and breakdown

Risk Factors
- Exposure to ultraviolet light
- Adverse medication effects
- Personal hygiene practices
- Conditions that ↑ risk for pressure ulcers

Nursing Interventions
- Teaching about self-care for healthy skin
- Teaching about detection and treatment of skin cancer
- Preventing and managing pressure ulcers

Wellness Outcomes
- Improved comfort
- Maintenance of intact and healthy skin
- Elimination of risk for skin cancer
- Absence (or quick healing) of pressure ulcers

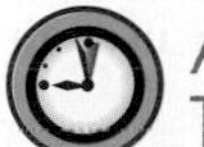

AGE-RELATED CHANGES THAT AFFECT THE SKIN

The skin is the largest, as well as the most visible, body organ. Structurally, the skin is composed of three layers: the epidermis, the dermis, and the subcutaneous tissue. Hair, nails, and sweat glands are also parts of the integumentary system. As with many other aspects of function, it is difficult to distinguish between changes that are strictly attributable to aging and those that occur because of risk factors. Most likely, lifestyle and environmental factors have a greater impact on skin aging than chronologic age alone. Genetic factors also may have a strong influence, especially with regard to baldness and gray hair.

Epidermis

The epidermis is the relatively impermeable outer layer of skin that serves as a barrier, preventing both the loss of body fluids and the entry of substances from the environment. Density of the epidermis varies, depending on the part of the body it covers. The epidermis consists of layers of cells that undergo a continual cycle of regeneration, cornification, and shedding. Corneocytes and melanocytes, respectively, account for approximately 85% and 3% of epidermal cells; both develop in the innermost layer of the epidermis, called the basal layer, or stratum germinativum. Corneocytes continually migrate to the surface of the skin, where they are shed. With increasing age, corneocytes become larger and more variable in shape; these changes are more marked in sun-exposed skin. In addition, the rate of epidermal turnover decreases by about 30% to 50% between the third and eighth decades of life (Yaar & Gilchrest, 2001).

Papillae give the skin its texture and connect the epidermis to the underlying dermis at the dermal–epidermal junction. With increased age, the papillae retract, causing a flattening of the dermal–epidermal junction and diminishing the surface area between the epidermis and dermis. This age-related change slows the transfer of nutrients between the dermis and epidermis. In contrast to other epidermal changes that are more prominent on exposed skin surfaces, this change occurs to some degree on all skin surfaces.

Melanocytes, cells located in the basal layer of the epidermis, give the skin its color and provide a protective barrier against ultraviolet radiation. Beginning around the age of 25 years, the number of active melanocytes decreases by 10% to 20% each decade. Although this decline occurs in both sun-exposed and sun-protected skin, the density of melanocytes in exposed skin is double or triple that in unexposed skin. With increased age the number of Langerhans cells, which serve as macrophages, also decreases in both sun-exposed and sun-protected skin; the decrease ranges from 50% to 70% in sun-exposed skin. Another age-related change is a decrease in the moisture content of the outer epidermal layer, also known as the stratum corneum.

Diversity Note

In women, skin changes in the epidermis occur sharply between the ages of 40 and 60 years, but in men the rate of decline is more constant throughout adulthood (Yaar & Gilchrest, 2001).

Dermis

The primary functions of the dermis are

- Provision of support for structures within and below this layer
- Nourishment of the epidermis, which has no blood supply of its own
- Coloration
- Sensory perception
- Temperature regulation

Collagen, which constitutes 80% of the dermis, confers elasticity and tensile strength, which help to prevent tearing and overstretching of the skin. Elastin, which constitutes 5% of the dermis, maintains skin tension and allows for stretching in response to movement. The dermal ground substance, which has a water-binding capacity, determines skin turgor and elastic properties. Blood vessels in the deep plexus play a role in thermoregulation, and those in the superficial plexus supply nutrients to the epidermal layer. Cutaneous nerves in the dermis receive information from the environment regarding pain, pressure, temperature, and deep and light touch.

Beginning in early adulthood, dermal thickness gradually diminishes, with collagen thinning at a rate of 1% per year. Elastin increases in quantity and decreases in quality because of age-related and environmentally induced changes. The dermal vascular bed decreases by about one third with increased age; this contributes to the atrophy and fibrosis of hair bulbs and sweat and sebaceous glands. Additional age-related changes in the dermis include a decrease in the number of fibroblasts and mast cells.

Subcutaneous Tissue and Cutaneous Nerves

The subcutis is the inner layer of fat tissue that protects the underlying tissues from trauma. Additional functions include storage of calories, insulation of the body, and regulation of heat loss. With increased age, some areas of subcutaneous tissue atrophy, particularly in the plantar foot surface and in sun-exposed areas of the hands, face, and lower legs. Other areas of subcutaneous tissue hypertrophy, however, with the overall effect being a gradual increase in the proportion of body fat between the third and eighth decades. This increased body fat is more pronounced in women than in men, and is most noticeable in the waists of men and the thighs of women. Age-related changes also affect the cutaneous nerves responsible for sensations of pressure, vibration, and light touch.

Sweat and Sebaceous Glands

Eccrine and apocrine sweat glands originate in the dermal layer and are most abundant in the palms of the hands, soles of the feet, and axillae. Eccrine glands, which are important for thermoregulation, open directly onto the skin surface and are most abundant on the palms, soles, and forehead. Apocrine glands are larger than eccrine glands and open into hair follicles, primarily in the axillae and genital area. The sole function of these glands is to produce secretions that are decomposed by skin bacteria to create a distinctive body odor. Both eccrine and apocrine glands decrease in both number and functional ability with increased age.

Sebaceous glands are present in the dermal skin layer over every part of the body except the palms of the hands and the soles of the feet. These glands continually secrete sebum, a substance that combines with sweat to form an emulsion. Functionally, sebum prevents the loss of water and serves as a mild retardant of bacterial and fungal growth. Secretion of sebum begins to diminish during the third decade, with women having a greater decline than men. In younger adults, sebum production is closely related to the size of the sebaceous glands; however, in older adults the sebaceous glands increase in size but produce less sebum.

Nails

The rate of nail growth is influenced by many factors, including age, climate, state of health, circulation to and around the nails, and activity of the fingers and toes. Nail growth begins to slow in early adulthood, with a gradual decrease of 30% to 50% over the life span. Other age-related changes affecting the nails include the development of longitudinal striations and a decrease in lunula size and nail plate thickness. Because of these changes, the nails become increasingly soft, fragile, and brittle, and are more prone to splitting. In appearance, the older nail is dull, opaque, longitudinally striated, and yellow or gray.

Hair

Hair color and distribution change to some degree in all older adults, with the most noticeable changes being baldness and gray hair. By the age of 50 years, about 50% of people have graying hair and about 60% of white men have a noticeable degree of baldness. Graying of the hair results from a decline in melanin production and the gradual replacement of pigmented hairs by nonpigmented ones. Age-related changes also affect hair distribution, with patches of coarse terminal hair developing over the upper lip and lower face in older women, and in the ears, nares, and eyebrows of older men. Most older adults experience an age-related, progressive loss of body hair, initially in the trunk, then in the pubic area and axillae. In addition, some men are genetically predisposed to baldness, which is attributable to a change in production from coarse terminal hair to fine vellus hair.

Diversity Note

Whites develop wrinkles and gray hair at an earlier age than do other ethnic groups in the United States. Gray hairs usually first appear in the mid-30s in whites, in the early 40s in the Japanese population, and in the mid-40s in African Americans (Hordinsky et al., 2002).

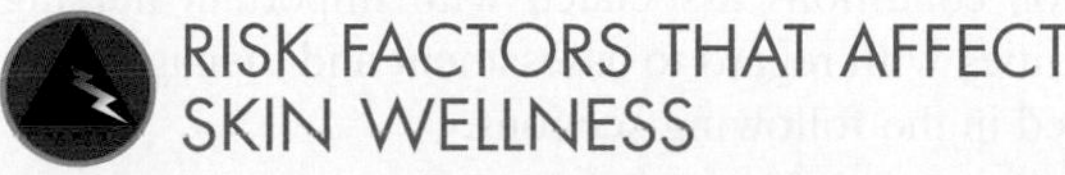

RISK FACTORS THAT AFFECT SKIN WELLNESS

The risk factors that influence the skin and hair of older adults include heredity, lifestyle and environmental factors, and adverse medication effects. Pathologic conditions also pose risks and are discussed in a separate section. Genetic influences have only a small impact on the skin, whereas lifestyle and environmental factors, which are the most amenable to interventions, have a significant impact. Thus, it is important to identify those risk factors, such as exposure to ultraviolet radiation, that can be alleviated through relatively simple interventions.

Genetic Influences

Heredity plays an important role in the development of pathologic and age-related skin and hair changes. People with fair skin, light hair, and light eyes are more sensitive to the effects of ultraviolet radiation than people with dark skin, as evidenced by the fact that skin cancers are common in light-skinned people of northern European ancestry but rare in African Americans.

Lifestyle and Environmental Influences

Smoking, sun exposure, emotional stress, and substance or alcohol abuse are the lifestyle and environmental factors that significantly affect skin wellness. Exposure to ultraviolet radiation is the most significant environmental factor, but adverse climate conditions also can cause negative functional consequences. For example, because the water content of the stratum corneum is influenced by relative humidity, **xerosis** (dry skin) is exacerbated when the relative humidity is below 30%.

Photoaging is the term used to describe skin changes that occur because of exposure to ultraviolet radiation, even at levels that do not cause any detectable sunburn. Distinct characteristics of ultraviolet radiation–damaged skin include

- Coarse, leathery, and ruddy or yellowed appearance
- Many deep wrinkles, particularly on the face and neck.
- The presence of pathologic lesions and seborrheic and actinic keratoses
- Thickened epidermis
- Enlarged sebaceous glands
- Marked loss of elasticity
- Dilated and tortuous blood vessels
- Decreased amounts of mature collagen
- Large quantities of thickened and tangled elastic fibers

Ultraviolet radiation–related skin changes are distinct from age-related changes, but these changes have often been viewed as premature or accelerated aging. One reason for the common misconception that photoaging is an age-related change is that the cumulative effects of ultraviolet radiation may not be evident until later adulthood. Another reason for the difficulty in distinguishing between age-related and environmental causes is that some environmentally induced skin changes, such as slowed wound healing, are thought to be accelerations or exacerbations of age-related processes.

Cigarette smoking is another factor that has been associated with detrimental skin changes, as well as with hair changes, such as balding and gray hair. The skin of people who smoke is likely to have more wrinkles and a grayish discoloration, and these changes are more pronounced in women. Cigarette smoking also diminishes the skin's ability to protect against ultraviolet radiation damage and increases the risk of skin cancer. Epidemiologic studies suggest that the carcinogens in cigarettes directly affect epidermal and dermal cells (Yaar & Gilchrest, 2001).

Cultural factors, societal attitudes, and advertising trends influence hygiene and skin care practices. People in industrialized societies place a high value on frequent bathing and the use of commercial products for hygienic and cosmetic purposes. Although most of the personal practices associated with these values are desirable or harmless in younger adults, they may adversely affect older adults. For example, frequent bathing with harsh deodorant soaps may cause or exacerbate dry skin problems in an older person.

Wellness Opportunity

From a holistic perspective, nurses need to nonjudgmentally consider the influence of cultural and societal attitudes on personal care practices and address any factors that negatively affect self-esteem.

Diversity Note

Hair loss patterns that commonly occur in older Hispanic and African American women (i.e., balding at the frontal and temporal hairline) may be associated with both biological factors, such as fewer elastic fibers to anchor hair follicles, and cultural practices, such as tight braids and ponytails (Taylor, 2002).

Medication Effects

Common adverse medication effects involving the skin include pruritus, dermatoses, and photosensitivity reactions. Less common adverse medication effects on the skin and hair include alopecia and pigmentation changes of the skin or hair. Medications may also exacerbate age-related skin changes. For example, fluid loss from diuretics can exacerbate xerosis and cause further discomfort or skin problems for the older adult. In addition, older adults taking anticoagulants are likely to bruise easily and have more extensive bruising because of the combination of age-related changes and medication effects.

Dermatoses, or rashes, are the most frequently cited adverse medication effect, and they can be caused by virtually any medication. Medication-related skin eruptions vary widely in their manifestations and have no specific characteristics. In contrast to dermatoses arising from other causes, however, medication-related dermatoses tend to be redder in appearance, more abrupt in onset, and more widespread and symmetric in distribution. Although adverse dermatologic reactions frequently occur early in the course of treatment with a new medication, they can occur at any time during an initial or subsequent treatment course. Penicillin and penicillin-based medications are the medications most often associated with skin eruptions. Other medications that are commonly associated with dermatoses include sulfonamides, cephalosporins, barbiturates, and salicylates.

Photosensitivity is an adverse medication effect that causes an intensified response to ultraviolet radiation. The inflammatory reaction initially is distributed over sun-exposed areas, but it may spread to nonexposed areas and persist even after a medication is discontinued. Photosensitivity may begin during a seasonal exposure to bright sunlight or during a vacation in an unusually hot climate. Thiazides, phenothiazines, tetracyclines, amiodarone, and sulfonamides are the medications most often associated with photosensitivity reactions. Some herbal preparations also may increase the risk of photosensitivity.

Risk for Skin Breakdown

Although most older adults do not have mobility or activity limitations that are serious enough to increase the risk of skin breakdown, for the small percentage of older people who do, this risk is a major problem with far-reaching negative functional consequences. Because the primary contributing factor in the development of pressure ulcers is persistent pressure, people who lack the ability to move around independently are most vulnerable (Fig. 23-1). Thus, the prevention of pressure ulcers is the focus of much of the nursing care for dependent older adults in any setting. Other risk factors that combine with activity limitations to cause pressure ulcers are moisture, friction, shearing force, poor hydration or nutrition (especially hypoproteinemia), and certain pathologic conditions (especially those that alter level of consciousness). Age-related changes in the skin and pathologic conditions that occur more commonly in older adults also increase the risk of pressure ulcers and delay wound healing once pressure ulcers develop.

PATHOLOGIC CONDITIONS AFFECTING SKIN AND NAILS

In addition to experiencing dry skin, the most common dermatologic conditions in older adults are dermatitis, pruritus, and viral, fungal, and bacterial infections (Yalcun et al., 2006). Older adults also are likely to have long-term onychomycosis (a fungal infection of the nail) or onychogryposis (a thickening, curving, and distortion of the nail), which is caused by trauma, infection, poor circulation, or ill-fitting shoes (Popoola et al., 2005). Skin cancer and pressure ulcers are common conditions associated with important nursing responsibilities with regard to assessment and management, as discussed in the following sections.

Skin Cancer

Skin cancer, defined as an abnormal growth of skin cells, is the most common type of cancer and accounts for about half of all cancers. Older adults are highly vulnerable to the two most common types of skin cancer, primarily because of the cumulative effects of sun exposure. Basal cell carcinoma, which is the most common type, occurs most often

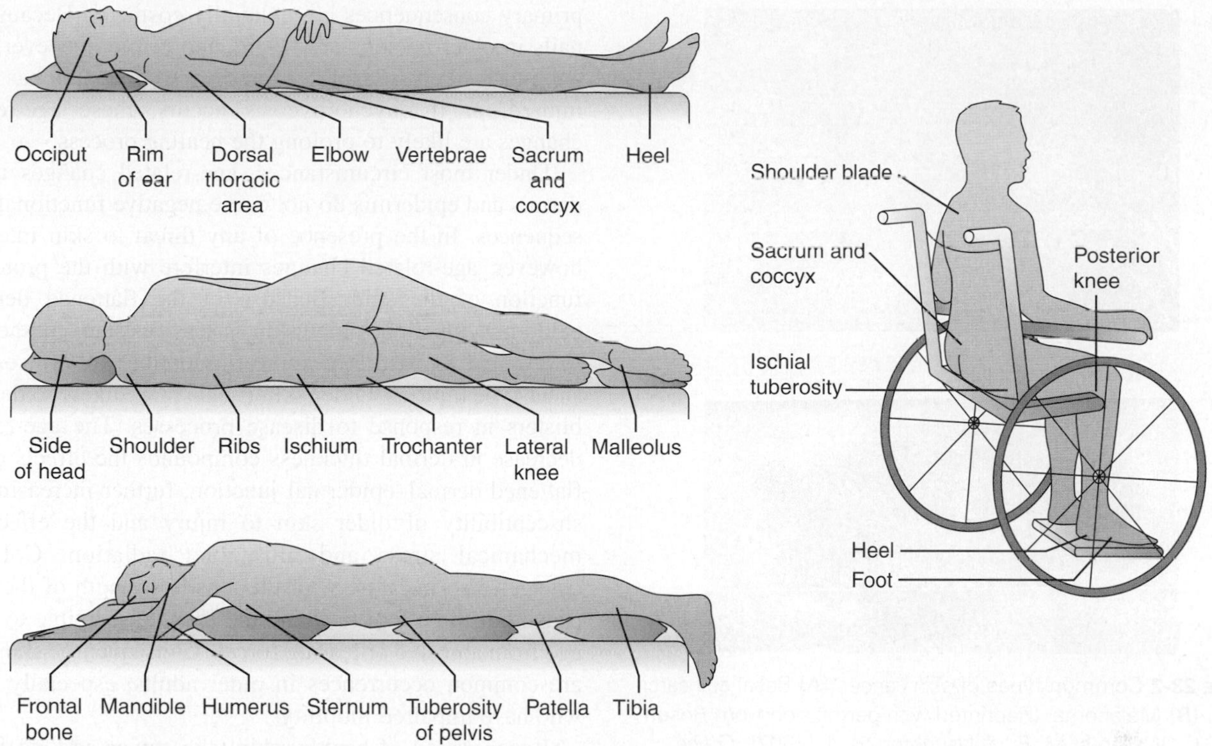

FIGURE 23-1 The risk for development of pressure ulcers is higher at these points.

on the head and neck (Fig. 23-2A). If diagnosed and treated during its early stage, the cure rate for basal cell carcinoma is close to 100%; however, if left untreated, it invades the surrounding tissue. Squamous cell carcinoma, the second most common type, occurs most commonly on the head, neck, forearms, and dorsal hands. Melanoma is the third most common—and the most serious—type (see Fig. 23-2B). Although melanoma is the most common cancer in younger women, the highest incidence is in older men, and 38% of cases are diagnosed in people over the age of 65 years (Loo & Gilchrest, 2004; Rager et al., 2005). Melanoma is the skin cancer most likely to metastasize and cause death, with almost half of all melanoma deaths occurring in white men 50 years of age and older (Loo & Gilchrest, 2004). Early detection and treatment are imperative for improving the outcomes of all types of skin cancer, and nurses have an essential role in assessing and teaching older adults about skin cancer, as discussed in the sections on Nursing Assessment and Nursing Interventions.

Nurses also need to be alert to risk factors so they consider these in their assessments and address them in health promotion. Chronic exposure to ultraviolet rays, including those from tanning booths, is a risk factor that is highly associated with skin cancers and that is most amenable to protective measures. Precancerous skin lesions occur more commonly with increased age, especially on sun-exposed areas of fair-skinned people.

Wellness Opportunity

Nurses promote self-care for wellness by teaching older adults to examine their skin for suspicious changes once a month.

Pressure Ulcers

A nursing definition of **pressure ulcers** is "localized areas of cellular necrosis that occur over bony prominences exposed to pressure for a sufficient period of time to cause tissue ischemia" (Frantz, 2001, p. 138). Although pressure ulcers are not a common problem for healthy older adults, they are a major problem for dependent older adults in any setting. A report from the National Pressure Ulcer Advisory Panel (NPUAP) found the following prevalence and incidence rates of pressure ulcers in various settings (Cuddigan et al., 2001):

- Acute care: 10% to 17% prevalence, 0.4% to 38% incidence
- Long-term care: 2.3% to 28% prevalence, 2.2% to 23.9% incidence
- Home health care: 0% to 29% prevalence, 0% to 17% incidence

These figures are based on a review of over 300 studies published between January 1, 1990, and December 31, 2000. Older adults account for about 70% of all patients

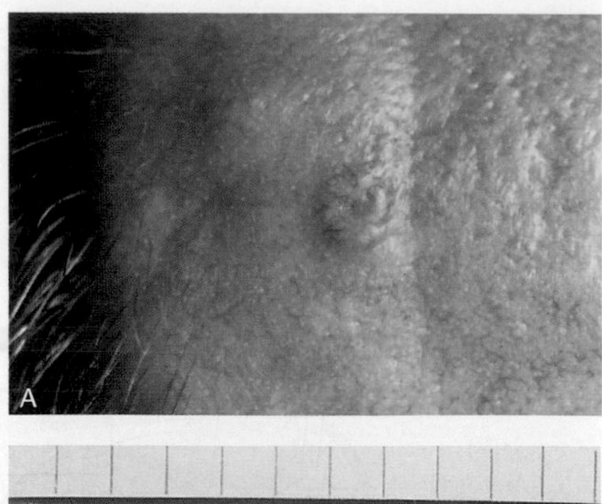

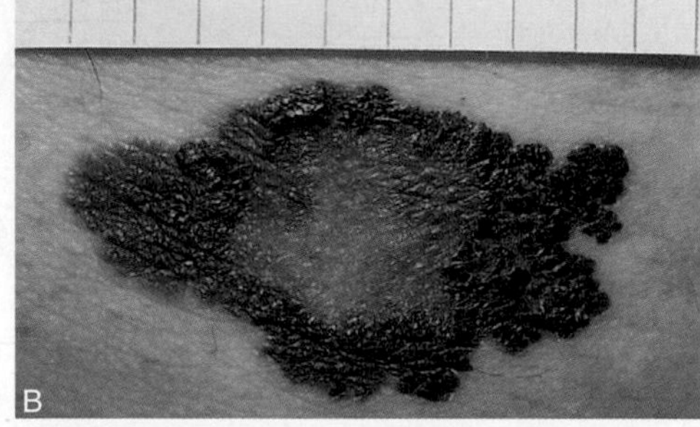

FIGURE 23-2 Common types of skin cancer. **(A)** Basal cell carcinoma. **(B)** Melanoma. (Reprinted with permission from Rosenthal, T. C., Williams, M. E., & Naughton, B. J. [2007]. *Office care geriatrics.* Philadelphia: Lippincott Williams & Wilkins.)

with pressure ulcers (Thomas, 2001). In recent years, much attention has focused on the cost of prevention as well as treatment of pressure ulcers (Courtney et al., 2006). Moreover, clinicians, residents, families, and policy makers regard the presence or absence of pressure ulcers as an indicator of the quality of nursing care in institutional settings (Bergstrom et al., 2005; Thomas, 2006). A goal of *Healthy People 2010* is to reduce the proportion of nursing home residents with a current diagnosis of pressure ulcers from a baseline of 16 diagnoses per 1000 residents in 1997 to a target of 8 diagnoses per 1000 residents (USDHHS, 2000). Pressure ulcers in older adults are discussed in more detail in the sections on Nursing Assessment and Interventions.

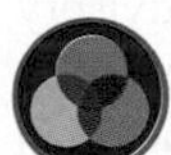

FUNCTIONAL CONSEQUENCES AFFECTING SKIN WELLNESS

Age-related changes and risk factors negatively affect many functions of the skin, including thermoregulation, tactile sensitivity, and response to injury. Psychosocial consequences may result when changes in the appearance of the skin and hair are associated with negative attitudes about visible indicators of aging.

Susceptibility to Injury

Under normal circumstances, age-related changes do not interfere with the protective function of the nails, and the primary consequences are generally cosmetic. Because the nails in older persons are fragile and brittle, however, they are more likely to split. Moreover, if the nail has been injured, or if onychomycosis occurs, these age-related changes are likely to prolong the healing process.

Under most circumstances, age-related changes in the dermis and epidermis do not cause negative functional consequences. In the presence of any threat to skin integrity, however, age-related changes interfere with the protective function of the skin. Because of the flattened dermal–epidermal junction, older skin is less resistant to shearing forces and is therefore more susceptible to bruises and shear-type injuries. Older skin is also more likely to develop blisters in response to disease processes. The age-related decrease in dermal thickness compounds the effects of the flattened dermal–epidermal junction, further increasing the susceptibility of older skin to injury and the effects of mechanical stress and ultraviolet radiation. Collagen changes also interfere with the tensile strength of the skin, causing it to be less resilient and more susceptible to damage from abrasive or tearing forces. Consequently, skin tears are common occurrences in older adults, especially those who have impaired mobility.

Regeneration of healthy skin takes twice as long for an 80-year-old person than for a 30-year-old person. In perfectly intact skin, this slowed regeneration does not have any noticeable effects. When skin integrity is compromised, however, this age-related change contributes to delayed wound healing, even for superficial wounds. Consequences of age-related changes that affect the healing of deep wounds include an increased risk for postoperative wound disruption, decreased tensile strength of healing wounds, and increased risk of secondary infections.

Response to Ultraviolet Radiation

The age-related decrease in melanocytes causes older adults to tan less deeply and more slowly when exposed to ultraviolet radiation, and the increased variability in the melanocyte density in exposed and unexposed skin may cause a mottled and irregular appearance in the overall pigmentation. A positive functional consequence of age-related melanocyte changes is a decrease in the occurrence of moles beginning around the fourth decade. Aside from these cosmetic effects, a more serious functional consequence of the age-related decrease in melanocytes is the increased incidence of skin cancers in older adults. Other factors that increase the susceptibility of older adults to skin cancers are increased age, decreased number of Langerhans cells, and cumulative exposure to ultraviolet radiation.

Comfort and Sensation

Dry skin is one of the most universal complaints of older adults; indeed, it has been observed in up to 85% of noninstitutionalized older people. Age-related changes, such as diminished output of sebum and eccrine sweat, contribute to a decrease in the moisture content of the skin. Risk factors that may contribute to dry skin include stress, smoking, sun exposure, dry environments, excessive perspiration, adverse medication reactions, excessive use of soap, and certain medical conditions (e.g., hypothyroidism).

Tactile sensitivity begins to decline around the age of 20 years, eventually causing older adults to have a diminished and less intense response to cutaneous sensations. This decline is attributable, at least in part, to age-related changes in pacinian and Meissner's corpuscles, which are the skin receptors that respond to vibration. Other contributing factors include lower body temperature and functional alterations in the central nervous system. Functionally, older adults are more susceptible to scald burns because of their diminished ability to feel dangerously hot water temperatures.

Thermoregulation also is affected by age-related reductions in eccrine sweat, subcutaneous fat, and dermal blood supply. These age-related changes interfere with sweating, shivering, peripheral vasoconstriction and vasodilation, and insulation against adverse environmental temperatures. Thus, older adults are more at risk for development of hypothermia and heat-related illnesses, as discussed in Chapter 25.

Quality of Life

The overall cosmetic effect of age-related skin changes is that the skin looks paler, thinner, more translucent, and irregularly pigmented. Additional indicators of age-related skin changes include sagging, wrinkling, and various growths and lesions. Skin coloration changes are attributable to decreased melanocytes and dermal circulation. Wrinkling and sagging of the skin are caused by age-related changes in the epidermis and dermis, particularly those changes that affect the collagen fibers. Decreased subcutaneous tissue contributes to sagging of the skin, especially over the upper arms, by allowing gravity to pull the skin downward.

Although these changes in appearance are gradual and do not interfere significantly with physiologic function, the psychosocial consequences of these changes can be significant because of the social value placed on personal appearance and negative attitudes that may be held about growing old. Regardless of age, one's physical appearance has been shown to be an important determinant of self-perception, and modern societies associate attractiveness with young-looking skin.

Wellness Opportunity

Nurses can promote positive attitudes about aging by challenging societal perspectives that associate beauty only with youth.

Because of the high visibility of the face and neck, any signs of increased age that are prominent around the eyes and mouth may be especially bothersome to the person who wants to avoid visible indications of age. Characteristic signs of advanced age that are evident around the eyes include increased pigmentation, crow's-feet wrinkles, and fat and fluid accumulation in the upper lid and under the eye. Also, because of diminished skin elasticity and loss and shifting of subcutaneous fat, the neck skin sags and a double chin may develop.

Table 23-1 summarizes the functional consequences resulting from age-related changes of the skin, hair, nails, and glands.

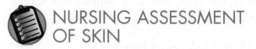

NURSING ASSESSMENT OF SKIN

Because the skin is the largest and most visible organ of the body, it is relatively easy to identify problems that affect it. In addition, the skin may yield clues to other areas of physiologic and psychosocial function, such as nutrition, hydration, and personal care. Nurses collect information about the skin, hair, and nails during an assessment interview and through physical examination procedures. Opportunities for

TABLE 23-1 Functional Consequences Affecting Skin and Appendages

Age-Related Change	Consequence
Decreased rate of epidermal proliferation	Delayed wound healing; increased susceptibility to infection
Flattened dermal–epidermal junction; thinning of dermis and collagen; increased quantity, but decreased quality, of elastin	Decreased resiliency; increased susceptibility to injury, bruising, mechanical stress, ultraviolet radiation, and blister formation
Reductions in dermal blood supply and the number of melanocytes and Langerhans cells	Decreased intensity of tanning; irregular pigmentation; increased susceptibility to skin cancer; diminished dermal clearance, absorption, and immunologic response
Reductions in eccrine sweat, subcutaneous fat, and dermal blood supply	Decreased sweating and shivering; increased susceptibility to hypothermia or hyperthermia
Decreased moisture content	Dry skin; discomfort
Decreased number of Meissner's and pacinian corpuscles	Diminished tactile sensitivity; increased susceptibility to burns
Slowed nail growth	Increased susceptibility to cracking and injury; delayed healing
Changes in hair color, quantity, and distribution	Negative impact on self-esteem in proportion to negative attitudes

direct examination also arise during routine nursing care activities, such as assisting with personal care or listening to the lungs and apical heart rate. Noting the characteristics of the skin, hair, and nails can also provide information to validate or raise questions about other areas of function. For example, the observation that an older man has a beard of several days' growth, when combined with assessment information about his overall function, may support conclusions about possible depression or the need for assistance with personal care activities.

Identifying Opportunities for Health Promotion

Assessment questions are aimed at identifying the person's perception of any problems, any risk factors that may contribute to skin problems, and the person's personal care behaviors that influence hair and skin status. Assessing these aspects of skin care can help identify opportunities for health education about risk factors and healthy skin care practices. Older adults often initiate a discussion about age spots or other noticeable skin changes, and they are usually very receptive to information about skin and hair care. Nurses obtain information about medications and other risk factors as part of the overall assessment, and they incorporate this information into the skin assessment. Likewise, other pertinent information obtained during a comprehensive assessment, such as information about fluid intake, nutritional status, and mobility and safety, is applicable to the assessment of the skin. Box 23-1 summarizes assessment questions about skin and nails.

Observing Skin, Hair, and Nails

Close inspection of the skin in a warm, private, and well-lit environment is an essential component of skin assessment. Examination of the skin is especially important because older adults may focus on benign conditions, such as xerosis, but not notice more serious conditions, such as skin cancer. Nurses observe skin color, turgor, dryness, overall condition, and any growths or pathologic conditions. Nurses also observe and document cultural variations. For example, older adults of Latin, Asian, or African ancestry may have faded **Mongolian spots** (i.e., irregular areas of blue coloration common on the buttocks and lower back, and sometimes on the arms, thighs, and abdomen) that might be mistaken for bruises. Also, when assessing for erythema or pressure areas, nurses should keep in mind that early skin changes may be difficult to detect in people with darkly pigmented skin.

Diversity Note

Mongolian spots occur in 90% of African Americans, 80% of Asians and Native Americans, and 9% of whites.

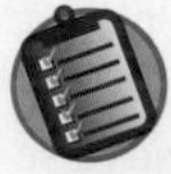

Box 23-1 Interview Questions for Assessing the Integument

Questions to Assess Risk Factors and Skin Problems

- Do you have any concerns about or trouble with your skin?
- Do you have any sores that will not heal?
- Do you bruise easily?
- Have you ever been treated for skin cancer or any other skin problems?
- How much time do you spend in the sun?
- Do you spend time in tanning booths?
- Do you do anything to protect yourself from the effects of the sun?
- Do you have any problems with rashes, itching, swelling, or dry skin?

Questions to Assess Personal Care Practices

- How do you manage your bathing?
- How often do you take a bath or shower?
- What temperature water do you use?
- Do you use soap every time you bathe?
- What kind of soap do you use?
- Do you use any kind of skin lotion, creams, or ointments? What kind do you use and how frequently do you use it? Where do you apply it?
- Do you have any problems with your fingernails or toenails?
- Do you get or need any help with nail care?

The common occurrence of various skin lesions complicates the assessment of skin in older adults. Although most of these changes are harmless, except in terms of their cosmetic consequences, some are cancerous or precancerous. An important aspect of health promotion is to reassure the older adult about the harmless changes and to encourage medical evaluation of the questionable ones. In general, the following characteristics of a skin lesion warrant medical evaluation:

- Redness
- Swelling
- Dark pigmentation
- Moisture or drainage
- Pain or discomfort
- Raised or irregular edges around a flat center

Also, any lesion that undergoes change, or any sore that does not heal within a reasonable time, should be evaluated further. Evaluation is also indicated when, because of its location, a mole or other skin lesion is subject to frequent rubbing or irritation. When nurses observe a questionable skin lesion, they assess and document all the following characteristics: size, shape, color, location, macular (flat) versus papular (raised), superficial versus penetrating, discrete versus diffuse borders, and the presence or absence of inflammation, redness, or discharge. Terminology related to various skin lesions in older adults is confusing, and many

TABLE 23-2 Common Skin Lesions in Older Adults

Common Term(s)	Description
Age spots, liver spots, senile lentigines, senile freckles	Pale to dark brown macules, occurring most frequently on exposed areas
Actinic keratosis, solar keratosis	Red, yellow, brown, or flesh colored papules or plaques; gritty texture; surrounded by erythema; *premalignant*
Senile purpura	Areas of brown or bluish discoloration that look like bruising
Seborrheic keratosis	Brown or black papules or plaques with sharp edges and a waxy or wart-like texture; appearing most frequently on trunk and face
Sebaceous hyperplasia	Yellowish, doughnut-shaped elevations; common on face, especially in men
Senile angiomas, cherry or ruby angiomas, telangiectasia	Bright, ruby-red, pinpoint, superficial elevations of small blood vessels
Spider angiomas	Tiny, red papules with radiating arms; *may indicate a pathologic condition*
Venous stars	Bluish, irregular, sometimes spider-shaped lesions, appearing mainly on legs or chest
Venous lakes, benign venous angiomas	Bluish papules with sharp borders, appearing mainly on lips or ears
Acrochordons, skin tags	Flesh-colored, pedunculated, or stalklike lesions
Corns, calluses	Hard masses of keratin caused by repeated pressure or irritation
Xanthelasma	Fatty deposits, usually around the eyes; *may be related to a pathologic condition*, especially if large or numerous

terms are used interchangeably. Table 23-2 describes some of the terms used in conjunction with skin lesions that are common in older adults; some of these lesions are shown in Figure 23-3.

Nursing assessment of the skin, hair, and nails can provide clues to a broad spectrum of physiologic functioning, particularly when nursing observations are combined with additional assessment information. For example, brown-stained fingertips are an indication of cigarette use, and feces under the fingernails and around the cuticle may be a clue to constipation. In some circumstances, toenails provide clues to mobility difficulties, especially when extremely long nails curl under the toes. Observations of the skin may provide the only objective evidence of serious functional problems that the older person might not otherwise acknowledge. For example, multiple bruises, especially in various stages of healing, may be a significant clue to falls, alcoholism, self-neglect, or physical abuse. Observation and documentation of these signs are especially important when neglect or abuse is suspected but the older adult or caregiver denies any such problems (see Chapter 10 for detailed description).

In assessing the skin for clues to broader aspects of function, it is important to understand that some of the usual manifestations may be altered in older adults. For example, nurses often assess skin turgor on the hands or arms as an indication of hydration status. Because of xerosis and decreased elasticity in the skin of older adults, however, skin turgor is not necessarily a reliable indicator of hydration status. Although the hands or arms may be convenient and socially acceptable sites of inspection, the skin over protected areas, such as the sternum or abdomen, is a more accurate indicator of hydration status in older adults. In non-medicated, older adults, the oral mucous membranes usually are reliable indicators of hydration. However, many medications, including over-the-counter preparations containing anticholinergic ingredients, cause dry mouth. Another age-related change that complicates assessment of the skin is delayed wound healing. This change makes it difficult to assess patterns of wound healing using the same standards that are applied to younger adults.

Observations of the hair, skin, and nails provide multiple clues to self-esteem and other aspects of psychosocial function. Physical limitations can interfere with personal grooming, as can psychosocial influences, such as lack of motivation or awareness. Thus, evidence of self-neglect in grooming may indicate depression, dementia, or social isolation. The use of hair coloring may reflect the person's attitudes about aging, and unusually deep hues of hair coloring or facial cosmetics may indicate impaired color perception. Nurses can use Box 23-2 as a guide to assessment observations regarding the integumentary system.

Ms. S. is an 84-year-old white woman who lives in her own home on the coast of Florida. She is quite active and healthy and enjoys golfing and "beach-combing." She attends the local senior center, where you are the Wellness Nurse. The local chapter of the American Cancer Society is co-sponsoring a skin cancer screening day at the senior center, and you have been asked to prepare a health education program titled "Checking Your Skin for Serious Changes." You are also assisting the dermatologist with the screening examinations. Ms. S. attends the health education part of your program and says she's not sure if she can stay for the screening. She just has one "age spot" and she knows it's not serious because she's "had a couple skin cancers removed and this one looks different."

(case study continues on page 500)

You look at the questionable spot and you assess it as a brown, raised, plaque with a gritty texture, about 1 cm in diameter.

THINKING POINTS

- What additional assessment information would you want to obtain from Ms. S.?
- How would you use Table 23-2 and Boxes 23-1 and 23-2 in your assessment?
- What advice would you give to Ms. S. about her skin?

Assessing Pressure Ulcers

Nurses are responsible for assessing risks for pressure ulcer development, the presence of pressure ulcers, and changes in the status of pressure ulcers. Several screening tools have been developed for assessing and rating risk factors for pressure ulcer development. In the United States, the Braden Scale (Fig. 23-4) is the most commonly used screening tool, and extensive testing supports its validity and reliability. The Hartford Institute for Geriatric Nursing recommends this tool as the best practice for identifying older adults who are at risk for development of pressure ulcers (Ayello, 2007). Rosenberg (2002) proposed a Checklist for Pressure Ulcer Prevention, which includes assessment of factors such as patient and caregiver knowledge about pressure ulcers. Because nutritional status is a factor in the development and healing of pressure ulcers, nurses need to consider nutrition as an essential component of pressure ulcer risk assessment.

Diversity Note

When using the Braden Scale to evaluate pressure ulcer risk in people with darkly pigmented skin, use a cut-off score of 18, rather than 16 (Ayello, 2007).

Recommended frequency of screening for pressure ulcers varies and depends on the person's acuity and the frequency of change in his or her condition. Recommended frequency also depends on the clinical setting and length of time in that setting. For example, because most pressure ulcers develop during the first 2 weeks of admission to a long-term care facility, it is imperative to use the screening tool frequently during that period. Recommended frequencies for using a screening tool in any setting are on admission and whenever

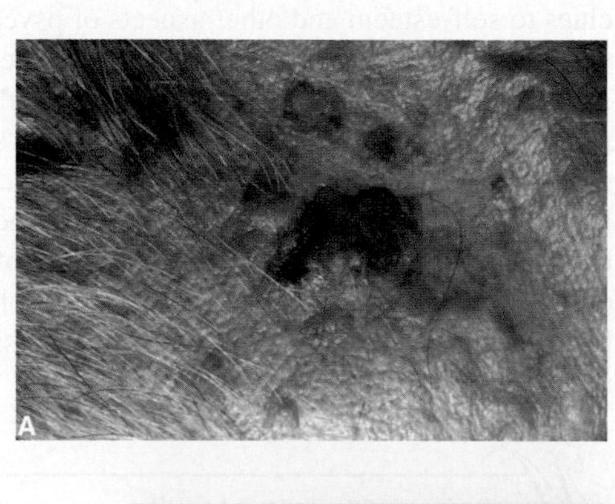

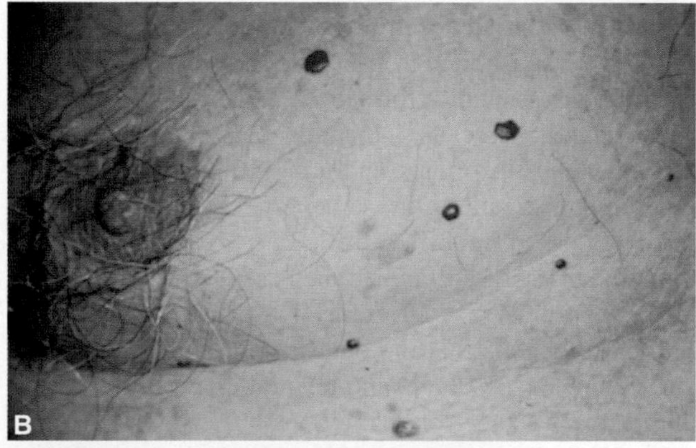

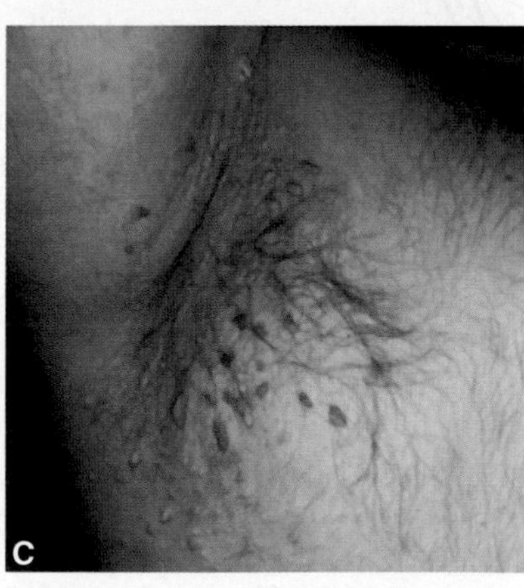

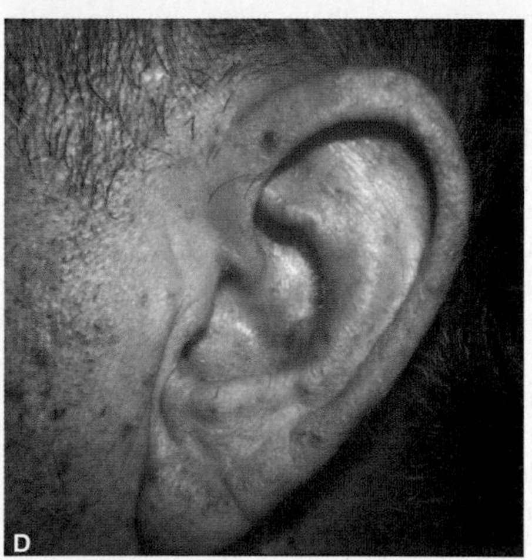

FIGURE 23-3 Common skin lesions in older adults. **(A)** Seborrheic keratosis. **(B)** Cherry angioma. **(C)** Skin tag. **(D)** Venous lakes, or benign venous angiomas. (**A** and **D,** Reprinted with permission from Rosenthal, T. C., Williams, M. E., & Naughton, B. J. [2007]. *Office care geriatrics.* Philadelphia: Lippincott Williams & Wilkins; **B,** Reprinted with permission from Weber, J., & Kelley, J. [2002]. *Health assessment in nursing* [2nd ed.]. Philadelphia: Lippincott Williams & Wilkins; **C,** Courtesy of Steifel Laboratories, Inc.)

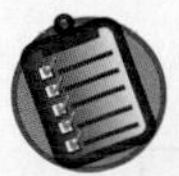

Box 23-2
Observations Regarding the Integument

Examination of the Skin

- What is the color?
- Are there any areas of irregular pigmentation?
- Are there any areas of sunburn or tan?
- Are there areas that are discolored in any way?
- Are there any indications of poor circulation, especially in the extremities (e.g., varicosities, or areas of red, blue, or brown discoloration indicative of chronic stasis problems in the lower extremities)?
- What is the skin temperature?
- Is there a marked difference between the temperature of the extremities and that of the rest of the body?
- How does the skin feel in terms of moisture? Is it dry? Clammy? Oily?
- What is the skin's texture? Is it smooth or rough?
- Does the skin look tissue-paper thin?
- What is the turgor of the abdominal skin?
- Are scars present? (If so, describe their location and appearance.) Are there any signs of falling or physical abuse?
- Are any of the lesions described in Table 23-2 present?

Examination of the Hair and Nails

- What are the color, texture, and general condition of the hair?
- What is the distribution pattern of the hair?
- Is there any evidence of dandruff, scaling, or other problems with the hair?
- What are the color, length, cleanliness, and general condition of the toenails and fingernails?
- What are the color and general condition of the nail beds of the toes and fingers?

Personal Care Practices

- What is the person's overall appearance with regard to grooming and attention to personal attractiveness?
- If grooming is poor, does the person express concern about this or provide an explanation?
- Are there any psychosocial factors that influence personal care practices (e.g., is the person socially isolated or overburdened with caregiving responsibilities and, therefore, inattentive to personal care)?
- Are any of the following signs of neglect evident: presence of a body odor; unkempt, uncut, or matted hair; unusually long and unkempt fingernails or toenails; patches of brown crust on the skin; bruises; or any pathologic skin conditions?

the person's condition changes. Additional recommendations for reassessment in specific settings are as follows: in acute care, every 48 hours; in critical care, every 24 hours; in home care, every RN visit; in long-term care, weekly for the first 4 weeks, then monthly to quarterly (Ayello, 2007).

Assessment of pressure ulcers is important for developing appropriate interventions and for monitoring the effectiveness of interventions. Since the 1980s, health care professionals commonly have categorized pressure ulcers by stages I through IV (Table 23-3). This staging system was first published in 1975 by an orthopedic surgeon and has been modified and widely promulgated by the NPUAP. In 1998, the definition of stage I was revised to reflect more up-to-date information about assessment variations in lightly and darkly pigmented skin. In recent years, the NPUAP has taken a leadership role in addressing questions about the reliability and validity of this widely used tool, particularly for stage I and stage II pressure ulcers. For example, it is difficult to distinguish between stage I pressure ulcers and deep tissue injury wounds, which are defined as areas of deep bruising under intact skin (Doughty et al., 2006). Nursing organizations such as the NPUAP and the Wound, Ostomy, and Continence Nurses Society (WOCN) are currently emphasizing the need for a staging system that is physiologically sound and valid. Moreover, they state that nurses need to understand that "ulcer stage is only one parameter in comprehensive wound assessment, and we should be particularly aware of the unresolved issues surrounding Stage 1 and Stage 2 ulcers and resist efforts to assign undue significance to staging" (Doughty et al., 2006, p. 130).

Appropriate assessment of pressure ulcers involves visual inspection and consideration of factors that can contribute to false conclusions. For example, darkly pigmented skin can mask stage I ulcers, and eschar can mimic hyperpigmented healthy skin. Lesions must be palpated to detect the softness of the tissue and differences in skin temperatures (Siegler & Ayello, 2001). The presence or absence of odors, and the type of odor detected, are additional factors that the nurse must assess and document.

Once a pressure ulcer develops and is assessed according to the four stages, it must be reassessed on an ongoing basis for changes. In the late 1980s, some nurses began documenting improvements in pressure ulcers by using a "reverse staging" method in which a stage IV pressure ulcer progressing through the healing sequence was documented as proceeding through stages III, II, and I. Since the mid-1990s, the NPUAP has advised against this practice and has stated that "pressure ulcer staging is only appropriate for defining the maximum anatomic depth of tissue damage" (NPUAP, 2000, p. 1). The NPUAP further emphasizes that stage IV pressure ulcers can never become stage III, II, or I pressure ulcers because there is a permanent replacement of epidermis, dermis, subcutaneous, muscle, and bone tissue with granulation tissue. Therefore, there are significant structural and anatomic differences between a healed or healing stage IV pressure ulcer and any other pressure ulcer (NPUAP, 1995). Since 1996, the NPUAP has encouraged the use of a standardized tool for assessing changes in pressure ulcers called the Pressure Ulcer Scale for Healing (PUSH) tool (NPUAP, 2000). The PUSH tool scores pressure ulcers according to

Braden Scale

FOR PREDICTING PRESSURE SORE RISK

Patient's Name ________________ Evaluator's Name ________________ Date of Assessment

SENSORY PERCEPTION Ability to respond meaningfully to pressure-related discomfort	**1. Completely Limited:** Unresponsive (does not moan, flinch, or grasp) to painful stimuli, due to diminished level of consciousness or sedation. OR limited ability to feel pain over most of body surface.	**2. Very Limited:** Responds only to painful stimuli. Cannot communicate discomfort except by moaning or restlessness. OR has a sensory impairment which limits the ability to feel pain or discomfort over 1/2 of body	**3. Slightly Limited:** Responds to verbal commands, but cannot always communicate discomfort or need to be turned. OR has some sensory impairment which limits ability to feel pain or discomfort in 1 or 2 extremities.	**4. No Impairment:** Responds to verbal commands. Has no sensory deficit which would limit ability to feel or voice pain or discomfort.	
MOISTURE Degree to which skin is exposed to moisture	**1. Constantly Moist:** Skin is kept moist almost constantly by perspiration, urine, etc. Dampness is detected every time patient is moved or turned.	**2. Very Moist:** Skin is often, but not always moist. Linen must be changed at least once a shift.	**3. Occasionally Moist:** Skin is occasionally moist, requiring an extra linen change approximately once a day.	**4. Rarely Moist:** Skin is usually dry, linen only requires changing at routine intervals.	
ACTIVITY Degree of physical activity	**1. Bedfast:** Confined to bed	**2. Chairfast:** Ability to walk severely limited or non-existent. Cannot bear own weight and/or must be assisted into chair or wheelchair.	**3. Walks Occasionally:** Walks occasionally during day, but for very short distances, with or without assistance. Spends majority of each shift in bed or chair.	**4. Walks Frequently:** Walks outside the room at least twice a day and inside room at least once every 2 hours during waking hours.	
MOBILITY Ability to change and control body position	**1. Completely Immobile:** Does not make even slight changes in body or extremity position without assistance.	**2. Very Limited:** Makes occasional slight changes in body or extremity position but unable to make frequent or significant changes independently.	**3. Slightly Limited:** Makes frequent though slight changes in body or extremity position independently.	**4. No Limitations:** Makes major and frequent changes in position without assistance.	
NUTRITION Usual food intake pattern	**1. Very Poor:** Never eats a complete meal. Rarely eats more than 1/3 of any food offered. Eats 2 servings or less of protein (meat or dairy products) per day. Takes fluids poorly. Does not take a liquid dietary supplement. OR is NPO and/or maintained on clear liquids or IVs for more than 5 days.	**2. Probably Inadequate:** Rarely eats a complete meal and generally eats only about 1/2 of any food offered. Protein intake includes only 3 servings of meat or dairy products per day. Occasionally will take a dietary supplement. OR receives less than optimum amount of liquid diet or tube feeding.	**3. Adequate:** Eats over half of most meals. Eats a total of 4 servings of protein (meat, dairy products) each day. Occasionally will refuse a meal, but will usually take a supplement if offered. OR is on a tube feeding or TPN regimen which probably meets most of nutritional needs.	**4. Excellent:** Eats most of every meal. Never refuses a meal. Usually eats a total of 4 or more servings of meat and dairy products. Occasionally eats between meals. Does not require supplementation.	
FRICTION AND SHEAR	**1. Problem:** Requires moderate to maximum assistance in moving. Complete lifting without sliding against sheets is impossible. Frequently slides down in bed or chair, requiring frequent repositioning with maximum assistance. Spasticity, contractures or agitation leads to almost constant friction.	**2. Potential Problem:** Moves feebly or requires minimum assistance. During a move skin probably slides to some extent against sheets, chair, restraints, or other devices. Maintains relatively good position in chair or bed most of the time but occasionally slides down.	**3. No Apparent Problem:** Moves in bed and in chair independently and has sufficient muscle strength to lift up completely during move. Maintains good position in bed or chair at all times.		
				Total Score	

Braden Scale Scores
1=Highly Impaired
3 or 4 = Moderate to Low Impairment
Total Points Possible: 23
Risk Predicting Score: 16 or Less

NPO: Nothing by Mouth
IV: Intravenously
TPN: Total parenteral nutrition

FIGURE 23-4 The Braden Scale is a widely used screening tool to identify people at risk for pressure ulcers. (© Barbara Braden and Nancy Bergstrom, 1988. Reprinted with permission. Permission to use this tool should be sought at www.bradenscale.com.)

size, exudates, and tissue type, with changes in the PUSH score over time indicating the progression or regression of the pressure ulcer. Studies of the validity of the PUSH model found that it provides a simple, accurate, and clinically useful method of measuring progress toward wound healing (Gardner et al., 2005). This tool and instructions for its use are available from the NPUAP at www.npuap.org.

NURSING DIAGNOSIS

For functionally impaired older adults, the nursing diagnosis of Impaired Skin Integrity (or Risk for Impaired Skin Integrity) might be applicable. This diagnosis is defined as a "state in which the individual experiences or is at risk for altered epidermal and/or dermis"

TABLE 23-3 Stages of Pressure Ulcer Development

Stage	Description
I	An observable pressure-related alteration of intact skin whose indicators, as compared with the adjacent or opposite area on the body, may include changes in one or more of the following: skin temperature (warmth or coolness), tissue consistency (firm or boggy feel), and sensation (pain, itching). The ulcer appears as a defined area of persistent redness in lightly pigmented skin, whereas in darker skin tones, the ulcer may appear with persistent red, blue, or purple hues.
II	Partial-thickness skin loss involving epidermis, dermis, or both. The ulcer is superficial and presents clinically as an abrasion, blister, or shallow crater.
III	Full-thickness skin loss involving damage to, or necrosis of, subcutaneous tissue that may extend down to, but not through, underlying fascia. The ulcer presents clinically as a deep crater with or without undermining of adjacent tissue.
IV	Full-thickness skin loss with extensive destruction, tissue necrosis, or damage to muscle, bone, or supporting structures (e.g., tendon, joint capsule). Undermining and sinus tracts also may be associated with stage IV pressure ulcers.

Source: National Pressure Ulcer Advisory Panel. (1995). Statement on reverse staging of pressure ulcers. *NPUAP Report, 4*(2).

(Carpenito-Moyet, 2006, p. 347). Some of the related factors that increase the risk for skin breakdown and that are commonly found in functionally impaired older adults include incontinence, malnutrition, dehydration, limited mobility, prolonged bed rest, or a combination of these factors.

If the older adult has any suspect skin lesion, the nursing diagnosis of Ineffective Health Maintenance might be applicable. This is defined as "the state in which an individual or group experiences or is at risk of experiencing a disruption in health because of an unhealthy lifestyle or lack of knowledge to manage a condition" (Carpenito-Moyet, 2006, p. 197).

This diagnosis also would be applicable for people who are exposed to ultraviolet radiation (from sunlight or tanning booths) and who do not use protective measures.

Wellness Opportunity

Nurses can use the wellness nursing diagnosis Readiness for Enhanced Knowledge: Skin Care for older adults who are interested in learning how to address risks for conditions such as dry skin and skin cancer.

PLANNING FOR WELLNESS OUTCOMES

When older adults have conditions that affect skin comfort or integrity, nurses identify wellness outcomes as an essential part of the nursing process. Similarly, when they have risks for conditions that can cause skin problems (e.g., skin cancer or pressure ulcers), nursing goals focus on prevention. For healthy older adults with risk factors (e.g., history of skin cancer) or minor skin problems (e.g., xerosis), applicable Nursing Outcomes Classification (NOC) terminology includes Comfort Level, Tissue Integrity: Skin and Mucous Membranes, Knowledge: Health Behavior, Health Seeking Behavior, Nutritional Status, Risk Control: Cancer, and Symptom Control.

For older adults with pressure ulcers or other types of wounds or skin breakdown, NOC terms include Impaired Skin Integrity, Wound Healing: Primary Intention, and Wound Healing: Secondary Intention. Outcomes are achieved through interventions discussed in the following section.

Wellness Opportunity

Nurses promote wellness when they plan outcomes to address skin comfort and the prevention of skin cancer.

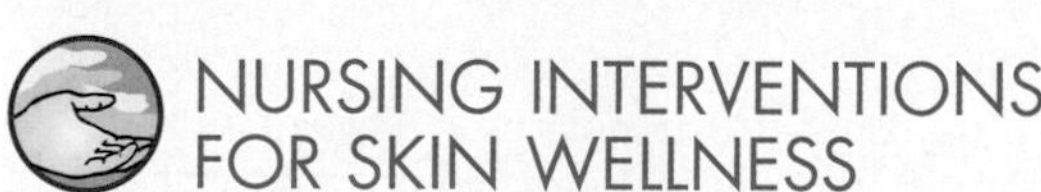

NURSING INTERVENTIONS FOR SKIN WELLNESS

Nurses have many opportunities for promoting wellness with regard to comfort, self-esteem, and maintenance of a healthy integumentary system. Nursing interventions for healthy older adults focus on teaching about self-care practices, such as promoting responsibility for identifying and seeking further evaluation for harmful or precancerous lesions. Interventions for physically compromised older adults focus on maintenance of intact skin and management of pressure ulcers. Nurses can use the following Nursing Interventions Classification (NIC) terminology in their care plans: Hair Care, Health Education, Health Screening, Nutrition Therapy, Positioning, Pressure Management, Pressure Ulcer Prevention, Pruritus Management, Risk Identification, Self-Esteem Enhancement, Skin Surveillance, and Wound Care.

Promoting Healthy Skin

Because the condition of the skin depends largely on the overall health of the person, the maintenance of optimal nutrition and hydration is an important intervention in the skin care of older adults. Because environmental conditions and personal care practices also influence the health of the skin, interventions include education of the older adult about these factors. Box 23-3 summarizes teaching points that should be included in the education of older adults, or caregivers of dependent older adults, regarding skin health. Although much of the gerontological nursing literature advocates limiting the number of baths or showers to one to three times weekly, it is not clear that there is a cause–effect relationship between bathing or showers and dry skin. Factors such as smoking, dehydration, sun exposure, low environmental humidity, and the use of harsh cleansing products are more likely than frequency of bathing to contribute to xerosis in older adults (Sheppard & Brenner, 2000).

Nurses have evaluated a variety of products and methods for bathing older adults. Dawson and colleagues (2001) compared the cost and effectiveness of a no-rinse skin cleanser with that of regular bathing soap and found that cost was the only difference between the two products, with the no-rinse product being twice as expensive. Sheppard and Brenner (2000) investigated the use of the Bag Bath/Travel Bath and concluded that this prepackaged bed bath kit provided an easy, convenient, and effective method of bathing that improved skin quality for long-term care residents. Institutional settings are now making their own bag bath kits and finding that this is cost effective because of reduced use of staff time and other resources. These kits generally contain all the supplies needed for a bed bath, and the washcloths and towels often are warmed in a microwave before being used for a bath. Some of these kits use disposable materials to eliminate the need for laundering. Prepackaged bed bath kits also are available at drugstores for home use. Nurses need to be sure that the temperature of anything warmed in a microwave is safe, especially for older adults with impaired sensory perception.

Preventing Skin Wrinkles

The best methods of preventing skin wrinkles are avoiding exposure to sunlight and using a sunscreen with a sun protection factor (SPF) of 15 or higher when exposure to the sun is unavoidable. Sunscreens also can prevent the occurrence of keratoses (Lawrence, 2000), and topical products containing alpha- or beta-hydroxy acids may be beneficial in reversing wrinkles and promoting the regression of solar keratoses. Nurses need to be alert to the possibility that older adults might develop an allergic or sensitivity reaction to some of the ingredients in topical products. Information about the harmful effects of sunlight should be included in health education about maintenance of healthy skin and pre-

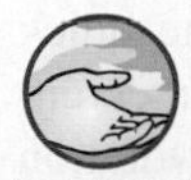

Box 23-3
Health Promotion Teaching About Skin Care for Older Adults

Maintaining Healthy Skin

- Include adequate amounts of fluid in the daily diet.
- Use humidifiers to maintain environmental humidity levels of 40% to 60%.
- Apply emollient lotions twice daily or more often.
- Use emollient lotions immediately after bathing, when the skin is still moist.
- Avoid massaging over bony prominences when applying lotions. Do not use rubbing alcohol.
- Avoid skin care products that contain perfumes or isopropyl alcohol.
- Avoid multiple-ingredient preparations because unnecessary additives may cause allergic responses.
- Inspect skin monthly for suspicious-looking changes.

Personal Care Practices

- When bathing or showering, use soap sparingly or use a mild, superfatted, nonperfumed soap (e.g., Castile, Dove, Tone, Basis).
- Maintain water temperatures for bathing at about 90°F to 100°F.
- Make sure skin is well rinsed after soap use. Whirlpool baths stimulate circulation, but moderate temperatures should be maintained.
- Apply emollient products after bathing, rather than using them in the bath water, to minimize the risk for falls on oily surfaces and to maximize the benefits of the emollient.
- Use emollient products containing petrolatum or mineral oil (e.g., Keri, Eucerin, Aquaphor).
- If you use bath oils, take extra safety precautions to prevent slipping.
- If emollient products are applied to the feet, don nonskid slippers or socks before walking.
- Make sure your skin is dried thoroughly, especially between your toes and in other areas where your skin rubs together.
- When drying your skin, use gentle, patting motions rather than harsh, rubbing motions.
- Obtain regular podiatric care.

Avoiding Sun Damage

- Wear wide-brimmed hats, sun visors, sunglasses, and long-sleeved garments when exposed to the sun.
- Wear clothing made of cotton, rather than polyester fabrics, because ultraviolet rays can penetrate polyester.
- Apply sunscreen lotions generously and frequently, beginning 1 hour before sun exposure.
- Use sunscreen lotions with an SPF of 15 or higher. Avoid exposure to the sun between 10:00 AM and 3:00 PM
- Protect yourself from ultraviolet rays even on cloudy days and when you are in the water.
- Artificial tanning booths use ultraviolet type A rays, which are advertised as harmless, but which have been found to cause damage in high doses.

Preventing Injury From Abrasive Forces

- Do not use starch, bleach, or strong detergents when laundering clothing or linens.
- Use knit or percale bed linens.
- Use soft terry or cotton washcloths.
- If plastic-lined pads are necessary, make sure that an adequate amount of soft, absorbent material is placed over the plastic.

Nutritional Considerations

- Include adequate intake of zinc, magnesium, and vitamins A, B-complex, C, and E.

Complementary and Alternative Care Practices

- Herbs for topical use as emollients include aloe vera and calendula.
- Herbs for itching and inflammation include burdock, chickweed, marigold, chamomile, purslane, pineapple, marshmallow, peppermint oil, witch hazel, walnut leaves, and evening primrose oil.
- Bergamot, chamomile, lavender, and geranium can be used for aromatherapy.

vention of undesirable cosmetic and pathologic skin changes. Also, nurses can encourage women who are concerned about wrinkles and dry skin to discuss medical interventions with their primary care provider.

Wellness Opportunity

Nurses promote wellness by teaching that exposure to ultraviolet light—by sunlight or tanning lights—is a major factor in the occurrence of skin wrinkles, skin cancer, and other skin changes.

Preventing Dry Skin

Dry skin discomfort may be alleviated with moisturizers, which can act either as occlusive agents that prevent evaporation of water from the skin or as humectant agents that attract water to the stratum corneum. Petrolatum is the most effective occlusive moisturizer, and silicones are the newest type of occlusive moisturizer. Lanolin is an effective occlusive moisturizer, but it is expensive and tends to cause allergic reactions. Honey, urea, and glycerin are examples of humectant moisturizers. Unless the environmental humidity is at least 70%, humectants alone are not effective in hydrating the skin because they draw moisture from the dermis to the epidermis (Draelos, 2000).

Emollients are skin care products that moisturize and lubricate the skin. Because the effectiveness of an emollient is based on its ability to prevent water evaporation, its beneficial effects will be enhanced when it is applied to skin that already has some degree of moisture. Thus, an emollient applied to moist skin immediately after bathing will trap moisture and be more effective than an emollient that is added to the bath water. See Box 23-3 for information on the use of emollients and other interventions designed to prevent or care for dry skin in older adults.

Detecting and Treating Harmful Skin Lesions

Early detection and treatment of cancerous or precancerous skin lesions are key factors in the prevention of serious functional consequences because the cure rate for most skin cancers approaches 100% with early excision. The nurse's role is to detect any suspicious-looking lesions and to encourage or facilitate further evaluation. Nurses can encourage all older adults to use the following guide to identify for themselves any skin changes that require further evaluation:

- **A**symmetric shape: irregular or different-looking sides
- **B**order that is irregular: ragged, notched, blurred, irregular
- **C**olor change: different shades, uneven distribution
- **D**iameter: larger than $^1/_4$ inch (6 mm), increasing

If the older adult or caregiver has avoided medical evaluation because of fears about cancer, the nurse can provide assurance about the high cure rate and the minimal chance of long-term problems if early treatment is sought. Similarly, if they have ignored suspicious changes because they attribute them to "normal aging," nurses can teach about the importance of further evaluation. Box 23-3 includes health promotion information about prevention and early detection of skin cancer.

Wellness Opportunity

Nurses address body–mind–spirit interrelationship by allaying unreasonable fears about skin cancer.

Preventing and Managing Pressure Ulcers

Preventing pressure ulcers is one of the most important responsibilities of any nurse caring for dependent older adults who have activity or mobility limitations. Because skin tissue breakdown is attributable to both impaired circulation and external pressure, the key intervention for preventing skin breakdown is to ensure adequate circulation and minimal external pressure. Thus, nurses make sure that older adults with mobility limitations change position at a minimum of 2-hour intervals and institute measures to relieve any external pressure areas. A review of studies found that pressure-reducing mattresses were superior to standard mattresses, with a 70% relative risk reduction, but there was no significant difference in the relative effectiveness of different devices, such as alternating air mattress and low–air-loss beds (Thomas, 2001). This review concluded that patients at risk for development of a pressure ulcer should be treated with a pressure-reducing device, with the choice of device based on cost, comfort, and availability. Gel, foam, and low–air-loss pressure-relieving overlays and cushions also should be used for wheelchairs and other chairs.

In addition to preventing persistent pressure on the skin, it is important to avoid any friction or shearing forces and to ensure that the skin is free of excess moisture. The nurse also should promote good skin circulation by applying moisturizing agents at frequent intervals, avoiding massage over bony prominences. Good personal hygiene and the quick removal of irritants, such as urine, are important interventions, as are measures aimed at promoting optimal hydration and nutrition. Many of the interventions summarized in Box 23-3 are effective in preventing pressure ulcers as well.

Guidelines for the treatment of pressure ulcers have been developed by the Agency for Healthcare Research and Quality, and a wealth of up-to-date information is available from the NPUAP; both resources are listed in the Educational Resources at the end of this chapter. Although a wide variety of interventions are used for wound healing, the National Pressure Ulcer Long-Term Care Study found that the following interventions are most strongly associated with improved healing (Bergstrom et al., 2005):

- Moist wound environments for stages II through IV
- Nutritional support of 30 kcal/kg of weight or more
- Pressure relief

Zinc or vitamin C supplements above the recommended daily allowance have not been found to improve pressure ulcer healing, and supplementation of more than 100 mg/day of zinc may be detrimental (Houston et al., 2001; Thomas, 2001). Similarly, the effectiveness of enteral feeding as an intervention for pressure ulcers has not been established (Thomas, 2001).

Recall that Ms. S. attends the senior center in Florida where you are responsible for presenting a health education program titled "Maintaining Healthy Skin." You plan to emphasize the importance of self-care techniques, such as checking for skin changes. Ms. S. is very interested in attending the program and tells you she will be bringing her 80-year-old sister, who also lives in Florida. Ms. S. worries about her sister because she uses a wheelchair and is very frail. You know that several of the participants at the senior program use wheelchairs, and you plan to include health education about prevention of pressure ulcers.

THINKING POINTS

- Outline your health education points for a half-hour program, including specific points about prevention of pressure ulcers.
- How would you use Table 23-2 and Box 23-3 in your program?
- Find additional information that you would consider using as educational materials for this program.

EVALUATING EFFECTIVENESS OF NURSING INTERVENTIONS

Nursing care for older adults with dry or itching skin is evaluated by determining the degree to which the interventions alleviate the person's complaints. It may take several weeks for older adults to feel the full effects of skin care interventions because of an age-related delay in dermal response to external stimuli. Also, there is a great deal of individual variation among older adults in their response to interventions. Thus, it may be necessary to evaluate the effects of one type of soap or lotion for several weeks before trying a different brand if the problem does not resolve. Because environmental humidity affects skin comfort, environmental conditions may also influence the evaluation of interventions.

Effectiveness of interventions for older adults at risk for skin breakdown is measured by the absence of pressure ulcers. Effectiveness of interventions for pressure ulcers that have developed is determined by rate of healing and prevention of complications, such as osteomyelitis. Because significant cost and quality-of-life issues are associated with pressure ulcers, the prevention of skin breakdown can have far-reaching positive consequences for older adults who are at risk for development of pressure ulcers.

Ms. S. is now 92 years old and lives in an assisted-living facility in Florida. She ambulates with a walker and needs assistance with meals, medications, and personal care. Three months ago, her doctor prescribed hydrochlorothiazide 25 mg every morning for isolated systolic hypertension. She has a history of arthritis but does not take any medication for it. Ms. S. attends your monthly nursing clinic for health education and blood pressure monitoring. When she comes to see you in January, she complains of dry skin and discomfort.

NURSING ASSESSMENT

You interview Ms. S. about her personal care practices and find out that she soaks in the tub in lukewarm water three times weekly and enjoys using bath salts and perfumed skin lotions. She spends much of her leisure time outdoors on the patio or in the air-conditioned solarium. She does not use sunscreens because she thinks they are unnecessary and too oily. She states that she has not had a sunburn for several years, and that she's built up a good tolerance to the sun. She does not wear sunglasses or sun hats. She reports that she has had three skin cancers removed in the past 10 years, one from her cheek, one from her arm, and one from her ear lobe. She says she does not worry about recurrent skin cancer because she no longer swims outside or sits by the swimming pool. Also, because she doesn't get sunburned, she believes she is not at risk for skin cancer.

Inspection of Ms. S.'s skin reveals dry, wrinkled skin on her face and arms, and unevenly tanned skin on her face, neck, and extremities. She has many age spots over the exposed skin areas but no suspicious-looking lesions. Ms. S. has blue eyes and fair skin.

NURSING DIAGNOSIS

Your nursing diagnosis is Ineffective Health Maintenance related to excessive sunlight exposure and insufficient knowledge of the effects of ultraviolet light. Evidence for this diagnosis comes from her misconceptions about risk factors for skin cancer and other skin problems. Also, you identify her lack of knowledge about the potential photosensitivity of hydrochlorothiazide as a factor that contributes to Ineffective Health Maintenance.

NURSING CARE PLAN FOR MS. S.

Expected Outcome	Nursing Interventions	Nursing Evaluation
Ms. S.'s discomfort from dry skin will be alleviated.	• Discuss and describe age-related skin changes. • Discuss risk factors that contribute to skin discomfort (e.g., bath salts, perfumed lotions, unprotected exposure to sunlight). • Use Box 23-3 to teach Ms. S. about skin care practices directed toward alleviating dry skin.	• Ms. S. will report that she no longer experiences skin discomfort and dryness.
Ms. S.'s knowledge about risk factors for skin cancer will be increased.	• Discuss the relationship between skin cancer and exposure to ultraviolet rays. • Explain that any exposure to ultraviolet rays is a risk factor for skin cancer.	• Ms. S. will verbalize an awareness of the risk factors for skin cancer.

(case study continues on page 508)

Expected Outcome	Nursing Interventions	Nursing Evaluation
	• Emphasize that a history of skin cancer increases the chance of recurrent skin cancer.	
The factors that increase Ms. S.'s risk of skin problems and skin cancer will be eliminated.	• Inform Ms. S. that hydrochlorothiazide may increase the risk for photosensitivity, making protective measures increasingly important. • Use Box 23-3 as a guide for discussing measures to avoid sun damage. • Emphasize the importance of using sunscreens and wearing wide-brimmed hats when in the solarium or outside.	• Ms. S. will use measures to reduce the risk for skin cancer and sun damage.

THINKING POINTS

- What risk factors would you address in your care plan?
- How would you promote Ms. S.'s personal responsibility for skin care, including addressing risks for skin cancer?

CHAPTER HIGHLIGHTS

Age-Related Changes That Affect Skin Wellness (Table 23-1)

- Decreased rate of epidermal proliferation
- Thinner dermis, flattened dermal–epidermal junction
- Diminished moisture content
- Decreased dermal blood supply
- Fewer sweat and sebaceous glands
- Decreased number of melanocytes and Langerhans cells
- Changes in patterns of hair distribution

Risks Factors That Affect Skin Wellness

- Genetic factors (hair color and distribution, skin cancer)
- Exposure to ultraviolet radiation (sunlight or tanning light)
- Adverse medication effects
- Personal hygiene practices
- Factors that increase the risk for skin breakdown (Fig. 23-1)

Pathologic Conditions Affecting Skin Wellness (Fig. 23-2, Table 23-3)

- Skin cancer
- Pressure ulcers

Functional Consequences Affecting Skin Wellness (Table 23-1)

- Xerosis (dry skin), discomfort
- Irregular pigmentation and other cosmetic changes
- Increased susceptibility to injury, mechanical stress, and effects of ultraviolet radiation
- Delayed wound healing, increased susceptibility to infection
- Decreased tactile sensitivity, increased susceptibility to burns
- Diminished sweating and shivering, increased susceptibility to hypothermia and heat-related conditions
- Increased risk for skin cancer
- Increased risk for skin breakdown and pressure ulcers

Nursing Assessment of Skin (Table 23-3, Boxes 23-1 and 23-2)

- Abnormal skin conditions
- Personal care practices
- Skin lesions common in older adults (Table 23-2, Fig. 23-3)
- Risk for pressure ulcers (Fig. 23-4)

Nursing Diagnosis

- Readiness for Enhanced Knowledge: Skin
- Impaired Skin Integrity (or Risk for)
- Ineffective Health Maintenance

Planning for Wellness Outcomes

- Comfort Level
- Tissue Integrity: Skin and Mucous Membranes
- Nutritional Status
- Risk Control: Cancer
- Wound Healing

Nursing Interventions for Skin Wellness (Box 23-3)

- Health promotion teaching about healthy skin
- Preventing skin wrinkles
- Preventing dry skin
- Detecting and treating suspect skin changes
- Preventing and managing pressure ulcers

Evaluating Effectiveness of Nursing Interventions

- Alleviation of complaints (e.g., dryness)
- Evaluation of suspect skin changes
- Absence of pressure ulcers in high-risk older adults
- Wound healing

CRITICAL THINKING EXERCISES

1. What changes would a healthy 85-year-old person notice with regard to his or her skin, hair, and nails?

2. Describe the questions you would ask and the observations you would make to assess the skin, hair, and nails of an 82-year-old person.
3. Describe at least eight skin lesions that are normal and three skin lesions that require further evaluation.
4. You are asked to give a 20-minute presentation on "Maintaining Healthy Skin" at a senior center. Outline the content of your health education program.
5. What would you teach the family caregivers of a 74-year-old woman who is confined to a wheelchair with regard to the prevention of pressure ulcers?

Clinical Tool Resources

Hartford Institute for Geriatric Nursing
Try This: Best Practices in Nursing Care to Older Adults
Issue Number 5 (Revised 2007), Predicting Pressure Ulcer Risk
www.hartfordign.org/resources/education/tryThis.html

Educational Resources

Agency for Health Care Policy and Research
www.ahrq.gov

American Cancer Society
www.cancer.org

Canadian Cancer Society
www.cancer.ca

National Arthritis and Musculoskeletal and Skin Diseases Information Clearinghouse (NAMSIC)
www.nih.gov/niams

National Pressure Ulcer Advisory Panel (NPUAP)
www.npuap.org

References

Ayello, E. A. (2007). Predicting pressure ulcer risk. *Try this: Best practices in nursing care to older adults*. Issue 5 (revised). New York University: Hartford Institute for Geriatric Nursing. Available at www.hartfordign.org/resources/education/tryThis.html.

Bergstrom, N., Horn, S. D., Smout, M. S., & Bender, S. A. (2005). The national pressure ulcer long-term care study: Outcomes of pressure ulcer treatment in long-term care. *Journal of the American Gerontological Society, 53*, 1721–1729.

Carpenito-Moyet, L. J. (2006). *Handbook of nursing diagnosis* (11th ed.). Philadelphia: Lippincott Williams & Wilkins.

Courtney, B. A., Ruppman, J. B., & Cooper, H. M. (2006). Save our skin: Initiative cuts pressure ulcer incidence in half. *Nursing Management, 37*(4), 36–45.

Cuddigan, J., Berlowitz, D. R., & Ayello, E. A. (2001). Pressure ulcers in America: Prevalence, incidence, and implications for the future. *Advances in Skin & Wound Care, 14*, 208–215.

Dawson, M., Pilgrim, A., Moonsawmy, C., & Moreland, J. (2001). An evaluation of two bathing products in a chronic care setting. *Geriatric Nursing, 22*, 91.

Doughty, D., Ramundo, J., Bonham, P., Beitz, J. & Erwin-Toth, P. (2006). Issues and challenges in staging of pressure ulcers. *Journal of Wound Ostomy Continence Nursing, 33*, 125–132.

Draelos, Z. D. (2000). Dermatologic aspects of cosmetics: Therapeutic moisturizers. *Dermatologic Clinics, 18*, 597–607.

Frantz, R. A. (2001). Impaired skin integrity: Pressure ulcer. In M. L. Maas, K. C. Buckwalter, M. D. Hardy, T. Tripp-Reimer, M. G. Titler, & J. P. Specht (Eds.), *Nursing care of older adults: Diagnoses, outcomes, and interventions* (pp. 137–144). St. Louis: Mosby.

Gardner, S. E., Frantz, R. A., Bergquist, S., & Shin, C. D. (2005). A prospective study of the pressure ulcer scale for healing (PUSH). *Journals of Gerontology: Series A, Biological Sciences and Medical Sciences, 60*, 93–97.

Hordinsky, M., Sawaya, M., & Roberts, J. L. (2002). Hair loss and hirsutism in the elderly. *Clinics in Geriatric Medicine, 18*, 121–133.

Houston, S., Haggard, J., Williford, J., Meserve, L., & Shewokis, P. (2001). Adverse effects of large-dose zinc supplementation in an institutionalized older population with pressure ulcers. *Journal of the American Geriatrics Society, 49*, 1130–1131.

Lawrence, N. (2000). New and emerging treatments for photoaging. *Dermatologic Clinics, 18*, 99–112.

Loo, D. S., & Gilchrest, B. A. (2004). Common skin disorders. In C. S. Landefeld, R. M. Palmer, M. A. Johnson, C. B. Johnston, & W. L. Lyons (Eds.), *Current geriatric diagnosis and treatment* (pp. 289–304). New York: McGraw-Hill.

National Pressure Ulcer Advisory Panel. (1995). Position statement on reverse staging of pressure ulcers. Available at www.npuap.org.

National Pressure Ulcer Advisory Panel. (2000). The facts about reverse staging in 2000: The NPUAP position statement. *NPUAP Report, 4*(2).

Popoola, M. M, Jenkins, L., & Griffin, O. (2005). Caring for the foot mobile. *Holistic Nursing Practice, 19*, 222–227.

Rager, E. L., Bridgeford, E. P., & Ollila, D. W. (2005). Cutaneous melanoma: Update on prevention, screening, diagnosis and treatment. *American Family Physician, 72*, 269–276.

Rosenberg, C. J. (2002). New checklist for pressure ulcer prevention. *Journal of Gerontological Nursing, 28*(8), 7–12.

Sheppard, C. M., & Brenner, P. S. (2000). The effects of bathing and skin care practices on skin quality and satisfaction with an innovative product. *Journal of Gerontological Nursing, 26*(10), 36–45.

Siegler, E. L., & Ayello, E. A. (2001). Pressure ulcer prevention and treatment. In M. D. Mezey (Ed.), *The encyclopedia of elder care* (pp. 521–523). New York: Springer.

Taylor, S. C. (2002). Understanding of skin color. *Journal of the American Academy of Dermatology, 46*(2 Suppl.), S41–S62.

Thomas, D. R. (2001). Issues and dilemmas in the prevention and treatment of pressure ulcers: A review. *Journals of Gerontology: Series A, Biological Sciences and Medical Sciences, 56*, M328–M340.

Thomas, D. R. (2006). Prevention and treatment of pressure ulcers. *Journal of the American Medical Directors Association, 7*, 46–59.

U.S. Department of Health and Human Services (USDHHS). (2000). *Healthy People 2010* (2nd ed.). Washington, DC: U.S. Government Printing Office.

Yaar, M., & Gilchrest, B. A. (2001). Skin aging: Postulated mechanisms and consequent changes in structure and function. *Clinics in Geriatric Medicine, 17*, 617–630.

Yalcun, B., Tamer, E., Toy, G. G., Oztas, P., Hayran, M., & Alli, N. (2006). The prevalence of skin diseases in the elderly: Analysis of 4099 geriatric patients. *International Journal of Dermatology, 45*, 672–676.

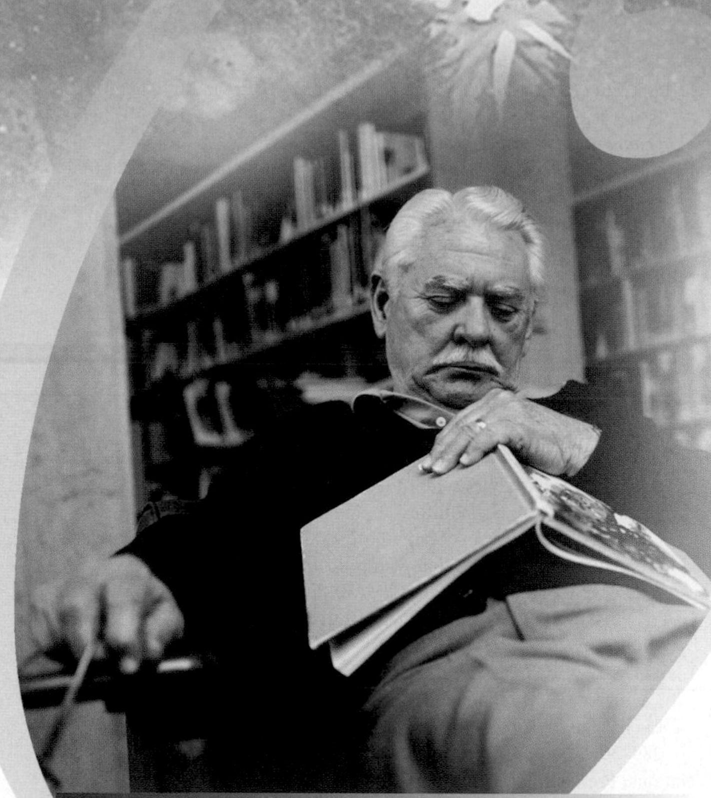

CHAPTER 24

Sleep and Rest

Learning Objectives

After reading this chapter, you will be able to:

1. Delineate age-related changes that affect sleep and rest patterns in older adults.
2. Identify psychosocial, environmental, and physiologic risk factors that influence sleep and rest in older adults.
3. Discuss sleep changes and problems common in older adults.
4. Assess sleep patterns in older adults to identify opportunities for health promotion to improve sleep.
5. Identify nursing interventions to promote optimal sleep and to address risks that interfere with sleep in older adults.

Key Terms

circadian rhythm
excessive daytime sleepiness
insomnia
obstructive sleep apnea
periodic limb movements in sleep (PLMS)
restless legs syndrome (RLS)

Approximately one third of a person's lifetime is spent in sleep and rest activities, yet little attention is paid to the essential physiologic and psychosocial functions accomplished through these activities. During periods of sleep and rest, many metabolic processes decelerate, production of growth hormone increases, and tissue repair and protein synthesis accelerate. During the deeper stages of sleep, cognitive and emotional information is stored, filtered, and organized. Thus, the quantity and quality of sleep affect physiologic function and psychosocial well-being.

Before the 1930s, research on sleep was nonexistent, and nocturnal sleep was viewed as the absence of daytime activity, rather than as an activity in its own right. In the 1950s, polygraphic measurements were used to identify sleep cycles, and our understanding of sleep patterns improved significantly. By the 1960s, rapid eye movement (REM), non–rapid eye movement (NREM), and waking stages were recognized as three distinct states of consciousness. In the 1970s, sleep disorder centers were established to conduct research on sleep and offer comprehensive evaluation and treatment programs for persons suffering from sleep disorders. By the late 1990s, the American Sleep Disorders Association, a professional organization of primary care providers involved in the diagnosis and treatment of sleep disorders, had more than 2000 members. In the early 2000s, print and broadcast media focused public attention on the detrimental effects of sleep deprivation and the large numbers of people in developed countries affected by inadequate sleep. Numerous Internet sites sprang up, and *sleep apnea syndrome* became part of the common language. Now, health care practitioners are likely to refer patients for comprehensive sleep studies as a health promotion intervention. Because older adults are as likely as younger adults to bene-

Promoting Sleep Wellness in Older Adults

Nursing Assessment
- Usual sleep patterns
- Perception of and satisfaction with sleep
- Pre-bedtime routines
- Risks that interfere with sleep
- Sleep assessment tools

Age-Related Changes
- ↓ time in deep sleep
- ↑ time in light sleep
- ↓ time spent dreaming

Negative Functional Consequences
- ↑ time to fall asleep
- Frequent arousals
- ↑ difficulty returning to sleep
- ↑ time in bed with ↓ sleep
- Poorer quality of sleep

Risk Factors
- Pain, discomfort, nocturia
- Beliefs, attitudes, myths
- Anxiety, depression
- Adverse medication effects
- Pathologic conditions
- Environmental factors

Nursing Interventions
- Teaching about interventions for sleep wellness
- Environmental modifications
- Relaxation and mental imagery
- Teaching about medications and risk factors
- Addressing obstructive sleep apnea

Wellness Outcomes
- Feeling rested and satisfied with sleep
- Improved scores on sleep assessment tools
- Improved quality of life
- Better overall health and functioning

fit from newer information and technology, it is important to understand the specific sleep problems of older adults so that they too can take advantage of the most recent approaches to addressing this health-related quality-of-life concern.

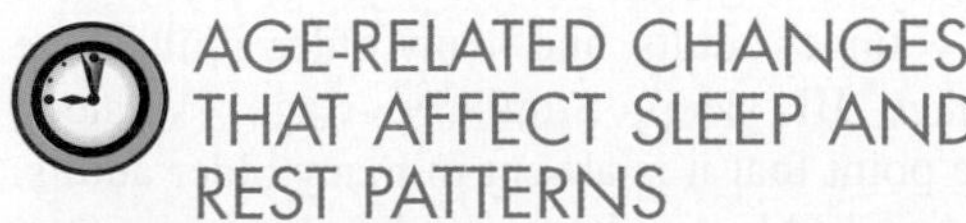

AGE-RELATED CHANGES THAT AFFECT SLEEP AND REST PATTERNS

Sleep research initially focused on identifying the characteristics of each phase of the sleep cycle across the life span, with some attention directed to the unique aspects of the sleep structure and patterns of older adults. Although age-related changes in the sleep cycle are now fairly well understood, many questions remain to be answered about sleep-related phenomena, such as apnea and circadian rhythms variations, that often affect older adults. A sleep cycle is characterized according to the quantity of time spent in bed while awake or asleep, and the depth and quality of sleep. Age-related changes have little impact on the overall quantity of sleep of older adults, but they do have a significant impact on the quality of sleep and the quantity of rest. The inability to initiate and maintain sleep is one of the most frequent complaints among older adults. One comprehensive review of sleep in community-dwelling older adults reported 15% to 45% had difficulty initiating sleep, 20% to 65% experienced disrupted sleep, 15% to 45% experienced early morning awakenings, and 10% experienced nonrestorative sleep (Ancoli-Israel & Ayalon, 2006). Although some complaints about the quality of sleep may be attributable to age-related changes, most sleep disturbances are the result of risk factors and external influences. A wide range of physiologic, environmental, and psychosocial factors interact to affect sleep patterns, and these interrelationships become even more complex with increasing age.

Time in Bed and Total Sleep Time

Researchers agree that older adults spend increasing amounts of time in bed, not always attempting to sleep, with a decreasing proportion of time in actual sleep. Both older and younger adults spend an average of 6.5 to 7.5 hours sleeping during a 24-hour period, but older adults spend an additional 3 to 4 hours resting in order to attain the same amount of sleep attained by younger adults. Compared with younger adults, older adults are more likely to spend more time napping as a way of compensating for not obtaining adequate restorative sleep at night (Avidan, 2005). Additional reasons for napping are to improve alertness and relieve excessive daytime sleepiness.

Sleep Efficiency and Number of Arousals

Sleep efficiency, or the percentage of time asleep during time in bed, influences perceived quality of sleep. Sleep efficiency ranges from 80% to 95% for younger people and is about 70% for older people. This diminished sleep efficiency is attributed both to prolonged sleep latency, which is the time required to fall asleep, and to an increased number of awakenings during the night. Beginning in the fourth decade, the number of awakenings during the night gradually increases to the point that, by later adulthood, as much as one fifth of the night may be spent in periods of wakefulness.

As with many other changes that commonly occur in older adults, there is much controversy about whether the changes are attributable to pathologic conditions or to age-related phenomena. The increased number of awakenings in older adults may be the result of any of the following factors: sleep apnea, physical discomfort, dementia or depression, pathologic processes, lower auditory arousal threshold, or increased levels of plasma norepinephrine. Whether these conditions are age related or pathologic, they occur with increased frequency in older adults and must be considered as risk factors for disturbed sleep.

Sleep Cycles and Stages

Nocturnal sleep patterns are described in terms of sleep cycles and sleep stages. Each sleep cycle, which lasts between 70 to 120 minutes, is a combination of sleep stages. Sleep stages are classified according to the presence (REM) or absence (NREM) of rapid eye movements. A typical cycle consists of four NREM stages (also called slow-wave stages) and one REM stage (also called the dream stage). At the beginning of each cycle, the NREM stages occur sequentially from stage I (lightest sleep) through stage IV (deepest sleep). These stages then occur in reverse order until stage I is reached again and is followed by REM sleep. The cycle repeats during the night, with the length of REM increasing and the length of stages III and IV gradually diminishing (i.e., more time is spent in dream stage and less time in deeper NREM stages as the night progresses). During the NREM stages, muscles gradually relax, body systems function at low levels, and heart and respiratory rates are slower and more regular than during REM or waking periods. Stages III and IV are the deepest stages, and essential restorative functions and the release of hormones take place during the fourth stage.

Although some dreaming takes place in NREM stages, most active and vivid dreaming takes place during REM sleep. In addition to rapid eye movement, REM sleep is characterized by the following physiologic changes:

- Flaccid muscles
- Fluctuating blood pressure
- Diminished thermoregulatory functions
- Increased gastric acid secretions
- Production of more highly concentrated urine
- An approximately 40% increase in cerebral blood flow
- Irregular and increased rate and rhythm of pulse and respirations
- Clitoral engorgement and increased vaginal blood flow (in women)
- Penile tumescence (in men)

The physiologic alterations that occur during REM may exacerbate some medical problems. For example, increased gastric acid secretion during REM sleep may precipitate gastrointestinal pain for people with peptic ulcer disease. Likewise, people with chronic obstructive pulmonary disease (COPD) may experience dyspnea or even a respiratory crisis because of decreased oxygen saturation during REM periods.

Throughout adulthood, the duration of stage I sleep increases gradually, from 5% of a younger adult's sleep to about 20% of an older adult's sleep. In the early part of the night, older adults experience longer periods of drowsiness without actual sleep compared with younger adults. During the night, older adults have more frequent shifts in and out of stage I sleep than do younger adults, but the length of stage II does not differ in older and younger adults. Stage III sleep shows a greater degree of variability in older adults compared with younger adults, and many older adults have little or no stage III sleep. Similarly, stage IV sleep decreases to the point that it is absent in many older adults. In both younger and older adults, stage IV sleep increases significantly during the night after sleep loss. Both older and

TABLE 24-1 Age-Related Changes in Sleep

Sleep Stage	Young Adults	Older Adults
NREM: slow eye movements, normal muscle tension		Increased number of shifts into NREM
Stage I	5% TST	Steady increase to 10%–20%
Stage II	50% TST	Generally unchanged
Stage III	10% TST	Little or no change
Stage IV	10% TST	Very short or absent, especially in men
REM: rapid eye movements, weak muscle tension, vivid dreams	25% TST	Shorter, less intense, more evenly distributed
OVERALL CHANGES		Longer time required to fall asleep
		More frequent arousals
		Different quality of sleep, with less time in deep sleep
		More time in bed
		Same quantity of sleep during a 24-hour period

NREM, non–rapid eye movement; REM, rapid eye movement; TST, total sleep time.

younger adults experience the same number of episodes of REM sleep, but each episode is shorter in older adults. Also, in older adults, REM sleep occurs more uniformly throughout the night, rather than occurring more predominantly during the second half of the night, as is the case in younger adults. Table 24-1 summarizes the usual adult sleep cycle and typical age-related changes in sleep patterns. Typical sleep cycles for younger and older adults are illustrated in Figure 24-1.

Circadian Rhythm

Sleep patterns are determined, in part, by an individual's **circadian rhythm**, also known as a *biological clock*. Body functions that have a circadian pattern include thermoregulation, sleep–wake cycles, and secretion of many hormones, including cortisol and melatonin. The sleep–wake circadian rhythm generally causes adults to become sleepy between 10 PM and midnight and to awaken feeling rested between 6 AM and 8 AM. With increasing age, the circadian rhythm advances, causing older adults to become sleepy earlier in the evening and to awaken earlier in the morning. Alterations in circadian rhythm may also account for difficulties maintaining sleep, as well as difficulty returning to sleep after awakening during the night. This phenomenon is sometimes called *advanced sleep phase*. Sleep disturbances associated with altered circadian rhythm are not necessarily caused by age-related changes alone, and are likely to be exacerbated by lack of exposure to bright light.

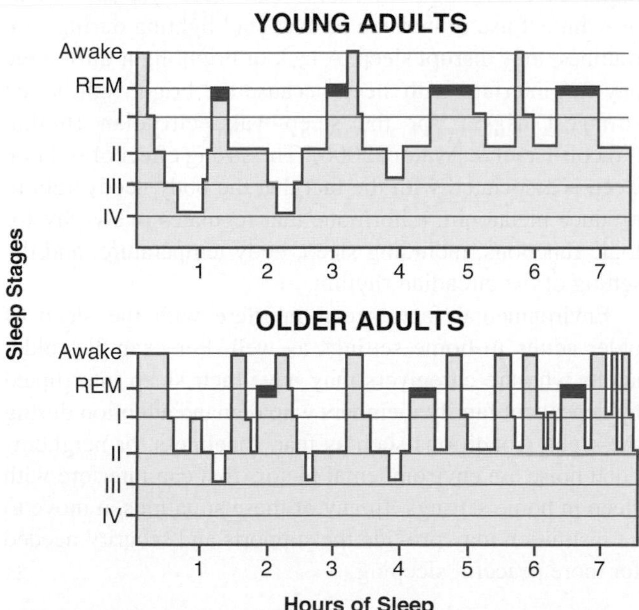

FIGURE 24-1 Changes in the sleep cycle with aging. Older adults typically take longer to fall asleep and experience more frequent arousals. Older adults also usually spend less time in deep sleep.

Gender-Related Differences in Sleep Patterns

Beginning at puberty, sleep patterns of men and women differ, with men having a relatively higher percentage of stage I sleep and more awakenings during the night. The gender differences in stage I sleep remain consistent throughout adulthood, but by the eighth decade, there are no gender differences in the number of awakenings during the night. Also, older men have shorter but more frequent REM episodes and decreased amounts of both total sleep time and stages III and IV sleep compared with women. At all ages, however, women consistently report more sleep complaints than men (Ancoli-Israel & Ayalon, 2006).

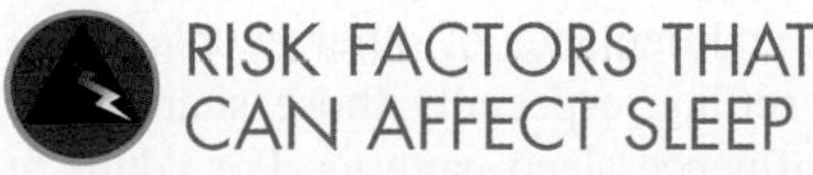

RISK FACTORS THAT CAN AFFECT SLEEP

The common complaint of sleep problems among older adults is associated not only with age-related changes that occur even in healthy older adults, but with the many psychosocial or physiologic risk factors that frequently affect older adults. In addition, environmental conditions, particularly in institutional settings, can significantly affect the sleep patterns of older adults.

Psychosocial Factors

Beliefs and attitudes about sleep can have a powerful impact, with many beliefs having a detrimental, anxiety-producing effect. For example, older adults who believe that arousals during the night are abnormal and unhealthy may think they have insomnia and seek treatment with medications. Rigid beliefs about the amount of sleep required during the night, or the need for the same amount of sleep every night, also can lead to false definitions of insomnia and inappropriate treatment. Likewise, worry about the quantity or quality of sleep can have a negative impact on sleep.

Anxiety, dementia, depression, and sensory impairments are psychosocial disorders associated with disrupted sleep. Anxiety and dementia are associated with difficulty falling asleep, and also cause frequent arousals during the night, after which it may be difficult to return to sleep. People with dementia have been found to have the following sleep alterations: no stage IV sleep, disrupted sleep–wake cycle, very little REM or stage III sleep, and frequent nighttime arousals and daytime napping. Compared with people unaffected by depression, people who are depressed typically take longer to fall asleep, have less deep sleep and more light sleep, awaken more frequently during the night and earlier in the morning, and feel less rested in the morning. In addition, the presence of dementia, depression, or sensory impairments may interfere with the person's ability to respond to time cues and environmental stimuli, thereby disrupting the overall sleep–wake pattern.

Older adults with few or no structured activities, work demands, social responsibilities, or environmental stimuli may find it particularly difficult to establish healthy sleeping patterns. Older adults with dementia or depression who are living alone are particularly susceptible to disturbed sleep patterns because of the tendency to stay in bed during the day out of boredom, lack of motivation, difficulty concentrating on interesting activities, or a desire to withdraw from stressful situations. Finally, in any setting, if an older adult spends all of his or her time in the same room, the lack of differentiation between space for waking and sleeping activities may interfere with sleep patterns.

Environmental Factors

Environmental circumstances are another factor that can significantly influence sleep patterns. For people who do not live alone, the actions and demands of other people in the home or institutional setting, especially those sharing the same sleeping area, influence sleep patterns. For adults at any age, a change in the sleeping environment usually requires a period of adjustment before optimal sleep patterns are established. Thus, older adults may have a particularly difficult time sleeping in institutional settings, especially during the first few nights in a new environment.

In institutional settings, lack of quiet and privacy, conflicting needs of various people, and sleeping in close proximity to others are all factors that can interfere with sleep. Older adults who are accustomed to sleeping alone or with close relations may feel their privacy is being violated in institutional settings where they are required to share a room with people from outside their family. Difficulty falling asleep also may arise if environmental circumstances do not allow the performance of usual pre-bedtime activities, such as listening to music or reading a book. Schedules of caregivers also may interfere with the sleeping habits of the older adult. For example, in institutional settings, the time for awakening patients/residents is often based on the most efficient use of nursing and dietary time, and patients/residents are expected to adjust their sleep routines accordingly. Likewise, in home settings, dependent older adults may have to adjust their sleep routines to the schedule of their caregivers, who may have work and other responsibilities.

Uncomfortable temperatures are another environmental factor that can interfere with sleep and often can be modified, especially in institutional settings. Uncomfortably low or high temperatures, which often are caused by inadequate heating or cooling systems, also contribute to decreased sleep efficiency. Hot and humid conditions can contribute to sleep disturbances in menopausal women by increasing the number of nighttime hot flashes.

Noise is a risk factor for sleeping problems because around the age of 40 years, people become more sensitive to noise when they are sleeping and can be awakened by less intense auditory stimuli. Studies have found that this is particularly problematic for residents of long-term care facilities (Ancoli-Israel & Ayalon, 2006).

Lighting exerts a strong influence on circadian rhythms and can affect sleep patterns in several ways. During the night, excessive light in rooms and hallways, as well as intermittent use of bedside or overhead lighting during care routines, may disrupt sleep. A lack of bright light during the day can interfere with sleep because the bright light is the strongest trigger for the sleep–wake circadian rhythm (Ancoli-Israel & Ayalon, 2006). The strong effect of light on sleep is associated with the fact that the body needs light to produce melatonin, a hormone that regulates many physiologic functions, including sleep, body temperature, and the setting of the circadian rhythm.

Environmental factors can interfere with the sleep of older adults in home settings as well. For example, older adults who are caregivers may have their sleep interrupted by dependent family members who demand attention during the night. Conditions such as fear, loneliness, or neighborhood noise are environmental factors that can interfere with sleep in home settings. In any of these situations, a move to an institution may provide the supports and security needed for more peaceful sleeping.

Physiologic Factors

Pathologic processes, physical pain or discomfort, neuromuscular disorders, and adverse effects of chemicals and medications are physiologic factors that can interfere with sleep. Although these risk factors are not unique to older adults, they are increasingly likely to occur in older adults, and are more detrimental in the presence of age-related changes and other risk factors.

Disease processes and physical discomfort interfere with sleep patterns in many ways, with some pathologic conditions being exacerbated during sleep, particularly during the REM sleep stage. Chronic insomnia is most likely to occur in older adults with fair to poor health, physical disability, or respiratory problems, and in those with a depressed mood (Ancoli-Israel & Ayalon, 2006). Disease conditions that are likely to be exacerbated during sleep include angina, hypertension, duodenal ulcers, coronary artery disease, and COPD. Acute and chronic pain and discomfort are significant factors contributing to sleep disturbances. Likewise, cramps in the calf or foot muscles are a nighttime problem for some older adults and may interrupt sleep patterns. Nocturia is another condition that has been found to contribute to both sleep deterioration and daytime sleepiness (Ohayon, 2005). Table 24-2 lists specific processes and their effects on sleep, including some processes that are not pathologic.

Wellness Opportunity

Nurses promote wellness by paying particular attention to risk factors such as pain and discomfort that are often overlooked and that can be addressed through many types of holistic nursing interventions.

Two neuromuscular disorders, **restless legs syndrome (RLS)** and **periodic limb movements in sleep (PLMS)**, have been topics of interest and research in sleep disorder centers since the mid-1970s. RLS is the experience of an almost irresistible urge to move the legs, usually accompanied by unpleasant leg sensations. RLS can interfere both with initiating and maintaining sleep. RLS prevalence ranges from 9% for younger adults to 20% for older adults (Ancoli-Israel & Ayalon, 2006; Ohayon, 2005). Conditions that can exacerbate RLS include peripheral neuropathy, rheumatoid arthritis, excessive caffeine intake, and iron-deficiency anemia (Avidan, 2005). Medications that can intensify the symptoms of RLS include phenytoin, antidepressants, tranquilizers, dopamine blockers, and cold and allergy agents.

Periodic limb movements in sleep, also known as *nocturnal myoclonus*, is the occurrence of brief muscle contractions, spaced at intervals of about 20 to 40 seconds, that cause leg jerks, or rhythmic movements of muscles in the foot or leg. They occur several times to more than 200 times nightly. Ancoli-Israel and Ayalon (2006) found a 45% prevalence of PLMS in older adults, compared with only 5% to 6% in younger adults. PLMS can contribute to complaints of insomnia, frequent arousals, and increased daytime sleepiness. In addition to increased age, risk factors for PLMS include caffeine, alcohol, and certain medications (e.g., benzodiazepines and antidepressants).

Adverse effects of medications and chemicals, such as caffeine, alcohol, and nicotine, can interfere with sleep in a number of ways. Caffeine is a central nervous system stimulant that lengthens the sleep latency period and causes awakening during the night. Although low doses of nicotine can have relaxing and sedative effects, higher doses interfere with sleep because of nicotine's stimulant effect as well as its effects on respiration. Alcohol may induce drowsiness as an initial effect, but it suppresses REM sleep and increases the number of awakenings, especially during the latter half of the sleep period. The end result of alcohol consumption is a decrease in total sleep time and an increase in daytime sleepiness. Moreover, people who have consumed alcohol over many years may experience alcohol-related insomnia for a few years after withdrawing from it. If obstructive sleep apnea is an underlying causative factor of insomnia, the use of alcohol, hypnotics, or other central nervous system depressants may exacerbate the sleep disorder and lead to increased doses of medication and further detrimental effects. These chemical effects are not unique to older adults; however, adverse effects of medication are more likely to occur in older adults, as discussed in detail in Chapter 8.

Contrary to their primary purpose, hypnotic medications often cause or contribute to sleep disturbances in the following ways:

TABLE 24-2 Physiologic Factors Affecting Sleep

Risk Factor	Sleep Alteration
Arthritis	Chronic pain and discomfort that interfere with sleep
COPD	Awakening as a result of apnea and respiratory distress
Diabetes mellitus	Awakening secondary to nocturia or poorly controlled blood glucose levels
Gastrointestinal disorders, ulcers	Nocturnal pain secondary to increased gastric secretions during REM sleep
Hypertension	Early morning awakening
Hyperthyroidism	Increased difficulty falling asleep
Nocturnal angina	Awakening without perception of pain, especially during REM sleep
PLMS, RLS	Awakening caused by periodic, involuntary leg movements
Altered circadian rhythm	Earlier sleep time; earlier awakening in the morning; difficulty returning to sleep after arousals
Parkinsonism	Increased time awake; decreased amount of sleep

COPD, chronic obstructive pulmonary disease, PLMS, periodic limb movements in sleep; REM, rapid eye movement; RLS, restless legs syndrome.

- Although the initial response to hypnotics may be good, tolerance to these medications usually develops, sometimes within several days.
- Because of central nervous system depression and the increased sensitivity of older adults to these medications, adverse effects are likely to occur, especially if the dose is increased to compensate for tolerance.
- Hypnotics tend to have paradoxical effects, including nightmares and agitation.
- Hypnotics interfere with REM and deep sleep stages.
- Rebound insomnia and nightmares occur after the withdrawal of many hypnotics.
- Some hypnotic medications, particularly those that have been in use for many years, tend to have very long half-lives, interfering with nighttime sleep by causing daytime drowsiness. For example, flurazepam is broken down to an active metabolite with an average half-life of 47 to 100 hours. When used nightly for 1 week, the blood level of flurazepam reaches a level five to six times that of the initial dose.

Other medications that have been associated with disturbed sleep include steroids, antidepressants, aminophylline preparations, thyroid extracts, antiarrhythmic medications, and centrally acting antihypertensives. Table 24-3 summarizes the effects of various medications and chemicals on sleep in older adults.

Diversity Note

Women are twice as likely as men, and whites are almost three times as likely as African Americans, to be taking sedative-hypnotic medications (Blazer et al., 2000).

PATHOLOGIC CONDITION AFFECTING SLEEP: OBSTRUCTIVE SLEEP APNEA

Although medical literature in the late 1880s referred to syndromes in which sleep disorders were associated with brief interruptions in respirations, this phenomenon received little attention until the mid-1970s. More recently, sleep apnea syndromes have received widespread attention in the literature, largely because of research in sleep disorder centers, where they currently are a dominant focus. In 1988, the U.S. Congress established the National Commission on Sleep Disorders Research to promote prevention, diagnosis, and treatment of obstructive sleep apnea and other sleep disorders. **Obstructive sleep apnea** is the involuntary cessation of airflow for 10 seconds or longer; the occurrence of more than five to eight of these episodes per hour is considered to be pathologic. This condition occurs because the muscles responsible for holding the throat open relax during sleep, narrowing the throat opening and blocking the passage of air. Symptoms of obstructive sleep apnea include daytime fatigue, morning headaches, diminished mental acuity, and loud snoring punctuated by brief periods of silence.

Obstructive sleep apnea is not exclusively a condition of older adults, but it is generally agreed that between one third and two thirds of adults aged 60 years or older experience five or more brief sleep interruptions per hour because of apnea episodes. The prevalence of apnea increases with advancing age, beginning around the fifth decade, and is higher in men than in women. One epidemiologic study determined that the prevalence of sleep apnea in the United States was 4% for older women and 13% for older men (Avidan, 2005). In addition to being associated with increased age, sleep apnea is associated with obesity, dementia, depression, hypertension, hypothyroidism, kyphoscoliosis, deformities of the jaw or nasal structures, and the use of nicotine, alcohol, and medications that depress the respiratory center.

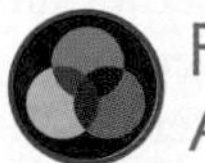

FUNCTIONAL CONSEQUENCES AFFECTING SLEEP WELLNESS

The functional consequences of age-related sleep changes can be summarized as follows: compared with younger adults, older adults have more difficulty falling asleep, awaken more readily and more frequently, and spend more

TABLE 24-3 The Effect of Various Medications and Chemicals on Sleep

Medication or Chemical	Sleep Alteration
Alcohol	Suppression of REM sleep; early morning awakening
Alcohol or hypnotic withdrawal	Sleep disturbances; nightmares
Anticholinergics	Hyperreflexia; overactivity; muscle twitching
Barbiturates	Suppression of REM sleep; nightmares; hallucinations; paradoxical responses
Benzodiazepines	Awakening secondary to apnea
Beta-blockers	Nightmares
Corticosteroids	Restlessness; sleep disturbances
Diuretics	Awakening for nocturia; sleep apnea secondary to alkalosis
Theophylline, levodopa, isoproterenol, phenytoin	Interference with sleep onset and sleep stages
Antidepressants	PLMS; suppression of REM sleep

PLMS, periodic limb movements in sleep; REM, rapid eye movement.

time in the drowsiness stage and less time in deep sleep. Functionally, these changes alone have little impact on the daily life of the older adult, especially because the total amount of sleep time is not significantly changed. However, the prevalence of risk factors that make the older adult more vulnerable to sleep disorders often gives rise to complaints of insomnia and feelings of excessive daytime sleepiness. Approximately two thirds of nursing home residents have a sleep disorder and half of community-living older adults express dissatisfaction with their sleep (Avidan, 2005). Factors that are associated with the increased likelihood of sleep complaints in older adults include angina, depression, white race, female sex, cognitive impairment, anxiety and worries, low educational level, poor self-rated health, and the presence of chronic health conditions.

Wellness Opportunity

Older adults who are significantly dissatisfied with their sleep need to identify the risk factors that can be addressed to improve sleep quantity and quality, rather than viewing this as an inevitable consequence of aging.

Common sleep complaints of older adults include daytime sleepiness, difficulty falling asleep, and frequent arousals during the night. In the late 1970s, sleep disorders were classified systematically, and standards were established to diagnose these disorders. **Insomnia** is classified as a disorder of initiating and maintaining sleep and is one of the most common sleep disorders of older adults. **Excessive daytime sleepiness**, defined as the inability to maintain alertness, is classified as hypersomnia and can be measured objectively with the Multiple Sleep Latency Test (MSLT). This test is based on polygraphic recordings of the speed of falling asleep at periodic intervals during a 24-hour period. Excessive daytime sleepiness differs from fatigue, which manifests as difficulty sustaining a high level of functioning. Two strong indicators of excessive daytime sleepiness are more time in bed during the day and less social activity (Martin et al., 2006).

Although sleep deprivation is not a normal consequence of age-related changes, it can arise from a combination of age-related changes and risk factors in older adults. Psychosocial consequences of short-term sleep loss include confusion, irritability, excessive daytime sleepiness, an inability to concentrate, and poor performance on psychometric tests. Studies have found chronic sleep disorders affect quality of life not only because they result in daytime sleepiness, but because they are associated with confusion, disturbed cognition, psychomotor retardation, and increased risk of injury (Avidan, 2005). Manifestations of prolonged sleep deprivation include fatigue, irritability, disorientation, persecutory feelings, attention deficits, perceptual disturbances, and transient neurologic symptoms, such as hand tremors. When manifestations such as these (e.g., disorientation, attention deficits, and persecutory feelings) occur in older adults, they may mistakenly be attributed to dementia or other pathologic conditions rather than being recognized as effects of sleep deprivation.

Diversity Note

A 3-year study of over 6000 older adults found that cognitive decline was associated with chronic insomnia in men, but in women cognitive decline was found only in those subjects who had both chronic insomnia and a high level of depression (Cricco et al., 2001).

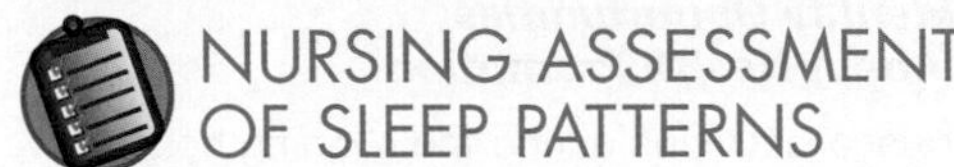

NURSING ASSESSMENT OF SLEEP PATTERNS

Identifying Opportunities for Health Promotion

Nurses assess sleep patterns to determine the adequacy of the person's usual sleep and rest pattern and to identify factors that either contribute to or interfere with the quality and quantity of sleep. During the assessment, the nurse listens for any indications of misinformation or a lack of knowledge that might contribute to sleep disorders. Identification of these factors will lay the groundwork for health promotion interventions. Box 24-1 provides guidelines for interviewing independent older adults and caregivers of dependent older adults about sleep and rest patterns.

Wellness Opportunity

Nurses pay particular attention to identifying any detrimental behaviors, such as the prolonged use of hypnotics, that are likely to be based on myths or misinformation.

In addition to obtaining subjective information from older adults and their caregivers, nurses observe behavioral cues of nighttime and daytime rest and activities. This is especially important when objective observations are contrary to subjective complaints. For example, older adults may complain of not sleeping at all, but when observed by caregivers, they may appear to be sleeping during the entire night. By contrast, older adults who deny any problems sleeping may nap frequently and readily fall asleep during daytime activities.

Using Sleep Assessment Tools

Nurses can perform a sleep history or ask older adults to keep a sleep–wake diary to help identify problem areas and plan appropriate interventions (Avidan, 2005). Nurses can use the Pittsburgh Sleep Quality Index (PSQI; Fig. 24-2) for initial and ongoing assessment of sleep quality and patterns in older adults in a variety of health care settings. They

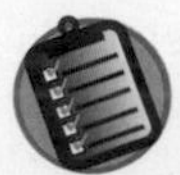

Box 24-1
Guidelines for Assessing Sleep and Rest

Questions to Assess the Perception of Quality and Adequacy of Sleep

- On a scale of 1 to 10, with 10 as the highest, how would you rate your sleep?
- When you awaken in the morning, do you feel like you are rested?
- Do you feel drowsy or sleepy during the day or early evening?
- Does fatigue interfere with your desired daytime activity level?

Questions to Identify Opportunities for Education About Health Promotion

- Describe your usual activities during the evening hours before you fall asleep.
- What is your usual time for getting into bed?
- What are the factors that help you fall asleep (e.g., food or drink, relaxation strategies, environmental influences)?
- Do you take any medicines to help you sleep?
- Do you take medicines to help you stay awake during the day?
- Do you drink alcoholic or caffeinated beverages, or take medicines that contain alcohol or caffeine during the late afternoon or evening? (If yes, how much and what kind?)
- What kind of activities do you engage in during the day and evening?

Questions to Assess Nighttime Sleep Pattern

- Where do you sleep at night (e.g., bed, couch, recliner chair)?
- How long does it usually take to fall asleep after you get into bed?
- Do you think you lie awake too long before falling asleep?
- After you fall asleep, do you wake up during the night? (If so, how many times?)
- What kinds of things disturb your sleep during the night (e.g., getting up to urinate; activities of roommates or other people in the setting; environmental factors, like noise or lighting)?
- If changes in living arrangements have occurred in the past few months: Has your sleep pattern changed since … (e.g., since you came to this nursing home; since your spouse passed away)?

also can encourage older adults to use this tool for self-assessment. In addition, the Hartford Institute for Geriatric Nursing suggests that nurses use the Epworth Sleepiness Scale to differentiate between average sleep and significant issues with sleep that require interventions (Smyth, 2007).

Mrs. Z. is 66 years old and recently retired from her job as office manager for a law firm. She considers herself to be in good health, although she has had hypertension for 20 years and osteoarthritis for the past several years. She self-monitors her blood pressure and takes atenolol, 100 mg daily. She occasionally takes an over-the-counter analgesic medication when her arthritis pain bothers her. She just started going to the local senior center once a week for lunch and social and educational activities. During one of your weekly Senior Wellness Clinics, Mrs. Z. comes to talk with you about her difficulty sleeping. She reports that since she has retired she often wakes up several times during the night and has difficulty returning to sleep. She used to sleep an average of 7 to 8 hours nightly and could easily return to sleep if she woke up during the night. Now she is lucky if she gets 6 hours of sleep because she lies in bed for several hours. She used to go to bed between 10 and 11 PM and get up promptly between 6:30 and 7 AM. Now that she is retired she goes to bed around 11 PM, but stays in bed until 10 AM if she wakes up during the night and does not get a full night's sleep.

THINKING POINTS

- What age-related changes may be contributing to Mrs. Z.'s dissatisfaction with her sleep?
- What risk factors might be contributing to Mrs. Z.'s dissatisfaction with her sleep?
- What further assessment information would you need to obtain, and how would you obtain it?

NURSING DIAGNOSIS

When older adults report dissatisfaction with their sleep or when nursing staff find that patients or residents have difficulty initiating or maintaining sleep, a nursing diagnosis of Disturbed Sleep Pattern is applicable. This diagnosis is defined as the "state in which an individual experiences or is at risk of experiencing a change in the quantity or quality of his rest pattern that causes discomfort or interferes with desired lifestyle" (Carpenito-Moyet, 2006, p. 453). Related factors common in older adults include pain, anxiety, depression, nocturia, incontinence, medication effects, menopausal hormonal changes, environmental changes or conditions, and pathologic conditions, such as dementia.

Wellness Opportunity

Nurses can use the wellness nursing diagnosis of Readiness for Enhanced Sleep for older adults who are willing to explore interventions that improve sleep quantity or quality.

PITTSBURGH SLEEP QUALITY INDEX

Instructions: The following questions relate to your usual sleep habits during the past month only. Your answers should indicate the most accurate reply for the majority of days and nights in the past month. Please answer all questions.

During the past month,
1. When have you usually gone to bed?_______
2. How long (in minutes) has it taken you to fall asleep each night?_______
3. When have you usually gotten up in the moring?_______
4. How many hours of actual sleep did you get that night? (This may be different than the number of hours you spend in bed)._______

5. During the past month, how often have you had trouble sleeping because you...	Not during the past month (0)	Less than once a week (1)	Once or twice a week (2)	Three or more times a week (3)
a. Cannot get to sleep within 30 minutes.				
b. Wake up in the middle of the night or early morning.				
c. Have to get up to use the bathroom.				
d. Cannot breathe comfortably.				
e. Cough or snore loudly.				
f. Feel cold.				
g. Feel too hot.				
h. Have bad dreams.				
i. Have pain.				
j. Other reason(s). Please describe, including how often you have had trouble sleeping because of this reason(s):				
6. During the past month, how often have you taken medicine (prescribed or over the counter) to help you sleep?				
7. During the past month, how often have you had trouble staying awake while driving, eating meals, or engaging in social activity?				
8. During the past month, how much of a problem has it been for you to keep up enthusiasm to get things done?				
	Very good (0)	Fairly good (1)	Fairly bad (2)	Very bad (3)
9. During the past month, how would you rate your sleep quality overall?				

Component 1 #9 Score. C1_______
Component 2 #2 score (≤15 minutes = 0; 16 to 30 minutes=1; 31 to 60 minutes = 2; > 60 minutes = 3) + #5a Score (if sum is equal 0 = 0; 1 to 2 = 1; 3 to 4 = 2; 5 to 6 = 3) C2_______
Component 3 #4 Score (>7 = 0; 6 to 7 = 1; 5 to 6 = 2; < 5 = 3) C3_______
Component 4 (total number of hours asleep)/ (total number of hours in bed) x 100 (>85% = 0; 75% to 84% = 1; 65% to 74% = 2; < 65% = 3) C4_______
Component 5 Number sum or scores #5b to #5j (0 = 0; 1 to 9 = 1;10 to 18 = 2; 19 to 27 = 3) C5_______
Component 6 #6 Score C6_______
Component 7 #7 Score + #8 Score (0 = 0; 1 to 2 = 1; 3 to 4 = 2; 5 to 6 = 3) C7_______
Add the seven component scores together _______ **Global PSQI Score** _______

FIGURE 24-2 The Pittsburgh Sleep Quality Index (PSQI) is a tool that can be used to assess sleep habits and sleep quality. (Adapted from Buysse, D. J., Reynolds III, C. F., Monk, T. H., Berman, S. R., & Kupfer, D. J. [1989]. The Pittsburgh Sleep Quality Index: A new instrument for psychiatric practice and research. *Psychiatric Research, 28*, 193–213. Reprinted with permission from Elsevier Science.)

PLANNING FOR WELLNESS OUTCOMES

When older adults experience sleep disturbances or have risk factors that affect sleep patterns, nurses identify wellness outcomes as an essential part of the nursing process. Nursing Outcomes Classification (NOC) terms that most directly relate to interventions to enhance sleep or address disturbed sleep pattern in older adults are Sleep, Rest, Comfort Level, and Personal Well-Being.

Wellness Opportunity

Quality of Life is a wellness outcome that is achieved through nursing interventions directed toward enhancing sleep.

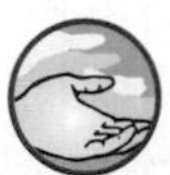

NURSING INTERVENTIONS FOR SLEEP WELLNESS

Nursing interventions to promote healthy sleep include health education and direct interventions, such as environmental modifications and comfort and relaxation strategies. As with other aspects of nursing care for older adults, it is essential that care be individualized for each person's identified needs. Nurses in community and long-term care settings have numerous opportunities to teach older adults and their caregivers about interventions that can improve sleep and quality of life. In hospital settings, nurses focus primarily on acute medical problems, but sleep disturbances should not be overlooked as quality-of-life concerns. Nurses can use the following pertinent Nursing Interventions Classification (NIC) terminology for documentation of interventions: Sleep Enhancement, Risk Identification, Environmental Management, Environmental Management: Comfort, Pain Management, Medication Management, and Exercise Promotion.

Promoting Healthy Sleep Patterns

Health promotion interventions begin with educating independent older adults and caregivers of dependent older adults about age-related changes that affect sleep. As discussed earlier, these changes can be summarized as follows: older adults may need more time to fall asleep, may awaken more readily and more often during the night, and may have greater difficulty falling back to sleep after awakening. A good understanding of the age-related changes in sleep patterns may alleviate anxiety about sleep problems. Also, nurses can emphasize the importance of establishing good sleep habits, even in older adults who do not report sleep problems. Older adults without sleep problems who participated in a year-long program of sleep hygiene education and modest bed restriction time reported an improved sense of well-being on awakening and improvements in sleep depth and continuity (Hoch et al., 2001). Box 24-2 summarizes some measures that can be taken by older adults to promote healthy sleep, as well as complementary and alternative care practices that may be used to promote sleep and rest.

Wellness Opportunity

Health education about sleep is particularly important in community and long-term care settings because nurses have more opportunities to focus on quality-of-life issues.

Nursing actions are directed toward eliminating risk factors and promoting sleep when risk factors cannot be eliminated. Nurses who work evening or night shifts in institutional or home care settings have many opportunities to engage in activities that promote good nighttime sleep. For dependent older adults, nursing responsibilities include assisting with positioning in bed and ensuring the most comfortable environment possible. If dementia or depression interferes with sleep onset, the nurse may simply stay with the older person to provide reassurance until the person is able to fall asleep. In addition, relief of pain and anxiety are nursing responsibilities that directly influence the sleep of older adults. Older adults who are cognitively impaired may not request analgesics but may give nonverbal cues that pain is interfering with sleep. Nurses should be alert to this possibility and assess for chronic or acute pain. An analgesic taken 30 minutes before bedtime may help induce sleep in people with chronic pain or discomfort.

Soft music and dim lighting are additional interventions to promote sleep. Comfort and relaxation measures, such as backrubs, afternoon baths, and the use of therapeutic touch, are particularly helpful when emotional stress or physical pain interfere with sleep. Music therapy is an empirically based intervention shown to improve sleep quality, duration, and efficiency, sleep latency, and daytime function in older people (Lai & Good, 2005). Older adults and caregivers of dependent older adults can be taught to use relaxation techniques as an effective method of inducing sleep without any adverse effects. Cassette tape or CD players with automatic shut-offs can be used to play soothing music or instructions for deep breathing, guided imagery, or relaxation exercises. These products are growing in popularity and can be purchased in many book and music stores or through the Internet. Nurses have many opportunities to teach about relaxation and mental imagery techniques designed to promote sleep, such as the ones summarized in Box 24-3.

Modifying the Environment to Promote Sleep

Environmental modifications are among the simplest and most effective interventions to improve sleep, especially in institutional settings. Activities such as closing bedroom doors and adjusting bedroom lighting may be quite effective in promoting adequate sleep for older adults. In long-term care settings, preferences for bedtime routines and measures

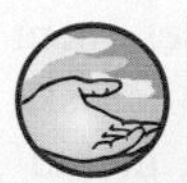

Box 24-2
Health Promotion Teaching About Sleep

Actions to Take

- Establish a bedtime ritual that is effective for you, and try to follow it every night.
- Maintain the same daily schedule for waking, resting, and sleeping.
- Take a warm, relaxing bath in the afternoon or early evening.
- After 1:00 PM, avoid foods, beverages, and medications that contain caffeine, including tea, cocoa, coffee, chocolate candy, hot chocolate, and some over-the-counter pain relievers and cold preparations. In addition, avoid alcohol, sugar, refined carbohydrates, and food additives and preservatives.
- Pre-bedtime foods that promote sleep include milk (warm), chamomile tea, and a light snack of complex carbohydrates (e.g., whole grains).
- Use one or more of the following relaxation methods: imagery, meditation, deep breathing, progressive relaxation, passive exercise, soothing music, body or foot massage, rocking in a chair, reading nonstimulating materials, or watching nonstimulating television.
- Perform daily moderate aerobic exercise, preferably before the late afternoon, but avoid vigorous exercise in the evening.

Actions to Avoid

- Do not drink alcohol before bedtime because it may cause early morning awakening. If you use alcohol, use only in small amounts.
- Do not smoke cigarettes in the evening because nicotine is a stimulant.
- If your bedtime is temporarily changed, try to keep your waking time as close to the usual time as possible, and avoid staying in bed beyond your usual waking time.
- Do not use your bed for reading or other activities not associated with sleeping.
- If you awaken during the night and cannot return to sleep, get out of bed after 30 minutes and engage in a nonstimulating activity, such as reading, in another room.
- Arise at your usual time, even if you have not slept well.

Nutritional Considerations

- L-Tryptophan probably has some hypnotic effects; it occurs naturally in milk, eggs, meat, fish, poultry, beans, peanuts, and green leafy vegetables.
- Provide adequate intake of zinc, calcium, magnesium, manganese, and vitamins B-complex and C.
- Vitamin E and folic acid may be helpful for restless leg syndrome.

Complementary and Alternative Care Practices

- Yoga, meditation, imagery, hypnotherapy, light therapy, progressive relaxation, and a warm bath or warm footbath may be effective in promoting sleep.
- Chamomile, coriander, lavender, and marjoram can be used as aromatherapy to promote sleep.
- Herbs commonly used for sleep problems include hops, ginseng, catnip, skullcap, lavender, chamomile, valerian, rose hips, lemon balm and passion flower.

Special Precautions

- Although widely promoted as sleep aids, herbs should be used with caution in older adults because of their possible adverse effects, and only under the supervision of a qualified health care provider.

that promote sleep can be documented on each resident's care plan and carried out by nursing staff. Elimination of unnecessary staff-initiated noise, especially conversations at the nursing station, is a helpful intervention for patients/residents located near the center of nursing activity. In long-term care settings, decisions about room assignments should be based partially on an assessment of sleep requirements and compatibility of individual needs. Once room assignments have been made, roommate behaviors that interfere with sleep may be addressed by a room change, if necessary.

If a noisy environment contributes to sleeping difficulties, and the noise cannot be controlled or eliminated, the older person may wish to use earplugs. Any person who lives alone, however, should be cautioned about the danger of blocking out protective noises, such as that of a smoke detector. Environmental noise that cannot be eliminated can be masked by white noise (e.g., using a fan, air conditioner, soft music, tape-recordings of such sounds as waves or rain, or white noise machines). If outside neighborhood noise is bothersome, heavy draperies can be installed over windows to filter it out. In addition to addressing noise in the environment, interventions address temperature in the sleeping area. The nighttime room temperature should be comfortable, and is usually slightly lower than during the day. In cooler environments, the older adult should wear a nightcap to prevent loss of heat through the head.

If the effects of lighting interfere with sleep, environmental modifications should be made to expose older adults to bright lights during daytime hours and to eliminate bright lights during nighttime hours. For example, nurses can pay particular attention to avoiding the use of overhead lights at night if they can perform tasks effectively with lower lighting. Studies have found that bright light therapy has been effective in reducing daytime sleepiness in nursing home residents who have dementia (Fetveit & Bjorvatn, 2005). However, bright light therapy may not be effective for people who have cataracts and it can be detrimental for people who have macular degeneration (Avidan, 2005).

Individualizing Care in Institutional Settings

Individualized care plans for older adults in residential settings focus on promoting better sleep for people with dis-

Box 24-3
Relaxation and Mental Imagery Techniques That Promote Sleep

Deep Breathing

- Focus your attention on your breathing; extend your belly and draw in a deep breath as you count.
- Hold your breath for 3 or 4 counts.
- Exhale completely.
- Repeat this pattern, focusing your total attention on breathing.
- Phrases, such as "I am sleepy," or counting may be repeated during each exhalation to help keep your attention focused on breathing.

Progressive Relaxation

- Start by focusing your attention on the muscles in your toes.
- Flex or tense these muscles, and then relax them.
- Repeat 2 or 3 times.
- Focus your attention on the muscles in your foot.
- Flex or tense, then relax these muscles, 2 or 3 times.
- Repeat this process, progressively focusing on different muscle groups and proceeding from your feet to your head.

Mental Imagery

- Begin with deep breathing exercises to relax yourself.
- Focus your attention on a serene and peaceful scene, visualize the setting, and imagine the sounds (e.g., a beach with waves gently washing ashore).
- Imagine yourself in the setting, lying relaxed, enjoying the environment.
- Keep your attention focused on the scene.
- Imagine repetitive motions, such as waves on the beach or sheep jumping over a fence.

turbed sleep patterns. Because daytime activities influence sleep patterns, they should be addressed in plans to improve sleep of older adults in residential settings. One study of cognitively impaired older adults demonstrated that timing activities in relation to peak napping times and prescribing activities that held the attention of the resident improved their nocturnal sleep and reduced their daytime napping (Richards et al., 2001). Another study showed that participation in light physical activity and structured social activity resulted in improved slow-wave sleep in older adults living in an assisted-living facility (Naylor et al., 2000).

Nighttime routines also need to be individualized to meet the needs of each resident. In one study the usual nighttime nursing care regimens at predetermined times were replaced with nondisruptive care routines, which included hourly flashlight checks of residents and provision of care only when the resident was awake. The nondisruptive routine resulted in increased total and consecutive sleep times and did not compromise skin condition in the participants (O'Rourke et al., 2001). Nurses in residential care facilities are encouraged to individualize nighttime care practices to meet the needs of each resident. An individualized care plan is based on a comprehensive assessment of the various needs of the older adult and weighs the risks and benefits of addressing needs that may conflict, including the need for a good night's sleep. Thus, for some older adults, the need for an uninterrupted night's sleep may outweigh the potential benefits of being awakened for nighttime care tasks. In many situations, the needs can be addressed during the person's usual waking time, rather than performing the tasks on a rigid schedule designed for the convenience of staff.

Educating Older Adults About Medications and Sleep

Hypnotics may be effective for short-term management of sleep disorders, especially in temporary circumstances, such as in acute care settings; however, the adverse effects of hypnotics usually outweigh their advantages in longer-term use. Guidelines and studies encourage the use of behavioral therapies rather than benzodiazepines for treatment of insomnia, especially in nursing home residents (Ruby & Kennedy, 2001; Holbrook et al., 2001).

Wellness Opportunity

Nurses have important roles in correcting misperceptions about sleep and teaching older adults about nonpharmacologic ways of improving sleep.

If a hypnotic agent is used for older adults, special attention should be paid to its half-life. The half-lives of the benzodiazepines vary, and some of these drugs have an extremely long half-life in older adults. Benzodiazepines with longer half-lives are associated with a higher risk of adverse effects, including risks for falls. Table 24-4 provides information about the half-life of hypnotics in younger and older adults. Newer nonbenzodiazepine medications (e.g., zolpidem, zaleplon) are less likely to have adverse effects such as tolerance, rebound insomnia, or withdrawal symptoms in older adults (Kamel & Gammack, 2006). Nurses can educate older adults and their caregivers about the effects of alcohol, medications, and certain chemicals on sleep. Box 24-4 summarizes the pertinent teaching points for older adults.

In addition to educating older adults about medications, nurses may need to address the use of other physiologically active substances (e.g., L-tryptophan and melatonin) because older adults are likely to be using these substances or asking questions about their use as sleep aids. L-tryptophan is an amino acid essential to the synthesis of serotonin in the brain. Approximately 0.5 to 2 g is consumed daily in the typical adult diet, primarily in protein and dairy products. L-tryptophan has natural sedative qualities, especially in its effect on sleep latency and slow-wave sleep. L-tryptophan, in doses of 1 g or less, shortens the sleep latency period for people who have difficulty falling asleep, but has no impact

TABLE 24-4 Half-Life of Benzodiazepines

Medication	Half-Life in Average Adult (hr)	Half-Life in Older Adult (hr)
Flurazepam (Dalmane)	47–100	120–160
Diazepam (Valium)	20–50	36–98
Estazolam (ProSom)	10–24	10–24*
Lorazepam (Ativan)	10–20	10–20*
Chlordiazepoxide (Librium)	5–20	15–30
Temazepam (Restoril)	9–13	8–20
Oxazepam (Serax)	5–20	5–20*
Alprazolam (Xanax)	6–20	6–20*
Triazolam (Halcion)	2–5	2–6

*Insufficient data available to determine a difference in younger and older adults.

on the number of awakenings during the night. Although doses of 1 g or less were thought to be harmless in humans, the U.S. Food and Drug Administration (FDA) declared a recall of synthetic L-tryptophan in late 1989, based on reports of an association between L-tryptophan and a rare, but potentially fatal, blood disorder. There is no contraindication to taking L-tryptophan in its natural form.

Melatonin is a hormone that is synthesized by the pineal gland as a byproduct of tryptophan. Serum levels of melatonin follow a circadian rhythm, with very low levels occurring during the day and peak levels occurring between 2 and 4 A.M. Melatonin levels diminish with increased age, but the clinical significance of this diminishing, if any, has not been identified. Melatonin has been found to be effective for the treatment of jet lag and circadian rhythm disruptions associated with blindness, but its effectiveness as a treatment for insomnia is not clear. Overall, exogenous melatonin has not shown significant effects on sleep quality, efficiency, or latency. However, in recent studies with patients with Alzheimer's disease and elderly people with insomnia and sleep disturbances, exogenous melatonin has been effective in improving sleep (Pandi-Perumal et al., 2005). Zhdanova and colleagues (2001) used polysomnography to investigate the effects of three doses of melatonin on people aged 50 years and older who complained of insomnia. These researchers found that lower doses (0.1 mg and 0.3 mg) of melatonin were effective in restoring sleep efficiency without adverse effects, but the pharmacologic dose of 3 mg induced hypothermia and caused plasma melatonin levels to remain abnormally elevated in the daylight hours (Zhdanova et al., 2001). Adverse effects of melatonin include drowsiness, hypothermia, and loss of libido. In 2005, the FDA approved a selective melatonin receptor agonist (ramelteon) as the first non-narcotic prescription sleep aid available in the United States. This new drug is safe and effective in older adults, but should not be used by people who have liver disease or are taking fluvoxamine, rifampin, fluconazole, or ketoconazole.

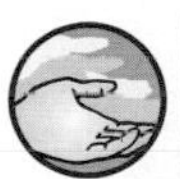

Box 24-4
Health Promotion Teaching About Medications and Sleep

- Older adults are more susceptible than younger adults to the adverse effects of sleeping medications.
- Hypnotic medications are not effective for long-term use because of increasing tolerance, which often develops within the first week and usually develops after a month of regular use.
- Hypnotics should not be used for more than 3 nights in a row.
- Sleeping medications, even over-the-counter ones, are likely to have adverse effects that interfere with daytime function and with the quality of nighttime sleep.
- Most hypnotics interfere with REM sleep. When hypnotics are discontinued, a rebound effect, characterized by nightmares and excessive dreaming, may occur.
- Over-the-counter sleeping preparations generally contain antihistamines and can have adverse effects, such as confusion, constipation, or blurred vision, either alone or in combination with other medications.
- Alcohol is likely to cause nightmares and awakenings during the latter part of the night.
- Medications that can interfere with sleep include steroids, diuretics, theophylline, anticonvulsants, decongestants, and thyroid hormone.
- Combining a sleeping medication with any other medication can be harmful and even fatal.

Addressing Obstructive Sleep Apnea

When older adults have sleep disturbances that do not respond to interventions and interfere with their quality of life, nurses should suggest referrals for further evaluation and treatment. One goal of *Healthy People 2010* is to increase the proportion of people with symptoms of obstructive sleep apnea who seek medical evaluation and receive medical care for long-term management of their condition (USDHHS, 2000). Many behavioral, mechanical, and surgical interventions are available for the treatment of obstructive sleep apnea, so obtaining a comprehensive evaluation and treatment at a sleep disorders clinic should be considered. A list of accredited sleep disorder centers is available from the American Academy of Sleep Medicine (listed in the Educational Resources section at the end of this chapter).

Wellness Opportunity

Nurses address the goals of *Healthy People 2010* by educating older adults about the importance of having any sleep disorder evaluated by a knowledgeable professional.

Mrs. Z. returns for further discussion of her sleep problem after filling out a sleep log for 5 days. You review the log with her and find out that when she is home she spends most of her time reading or doing crossword puzzles. She attends the senior center weekly, plays bridge two evenings a week, and goes to lunch with friends a few times every week. She enjoys gardening during the summer but has no other interest in physical activities. She avoids exercise because she is afraid that physical activity "will get the old arthritis all stirred up." On further questioning, she estimates that when she worked she walked about one half mile daily. She drinks about "a pot" of coffee daily, and has coffee and cookies at bridge games. She enjoys a glass of wine in the evenings. When she wakes up during the night, she usually gets up and goes to the bathroom, then returns to bed and lies there "thinking" until she returns to sleep. Her sleep log reflects that she often stays awake for as long as 2 hours before returning to sleep. She says she's heard that melatonin is good for insomnia and asks your opinion about trying it.

THINKING POINTS

- What myths and misunderstandings about sleep would you address?
- What risk factors might you address through health education?
- Because you can see Mrs. Z. weekly at the Wellness Clinic, you can develop a long-term teaching plan. How would you establish priorities for immediate and long-term goals?
- What information from Boxes 24-2, 24-3, and 24-4 would you use for health education with Mrs. Z.?

EVALUATING EFFECTIVENESS OF NURSING INTERVENTIONS

The effectiveness of interventions for the nursing diagnosis of Disturbed Sleep Pattern can be measured subjectively or objectively. A subjective measurement would be that the older adult reports that he or she feels rested and refreshed upon awakening in the morning. If a sleep assessment tool is used during the initial assessment, it can be used again for a reassessment after interventions have been implemented. An example of an objective measurement would be that the older adult is able to sleep for 6 to 8 hours at night with only brief interruptions, and that the person looks and acts rested during the day.

Mrs. Z. is now 79 years old and is being admitted to a long-term care facility for skilled care after a total hip replacement. Her diagnoses include osteoarthritis and osteoporosis. After a few weeks in the facility, she plans to return to her ranch-style home where she lives with her husband. Before surgery, she was independent in her activities of daily living, and she expects to regain her independence and walk with a walker. The hospital transfer form has orders for nabumetone, 750 mg, every morning and temazepam, 15 mg, at bedtime as needed.

NURSING ASSESSMENT

During the admission interview, you ask Mrs. Z. about her sleep patterns. She states that for the past few years she has been awakened frequently at night by her hip pain and other arthritic discomforts. Also, she reports that she would usually get up three or four times during the night to go to the bathroom. When questioned further, she explains that the pain and discomfort would wake her, and so she would go to the bathroom because she wanted to move around, not because she felt an urge to urinate that often. Although her doctor had advised her to take ibuprofen four times daily, she tried not to take this medication more than two times a day because the pills upset her stomach. She avoided taking any medications at night because she thought she shouldn't take the medications on an empty stomach. During her 1-week hospitalization, she had taken a sleeping pill several

(case study continues on page 525)

times. She had also taken Darvocet-N, 100 mg every 4 hours while she was in the hospital, but said that her doctor wanted her to start taking a nonsteroidal anti-inflammatory drug on a regular basis for her arthritis and hip pain. She said he had prescribed a new drug that would not upset her stomach, but she had not yet begun to take it. Mrs. Z. expresses anxiety about sleeping in the long-term care facility because she says that the noise in the hospital was very disruptive to her sleep. She reports that she feels rested in the morning if she gets at least 6 hours of sleep during the 8 hours she spends in bed. During her hospitalization, she never felt rested in the morning, and was unable to sleep for 6 hours except when she took sleeping pills. Mrs. Z. says that listening to relaxing music helps her to fall asleep.

NURSING DIAGNOSIS

In addition to nursing diagnoses related to Mrs. Z.'s osteoarthritis and hip surgery, you identify a nursing diagnosis of Disturbed Sleep Pattern. Related factors are pain, age-related changes, and environmental conditions. You decide that you will not list nocturia as an associated factor because Mrs. Z. does not feel an urge to void during the night. Rather, she wakes up with pain and then goes to the bathroom. You decide to list age-related changes as a related factor because it is important for Mrs. Z. to understand that, even though she may not awaken with pain, she may awaken because of age-related changes.

NURSING CARE PLAN FOR MRS. Z.

Expected Outcome	Nursing Interventions	Nursing Evaluation
Mrs. Z. will identify factors that influence her sleep pattern.	• Describe age-related changes in sleep patterns. • Discuss the important role of pain-relieving measures in promoting good sleep.	• Mrs. Z. will be able to describe the age-related changes and other conditions that affect her sleeping pattern.
Mrs. Z. will consistently obtain 6 hours of sleep nightly without the aid of sleeping medications.	• Administer nabumetone as ordered and evaluate its effectiveness in controlling Mrs. Z.'s pain. • Explain that sleeping medications should be avoided, except for periodic use in short-term situations. • Assign Mrs. Z. to a room that is not close to the nursing station. • Make sure Mrs. Z.'s door is closed at night. • Encourage Mrs. Z. to use her tape recorder to play quiet music at bedtime. • Give Mrs. Z. a copy of Boxes 24-3 and 24-4 and discuss additional nonpharmacologic methods for promoting sleep.	• Mrs. Z. will report that she is not awakened by pain. • Mrs. Z. will report that she feels rested upon awakening in the morning.

THINKING POINTS

- What additional assessment information pertinent to Mrs. Z.'s sleep patterns would you like to have, and how would you obtain this information?
- What additional nursing interventions would you include in the care plan to address Mrs. Z.'s disturbed sleep pattern? Would you use any of the information in Box 24-2 or give her a copy of it?
- What concerns specifically related to sleep would you have about Mrs. Z. after she is discharged from the skilled nursing facility to her own home? How would you address these concerns in your health promotion interventions?

Chapter Highlights

Age-Related Changes That Affect Sleep and Rest Patterns (Fig. 24-1, Table 24-1)

- Time in bed and total sleep time
- Diminished sleep efficiency
- Alterations in sleep cycles and stages
- Shifts in circadian rhythm

Risks Factors That Affect Sleep Wellness (Tables 24-2 and 24-3)

- Psychosocial factors: beliefs, attitudes, anxiety, depression, boredom
- Environmental factors: noise, light, lack of privacy
- Physiologic factors: pain and discomfort, medication effects, physiologic disorders

Pathologic Condition Affecting Sleep Wellness

- Obstructive sleep apnea

Functional Consequences Affecting Sleep Wellness

- Longer time needed to fall asleep
- Frequent arousals during the night
- More time in bed to achieve same quantity of sleep
- Diminished quality of sleep (less dreaming and deep sleep)

Nursing Assessment of Sleep Patterns (Fig. 24-2, Box 24-1)

- Perception of quantity and quality of sleep
- Factors that affect sleep
- Usual sleep pattern and behaviors that affect it
- Actual sleep pattern (observed in institutional settings)
- Sleep assessment tool

Nursing Diagnosis

- Readiness for Enhanced Sleep
- Disturbed Sleep Pattern

Planning for Wellness Outcomes

- Sleep
- Rest
- Comfort Level
- Personal Well-Being

Nursing Interventions for Sleep Wellness (Boxes 24-2 through 24-4)

- Teaching about interventions to promote healthy sleep patterns
- Modifying the environment
- Individualizing care in institutional settings
- Relaxation and mental imagery techniques
- Teaching about medications that affect sleep
- Addressing obstructive sleep apnea

Evaluating Effectiveness of Nursing Interventions

- Expressed feelings of being rested upon awakening
- Improved score on sleep assessment tool
- Observations that the person is sleeping at night

Critical Thinking Exercises

1. What is an older adult likely to experience with regard to sleep and rest patterns? How would you explain these changes to an older adult?
2. Identify three specific factors in each of the following categories that might interfere with sleep: environmental influences, physiologic disturbances, and psychosocial factors.
3. How would you assess an 82-year-old person who comes to the nursing clinic at the senior wellness center complaining of feeling tired all the time and not getting enough sleep?
4. What would you include in a half-hour presentation on Tips for Good Sleep for participants in a senior wellness program at a community-based center?
5. What information about sleep and rest would you include in an in-service program for evening and night shift nursing assistants employed in a long-term care facility?

Clinical Tool Resources

Hartford Institute for Geriatric Nursing
Try This: Best Practices in Nursing Care to Older Adults
Issue Number 6 (Revised 2007), The Epworth Sleepiness Scale (ESS)
www.hartfordign.org/resources/education/tryThis.html

Educational Resources

American Academy of Sleep Medicine
(formerly called the American Sleep Disorders Association)
www.sleepcenters.org

American Sleep Apnea Association
www.sleepapnea.org

Better Sleep Council
www.bettersleep.org

Canadian Sleep Society
www.css.to

National Center on Sleep Disorders NHLBI Information Center
www.nhlbi.nih.gov/about/ncsdr/

National Sleep Foundation
www.sleepfoundation.org

References

Ancoli-Israel, S., & Ayalon, L. (2006). Diagnosis and treatment of sleep disorders in older adults. *American Journal of Geriatric Psychiatry, 14*(2), 95–103.

Avidan, A. Y. (2005). Sleep in the geriatric patient population. *Seminars in Neurology, 25*(1), 52–63.

Blazer, D., Hybels, C., Simonsick, E., & Hanlon, J. T. (2000). Sedative, hypnotic, and antianxiety medication use in an aging cohort over ten years: A racial comparison. *Journal of the American Geriatrics Society, 48*, 1073–1079.

Carpenito-Moyet, L. J. (2006). *Handbook of nursing diagnosis* (11th ed.). Philadelphia: Lippincott Williams & Wilkins.

Cricco, M., Simonsick, E. M., & Foley, D. J. (2001). The impact of insomnia on cognitive functioning of older adults. *Journal of the American Geriatrics Society, 49*, 1185–1189.

Edinger, J. D., Wohlgemuth, W. K., Krystal, A. D., & Rice, J. R. (2005). Behavioral insomnia therapy for fibromyalgia patients. *Archives of Internal Medicine, 165*, 2527–2535.

Fetveit, A., & Bjorvatn, B. (2005). Bright-light treatment reduces actigraphic-measured daytime sleep in nursing home patients with dementia. *American Journal of Geriatric Psychiatry, 13*, 420–423.

FitzGerald, M. P., Mulligan, M., & Parthasarathy, S. (2006). Nocturic frequency is related to severity of obstructive sleep apnea, improves with continuous positive airways treatment. *American Journal of Obstetrics and Gynecology, 194*, 1399–1403.

Gais, S., Hullemann, P., Hallschmid, M., & Born, H. (2006). Sleep-dependent surges in growth hormone do not contribute to sleep-dependent memory consolidation. *Psychoneuroendocrinology, 31*, 786–791.

Groth, M. (2005). Sleep apnea in the elderly. *Clinics in Geriatric Medicine, 21*, 701–712.

Hoch, C. C., Reynolds, C. F. III, Buysse, D. J., Monk, T. H., Nowell, P., Begley, A. E., et al. (2001). Protecting sleep quality in later life: A pilot study of bed restriction and sleep hygiene. *Journals of Gerontology: Series B, Psychological Sciences, 56*, P52–P59.

Holbrook, A. M., Crowther, R., Lotter, A., & Endeshaw, Y. (2001). The role of benzodiazepines in the treatment of insomnia. *Journal of the American Geriatrics Society, 49*, 824–926.

Kamel, N. S., & Gammack, J. K. (2006). Insomnia in the elderly: Cause, approach, and treatment. *American Journal of Medicine, 119*, 463–469.

Lai, H., & Good, M. (2005). Music improves sleep quality in older adults. *Journal of Advanced Nursing, 49*, 234–244.

Martin, J. L., Webber, A. P., Alam, T., Harker, J. O., Josephson, K. R., & Alessi, C. A. (2006). Daytime sleeping, sleep disturbance, and circadian rhythms in the nursing home. *American Journal of Geriatric Psychiatry, 14*, 121–129.

McCall, W. V. (2005). Diagnosis and management of insomnia in older people. *Journal of the American Geriatrics Society, 53*(7 Suppl.), S272–S277.

Naylor, E., Penev, P. D., Orbeta, L., Janssen, I., Ortiz, R., Colecchia, E. F., et al. (2000). Daily social and physical activity increases slow-wave sleep and daytime neuropsychological performance in the elderly. *Sleep, 23*, 87–95.

Newman, A. B., Foster, G., Givelber, R. Nieto, F. J., Redline, S., & Young, T. (2005). Progression and regression of sleep-disordered breathing with changes in weight: The sleep heart health study. *Archives of Internal Medicine, 165*, 2408–2413.

Ohayon, M. M. (2005). Relationship between chronic painful physical condition and insomnia. *Journal of Psychiatric Research, 39*, 151–159.

Ohayon, M. M., Carskadon, M. A., Guilleminault, C., & Vitiello, M. V. (2004). Meta-analysis of quantitative sleep parameters from childhood to old age in healthy individuals: Developing normative sleep values across the human lifespan. *Sleep, 27*, 1255 1273.

O'Rourke, D. J., Klaasen, K. S., & Sloan, J. A. (2001). Redesigning nighttime care for personal care residents. *Journal of Gerontological Nursing, 27*(7), 30–37.

Pandi-Perumal, S. R., Zisapel, N., Srinivasan, V., & Cardinali, D. P. (2005). Melatonin and sleep in aging population. *Experimental Gerontology, 40*, 911–925.

Phillips, B., Hening, W., Britz, P., & Mannino, D. (2006). Prevalence and correlates of restless legs syndrome: Results from the 2005 National Sleep Foundation poll. *Chest, 129*, 76–80.

Richards, K. C., Sullivan, S. C., Phillips, R. L. Beck, C. K., & Overton-McCoy, A. L. (2001). The effects of individualized activities on the sleep of nursing home residents who are cognitively impaired: A pilot study. *Journal of Gerontological Nursing, 27*(9), 30–37.

Robinson, S. B., Weitzel, T., & Henderson, L. (2005). The Sh-h-h-h Project: Nonpharmacological interventions. *Holistic Nursing Practice, 19*, 263–266.

Ruby, C. M., & Kennedy D. H. (2001). Psychopharmacologic medication use in nursing-home care: Indicators for surveyor assessment of the performance of drug-regimen reviews, recommendations for monitoring, and nonpharmacologic alternatives. *Clinics in Family Practice, 3*, 577–598.

Smyth, C. (2007). The Epworth Sleepiness Scale (ESS). *Try this: Best practices in nursing care to older adults*, Issue 6 (revised). New York University, Hartford Institute for Geriatric Nursing.

Stierer, T., & Punjabi, N. M. (2005). Demographics and diagnosis of obstructive sleep apnea. *Anesthesiology Clinics of North America, 23*, 405–420.

Tworoger, S. S., Lee, S., Schernhammer, E. S., & Grodstein, F. (2006). The association of self-reported sleep duration, difficulty sleeping and snoring with cognitive function in older women. *Alzheimer's Disease and Associated Disorders, 20*, 41–48.

U.S. Department of Health and Human Services (USDHHS). (2000). *Healthy People 2010* (2nd ed.). Washington, DC: U.S. Government Printing Office.

Zhdanova, I. V., Wurtman, R. J., Regan, M. M., Taylor, J. A., Shi, J. P., & Leclair, O. U. (2001). Endocrine care: Of special interest to the practice of endocrinology. *Journal of Clinical Endocrinology and Metabolism, 86*, 4727–4730.

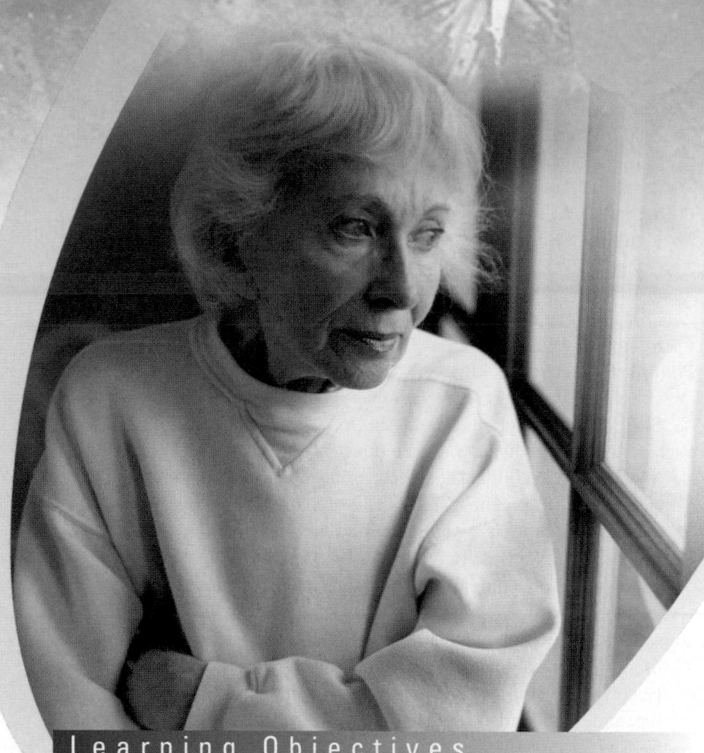

CHAPTER 25

Thermoregulation

Learning Objectives

After reading this chapter, you will be able to:

1. Describe age-related changes that affect an older adult's normal body temperature, febrile response to illness, and response to hot and cold environmental temperatures.
2. Identify risk factors that affect thermoregulation in older adults and increase the potential for hypothermia or hyperthermia.
3. Discuss the functional consequences of altered temperature regulation in older adults.
4. Assess the following aspects of thermoregulation: baseline temperature, risks for altered thermoregulation, hypothermia, hyperthermia, and febrile response to illness.
5. Implement health promotion interventions for preventing hypothermia and hyperthermia in older adults.

Key Terms

accidental hypothermia
acclimatize
heat exhaustion
heat stroke
hyperthermia
hypothermia

The primary function of thermoregulation is to maintain a stable core body temperature in a wide range of environmental temperatures. In the presence of infections, thermoregulation also assists in maintaining homeostasis. Under normal circumstances, the core body temperature is maintained at 97°F (36.1°C) to 99°F (37.2°C) through complex physiologic mechanisms governing heat production and dissipation. Age-related changes alone affect the older adult's thermoregulation. When risk factors are also present, the older adult may develop serious problems. Nurses play an important role in promoting healthy thermoregulation and comfort for older adults.

 AGE-RELATED CHANGES THAT AFFECT THERMOREGULATION

With increased age, subtle alterations in thermoregulation occur, and these become important considerations in caring for healthy, as well as frail, older adults. Because thermoregulation is a complex process involving many body systems, adaptive responses to environmental temperatures can be altered by many internal and external influences. Internal conditions that affect temperature regulation include metabolic rate; pathologic processes; muscle activity; peripheral blood flow; amount of subcutaneous fat; function of the cutaneous nerves; ingestion of fluid, nutrients, and medications; and the temperature of the blood flowing through the hypothalamus. External influences on thermoregulation include environmental temperature, humidity level, air flow, and the type and amount of clothing and covering used. The following sections address these factors in relation to the ability of older adults to respond to environmental temperatures and in relation to normal body temperature.

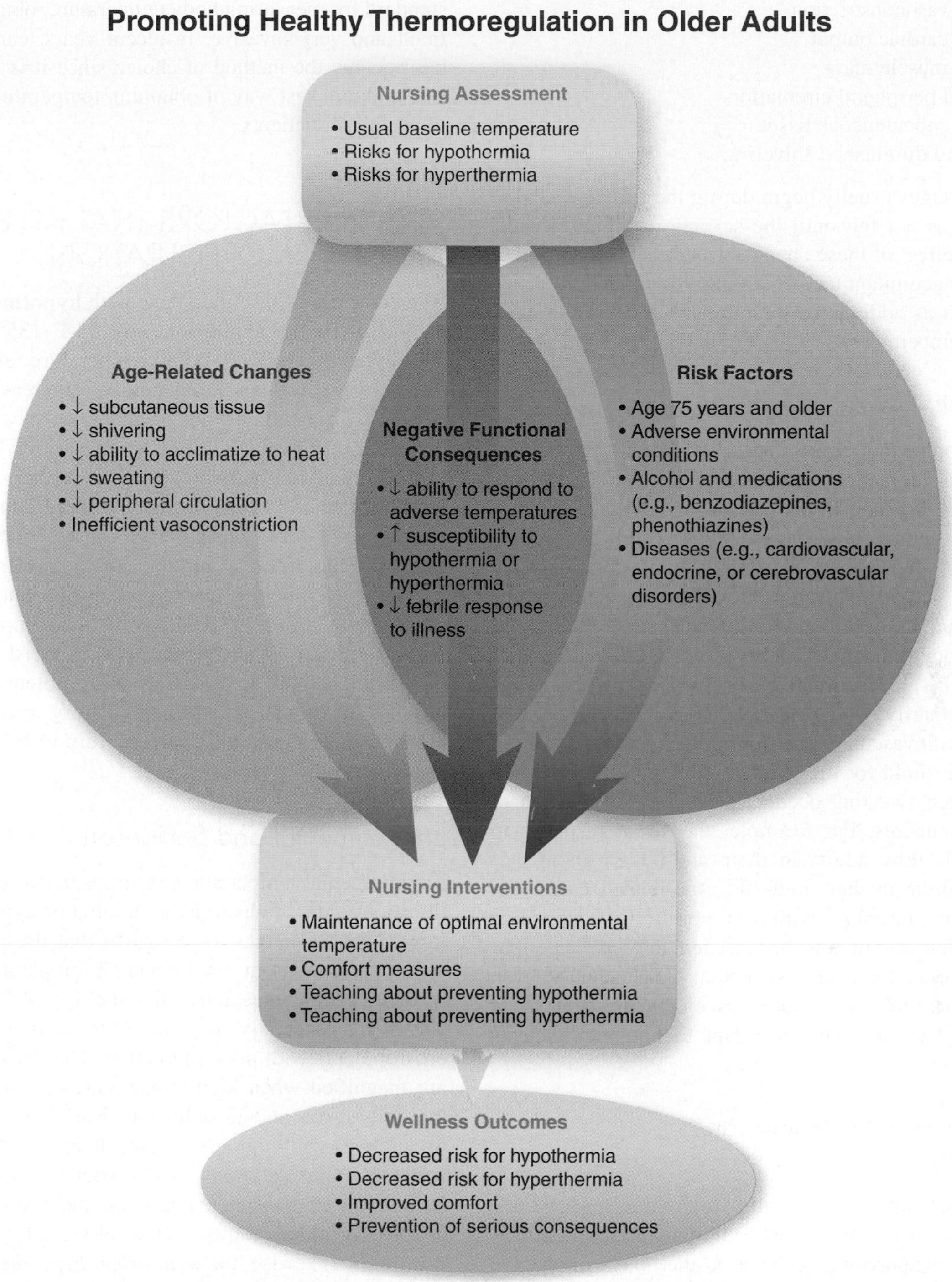

Promoting Healthy Thermoregulation in Older Adults

Nursing Assessment
• Usual baseline temperature
• Risks for hypothermia
• Risks for hyperthermia
Age-Related Changes
• ↓ subcutaneous tissue
• ↓ shivering
• ↓ ability to acclimatize to heat
• ↓ sweating
• ↓ peripheral circulation
• Inefficient vasoconstriction
Negative Functional Consequences
• ↓ ability to respond to adverse temperatures
• ↑ susceptibility to hypothermia or hyperthermia
• ↓ febrile response to illness
Risk Factors
• Age 75 years and older
• Adverse environmental conditions
• Alcohol and medications (e.g., benzodiazepines, phenothiazines)
• Diseases (e.g., cardiovascular, endocrine, or cerebrovascular disorders)
Nursing Interventions
• Maintenance of optimal environmental temperature
• Comfort measures
• Teaching about preventing hypothermia
• Teaching about preventing hyperthermia
Wellness Outcomes
• Decreased risk for hypothermia
• Decreased risk for hyperthermia
• Improved comfort
• Prevention of serious consequences

Response to Cold Temperatures

In cold environmental temperatures, the body normally initiates physiologic mechanisms to prevent loss of body heat and increase heat production. At the same time, individuals usually initiate protective behaviors to warm the body and protect themselves from adversely cold temperatures. Physiologic mechanisms that prevent heat loss and increase heat production include shivering, muscle contraction, increased heart rate, peripheral vasoconstriction, dilation of the blood vessels in the muscles, insulation of deeper tissues by subcutaneous fat, and release of thyroxine and corticosteroid by the pituitary gland. Protective actions that people commonly initiate in cold temperatures include seeking of shelter, ingestion of warm fluids, use of warm clothing or covering, and an increase in activity to stimulate circulation.

The following age-related changes, which can affect processes involved with heat loss or production, are likely to interfere with an older person's ability to respond to cold temperatures:

- Inefficient vasoconstriction
- Decreased cardiac output
- Decreased muscle mass
- Diminished peripheral circulation
- Decreased subcutaneous tissue
- Delayed and diminished shivering

These changes usually begin during the fifth decade, but their impact is not felt until the seventh or eighth decade. The overall effect of these changes is a dulled perception of cold and a concomitant lack of stimulus to initiate protective actions, such as adding more clothing or raising the environmental temperature.

Response to Hot Temperatures

In hot environmental temperatures, or when metabolic heat production is high, the normal mechanisms for heat dissipation are the production of sweat to facilitate evaporation and the dilation of peripheral blood vessels to facilitate heat radiation. When exposed to hot climates or engaged in strenuous activity daily for 7 to 14 days, healthy adults are able to **acclimatize** (i.e., gradually increase their metabolic efficiency to adapt to higher temperatures). The older person's ability to acclimatize and respond to heat stress is altered primarily by age-related changes affecting sweating and cardiovascular function. Older adults have an increased threshold for the onset of sweating, a diminished response when sweating occurs, and a dulled sensation of warm environments. For example, the sweat response to exercise in healthy adults in their mid-60s is about half of that in adults in their mid-20s. Age-related cardiovascular changes interfere with the ability to acclimatize because cardiac output must be sufficient to produce peripheral vasodilation for heat dissipation. Consequently, even healthy older adults are more susceptible to heat stress because they are less able to adapt to hot environments (Vicario, 2006).

Normal Body Temperature and Febrile Response to Illness

Body temperature is normally maintained at 98.6°F (36.7°C), plus or minus 1°F, with diurnal variations of 2°F. An elevated temperature, or fever, is the body's protective response to pathologic conditions such as cancer, infection, dehydration, or connective tissue disease. Normal body temperature decreases with increased age, particularly in people older than 75 years. Studies in healthy older adults have found mean oral temperatures of 97.4 to 97.9, with temperatures above 98.6 being the exception (Gomolin et al., 2005).

Oral and axillary temperatures may be questionable as a measurement of core temperature in older adults because the difference between their core and skin temperatures is greater and more variable than in younger people. Although rectal temperature has long been viewed as the established standard for measuring body temperature, obtaining it is difficult and very invasive. In recent years, ear thermometry has become the method of choice since it is the least invasive and quickest way of obtaining temperatures, especially in acutely ill patients.

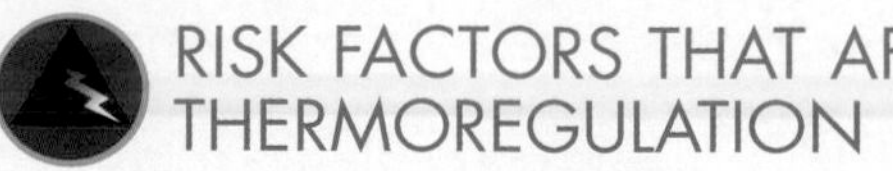

RISK FACTORS THAT AFFECT THERMOREGULATION

Age alone predisposes people to both **hypothermia**, defined as a core body temperature of 95°F (35°C) or lower, and **hyperthermia**, a body temperature elevated above the person's normal temperature. Whereas hypothermia develops in healthy young adults only when they are exposed to adversely cold temperatures, older adults can become hypothermic even in moderately cool environments, especially in the presence of additional risk factors. Likewise, healthy young adults can tolerate hot environmental temperatures without adverse effects, whereas heat-related illnesses or hyperthermia may develop in older adults even in moderately hot temperatures. Any combination of environmental and other risk factors in the older adult is likely to lead to serious problems or even death because of impaired thermoregulatory mechanisms that increase the older adult's vulnerability to hypothermia and hyperthermia.

Environmental and Socioeconomic Influences

Environmental temperatures significantly affect the susceptibility of older adults to hyperthermia or hypothermia. It is imperative for nurses to recognize that the impact of seasonal fluctuations in environmental temperatures increases in older adults, especially after the age of 75 years. Heat waves are especially hazardous for older adults living in environments with poor ventilation. The detrimental effects are magnified when high temperatures combine with high humidity levels and air pollutants. For older adults living in urban areas with high crime rates, keeping windows closed for safety considerations may restrict ventilation. In Great Britain, the term *urban hypothermia* has been used with reference to older adults living alone in poorly heated dwellings. Likewise, the term *urban hyperthermia* could be applied to older adults living in poorly ventilated houses and apartments, particularly public housing, in cities where heat waves and air pollution are common.

In addition to the obvious influence of hot or cold temperatures, substandard living conditions and diets deficient in protein and calories have been associated with hypothermia and hyperthermia. Because hypothermia and hyperthermia usually are not self-reported disorders, social isolation and living alone are conditions that increase the risk for progression of these conditions if they do occur. Homelessness is another socioeconomic factor that increases the risk for both hypothermia and hyperthermia.

Wellness Opportunity

Although the weather cannot be controlled, it is important to identify the environmental factors that affect thermoregulation and that can be addressed through health education about protective actions.

Behaviors Based on Lack of Knowledge

Lack of knowledge about age-related vulnerability to hypothermia and hyperthermia may create risks secondary to inadequate protective measures. For example, when the use of heating or air conditioning is curtailed as a cost-saving measure, younger adults may be able to adjust to the moderately hot or cool temperature, whereas an older adult might become hyperthermic or hypothermic under the same circumstances. If older adults and their caregivers are not aware of the age-related decrease in the perception of environmental temperatures, they may not take appropriate protective measures, such as removing or adding clothing.

In the presence of infection, lack of knowledge about age-related thermoregulatory changes may result in undetected illnesses. For example, if caregivers of older adults believe that an infectious disease is always accompanied by an elevated temperature, they may assume that no infection is present if there is no fever. Similarly, if they believe that the baseline temperature for all adults is 98.6°F (36.7°C), they may not recognize an elevated temperature in someone whose baseline temperature is lower than this. Lack of knowledge about diurnal temperature variations, the age-related decrease in body temperature, and the age-related increase in the difference between core and skin temperature also may contribute to false expectations and undetected illness.

Conditions That Predispose to Hypothermia or Hyperthermia

The risk for development of hypothermia is increased by conditions that decrease heat production (e.g., inactivity, malnutrition, endocrine disorders, neuromuscular conditions), increase heat loss (e.g., burns, vasodilation), or affect the normal thermoregulatory process (pathologic conditions of the central nervous system). Medications and alcohol are additional factors that can predispose to hypothermia by suppressing shivering or inducing vasodilation (e.g., alcohol, benzodiazepines, cyclic antidepressants). Excessive use of alcohol further increases the risk for hypothermia by dulling sensory perceptions and interfering with cognitive skills necessary for initiating protective behaviors. Infections (e.g., pneumonia, gram-negative sepsis) and pathologic conditions such as carcinoma and severe cerebrovascular disease may cause hypothermia in older adults, even though these conditions are more commonly associated with fever in younger adults.

The risk for development of hyperthermia is increased by physiologic alterations that increase internal heat production (e.g., hyperthyroidism, diabetic ketoacidosis) or interfere with the ability to respond to heat stress (e.g., cardiovascular disease, fluid or electrolyte imbalance). Medications can predispose to hyperthermia by increasing diuresis (e.g., diuretics), increasing heat production (e.g., salicylate intoxication), or interfering with sweating (e.g., anticholinergics) or peripheral vasodilation (e.g., beta-adrenergic blocking agents). Alcohol increases the risk for hyperthermia by inducing diuresis, and excessive alcohol can increase the risk by increasing heat production.

Older adults are predisposed to development of hypothermia or hyperthermia in direct relation to the number of risk factors present for either condition. Degree of risk also is affected by seasonal fluctuations in environmental temperatures, especially during winter months or heat waves. For example, heat-related illness can be precipitated by even moderate exercise in hot and humid weather, especially if fluid intake is not adequate. If older adults rely solely on their sensation of thirst to signal the need for fluid intake, they can become underhydrated or dehydrated because of the age-related diminished thirst sensation. Box 25-1 lists some of the conditions that most commonly increase the risk for hypothermia or hyperthermia in older adults.

In addition to factors that directly predispose older adults to hypothermia or hyperthermia, other factors increase the risk for serious consequences. For example, older adults who live alone or are socially isolated are at risk of not getting help if they experience hypothermia or hyperthermia, especially if the condition interferes with their problem-solving skills. Likewise, people who live alone and have dementia may be at increased risk if they do not have the cognitive skills to adjust the thermostat and wear proper clothing. Studies indicate that people who develop hypothermia while indoors have a significantly higher mortality rate than their outdoor counterparts. This is attributable to increased age and delayed discovery and treatment (McCullough & Arora, 2004).

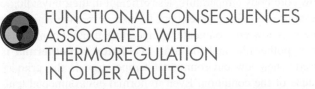

FUNCTIONAL CONSEQUENCES ASSOCIATED WITH THERMOREGULATION IN OLDER ADULTS

A healthy older adult in a comfortable environment will experience few, if any, functional consequences of altered thermoregulation. In the presence of any risk factor, however, hypothermia or hyperthermia may develop in an older adult. Even moderately adverse environmental temperatures can precipitate hypothermia or hyperthermia in an older adult, especially in the presence of additional predisposing factors, such as certain medications or pathologic conditions. For older adults in whom hypothermia or hyperthermia develops, the risk of subsequent morbidity or mortality from this condition is greater than that for their younger counterparts.

Box 25-1
Risk Factors for Hypothermia or Hyperthermia in Older Adults

Risks for Hypothermia and Hyperthermia

- Age 75 years and older
- Adverse environmental temperatures
- Infections or sepsis
- Cardiovascular disorders
- Cerebrovascular disease
- Peripheral neuropathy
- Uremia
- Medications: barbiturates, benzodiazepines, cyclic antidepressants, and phenothiazines

Risks for Hypothermia

- Alcohol
- Carcinoma
- Diabetes or hypoglycemia
- Hypoadrenalism
- Hypothalamic dysfunction
- Hypopituitarism
- Hypothyroidism
- Inactivity
- Malnutrition
- Parkinson's disease

Risks for Hyperthermia

- Alcohol and alcohol withdrawal
- Dehydration
- Diabetic ketoacidosis
- Hyperthyroidism
- Excessive exercise or even moderate exercise in hot environments
- Pheochromocytoma
- Medications: alpha-adrenergic blocking agents; anticholinergic agents (including antihistamines, phenothiazines, tricyclic antidepressants); benzodiazepines, beta-adrenergic blocking agents, calcium channel blockers, diuretics, and laxatives

Data from Danzl (2006); Glazer (2005); McCullough & Arora (2004); and Vicario (2006).

In the United States, hypothermia and hyperthermia usually are seasonal hazards that occur during heat waves and cold spells, and these weather-related problems most often affect older adults who live in climates with extremes of weather. States with the highest death rates for hypothermia between 1999 and 2002 are Alaska, Montana, Wyoming, New Mexico, and North Dakota. Hypothermia-related deaths also occur in states, such as North and South Carolina, where there are rapid temperature changes, and in states like Arizona with high elevations and colder nighttime temperatures (Fallico et al., 2005; Murphy et al., 2006).

Altered Response to Cold Environments

Increased age is associated with an increased vulnerability to hypothermia because most older adults are less aware of a low core body temperature, less efficient in their physiologic response to cold, and less apt to take corrective actions in them. A low environmental temperature usually contributes to hypothermia, and the term **accidental hypothermia** is used when low environmental temperature is the primary cause of the condition. Even in normal environmental temperatures, however, the condition can result from serious alterations in homeostasis, such as can occur with anesthesia or endocrine or neurologic disorders. Accidental hypothermia can occur in older adults as a consequence of exposure to moderately cool temperatures, and is thought to affect as many as 10% of older adults living in winter climates (e.g., Great Britain, Canada, and parts of the United States).

In the early stages of hypothermia, the older adult probably will not shiver or complain of feeling cold. In the absence of any protective measures, hypothermia will progress, clouding mental function. The effects of impaired thermoregulation are cumulative, and hypothermia progresses rapidly after the core body temperature falls to 93.2°F (33.9°C). The age-related diminished ability of the kidney to conserve water and the common occurrence of inadequate fluid intake in older adults exacerbate the effects of hypothermia. If the process is not reversed, death from hypothermia will result from the myocardial effects of seriously impaired thermoregulation.

Altered Response to Hot Environments

Functional consequences that affect an older adult's ability to respond to hot environments include delayed and diminished sweating and inaccurate perception of environmental temperatures. Because of these functional consequences, the older adult is more likely to have heat-related illnesses, including heat stroke and heat exhaustion. Although the term *hyperthermia* is often used to refer to heat-related illnesses in older people, this term more accurately refers to any condition in which the body temperature is elevated above normal. In addition to impaired thermoregulation and environmental factors, pyrogens and other pathologic conditions can cause hyperthermia.

Heat exhaustion is a condition that develops gradually from depletion of fluid, sodium, or both. It can occur in active or immobilized older people who are dehydrated or underhydrated and exposed to hot environments. **Heat stroke** is an even more serious condition that is likely to occur in active older adults because of a combination of age-related thermoregulatory changes and risk factors, such as overexertion and warm environments. Heat stroke can also occur in immobilized older adults in hot environments, either as a progression of untreated heat exhaustion or as a result of a combination of risk factors, such as diabetes and certain medications. The underlying mechanism in heat stroke is an inability to balance the rates of heat production and dissipation. This balance depends primarily on sweating and cardiac output.

In hot environments, the effects of altered thermoregulation are cumulative, and heat-related illnesses progress rapidly after the body temperature reaches 105.8°F (40.6°C). If fluid volume is not adequate to meet the requirements for effective sweating, then hyperthermia will progress even more rapidly. The age-related decrease in thirst sensation can contribute to inadequate fluid intake and diminished thermoregulation. If hyperthermia is not reversed, death will result from respiratory depression.

Altered Thermoregulatory Response to Illness

Age-related changes in the thermoregulatory centers of the hypothalamus diminish the older adult's febrile response to illness and infections. Thus, infections are likely to be undetected until they progress and manifest as a functional decline or change in mental status. Older adults with infections commonly have a normal or even lower than normal temperature, but when their temperature is compared with their baseline temperature, at least a slight elevation is evident. Thus, elevated temperature in older adults can be detected only in relation to their normal baseline temperature.

Altered Perception of Environmental Temperatures

Older adults often report feeling cool or cold, even in very warm environments, and they generally prefer environmental temperatures that are at least 75°F (23.9°C). Inaccurate perceptions of environmental temperatures are associated with pathophysiologic conditions, such as dementia, thyroid disorders, or cardiovascular inefficiency, rather than with age-related changes alone.

Psychosocial Consequences of Altered Thermoregulation

Psychosocial consequences are associated with hypothermia, hyperthermia, or diminished fever response. If hypothermia or hyperthermia is overlooked, or if interventions are not initiated at an early stage, the condition may progress to the point of impairing cognitive function. Likewise, if a diminished or delayed febrile response to an infection is not recognized, a treatable condition may be overlooked and treatment may unintentionally be delayed or denied. Untreated infections are likely to progress in severity and, in older adults, may manifest primarily as a functional decline, such as impaired cognition.

Mrs. T. is 76 years old and lives alone in a large farmhouse in a rural county in central Ohio. She has lived on this 20-acre farm for 49 years and has been a widow for 2 years. She has four children and eight grandchildren, but they all live in other states. Mrs. T. has been able to manage her farm with a part-time farmhand who comes a couple times a week to help feed the several dozen chickens and collect eggs. When her farmhand doesn't come, she manages the chores by herself. She has hypertension and type 2 diabetes, and manages reasonably well medically. She adheres to her diabetic diet and takes her medications daily. She sends her farmhand to the city once weekly for groceries and drives to the nearby church on Sundays. Once a month she attends the county senior center, where you are the nurse. It is the middle of July and summer in Ohio this year has been unusually hot and humid. A drought and heat wave are predicted for central Ohio and you are planning to present a health education program called "Hot Tips for Surviving the Summer." You are particularly concerned about Mrs. T. and several other participants who live in isolated areas and have little contact with others.

THINKING POINTS

- What factors increase the risk of Mrs. T. developing a heat-related illness? Which ones would you discuss in your health education program?
- In your health education program, how would you explain heat-related illnesses and the associated signs and symptoms?

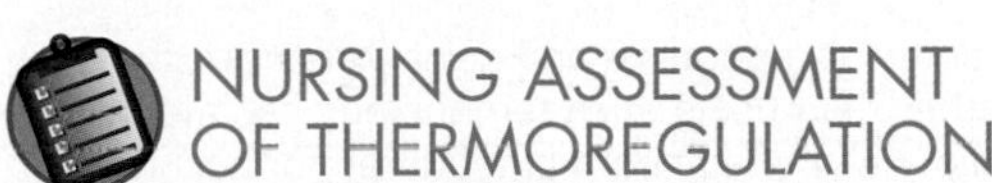

NURSING ASSESSMENT OF THERMOREGULATION

Nursing assessment of thermoregulation addresses the older person's baseline body temperature, any risk factors for altered thermoregulation, manifestations of hypothermia or hyperthermia, and febrile response to illness. Nurses use this information for planning health education interventions to prevent hypothermia and hyperthermia. Nurses also use the assessment information to detect hypothermia or heat-related illnesses as quickly as possible so that appropriate interventions can be initiated before serious or irreversible effects occur. Assessment information also is important in detecting infections at an early stage. Nurses obtain much of the pertinent information about risk factors as part of the overall assessment; they also obtain information by observing the environment, measuring the person's body temperature, and interviewing the older adult and the caregivers of dependent older adults.

Assessing Baseline Temperature

Body temperature measurements show a diurnal fluctuation of 1°F to 2°F, with lower temperatures during sleeping and greater fluctuations during periods of fever-inducing illness. Because older adults normally have a lower body temperature and may have a diminished febrile response to infection, it is especially important to determine the person's usual temperature, as well as to characterize the usual pattern of diurnal variation. Because many types of thermometers are now available (e.g., oral, rectal, tympanic, and bladder probes), it is important to document the method used for assessing temperature. Also, when assessing for hypothermia, it is advisable to use several methods and to make sure that the thermometers are able to detect low body temperatures.

Nurses can encourage older adults in home settings to determine their usual temperature by recording their temperature at different times of the day for several days when they are feeling well. Doing this seasonally by people who live in fluctuating climates and annually by those who live in stable climates, provides a baseline for comparison when symptoms of illness or functional decline occur. Nurses can follow this procedure in long-term care settings and record the results as baseline data on the chart. Box 25-2 summarizes the principles underlying nursing assessment of thermoregulation in older adults.

Identifying Risk Factors for Altered Thermoregulation

Anyone older than 75 years is at risk for altered thermoregulation, as are older adults who have one or more of the risk factors listed in Box 25-1. Because so many of the risk factors for altered thermoregulation are modifiable, it is important to identify those that can be addressed through health promotion interventions. Nurses usually identify risk factors involving medications and physiologic disturbances during the overall assessment, and it is important to consider any conditions predisposing the person to hypothermia or hyperthermia. In addition to assessing for risks for hypothermia or heat-related illnesses, nurses must consider a low baseline body temperature as a risk for undetected fever. It is important to document the person's baseline temperature and note this as a risk factor for both hypothermia and undetected febrile conditions if it is below 98°F (36.7°C).

Most nurses do not have the opportunity to observe and assess the older adult's home environment, but they can ask

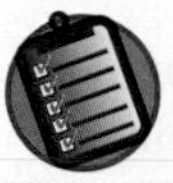

Box 25-2 Guidelines for Assessing Thermoregulation

Principles of Temperature Assessment

- Document the person's baseline body temperature and its diurnal and seasonal variations.
- Assume that even a small elevation above the baseline temperature is a clue to the presence of a pathologic process.
- Document actual temperature and deviations from the baseline, rather than using such terminology as "afebrile."
- Carefully follow all the standard procedures for accurate temperature measurement. Use a thermometer that registers temperatures lower than 95°F (35°C).
- Consider the influence of temperature-altering medications when evaluating a temperature reading (e.g., medications that mask a fever).
- Do not assume that an infection will necessarily be accompanied by an elevated temperature.
- Remember that, in the presence of an infection, a decline in function or change in mental status may be an earlier and more accurate indicator of illness than an alteration in temperature.
- Do not assume that an older adult will initiate compensatory behaviors or complain of discomfort when exposed to adverse environmental temperatures.

Questions to Assess Risk Factors for Hypothermia or Hyperthermia

- Do you have any particular health problems that occur in hot or cold weather?
- Are you able to keep your house or room at a comfortable temperature in both summer and winter months?
- What do you do to cope with hot temperatures in the summer?
- Do you have any difficulty paying your utility bills?
- What forms of protection against the cold do you use in the winter months (e.g., electric blanket, supplemental sources of heat)?
- Have you ever received medical care for exposure to heat or cold?
- Have you ever fallen and not been able to get up or get help?

Observations to Assess Risk Factors for Hypothermia or Hyperthermia

- Does the older person live in a house where the temperature is kept below 70°F (21.1°C) during the winter?
- Does the person drink alcohol or take temperature-altering medications (see Box 25-1)?
- Does the person live alone? If so, what is the frequency of outside contacts?
- Does the person have any pathologic conditions that predispose him or her to hypothermia (e.g., endocrine, neurologic, or cardiovascular disorders)?
- Is the person's fluid and nutritional intake adequate?
- Does the person have postural hypotension? (See Table 20-2 and Boxes 20-1 and 20-2 for assessment criteria relating to postural hypotension.)
- Is the person immobilized or sedentary? Is the person's judgment impaired because of dementia, depression, or other psychosocial disorders?
- Does the person live in a poorly ventilated dwelling without air conditioning?
- Are atmospheric conditions very hot, humid, or polluted?
- Does the person engage in active exercise during hot weather?
- Does the person have chronic illnesses, such as diabetes or cardiovascular disorders, that predispose him or her to hyperthermia?
- Is the person at risk for hyponatremia or hypokalemia because of medications or chronic illnesses?

pertinent questions and listen for clues to detect environmental risk factors. For example, older adults who live alone and express concern about keeping the house warm in winter should be considered to be at risk for hypothermia. Likewise, older adults who live in poor housing conditions, or with family members who keep the house at low temperatures during winter months, should be considered to be at risk for hypothermia. Older adults who live in poorly ventilated houses without air conditioning should be considered to be at risk for hyperthermia during heat waves. Interview questions aimed at identifying risk factors for altered thermoregulation are listed in Box 25-2.

Wellness Opportunity

From a holistic perspective, nurses consider that fears about paying utility bills in the winter or about personal safety when windows are open can increase the risk for hypothermia or heat-related conditions.

Assessing for Hypothermia

Hypothermia is best detected by measuring core body temperature with a thermometer that registers below 95°F (35°C). Cool skin in unexposed areas, such as the abdomen and buttocks, is a distinguishing characteristic of hypothermia. The environmental temperature may be only moderately cool and the older person will not necessarily shiver or complain of feeling cold. Even in environmental temperatures of 68°F (20°C) or 69°F (20.6°C), an older person may become hypothermic, especially if other risk factors, such as immobility or hypothermia-inducing medications, are present. Early signs of hypothermia are subtle, and the most objective assessment tool is a comparison of the person's body temperature with their usual baseline temperature. As untreated hypothermia progresses, additional signs may include lethargy, slurred speech, mental changes, impaired gait, puffiness of the face, slowed or irregular pulse, low blood pressure, slowed tendon reflexes, and slow, shallow respirations. Severe stages of hypothermia are characterized by muscular rigidity, diminished urinary function, and a progression of all other manifestations to the point of stupor and coma. The skin will feel very cool, and, contrary to what might be expected, the color of the skin will be pink. Also contrary to what might be expected, a hypothermic person may not shiver, particularly if the body temperature is below 90°F (32.2°C).

Assessing for Hyperthermia

Manifestations of heat-related illnesses range from mild headache to life-threatening respiratory and cardiovascular disturbances. In the early stages of heat-related illness, the person will feel weak and lethargic and may complain of headache, nausea, and loss of appetite. The skin will be warm and dry, and the sweating response may be absent, especially if the person's fluid intake is low. As the heat-related condition progresses, these manifestations will be exacerbated, and the following signs will become evident: dizziness, dyspnea, tachycardia, vomiting, diarrhea, muscle cramps, chest pain, mental impairment, and a wide pulse pressure.

Assessing the Older Adult's Febrile Response to Illness

Because the manifestations of delayed or diminished febrile response to infections are likely to be very subtle, nurses assess for any temperature changes from the person's baseline as well as for additional signs of illness, such as a decline in function. Nurses also should examine assumptions about temperature regulation that may apply to younger adults but not to older adults. For example, the expectation that pneumonia is accompanied by an elevated temperature is not necessarily applicable to older adults, as discussed in Chapter 21. Thus, nurses in long-term care facilities need to be particularly vigilant about subtle temperature changes and other manifestations of fever. A more reliable indicator of elevated temperature in older adults would be an increase of 2°F (1°C) above the person's baseline. See Box 25-2 for a summary of some of these considerations.

Wellness Opportunity

A holistic assessment for febrile conditions requires that nurses identify subtle manifestations such as behavior changes and slight elevations above the person's baseline temperature, even if the temperature is within the so-called normal range.

NURSING DIAGNOSIS

If the nursing assessment identifies risks for impaired thermoregulation in an older adult, pertinent nursing diagnoses include Hypothermia, Hyperthermia, or Risk for Imbalanced Body Temperature. Hypothermia, as a nursing diagnosis, is defined as "the state in which an individual has or is at risk of having a sustained reduction of body temperature of <35.5°C (96°F) rectally because of increased vulnerability to external factors" (Carpenito-Moyet, 2006, p. 26). The definition of the nursing diagnosis Hyperthermia is "the state in which an individual has or is at risk of having a sustained elevation of body temperature >37.8°C (100°F) orally or 38.8°C (101°F) rectally because of external factors" (Carpenito-Moyet, 2006, p. 23).

If conditions increase the risk for hypothermia, hyperthermia, and ineffective thermoregulation, the nursing diagnosis of Risk for Imbalanced Body Temperature may be appropriate. For example, an 83-year-old woman with diabetes, dementia, and hypertension who is taking a diuretic, an antipsychotic, and an oral hypoglycemic would have many risk factors for both hypothermia and hyperthermia. Related factors that are common in older adults include immobility, advanced age, medication effects, adverse environmental conditions, and acute and chronic illnesses. For older adults living alone, social isolation may be a related factor that increases the risk for experiencing more serious consequences if hypothermia or hyperthermia occurs.

Wellness Opportunity

Nurses can use the nursing diagnosis Readiness for Enhanced Knowledge: Prevention of Hypothermia (or Hyperthermia) for older adults and their caregivers who are interested in learning to address risks for these conditions.

PLANNING FOR WELLNESS OUTCOMES

When caring for older adults with risks for hypothermia or hyperthermia, nurses identify wellness outcomes as an essential component of the nursing process. Nurses can use the following Nursing Outcomes Classification (NOC) terminology in their care plans addressing risks for altered thermoregulation: Health Promoting Behavior, Hydration, Knowledge: Health Behavior, Knowledge: Personal Safety, Risk Detection, Risk Control, Safe Home Environment, Thermoregulation, and Vital Signs: Body Temperature.

Outcomes vary depending on the setting. In acute care settings, nurses are more likely to focus on outcomes that pertain to the patient's immediate physical condition (e.g., Hydration, Thermoregulation, and Vital Signs: Body Temperature). A focus of nursing care in long-term care settings is early detection of infections. In home and other community settings, nurses might be able to provide group or individual health education for older adults who are at risk for development of hypothermia or heat-related illness, especially during times of extreme weather conditions. In these situations, nurses focus more on teaching about self-care and environmental modifications to prevent hypothermia or hyperthermia.

Wellness Opportunity

Nurses promote wellness when their care plans include health-promoting behaviors to prevent hypothermia and hyperthermia.

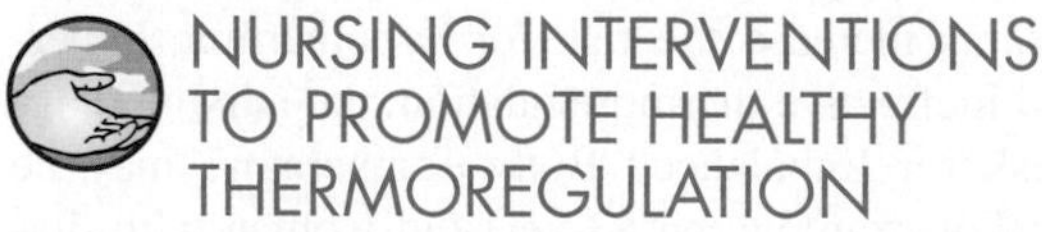

NURSING INTERVENTIONS TO PROMOTE HEALTHY THERMOREGULATION

Health promotion interventions to address altered thermoregulation are directed toward primary prevention of hypothermia and heat-related illness. Health promotion interventions also address early detection of altered thermoregulation and prompt initiation of interventions to restore thermal balance and to prevent detrimental effects. Comfort interventions are initiated to promote well-being in older adults. Nurses can use the following Nursing Interventions Classification (NIC) terminology to document interventions: Environmental Management, Environmental Risk Protection, Health Education, Risk Identification, Surveillance: Safety, Teaching: Individual, and Temperature Regulation.

Addressing Risk Factors

Maintenance of an environmental temperature of around 75°F (23.9°C) is the single most important intervention to prevent hypothermia or hyperthermia. In addition, relative humidity can be altered to minimize the discomfort and detrimental effects associated with extremely warm or cool environments. With comfortable indoor temperatures, the ideal humidity is between 40% and 50%, although an acceptable range is between 20% and 70%. Older adults can be encouraged to humidify the air in their homes during the dry winter months by using humidifiers, either alone or with their heating systems. Simpler measures, such as keeping wet towels near heating vents or using a vaporizer near the bed at night, may be appropriate if a humidifier is unavailable. Older adults living in hot, humid climates may need assistance in applying to elder care community programs that provide window air conditioners, fans, and assistance with summer electric bills.

In many areas of the United States and Canada in which cold winters are the norm, financial assistance for heating bills may be available through government-sponsored programs, such as the Low Income Home Energy Assistance Program's (LIHEAP) Fuel Assistance Program. Other government-sponsored programs provide financial assistance, such as low-interest loans, for home winterization and modernization measures to protect against adverse weather conditions. Older people and their family caregivers should be encouraged to take advantage of these programs, applications for which can be obtained from the LIHEAP contact listed in the Educational Resources at the end of this chapter.

Wellness Opportunity

Nurses promote wellness for socially isolated older adults by identifying ways of developing a system of social contact, such as a friendly phone call program, that ensures daily contact during periods of adversely hot or cold weather.

Promoting Healthy Thermoregulation

In cool environmental temperatures, interventions to prevent hypothermia include using adequate clothing and covering. Nurses can encourage older adults to wear several layers of warm clothing during the daytime, and caps and warm socks while sleeping. Electric blankets used during the night are a relatively inexpensive form of protection in cool environments, but proper safety precautions must be taken. Space heaters often are used to provide intense heat in a small area, but they can create serious fire and safety hazards. In addition to environmental considerations, special attention must be directed toward ensuring adequate nutrition, including fluid intake, and toward the treatment of any pathologic conditions.

During heat waves, hyperthermia can affect older adults living in their own homes or in long-term care settings that are not air-conditioned. In long-term care facilities without air conditioning, nurses need to ensure that all residents have adequate fluid intakes. Nurses also must observe for early signs of hyperthermia, especially in residents who are immobile or who have medical problems, such as endocrine or circulatory disorders, that predispose to hyperthermia. If only parts of the facility are air-conditioned, nurses can encourage residents to spend time in those areas and can provide assistance for residents who have mobility limitations.

Nurses can teach older adults living in community settings about measures to cool the environment, such as those summarized in Box 25-3. Older adults may be reluctant to use fans or air conditioners because of a desire to save money on utility bills; however, if they understand the health risks associated with hyperthermia, they may use these appliances judiciously. If the home setting cannot be cooled adequately during heat waves, nurses can encourage older adults to spend time in air-conditioned public places. Additional self-care actions to prevent hyperthermia during heat waves include the provision of adequate fluids and the avoidance of heavy meals and strenuous exercise. Nurses can use Box 25-3, which summarizes interventions for the prevention of hyperthermia, as an educational tool for older adults.

Promoting Comfort

Nurses have many opportunities to improve the comfort of older adults who live in environments where they frequently feel cold. Interventions directed toward warming the hands, feet, and head are particularly effective because these areas

Box 25-3
Health Promotion Teaching About Hypothermia and Heat-Related Illness

Environmental and Personal Protection Considerations for Preventing Hypothermia

- Maintain a constant room temperature as close to 75°F (23.9°C) as possible, with a minimum temperature of 70°F (21.1°C).
- Use a reliable, clearly marked thermometer to measure room temperature.
- Wear close-knit, but not tight, undergarments to prevent heat loss; wear several layers of clothing.
- Wear a hat and gloves when outdoors; wear a nightcap and socks for sleeping.
- Wear extra clothing in the early morning when your body metabolism is at its lowest point.
- Use flannel bed sheets or sheet blankets.
- Use an electric blanket set on a low temperature.
- Take advantage of programs that offer assistance with utility bills and home weatherization.

Environmental and Personal Protection Action to Prevent Heat-Related Illnesses

- Maintain room temperatures at below 85°F (29.4°C).
- If your residence is not air-conditioned, use fans to circulate the air and cool the environment.
- During hot weather, spend time in public air-conditioned settings, such as libraries or shopping malls.
- Drink extra noncaffeinated, nonalcoholic liquids, even if you don't feel thirsty.
- Wear loose-fitting, lightweight, light-colored, cotton clothing.
- Wear a hat or use an umbrella to protect yourself against sun and heat when you are outside.
- Avoid outdoor activities during the hottest time of the day (i.e., between 10:00 A.M. and 2:00 P.M.); perform them during the cooler hours of the morning or evening.
- Place an ice pack or cold, wet towels on your body, especially on the head, the groin area, and armpits. Take cool (about 75°F [23.9°C]) baths or showers several times daily during heat waves, but do not use soap every time.

Health Promotion Actions for Maintaining Optimal Body Temperature

- Maintain adequate fluid intake by drinking 8 to 10 glasses of noncaffeinated, nonalcoholic liquid daily.
- Do not rely on your thirst sensation as an indicator of the need for fluid.
- Eat small, frequent meals rather than heavy meals.
- Avoid drinking caffeinated beverages, such as cola and coffee.
- Avoid drinking alcohol.
- In cold weather, engage in moderate physical exercise and indoor activities to increase circulation and heat production.

Nutritional Considerations

- Maintain good nutrition, especially zinc, selenium, and vitamins A, C, and E.

Preventive Measures and Additional Approaches

- Know your normal temperature in the morning and in the evening.
- Know the difference in your temperature in the winter and the summer.
- Obtain pneumonia and influenza immunizations (as discussed in Chapter 21).
- Obtain tetanus and diphtheria vaccinations every 10 years.
- Be aware that melatonin and other bioactive substances (see Box 25-1) might alter temperature regulation; use these substances only under the advice of a health care professional.

of the body have the heaviest concentration of nerve endings that are sensitive to heat loss. Nurses can encourage older adults to wear caps, thermal socks, and leg warmers. Additional measures to increase comfort are summarized in Box 25-3, along with nutritional considerations and other practices that also may improve quality of life by preventing infections.

Wellness Opportunity

Nurses can use comfort measures to diminish the sensation of being cold, even if the interventions have no effect on core body temperature.

Recall that Mrs. T. is 76 years old and a participant at the county senior center where you will be presenting a health education program.

THINKING POINTS

- How would you incorporate assessment information into your health education program?
- How would you use information from Box 25-3 to teach about preventing heat-related illnesses?
- What specific suggestions would you make about early detection of heat-related illnesses to the participants at this rural senior center?
- How would you find health education materials to use for your program?

EVALUATING EFFECTIVENESS OF NURSING INTERVENTIONS

Nurses evaluate care of older adults diagnosed with Risk for Hypothermia/Hyperthermia or Imbalanced Body Temperature according to the extent to which the risks are eliminated. It is not always possible to know whether risk factors were eliminated, but nurses can evaluate the effectiveness of their teaching by asking for feedback from older adults and their caregivers. Nurses also can suggest referrals for resources and ask the older adult about his or her intent to follow through. For example, if housing and financial factors increase the risk of hypothermia and heat-related illnesses, nurses can refer the older adult to a program such as LIHEAP and document the person's response to this information. When nurses teach about preventing hypothermia and heat-related illnesses, effectiveness is evaluated based on the person's ability to describe ways of decreasing the risk factors for hypothermia or heat-related illnesses.

Mrs. T. is now 87 years old and continues to live alone in her own home in a rural area of central Ohio. She has a history of hypertension and diabetic retinopathy, and was recently hospitalized for uncontrolled diabetes. Upon discharge from the hospital in November, she was referred to the Visiting Nurses Association for teaching about insulin administration and monitoring of her diabetic care.

NURSING ASSESSMENT

During your initial visit, you observe that Mrs. T.'s house is poorly maintained and has no insulation or other weatherization. Mrs. T. tells you that she has lived in this house for 60 years and that, in recent years, she has had difficulty keeping up with its maintenance because of her poor eyesight and limited income. She has few social contacts, but her daughter visits her every other week and a neighbor visits weekly and brings her groceries. About once a month, friends pick her up and take her to church. Your assessment reveals that although Mrs. T. has difficulty preparing meals because of her poor eyesight, she is independent in all other activities of daily living.

During your initial visit, you identify several risk factors for hypothermia, so during subsequent visits you follow up with further assessment. You learn that Mrs. T. was taken to the emergency department in January 2 years ago to be treated for hypothermia. She recalls that her daughter had come for her usual visit and had found her in a very weak and confused state. Her description of the situation is that "they just warmed me up at the hospital and sent me home again. I could have done that myself if my daughter would have just let me be." It is apparent that she did not consider her condition to be of particular concern. In the winter, she keeps her utility bills low by using a small, portable

(case study continues on page 539)

heater in the living room during the day and moving it into the bedroom at night. Mrs. T. keeps her thermostat at 65°F (18.3°C) during the day and 60°F (15.6°C) at night. A neighbor told her that the county office on aging had a program to assist with utility bills, but she is embarrassed to ask her daughter to drive her to the county office to apply for this "welfare help."

NURSING DIAGNOSIS

In addition to addressing the nursing diagnoses related to Mrs. T.'s diabetes, you identify a nursing diagnosis of Risk for Imbalanced Body Temperature, Hypothermia. Related factors include advanced age, diabetes, social isolation, poor housing conditions, low environmental temperatures, and a history of hypothermia.

NURSING CARE PLAN FOR MRS. T.

Expected Outcome	Nursing Interventions	Nursing Evaluation
Mrs. T.'s knowledge about risk factors for hypothermia will be increased.	• Discuss risk factors for hypothermia, with emphasis on Mrs. T.'s diabetes, social isolation, environmental conditions, and history of hypothermia.	• Mrs. T. will be able to state at least four factors that place her at risk for hypothermia.
Mrs. T.'s knowledge about ways of preventing hypothermia will be increased.	• Use Box 25-2 to discuss interventions to prevent hypothermia and to explore ways of applying these interventions to Mrs. T.'s situation.	• Mrs. T. will implement strategies aimed at reducing her risk for hypothermia.
The risk factor of low temperatures in Mrs. T.'s house will be eliminated.	• Inform Mrs. T. that she is eligible for the Low Income Home Energy Assistance Program (LIHEAP) and can qualify for assistance with utility bills as well as help with weatherization. • Emphasize that LIHEAP is an important health-related program aimed at preventing hypothermia in older adults. • Ask Mrs. T.'s permission to arrange for a home assessment by a LIHEAP staff person.	• Mrs. T. will accept assistance from the LIHEAP program. • Mrs. T. will have her house weatherized. • Mrs. T. will keep her thermostat at 70°F (21.1°C) during the winter.
The risk factor of social isolation will be eliminated.	• Suggest home-delivered meals to Mrs. T. as a means of providing prepared meals and daily contact. • Emphasize that one of the purposes of such programs is to ensure that socially isolated older adults have daily contact with someone who can monitor their well-being. • Ask Mrs. T. for permission to contact her daughter to suggest that she call her mother daily during cold spells to make sure she is okay.	• Mrs. T. will accept home-delivered meals. • Mrs. T.'s daughter will phone daily during cold spells.

THINKING POINTS

- How would you address Mrs. T.'s perception that hypothermia does not have serious health-related implications?
- What additional interventions might you consider to address Mrs. T.'s risk for hypothermia?

CHAPTER HIGHLIGHTS

Age-Related Changes That Affect Thermoregulation
- Inefficient vasoconstriction
- Decreased cardiac output
- Diminished subcutaneous tissue and muscle mass
- Decreased peripheral circulation
- Delayed and diminished shivering
- Diminished ability to acclimatize to heat

Risks Factors That Affect Thermoregulation (Box 25-1)
- Environmental factors (e.g., temperatures, humidity)
- Socioeconomic and housing factors (e.g., poor ventilation, inadequate heat, lack of air conditioning)
- Insufficient knowledge about altered thermoregulation
- Medications and alcohol
- Chronic and acute conditions (e.g., infections; cardiovascular, endocrine, and neurologic conditions)
- Inactivity
- Social isolation

Functional Consequences Affecting Thermoregulation
- Compromised ability to respond to hot or cold environments
- Increased susceptibility to hypothermia and hyperthermia
- Lower baseline temperature
- Diminished febrile response to infections
- Dulled perception of environmental temperatures

Nursing Assessment of Thermoregulation (Box 25-2)
- Establish baseline temperature, including diurnal variations
- Identify risks for hypothermia or hyperthermia
- Observe for additional manifestations of infections

Nursing Diagnosis
- Readiness for Enhanced Knowledge: Prevention of Hypothermia (or Hyperthermia)
- Risk for Hypothermia
- Risk for Hyperthermia
- Risk for Imbalanced Body Temperature

Planning for Wellness Outcomes
- Health Promoting Behaviors
- Knowledge: Personal Safety
- Risk Detection
- Risk Control
- Safe Home Environment
- Thermoregulation

Nursing Interventions to Promote Healthy Thermoregulation (Box 25-3)
- Maintaining healthy environmental conditions
- Teaching about measures to protect from hypothermia
- Teaching about measures to prevent hyperthermia
- Instituting comfort measures

Evaluating Effectiveness of Nursing Interventions
- Evidence that risk factors are eliminated
- Feedback about improved knowledge regarding prevention of hypothermia and hyperthermia
- Feedback about referrals for community resources

CRITICAL THINKING EXERCISES

1. Describe four major functional consequences that an older adult is likely to experience with regard to thermoregulation. How would you explain these changes to an older adult?
2. Explain how each of the following factors might affect an older person's thermoregulation: medications, pathologic conditions, environmental conditions, socioeconomic factors, and lack of knowledge.
3. What would you include in an assessment of thermoregulation in an older adult?
4. What would you teach older adults about hypothermia and its prevention?
5. What would you teach older adults about heat-related illnesses and their prevention?
6. Find appropriate health education materials on the Internet to use in teaching older adults about hypothermia and heat-related illnesses.

EDUCATIONAL RESOURCES

Health Canada, Canada Health Portal
http://chp-pcs.gc.ca

Low-Income Home Energy Assistance Program (LIHEAP)
www.liheap.ncat.org

National Energy Assistance Referral Hotline (NEAR)
1-866-674-6327

National Institute on Aging (NIA)
www.nihseniorhealth.gov

REFERENCES

Carpenito-Moyet, L. J. (2006). *Handbook of nursing diagnosis* (11th ed.). Philadelphia: Lippincott Williams & Wilkins.

Danzl, D. F. (2006). Accidental hypothermia. In J. A. Marx, R. Hockberger, & R. Walls (Eds.), *Rosen's emergency medicine* (6th ed., pp. 2236–2252). St. Louis: Mosby.

Fallico, F., Nolte, K., Siciliano, L., & Yip, F. (2005). Hypothermia-related deaths: United States, 2003–2004. *MMWR Weekly, 54*(7), 173–175.

Glazer, J. L. (2005). Management of heatstroke and heat exhaustion. *American Family Physician, 71*, 2133–2142.

Gomolin, I. H., Aung, M. M., Wolf-Klein, G., & Auerbach, C. (2005). Older is colder: Temperature range and variation in older people. *Journal of the American Geriatrics Society, 53*, 2170–2172.

McCullough, L., & Arora, S. (2004). Diagnosis and treatment of hypothermia. *American Family Physician, 70*, 2325–2332.

Murphy, T., Zumwalt, R., Fallico, F., Sanchez, C., Belson, M., Rubin, C., et al. (2006). Hypothermia-related deaths: United States, 1999–2002 and 2005. *MMWR Weekly, 55*(10), 282–284.

Vicario, S. (2006). Heat illness. In J. A. Marx, R. Hockberger, & R. Walls (Eds.), *Rosen's emergency medicine* (6th ed., pp. 2253–2269). St. Louis: Mosby.

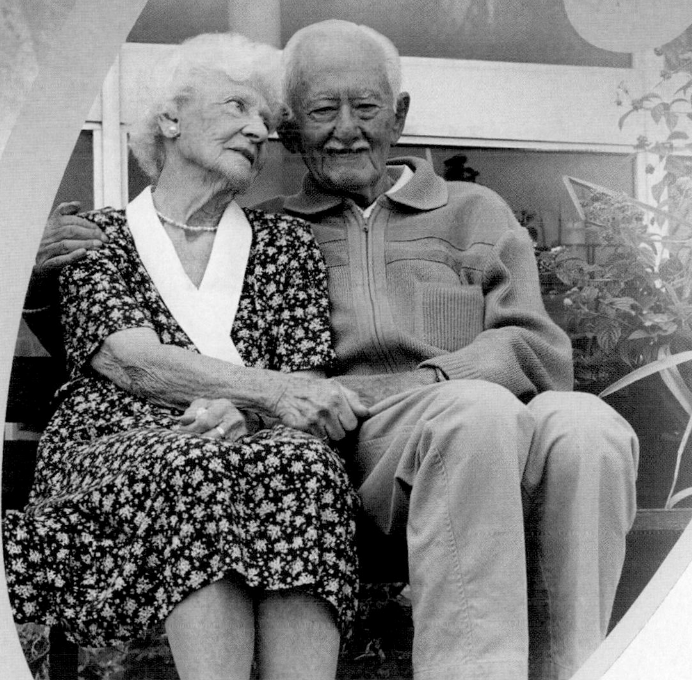

CHAPTER 26

Sexual Function

Learning Objectives

After reading this chapter, you will be able to:

1. Describe age-related changes that affect sexual function in older adults.
2. Discuss risk factors that influence older adults' interest in, opportunities for, and performance of sexual activities.
3. Discuss the functional consequences affecting sexual wellness in older adults.
4. Assess your own attitudes about sexual function in older adults.
5. Apply assessment guidelines in clinical settings when it is appropriate to address sexual wellness.
6. Teach older adults about interventions to promote sexual wellness.

Key Terms

andropause
erectile dysfunction
menopause
prostatic hyperplasia
urethritis
vaginitis

Because sexual function in older adults encompasses many physiologic and psychosocial aspects of sexuality and intimate relationships, this chapter's perspective is broad. Although sexual function is not a dominant focus of gerontological nursing care in most situations, it is a very important component of quality of life for many older adults. Thus, in situations in which quality of life is a focus of care (especially long-term care settings), nurses need to be prepared to assess sexual function and implement nursing interventions that promote sexual wellness.

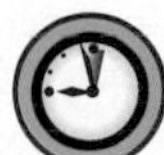

AGE-RELATED CHANGES THAT AFFECT SEXUAL FUNCTION

A loss of reproductive ability at the onset of menopause in women is the age-related change in sexual function that is most easily delineated. Erectile dysfunction in older men, often addressed as an age-related change, is more strongly associated with risk factors than with age-related changes and is discussed in the Risk Factors and Pathologic Conditions sections. Other, more subtle age-related changes in sexual function include diminished reproductive abilities in older men and alterations in both male and female responses to sexual stimulation. In the absence of risk factors, these changes have little impact because older adults generally do not desire high levels of reproductive ability and can readily compensate for any altered physiologic response to sexual stimulation. In the presence of risk factors, however, the sexual function of older adults may be severely compromised. This is because the risk factors, not the age-related changes, are the strongest determinants of sexual function in older adults.

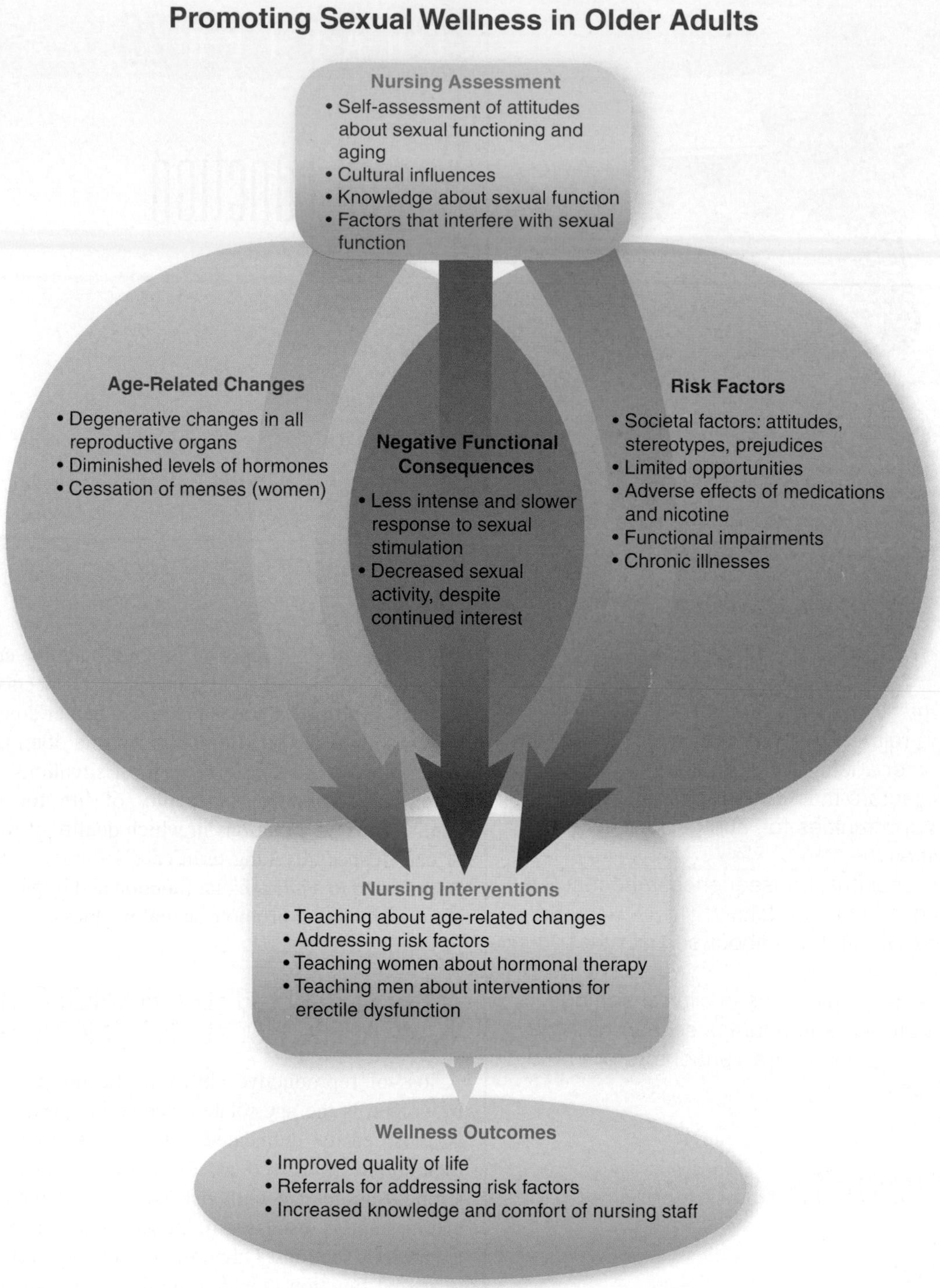

Promoting Sexual Wellness in Older Adults

Nursing Assessment
- Self-assessment of attitudes about sexual functioning and aging
- Cultural influences
- Knowledge about sexual function
- Factors that interfere with sexual function

Age-Related Changes
- Degenerative changes in all reproductive organs
- Diminished levels of hormones
- Cessation of menses (women)

Negative Functional Consequences
- Less intense and slower response to sexual stimulation
- Decreased sexual activity, despite continued interest

Risk Factors
- Societal factors: attitudes, stereotypes, prejudices
- Limited opportunities
- Adverse effects of medications and nicotine
- Functional impairments
- Chronic illnesses

Nursing Interventions
- Teaching about age-related changes
- Addressing risk factors
- Teaching women about hormonal therapy
- Teaching men about interventions for erectile dysfunction

Wellness Outcomes
- Improved quality of life
- Referrals for addressing risk factors
- Increased knowledge and comfort of nursing staff

Changes Affecting Older Women

Hormonally regulated cycles, called *menses*, control female reproductive abilities. With the onset of menses during adolescence, the cyclic release of ova marks the beginning of female reproductive abilities. Reproductive abilities decline around the fifth decade, when the frequency of ovulation diminishes and menstrual cycles become shorter and irregular. **Menopause** (the cessation of menses), which typically occurs around the age of 49 to 51 years, is a clear indicator that reproduction is no longer possible.

In addition to affecting reproductive ability, menopause influences other aspects of sexual function, predominantly because of the accompanying decline in endogenous estrogen levels. Production of estradiol by the ovaries is the primary source of estrogen before menopause, but after menopause the primary source is estrone, which is converted from androstenedione in skin and fat tissue. Endogenous estrogen levels decline in all postmenopausal women, but the extent and manifestations of estrogen deficiency vary. Factors that affect postmenopausal levels of endogenous estrogen include the interval since the onset of menopause; the production of hormones by the adrenal cortex; changes in the clearance rates of androgens and estrogens; and body weight, with higher body fat being positively correlated with higher levels of estrogen.

Diminished estrogen levels contribute to many age-related changes that indirectly or directly influence sexual function for older women. For example, breasts become more pendulous and have more fat and less mammary tissue. Effects of diminished estrogen on sexual organs include the following:

- The cervix, uterus, and fallopian tubes atrophy.
- The vaginal wall and mucosa become thinner.
- The vagina becomes shorter and narrower.
- Bartholin's glands atrophy and secrete less fluid.
- There is less vaginal lubrication during periods of sexual excitement.
- The labia lose their fullness.
- The amount of pubic hair diminishes.

Changes Affecting Older Men

Male reproductive function depends on the secretion of hormones, the production and release of sperm, and the motility of sperm through the urethra. Luteinizing and follicle-stimulating hormones are gonadotropins that regulate the production of testosterone and sperm. For many decades, researchers and gerontologists have debated the extent to which diminished testosterone in older men is due to age-related changes or risk factors. Recent research reviews conclude that when risk factors, such as medications and pathologic conditions, are controlled for, systemic testosterone levels decrease by 1% to 2% per year beginning around the age of 30 years (Liu et al., 2005). **Andropause** is a term that is used to describe the age-related decline in testosterone in men that is analogous to the age-related decline in estrogen in women (Anderson et al., 2002; Matsumoto, 2002). Even with the progressive decline, however, there is significant individual variation among older men, with many older men maintaining serum testosterone levels that are equal to or only slightly lower than those of healthy younger men (Orwoll et al., 2006; T'Sjoen & Kaufman, 2006). Researchers currently are addressing questions about any cause–effect relationship between age-related androgen deficiency and male sexual function (Liu et al., 2005).

The testes, paired oval-shaped organs in the scrotal sac, contain hundreds of seminiferous tubules that produce sperm and secrete testosterone. The seminiferous tubules undergo the following age-related changes:

- Increased fibrosis
- Thinning of the epithelium
- Thickening of the basement membrane
- Narrowing of the lumen, eventually to the point of obliteration of some of the tubules
- Diminished production of viable sperm

Despite these degenerative changes, however, some men never lose their reproductive abilities.

The seminal vesicles, prostate gland, and Cowper's (or bulbourethral) glands are accessory structures that produce semen, a mixture of sperm cells and secretions whose primary function is to nourish and transport sperm and facilitate reproductive functions. The following degenerative changes affect the seminal vesicles and prostate gland:

- The mucosa becomes smoother.
- The epithelium becomes thinner.
- Connective tissue replaces the muscle tissue.
- The fluid-retaining capacity is reduced.
- Secretions diminish.
- Gland cells atrophy.
- Firm masses form around the prostatic urethra.

Age-related changes in the Cowper's glands have not been documented.

Beginning around the fourth decade, the penis undergoes age-related changes. These degenerative changes do not affect reproduction, but they can affect sexual pleasure and contribute to erectile dysfunction (discussed in the section on Functional Consequences). The primary age-related penile changes are venous and arterial sclerosis and fibroelastosis of the corpus spongiosum. The weight and volume of the testes may decrease, but this is associated with pathologic conditions rather than age-related changes.

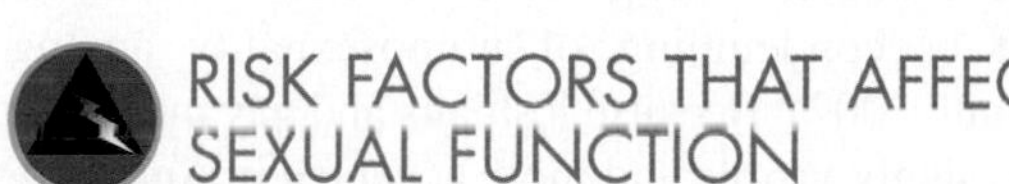

RISK FACTORS THAT AFFECT SEXUAL FUNCTION

Societal Influences

Societal influences can, in part, shape personal attitudes about sexuality and can affect a person's sexual behaviors and enjoyment of sexual activity. Thus, it is important to consider the societal context of attitudes about aging and sexuality. As long ago as the Middle Ages, Western cultural beliefs "have held that sexual drive disappears with old age, that sex is perverse in old age, and that those elderly who attempt it practice self-deception. In addition, traditional concepts related to sexuality, such as beauty, attractiveness, sexual potency, and female orgasm, did not refer to elderly people, but excluded them" (Covey, 1989, p. 93). In the early 20th century, strict Victorian standards of morality in Europe and North America strongly influenced the attitudes and behaviors of people who currently are older adults. According to Victorian standards, masturbation, homosexual activity, public displays of affection, and sex with anyone except a marital partner were totally taboo. Moreover, masturbation was considered to be more detrimental than sex outside of marriage, as evidenced by the Victorian norm of tolerating prostitution for the purpose of obviating the need for men to practice masturbation (Brecher, 1984).

Currently, people in Western societies associate sexual attractiveness with physical attractiveness in very gender-specific and stereotypical ways. For example, male sexuality is associated with the image of a tanned, muscular, and youthful man, and female sexuality is associated with the image of a thin, but adequately endowed, young woman. Because these images contrast sharply with typical portrayals of older adults as physically unattractive, they foster a stereotype of "sexless seniors."

These societal influences create a risk for the false perception that older adults are no longer interested in, or capable of engaging in, sexual activity. This can become a self-fulfilling prophecy if older adults believe this stereotype. If older adults do not believe these stereotypes and societal perceptions, they may be embarrassed to acknowledge their sexual desires and activities for fear of being ridiculed or considered abnormal.

Wellness Opportunity

Nurses need to avoid reinforcing, or even buying into, the pervasive societal attitudes about "sexless seniors."

Prejudiced societal attitudes have additional significant influences on lesbians' and gay men's sexual activity and relationships and can seriously interfere with their freedom to cultivate and express satisfying sexual relationships. This may be particularly problematic for lesbians and gay men who live in institutional settings because staff are likely to be intolerant or condemning of homosexuality among residents (Cahill, 2002). Because lesbians and gay men have become increasingly visible and more accepted in American society only recently, older adults who have experienced decades of feeling stigmatized may find it particularly difficult to meet partners and enjoy satisfying sexual activities and relationships. Despite their experience of long-term prejudice, however, older lesbians and gay men report levels of emotional well-being similar to those of older heterosexual people. Similarly, the social support they receive is comparable to that of heterosexual people, but the sources of support differ in that older lesbians and gay men are likely to receive assistance from friends, selected relatives, and current or former lovers (Cooney & Dunne, 2001).

Wellness Opportunity

Nurses holistically address sexual wellness by being nonjudgmental about choices of close personal relationships.

Attitudes and Behaviors of Families and Caregivers

In addition to societal influences, the attitudes and behaviors of family members and caregivers who are closest to the older adult can negatively affect the older adult's sexual function. Adult children of older people often find it difficult to deal with the sexuality of their parents because they are influenced by the common stereotype that older adults are asexual. In addition, children of older adults who are widowed may discourage their parent from having intimate relationships because they fear that a serious relationship could jeopardize their inheritance (Cooney & Dunne, 2001).

In institutional settings, attitudes of staff can significantly affect the way in which residents express or repress their sexual needs. Researchers have consistently found that nursing home staff hold negative or patronizing attitudes about sexual expression among older adults and that these attitudes are based largely on insufficient knowledge about sexuality and aging (Walker & Harrington, 2002). Staff in long-term care facilities are gradually developing more accepting and permissive attitudes; however, they tend to ignore the sexual needs of older adults. When staff does acknowledge sexual needs, it is usually because they find a resident engaging in sexual activity that they judge as inappropriate.

Typically, the only expression of sexual needs by residents of long-term facilities that is considered appropriate and socially acceptable is a private, medically approved visit by a spouse. Sexual activities in which a solitary resident or two unmarried people engage usually are not tolerated, even when done in private. Nonheterosexual relationships are often stigmatized if they are acknowledged at all (Ward et al., 2005). When the staff become aware of sexual activities that they consider inappropriate, they often ask family members to intervene, even when the resident is competent. Decisions regarding sexual activity, even between spouses, usually are treated as medical matters. In addition to the prerequisite of medical approval for sexual activity, staff in long-term care facilities may seek the permission of family members before allowing residents to enjoy sexual activity.

When older adults have dementia, issues related to sexual expression are compounded by questions about competency and the meaning of behaviors. Spouses often are overwhelmed with concerns about caregiving issues that take precedence over sexual relationships and expressions and other quality-of-life concerns. Families often question the ability of the person with dementia to make decisions about intimate relationships and sexual expressions, and this is particularly problematic with regard to nonmarital relationships. In institutional settings, staff are likely to view sexual expressions as disruption to routines, and they rarely consider that it could be beneficial or positive for the resident (Ward et al., 2005).

Limited Opportunities for Sexual Activity

Researchers have tried to identify factors that affect the level of sexual activity of older adults and have identified relative influences that differ for men and women. For older men, a decline in sexual activity is usually related to health problems and factors that contribute to erectile dysfunction such as medications and medical conditions (Avis, 2000; Beutel, 2002). For older women, however, health is less important; the most important variable is having a functioning and sexually interested partner (Avis, 2000; Weismiller, 2002). A study of married men between the ages of 50 and 80 years found that declines in sexual activity were most closely related to the wife's desire for intercourse and the man's ability to maintain an erection (Mazur, 2002).

The availability of an acceptable and desirable partner is a factor that can influence opportunities for sexual activity at any age, and especially in older adulthood. For older adults, particularly older women, social circumstances often are the strongest determinants of sexual activity because level of sexual activity for older women is directly related to their marital status, whereas the level of sexual activity for older men is not as closely associated with marital status. Men at all ages report a higher frequency of extramarital sexual relationships, and older widowers have the advantage of a higher likelihood of remarriage compared with older widows. Statistics on the ratio of women to men provide one logical explanation for the gender differences in availability of sexual partners. With increasing age, the ratio of men to women gradually changes, from a ratio of 86 men per 100 women between ages 65 and 69 years to a ratio of 41 men per 100 women in the age group of 85 years and older (He et al., 2005). The frequency and enjoyment of sexual activities during older adulthood is strongly associated with the importance assigned to sexual activity in the past. As a group, never-married women have the lowest rate of sexual activity compared with other categories of older adults. Although women of all ages are less sexually active than men in their cohort, the difference in their levels of sexual activity widens with increasing age.

In addition, lack of privacy can limit the older adult's opportunities for sexual activity. Privacy is generally considered a requisite for sexual activity, and adults who live in their own homes are usually able to arrange for this. However, older adults who live in institutions, group settings, or family homes may find it difficult or impossible to arrange for privacy, especially if their sexual needs are ignored or considered abnormal or even morally deviant. Even if some privacy is possible in institutional settings, additional environmental constraints include the inability to lock doors and ensure total privacy and the unavailability of anything larger than a single bed.

Wellness Opportunity

Nurses in long-term care settings need to create opportunities for privacy if a resident desires this.

Adverse Effects of Medication, Alcohol, and Nicotine

The role of medication as a cause of sexual dysfunction was first brought to the public's attention more than 2 decades ago in a *New York Times* article that cited medications as the single largest cause of erectile dysfunction in men and listed more than 50 medications with potentially adverse sexual effects (Brody, 1983). Brody cited a study published in the *Journal of the American Medical Association* (Slag et al., 1983) of 1180 male patients in a medical clinic. Thirty-four percent of these subjects were impotent, and 25% of the 188 subjects who subsequently underwent further evaluation were found to have medication-induced erectile dysfunction.

Recently, medication effects that adversely affect sexual function have been viewed increasingly as quality-of-life concerns. Most studies have focused on men, but the lack of attention to medication-induced sexual dysfunction in women and older adults is not because there are no problems in these groups. Rather, younger men are usually selected for studies because of cultural biases and the relative ease with which male sexual response is measured. Although researchers are only beginning to address this issue, it is likely that adverse medication effects can interfere with sexual function of women just as they do in men. For example, sexual dysfunction is a common adverse effect of antidepressants in older women, especially in combination with other risk factors such as concomitant medications (Basson, 2005).

Medications adversely affect sexual function through a variety of mechanisms, including their influence on the release of hormones and their actions on the autonomic and central nervous systems. For example, with the exception of trazodone and bupropion, all antidepressants are likely to cause erectile dysfunction (Thomas et al., 2003). Specific adverse medication effects that interfere with sexual function in men include a decreased or absent libido; difficulty obtaining or maintaining an erection; dry, premature, or retrograde ejaculation; and inability to achieve orgasm. A less common adverse medication effect is priapism, an erection that persists beyond or is unrelated to sexual stimulation, which can lead to permanent erectile dysfunction (Berger, 2001). Medications that can cause this condition include antipsychotics (e.g., quetiapine), antidepressants (e.g., trazodone), anticoagulants, antihypertensives, and medications used for the treatment of erectile dysfunction (Davol & Rukstalis, 2005; Thomas et al., 2003). Women may experience the following medication-induced limitations in sexual function: diminished vaginal lubrication, decreased or absent libido, and inability to achieve orgasm. Box 26-1 lists

Box 26-1
Medications That Can Interfere With Sexual Function

Antihypertensives and Cardiovascular Agents

Alpha-adrenergic blockers
Beta-blockers
Calcium channel blockers
Digoxin
Hydralazine
Spironolactone
Thiazide diuretics
Cyclic antidepressants
Lithium
Monoamine oxidase inhibitors (MAOIs)
Selective serotonin reuptake inhibitors (SSRIs)

Agents That Act on the Central Nervous System

Benzodiazepines
Phenothiazines
Antihistamines
Chlorpheniramine
Diphenhydramine

Antiparkinson Agents

Benztropine
Trihexyphenidyl

Gastrointestinal Agents

Anticholinergics
Histamine H_2 antagonists (e.g., cimetidine)

Miscellaneous Medications

Alcohol
Allopurinol
Colchicine
Cytotoxic agents

some of the medications that are commonly associated with sexual dysfunction. These effects usually disappear when the medication is discontinued; occasionally, the effects will disappear with a mere decrease in the dose.

Because alcohol is a central nervous system depressant, it can interfere with sexual function. In men, chronic alcohol use affects testosterone and gonadotropin production and can cause impotence and reduced libido (Nudell et al., 2002). Although in social settings alcohol can decrease inhibitions and heighten sensual and sexual interest, in excessive amounts, the central nervous system depressant effect of alcohol usually counteracts any beneficial effects and interferes with sexual performance. Moderate amounts of alcohol normally do not interfere with sexual performance; however, in combination with other risk factors, such as medications or pathologic conditions, even small amounts of alcohol may be detrimental to the sexual performance of older adults.

Cigarette smoking was first identified as a cause of erectile dysfunction in the mid-1980s. In recent years, studies have confirmed this association, with some finding a dose-dependent relationship between number of cigarettes and erectile dysfunction (Austoni et al., 2005; Corona et al., 2005; Gades et al., 2005; Millett et al., 2006; Shiri et al., 2005). Nicotine interferes with circulation to the sexual organs and accentuates the effects of other risk factors, such as hypertension and vascular disease.

Chronic Conditions and Functional Impairments

Chronic conditions and functional impairments can interfere with enjoyment of sexual activity in many ways, as in the following examples:

- Chronic obstructive pulmonary disease may cause hypoxia and severe shortness of breath in response to the high physiologic demands of sexual activity.
- Arthritis and other musculoskeletal disorders are likely to be associated with pain, stiffness, muscle spasms, and limited flexibility.
- Urinary incontinence can interfere with satisfying sexual relationships in people of any age, but this condition is more common in older adults.

In addition, diabetes mellitus and cardiovascular disease are two of the most common risk factors causing sexual dysfunction in both men and women (Ginsberg, 2006).

In people with diabetes, prevalence of sexual dysfunction ranges from 35% to 75%, with increased rates strongly associated with older age, longer duration of diabetes, and the presence of concurrent conditions such as heart disease or hypertension (Buvat & Lemaire, 2001; Sasaki et al., 2003). Men with diabetes are likely to experience retrograde ejaculation, whereas women experience delayed and diminished vaginal lubrication.

Cardiovascular disease is associated with many aspects of sexual dysfunction, including decreased libido, impaired performance and pleasure, and decreased frequency of sexual activities. For example, people who have had myocardial infarctions may avoid sexual activities, even when no physiologic basis exists for abstaining from sexual intercourse with a regular partner. Studies indicate that sexual activity with a marital partner can be resumed when the affected person can perform moderate exercise—such as climbing two flights of steps—without experiencing harmful cardiac effects (Steinke, 2005). Thus, a major barrier to sexual function after a heart attack is the influence of psychological factors, such as fatigue, depression, partner's decision, lack of information, fears and anxiety, and diminished sexual desire.

Although they are not unique to older adults, functional limitations increase with advancing age and are likely to combine with other risk factors to interfere with sexual function. In addition to direct effects, disabilities can indirectly affect sexual function because of the common misperception equating disability with lack of sexual function. This cultural bias, along with other effects of disabilities on self-image, can have a negative impact on sexual function. This may be more problematic for men because society tends to associate male sexual performance with physical vigor.

Sensory impairments can also interfere with sexual function because sensory stimulation is an important part of sexual pleasure and intimate communication. For example, an older adult with impaired hearing may find it difficult or impossible to carry on the intimate conversations that are often a part of sexual interactions. Similarly, hearing impairments can interfere with professional efforts to assess and counsel older adults on this sensitive topic. Likewise, impairments affecting vision, smell, or touch can interfere with some of the usual sensual stimulation associated with sexual activities.

In recent years, gerontologists and clinicians have focused attention on sexual function and intimate relationships in people with dementia. Although the majority of people with dementia are indifferent about sex by the later stages of the disease, issues related to sexual function and intimate relationships often arise during early and middle stages (Kuhn, 2002; Mace & Rabins, 2006). Loss of sexual desire is the most common effect of dementia on sexual function; however, some people with dementia experience hypersexuality and demand frequent sexual intercourse, especially men and especially during the middle stages. Hypersexuality in people with dementia may be caused by neuropathologic changes, particularly those that affect the temporal and frontal lobes of the brain (Robinson, 2003). Between 7% and 17% of nursing home residents with dementia exhibit behaviors that are considered sexually inappropriate; however, some of these behaviors, such as removing clothing or getting into bed with someone, are caused by cognitive impairments rather than sexual impulses (Velez & Peggs, 2001).

PATHOLOGIC CONDITIONS AFFECTING SEXUAL WELLNESS

Gender-Specific Conditions

Prostatic hyperplasia, or enlargement of the prostate, is a pathologic condition that affects 50% of 50-year-old men and 90% of 90-year-old men and that is caused, at least in part, by age-related hormonal changes. This condition is a common cause of urinary incontinence, which can interfere with enjoyment of sexual activities. Another condition that commonly affects older men is diminished frequency and rigidity of nocturnal penile tumescence, which is a reflex erection that occurs during sleep.

A condition that commonly affects sexual function in older women is increased susceptibility to **urethritis** and **vaginitis** because of the thinning of the vaginal tissue and the decreased acidity and quantity of vaginal secretions. These conditions can occur after intercourse and cause urinary urgency and burning that persists for several days. Fibroid cysts also are more likely to develop in older women than in younger women.

Sexual Dysfunction

Since the 1990s, knowledge about erectile dysfunction has been growing at a rapid pace, and much of the information that was thought to be accurate has been disproved. For example, erectile dysfunction is no longer viewed as an inevitable consequence of aging, and physiologic, rather than psychological, factors are recognized as the most common cause. In the early 1990s, the National Institutes of Health proposed that the term *impotence* be replaced by ***erectile dysfunction***, defined as the inability to achieve or maintain an erection sufficient for satisfactory sexual function (National Institutes of Health, 1993). About half of men older than 40 years of age have some degree of erectile dysfunction, and the incidence rate doubles during each decade after 40 (Grover et al., 2006; Johannes et al., 2000). Erectile dysfunction is strongly associated with increasing age, but it is caused by risk factors that occur more commonly in older men rather than by age-related changes alone (Rosen et al., 2005). It is currently viewed as a complex disease associated with several interacting factors, the most common physiologic causes being adverse medication effects and pathologic conditions, as discussed in the section on Risk Factors. Much progress has been made in understanding and addressing erectile dysfunction, but researchers estimate that more than 70% of men with erectile dysfunction are not diagnosed because of reluctance to discuss it with health care professionals (Chun & Carson, 2001). The trend in promoting medications for treatment of erectile dysfunction is likely to prompt more men and health care practitioners to discuss this topic and identify causes and treatments.

Diversity Note

One study found that Hispanic men had a disproportionately high risk for erectile dysfunction (Saigal et al., 2006)

In recent years, health care practitioners and pharmaceutical companies have started addressing female sexual dysfunction, similar to the way in which erectile dysfunction has been addressed since the early 1990s. Female sexual dysfunction causes significant personal distress and negatively affects interpersonal relationships and quality of life (Munarriz et al., 2002). Any of the four phases of sexual function—libido, arousal, orgasm, and satisfaction—can be affected. A current view is that three factors interact to contribute to female sexual dysfunction (Basson, 2005):

- Past psychosexual development
- Current life context
- Medical factors, including illness, medications, and previous surgery

Many of the same physiologic risk factors associated with erectile dysfunction also are associated with female sexual dysfunction: hypertension, hypercholesterolemia, cigarette smoking, pelvic surgeries, and adverse medication effects. In addition, diminished estrogen levels in menopausal women who are not taking hormonal therapy are a major contributing factor. Urinary incontinence, disorders of the pelvic floor (cystocele, vaginal prolapse), and any type of pelvic surgery (e.g., hysterectomy or procedures for urinary incontinence) increase the risk for female sexual dysfunction (Pauls & Berman, 2002). Depression and a history of sexual trauma are two psychological factors that may cause female sexual dysfunction (Kaplan, 2002).

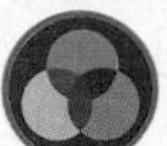

FUNCTIONAL CONSEQUENCES AFFECTING SEXUAL WELLNESS

Sexual function involves reproduction, response to sexual stimulation, and interest and participation in sexual activity. Whereas reproduction is directly affected by age-related changes, the other two aspects of sexual function are affected more directly by risk factors. In addition, andropause and menopause are considered in the context of functional consequences associated with sexual function in older adults.

Reproductive Ability

For women, loss of reproductive ability is a functional consequence of menopause, caused by the cessation of ova production within 1 year of the last menstrual cycle. Another functional consequence affecting reproduction in women is the increased risk that a fetus will be defective if ova are fertilized during the premenopausal years. The reproductive ability of men, by contrast, gradually declines with age but does not cease completely.

Response to Sexual Stimulation

The Masters and Johnson (1966) investigation is recognized as the landmark study of human physiologic response to sexual stimulation. This study of 694 adults in a laboratory setting identified four phases of physiologic response to sexual stimulation in men and women. An analysis of data on older subjects led to the following conclusions:

- Older adults maintain their ability to respond to sexual stimulation, but their response is slower and less intense.
- Regularly engaging in sexual activity helps older adults respond to sexual stimulation.
- Any major changes in response to sexual stimulation are associated with risk factors rather than aging, per se.

Although older adults were greatly underrepresented in this study, the findings of Masters and Johnson have been widely accepted as the knowledge base about age-related changes in physiologic response to sexual stimulation. Normal age-related changes in male and female responses to sexual stimulation and the associated consequences are discussed in the following sections and summarized in Table 26-1.

Female Response

During the initial excitement phase of sexual stimulation, the following physiologic changes occur in women: the breasts enlarge and the nipples become erect; the skin over the upper

TABLE 26-1 Functional Consequences for Response to Sexual Stimulation

	Changes in Female Response	Changes in Male Response
Excitement Phase	Breasts not as fully engorged Sexual flush absent or diminished Delayed or diminished vaginal lubrication Decreased expansion of vaginal wall Decreased vasocongestion of labia	Longer time required to attain erection Less firm erection Longer maintenance of erection before ejaculation Increased difficulty regaining an erection if lost Reduced or absent scrotal and testicular vasocongestion
Plateau Phase	Decreased areolar engorgement Less intense sexual flush Less intense myotonia Decreased degree of deepening of labial color Decreased vasocongestion of labia Reduced Bartholin's gland secretions Slower/less marked uterine elevation	Diminished or absent nipple turgidity and sexual flush Less intense muscle tension Slower penile erectile response No color change in glans penis Delayed and diminished testicular elevation
Orgasmic Phase	Decreased frequency of rectal sphincter contractions Decreased number and intensity of orgasmic contractions	Decreased frequency of rectal sphincter contractions Diminution of ejaculatory expulsion force by about 50% Absent or diminished sense of ejaculatory inevitability Fewer and less intense ejaculatory contractions
Resolution Phase	Slower loss of nipple erection Quicker return to pre-excitement stage	Slower loss of nipple erection Longer refractory period Very rapid penile detumescence Very rapid testicular descent

chest becomes flushed; voluntary muscles become tense; the heart rate and blood pressure increase; the labia and clitoris enlarge and become vasocongested; the vaginal barrel expands, distends, and becomes lubricated and vasocongested; and the uterus elevates slightly. During the plateau phase, the following responses normally occur: the breasts enlarge to a greater degree and the areola become engorged; the sexual flush spreads over the body and becomes more intense; the voluntary muscles become more tense; the rectal sphincter is voluntarily contracted; the blood pressure, heart rate, and respiratory rate increase; the clitoral shaft and glans withdraw; the vaginal barrel increases further in width and depth; the uterus elevates fully and the cervix elevates; the labia become more vasocongested; and Bartholin's glands secrete mucoid material. Older women experience these same responses, but with less intensity (see Table 26-1).

The orgasmic phase of female sexual response is characterized by the following: sexual flush increases in intensity, parallel to the intensity of orgasm; muscle groups contract involuntarily; the rectal sphincter contracts involuntarily; pulse, blood pressure, and respirations increase further; the orgasmic platform contracts at intervals, with gradual lengthening of the intervals and weakening of the contractions; and the uterus contracts with an intensity parallel to that of the orgasm. As with other phases of sexual excitement, all the responses of the orgasmic phase are less intense in older women. In addition, the involuntary rectal sphincter contractions occur only with high tension levels, and the number of orgasmic contractions decreases by about 50%. Because postmenopausal women are no longer concerned about the reproductive consequences, however, their capacity for orgasm may actually be increased. Some women experience orgasm or multiple orgasms for the first time during their postmenopausal years.

The resolution phase involves a gradual return to the pre-excitement state, beginning with a loss of deep vasocongestion. The breasts return to their normal appearance, the sexual flush disappears, muscle tone returns to a normal state within 5 minutes, vital signs return to normal, and all pelvic organs resume their pre-excitement characteristics. With the exception of a slower loss of nipple erection, the resolution phase occurs more rapidly in older women.

Male Response

During the excitement phase of sexual stimulation, men experience the following physiologic changes: nipples may become erect; voluntary muscles become more tense; heart rate and blood pressure increase; the penis becomes erect; the scrotal sac flattens and elevates; and the testes become partially elevated. The most noticeable change in this phase is the need for longer or more intense stimulation before attaining an erection. In addition, the erection may be less firm, but it can be maintained longer before ejaculation. If the erection subsides before ejaculation, however, a refractory period occurs and older men may have greater difficulty than younger men regaining a full erection. Scrotal and testicular vasocongestion is markedly reduced in older men, as is testicular elevation. In general, all responses of the excitement phase are less intense and are influenced more by arousal conditions than by autonomic nervous system responses.

During the plateau phase, men experience the following: the nipples become erect and turgid; the skin over the head and trunk becomes flushed; voluntary and involuntary muscle tone increases; the rectal sphincter is voluntarily contracted; the pulse, respirations, and blood pressure are increased; penile circumference increases at the coronal ridge; the testes elevate and enlarge by 50%; and Cowper's glands emit pre-ejaculatory fluid. During this phase, older men are likely to experience reduced or absent sexual flush, nipple erection, and muscle tension. Full penile erection often occurs later in this stage, just before ejaculation, and testicular elevation is delayed or diminished because of less intense vasocongestion.

The orgasmic phase is characterized by the following changes: the skin flush is well developed and parallels the intensity of excitement; there is a loss of voluntary control of muscles, and the rectal sphincter and some muscle groups involuntarily contract; heart rate, blood pressure, and respirations increase above normal; the penis contracts at intervals and with an expulsive force; and a sensation of ejaculatory inevitability is experienced and the ejaculatory process is initiated. Older men typically experience the following changes in the orgasmic phase: ejaculation is less powerful; seminal fluid emerges under less pressure; penile contractions are fewer and less intense; rectal sphincter contractions occur less frequently; and intercontractile intervals lengthen rapidly after the second expulsive contraction. Older men also reported a decreased sense of ejaculatory inevitability.

During the resolution phase, the manifestations of sexual excitement gradually disappear, and all physiologic responses return to the pre-excitement state. A refractory period occurs, during which the man is unable to redevelop an erection that is accompanied by ejaculation. The refractory period in older men may last for a day or two, but they may be able to achieve erection without ejaculation during this time. With the exception of a slower loss of nipple erection, all other responses to sexual stimulation return to their pre-excitement state more rapidly in older men.

Sexual Interest and Activity

During the 1940s and 50s, the Kinsey surveys first brought information about sexual behaviors of older adults to public attention. Since then, other reports have confirmed that the frequency of sexual activity gradually declines with increasing age; however, sexual interest and competence of older adults do not necessarily decline. Sexual interest, attitudes, activity, and satisfaction are a continuation of lifelong patterns, and they remain stable in older adulthood unless risk factors interfere with sexual function. Factors that most commonly affect sexual interest and activity in older adults include social circumstances, pathologic conditions, adverse medication effects, and influences of family and caregivers.

The social circumstances that most frequently lead to decreased sexual activity are spousal death or illness and lack of an available partner. The sexual needs and interest of older adults, including residents of long-term care facilities, do not necessarily decrease, but their opportunities for sexual activity are often limited.

In recent decades, studies of sexuality and aging have focused on broader aspects, such as affection, friendships, and intimacy. For older adults, these aspects of sexual function may become more important as the number of acceptable opportunities for sexual activities diminishes. For example, in one of the first studies addressing sexual behaviors other than intercourse and masturbation, Bretschneider and McCoy (1988) found that the most common sexual activities in a sample of 202 adults aged 80 to 102 years were touching and caressing without sexual intercourse. Similarly, Johnson (1996) found that older adults (mean age 66 years) reported that the sexual activities of kissing, hugging, and hearing loving words were more important than masturbation, oral sex, or sexual conversation. In this study, older women ascribed greater importance to sexual activities of sitting and talking, making oneself more attractive, and saying loving words than did men. By contrast, older men reported greater interest in sexual activities, such as erotic movies and readings, sexual daydreams, and physically intimate activities. Studies of nursing home residents suggest that it would be more appropriate to view intimacy and sexual function as a continuum, ranging from social intimacy to sexual–physical intimacy (Lichtenberg, 1997).

In summary, older adults do not lose their interest in or capacity for sexual activity because of age-related changes, but risk factors such as misinformation, social circumstances, pathologic conditions, environmental constraints, and adverse medication effects do commonly interfere with sexual function. A normal consequence of aging, however, is that the response of older men and women to sexual stimulation is slower, less intense, and of shorter duration. As one 79-year-old man confided to this author, "It's like sparklers, not fireworks."

Wellness Opportunity

Nurses need to recognize that many interacting physical and psychosocial factors affect sexual wellness in a unique way for each older adult.

Menopause and Andropause

In addition to the consequences of changes in reproduction, sexual response, and sexual interest, older adults may experience consequences in sexual function and quality of life related to the hormonal changes associated with menopause and andropause. Diminished estrogen levels that occur during menopause affect sexual function and many other aspects of functioning. One of the most noticeable effects of estrogen deficiency in menopausal women is the occurrence of hot flashes, described as "the sudden, transient sensation of heat spreading over the upper body, usually starting in the neck and face, then extending to the chest, back, and arms, the hot flash may also bring on flushing and sweating, and then a sensation of chilling" (Taylor, 2002, p. 559). Hot flashes are commonly accompanied by nausea, anxiety, palpitation, air hunger, and head stuffiness or fullness. Additional functional consequences include embarrassment, discomfort, and interruptions in activities, including sexual activities. Hot flashes affect up to 85% of all menopausal women, with as much as 57% reporting persistent but less severe hot flashes for 10 years after their last menstrual period (Taylor, 2002). Factors that increase the intensity and frequency of hot flashes during menopause include obesity and cigarette smoking (Whiteman et al., 2003). For some women, hot flashes may occur frequently throughout the day and night and last for as long as half an hour. About 25% of women characterize their hot flashes and sweats as severe and disruptive of their quality of life (Taylor, 2002). Another effect of diminished estrogen is significantly diminished vaginal secretions, which can affect sexual intercourse unless compensatory interventions, such as a lubricant, are used.

Manifestations of andropause that affect sexual function and quality of life include fatigue, depression, and diminished sexual desire and erectile capacity (Haren et al., 2006; Matsumoto, 2002). Researchers currently are investigating the use of testosterone therapy, as discussed in the section on Interventions.

You are the "wellness nurse" at the senior center where Mr. and Mrs. S. come for the meal program and social interaction. Mr. S. is 73 years old and has hypertension and a history of a heart attack. He takes atenolol, 100 mg daily; hydrochlorothiazide, 25 mg daily; and digoxin, 0.125 mg daily. Mrs. S., who is 71 years old, describes herself as generally healthy, but with a history of depression and some arthritis. She takes ibuprofen, 400 mg four times daily, and sertraline, 50 mg daily. During your nursing clinics, Mr. S. and several other men have asked you about the drug that is advertised on television for men who have trouble satisfying their partners. The senior center director also has noticed an increased interest in this topic and has asked that you plan a group health information session about "Sexuality and Aging."

THINKING POINTS

- Develop a plan for teaching older adults about the normal changes in sexual function that they are likely to experience.
- What risk factors would you discuss in relation to sexuality and aging?
- What educational materials would you use?
- What teaching would you do about interventions?

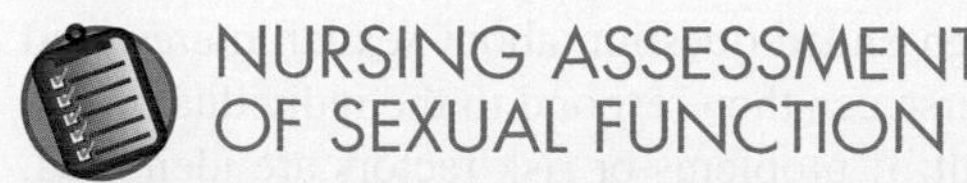

NURSING ASSESSMENT OF SEXUAL FUNCTION

Nurses do not necessarily include sexual function in every assessment, but they should assess it whenever they are addressing quality of life issues that affect day-to-day function. Thus, assessment of sexual function is especially important in home care and long-term care settings (e.g., nursing facilities, group homes, and assisted living facilities). Sexual function is often neglected in nursing assessments because of the high degree of privacy associated with sexual function and the stereotype of the "sexless senior" that is prevalent in our society. In addition, gender or generational differences between the health professional and the older person may interfere with an assessment of sexual function. Although all of these factors may explain why sexual function in older adults is so often overlooked, they do not justify its exclusion.

Self-Assessment of Attitudes About Sexual Function and Aging

Because of the private nature of sexual function and its associated emotional responses and cultural factors, nurses are often uncomfortable discussing it. Additional discomfort occurs because nurses are not confident in dealing with concerns about human sexuality in nursing practice (Reynolds & Magnan, 2005). Thus, an assessment of personal attitudes about sexuality and aging is a prerequisite to addressing sexual wellness. Box 26-2 lists some of the questions nurses can use to examine their attitudes toward the sexual function of older adults. Some questions are specific to long-term care facilities because of the dominant role of nurses in addressing sexual function as a quality-of-life issue for residents. Kuhn (2002) developed a self-assessment tool, called the Staff Attitudes about Intimacy and Dementia (SAID), that can be used by staff in long-term care facilities to identify personal attitudes about aging, intimacy, sexuality, and dementia.

Wellness Opportunity

Nurses should take time for self-assessment to increase their comfort with, openness to, and sensitivity about issues related to sexual wellness for older adults.

Significant cultural differences between the nurse and the older adult may increase the difficulty of discussing sexual function. Cultural Considerations 26-1 summarizes some cultural aspects of sexual function that may be applicable to nursing assessment. Nurses also may be uncomfortable discussing sexual function with older adults who are involved

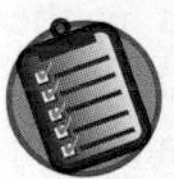

Box 26-2
Assessing Personal Attitudes Toward Sexuality and Aging

What do I believe about sexuality and aging?

- Do I believe that older people, especially unmarried ones, are no longer interested in or capable of sexual activities?
- Do I believe the subtle messages associating sexual activities with youth and attractiveness?
- Do I hold age-specific standards regarding sexual activity and romantic relationships? (For example, do I think it is okay for young adults to kiss or hold hands, but inappropriate or "cute" for older people to do this?)

What do I believe about the nurse's role with regard to the sexual function of older adults?

- Do I believe that sexual function is strictly a private matter that should not be addressed by health professionals?
- Do I view sexual function as an activity of daily living that should be included in a comprehensive assessment of long-term care needs of older adults?
- Do I feel more comfortable discussing sexual function with people who are of the same gender and age range as myself, but very uncomfortable in discussing this matter with people who are old enough to be my parents or grandparents?
- Do I avoid discussion of sexual function with older adults because I believe they are not interested in sexual activity or are uncomfortable discussing this topic?
- Do I avoid discussing sexual function with older adults who are not in traditional marital relationships?
- Do I hold different beliefs about the assessment of sexual function based on the age of the person? For example, do I think sexual function should be assessed in sexually active teenagers who are at risk for unwanted pregnancy, but not older people?

What is my attitude about various expressions of sexual activity?

- How do I view sexual activity and romantic relationships between unmarried people, or between people of the same gender?
- How do I view masturbation?
- Do my views about masturbation or sexual activity between unmarried or same-gender people influence my assessment of and interventions for people who engage in these activities?
- Am I tolerant and nonjudgmental toward people whose views and practices are nontraditional or different from mine?

For nurses in settings where long-term needs are addressed:

- How do I feel about the rights of residents to engage in sexual activity in private, either with themselves or people of their own choosing?
- Do I try to ensure privacy for those residents who desire it?
- If I am aware of the sexual activities of a resident, do I think that I should inform the administrator, a family member, or another "responsible adult?"

Cultural Considerations 26-1

Cultural Aspects of Sexual Function

Expressions of Sexuality and Intimacy

- In some cultures, direct eye contact, especially between a man and woman, is interpreted as an expression of intimacy.
- In some cultures, it is taboo for a man to be alone with a woman other than his wife.
- Touching another person (particularly of the opposite sex) is considered taboo in many cultures.
- In some cultures, heterosexual men and women commonly hold hands with another person of the same gender.
- Only a few cultures value sexual equality between men and women.
- Homosexuality is accepted in some cultures but is considered taboo or is kept secret among family members in others.

Assessment Considerations

- In some cultures, it is considered taboo for postmenopausal women to have their breasts or vagina examined, even by a health care provider.
- Menopausal manifestations may vary in different cultural groups (e.g., most Japanese women do not experience hot flashes).

in same-sex or other nontraditional relationships. Thus, an important aspect of self-assessment is to identify attitudes toward nontraditional sexual activities because these attitudes can influence the assessment and care of people who do not conform to the nurse's expectations. When assessing sexual function, it is important that nurses be nonjudgmental, have an awareness of gay and lesbian culture, and understand the importance of relationships for older lesbians and of sexual activity for older gays (Pope, 1997). In addition, it is important to use gender-neutral pronouns when asking questions about significant relationships. For example, ask if the person has anyone who is a confidant or is very important, rather than asking if the person is married.

Assessing Sexual Function in Older Adults

The goals of assessment of sexual function in older adults are (1) to provide an opportunity for the older adult to address any issues related to sexual function that are important or relevant; and (2) to identify risk factors, particularly attitudinal influences and lack of information, that interfere with the older person's sexual function and quality of life. Although the extent of the assessment varies according to individual circumstances, it should include, at a minimum, questions about the gynecologic aspects of female sexual function and the genitourinary aspects of male sexual function. These questions are easily incorporated into a routine assessment of overall function. If these questions are followed by an open-ended question about sexual interest and activities, the nurse can then respond to the individual needs of the older adult. If problems or risk factors are identified, the nurse is not expected to conduct an in-depth assessment of all aspects of sexual function, but should obtain enough information to suggest appropriate resources for further evaluation. Box 26-3 summarizes guidelines for assessing sexual function in older adults. The Hartford Institute for Geriatric Nursing recommends that nurses use the PLISSIT assessment model as a routine nursing assessment for older adults (Wallace, 2007). The four components of this model are

- Obtaining ***P**ermission* from the client to initiate sexual discussion
- Providing ***L**imited **I**nformation* about sexual function
- Giving ***S**pecific **S**uggestions* for the individual to proceed with sexual relations
- Providing ***I**ntensive **T**herapy* surrounding the issues of sexuality for the client

NURSING DIAGNOSIS

When nurses identify risks that interfere with sexual function, or when older adults express an interest in discussing sexual function, the appropriate nursing diagnosis is Ineffective Sexuality Pattern. This is defined as "the state in which an individual experiences, or is at risk of experiencing, a change in sexual health. Sexual health is the integration of somatic, emotional, intellectual, and social aspects of sexual being in ways that are enriching and that enhance personality, communication, and love" (Carpenito-Moyet, 2006, p. 443). Related factors commonly identified in older adults include medication effects (e.g., from antihypertensive medications); endocrine diseases (e.g., diabetes); cardiovascular diseases (e.g., congestive heart failure); genitourinary conditions (e.g., vaginitis, prostatitis, incontinence); functional impairments secondary to chronic conditions (e.g., limited range of motion as a result of arthritis); psychosocial circumstances (e.g., lack of a partner); and myths and misunderstandings about age-related changes. The case example at the end of this chapter addresses this nursing diagnosis.

Wellness Opportunity

The nursing diagnosis of Readiness for Enhanced Knowledge: Sexual Functioning would be applicable to older adults who express an interest in learning about the effects of aging or risk factors on sexual wellness.

PLANNING FOR WELLNESS OUTCOMES

Increased knowledge about sexual function is an expected outcome for older adults who lack accurate information

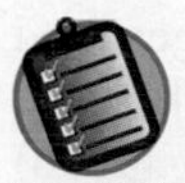

Box 26-3
Guidelines for Assessing Sexual Function in Older Adults

Interview Atmosphere and Communication Techniques

- Ensure both privacy and comfort.
- Be nonjudgmental and matter-of-fact in verbal and nonverbal communication.
- If feasible, sit face-to-face in chairs, rather than conducting the interview while the person being interviewed is in bed.
- If feasible, allow the person being interviewed to wear usual daytime clothing, rather than a hospital gown.

Initiation and Discussion of the Topic

- Begin by acknowledging feelings of discomfort and by stating the reason for discussing this topic. (For example, "I know that sexuality is a private matter and people are often uncomfortable discussing this topic. However, as a nurse, I consider sexuality to be an aspect of health and well-being, and it may have a significant bearing on your overall care.")
- Include statements that address stereotypes and require a response from the older adult. (For example, "Our society tends to view old people as being uninterested in sex, but for most older people, this is not true. Many older people are less sexually active than when they were younger, but this is not because of age-related changes. Have you experienced any changes in your sexual activities in the past few years?")
- Initiate the topic near the end of a comprehensive assessment interview, and begin with questions about the physiologic aspects of male or female function, such as those that follow.

Interview Questions to Assess Male Sexual Function

- Have you ever had prostate problems or related surgery? Have you ever been told that you have or had an enlarged prostate?
- How often do you undergo a complete medical examination? When was your last complete physical?
- Do you ever experience dribbling of urine or have problems holding your water?
- Do you have any trouble initiating the stream of urine?
- After you have urinated (passed water), do you still feel like you haven't emptied your bladder completely?
- Do you have to get up during the night to empty your bladder? If so, how many times?
- Have you ever noticed any blood in your urine?
- Do you ever have any discharge from your penis?
- Do you have any sores, lumps, ulcers, irritations, or areas of inflammation on your penis or scrotum?
- Do you have any trouble with erection or ejaculation?

Interview Questions to Assess Female Sexual Function

- How many children, if any, have you had? How many pregnancies?
- At what ages did your menstrual periods begin and end?
- Have you ever had a Pap (Papanicolaou) test? When was your most recent Pap test and gynecologic examination?
- Have you ever had a mammogram? When was the most recent one?
- Have you ever been taught to examine your breasts for lumps?
- Do you examine your breasts for lumps? How often?
- Have you noticed any changes in your breasts? Do you ever have any discharge from your nipples?
- Do you have any burning, itching, or irritation in the vaginal area?
- Do you ever have any vaginal discharge or bleeding?
- Do you have any difficulties with sexual intercourse?

Principles for Assessing Sexual Interest and Activities

- If the older adult makes a clear statement that this topic is irrelevant, do not insist on further questions. If the older adult responds to questions, however, do not discontinue the interview because of your own discomfort.
- Do not assume that an assessment of sexual function is irrelevant to unmarried people.
- For both married and unmarried older adults, use open-ended questions to elicit information about intimate relationships (e.g., "Is there anything you would like to ask or discuss about intimate relationships?").
- For a married person, open-ended questions may be asked about the partner's influence on sexual activities (e.g., "Has your husband experienced any changes in his health that have affected your sexual activities?").
- Listen for statements that reflect myths, a negative self-image, or self-fulfilling prophecies, such as "Of course I stopped being interested in sex after menopause," or "I can't have an erection because I have prostate trouble."
- If risk factors, such as certain medications or pathologic conditions, have been identified earlier in the interview, ask additional questions, such as, "Have you had any difficulties with sexual activities since your heart attack?" or "Do you have any questions about the possible effects of diabetes on sexual activity?"
- Emphasize the clinical reason for the questions. ("Sometimes certain illnesses or medications interfere with sexual function, and we want to identify any problems you might be having in this area.")
- Use open-ended questions that allow for either closure of the topic or a further discussion of issues. ("Is there anything you would like to discuss with regard to your sexual relationships?")

about age-related changes and risk factors. An outcome for residents of long-term care facilities would be Client Satisfaction: Protection of Rights. For a long-term care resident who is gay or lesbian, an applicable outcome would be Client Satisfaction: Cultural Needs Fulfillment, defined as "the extent of positive perception of integration of cultural beliefs, values, and social structures into nursing care" (Johnson et al., 2005, p. 624). Nurses can use the following additional Nursing Outcomes Classification (NOC) terminology in care plans to promote sexual wellness for older adults: Body Image, Health Beliefs, Knowledge: Sexual Functioning, Personal Well-Being, Self-Esteem, and Sexual Functioning.

Wellness Opportunity

Quality of Life is a wellness outcome for older adults who achieve more satisfying relationships through a variety of expressions of intimacy.

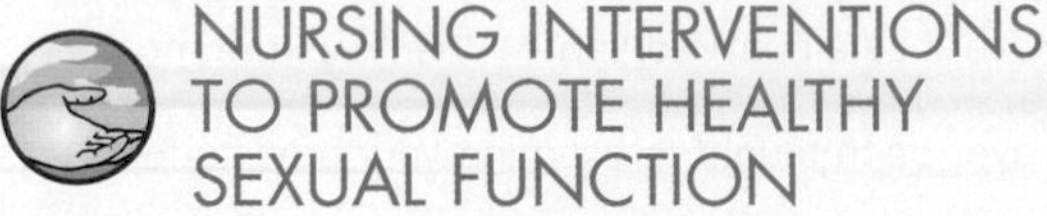

NURSING INTERVENTIONS TO PROMOTE HEALTHY SEXUAL FUNCTION

Nurses have many opportunities to teach older adults about healthy sexual function as an important aspect of quality of life, particularly in home and long-term care settings. Nurses have an important teaching role because many older adults, as well as family and caregivers, hold stereotypes or have little accurate information about sexuality and aging. Nurses can use the following Nursing Interventions Classification (NIC) terminology in their care plans: Body Image Enhancement, Energy Management, Health Education, Patient Rights Protection, Risk Identification, Role Enhancement, Self-Awareness Enhancement, Self-Esteem Enhancement, and Teaching: Sexuality.

Teaching Older Adults About Sexual Wellness

Unlike sex therapists or primary health care providers, nurses are not expected to provide sex education or direct interventions; however, nurses are expected to address sexual function as a quality-of-life concern. Health education about sexual wellness for older adults includes the following information:

- Acknowledgment that sexual function is within the usual realm of health promotion for older adults, especially in long-term care settings
- Effects of age-related changes on sexual function
- Risk factors that cause or contribute to problems with sexual function
- Resources for addressing identified problems and risk factors

In addition, nurses in long-term care settings often need to address attitudes of staff, families, and residents by providing accurate information and role modeling nonjudgmental behaviors.

In some situations, it is appropriate for nurses to teach older adults, as well as their caregivers, about age-related changes and risk factors that affect sexual function. However, the privacy of this topic, particularly on the part of older adults, requires that nurses use excellent communication skills when teaching about sexual wellness. A survey of older adults found that they prefer that health care professionals use open, respectful, nonjudgmental, and plain English communication when discussing sexuality (Johnson, 1997). Group sex education programs for older adults can be effective in achieving positive attitudinal changes and improving knowledge, confidence, and sensitivity of participants (Wiley & Bortz, 1996). Tunstull and Henry (1996) describe a nursing model of a group education program, called the Intimacy Group, that can be used for long-term care residents.

Nurses can use printed information written in nontechnical terms, such as the teaching tool in Box 26-4, as a basis of discussion about sexual function for older adults and caregivers. Nurses can emphasize that any major changes in sexual function are not due to age-related changes alone, and they can use Table 26-1 for further discussion of sexual function in healthy older adults. Many excellent resources for professionals and laypeople are available in bookstores and on the Internet.

Wellness Opportunity

Nurses promote personal responsibility for sexual wellness by suggesting sources of accurate information that older adults can use.

Addressing Risk Factors

If an older adult with significant changes in sexual function also has a pathologic condition, takes a medication, or uses any substance that might be a contributing factor, nurses can teach about the potential influence of these risk factors. This is particularly important when nurses identify pertinent risk factors but the older adult attributes sexual problems to old age. For example, an older man may attribute a problem with attaining an erection to age-related changes, when, in fact, he has diabetes and takes an antihypertensive medication that is associated with erectile dysfunction. Nurses can use Box 26-1 to identify some of the medications and substances that can interfere with sexual function. When nurses identify a potential relationship between a risk factor and sexual problems, it is appropriate to suggest that the older adult seek professional advice. A complete medical evaluation by a primary care provider who is knowledgeable about the sexual problems of older adults is usually the best starting point. If medications are causing or contributing to sexual dysfunction, the primary care provider should consider alternative medications or reduced doses if medically feasible. For example, people with hypertension are less likely to have sexual dysfunction when treated with calcium channel blockers, angiotensin-converting enzyme inhibitors, or peripheral alpha-adrenergic receptor blockers. After any medical problems are addressed, a mental health professional may be an appropriate resource if problems with sexual function persist.

Arthritis is one of the most common pathologic conditions affecting older adults, and it is often self-managed with little or no medical supervision. Often, the symptoms are not severe enough to motivate the older adult to seek medical evaluation and treatment, but they may interfere with sexual activities. In such cases, nurses can use Box 26-5 to teach

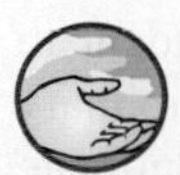

Box 26-4
Health Education About Sexual Activity for Older People

- Older people remain fully capable of enjoying orgasm, but their response to sexual stimulation usually is slower, less intense, and of shorter duration. Increasing the amount and diversity of sexual stimulation and experimenting with different positions can compensate for these changes and increase sexual enjoyment.
- The "use it or lose it" principle applies to sexual activity.
- Sexual problems in older people occur for the same reasons they occur in younger people. That is, they may be related to illness or disability, medications or alcohol, or psychological and relationship factors. The only cause of sexual problems that is unique to older people is the self-fulfilling prophecy of the "sexless senior" stereotype.
- The following habits enhance sexual enjoyment: exercising regularly, avoiding or limiting consumption of alcohol, maintaining optimal health and nutrition, using hearing aids and corrective lenses as needed, and engaging in sexual activities when you are relaxed and your energy level is at its peak.
- If you experience problems with sexual function, seek advice from a professional who is skilled in working with older people. Medical help can be obtained from a urologist, gynecologist, or other medical specialist. If there is no medical basis for the problem, a sex therapist or marriage counselor might be helpful.

Facts Specific to Older Men

- Periodic difficulties with erection and ejaculation do not necessarily indicate that you are impotent.
- After you've reached orgasm, it may be 1 or 2 days before you are able to reach full orgasm again.
- Many new treatment options are available for treating erectile dysfunction (impotence). If your health care provider cannot provide up-to-date information about these options, ask for a referral for an appropriate evaluation and discussion of various options.

Facts Specific to Older Women

- Using a water-soluble lubricant will compensate for decreased vaginal lubrication. Do *not* use petroleum jelly because it is not a very effective lubricant for this purpose and can predispose you to infection.
- Estrogen is beneficial in preventing some problems with sexual function, but the relative risks and benefits of such therapy should be considered and discussed thoroughly with your primary care provider.
- You may have vaginal irritation or urinary tract infections, especially after sexual intercourse, because of age-related thinning of the vaginal wall. Such problems may be avoided by the following interventions:
  - Drink plenty of fluids.
  - Use an estrogen cream or vaginal lubricant.
  - Maintain good hygiene in the vaginal area.
  - If you have a male partner, have him thrust his penis downward, toward the back of your vagina.
  - Empty your bladder before and after intercourse.

about self-care interventions that may be effective in improving the quality of sexual activities for the older adult with arthritis. Nurses can also suggest that older adults who have arthritis obtain pamphlets from local chapters of the Arthritis Foundation.

Another pathologic condition often associated with sexual dysfunction is coronary artery disease, especially in those who have had myocardial infarctions or who have undergone coronary artery bypass surgery. Although cardiac rehabilitation programs usually provide information about sexual function, many older adults do not receive this and would benefit from additional information about sexual function. Nurses can encourage older adults to discuss these concerns with their primary care practitioner and can provide health education using the general guidelines outlined in Box 26-6.

Promoting Sexual Wellness in Long-Term Care Settings

Responsibilities of nurses in long-term care settings to address sexual needs differ from those responsibilities of nurses in acute care or home settings in the following ways:

- Intense medical needs of patients in acute care settings take precedence over sexual needs.

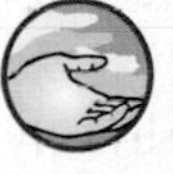

Box 26-5
Health Education About Sexual Activity for People With Arthritis

The pain, fatigue, and joint limitations of arthritis may interfere with, but do not have to curtail, your enjoyment of sexual activity. In fact, sexual activity can be beneficial to you because it stimulates the release of cortisone, adrenalin, and other chemicals that are natural pain relievers. The following actions may enhance your sexual enjoyment and minimize the effects of arthritis:

- Engage in sexual activity when you feel least fatigued and most relaxed.
- Use analgesic medications and other methods of pain relief before engaging in sexual activity.
- Use relaxation techniques before engaging in sexual activity. Relaxation techniques that may be helpful for arthritis include warm baths or showers and the application of hot packs to the affected joints.
- Maintain optimal health through good nutrition and a proper balance of rest and activity.
- Experiment with different sexual positions and use pillows for comfort and support.
- Increase the time spent in foreplay.
- Use a vibrator if your ability to massage is limited by arthritis.
- Use a water-soluble jelly for vaginal lubrication.

Box 26-6
Health Education About Sexual Activity for People With Cardiovascular Disease

- Participation in a medically supervised exercise program can reduce oxygen requirements during sexual activity and improve the quality of your sex life.
- The typical energy expenditure for sexual intercourse is equivalent to that used for climbing two flights of steps.
- Do not engage in sexual activity in extremely hot and humid environments.
- Wait 3 hours after consuming alcohol or a large meal before initiating sexual activity.
- Engage in sexual activity when your energy is at its peak and you are feeling rested and relaxed.
- Avoid sexual activity during times of intense emotional stress.
- Avoid engaging in sexual activity with a partner with whom you are uncomfortable (e.g., an extramarital partner).
- Experiment with different positions to find one that is least demanding of your energy.
- Consider using nitroglycerin, if ordered by your primary care provider, as needed before sexual activity.
- Consult your primary care provider if you experience chest pain during or after sexual activity, or breathlessness or heart palpitations persisting for 15 minutes after orgasm.
- Know that many types of oral medications for erectile dysfunction can cause serious (even fatal) interactions with nitrates.

- The short duration of stay in acute care settings is not conducive to addressing long-term sexual needs of patients.
- Because of the high degree of privacy and autonomy for people in their own homes, home care nurses are not routinely concerned about sexual needs.

Residents in long-term care facilities, however, usually are not acutely ill, are planning to stay in the facility for a long time, and do depend on the nursing staff to ensure the privacy necessary to meet their personal needs. Thus, the nurse in long-term care facilities must address the sexual needs of residents as an integral part of the overall care plan.

Because many of the barriers to meeting the sexual needs of older adults in long-term care facilities are based on myths and attitudes of the staff, education of the staff is the most effective starting point for addressing these issues (Kuhn, 2002; Walker & Harrington, 2002). In-service programs should address various aspects of sexual function, including the lifelong interest in and need for sexual activity and intimate relationships. Audiovisual materials can be used to stimulate discussion about the unique aspects of meeting sexual needs in institutional settings and about the responsibilities and limitations of staff. Nurses generally participate in such in-services as part of the interdisciplinary team, which also includes social service and administrative staff. Presenters and discussion leaders should be nonjudgmental and matter-of-fact so they role model the most effective approach for addressing this sensitive topic.

When the ability of a cognitively impaired resident to give informed consent is questionable, an interdisciplinary team can assess competence to participate in an intimate relationship (e.g., see Lichtenberg, 1997). Emphasis should be placed on the Residents' Rights bill, as defined by the federal government in the 1987 Nursing Home Reform Law. Sexual needs of residents of long-term care facilities are protected through the rights to

- Self-determination
- Participation in their own care
- Independence in making personal decisions
- Reasonable accommodation of their needs and preferences
- Privacy and unrestricted communication with any person of their choice
- Immediate access by their relatives and for others subject to reasonable restriction with the resident's permission

In addition to educating staff members about the sexual needs and rights of residents, nurses are responsible for ensuring privacy for those residents who desire it. If a resident does not have a private room, staff try to provide privacy, while still respecting the rights of any roommates. Sometimes, the role of the nurse will be that of a negotiator, assisting residents in reaching mutually acceptable agreements about privacy and shared space.

Wellness Opportunity

Nurses respect autonomy by working with other staff to assess the ability of someone with dementia to make decisions about expressions of sexuality.

Teaching About Hormonal Therapy for Women

Nurses need to be familiar with results of recent studies on hormonal therapy and explanations of why these results differed so significantly from previous studies so they can provide health education about hormonal therapy and other aspects of menopause and sexual function in older women. Nurses also need to be familiar with recommendations about nonhormonal interventions for menopausal symptoms in order to teach older women.

Research on Hormonal Therapy

Since the 1940s, when estrogen was first prescribed for treatment of menopausal symptoms, the relative risks and benefits of hormonal therapy have been hotly debated. Researchers and health care practitioners agree that estrogen is an effective intervention for alleviating hot flashes, vaginal atrophy, and other manifestations of menopause that interfere with comfort, sexual function, and quality of life. However, there have been mounting concerns about risks and increasing controversy about any additional potential benefits. Questions about the safety of estrogen therapy were first raised during the 1970s, when studies began showing an association between estrogen therapy and increased rates of breast cancer and endometrial cancer and hyperplasia. Although initial studies raised questions about the risk-to-benefit ratio of estrogen therapy, later studies suggested that the administration of a combination of estrogen and progestin could reduce or eliminate such risks for most women. Around the same time, studies found that estrogen was effective in preventing osteoporosis and fractures in postmenopausal women. By the 1980s, studies indicated that hormonal therapy had far-reaching benefits and might even reduce mortality, prevent skin aging, and decrease the incidence of dementia, depression, urinary incontinence, and cardiovascular disease. By the late 1990s, hormonal therapy was widely recommended not only for menopausal symptoms but for preventing osteoporosis, fractures, and heart disease.

By the early 2000s, however, findings from two major long-term studies—the Women's Health Initiative and the Heart and Estrogen/Progestin Replacement Study—contradicted many of the findings of earlier studies. In July 2002, a major part of the Women's Health Initiative study was suddenly halted and study participants were advised to discontinue using the same hormonal therapy regimen that millions of women worldwide had been using for many decades. Results of this study—which "caused a leap in knowledge"—and its premature discontinuation had enormous implications for women and health care practitioners, who began to ask "How could we have been so wrong?" (Laine, 2002, p. 290).

The Women's Health Initiative and the Heart and Estrogen/Progestin Replacement Study concluded that the most commonly prescribed hormonal therapy regimen, called continuous–combined estrogen–progestin (i.e., daily administration of 0.625 mg of conjugated equine estrogens plus 2.5 mg of medroxyprogesterone acetate), increased the risk for all of the following: heart disease, blood clots, stroke, breast cancer, and symptomatic gallbladder disease (Grady et al., 2002; Hulley et al., 2002; Women's Health Initiative Investigators, 2002). Positive effects of hormonal therapy identified in these studies included a decreased risk of colorectal cancer, improved bone mineral density, and decreased rates of fractures. After weighing both risks and benefits, the researchers concluded that the risks exceeded the benefits, even though the risk of experiencing an adverse effect was relatively small. For example, based on the findings of the Women's Health Initiative study, 100 women would have to take hormonal therapy for 5 years to experience one additional adverse effect (Sherman, 2002). Because of these studies, organizations such as the U.S. Preventive Services Task Force (USPSTF) updated their guidelines and cautioned against the long-term use of combined estrogen and progestin therapy because the harmful effects are likely to exceed the chronic disease prevention benefits in most women (USPSTF, 2005).

In January 2003, the U.S. Food and Drug Administration (FDA) mandated that the label on all medications containing estrogen must warn about the increased risk for heart disease, heart attacks, stroke, and breast cancer. Labels on hormonal therapy products also should do the following:

- Suggest that topical vaginal products be used for treatment of vulvar or vaginal atrophy
- Suggest that nonestrogen treatments be considered for prevention of postmenopausal osteoporosis
- Encourage practitioners to prescribe the lowest dose for shortest duration
- Emphasize that decisions about hormonal therapy should be individualized, based on an evaluation of potential risks and benefits
- Suggest that menopausal women may still want to rely on these products for relief of severe vasomotor symptoms

In summary, hormonal therapy is no longer recommended for prevention of any chronic condition (including osteoporosis and cardiovascular disease). It continues to have a place in the treatment of menopausal symptoms such as hot flashes, but its use should be limited to the lowest dose for the shortest duration.

Differences Between Early and Recent Studies

Many questions have been raised about how these recent studies could so blatantly contradict earlier findings and lead to major reversals of recommendations made by highly respected health care organizations. It is important to recognize that conclusions were based on different types of studies. Until the early 2000s, conclusions about hormonal therapy were based on observational studies (e.g., the Nurses' Health Study) that found that women taking hormonal therapy had lower rates of cardiovascular disease than women who were not taking estrogen. Observational studies also found that women taking hormonal therapy had decreased serum levels of low-density lipoproteins and increased serum levels of high-density lipoproteins, two factors that reduce the risk for cardiovascular disease (Gupta & Aronow, 2002). By the early 2000s, "a large body of observational data" suggested that hormonal therapy caused a "sizable reduction in the risk for coronary events" in postmenopausal women (Humphrey et al., 2002; Laine, 2002). Researchers then speculated that there was a possible cause–effect relationship between the use of hormonal therapy and improved cardiovascular health, so they designed longitudinal and well-controlled prospective studies (e.g., the Women's Health Initiative and Heart and Estrogen/Progestin Replacement Study) to shed additional light on these issues. Contrary to what was expected, however, the well-controlled studies did not support findings from observational studies, and, in fact, contradicted many conclusions of earlier studies. An explanation for this contradiction is that the Nurses' Health Study did not control for the fact that women taking hormonal therapy were more likely to be better educated, have better access to medical care, and lead healthier lifestyles. This so-called "healthy woman effect" accounted for the decreased rate of cardiovascular disease in subjects who took hormonal therapy. In summary, the observational data were misleading because they did not adequately account for socioeconomic status; rather than hormonal therapy keeping women healthy, healthy women were taking hormonal therapy (Laine, 2002).

Recommendations About Interventions for Menopausal Symptoms

Currently, an advisory panel of the Women's Health Initiative is investigating the following questions:

- Do lower doses of estrogen plus progestin reduce the risk of adverse events?
- Is the risk of adverse effects changed with the use of transdermal estrogen and progestin?
- What is the best way of discontinuing hormonal therapy?
- Which risks are associated with estrogen and which are associated with progestin?

Until these questions are answered, women who have taken hormonal therapy for more than 3 to 5 years are advised to talk with their primary care practitioner about discontinuing the medication and seeking other treatments for the menopausal symptoms that need to be addressed. Although some women have no major adverse effects from abruptly discontinuing hormonal therapy, many find that a process of gradual tapering off is more comfortable and allows their body to adjust better to the changes. Some women who discontinue hormonal therapy find that the benefits of the therapy outweigh the risks, and choose to resume hormonal therapy because they cannot find effective ways of managing menopausal symptoms. Women need to understand that decisions about hormonal therapy are highly individualized and should be made only after careful consideration by the woman and her health care practitioner.

Researchers and health care practitioners are trying to identify interventions (e.g., medications, herbal and botanical products) that are both safe and effective for managing menopausal symptoms. For example, a recent study found that testosterone patches were well tolerated and effective in increasing the frequency of sexual desire and activity in naturally menopausal women with hypoactive sexual desire disorder (Shifren et al., 2006). Other studies support the use of topical estrogen cream as a safe and effective intervention for vaginal dryness (Long, et al., 2006). Because information about the use of hormonal therapy and other interventions for menopausal symptoms is rapidly evolving, nurses need to keep up to date about these issues so that they can provide accurate, complete, and objective information. The Women's Health Initiative is investigating many of these issues, and ongoing findings and recommendations can be found on their website (www.whi.org). The North American Menopause Society (www.menopause.org) is another excellent source of up-to-date information about interventions for menopausal symptoms. Box 26-7 can be used for educating older women about menopause and hormonal therapy.

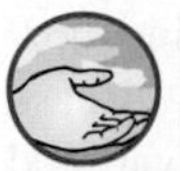

Box 26-7 Health Education About Interventions for Menopause

Health promotion interventions to reduce the frequency or intensity of hot flashes:

- Engage in regular exercise (especially aerobic exercise).
- Avoid caffeine, alcohol, hot beverages, spicy foods.
- Perform relaxation techniques (e.g., slow, deep breathing) several times daily and at the onset of a hot flash.
- Wear layers of lightweight clothing.
- Keep environmental temperatures cool.

Over-the-counter products that may be effective in reducing the frequency or intensity of hot flashes:

- Isoflavones (e.g., soy protein)
- Progesterone cream

Prescription medications that may be effective in reducing the frequency or intensity of hot flashes:

- Progesterone and progestational agents (e.g., megestrol, 20–40 mg daily)
- Antidepressants (e.g., venlafaxine, 75 mg daily; fluoxetine, 20 mg daily; paroxetine, 12.5–25 mg daily; sertraline, 50–100 mg daily)
- Clonidine, 0.1 mg daily
- Gabapentin, 100–900 mg daily

Clinical trials have* not *supported the use of any of the following interventions for hot flashes:

- Vitamin E
- Herbal products: sage, ginseng, licorice, sarsaparilla, dong quai, fish oil, wild yam, flaxseed oil, gotu kola, ginkgo biloba, valerian root, evening primrose oil

Interventions that need further investigation of their potential effectiveness for hot flashes:

- Chasteberry
- Hypnosis
- Acupuncture
- Biofeedback

Health promotion interventions for other symptoms of menopause:

- Engage in regular weight-bearing exercises for prevention of osteoporosis.
- Provide daily intake of 1500 mg calcium and 600 IU vitamin D for prevention of osteoporosis.
- Talk with your primary care practitioner about assessment of and interventions for osteoporosis.
- Perform pelvic muscle exercises for prevention of urinary incontinence.
- Use water-soluble lubricants or estrogen cream (prescription) for vaginal dryness.

Teaching About Interventions for Men

Attention to sexual wellness in men initially focused on erectile dysfunction, but, until recently, even that condition was viewed as a relatively inevitable and untreatable consequence of aging. The development of sildenafil and other oral agents that are relatively safe, effective, and easy to use has significantly increased the interest of researchers, clinicians, and pharmaceutical companies in men's sexual health. There is also increased interest in testosterone therapy for treating symptoms of andropause. Nurses need to be familiar enough with both of these emerging issues so they can provide health education to older men and facilitate appropriate referrals.

Testosterone Therapy

Researchers and practitioners are addressing questions about testosterone therapy for treating andropausal symptoms and erectile dysfunction. Studies indicate that testosterone therapy in healthy older men may have beneficial effects on libido, muscle strength, cognitive function, cardiovascular function, body composition, bone mineral density, and general well-being (Kenny et al., 2002; Matsumoto, 2002). These effects may be greater in younger rather than older men and are most significant in men who have low serum levels of testosterone because there is a "threshold effect" (i.e., a level at which no further benefits are seen) (Vermeulen, 2001). Because detrimental effects of testosterone therapy, including prostatic hyperplasia and increased risks of prostate cancer, may outweigh the benefits, it is not widely recommended for management of andropause or sexual dysfunction and is contraindicated in men with breast cancer or prostate cancer. Current studies are examining the risks, benefits, and optimal routes of administration of testosterone therapy, with particular emphasis on older men (Gore et al., 2005). Currently approved methods of administering testosterone therapy in the United States include gels, patches, and intramuscular injections; a buccal preparation is under investigation. Testosterone pills are available outside the United States, but they are not recommended because they are less effective and are associated with potentially serious adverse effects (e.g., hepatotoxicity and cardiovascular disease). Information about testosterone therapy is rapidly evolving; however, some of the information is disseminated by companies whose primary goal is to sell testosterone products, so there is a great need for well-controlled studies of testosterone therapy.

Interventions for Erectile Dysfunction

In recent years, health care professionals have recognized erectile dysfunction as a very common and treatable condition that should be evaluated and treated. Many medical and surgical interventions are now available for erectile dysfunction, ranging from surgical procedures (e.g., penile prostheses) to oral medications (Table 26-2). In 1998, FDA approval of the first oral medication for erectile dysfunction,

TABLE 26-2 Interventions for Erectile Dysfunction

Intervention	Mode of Action	Comment
Oral medication (e.g., sildenafil, vardenafil, tadalafil)	Causes penile engorgement by increasing the blood flow and relaxing the smooth muscles	**Cannot be used by men taking nitrate medications.** Adverse effects include headache, indigestion, and facial flushing
Sublingual apomorphine	Acts on the dopamine receptors in the brain to stimulate erection	Can be used by men taking nitrate medications. Adverse effects include nausea, sweating, dizziness, and somnolence
Testosterone therapy (oral, sublingual, or injectable preparations)	Increases serum testosterone in the small number (1% to 5%) of men who have testosterone deficiency	May worsen prostate problems and increase the risk for prostate cancer
Vacuum pumps and constriction devices	Stimulate an erection by using an airtight plastic cylinder to create a vacuum; a constriction band is then placed around the base of the penis to retain the erection, and the cylinder is removed	Requires a high degree of manual dexterity; is intrusive and cumbersome; may cause ejaculatory discomfort
Intracavernosal injection of vasoactive drug (e.g., alprostadil)	Injects medication directly into the erectile tissue to cause vasodilation and relaxation of the smooth muscles of the penis	Adverse effects include priapism, bruising, and local pain
Transurethral alprostadil suppository	Aids erection by causing vasodilation and relaxation of smooth muscle tissue after the active agent is absorbed from the urethral tissue	Adverse effects include hypotension, syncope, and transient burning sensation in the urethra
Topical medication (e.g., herbal combinations, vasodilators)	Enhance erections by increasing blood flow	Not approved by the Food and Drug Administration; vasodilators should not be used by men with cardiovascular disease
Yohimbine (alone or in combination with L-arginine or trazodone)	Stimulates receptors in the brain associated with libido and erections	Low success rate (not proven effective in clinical trials); adverse effects include nausea, insomnia, nervousness, dizziness, and hypertension
Penile prosthesis (requires a surgical procedure)	Facilitates erection by improving penile rigidity without affecting urination, ejaculation, or orgasm	High rate of success, is the only intervention that is permanent

sildenafil (Viagra), simplified the treatment of this disorder and stimulated much public debate and attention. Two additional drugs in this class of phosphodiesterase inhibitors have been approved by the FDA: vardenafil (Levitra) and tadalafil (Cialis). Many recent, large-scale studies have evaluated these drugs and concluded that they are safe and effective as first-line therapies for erectile dysfunction in older adults (Dinsmore, 2005; Salonia et al., 2005). In particular, studies have not found any association between these drugs and increased risk of cardiovascular events, even in men who have compromised cardiac function (Katz et al., 2005; Mittleman et al., 2005). These drugs, however, can cause serious and even fatal adverse effects when they interact with nitrate medications. Apomorphine, a dopamine receptor agonist, is a sublingual oral agent that is safe and effective for erectile dysfunction and can be used concomitantly with nitrates. Common adverse effects of apomorphine include nausea, dizziness, and headache.

Interventions also need to address risk factors that cause or contribute to sexual dysfunction. For example, smoking cessation and optimal management of diabetes can improve erectile dysfunction in men with these contributing factors. If blood flow is blocked, vascular surgery to restore normal circulation to the penis may be an appropriate intervention. Psychotherapy and behavioral therapy may be used as primary or adjunctive treatment options to address the psychosocial issues that may be contributing to erectile dysfunction. Pelvic muscle exercises, commonly performed as a treatment for urinary incontinence, may also be useful in the treatment of erectile dysfunction. The technique for performing these exercises is described in Chapter 19. Decisions about appropriate treatment options must be based on a comprehensive evaluation by a urologist or by a primary care provider who is knowledgeable about erectile dysfunction. The primary responsibility of nurses is to keep up to date on the types of interventions that are available and to teach about the importance of seeking help for erectile dysfunction.

EVALUATING EFFECTIVENESS OF NURSING INTERVENTIONS

Nursing care for older adults with the diagnosis of Altered Sexuality Patterns is evaluated by the degree to which risk factors are eliminated, particularly through the provision of accurate information. For example, older adults may verbalize an improved understanding of the age-related changes that affect their response to sexual stimulation. In turn, this information can alleviate anxiety about sexual performance and improve quality of life. Interventions to alleviate risk factors, such as medical conditions or adverse medication/chemical effects, would be considered successful if the older adult follows through with a referral to an appropriate resource. One measure of successful intervention in long-term care settings would be that staff members increase their understanding of the sexual needs of older adults and are more comfortable allowing appropriate sexual expressions by the residents.

Mr. and Mrs. S. are now 75 and 73 years old, respectively, and they have moved to an assisted-living facility where you are the nurse. Their health conditions have not changed significantly in the past 2 years, with the exception of Mrs. S. having more difficulty walking because of her arthritis. Mr. and Mrs. S. recently moved to the facility because they needed help with transportation and wanted to live in a place where they had fewer responsibilities and more time to enjoy life. During one of their appointments, Mrs. S. becomes tearful and says she has been disappointed in their move from their own home. She says, "Now we have the time to enjoy our life together, but we seem to be in each other's way all the time. When we lived in our own home we were so busy with the yard and the housekeeping and all the daily chores, we never had time to think about what we enjoy together. Now I don't have to cook meals and worry about getting to the grocery store, but we aren't enjoying the time we have together."

NURSING ASSESSMENT

On further discussion, Mrs. S. acknowledges that she has talked with her husband about having more "intimate time and resuming sexual activities that have petered out in the past few years because we were always so tired and never seemed to have much time." In reply, Mr. S. has stated that "We're probably too old to do those things, and old people shouldn't expect to have the fun we used to have." Mrs. S. says she used to believe that, but recently she's been talking with some of the other women in the assisted-living facility who seem to be enjoying sexual activities. Mr. and Mrs. S. relate that they had a good

(case study continues on page 561)

sexual relationship until Mr. S.'s heart attack 5 years ago. After that, he lost interest in sexual activities, even though he was told he could resume all his usual activities except for very strenuous activity, such as shoveling snow. Mrs. S. says she masturbates occasionally, but she doesn't find that very satisfying. Mrs. S. expresses concern about being comfortable in the sexual position they used previously because her arthritis has gotten worse in the past few years.

NURSING DIAGNOSIS

You address Ineffective Sexuality Patterns as your nursing diagnosis for Mr. and Mrs. S. Related factors include myths and lack of information about the age-related changes and risk factors that influence sexual function. Potential risk factors that you identify are Mr. S.'s medications and his lack of information about sexual function after a heart attack.

NURSING CARE PLAN FOR MR. AND MRS. S.

Expected Outcome	Nursing Interventions	Nursing Evaluation
Mr. and Mrs. S.'s knowledge about age-related changes and risk factors that affect sexual function will be increased.	• Use Box 26-4 as a basis for discussion of sexual function in later adulthood.	• Mr. and Mrs. S. will verbalize correct information about sexual function in older adulthood.
The risk factors associated with Mr. S.'s heart attack and medication regimen will be addressed.	• Explain that many medications for heart problems and high blood pressure are associated with problems with sexual function. • Use Box 26-6 as a basis for discussing sexual activity as it relates to people with heart problems. • Encourage Mr. S. to talk with his primary care provider about his medication regimen and about his heart condition. Suggest that he inquire whether a different medication would effectively treat his high blood pressure without interfering with sexual function.	• Mr. S. will agree to talk with his primary care provider about the potential relationship between his medications and heart condition and his lack of sexual activity.
The risk factors associated with Mrs. S.'s arthritis will be addressed.	• Use Box 26-5 to discuss sexual activity as it relates to people with arthritis.	• Mrs. S. will identify ways to increase her comfort during sexual activities.

THINKING POINTS

- What risk factors are likely to influence Mrs. S.'s enjoyment of sexual activity?
- What risk factors are likely to affect Mr. S.'s enjoyment of sexual activity?
- What health education would you provide for Mrs. S., and what would you use for patient teaching tools?
- What health education would you provide for Mr. S., and what would you use for patient teaching tools?

Chapter Highlights

Age-Related Changes That Affect Sexual Wellness

- Diminished levels of hormones
- Degenerative changes of reproductive organs
- Cessation of menses and onset of menopause in women

Risk Factors That Affect Sexual Wellness

- Societal influences, especially on attitudes, stereotypes, and prejudices
- Effects of attitudes and behaviors of families and caregivers, especially on dependent older adults
- Limited opportunities for sexual activity: lower ratio of men to women with increasing age, psychosocial factors, privacy
- Adverse effects of medication, alcohol, and nicotine (Box 26-1)
- Functional impairments and chronic conditions (e.g., disabilities, diabetes, cardiovascular disease, sensory impairments)

Pathologic Conditions Affecting Sexual Wellness
- Men: prostatic hyperplasia
- Women: urethritis, vaginitis
- Sexual dysfunction in men and women

Functional Consequences Affecting Sexual Wellness
- Reproductive ability: ceases in women, diminishes in men
- Response to sexual stimulation: slower and less intense (Table 26-1)
- Sexual interest and activity: maintenance of interest and capacity in most older adults, but diminished sexual activity due to risk factors
- Menopause and andropause

Nursing Assessment of Sexual Function
- Self-assessment of attitudes about sexual function and aging (Box 26-2)
- Assessment of cultural influences (Cultural Considerations 26-1)
- Assessing sexual function: general principles and specific interview questions (Box 26-3)

Nursing Diagnosis
- Readiness for Enhanced Knowledge: Sexual Functioning
- Ineffective Sexuality Pattern

Planning for Wellness Outcomes
- For residents in long-term care facilities, Client Satisfaction: Protection of Rights or Client Satisfaction: Cultural Needs Fulfillment
- Body Image
- Personal Well-Being
- Self-Esteem
- Sexual Functioning

Nursing Interventions to Promote Sexual Wellness (Boxes 26-4 through 26-7)
- Teaching older adults about sexual wellness: age-related changes and risk factors
- Addressing risk factors: teaching about sexual activity for people with arthritis or cardiovascular disease
- Promoting sexual wellness in long-term care facilities: staff education, protection of rights, ensuring privacy
- Teaching about hormonal therapy for women: research and recommendations
- Teaching about interventions for men: testosterone therapy, interventions for erectile dysfunction

Evaluating Effectiveness of Nursing Interventions
- Provision of accurate information to dispel myths and misconceptions
- Improved quality of life
- Referrals to health care professionals for addressing risk factors
- Increased knowledge and comfort of staff in long-term care facilities

Critical Thinking Exercises

1. Describe the attitudinal risk factors on the parts of society, older adults, and health care providers that can interfere with healthy sexual function in older adults.
2. Summarize the functional consequences that are likely to affect sexual function in healthy older men and women.
3. What are the responsibilities of nurses in each of the following settings related to assessment of sexual function in older adults: community setting, acute care facility, and long-term care facility?
4. Describe the assessment and health education approaches you might use for a 73-year-old married man who confides that he has difficulty making his wife "happy in bed."
5. Spend a few minutes answering all the questions included in Box 26-2, Assessing Personal Attitudes Toward Sexuality and Aging. What did you learn about yourself?

Clinical Tool Resources

Hartford Institute for Geriatric Nursing
Try This: Best Practices in Nursing Care to Older Adults
Issue Number 10 (Revised 2007), Sexuality Assessment for Older Adults
www.hartfordign.org/resources/education/tryThis.html

Educational Resources

American Association of Sex Educators, Counselors and Therapists
www.aasect.org

American Menopause Foundation, Inc.
www.americanmenopause.org

North American Menopause Society
www.menopause.org

Senior Action in a Gay Environment (SAGE)
www.sageusa.org

Sexuality Information and Education Council of the United States
www.siecus.org

References

Anderson, J. K., Faulkner, S., Cranor, C., Briley, J., Gevirtz, F., & Roberts, S. (2002). Andropause: Knowledge and perceptions among general public and health care professionals. *Journals of Gerontology: Series A, Biological Sciences and Medical Sciences, 57*, M793–M796.

Austoni, E., Mirone, V., Parazzini, F., Fasolo, C. B., Turchi, P., Pescatori, E. S., et al. (2005). Smoking as a risk factor for erectile dysfunction: Data from Andrology Preventions Weeks 2001–2002. *European Urology, 48*, 810–817.

Avis, N. E. (2000). Sexual functioning and aging in men and women: Community and population-based studies. *Journal of Gender-Specific Medicine, 3*(2), 37–41.

Basson, R. (2005). Women's sexual dysfunction: Revised and expanded definitions. *Canadian Medical Association Journal, 172*, 1327–1333.

Berger, R. (2001). Report of the American Foundation for Urologic Disease Thought Leader Panel for evaluation and treatment of priapism. *International Journal of Impotence Research, 13*(Suppl. 5), S39–S43.

Beutel, M. E. (2002). Sexual activity, sexual and partnership satisfaction in ageing men: Results from a German representative community study. *Andrologia, 34*, 22–28.

Brecher, E. M. (1984). *Love, sex, and aging: A Consumers Union report.* Boston: Little, Brown.

Bretschneider, J. G., & McCoy, N. L. (1988). Sexual interest and behavior in healthy 80- to 102-year-olds. *Archives of Sexual Behavior, 17*, 109–129.

Brody, J. E. (1983, September 28). Drugs can be bad medicine for lover. *New York Times*, p. III, 1:1.

Buvat, J., & Lemaire, A. (2001). Sexuality of the diabetic woman [in French]. *Diabetes and Metabolism, 27*(4 Pt. 2), S67–S75.

Cahill, S. (2002). Long term care issues affecting gay, lesbian, bisexual and transgender elders. *Geriatric Care Management Journal, 12*(3), 4–8.

Carpenito-Moyet, L. J. (2006). *Handbook of nursing diagnosis* (11th ed.). Philadelphia: Lippincott Williams & Wilkins.

Chun, J., & Carson, C. C. (2001). Physician-patient dialogue and clinical evaluation of erectile dysfunction. *Urologic Clinics of North America, 28*, 249–258.

Cooney, T. M., & Dunne, K. (2001). Intimate relationships in later life. *Journal of Family Issues, 22*, 838–858.

Corona, G., Mannucci, E., Petrone, L., Ricca, V., Mansani, R., Cilotti, A., et al. (2005). Psychobiological correlates of smoking in patients with erectile dysfunction. *International Journal of Impotence Research, 17*, 527–534.

Covey, H. C. (1989). Perceptions and attitudes toward sexuality of the elderly during the middle ages. *The Gerontologist, 29*(1), 91–103.

Davol, P., & Rukstalis, D. (2005). Priapism associated with routine use of quetiapine: Case report and review of the literature. *Urology, 66*, 880.e13–880.e14.

Dinsmore, W. W. (2005). Available and future treatments for erectile dysfunction. *Clinical Cornerstone, 7*, 37–45.

Gades, N. M., Nehra, A., Jacobson, D. J., McGree, M. E., Girman, C. J., Rhodes, T., et al. (2005). Association between smoking and erectile dysfunction: A population-based study. *American Journal of Epidemiology, 161*, 346–351.

Ginsberg, T. B. (2006). Aging and sexuality. *Medical Clinics of North America, 90*, 1025–1036.

Gore, J. L., Swerdloff, R. S., & Rajfer, J. (2005). Androgen deficiency in the etiology and treatment of erectile dysfunction. *Urologic Clinics of North America, 32*, 457–468.

Grady, D., Herrington, D., Bittner, V., Blumenthal, R., Davidson, M., Hlatky, M., et al. (2002). Cardiovascular disease outcomes during 6.8 years of hormone therapy: Heart and Estrogen/Progestin Replacement Study follow-up (HERS II). *Journal of the American Medical Association, 288*, 49–57.

Grover, S. A., Lowensteyn, I., Kaouache, M., Marchand, S., Coupal, L., DeCarolis, E., et al. (2006). The prevalence of erectile dysfunction in the primary care setting. *Archives of Internal Medicine, 166*, 213–219.

Gupta, G., & Aronow, W. S. (2002). Hormone replacement therapy: An analysis of efficacy based on evidence. *Geriatrics, 57*(8), 18–24.

Haren, M. T., Kim, H. J., Tariq, S. H., Wittert, G. A., & Morley, J. E. (2006). Andropause: A quality-of-life issue in older males. *Medical Clinics of North America, 90*, 1005–1023.

He, W., Sengupta, M., Velkoff, V. A., & DeBarros, K. A. (2005). *65+ in the United States: 2005*. Current Population Reports: Special Studies, P23-209. U.S. Department of Health and Human Services, National Institute on Aging, and U.S. Department of Commerce, U.S. Census Bureau. Available at www.census.gov/prod/2006pubs/p23-209.pdf.

Hulley, S., Furberg, C., Barrett-Connor, E., Cauley, J., Grady, D., Haskell, W., et al. (2002). Noncardiovascular disease outcomes during 6.8 years of hormone therapy: Heart and Estrogen/progestin Replacement Study follow-up (HERS II). *Journal of the American Medical Association, 288*, 58–66.

Humphrey, L. L., Chan, B. K. S., & Sox, H. C. (2002). Postmenopausal hormone replacement therapy and the primary prevention of cardiovascular disease. *Annals of Internal Medicine, 137*, 273–284.

Johannes, C. B., Araujo, A. B., Feldman, H. A., Derby, C. A., Kleinman, K. P., & McKinlay, J. B. (2000). Incidence of erectile dysfunction in men ages 40–69: Longitudinal results from the Massachusetts Male Aging Study. *Journal of Urology, 163*, 460–463.

Johnson, B. (1997). Older adults' suggestions for health care providers regarding discussions of sex. *Geriatric Nursing, 18*(2), 65–66.

Johnson, B. K. (1996). Older adults and sexuality: A multidimensional perspective. *Journal of Gerontological Nursing, 22*(2), 6–15.

Johnson, M., Bulechek, G., Butcher, H., Dochterman, J. M., Maas, M., Moorehead, S., et al. (2005). *NANDA, NOC, and NIC linkages: Nursing diagnoses, outcomes, & interventions* (2nd ed.). St. Louis: Mosby Elsevier.

Kaplan, M. J. (2002). Approaching sexual issues in primary care. *Primary Care: Clinics in Office Practice, 29*(1), 113–124.

Katz, S. D., Parker, J. D., Glasser, D. B., Bank, A. J., Sherman, N., Wang, H., et al. (2005). Efficacy and safety of sildenafil citrate in men with erectile dysfunction and chronic heart failure. *American Journal of Cardiology, 95*, 36–42.

Kenny, A. M., Bellantonio, S., Gruman, C. A., Acosta, R. D., & Prestwood, K. M. (2002). Effects of transdermal testosterone on cognitive function and health perception in older men with low bioavailable testosterone levels. *Journals of Gerontology: Series A, Biological Sciences and Medical Sciences, 57*, M321–M325.

Kuhn, D. (2002). Intimacy, sexuality, and residents with dementia. *Alzheimer's Care Quarterly, 3*, 165–176, Appendix A.

Laine, C. (2002). Postmenopausal hormone replacement therapy: How could we have been so wrong? *Annals of Internal Medicine, 137*, 290.

Lichtenberg, P. A. (1997). Clinical perspectives on sexual issues in nursing homes. *Topics in Geriatric Rehabilitation, 12*(4), 1–10.

Liu, P. Y., Swerdloff, R. S., & Wang, C. (2005). Relative testosterone deficiency in older men: Clinical definition and presentation. *Endocrinology and Metabolism Clinics of North America, 34*, 957–972.

Long, C.-Y., Liu, C.-M., Hsu, S.-C., Wu, C.-H., Wang, C.-L., & Tsai, E.-M. (2006). A randomized comparative study of the effects of oral and topical estrogen therapy on the vaginal vascularization and sexual function in hysterectomized postmenopausal women. *Menopause, 13*, 737–743.

Mace, N. L., & Rabins, P. V. (2006). *36-Hour day* (4th ed.). Baltimore: The Johns Hopkins University Press.

Masters, W. H., & Johnson, V. E. (1966). *Human sexual response*. Boston: Little, Brown.

Matsumoto, A. M. (2002). Andropause: Clinical implications of the decline in serum testosterone levels with aging in men. *Journals of Gerontology: Series A, Biological Sciences and Medical Sciences, 57*, M76–M99.

Mazur, A. (2002). Causes of sexual decline in aging married men: Germany and America. *International Journal of Impotence Research, 14*(2), 101–106.

Millett, C., Wen, L. M., Rissel, C., Smith, A., Richters, J., Grulich, A., et al. (2006). Smoking and erectile dysfunction: Findings from a representative sample of Australian men. *Tobacco Control, 15*, 73–74.

Mittleman, M. A., Maclure, M., & Glasser, D. B. (2005). Evaluation of acute risk for myocardial infarction in men treated with sildenafil citrate. *American Journal of Cardiology, 96*, 443–446.

Munarriz, R., Kim, N. M., Goldstein, I., & Traish, A. M. (2002). Biology of female sexual function. *Urologic Clinics of North America, 29*, 685–693.

National Institutes of Health. (1993). Consensus statement, National Institutes of Health: Impotence. December 7–9, 1992. *International Journal of Impotence Research, 5*, 181–284.

Nudell, D. M., Monoski, M. M. & Lipshultz, L. I. (2002). Common medications and drugs: How they affect male fertility. *Urologic Clinics of North America, 29*, 347–354.

Orwoll, E., Lambert, L. C., Marshall, L. M., Blank, J., Barrett-Connor, E., Cauley, J., et al. (2006). Testosterone and estradiol among older men. *Journal of Clinical Endocrinology and Metabolism, 91*, 1336–1344.

Pauls, R. N., & Berman, J. R. (2002). Impact of pelvic floor disorders and prolapse on female sexual function and response. *Urologic Clinics of North America, 29*, 677–683.

Pope, M. (1997). Sexual issues for older lesbians and gays. *Topics in Geriatric Rehabilitation, 12*(4), 53–60.

Reynolds, K. E., & Magnan, M. A. (2005). Nursing attitudes and beliefs toward human sexuality: Collaborative research promoting evidence-based practice. *Clinical Nurse Specialist, 19*, 255–259.

Robinson, K. M., (2003). Understanding hypersexuality: A behavioral disorder of dementia. *Home Healthcare Nurse, 21*(1), 43–47.

Rosen, R. C., Wing, R., Schneider, S., & Gendrano III, N. (2005). Epidemiology of erectile dysfunction: The role of medical comorbidities and lifestyle factors. *Urologic Clinics of North America, 32*, 403–417.

Saigal, C. S., Wessells, H., Pace, J., Schonlau, M., & Wilt, T. J. (2006). Predictors and prevalence of erectile dysfunction in a racially diverse population. *Archives of Internal Medicine, 166*, 207–212.

Salonia, A., Briganti, A., Montorsi, P., Maga, T., Deho, F., Zanni, G., et al. (2005). Safety and tolerability of oral erectile dysfunction treatments in the elderly. *Drugs & Aging, 22*, 323–338.

Sasaki, K., Yoshimura, N., & Chancellor, M. B. (2003). Implications of diabetes mellitus in urology. *Urologic Clinics of North America, 30*, 1–12.

Sherman, F. T. (2002). Hormone replacement therapy: The sudden halt of a clinical trial shakes long held beliefs. *Geriatrics, 57*(8), 7–8.

Shifren, J. L., Davis, S. R., Moreau, M., Waldbaum, A., Bouchard, C., DeRogatis, L., et al. (2006). Testosterone patch for the treatment of hypoactive sexual desire disorder in naturally menopausal women: Results from the INTIMATE NM1 Study. *Menopause, 13*, 770–779.

Shiri, R., Hakama, M., Hakkinen, J., Tammela, T. L., Auvinen, A., & Koskimaki, J. (2005). Relationship between smoking and erectile dysfunction. *International Journal of Impotence Research, 17*, 164–169.

Slag, M., Morley, J. E., Elson, M. K., Trence, D. L., Nelson, C. J., Nelson, A. E., et al. (1983). Impotence in medical clinic patients. *Journal of the American Medical Association, 249*, 1736–1740.

Steinke, E. E. (2005). Intimacy needs and chronic illness. *Journal of Gerontological Nursing, 31*(5), 40–50.

Taylor, M. (2002). Alternative medicine and the perimenopause: An evidence-based review. *Obstetrics and Gynecology Clinics, 29*, 555–573.

Thomas, A., Woodard, C., Rovner, E. S., & Wein, A. J. (2003). Urologic complications of nonurologic medications. *Urology Clinics of North America, 30*, 123–131.

T'Sjoen, G. G., & Kaufman, J.-M. (2006). Androgen deficiency in aging men. *Current Opinion in Endocrinology and Diabetes, 13*, 254–261.

Tunstull, P., & Henry, M. E. (1996). Approaches to resident sexuality. *Journal of Gerontological Nursing, 22*(6), 37–42.

U.S. Preventive Services Task Force (USPSTF). (2005). Clinical guidelines: Hormone therapy for prevention of chronic conditions in postmenopausal women: Recommendations from the U. S. Preventive Services Task Force. *Annals of Internal Medicine, 142*, 855–860.

Velez, L., & Peggs, J. (2001). Managing behavioral problems in long-term care. *Clinics in Family Practice, 3*, 561–576.

Vermeulen, A. (2001). Special articles: Hormones and reproductive health. *Journal of Clinical Endocrinology and Metabolism, 86*, 2380–2390.

Walker, B. L., & Harrington, D. (2002). Effects of staff knowledge and attitudes about sexuality. *Educational Gerontology, 38*, 639–654.

Wallace, M. (2007). Sexuality assessment of older adults. *Try this: Best practices in nursing care to older adults,* Issue 10. New York University College of Nursing, Hartford Institute for Geriatric Nursing. Available at www.hartfordign.org/resources/education/tryThis.html.

Ward, R., Vass, A. A., Aggarwal, N., & Garfield, C. (2005). A kiss is still a kiss?: The construction of sexuality in dementia care. *Dementia, 4*, 49–72.

Weismiller, D. G., (2002). The perimenopause and menopause experience. *Clinics in Family Practice, 4*, 1–12.

Whiteman, M. K., Staropoli, C. A., Langenberg, P. W., McCarter, R. J., Kjerulff, K. H., & Flaws, J. A. (2003). Smoking, body mass, and hot flashes in midlife women. *Obstetrics and Gynecology, 101*, 264–272.

Wiley, D., & Bortz, W. M. (1996). Sexuality and aging: Usual and successful. *Journals of Gerontology: Series A, Biological Sciences and Medical Sciences, 51*, M142–M146.

Women's Health Initiative Investigators. (2002). Risks and benefits of estrogen plus progestin in healthy postmenopausal women: Principal results from the Women's Health Initiative randomized controlled trial. *Journal of the American Medical Association, 288*, 321–333.

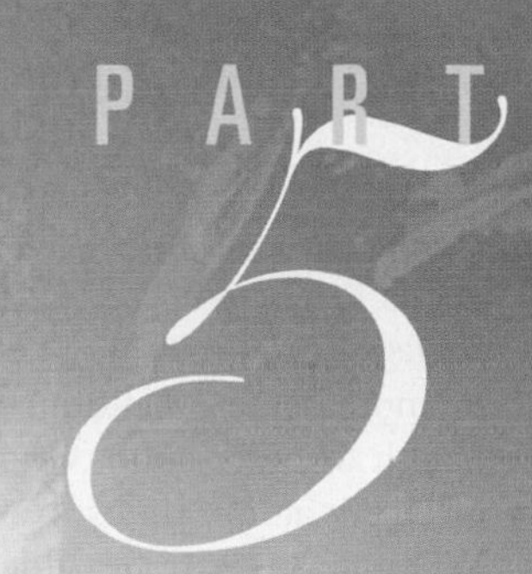

Promoting Wellness in All Stages of Health and Illness

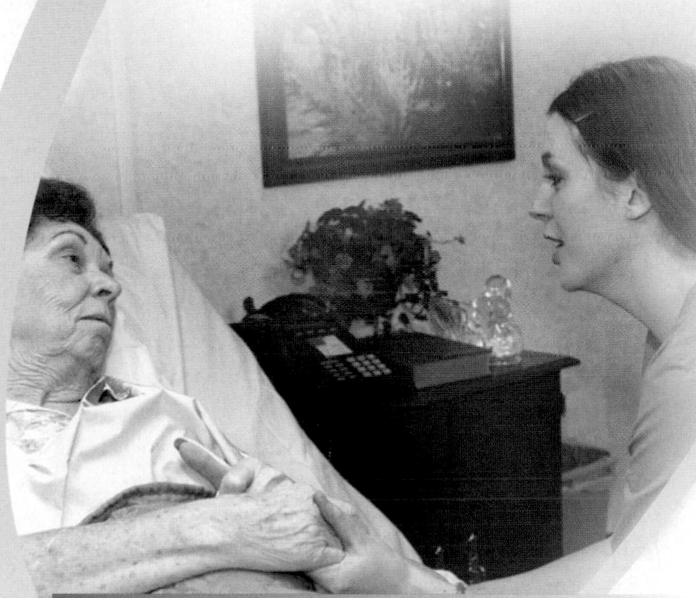

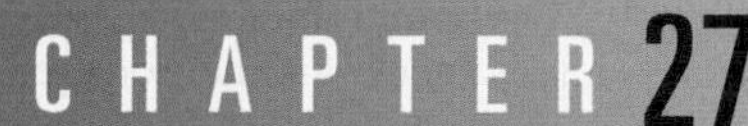

CHAPTER 27

Caring for Older Adults During Illness

Learning Objectives

After reading this chapter, you will be able to:

1. Describe characteristics of illness in older adults.
2. Discuss the role of nurses in promoting wellness in older adults who are ill.
3. Describe the palliative care model for addressing the needs of older adults during illness.
4. Apply wellness concepts to nursing care of older adults who have cancer, diabetes, or heart failure.
5. Describe the role of nurses in holistically addressing needs of families and caregivers.

Key Terms

caregiver burden
palliative care

Several factors differentiate care of older adults from that of other populations and add to the challenge of promoting wellness. Foremost among these is the reality that most older adults—and all of those whom nurses care for in acute and long-term care settings—are coping with several or even many pathologic conditions that threaten their wellness. Despite the presence of pathologic conditions, however, nurses can identify numerous opportunities to promote wellness, especially by addressing the whole person instead of focusing only on physiologic processes. This chapter discusses a philosophy of holistic care that is applicable for older adults who have chronic or progressively declining conditions. Concepts are applied to nursing care for older adults who have cancer, diabetes, and heart failure.

CHARACTERISTICS OF ILLNESS IN OLDER ADULTS

Older adults commonly have one or more chronic conditions that gradually accumulate and affect their daily functioning and quality of life. As discussed in Chapter 7, these chronic conditions, rather than acute conditions, account for most of the health care needs of older adults. Older adults typically receive health care on a continuing basis for a combination of chronic conditions, with the periodic acute episode that needs to be addressed. Even when acute conditions are the focus of care, interplay between chronic conditions and one or more acute conditions is likely to affect care. Thus, the health of older adults often fluctuates unpredictably and is affected at all times by multiple interacting conditions. When nurses care for older adults who are experiencing illness, then, they address not only the acute conditions but the interaction among acute and chronic conditions.

In addition to having more chronic conditions, older adults are more likely than their younger counterparts to have serious pathologic conditions (e.g., cancer) and neurodegenerative conditions (e.g., dementia) that seriously compromise their health. The diseases most prevalent among older adults are musculoskeletal conditions, stroke, hypertension, cardiovascular disease, cancer, dementia, diabetes, lung conditions, and hearing and vision impairments. They are also more likely to experience adverse effects from the medications they take for these conditions, as discussed in Chapter 8.

Consequences of illness in older adults are often far reaching and likely to affect both functioning and quality of life. For example, older adults with heart failure are often hospitalized when their condition becomes unstable and they are likely to be discharged to skilled care facilities for ongoing care before returning to independent living. These intermittent periods of care in institutional settings are likely to interfere with the person's ability to function independently. Eventually, they can lead to long-term placement in an assisted-living or other type of nursing facility, especially if the older adult does not have adequate supports for managing the condition at home. In addition, an illness that threatens the older adult's independence in this way may have serious psychosocial consequences. For example, in the United States, fear of being "put away" in a nursing home is a common—although often unfounded—worry among older people. Because of this anxiety, older people may deny symptoms of illness for fear that the solution will result in a loss of independence; they also may avoid the health care system and experience unnecessary anxiety about minor or treatable illnesses.

The combined and cumulative effects of aging (which diminish physiologic reserves) and disease (which place additional physiologic demands on the person) make it more difficult for older adults to adapt to the burden of acute illness or other additional physiologic stresses. Because even healthy older adults usually have many psychosocial stressors that require coping resources, coping with acute and chronic illnesses becomes even more stressful.

The cumulative effects of all these intermittent and interacting forces often leads to a "yo-yoing" effect: the person experiences a cycle of ups and downs in health, with the "yo-yo" failing to return to the height of its previous cycle. With diminishing resiliency during subsequent cycles, the yo-yo eventually loses its ability to bounce back. Promoting wellness involves holistically addressing the changing needs of older adults as they progress through these cycles of ups and downs. Thus, when nurses care for older adults, they typically address several nursing diagnoses simultaneously, reassessing the situation frequently so they can modify their goals accordingly. When nurses care for older adults holistically, they should be able to identify at least one wellness outcome in every situation.

Wellness Opportunity

By attending to the body–mind–spirit interconnectedness of older adults, nurses can identify opportunities to provide physical comfort and support emotional and spiritual growth even in situations involving inevitable physical decline.

A Student's Perspective

I learned a lot from my interview this past week. The woman I spoke with has gone through a lot of hardships in her life—and is still going through hardships—but she continues to move forward despite setbacks. She is suffering physical ailments, but her faith in God keeps her head above water. This woman was open to questioning and insightful with her answers. For being a quiet woman, she has a lot of inner strength she pulls on.

For a while after she was diagnosed with multiple sclerosis, she suffered depression and lost five dress sizes unintentionally. She also became fatigued and withdrawn. This was in line with how it has been shown that physical ailments can cause stress in a person, and that this in turn can cause other physical ailments. She was fortunate (if it can be called so) to be able lose the amount of weight that she did and not have severe consequences. If this were to happen to someone of lesser weight, the results may have been more serious. This is a first-hand experience of how depression can cause more than just sad feelings as effects. Once she accepted her fate, she gained back two dress sizes and is holding there, which she is content with.

Her daughter has also been diagnosed with MS, which is a blessing and burden at the same time. Her daughter has been diagnosed at a much younger age and has more serious problems with it, causing her to be periodically hospitalized. It is difficult for a mother to watch a daughter go through this, but it's a blessing that she has someone to share the experience with.

As stated earlier, her faith in God keeps her head above water. She still has her bouts with frustration, but she believes that God only gives what we can handle and that He is always there for her. Her strength is encouraging to the people around her. I know it has given me strength.

Anita M.

CONNECTING THE CONCEPTS OF WELLNESS, AGING, AND ILLNESS

Although the concepts of wellness and aging may seem almost contradictory, it is relatively easy to apply wellness to older adults who are healthy, functional, and satisfied with their lives. The greater challenge is to apply the concept of wellness to the nursing care of people who not only are in their 80s, 90s, or even older, but are seriously ill or even dying. It is necessary in these circumstances to understand wellness in the context of the body–mind–spirit interrelationship as well as one's relationships with self, others, and all that is sacred to the individual. When caring for older adults who are ill, nurses have unique opportunities to promote wellness by addressing needs related not only to physical comfort, health, and function, but also to emotional comfort and spiritual well-being. For example, nurses can promote wellness during illness through nursing actions such as the following:

- Helping older adults identify personal strengths that are not dependent on their physical health and functioning (e.g., emotional, interpersonal, and spiritual qualities), then identifying strategies that build on or improve these personal characteristics
- Supporting and promoting interpersonal relationships, including the development of new relationships and support resources, that can improve the older adult's health, functioning, and quality of life
- Helping older adults identify realistic goals for quality of life, which can be identified in any situation when wellness is conceptualized in the context of the body–mind–spirit interrelationship
- Facilitating the use of new resources and strengthening the support resources that already are in place for older adults, their families, and caregivers
- Identifying ways of supporting wellness for families and caregivers of dependent older adults

Personal responsibility for health is an important aspect of wellness for older adults because self-care is essential for achieving optimal health in people who have chronic illnesses. Nurses can help older adults identify ways to assume personal responsibility for their health, even when they are dependent on others for their care. Because personal responsibility for health—with regard to both general wellness and specific chronic conditions—often requires that a person address health-related behaviors, nurses can apply principles of behavior change as discussed in Chapter 5. Nurses and other health care professionals must be careful not to be influenced by ageist attitudes that would suggest that older adults are too old to learn or change behaviors.

Health promotion is an important aspect of wellness that should not be overlooked in the care of older adults suffering from illness. Unfortunately, ageist attitudes of health professionals, older adults, and family members create barriers to health promotion. For example, health care professionals may falsely believe that there is little or no benefit from improving health behaviors in later life. Moreover, ageist attitudes contribute to the low rate of cancer screening for older adults (Bourbonniere & Van Cleave, 2006). Fortunately, studies have debunked many of the myths that influence these ageist attitudes, as the following evidence indicates:

- Eliminating a risky behavior or initiating a health-protective behavior, even in later life, in most cases has positive effects on longevity, functional ability, and quality of life (Ferraro, 2006).
- In women 65 years of age and older, mammography is the most effective method for reducing breast cancer mortality and metastasis by detecting the disease at an early stage when cure is most likely (Greco, 2006).
- A study of chronically ill adults aged 50 years and older found that those who read health promotion materials about their chronic illnesses were twice as likely to engage in exercise self-care as the nonreaders (Chou & Wister, 2005).
- For adults of all ages, lifestyle interventions, such as diet, exercise, and weight loss, can reverse glucose intolerance, delay the onset of diabetes, and prevent many of its complications (Aldwin et al., 2006; Kelly et al., 2004).
- Quitting smoking is beneficial for people at any age, and smoking cessation programs are as effective in older people as in younger ones (Aldwin et al., 2006; Hajjar, 2004).

Although it is challenging to promote wellness for older adults when their health, functioning, and quality of life are compromised by illness, nurses can usually identify wellness-oriented outcomes and interventions if they use a holistic perspective. Table 27-1 lists examples of Nursing Outcomes Classification (NOC) and Nursing Interventions Classification (NIC) labels that are applicable to addressing psychosocial, comfort, health promotion, and spiritual needs. Nurses can incorporate these outcomes and interventions into care plans in conjunction with addressing the needs that are directly related to the primary health conditions.

HOLISTICALLY CARING FOR OLDER ADULTS WHO ARE ILL: FOCUSING ON CARING AND COMFORTING

Care and comfort are core components of all nursing, but they become even more important when a cure is not feasible. Equating aging with inability to cure not only is inaccurate, it is a great disservice to older adults. However, it also is a disservice to older adults to focus only on curing disease when they reach the point at which treatments are more detrimental than the underlying conditions. Moreover, because of the complexity of illness in older adults, the "turning point" when the focus changes from cure to care is rarely clearly defined. Thus, geriatricians, gerontologists,

TABLE 27-1 Nursing Outcomes and Nursing Interventions Classifications for Promoting Wellness in Older Adults During Illness

Type of Needs	Nursing Outcomes Classification (NOC)	Nursing Interventions Classification (NIC)
Psychosocial needs	Anxiety Level, Coping, Decision Making, Fear Level, Participation in Health Care Decisions, Personal Autonomy, Personal Well-Being, Self-Direction of Care, Self-Esteem, Social Involvement, Stress Level, Suffering Severity	Anxiety Reduction, Counseling, Coping Enhancement, Decision-Making Support, Emotional Support, Patient Rights Protection, Resiliency Promotion, Support Group, Simple Guided Imagery, Touch
Comfort needs	Comfort Level, Pain Control, Pain: Disruptive Effects, Sleep, Symptom Control, Thermoregulation	Pain Management, Positioning, Simple Massage, Temperature Regulation, Therapeutic Touch
Health promotion needs	Fall Prevention Behavior; Health Promoting Behavior; Immunization Behavior; Knowledge: Diet, Disease Process, Health Behavior, Health Resources, Illness Care, Medication; Nutritional Status; Physical Fitness; Risk Control; Risk Detection; Self-Care Status; Safe Home Environment	Anticipatory Guidance, Environmental Management: Comfort/Safety, Exercise Promotion, Fall Prevention, Health Education, Immunization Management, Nutrition Management, Risk Identification, Self-Responsibility Facilitation, Simple Relaxation Therapy, Skin Surveillance, Sleep Enhancement, Surveillance: Safety
Spiritual needs	Hope, Spiritual Health	Active Listening, Forgiveness Facilitation, Guilt Work Facilitation, Hope Instillation, Presence, Reminiscence Therapy, Religious Ritual Enhancement, Self-Awareness Enhancement, Spiritual Growth Facilitation, Spiritual Support
Quality-of-life needs	Leisure Participation, Personal Well-Being, Quality of Life	Animal-Assisted Therapy, Aromatherapy, Family Involvement Promotion, Humor, Music Therapy

ethicists, and gerontological nurses increasingly are trying to identify ways to improve quality of life for people whose quantity of life is limited.

The emergence of palliative care programs in recent years provides a framework for promoting wellness during serious illness, and palliative care is increasingly being incorporated into the care of older adults. For example, articles and entire books address palliative care for people with dementia in long-term care settings (e.g., Evans, 2002; Purtilo, 2004; Winn & Dentino, 2005). Professional literature, including nursing journals, also describes models of palliative care for chronic medical conditions such as heart failure (Davidson et al., 2004), orthopedic conditions (Watters et al., 2005), and in a variety of settings including homes, long-term care facilities, and medical intensive care units (e.g., Billings et al., 2006; Byock, 2006; Green & Wakefield, 2006; Pfeifer et al., 2006). Health care professionals increasingly are recognizing the value of applying palliative care principles to people who are experiencing the cumulative effects of conditions for which there is no cure.

The World Health Organization (1990) defined **palliative care** as a holistic approach to caring for patients with advanced progressive illnesses through prevention, assessment, and treatment of pain and other physical, psychosocial, and spiritual problems. Some articles state that palliative care is for people whose quantity of life is certain to be limited (e.g., Hopkins, 2004); however, the Clinical Practice Guidelines for Quality Palliative Care emphasize that these services are for people of all ages and with a broad range of persistent or recurring conditions that adversely affect their daily functioning or will predictably reduce life expectancy (National Consensus Project for Quality Palliative Care, 2004). Consistent with these guidelines, palliative care programs can effectively and holistically address the care and comfort needs of older adults with complex and declining conditions. Palliative care is always a part of hospice care, but the programs differ in that entry into hospice requires that the patient be in a terminal state (discussed in Chapter 29), whereas palliative care services can be provided at any point during the course of a chronic declining condition.

Increasing attention is being given to the use of palliative care to specifically address the needs of older adults. For example, a review of studies found that finding meaning and purpose in life is an aspect of quality of life that is very important to older patients receiving palliative care—and that can be addressed by nurses (Duggleby & Raudonis, 2006). Some characteristics of palliative care programs that are particularly pertinent to promoting wellness in older adults include

- A primary focus on ensuring comfort and psychosocial and spiritual well-being rather than on physical functioning
- Management of distressing symptoms (e.g., pain, thirst, nausea, dyspnea, constipation, dry mouth)
- Education and support of families and all support people (e.g., friends, volunteers, significant others)
- Consultation, education, and support of professional caregivers (e.g., nurses, nursing assistants, primary care providers)

Nurses have an important responsibility to recognize the appropriateness of a referral for palliative care and to initiate discussion of this option with older adults and their families. Although palliative care can be initiated at any time during the course of a serious illness, programs are usually provided in conjunction with hospice services, which are considered the established and proven model of palliative care (National Consensus Project for Quality Palliative Care, 2004). When discussing palliative care services with older adults or their families, nurses need to make sure they understand that although these services are provided in conjunction with hospice, they focus on management of symptoms rather than on care of dying, and they are generally short-term. Thus, nurses can contact local hospice organizations or provide referral information to families about palliative care services. Information also is available from the Hospice and Palliative Nurses Association, the National Hospice and Palliative Care Organization, and other organizations listed in the Educational Resources section at the end of this chapter.

APPLYING WELLNESS CONCEPTS IN SPECIFIC PATHOLOGIC OR CHRONIC CONDITIONS

Although it is beyond the scope of this book to address specific pathophysiologic conditions in depth, the next sections highlight some considerations that are more specific to promoting wellness in older adults who have cancer, diabetes, or heart failure. These three conditions are selected as examples and are discussed within the framework of the Functional Consequences Theory. The text identifies opportunities for nurses to focus on health promotion, self-management, and holistic aspects of care.

Promoting Wellness for Older Adults With Cancer

Because cancer is a condition that requires the passage of time before it reaches the stage of being a diagnosable disease, an increased risk of cancer is an unavoidable consequence of aging (Hajjar, 2004; Masoro, 2006). Thus, older adults are disproportionately affected by cancer, with 60% of all cancers and 70% of cancer-related deaths occurring in people 65 years of age and older (Greco, 2006). Compared with younger adults, those 65 years of age and older are less likely to be screened for cancer and are diagnosed at a later stage (Oncology Nursing Society and Geriatric Oncology Consortium, 2004).

Types of cancer that most commonly occur in older adults are skin, breast, prostate, lung, ovarian, cervical, brain, and non-Hodgkin's lymphoma. Cancer is an important focus of health promotion efforts because nearly two thirds of cancer deaths are from potentially preventable causes (Greco, 2006). In addition, cancer is one of the most correctable sources of disparities among minority elders who have excess morbidity and mortality in all phases (i.e., screening or diagnostic, treatment, and postcancer survival) (Miles, 2005). Thus, nurses have important health promotion roles with regard to teaching about cancer prevention and early detection.

Although cancer is highly prevalent among older adults, research, education, treatment, and public policy are limited, so there is a scarcity of evidence-based data specific to the older adult population (Oncology Nursing Society and Geriatric Oncology Consortium, 2004; Walter et al., 2005). This lack of data may be the result of ageist beliefs that older adults will not respond to treatment or health education. In addition, older adults themselves are likely to be influenced by their own misperceptions based on outdated beliefs. For example, they may have anxieties and fears based on inaccurate or outdated perceptions of a diagnosis of cancer being a "death sentence." Myths and ageist attitudes also can interfere with symptom management, especially with pain management (see Chapter 28).

Care of older adults with cancer is complicated not only by the pathologic processes of cancer itself, but also by the many interacting conditions that make their response to treatments riskier and less predictable. Moreover, cancer has evolved from an inevitably fatal disease to a chronic, progressive condition, and it often leads to permanent or temporary admission to a long-term care facility (Bourbonniere & Van Cleave, 2006). Thus, decisions about screening and treatment of cancer are more complex and need to be based not on chronologic age alone, but on a multidimensional assessment that considers all the following: effects of normal age-related changes, physical and psychosocial health and functioning, effects of accumulated chronic conditions, life expectancy, potential benefits versus harms, and the individual's values and preferences (Greco, 2006; White & Cohen, 2006).

Decisions about screening and treatment of cancer in older adults can be complicated for several reasons. When older adults have pathophysiologic conditions that compromise cognitive abilities, these decisions must be made by health care proxies. Although this holds true for many situations with older adults, it is particularly problematic when older adults have cancer because evidence-based guidelines for screening or treatment are often lacking. Treatment-related decisions are also complicated by the presence of medical conditions that affect the older adult's ability to tolerate treatments. In addition, older adults are less likely to have family and caregiver supports to assist with complex treatment regimens (e.g., transportation for radiation, assistance with dealing with chemotherapy treatments and effects), and this may affect treatment decisions.

Nursing Assessment

From a health promotion perspective, nurses assess older adults to identify their knowledge and attitudes about screening for the types of cancer most likely to develop. For example, skin cancer is one of the most commonly occurring types, and it can be readily detected through self-examination. Thus, nurses can assess whether older adults understand how important it is to check for skin cancer and what they need to look for (as discussed in Chapter 23). Nurses also assess level of knowledge about prevention of cancer because this provides a base for identifying health promotion goals. When caring for an older adult who has cancer, nurses holistically assess psychosocial aspects such as the meaning of cancer for the individual, coping strengths and supports, and the person's ability to participate in decisions about screening and care.

Wellness Nursing Diagnoses and Wellness Outcomes

Readiness for Enhanced Knowledge is a wellness nursing diagnosis applicable for older adults who are interested in learning about screening and prevention of cancer. This diagnosis would also be applicable if the person is interested in learning more about holistically oriented resources such as hospice services (discussed in Chapter 29). The wellness nursing diagnosis of Readiness for Enhanced Self-Care would be applicable for increasing personal responsibility for older adults who have cancer. For example, this would be particularly applicable with regard to complex decision making regarding treatment of cancer.

Two outcomes applicable to prevention and early detection of cancer are Health Promoting Behavior and Knowledge: Health Behavior. Outcomes that are pertinent to holistically caring for older adults with cancer include Comfort, Coping, and Quality of Life.

Nursing Interventions

Health promotion interventions focus on teaching older adults about primary prevention and early detection of cancer through screening, as summarized in Box 27-1. Nurses can encourage older adults and surrogate decision makers to discuss cancer detection and treatment options with their primary care providers with an emphasis on quality of life.

For older adults already diagnosed with cancer, nurses address all aspects of pain and comfort (see Chapter 28). Also, because people with cancer commonly use complementary and alternative therapies, nurses can teach them to obtain information from reliable sources (e.g., the National Cancer Institute and the National Center for Complementary and Alternative Medicine, listed under Educational Resources). In addition, nursing interventions include offering hope, support, and encouragement and considering referrals for hospice and palliative care. Nurses can find additional information about cancer in older adults through the Oncology Nursing Society and Geriatric Consortium and the Hospice and Palliative Care Nurses Association.

Wellness Opportunity

Nurses can promote personal responsibility for wellness by teaching older adults about screening and preventive actions they can take.

Box 27-1 Health Promotion Interventions Related to Cancer and Older Adults

Teaching About Primary Prevention

- Tobacco cessation (if applicable)
- Avoid secondhand smoke
- Maintain ideal body weight
- Consume at least five servings of fresh fruit and vegetables and 25 to 30 g of fiber daily
- Limit intake of fats, red meats, and fried foods
- Avoid exposure to sunlight
- Avoid excessive alcohol consumption

Screening Recommendations of the American Cancer Society for Older Adults

- Annual fecal occult blood
- Flexible sigmoidoscopy and double contrast barium enema every 5 years
- Colonoscopy every 10 years
- Annual prostate-specific antigen and digital rectal examination for men
- Annual mammogram, and Pap test every 2 to 3 years for women
- Annual checkup by primary care practitioner to examine skin, thyroid, oral cavity, breasts, ovaries, and testicles

Promoting Wellness for Older Adults With Diabetes Mellitus

Diabetes mellitus is one of the most common chronic conditions in older adults, and it affects at least 20% of people 65 years of age and older. Age-related changes that increase the risk for development of diabetes include declining beta cell function and increased insulin resistance (glucose intolerance). In addition to age-related changes, risk factors for diabetes include obesity, hypertension, family history, physical inactivity, high levels of triglycerides, and low levels of high-density lipoproteins. The prevalence of diabetes is disproportionately high among American Indians/Alaskan Natives, African Americans, Hispanic/Latino Americans, and Asian/Pacific Island Americans.

Disease management and nursing care related to diabetes are complicated by the common occurrence of concomitant conditions in older adults. For example, infections can affect the optimal doses of insulin and hypoglycemic agents, and chronic arthritis or periodic flare-ups of gout are likely to affect the older adult's level of activity. Another complicating factor is that older adults are likely to be taking medications that can lead to disease instability. For example, older adults are likely to have acute or chronic conditions that require treatment with prednisone, which, in turn, affects control of blood glucose. Conditions that occur more commonly in older adults such as dementia, depression, and functional limitations can interfere with self-management of diabetes, as can dependence on others who interfere with meals or financial constraints that affect ability to purchase medications and appropriate foods.

Older adults with diabetes are at greater risk for frailty, injurious falls, and a decline in functional status owing to complications such as the following: cognitive dysfunction, peripheral neuropathy, peripheral vascular disease, decreased pain threshold, and autonomic neuropathy (causing orthostatic and postprandial hypotension) (Morley et al., 2006). Negative functional consequences of diabetes in older adults include higher rates of premature death and concomitant conditions such as stroke, hypertension, and heart disease.

Nursing Assessment

Although nurses are not expected to diagnose diabetes, they are expected to know about variations in diagnostic indicators that are specific to older adults. For example, the renal threshold for glucose increases in older adults, so glycosuria is not an accurate indicator. A glucose tolerance test (GTT) is the most accurate diagnostic test, but the normal range is adjusted upward by 10 mg/dL at the first, second, and third hours for each decade after age 55 years. Diagnostic criteria for diabetes in older adults include any of the following: fasting blood glucose of at least 136 mg/dL on two occasions or plasma glucose concentrations (either random or after oral glucose intake) of at least 200 mg/dL.

In addition to the usual nursing assessment parameters for diabetes, a holistic nursing approach for older adults addresses issues such as the meaning of the condition to the person, identification of ageist attitudes that may affect management, and socioeconomic and cultural influences. Box 27-2 summarizes some questions that are more specific to assessment of diabetes in older adults from a wellness perspective.

Box 27-2
Assessment Guidelines for Older Adults With Diabetes

Considerations About the Meaning of Diabetes

- What terminology is appropriate for discussing the condition (e.g., older adults may refer to diabetes as "sugar")?
- What is the person's understanding of diabetes?

Considerations for Disease Management

- What is the person's understanding of personal responsibility for managing diabetes?
- Socioeconomic influences: Who does grocery shopping and meal preparation? What is the usual "budget" for food? Where does the person eat meals?
- What cultural factors affect health beliefs, disease management, food preparation, eating patterns, and health-related behaviors, such as exercise?
- What concomitant conditions affect the older adult's self-care abilities?

Considerations Regarding the Influence of Ageist Attitudes

- Do ageist attitudes (of the older adult, caregiver, or health care professionals) interfere with setting wellness-oriented goals? (e.g., "I've been eating donuts for breakfast all my life, why should I worry about that now at my age?")
- Does the older adult (or do others) inaccurately associate a sense of hopelessness with his or her condition because of advanced age? (e.g., "At my age, I can't do anything about my sugar levels.")

Wellness Nursing Diagnoses and Wellness Outcomes

Readiness for Enhanced Knowledge is a wellness nursing diagnosis applicable for older adults who are interested in learning about diabetes, especially with regard to improved understanding of how this condition affects their health. Nurses can use the wellness nursing diagnosis of Readiness for Enhanced Self-Care when they care for older adults who are interested in improving personal responsibility for management of their condition, including preventing complications.

Outcomes that would be pertinent to promoting wellness in older adults with diabetes include the following:

- Diabetes Self-Management
- Blood Glucose Level
- Health Promoting Behavior
- Knowledge: Diabetes Management
- Self-Care Status

Nursing Interventions

Care plans for older adult with diabetes include all the usual interventions that apply to all adults with diabetes (e.g., teaching about nutrition, exercise, medications, glucose monitoring and other aspects of self-care). Nurses should emphasize the importance of ophthalmologic care, podiatric care, prevention of injury, and observations of wound healing. In addition, nurses often need to address factors that are more common among older adults, such as involving and teaching caregivers, compensating for memory deficits, and identifying the most cost-effective ways of obtaining medications and glucometer supplies. Older adults with diabetes may benefit from referrals for community-based services, including home-delivered meals, assistance with grocery shopping or meal preparation, participation in group meal programs, transportation to appointments, and assistance with medication management or glucose monitoring. Provision of such services for an older adult with diabetes is often an essential element in both ensuring optimal control and supporting the person's ability to remain in his or her own home.

Nurses also may need to address fear and anxiety in older adults and caregivers and to encourage discussion of feelings about diabetes and the impact of this chronic condition on the person's health and lifestyle. Nurses can help older adults identify safe and enjoyable ways of engaging in physical activity, especially if they have concomitant conditions that affect their ability to exercise. For example, swimming or aquatherapy classes may be more appropriate than walking for an older adult who has arthritis or problems with balance.

Wellness Opportunity

Nurses can teach all older adults about actions they can take to prevent diabetes by using resources such as the tools adapted from the Diabetes Prevention Program, which is available from the National Diabetes Education Program at www.ndep.nih.gov.

Promoting Wellness for Older Adults With Heart Failure

Although only 10% of people 70 years of age and older have heart failure, this condition is the leading indication for hospitalization in older adults (Deaton et al., 2004; Rich, 2006). Moreover, it is the most expensive medical diagnosis in the United States for people 65 years of age and older, but it is estimated that one third to one half of hospital readmissions could be prevented through better health education (Clark et al., 2006). In addition to recurrent hospitalizations, other common consequences of heart failure in older adults include the following:

- Increased likelihood of development of arrhythmias, which can be life-threatening or cause syncopal episodes
- Increased risk for hypotension and falls because of compromised cardiovascular function and adverse medication effects
- Increased risk for hospital-acquired iatrogenic conditions, such as *Clostridium difficile* infection
- Increased risk for drug interactions and adverse medication effects, especially if the older adult has concomitant conditions and requires several types of medications
- High incidence of sleep disorders
- Shorter life expectancy

Because of consequences such as these, which make it a major source of chronic disability and impaired quality of life, heart failure in older adults has emerged as a major focus of health promotion (Rich, 2006).

Nursing Assessment

Nurses assess for signs and symptoms of heart failure in older adults using the same assessment techniques that apply to adults of any age. However, older adults are more likely to have concomitant conditions that can affect the assessment. For example, because older adults with mobility limitations may not exert themselves enough to experience dyspnea, nurses need to consider other limiting factors when they assess the effects of heart failure on respirations. Another assessment consideration is that older adults with heart failure are likely to have some degree of chronic renal failure, which often fluctuates within an abnormal range. Thus, nurses need to identify and document the older adult's usual indicators of renal function (i.e., ranges of blood urea nitrogen and creatinine that are typical for that individual). Because older adults with heart failure and renal failure are at increased risk for electrolyte imbalance and adverse medication effects, nurses need to assess for these and other consequences. If the older adult with heart failure also has dementia, nurses need to assess mental status, recognizing that it may be influenced by the degree to which the heart failure is controlled.

In addition to assessing signs and symptoms of heart failure, nurses assess risk factors, paying particular attention to those that can be addressed through health promotion interventions. Factors that increase the risk for heart failure include hypertension, coronary artery disease, myocardial infarction, family history of heart failure, hyperthyroidism, diabetes, smoking, obesity, and cardiotoxic drugs (e.g., some cancer chemotherapy agents). Even though older adults may have long-term patterns of behavior that affect disease management (e.g., smoking, inadequate physical activity, or high-sodium diets), nurses need to assess their attitudes about changing these behaviors so they can address this in health promotion teaching.

Additional wellness-focused assessment considerations that are important for older adults who have heart failure are outlined in Box 27-3.

Wellness Nursing Diagnoses and Wellness Outcomes

Nurses can use the wellness nursing diagnosis of Readiness for Enhanced Therapeutic Regimen Management to promote increased personal responsibility for management of heart failure and prevention of hospitalizations and other complications. The wellness nursing diagnosis of Readiness

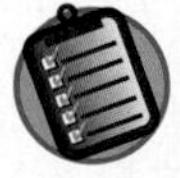

Box 27-3
Assessment Guidelines for Older Adults With Heart Failure

Considerations About the Meaning of Heart Failure

- What is the older adult's understanding of heart failure?
- What terminology is appropriate for discussing the condition? Does the term *failure* cause anxiety or fear?
- What personal experiences or those of significant others are influencing the older adult's response to cardiovascular disease? (e.g., How life-threatening does the person perceive this to be?)

Considerations Regarding the Influence of Ageist Attitudes

- Do ageist attitudes interfere with health promotion interventions? (e.g., Do health care providers avoid teaching about smoking cessation because they think the person is too old to quit or to benefit from quitting?)

Considerations Regarding Disease Management

- Does the older adult have questions or fears about engaging in therapeutic or enjoyable activities (e.g., exercise, swimming, sexual relationships)? If so, would he or she benefit from health education about this?
- Do socioeconomic factors affect disease management (e.g., limited income that interferes with ability to purchase needed medications or healthy foods)?

for Enhanced Fluid Balance might be applicable when older adults with heart failure are interested in learning about actions they can take to improve and maintain fluid and electrolyte balance.

Outcomes that are pertinent to promoting wellness in older adults with heart failure include the following:

- Cardiac Disease Self-Management
- Energy Conservation
- Health Promoting Behavior
- Knowledge: Cardiac Disease Management

Nursing Interventions

In addition to providing the usual patient teaching about medications, nurses caring for older adults with heart failure must monitor for digoxin toxicity (because there is a very narrow therapeutic range) and provide patient education about drug interactions and the effect of drugs and other concomitant conditions. For example, nonsteroidal anti-inflammatory agents, including over-the-counter ones, are associated with development of heart failure and can interfere with antihypertensives and angiotensin-converting enzyme inhibitors.

Wellness-oriented care plans for older adults with heart failure focus on teaching about actions the person can take to achieve the best possible level of functioning and quality of life despite the chronic condition. For example, nurses can teach older adults about planning appropriate rest and "energy management" techniques to achieve optimum quality of life with limited energy. Nurses also need to address psychosocial consequences associated with heart failure, such as fear, anxiety, loneliness, and depression (discussed in Chapters 12, 13, and 15). Another health promotion intervention is to encourage older adults who have risks for falls to perform exercises while seated. Nurses also can suggest participation in t'ai chi as a holistic exercise modality.

Wellness Opportunity

Because stress reduction activities are especially important when older adults have chronic conditions such as heart failure, nurses can suggest relaxation and health promotion activities such as breathing, meditation, and guided imagery.

ADDRESSING NEEDS OF FAMILIES AND CAREGIVERS

During periods of illness, whether acute, chronic, or declining, the importance of relationships increases in proportion to the need not only for physical care but for emotional and spiritual care. Thus, when nurses care for older adults during illness, families and caregivers are an integral focus of care. Even with the increasing availability of formal services for older adults in the United States, families and friends continue to provide 80% to 90% of the care given to dependent older adults in the community. For older adults who have dementia or other conditions that cause progressive declines in functioning, the role of caregiver usually evolves gradually and can last for years. Even in situations in which older adults do not have progressively declining conditions, families of older adults frequently deal with intermittent and cumulative conditions that require intense medical care or rehabilitative services. It is not uncommon for families of older adults to take on roles of care managers and find themselves negotiating health care services for at least one and sometimes several parents, grandparents, aunts, uncles, and other relatives and "significant others."

The term **caregiver burden** is commonly used to describe the financial, physical, and psychosocial problems that family members experience when caring for older adults who are impaired or suffering from illness. Most studies of caregiver burden focus on stresses related to caring for people in home settings, but some studies suggest that moving the dependent person to a nursing home does not alleviate or even diminish the stress (Larrimore, 2003). Researchers have identified the following specific functional consequences of caregiving (Acton, 2002; Larrimore, 2003; Narayan et al., 2001):

- Depression
- Disturbed sleep
- Social isolation
- Family discord
- Career interruptions
- Financial difficulties
- Lack of time for self
- Poor physical health
- Impaired immune function
- Mental, physical, and emotional strain
- Feelings of anger, guilt, grief, anxiety, hopelessness, helplessness, and chronic fatigue

Although most gerontologists have focused on the burdens of caregiving, there is increasing recognition that caregivers experience positive as well as negative consequences. For example, Narayan and colleagues (2001) found that spouse caregivers of people with dementia experienced their caregiving role as self-fulfilling and affirming, while at the same time experiencing the losses and hardships of their role. The caregiving experience can cause anger, ambivalence, and emotional fragility; however, it can also be a source of strength and personal growth (Acton, 2002). Gerontologists currently emphasize the need to assess the caregiving experience in the context of the caregiver's whole life and to identify burdensome as well as beneficial aspects (Suwa, 2002). The Hartford Institute for Geriatric Nursing recommends the Caregiver Strain Index (Sullivan, 2002) as a best practice tool that has high reliability and validity.

Nurses address teaching needs of older adults' families and significant others as an essential nursing responsibility, particularly in home care and community settings and as part of plans for discharging patients from any institutional

TABLE 27-2 Nursing Outcomes and Nursing Interventions Classifications for Promoting Wellness in Caregivers

Type of Needs	Nursing Outcomes Classification (NOC)	Nursing Interventions Classification (NIC)
Needs related to caregiver role	Caregiver Adaptation to Patient Institutionalization, Caregiver Emotional Health, Caregiver Endurance Potential, Caregiver Home Care Readiness, Caregiver Lifestyle Disruption, Caregiver–Patient Relationship, Caregiver Performance: Direct/Indirect Care, Caregiver Physical Health, Caregiver Stressors, Caregiver Well-Being	Caregiver Support, Case Management, Counseling, Energy Management, Family Support, Family Integrity Promotion, Resiliency Promotion, Role Enhancement, Self-Awareness Enhancement, Support Group
Needs related to using resources and managing care	Information Processing, Knowledge: Health Resources, Participation in Health Care Decisions, Role Performance	Decision-Making Support, Health Education, Health System Guidance, Referral, Respite Care, Support System Enhancement, Teaching: Individual, Telephone Consultation
Psychosocial needs	Anxiety Level, Coping, Decision Making, Depression Level, Family Coping, Family Resiliency, Fear Level, Grief Resolution, Loneliness Severity, Self-Esteem, Stress Level	Active Listening, Anticipatory Guidance, Anxiety Reduction, Cognitive Restructuring, Coping Enhancement, Emotional Support, Grief Work Facilitation, Mood Management, Presence, Simple Guided Imagery
Spiritual and quality-of-life needs	Hope, Leisure Participation, Quality of Life, Sleep, Social Involvement, Social Support, Spiritual Health	Forgiveness Facilitation, Guilt Work Facilitation, Hope Instillation, Humor, Sleep Enhancement, Spiritual Support

setting or formal health care programs (e.g., inpatient, outpatient, or long-term care settings). Consistent with this responsibility, nurses follow standards of care and document the teaching they provide regarding caregiving instructions, but they do not necessarily address the broader needs of caregivers because of barriers such as time constraints and not perceiving this as an essential aspect of care. However, when nurses care for dependent older adults, it is important to recognize that even the basic needs of the older adult cannot be met without a strong support system. Thus, nurses need to identify outcomes and interventions to prevent caregiver burnout and enhance the ability of families and other caregivers to provide the necessary care. Although it is beyond the scope of this book to comprehensively discuss ways of addressing caregiver needs, Table 27-2 lists NOC and NIC terms that are applicable to promoting wellness for families and caregivers who are involved with care of ill or dependent older adults.

Chapter Highlights

Characteristics of Illness in Older Adults

- Presence of many interacting conditions and factors (e.g., acute illness, chronic conditions, psychosocial factors, environmental conditions, age-related changes, medication effects)
- Complexity of interpreting signs and symptoms (e.g., vague or atypical manifestations)
- Far-reaching consequences (e.g., loss of independence due to fractured hip)
- Cumulative effects of aging and illness make it difficult to adapt
- Older adults are likely to experience a “yo-yoing” pattern of health, with gradually diminishing resiliency

Connecting the Concepts of Wellness, Aging, and Illness

- A holistic perspective enables nurses to identify ways of promoting wellness by addressing needs related to physical health and functioning and emotional and spiritual well-being.
- Nurses promote personal responsibility for managing illness, especially chronic conditions.
- Nurses challenge ageist attitudes and provide health education to foster behavior change when appropriate.
- Many NIC and NOC terms are applicable in care plans that address psychosocial, comfort, health promotion, and spiritual needs (Table 27-1).

Holistically Caring for Older Adults Who Are Ill: Focusing on Caring and Comforting

- Palliative care is a holistic approach to caring for patients with advanced progressive illnesses through prevention, assessment, and treatment of pain and other physical, psychosocial, and spiritual problems.
- Nurses have important roles in suggesting referrals for palliative care and talking with older adults and their families about the scope of these services.

Promoting Wellness for Older Adults With Cancer

- Older adults are disproportionately affected by cancer, they are less likely to be screened for cancer, and they are diagnosed at a later stage.
- From a health promotion perspective, nurses assess older adults to identify their knowledge and attitudes about screening for the types of cancer that they are most likely to develop.

- Nurses can teach older adults about primary prevention interventions and about screening recommendations (Box 27-1).

Promoting Wellness for Older Adults With Diabetes

- Diabetes affects at least 20% of older adults.
- Disease management and nursing care related to diabetes are complicated by the common occurrence of concomitant conditions and by the increased vulnerability of older adults to complications.
- In addition to usual assessment parameters, nurses identify ageist attitudes and the meaning of diabetes (Box 27-2).
- Care plans for older adults with diabetes include all the usual interventions and additional teaching points (e.g., teaching caregivers, referring for community-based services, and appropriate ways of engaging in physical activity).

Promoting Wellness for Older Adults With Heart Failure

- Heart failure affects only 10% of older adults, but it is the leading cause of hospitalization. It is the most expensive medical diagnosis, but one third to one half of hospitalizations could be prevented through better health education.
- In addition to assessing all the usual signs and symptoms of heart failure, nurses assess effects of other conditions, risk factors that can be addressed through health promotion, and other aspects that are specific to older adults (e.g., the effects of ageist attitudes).
- In addition to all the usual teaching points, wellness-oriented care plans focus on teaching about actions the person can take to achieve the best possible level of functioning and quality of life, despite the effects of heart failure.

Addressing Needs of Families and Caregivers

- Functional consequences of caregiving (burdens and benefits)
- Many NIC and NOC terms are applicable in care plans that address caregivers with regard to role performance; use of resources and management of care; and psychosocial, spiritual, and quality-of-life needs (Table 27-2).

Critical Thinking Exercises

1. Identify an older person (in your personal life or clinical experience) who has recently been hospitalized and address the following in relation to that person:
   - How many different conditions (e.g., acute and chronic illness, functional limitations, support resources, psychosocial factors, or environmental factors) affected how the person was able to adapt to the hospitalization?
   - How did these factors affect the outcome for the person (e.g., longer hospitalization, increased dependency on others, discharge plans)?
   - Select two NOC and NIC terms from Table 27-1 that you could apply to a care plan to promote wellness for this person.
2. Think about your expectations for older adults who are affected by multiple interacting conditions and identify any ageist attitudes or assumptions that are likely to affect your care.
3. Identify a situation in your personal life or clinical experience that requires caregiving assistance from a family member at least once weekly and address the following in relation to this situation:
   - What benefits (rewards) and stresses is the caregiver likely to experience?
   - Select two NOC and NIC terms from Table 27-2 that you could apply to a care plan to address the needs of this caregiver.

Clinical Tool Resources

Hartford Institute for Geriatric Nursing
Try This: Best Practices in Nursing Care to Older Adults
Issue Number 13 (Revised 2007), Caregiver Strain Index (CSI)
www.hartfordign.org/resources/education/tryThis.html

Educational Resources

Hospice and Palliative Nurses Association
www.HPNA.org

National Diabetes Education Program
www.ndep.nih.gov

National Hospice and Palliative Care Organization
www.nhpco.org

Oncology Nursing Society
www.ons.org

References

Acton, G. J. (2002). Self-transcendent views and behaviors: Exploring growth in caregivers of adults with dementia. *Journal of Gerontological Nursing, 28*(12), 22–30.

Aldwin, C. M., Spiro, A., & Park, C. L. (2006). Health, behavior, and optimal aging: A life span developmental perspective. In J. E. Birren & K. W. Schaie (Eds.), *Handbook of the psychology of aging* (6th ed., pp. 85–104). San Diego: Academic Press.

Billings, J. A., Keeley, A., Bauman, J., Cist, A., Coakley, E., Dahlin, C., et al. (2006). Merging cultures: Palliative care specialists in the medical intensive care unit. *Critical Care Medicine, 34*(11), S388–S393.

Bourbonniere, M., & Van Cleave, J. H. (2006). Cancer care in nursing homes. *Seminars in Oncology Nursing, 22*, 51–57.

Byock, I. (2006). Where do we go from here? A palliative care perspective. *Critical Care Medicine, 34*(11), S416–S420.

Chou, P. H. B., & Wister, A. V. (2005). From cues to action: Information seeking and exercise self-care among older adults managing chronic illness. *Canadian Journal on Aging, 24*, 395–408.

Clark, A. P., Stuifbergen, A., Gottlieb, N. H., Voelmeck, W., Darby, D., & Delville, C. (2006). Health promotion in heart failure: A paradigm shift. *Holistic Nursing Practice, 20*, 73–79.

Davidson, P. M., Paull, G., Introna, K., Cockburn, J., Davis, J., Rees, D., et al. (2004). Integrated, collaborative palliative care in heart failure: The St. George Heart Failure Service Experience 1999–2002. *Journal of Cardiovascular Nursing, 19*(1), 68–75.

Deaton, C., Bennett, J. A., & Riegel, B. (2004). State of the science for care of older adults with heart disease. *Nursing Clinics of North America, 39*, 495–528.

Duggleby, W., & Raudonis, B. (2006). Dispelling myths about palliative care and older adults. *Seminars in Oncology Nursing, 22*, 58–64.

Evans, B. D. (2002). Improving palliative care in the nursing home: From a dementia perspective. *Journal of Hospice and Palliative Care, 4*, 91–99.

Ferraro, K. F. (2006). Health and aging. In R. H. Binstock & L. K. George (Eds.), *Handbook of aging and the social sciences* (6th ed., pp. 238–256). San Diego: Academic Press.

Greco, K. (2006). Cancer screening in older adults in an era of genomics and longevity. *Seminars in Oncology Nursing, 22*, 10–19.

Green, A., & Wakefield, A. (2006). A unique approach to supportive palliative care. *Journal of Hospice and Palliative Nursing, 8*, 164–171.

Hajjar, R. R. (2004). Cancer in the elderly: Is it preventable? *Clinics in Geriatric Medicine, 20*, 293–416.

Hopkins, K. (2004). BAPEN Symposium 2: Nutrition in palliative care. *Proceedings of the Nutrition Society, 63*, 427–429.

Kelly, J. M., Marrero, D. G., Gallivan, J., Leontos, C., & Perry, S. (2004). Diabetes prevention: A game plan for success. *Geriatrics, 59*(7), 26–32.

Larrimore, K. L. (2003). Alzheimer disease support group characteristics: A comparison of caregivers. *Geriatric Nursing, 24*, 32–35, 49.

Masoro, E. J. (2006). Are age-associated diseases an integral part of aging? In E. J. Masoro & S. N. Austad (Eds.), *Handbook of the biology of aging* (6th ed., pp. 43–62). San Diego: Academic Press.

Miles, T. P. (2005). Correctable sources of disparities in cancer among minority elders. *Medical Clinics of North America, 89*, 869–894.

Morley, J. E., Haren, M. T., Rolland, Y., & Kim, M. J. (2006). Frailty. *Medical Clinics of North America, 90*, 837–847.

Narayan, S., Lewis, M., Tornatore, J., Hepburn, K., & Corcoron-Perry, S. (2001). Subjective responses to caregiving for a spouse with dementia. *Journal of Gerontological Nursing, 27*(2), 19–28.

National Consensus Project for Quality Palliative Care. (2004). *Clinical practice guidelines for quality palliative care*. Available at www.nationalconsensusproject.org. Accessed January 17, 2007.

Oncology Nursing Society and Geriatric Oncology Consortium. (2004). Joint position on cancer care in older adults. *Oncology Nursing Forum, 21*(3), 1–2.

Pfeifer, M. P., Ritchie, C., Scharfenberger, J., Keeney, C., Hermann, C., Berwick, M., et al. (2006). The caring connections project: Providing palliative care to Medicaid patients with advanced cancer. *Lippincott's Case Management, 11*, 318–326.

Purtilo, R. B. (2004). Social marginalization of persons with disability. In R. B. Purtilo & H. tenHave (Eds.), *Ethical foundations of palliative care for Alzheimer's disease* (pp. 290–304). Baltimore: Johns Hopkins University Press.

Rich, M. W. (2006). Heart failure in older adults. *Medical Clinics of North America, 90*, 863–885.

Sullivan, M. T. (2002). Caregiver Strain Index (CSI). *Try this: Best practices in nursing care to older adults*, Issue 14. New York University, Hartford Institute for Geriatric Nursing. Available at www.hartfordign.org/resources/education/tryThis.html.

Suwa, S. (2002). Assessment scale for caregiver experience with dementia. *Journal of Gerontological Nursing, 28*(12), 2–12.

Walter, L. C., Lewis, C. L., & Barton, M. B. (2005). Screening for colorectal, breast, and cervical cancer in the elderly: A review of the evidence. *American Journal of Medicine, 118*, 1078–1086.

Watters, C. L., Harvey, C. V., Meehan, A. J., & Schoenly, L. (2005). Palliative care: A challenge for orthopaedic nursing care. *Orthopaedic Nursing, 24*(1), 4–7.

Winn, P. A. S., & Dentino, A. N. (2005). Quality palliative care in long-term care settings. *Journal of the American Medical Directors Association, 6*, S89–S98.

White, H. K., & Cohen, H. J. (2006). The older cancer patient. *Medical Clinics of North America*, 90, 967–983.

World Health Organization. (1990). *Cancer pain relief and palliative care* (pp. 11–12). Geneva: Author.

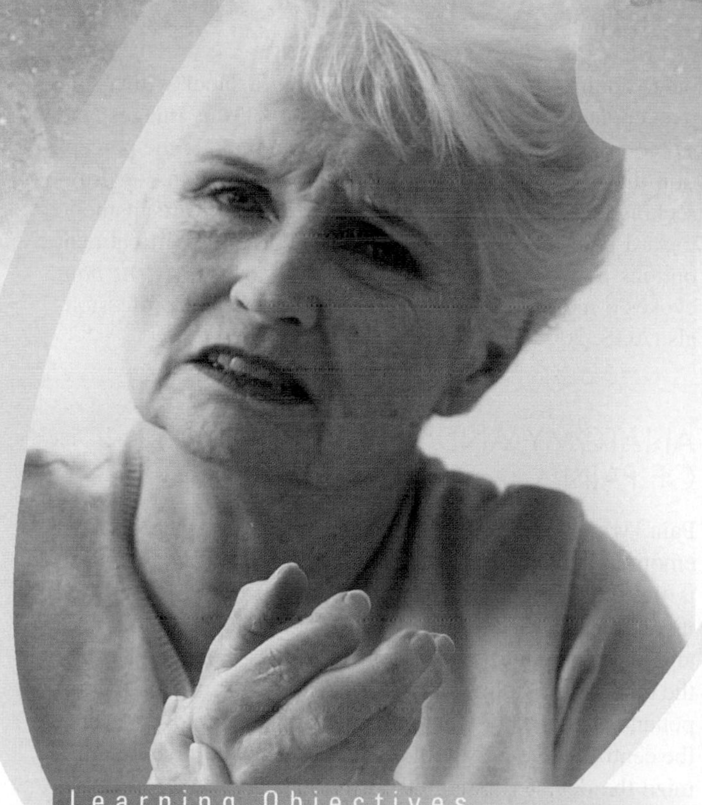

CHAPTER 28

Caring for Older Adults Experiencing Pain

Learning Objectives

After reading this chapter, you will be able to:

1. Define acute versus persistent pain, and identify the scope of the problem of pain and barriers to effective pain management.
2. Explain the physiology of pain and identify treatment options.
3. Examine and dispel commonly held myths and beliefs about persistent pain in older adults.
4. Provide age-appropriate assessment techniques for effective pain management and patient advocacy for pain management issues.
5. Describe principles of analgesic medication use in older adults.

Key Terms

acute pain
addiction
adjuvant analgesics
cancer pain
dependence
modulation
neuropathic pain
nociception
nociceptive pain
nonopioid analgesics
opioid analgesics
pain
pain intensity
pain receptors
perception
persistent pain
primary afferent nociceptors
somatic pain
tolerance
transduction
transmission
visceral pain

The experience of pain is not unique to older adults, but the higher rate of chronic conditions in this patient population places them at increased risk for pain. Nurses who care for older adults have an important responsibility to assess pain in order to plan appropriate pain management interventions. In addition, nurses need to be able to address common misconceptions about pain in older adults and implement effective pain management plans. This chapter provides a base of information about common types of pain and discusses assessment and pain management interventions that are important for addressing pain in older adults.

DEFINITIONS: ACUTE VERSUS PERSISTENT PAIN

Pain is defined as an unpleasant sensory and emotional experience associated with actual or potential tissue damage (Gordon et al., 2005; International Association for the Study of Pain, 1986). McCaffery (1968) presented the most commonly used definition of pain as being whatever the person experiencing it says it is, existing whenever she or he says it does.

Acute pain is sharp, immediate pain from an injury to tissue, but it can also be triggered by physiologic malfunction or severe illness. It is a warning signal of possible or actual tissue damage, and is the normal, predicted physiologic response to an adverse chemical, thermal, or mechanical stimulus. It is generally time limited and responsive to anti-inflammatory and opioid medications, as well as other treatments. Acute pain may be caused by trauma or an acute medical or orthopedic problem. Additional types of acute pain are postoperative pain, acute exacerbations of pain associated with chronic medical problems (e.g., cancer or postherpetic neuralgia), and pain associated with medical procedures.

The importance of effectively treating acute pain and providing greater comfort with the use of new medications and techniques must be emphasized not only with regard to the needs and quality of life of the individual, but in relation to broader effects. For example, recent research indicates that the failure to effectively treat acute pain can lead to prolonged hospital stays and delayed recovery, both of which ultimately drive up health care costs and adversely affect medical and social outcomes (Chin et al., 2001; McDonnell et al., 2003). More important for older adults, however, is the potential for acute pain to develop into persistent pain (Shipton & Tait, 2005).

Clinical practice guidelines, established by professional groups such as the American Pain Society (APS), the International Association for the Study of Pain (IASP), and the American Geriatrics Society (AGS), define **persistent pain** as a multidimensional phenomenon characterized by unpleasant sensory and emotional experiences. Persistent pain is a state in which pain persists beyond the usual course of an injury or acute disease, and is associated with actual or potential tissue damage that continues for a prolonged period and that may or may not be associated with a recognizable disease process (AGS, 2002; Gordon et al., 2005; IASP, 1986). Some experts, such as the IASP, use a period of 3 months to designate persistent pain (IASP, 1986), and others, including the APS, use 6 months (Gordon et al., 2005). Although the terms *persistent* and *chronic* are often used interchangeably, for many older adults, *chronic pain* has become a label with negative connotations. Examples of some of the images and stereotypes associated with chronic pain include the perception that these patients have psychiatric problems or drug-seeking behaviors, that health care practitioners are apathetic toward pain management, and that in general the treatment options available are ineffective. The term *persistent pain* evokes a more positive reaction by patients and professionals (AGS, 2002).

ANATOMY AND PHYSIOLOGY OF PAIN

Pain, which is a subjective experience, involves both an emotional quality and a physiologic sensation. **Nociception** is the physiologic occurrence of a measurable pain signal involving the transmission of information to the spinal cord and brain about inflammation or tissue damage. Despite the unpleasant feeling of pain, nociception is a critical component of the body's defense mechanism, rapidly warning the central nervous system to initiate motor neurons to minimize the detected potential for harm. Four basic processes occur with nociception: (1) transduction, (2) transmission, (3) perception, and (4) modulation (Fig. 28-1).

Transduction is the conversion of one energy form to another. A noxious stimulus of a mechanical, thermal, or chemical nature causes tissue damage, resulting in a release of substances that activate nociceptors and lead to the generation of an impulse known as an *action potential*. Primary afferent nociceptors are classified according to their diam-

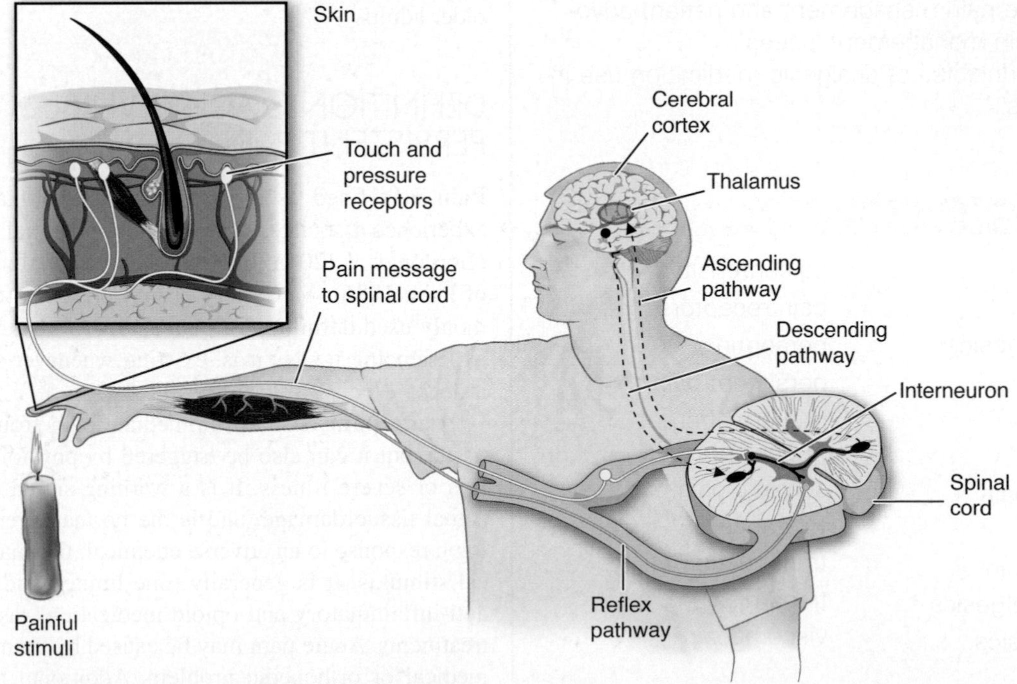

FIGURE 28-1 Processes involved in the physiology of pain.

eter, degree of myelination, and conduction velocity. The largest-diameter fibers, A-beta fibers, respond maximally to light touch or moving stimuli. They are present primarily in nerves that innervate the skin. In healthy individuals, the activity of these fibers does not produce pain. There are two other classes of primary afferents: the small-diameter myelinated A-delta (A fibers) and the unmyelinated (C fiber) axons. These fibers, known as **primary afferent nociceptors** or **pain receptors**, are present in nerves to the skin and to deep somatic and visceral structures. Most A and C afferents respond maximally only to intense or pain-inducing stimuli and produce the subjective experience of pain when they are electrically stimulated. This stimulation occurs when damaged cells release sensitizing substances, such as substance P, histamine, and prostaglandins, which trigger changes in the neuron cell membrane that permit an influx of sodium ions (Na^+) as well as other ion transfers. The resulting change in electrical charge generates an action potential, and the signal is transmitted to the central nervous system.

Transmission is the continuation of the action potential from the site of damage to the spinal cord and then to the brain. Transmission occurs in three phases. First, the action potential generated at the site of damage travels to the termination site of the nociceptors in the spinal cord. It travels across the synaptic cleft between the nociceptors and the dorsal horn neurons of the spinal cord through the release of neurotransmitters, such as substance P, serotonin, and histamine. Next, the action potential impulse continues through the spinal cord and up to the brain. From the dorsal horn, neurons form several tracts, including the spinothalamic tract, and ascend to the brain stem and thalamus. In the third phase, the impulse moves through the thalamus, a sort of "relay station," and continues to the cortex and central brain structures for signal processing.

Perception, the third process of nociception, is the point at which pain becomes a conscious experience. Although it is still unclear if there is an exact location in the brain where pain is perceived, it is known that there are a number of central structures involved in the perception of pain. The reticular system is responsible for the autonomic response to pain, whereas the somatosensory cortex localizes and characterizes pain, and the limbic system regulates the emotional and behavioral responses to pain. (See the section on Functional Consequences of Pain in Older Adults for further discussion of the emotional and behavioral responses to pain in older adults.)

The final process of nociception, **modulation**, refers to the body's responses to painful stimuli. The descending tracts from the brain to the periphery follow the same pathway down the spinal cord to the dorsal horn. The descending tract neurons release substances such as endogenous opioids, serotonin, and norepinephrine that are capable of inhibiting the transmission phase of the noxious impulse, resulting in analgesia. These modulatory systems explain the action of tricyclic antidepressants for pain management.

The physiology of pain perception as described is the "normal" process by which acute pain is experienced. Although persistent pain follows the same basic principles, there are several key differences between the physiology of acute pain and persistent pain. Persistent pain is multifactorial in origin and can be affected by age, sex, ethnicity, and previous experiences with pain. Persistent pain often cannot be explained by objective clinical measures alone; its cause may be idiopathic and influenced by the patient's psychological makeup. Thus, recognition of the potential combination of physiologic and psychological processes at work in persistent pain may assist in guiding the development of appropriate pain management regimens. The etiology of persistent pain is not well understood; it can occur in the absence of apparent illness or after incomplete healing from injury. With persistent pain, the central nervous system continues to process pain signals as though new injuries were occurring. The perception of persistent pain is associated with the up-regulation of genes for sensory neuron–specific channels in which regulating proteins for signaling pain contain genetic components that, when continuously exposed to pain signals, can predispose certain persons to persistent pain. Because physiologic changes that occur during pain signal processing involve many neurotransmitters (e.g., substance P, serotonin, prostaglandins, bradykinin, leukotrienes, histamine, norepinephrine) and receptors (e.g., opioid, serotonin, acetylcholine, dopamine, norepinephrine), drug therapy can target a variety of pain pathways.

TYPES OF PAIN

Although clear distinctions between types of pain are not always possible, general classifications help nurses understand the source of and most appropriate interventions for pain. Pain is often defined in terms of acute and persistent pain (as previously described); however, other classifications include nociceptive and neuropathic pain. **Nociceptive pain** is caused by the normal processing of stimuli from damaged somatic and visceral structures. **Somatic pain**, which usually is well localized, arises from bone, joint, muscle, or skin tissues and is often described as aching, deep, sharp, or throbbing. **Visceral pain** originates in visceral organs, such as the kidney, gallbladder, and pancreas, usually from obstruction of the hollow viscus, and is often referred to other sites. Kidney stones, gallstones, or pancreatitis are common examples of visceral pain, which can be described as cramping, squeezing, or pressure.

Neuropathic pain originates from stimuli that are abnormally processed by both the central and peripheral nervous systems. Centrally generated pain is caused by either injury to the nervous system (e.g., phantom pain from an amputation) or dysregulation of the autonomic nervous system (e.g., burning pain below the level of a spinal cord lesion). Peripherally generated pain has two causes: mononeuropathies or polyneuropathies. Mononeuropathy results in pain along a known peripheral nerve pathway (e.g., nerve root compression or trigeminal neuralgia), and polyneuropathy occurs along the distribution of many peripheral nerves (e.g., diabetic neuropathy or Guillain-Barré syndrome).

One final classification of pain that is often used is that of cancer pain. Although **cancer pain** is not a physiologic classification, it has distinct characteristics. Cancer pain is a complex phenomenon in which pain can be acute, persistent, nociceptive, or neuropathic. Cancer pain can be caused by tumor progression, treatments and medications administered for the cancer, or even treatments for the side effects of the cancer treatments.

CAUSES OF PAIN IN OLDER ADULTS

Pain is a widespread problem for older adults, affecting 57% to 88% of those who live in community settings, with 80% to 85% of persons older than 65 years of age experiencing at some point in time a significant health problem that predisposes them to pain (Borglin et al., 2005; Rustoen et al., 2005; Tsai & Means, 2005). Persons older than the age of 65 years have an increased rate of chronic medical conditions predisposing them to associated pain and declining physical function, and they are disproportionately more likely to suffer from diseases that cause musculoskeletal pain, such as osteoporosis and arthritis, than their younger counterparts (Federal Interagency Forum on Aging-Related Statistics, 2004; Gallagher et al., 2000). Arthritis, the most common cause of persistent pain in older adult populations, currently affects between 49% to 59% of older adults (Bolen et al., 2002). It is projected that the occurrence of arthritis will double from 21.4 million older adults today to over 41 million by the year 2030. Osteoporosis shows a significant increase in occurrence with increased age, with an estimated 25 million older adults currently affected by this disease (Kotz et al., 2004). Other common causes of pain in older adults include postherpetic neuralgia, experienced by as much as 20% of those living to 85 years of age (Jung, et al., 2004; Opstelten et al., 2002); back problems, with prevalence rates in older adult populations reaching as high as 25% (Hartvigsen et al., 2003; Webb et al., 2003); fibromyalgia, experienced by as much as 9% of older adults (Gowin, 2000; Wolfe et al., 1995); and diabetic peripheral neuropathy, with a prevalence rate of approximately 15% of older adults, increasing in direct proportion to advancing age (Gregg et al., 2004).

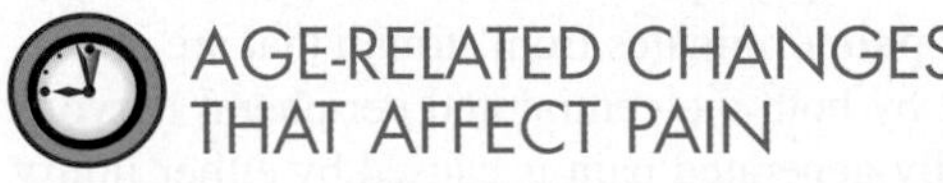

AGE-RELATED CHANGES THAT AFFECT PAIN

Although age-related changes in pain perception are not well understood, the process is altered by underlying neurochemical, neuroanatomic, and neurophysiologic mechanisms. Moreover, pain management is affected by age-related changes in the pharmacokinetics and pharmacodynamics of analgesic medications. Some age-related changes that can affect the pharmacologic treatment of pain include decreased renal function, decreased lean body weight, decreased liver mass and hepatic blood flow, decreased serum protein concentrations, and decreased pulmonary function. These physiologic changes can alter the absorption, distribution, metabolism, elimination, and side effects of analgesic medications in older adults. However, little is known about changes in the perception of pain due to the aging process. The misconception that older adults are not able to feel pain as intensely as younger adults should not reduce the aggressiveness of pain management in this population. The undertreatment of pain is a much greater concern.

The typical pain symptoms manifested in younger adults may not always be present in older adults. Older adults may be less likely to report pain because they do not want to "complain," or they believe that it is a part of the natural aging process. In older adults, pain is likely to manifest as:

- Confusion
- Restlessness
- Aggression
- Fatigue

The lack of "expected" symptoms might lead to a misdiagnosis or delay in treatment, especially if the older adult is reluctant to admit to having pain.

BARRIERS TO PAIN MANAGEMENT

Despite the progress in understanding the physiology of pain and the advances in its assessment and treatment, there are many barriers nationwide to the appropriate recognition and management of pain. These obstacles exist at many levels, from health care systems to insurance providers, and from health care providers to patients and family members. Nurses need to recognize these barriers so they can not only assess and manage pain, but also advocate for the needs of patients. Table 28-1 lists some of the barriers to pain management, along with problems and possible solutions that nurses can address.

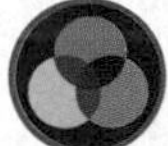

FUNCTIONAL CONSEQUENCES OF PAIN IN OLDER ADULTS

The functional consequences of pain in older adults include diminished physical function, loss of mobility, and higher levels of disability, as indicated by the following statistics:

- Older adults with persistent pain experience two to three times as many problems with walking and up to two times as many problems with impaired mobility (Jakobsson et al., 2004).
- Older adults with pain consistently have greater declines in function than those without pain (Al Snih et al., 2005; Croft et al., 2005; Jakobsson et al., 2004).

TABLE 28-1 Barriers to Effective Pain Management

Source of the Barrier	Problems Contributing to the Barrier	Possible Solutions to Overcoming the Barrier
Patients and families	• Attitude that pain cannot be effectively managed and is a normal part of aging • Family burnout (families are often involved in educating, goal setting, and primary caregiving) • Belief that pain is an atonement for past actions that must be endured • Belief that pain is inevitable • Belief that "complaining" equals "burden," or results in retribution • Belief that health care providers are "always right"; self-advocacy is not appropriate • Belief that morphine is used only at the end of life • Fear of addiction to medication • Stigma of opiate use • Side effects, which may be difficult to manage or impossible to treat • Fear of the underlying meaning of the pain (e.g., that it indicates worsening of the disease process)	• Provide education about the treatments for side effects. • Explain the mechanism of action of morphine and its appropriate use for pain management. • Explain the differences between "addiction" and "tolerance". • Present nonpharmacologic alternatives: ◦ Physical therapy ◦ Massage ◦ Body/energy work ◦ Acupuncture ◦ Chiropractic or naturopathic care ◦ Behavioral or mental health therapies ◦ Biofeedback ◦ Pilates, yoga
Health care providers	• Belief that older adults have a higher pain tolerance • Belief that patients with dementia do not experience pain • Belief that older adults cannot tolerate potent opioid analgesic medication • Fear of being investigated for excessive prescribing of opioids • Fear of the consequences of hospital policies for aggressive pain treatment • Lack of resources in rural/outlying areas • Insufficient communication between members of the health care team • Inadequate knowledge about pain and how best to manage it	• Complete continuing education in pain management (as for licensure renewal). • Attend educational seminars provided to health care workers by hospitals on prescription regulations with strategies for providing safe, structured pain management. • Participate in a pain management clinic or team for referral of complex pain management cases.
Health care system/ institution	• Cultural and political climate resistant to change in the standards of care • Systems do not encourage a multidisciplinary approach to pain management • Lack of a shared language among disciplines for communicating about pain • Lack of motivation to improve pain management standards (belief that the problem is already being adequately addressed) • Lack of health care provider accountability for effective pain relief	• Encourage institutions to: ◦ Identify key players among upper management and clinicians to include in discussions for change to standards of care ◦ Select a system-wide pain rating system, using clear, concise terminology for routine pain assessment and documentation ◦ Offer education from a policy perspective on the implications of unrelieved pain (e.g., increased length of stay and health care costs) ◦ Implement measures to hold individual providers responsible for appropriate pain assessment and treatment
Insurance companies/ payment plans	• Lack of reimbursement for opioid treatment • Lack of reimbursement for multidisciplinary pain centers • Lack of reimbursement for nonpharmacologic interventions	• Advocate for patients by contacting insurance companies that refuse to pay for treatment. • Advocate for policy-level changes to reimbursement formularies. • Assume a leadership or consultation position in an insurance company.

- A decline in physical function results in a greater risk for disability, increased financial burden, and the loss of independence in the community.
- Pain is significantly correlated with psychosocial consequences, including depression, sleep disturbances, fatigue, and anxiety (Call-Schmidt & Richardson, 2003; Elliott et al., 2003; Jakobsson et al., 2003; Reid et al., 2003; Tamiya et al., 2002).

Consequences associated with the undertreatment of pain include

- Decreased quality of life
- Social isolation and negative effects on relationships
- Impaired function
- Physical deconditioning
- Sleep disturbances
- Exhaustion or fatigue
- Depression
- Anxiety
- Suicide
- Excessive health care expenditures

These consequences are not unique to older adults; however, their effects can be particularly devastating in this population, causing unnecessary suffering and compounding the inherent toll of persistent pain. Anxiety, depression, and even suicide are correlated with persistent pain, but they are not inevitable outcomes. However, nurses must be aware that depression may indeed accompany ongoing pain, and when it is suspected, they are responsible for assessment and interventions, as detailed in Chapter 15.

An essential aspect of optimal pain management is recognizing the unique way in which each individual experiences pain. Pain is interpreted differently by each person and is influenced by many factors. Past pain experiences can influence one's current perception of pain by triggering "memories" in the pain pathways. In addition, age, sex, beliefs, values, and culture can influence the meaning and interpretation of pain for each individual. Moreover, expectations of what the pain means and attitudes about the pain can affect the degree to which patients tolerate it. Box 28-1 lists specific factors that can worsen or improve pain for older adults.

Box 28-1
Factors Affecting the Experience of Pain

Factors That Worsen Pain

- Insomnia/fatigue
- Anxiety
- Fear
- Isolation
- Boredom
- Anger
- Sadness
- Depression

Factors That Improve Pain

- Nonpharmacologic approaches
- Medications
- Sleep/rest
- Understanding/validation
- Companionship
- Diversional activity
- Reduction in anxiety
- Elevation of mood

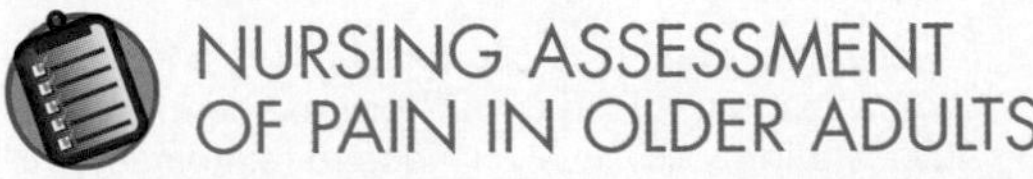

NURSING ASSESSMENT OF PAIN IN OLDER ADULTS

A basic pain assessment is a simple task to perform; however, a comprehensive pain assessment is one of the most complex, and important, nursing responsibilities. Unrelieved pain and unnecessary suffering for older adults result from an incomplete or inaccurate pain assessment, or from failure to perform one at all. The major mistakes associated with a pain assessment include failure to assess pain, failure to accept a patient's report of pain, and failure to act on the patient's report of pain. A pain assessment *is*: asking and believing the patient, assessing the critical components of the pain experience, assessing the cause of the pain, and communicating the findings of the pain assessment to the health care team. Pain assessment *is not*: relying only on changes in vital signs; deciding that the patient does not "look in pain"; basing pain assessment only on how much the nurse believes a procedure or disease "should" hurt; assuming sleeping patients do not have pain; and assuming a patient will tell the nurse when he or she is in pain. Box 28-2 summarizes assumptions that should and should not be made when assessing pain in older adults.

Several organizations have proposed guidelines for the assessment of pain in older adults, including The Hartford Institute for Geriatric Nursing, the National Gerontological Nursing Association, and the AGS. The Educational Resources section at the end of this chapter lists Internet sites for additional information on pain assessment and management strategies. This section synthesizes information from these organizations' guidelines for a comprehensive pain assessment.

Collecting Pertinent Information

An essential first step in assessing pain is recognizing that many older adults refer to pain by using words such as:

- Burning
- Discomfort
- Aching
- Soreness
- Hurting

The nurse should also observe for physical indicators of pain, which include grimacing, muscle tension, rubbing or protecting body parts, rapid or excessive eye blinking, or

Box 28-2
Assumptions Made by Nurses Regarding Pain Assessment

Assumptions that* should *be made in* all *situations:

- Self-report is the gold standard for pain assessment.
- Pain assessment must be regular, systematic, and documented in order accurately to evaluate treatment effectiveness.
- Both patients and health care providers have personal beliefs, prior experiences, insufficient knowledge, and mistaken beliefs about pain and pain management that
    - Influence the pain management process
    - Must be acknowledged and addressed before optimal pain relief can be achieved

Assumptions that* should *be made in* specific *situations:

- The majority of hospitalized older adults suffer from both acute and chronic pain.
- People with dementia have the same physiologic experience of pain as those who do not have any cognitive impairment.
- People with cognitive impairment experience pain, but are often unable to verbalize it; however, there may be nonverbal indicators.
- People with dementia have pain if they have conditions or are in situations that typically cause pain; therefore, medicate for pain even if they are unable to report it.

Assumptions that* should not *be made:

- All older adults complain about pain.
- Older adults cannot or will not comply with complex or alternative therapies.
- Older adults are unreliable historians and will not accurately report their pain.
- Older adults will under-report their pain because they believe that pain is an inevitable aspect of aging.

Sources: National Gerontological Nursing Association. (2002). Innovations in clinical practice: Chronic pain management in older adults. Available at www.ngna.org/pdfs/Chronic%20Pain%20ICP.pdf; The Hartford Institute for Geriatric Nursing. (2000). Assessing pain in older adults. *Try This: Best Practices in Nursing Care to Older Adults, 7*; and The Hartford Institute for Geriatric Nursing. (2003). Assessing pain in persons with dementia. *Try This: Best Practices in Nursing Care for Older Adults With Dementia, 1*(2), both available at www.hartfordign.org/resources/education/tryThis.html.

a sad or frightened facial expression (see the section on Assessment in Cognitively Impaired Older Adults for further discussion of the nonverbal indicators of pain). Verbalizations and vocalizations can also indicate the presence of pain, and can include sighing or moaning, chanting or calling out "Help," noisy breathing, yelling "Ow" or "Ouch," swearing or cursing, or stop commands like "Stop" or "Don't do that."

If nurses are not familiar with the older adult, they need to elicit a history of recent changes in function from the patient, family members, or caregivers because these changes can be indicators of pain. Information about the usual activities of daily living (ADLs) and baseline measures of functioning are useful in assessing changes that are indicative of pain. It is also important to recognize the relationship between pain and the person's mood and psychological function. For example, nurses can use age-specific and cognitive-appropriate scales such as the Geriatric Depression Scale (see Chapter 15) and the tools recommended by the Hartford Institute for Geriatric Nursing listed in the Clinical Tools Resources at the end of this chapter. Finally, the nurse must recognize that medication effects and chronic medical conditions can influence both the experience of pain and the treatment of that pain. Nurses can use the questions in Box 28-3 as a guide for collecting pertinent information throughout the pain assessment.

Assessment of Pain Components

Nurses assess the following components of the pain experience: intensity, impact on ADLs, quality, location, physical findings, temporal characteristics, aggravating and alleviating factors, analgesic history, patient goals and expectations, and the meaning of pain and the patient's attitudes. **Pain intensity** is the state of being unpleasant, or the subjective determination of the strength, concentration, or force of the symptom of pain. The subjective report of the intensity is the component most often addressed in pain assessment because it is the most easily identified indicator of improvement or

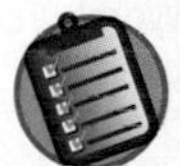

Box 28-3
Sample Questions for Pain Assessment in Older Adults

- How strong is your pain right now?
- What was the worst/average pain over the past week?
- How many days over the past week have you been unable to do what you would like to do because of your pain?
- How often do you participate in pleasurable activities such as hobbies, socializing with friends, travel? Over the past week, how often has pain interfered with these activities?
- How often do you exercise? Over the past week, how often has pain interfered with your ability to exercise?
- How often does pain interfere with your ability to think clearly?
- How often does pain interfere with your appetite? Have you lost weight as a result?
- How often does pain interfere with your sleep? How often over the past week has this scenario occurred?
- Has pain interfered with your energy, mood, personality, or relationships with other people?
- Over the past week, how often have you taken pain medication?
- How would you rate your health at the present time?

worsening. Intensity is the component that is often considered the "fifth vital sign" and it is addressed by a numerical rating scale (NRS) of 0 to 10. Nurses begin assessing pain intensity by establishing one rating scale for use over time, and ensure that the entire health care team uses that same scale. Nurses also ensure that alternate scales are available for patients who cannot use the standard scale because of language barriers or cognitive impairment. Scales that have been found to be appropriate for older adults include the Verbal Descriptor Scale (VDS), the NRS, as well as most other pain scales (Herr & Mobily, 1993). The VDS rates pain on a continuum with verbal cues ranging from no pain, to mild pain, moderate pain, severe pain, very severe pain, to the worst pain possible. Often this scale is used in conjunction with the NRS (Fig. 28-2). Always document the patient's self-report of his or her pain rating, not your personal impression of what you think the rating "should" be. In addition to consistently using the same tool each time, nurses should document additional assessment comments in the chart when appropriate.

Assessing the effects of pain on ADLs not only provides additional information for the nurse, it may help older adults recognize subtle ways in which pain interferes with their lives. Thus, nurses should ask how often in the past week the pain or discomfort has interfered with self-care or the usual ability to perform activities such as bathing, eating, dressing, and going to the toilet. Limiting the time frame to the past week helps the patient to focus attention on the present, rather than recalling how pain has fluctuated over the course of months or years. Nurses should also ask about the effects on complex activities such as driving, paying bills, preparing meals, shopping for groceries, and taking care of home-related chores.

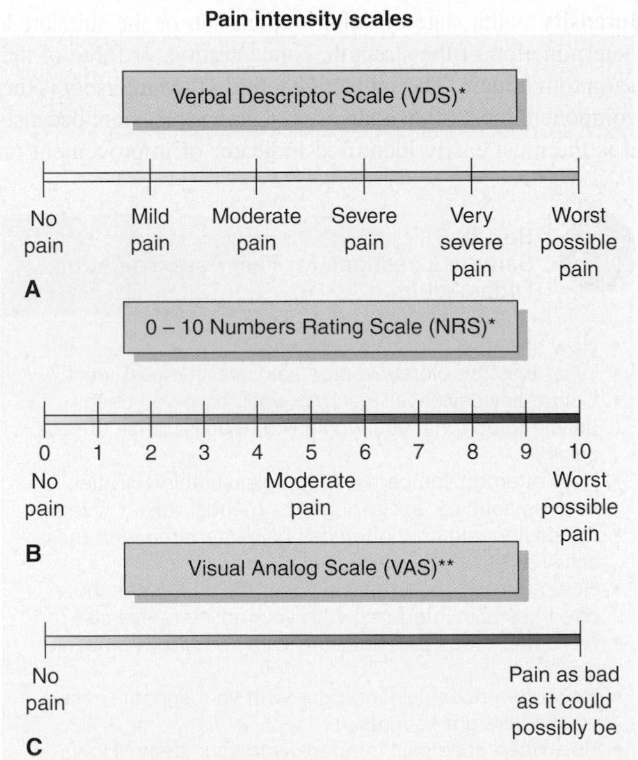

FIGURE 28-2 Examples of pain rating scales: **(A)** Verbal Descriptor Scale, **(B)** Numerical Rating Scale, and **(C)** Visual Analog Scale.

Assessing the quality of the pain based on specific descriptors used by older adults is helpful in determining the underlying pain mechanism as somatic, visceral, or neuropathic. Somatic pain, which is associated with muscle, joint, tendon, skin, or bone injuries, is localized and may be described as aching, deep, dull, gnawing, throbbing, sharp, or stabbing. Visceral pain results from injury to visceral organs, such as the pain from gallstones, kidney stones, gastrointestinal tract disorders, or pancreatitis. Visceral pain can be described as cramping, squeezing, shooting, or pressure, and can be referred to distant sites. Finally, neuropathic pain results from an abnormal processing of sensory input by the peripheral or central nervous system, such as with spinal cord injuries, herpes zoster, or peripheral neuropathies. Descriptors characteristic of neuropathic pain include burning, numbness, radiating, shooting, stabbing, tingling, or hypersensitivity to touch.

Nurses should document the location of the pain on a figure drawing in the patient's chart. Location can be identified simply by asking the patient to mark the location on a figure drawing, or by having the patient point to the location on his or her own body. If there is more than one site, letters may be used for distinguishing the different sites for documentation, (e.g., A, B, C, and so forth). This step of assessment is critical for delineating different areas of pain because they may be different types of pain. Each location may require an individual approach to management.

Physical findings may also aid in assessing the location of the pain. While pain assessment cannot rely only on physical findings, the nurse must observe the site of pain; note any changes in skin color, warmth, irritation, or integrity; and review any pertinent physical assessment data.

Temporal characteristics describe the course of the pain experience using the following parameters: onset, duration of episodes, frequency (i.e., constant or intermittent), and variations with time of day or certain activities. It is logical to assess aggravating and alleviating factors in conjunction with temporal characteristics. This goal is accomplished by inquiring about what makes the pain better or worse, if the pain is affected by movement or changing position, and if any nonpharmacologic methods help to alleviate the pain. Analgesic history can also be taken at this time and should include information on the patient's current medication use, the onset and duration of maximal analgesia with medication use, and the number of medications that are being taken on a set schedule versus those taken only as needed (p.r.n.).

The nurse must also thoroughly assess and document analgesic use within the previous 24 hours because a patient can have very different pain ratings depending on whether analgesics have been taken on the day of the assessment. This point is also the time to inquire about problems the patient has had with side effects of medications, as well as any fears of potential side effects or addiction to pain medication.

When assessing pain, nurses must evaluate the patient's goals and expectations, as well as the meaning he or she associates with the pain. Some older adults may fear the onset of pain as an indicator of a progressive terminal illness or disease process, and others may view pain as a positive sign that they are still alive for another day. Nurses assess the meaning and context of the pain in relation to actual and potential effects on functional and psychosocial activities, such as sleep, physical activities, recreational activities, personal relationships, and work. These areas can influence older adults' perception of the severity of the pain and their willingness to participate in a pain management regimen. This time is also the point at which to gain an understanding of the patient's short- and long-term goals of treatment. Does the patient expect to return to baseline functioning, or is he or she expecting to continue to experience some pain? Another important issue to determine is the patient's acceptable level of pain and to incorporate this acceptable level as a goal of the pain management regimen. Is a pain level of 5 on the 0-to-10 NRS acceptable to the patient, or is 3 the target pain level?

A crucial step that is often overlooked is the reassessment of pain frequently and regularly. In acute care settings, nurses should assess the effectiveness of the treatment shortly after the administration of pain medication (30 to 60 minutes) and whenever pain management interventions are changed. Nurses also need to reassess whenever patients experience changes in any of the critical components of pain. This reassessment includes questions regarding pain severity and length of time the pain was relieved with the previous intervention.

Assessment in Cognitively Impaired Older Adults

Damage to the central nervous system can affect memory, language, and the higher-order cognitive skills necessary for communicating the experience of pain. Despite these changes, people with dementia still experience pain sensations to a degree similar to that of cognitively intact older adults (Schuler et al., 2004). However, pain assessment in this population can be a difficult task for nurses because the disease interferes with the patient's ability to interpret the pain stimulus through the step of perception in the pain pathway. The affective response to the pain sensation that occurs in both the perception and modulation phases is affected by this central nervous system damage (Scherder et al., 2005). Although difficult, it is possible to obtain a comprehensive pain assessment in older adults with cognitive impairment by using the right information and tools.

According to the hierarchy of pain assessment principles, self-report is the gold standard for pain assessment, and all attempts should be made to obtain this self-report from the patient (McCaffery & Pasero, 1999). Patients with mild to moderate cognitive impairment often are able to provide an accurate self-report of pain. However, in advanced stages of cognitive disease, the ability to self-report decreases, and eventually self-reporting is no longer possible. When nurses cannot obtain a self-report, as with nonverbal older adults or those with cognitive impairments, they should take the following steps:

- Look for clues to the potential causes of pain.
- Observe the patient's behaviors.
- Obtain pertinent information about pain and behaviors from family members or caregivers.
- Attempt an analgesic trial.

If the nurse is not familiar with the cognitively impaired patient, information should be obtained from someone who does know him or her, such as a family member or caregiver. Always ask the patient to rate his or her pain (Table 28-2). The nurse must also search for potential causes of pain or discomfort. A thorough medical history should be gathered, with particular attention paid to conditions associated with chronic pain common in older persons (i.e., a history of arthritis, diabetic neuropathies, fibromyalgia, or low back pain). Note if the patient has a history of any musculoskeletal or neurologic disorders that could potentially be a cause of pain. Also, family members or caregivers should report any recent falls or other acute problems that could cause pain, such as urinary tract infections, skin tears or injuries, or bacterial infections (e.g., pneumonia), as well as chronic conditions.

After gathering information on potential causes of pain in the nonverbal older adult, the nurse must observe the patient's behaviors for any subtle changes, and seek a surrogate report of pain and behavior or activity changes from family members or caregivers. Behavioral indicators of pain include facial expressions, verbalizations, vocalizations, body movements, an alteration in interpersonal interactions, or mental status changes (AGS, 2002). Some behaviors are more obviously associated with pain (e.g., facial grimacing, moaning, groaning, or rubbing a suspected painful body part); others, however, have a more subtle association and may be labeled as behavioral disorders (e.g., agitation, restlessness, irritability, confusion, and combativeness), particularly when they occur with care activities or treatments. Changes in appetite, functional level, or usual activities also can be clues to pain. Thus, nurses need to document behaviors as well as changes in patterns that might be indicative of pain exacerbation. Two of the most widely recommended of the many published pain assessment tools for nonverbal or cognitively impaired patients are the

TABLE 28-2 Principles of Pain Assessment in Older Adults With Cognitive Impairment

Principle	Steps to Achieve in Pain Assessment
Know the person	• Develop a relationship with the patient. • Include family members or caregivers in obtaining history of the patient's painful conditions and behavior or activity changes.
Ask the person	• Always assume the person can communicate with you and understand a rating scale. • If at first you don't succeed, try, try again. • Use the same words they use: "hurting," "uncomfortable," "sore," "tender," "achy," etc. • Try asking, "Are you comfortable?" • Gently touch the suspected painful area and ask again about the specific site. • Document and communicate with the health care team what works and what language is used by the person.
Use multiple resources	• Review the chart for a current or past history of painful diagnoses. • Talk with direct caregivers. • Talk with family and close friends. • Communicate with other nurses, pharmacists, and physical and occupational therapists.
Individualize pain care plans	Include the following: • Pain-related diagnoses • Pain-related medication use and bowel care • Unique expressions of pain • Unique expressions of comfort • Individualized strategies for promoting comfort and reducing pain
Promote comfort	Take the following steps during pain assessment: • Ask for assistance from caregivers. • Use warm supplies. • Keep the person warm and covered. • Provide timely warnings. • Maximize the person's control. • Respond to evidence of pain with sincere apology and reassurance.
Prevent discomfort	Ensure the following during pain assessment: • Toileting and personal hygiene needs are met. • Clothing is slightly oversized and not restrictive, and shoes fit well (not rubbing on toes). • Movement and seating are conducted with great care to avoid any sudden or jarring movements that could initiate pain.

Discomfort Scale—Dementia of the Alzheimer's Type (DS-DAT) (Hurley et al., 1992) and the Checklist of Nonverbal Pain Indicators (CNPI) (Feldt, 2000). A task force of the American Society for Pain Management Nursing has developed a position statement with clinical practice recommendations pertinent to older adults with dementia as well as patients who are intubated or unconscious (Herr et al., 2006).

Finally, nurses should attempt an analgesic trial to investigate any changes in behavior or activity that are thought to be a result of pain. Using data collected during a comprehensive pain assessment, the nurse estimates the intensity of pain and selects an appropriate analgesic based on the principles of analgesic medication discussed in the following section. For example, acetaminophen 500 to 1000 mg every 8 hours may be an appropriate first step when mild to moderate pain is suspected in a patient with a history of mild osteoarthritis. If behaviors continue to indicate potential pain, it may be appropriate to begin low-dose opioids and titrate (increase the dose) upward as indicated, because these medications are effective in decreasing pain-related agitation (Manfredi et al., 2003).

PRINCIPLES OF ANALGESIC MEDICATION

The rapid pace of change in the world of analgesic development makes it difficult to maintain proficiency in pain management medications unless one specializes in this field. However, if nurses have a basic understanding of the principles of analgesic medication administration, and learn a few medications well, they will know where to go to find more specific information about developing complex pain management regimens. This section presents the basic information needed for understanding the administration of analgesics, covers medication cautions specific to older adults, discusses the issues surrounding fear of addiction and side effects, and provides some disease-specific treatment recommendations.

Classifications of Analgesics

Analgesics are divided into three different groups: nonopioids, opioids, and adjuvants. The term *narcotic* has become obsolete and should not be used in clinical practice because the media and general population apply the term to substances that have the potential for abuse, such as cocaine, that actually have no analgesic properties. The terms *non-opioid* and *opioid* analgesics should be used in place of *non-narcotic* and *narcotic*.

Nonopioid analgesics include acetaminophen; non-aspirin, nonsteroidal anti-inflammatory drugs (NSAIDs); and aspirin. Nonopioids act at the site of the injury to decrease pain; NSAIDs, for example, inhibit the release of prostaglandin from damaged cells. **Opioid analgesics** are natural, semisynthetic, or synthetic drugs that relieve pain by binding to multiple types of opioid receptors in the central nervous system. As a result of this action, the release of neurotransmitters is blocked and the pain impulse cannot cross the synapse into the dorsal horn during the transmission phase of the pain pathway. Examples of opioids are codeine, morphine, tramadol, fentanyl, and methadone. **Adjuvant analgesics** are medications that have a primary indication other than the treatment of pain, such as an antidepressants or anticonvulsants, but relieve pain in some conditions. Adjuvants most often act on the modulation phase of the pain pathway by interfering with the reuptake of serotonin and norepinephrine, which inhibit the transmission of nociceptive impulses. All three groups are effective in the perception phase, acting in different ways to decrease the conscious experience of pain perception.

The World Health Organization's Three-Step Pain Relief Ladder for Pain Management

The AGS has endorsed the use of the World Health Organization's (WHO) pain relief ladder as a guide for the treatment of persistent pain in older adults (AGS, 2002). Nurses can apply this approach for selecting analgesics on the basis of the intensity of the pain, using analgesics from each of the three different classifications, and building on previously effective treatments. The three steps of the WHO's pain relief ladder (Fig. 28-3) address different levels of pain intensity, and also allow for the fact that not all people experience pain in the same way along the same trajectory. Therefore, tailoring therapeutic regimens to individual needs is considered the gold standard of pain management for older adults (AGS, 2002). Based on this AGS guideline, treatment does not necessarily begin at Step 1 and progress sequentially. For example, it may be appropriate to begin at Step 3 or titrate more rapidly for an older adult who is experiencing excruciating pain.

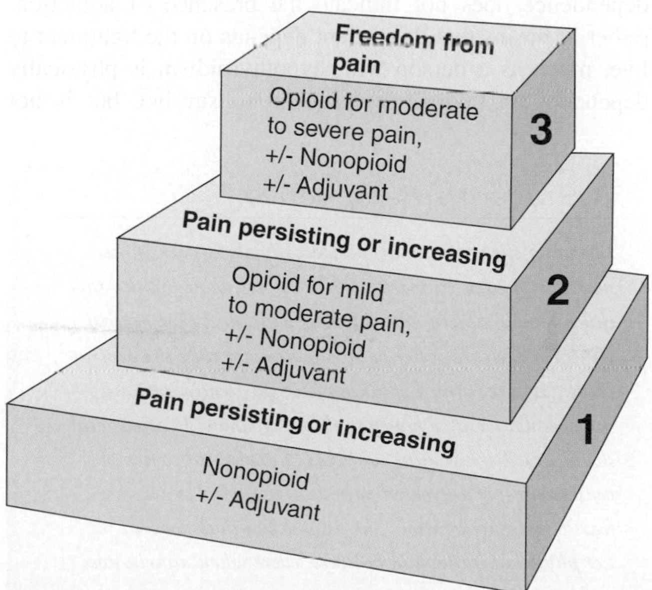

FIGURE 28-3 World Health Organization pain relief ladder. (©World Health Organization 2005. Redrawn with permission.)

Step 1 of the WHO pain relief ladder addresses mild pain (i.e., ranging from 1 to 3 out of 10 on an NRS) by recommending the use of nonopioid analgesics initially, with the addition of an adjuvant if it is deemed appropriate. Although nonopioids are generally viewed as having fewer risks of side effects than opioids, this misconception is a dangerous one. The use of NSAIDs poses many serious side effects for older adults because they can cause significant end-organ toxicity; thousands of hospitalizations occur annually as a result of gastric bleeding caused by these drugs. Excessive use of NSAIDs can also result in renal insufficiency, decreased platelet aggregations, and even death. Acetaminophen is often considered a "safe" alternative to NSAIDs because it is a very effective analgesic with few side effects and does not cause problems with the stomach, kidneys, or platelets. However, the most common side effect associated with the overuse of acetaminophen is a deadly one: hepatotoxicity. It is important to recognize that the recommended ceiling dose for acetaminophen (i.e., 4 g daily) is for *healthy individuals* with no previous liver or metabolic complications. *Extreme caution* must be taken with older adults using any nonopioid medication. Levels of acetaminophen must also be carefully monitored if an older adult is using a combination medication (an opioid plus acetaminophen) for breakthrough pain because levels greater than the safe maximum can easily be reached. This principle is critically important for patient teaching because older adults may not realize that many over-the-counter products (e.g., arthritis pain relievers, Tylenol PM) contain acetaminophen that must be factored into the daily maximum dose.

If the pain continues to be in the mild to moderate range (e.g., it worsens from a 3 to a 5 of 10 on an NRS), and is not adequately relieved by the use of a nonopioid, then Step 2 suggests adding a weak opioid, or opioid combination, to the regimen. This step *builds on* the previous one; it does not replace the use of the Step 1 nonopioid analgesics. Step 2 should also include a method of providing around-the-clock analgesia by using a breakthrough medication. For example, a patient would take acetaminophen 500 mg every 6 hours, and use one tablet of Percocet (i.e., 5 mg oxycodone plus 325 mg acetaminophen) every 4 hours as needed for breakthrough pain. This combination of acetaminophen and Percocet contains only half the maximum recommended dose of acetaminophen for older adults.

If the pain persists or worsens (i.e., ranging from 7 to 10 on an NRS), the interventions in Step 3 should be considered. Although both Steps 2 and 3 include the use of an opioid, different type of opioids are used in each step. Because Step 2 opioid drugs (e.g., Lortab 5/500, Tylenol #3, or Percocet) also have fixed doses of acetaminophen, the extent to which these opioids can be used is limited by the recommended maximum daily dose of acetaminophen for older adults. Thus, the use of stronger opioids is the appropriate next step. Step 3 builds on Steps 1 and 2, with the continued use of nonopioids and adjuvants. Opioid use in Step 3 must be scheduled around the clock and still include some type of breakthrough pain medication. Opioids prescribed for breakthrough pain should also have a short half-life so that they can be rapidly titrated for severe pain episodes. Opioids for around-the-clock administration should be delivered in a controlled-release formula, ensuring that the administration rate remains constant.

Box 28-4
Recommendations for Maintaining Bowel Function in Patients Taking Opioid Medications

Points to remember:
- *Tolerance* is your ally with regard to all side effects except constipation.
- The hand that writes the opioid order should also write the bowel regimen order.
- Constipation is an expected adverse effect that should be dealt with from the start.

Before requesting a laxative:
- Rule out other causes of constipation.
- Do not give laxatives if abdominal pain is present.
- Reassess daily for responses.

A bowel program can include:
- Senna + docusate tablets (Senokot-S)
- Lactulose
- Bisacodyl (Dulcolax)
- Magnesium hydroxide (Milk of Magnesia)
- Nonpharmacologic remedy: daily administration of a fruit paste (including such ingredients as senna tea leaves, prunes, raisins, or figs)

Management of Side Effects and Risks of Tolerance, Dependence, and Addiction

Because the fear of side effects and addiction is one of the greatest barriers to effective pain management in older adults, nurses may need to address this fear appropriately when developing a pain management regimen. In addition, side effects, especially constipation, are often limiting and potentially quite dangerous. All potential side effects of medications must be addressed in the plan, and the patient must be reassured that most side effects can be managed safely. When nurses care for patients who are taking opioid analgesics, they must incorporate a regimen for maintaining bowel function in the care plan because constipation is an expected side effect that should be dealt with proactively. Constipation, which occurs in 90% of patients treated with opioids, is caused by the following combination of physiologic effects: reduced secretions, increased intestinal fluid absorption, and increased intestinal blood flow (Yennurajalingam et al., 2005). Although medication tolerance can be considered a physiologic protective mechanism that helps the body become accustomed to the medication so that adverse effects gradually diminish, this mechanism does not extend to constipation. Therefore the risk will not diminish, and in fact can increase. Box 28-4 summarizes a recommended regimen for maintaining bowel function in people taking opioid analgesics.

Nurses need to teach patients and their families about the differences between tolerance, dependence, and addiction to help them understand that the risk of addiction is minimal and the effective management of pain can improve quality of life and decrease the negative sequelae of unmanaged pain. Many older adults fear addiction to opioids, and many of their family members may stigmatize the use of opioids. Tolerance to and dependence on opioids are not the same as addiction to opioids, but the three terms are often confused. The APS defines **tolerance** as a pharmacodynamic response at the neurophysiologic level due to chronic drug administration (Gordon et al., 2005). Tolerance is manifested by a decrease in one or more therapeutic effects of the medication (e.g., less analgesia) or its side effects (e.g., sedation, respiratory depression, or nausea). Tolerance should be viewed as a descriptive term that refers to a change in the relationship between the therapeutic effect and the dose, not as a negative label implying addictive behavior. **Dependence** is defined as a physiologic phenomenon manifested by the development of withdrawal symptoms on sudden discontinuation of the medication. The best approach to withdrawal symptoms is to reduce the dose gradually, rather than abruptly discontinuing the drug. Again, physical dependence does not indicate the presence of addiction; rather, it means that the patient depends on the treatment to live, much as a person with hypothyroidism is physically dependent on thyroid replacement to survive, but is not

A Student's Perspective

My aging client complains periodically about pain in her shoulder. She has stated that she does not want to take anything besides aspirin when she has pain, and that aspirin seems to take care of her pain. She does not take the aspirin every day. She's afraid of taking pain medications because she does not want to have to rely on strong medications and she is afraid of becoming addicted. I explained to her the consequences of untreated pain and also tried to ease her fears of pain medication. She assured me that she will see her physician if the pain becomes severe when aspirin does not help her.

Thelma M.

addicted to thyroid replacement. This distinction should be made very clear to the patient and the family.

In contrast to dependence and tolerance, **addiction** is a *psychological* dependence on the medication (Gordon et al., 2005). Addiction is no longer narrowly defined in relation to the symptoms of withdrawal; instead, it is described according to the following three behavioral characteristics:

- Compulsive use of the drug
- Loss of control over the use of the drug
- Use of the drug in spite of harm

Based on this definition, it is clear that the continued use of opioids for pain relief does not indicate addiction, regardless of the dose or length of time the person has been using the medication. In fact, several studies indicate that fewer than 1% of patients who use opioids are addicted to them (Friedman, 1990; Porter & Jick, 1980).

Development of a Pain Management Regimen

The following are key points to remember with analgesic administration:

- Use the nursing process to manage pain in older adults.
- Work closely with the interdisciplinary team, especially the pharmacist and the prescriber.
- Recognize that prescribers, like nurses, have their own values, beliefs, and potential biases about pain.
- Approach the prescriber as a colleague with mutual goals for the patient.
- When communicating with other members of the health care team, formulate a plan that addresses the patient's pain goals, anticipated side effects, and proposed interventions for those side effects. Proposed interventions should be based on analgesic guidelines (i.e., the WHO pain relief ladder) and should include nonpharmacologic interventions, when appropriate.
- Document objectively and frequently to establish evidence and justify requests.
- Collaboratively establish the pain relief goal and use it as the standard for assessing the response to medication adjustments.
- Include both the patient and family as members of the decision-making team.
- Nurses cannot be expected to know all the implications of all analgesics; learn a few drugs well and keep references handy for the rest.
- Develop your own expertise in nonpharmacologic interventions, which can often be the most effective and comforting interventions for your patients.

For specific recommendations for managing pain in some common chronic conditions, see Table 28-3.

TABLE 28-3 Managing Pain in Older Adults With Common Chronic Conditions

Type of Pain	Characteristics of Pain	Nonpharmacologic Treatments	Pharmacologic Treatments
Persistent back pain	• Difficult to manage • Up to 85% of back pain has no obvious etiology • Often more than one etiology	• Cognitive–behavioral therapy • Physical therapy • Yoga • Instructed stretching	• NSAIDs with caution for GI bleeds • Opioids in conjunction with nonpharmacologic methods • Adjuvant analgesics, such as tricyclic antidepressants in patients also diagnosed with depression
Osteoporosis pain	• Intensifies with sitting or standing and is relieved by bed rest • Exacerbated by sudden movements • May be an indirect consequence of multiple vertebral compression fractures	• Bed rest and bracing (for acute pain) • Rehabilitative physical therapy • Supportive pillows • Ice massage • Patient education • Social support	• NSAIDs with caution for GI bleeds • Opioid–nonopioid combination with short-acting opioids, or controlled-release opioids, with caution because sedation can increase risk of falls and fractures • Opioid-induced constipation can lead to straining, thereby increasing risk of osteoporotic fractures; carefully titrate dosage and prescribe a laxative
Osteoarthritis pain	• Characterized as deep, aching, poorly localized • Usual sites of involvement are the interphalangeal joints, lumbar and cervical spine, and weight-bearing joints	• Exercise • Weight control • Rest • Joint care	• Acetaminophen has been shown to relieve pain as effectively as NSAIDs for many patients with osteoarthritis. • NSAIDs with caution for GI bleeds (although all NSAIDs work similarly, each has a different chemical compound with slightly different side effects) • Celecoxib (Celebrex), a COX-2 inhibitor, is still being prescribed although other COX-2 inhibitors have been taken off the market. • Topical pain-relieving creams, rubs, and sprays (e.g., capsaicin cream) • Corticosteroids

GI, gastrointestinal; NSAID, nonsteroidal anti-inflammatory drug.

Chapter Highlights

Definitions: Acute Versus Persistent Pain

- Two commonly accepted definitions of pain are (1) an unpleasant sensory and emotional experience associated with actual or potential tissue damage; and (2) whatever the person experiencing it says it is, existing whenever she or he says it does.
- Acute pain is time-limited and responsive to analgesics, whereas persistent pain continues for a prolonged period and may or may not be associated with a recognizable disease process.

Anatomy and Physiology of Pain

- Nociception, which is the physiologic occurrence of a measurable pain signal, involves the four processes of transduction, transmission, perception, and modulation (Fig. 28-1).

Types of Pain

- Pain can be classified as nociceptive or neuropathic pain; nociceptive pain is further classified as either somatic or visceral pain.
- Cancer pain is a complex phenomenon in which pain can be acute, persistent, nociceptive, or neuropathic.

Causes of Pain in Older Adults

- For 80% to 85% of people age 65 years and older, a significant health problem is associated with pain.

Age-Related Changes That Affect Pain

- Age-related changes can affect pain perception and pain management, and pain symptoms may present differently in older and younger adults.

Barriers to Pain Management

- Nurses need to identify and address problems that create barriers to effective pain management in older adults (Table 28-1).

Functional Consequences of Pain in Older Adults

- The functional consequences of pain in older adults include diminished physical function, loss of mobility, higher levels of disability, and decreased quality of life.
- Untreated pain can lead to anxiety, depression, or even suicide.

Nursing Assessment of Pain in Older Adults

- Nurses need to assess factors that can worsen or improve pain for older adults (Box 28-1).
- Nurses can base their assessment of pain in older adults on certain assumptions (Box 28-2).
- Box 28-3 summarizes sample questions for pain assessment.
- Nurses need to apply specific principles of pain assessment for older adults who are cognitively impaired (Table 28-2).
- Figure 28-2 illustrates some of the commonly used pain scales that are applicable to assessing pain in older adults.

Principles of Analgesic Medication

- Principles of analgesic administration are outlined in the World Health Organization's pain relief ladder (Fig. 28-3) and applied to some common chronic conditions in Table 28-3.
- Nurses need to address adverse effects of analgesics, with particular attention to maintaining bowel function (Box 28-4).
- Nurses need to teach patients and their families about the differences between tolerance, dependence, and addiction.

Critical Thinking Exercises

1. Identify an older person in your recent clinical experience who has talked with you about persistent pain and address the following in relation to that person:
   - What factors listed in Box 28-1 affect the person's experience of pain?
   - What assumptions from Box 28-2 are applicable to assessment of pain in that person?
2. Review the barriers to effective pain management related to patients and families (Table 28-1) and identify ways in which you could overcome these barriers when you care for older adults in clinical practice.
3. Review the information about tolerance, dependence, and addiction, and write a sentence for each of these concepts in terms that you could use for teaching older adults and their caregivers.

Clinical Tool Resources

Hartford Institute for Geriatric Nursing

Try This: Best Practices in Nursing Care to Older Adults
Issue Number 7 (Revised 2007), Assessing Pain in Older Adults
www.hartfordign.org/resources/education/tryThis.html
Try This: Best Practices in Nursing Care for Older Adults With Dementia
Issue Number D2 (Revised 2007), Assessing Pain in Persons With Dementia
www.hartfordign.org/resources/education/tryThis.html

City of Hope, Pain Resource Center

Numerous clinical resources, including multilingual assessment tools
www.cityofhope.org/PRC/pain_assessment.asp

Educational Resources

American Society for Pain Management Nursing
http://aspmn.org

GeroNurseOnline
www.geronurseonline.org

Partners Against Pain
www.partnersagainstpain.com

References

Al Snih, S., Raji, M. A., Peek, M. K., & Ottenbacher, K. J. (2005). Pain, lower-extremity muscle strength, and physical function among older Mexican Americans. *Archives of Physical Medicine and Rehabilitation, 86*, 1394–1400.

American Geriatrics Society (AGS). (2002). The management of persistent pain in older persons. *Journal of the American Geriatrics Society, 50*(6 Suppl.), S205–224.

Bolen, J., Helmick, C. G., Sacks, J. J., & Langmaid, G. (2002). Prevalence of self-reported arthritis and chronic joint symptoms among adults: United States, 2001. *MMWR Morbidity and Mortality Weekly Report, 51*(42), 948–950.

Borglin, G., Jakobsson, U., Edberg, A., & Hallberg, I. R. (2005). Self-reported health complaints and their prediction of overall and health-related quality of life among elderly people. *International Journal of Nursing Studies, 42*, 147–158.

Call-Schmidt, T. A., & Richardson, S. J. (2003). Prevalence of sleep disturbance and its relationship to pain in adults with chronic pain. *Pain Management Nursing, 4*, 124–133.

Chin, J. J., Sahadevan, S., Tan, C. Y., Ho, S. C., & Choo, P. W. (2001). Critical role of functional decline in delayed discharge from an acute geriatric unit. *Annals of the Academy of Medicine, Singapore, 30*, 593–599.

Croft, P., Jordan, K., & Jinks, C. (2005). "Pain elsewhere" and the impact of knee pain in older people. *Arthritis and Rheumatism, 52*, 2350–2354.

Elliott, T. E., Renier, C. M., & Palcher, J. A. (2003). Chronic pain, depression, and quality of life: Correlations and predictive value of the SF-36. *Pain Medicine, 4*, 331–339.

Federal Interagency Forum on Aging-Related Statistics. (2004). *Older Americans 2004: Key indicators of well-being*. Available at www.agingstats.gov/Agingstatsdotnet/Main_Site/Data/2004_Documents/entire_report.pdf. Accessed December 4, 2004.

Feldt, K. S. (2000). The Checklist of Nonverbal Pain Indicators (CNPI). *Pain Management Nursing, 1*(1), 13–21.

Friedman, D. P. (1990). Perspectives on the medical use of drugs of abuse. *Journal of Pain and Symptom Management, 5*(1 Suppl.), S2–S5.

Gallagher, R. M., Verma, S., & Mossey, J. (2000). Chronic pain: Sources of late-life pain and risk factors for disability. *Geriatrics, 55*(9), 40–44.

Gordon, D. B., Dahl, J. L., Miaskowski, C., McCarberg, B., Todd, K. H., Paice, J. A., et al. (2005). American Pain Society recommendations for improving the quality of acute and cancer pain management: American Pain Society Quality of Care Task Force. *Archives of Internal Medicine, 165*, 1574–1580.

Gowin, K. M. (2000). Diffuse pain syndromes in the elderly. *Rheumatic Diseases Clinics of North America, 26*, 673–682.

Gregg, E. W., Sorlie, P., Paulose-Ram, R., Gu, Q., Eberhardt, M. S., Wolz, M., et al. (2004). Prevalence of lower-extremity disease in the US adult population ≥40 years of age with and without diabetes: 1999–2000 National Health and Nutrition Examination Survey. *Diabetes Care, 27*, 1591–1597.

Hartvigsen, J., Christensen, K., & Frederiksen, H. (2003). Back pain remains a common symptom in old age: A population-based study of 4486 Danish twins aged 70–102. *European Spine Journal, 12*, 528–534.

Herr, K., Coyne, P. J., Key, T., Manworren, M., McCaffery, M., Merkel, S., et al. (2006). Pain assessment in the nonverbal patient: Position statement with clinical practice recommendations. *Pain Management Nursing, 7*, 44–52.

Herr, K. A., & Mobily, P. R. (1993). Comparison of selected pain assessment tools for use with the elderly. *Applied Nursing Research, 6*(1), 39–46.

Hurley, A. C., Volicer, B. J., Hanrahan, S. H., & Volicer, L. (1992). Assessment of discomfort in advanced Alzheimer patients. *Research in Nursing & Health, 15*, 369–377.

International Association for the Study of Pain (IASP). (1986). Classification of chronic pain: Descriptions of chronic pain syndromes and definitions of pain terms. *Pain, 24*(Suppl. 1), S1–S226.

Jakobsson, U., Hallberg, I. R., & Westergren, A. (2004). Overall and health related quality of life among the oldest old in pain. *Quality of Life Research, 13*(1), 125–136.

Jakobsson, U., Klevgard, R., Westergren, A., & Hallberg, I. R. (2003). Old people in pain: A comparative study. *Journal of Pain and Symptom Management, 26*, 625–636.

Jung, B. F., Johnson, R. W., Griffin, D. R., & Dworkin, R. H. (2004). Risk factors for postherpetic neuralgia in patients with herpes zoster. *Neurology, 62*, 1545–1551.

Kotz, K., Deleger, S., Cohen, R., Kamigaki, A., & Kurata, J. (2004). Osteoporosis and health-related quality-of-life outcomes in the Alameda County Study population. *Preventing Chronic Disease, 1*(1). Available at www.cdc.gov/pcd/issues/2004/jan/2003_0005.htm.

Manfredi, P., Breuer, B., Wallenstein, S., Stegmann, M., Bottomley, G., & Libow, L. (2003). Opioid treatment for agitation in patients with advanced dementia. *International Journal of Geriatric Psychiatry, 18*, 700–705.

McCaffery, M. (1968). *Nursing practice theories related to cognition, bodily pain and man-environmental interactions*. Los Angeles: UCLA Students Store.

McCaffery, M., & Pasero, C. (1999). Assessment: Underlying complexities, misconceptions, and practical tools. In M. McCaffery & C. Pasero (Eds.), *Pain: Clinical manual for nursing practice* (2nd ed., pp. 35–102). St. Louis: Mosby.

McDonnell, A., Nicholl, J., & Read, S. M. (2003). Acute pain teams and the management of postoperative pain: A systematic review and meta-analysis. *Journal of Advanced Nursing, 41*, 261–273.

Opstelten, W., Mauritz, J. W., de Wit, N. J., van Wijck, A. J., Stalman, W. A., & van Essen, G. A. (2002). Herpes zoster and postherpetic neuralgia: Incidence and risk indicators using a general practice research database. *Family Practice, 19*, 471–475.

Porter, J., & Jick, H. (1980). Addiction rare in patients treated with narcotics. *New England Journal of Medicine, 302*, 123.

Reid, M. C., Williams, C. S., & Gill, T. M. (2003). The relationship between psychological factors and disabling musculoskeletal pain in community-dwelling older persons. *Journal of the American Geriatrics Society, 51*, 1092–1098.

Rustoen, T., Wahl, A. K., Hanestad, B. R., Lerdal, A., Paul, S., & Miaskowski, C. (2005). Age and the experience of chronic pain: Differences in health and quality of life among younger, middle-aged, and older adults. *Clinical Journal of Pain, 21*, 513–523.

Scherder, E., Oosterman, J., Swaab, D., Herr, K., Ooms, M., Ribbe, M., et al. (2005). Recent developments in pain in dementia. *British Medical Journal, 330*, 461–464.

Schuler, M., Njoo, N., Hestermann, M., Oster, P., & Hauer, K. (2004). Acute and chronic pain in geriatrics: Clinical characteristics of pain and the influence of cognition. *Pain Medicine, 5*, 253–262.

Shipton, E. A., & Tait, B. (2005). Flagging the pain: Preventing the burden of chronic pain by identifying and treating risk factors in acute pain. *European Journal of Anaesthesiology, 22*, 405–412.

Tamiya, N., Araki, S., Ohi, G., Inagaki, K., Urano, N., Hirano, W., et al. (2002). Assessment of pain, depression, and anxiety by visual analogue scale in Japanese women with rheumatoid arthritis. *Scandinavian Journal of Caring Sciences, 16*, 137–141.

Tsai, P., & Means, K. M. (2005). Osteoarthritic knee or hip pain: Possible indicators in elderly adults with cognitive impairment. *Journal of Gerontological Nursing, 31*(8), 39–45.

Webb, R., Brammah, T., Lunt, M., Urwin, M., Allison, T., & Symmons, D. (2003). Prevalence and predictors of intense, chronic, and disabling neck and back pain in the UK general population. *Spine, 28*, 1195–1202.

Wolfe, F., Ross, K., Anderson, J., Russell, I. J., & Hebert, L. (1995). The prevalence and characteristics of fibromyalgia in the general population. *Arthritis and Rheumatism, 38*, 19–28.

Yennurajalingam, S., Braiteh, F., & Bruera, E. (2005). Pain and terminal delirium research in the elderly. *Clinics in Geriatric Medicine, 21*, 93–119.

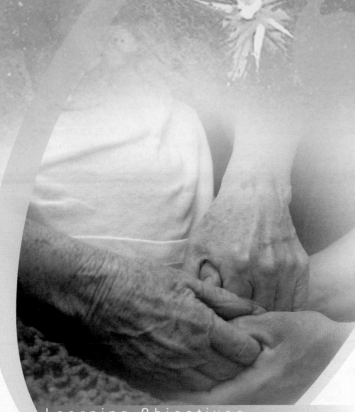

CHAPTER 29

Caring for Older Adults at the End of Life

Learning Objectives

After reading this chapter, you will be able to:

1. Identify factors that influence attitudes toward death.
2. Describe cultural and historical approaches to end-of-life care.
3. Explain the nurse's role in end-of-life care.
4. Identify the common characteristics of "quality of life" and a "good death."
5. Describe palliative care and hospice nursing.
6. Assess physical, psychological, social, and spiritual care needs for older adults at the end of life.
7. Identify appropriate nursing interventions to address symptoms commonly experienced by older adults at the end of life.

Key Terms

death
death with dignity
dying
end of life
hospice
medicalization
palliation
rehumanizing
spiritual well-being

END-OF-LIFE TRANSITIONS

Despite the fact that dying is a phenomenon that affects all living beings, many people fear death. This fear stems partially from associating death with inevitable pain, suffering, and loneliness. In recent decades, advances in medical knowledge and technology have shifted the focus of care to prolonging and sustaining life at all costs. Many illnesses that once were fatal are now chronic conditions to be managed over time. Because of these changes, the goals of health care are the cure of disease and management of chronic illness in efforts to prolong life. However, it has become evident in recent years that improving the quality of this resulting longer life is more difficult to achieve (Meier, 2004).

The Dying Process and Death

Although life and death appear to be clear concepts, the lack of an exact definition of the terms *life, dying*, and *death* can at times cloud the goals of care. According to the American Geriatrics Society's (AGS) position statement on *The Care of Dying Patients* (AGS, 2002), birth and death give definition to life as the period of time in between. **Death** is an irreversible lifeless state in which the physiologic functions of life are absent. **Dying** is regarded as a less specific, individualized process in which an organism's life comes to an end (i.e., the final portion of the life cycle). When does the dying process begin? People are considered to be dying when they are ill with a progressive condition that is expected to end in death and for which there is no treatment that can substantially alter the outcome (AGS, 2002). The length of the dying process is variable and dependent on the individual's holistic situation. Its duration may be a matter of minutes, hours, weeks, or months.

The **end of life** is the period for patients in which "there is little likelihood of cure for their disease(s); further aggressive therapy is judged to be futile; and comfort is the primary goal" (Wilke & TNEEL Investigators, 2003, p. 9). This period can last from hours to months and it encompasses the time during which a person is actively dying. **Palliation** is defined as "the relief of suffering when cure is impossible" (Wilke & TNEEL Investigators, 2003, p. 41). Palliative care is an evolving professional specialization, defined by the Robert Wood Johnson Foundation Last Acts Task Force (2002) as the "comprehensive management of the physical, psychological, social, spiritual, and existential needs of patients, particularly those with incurable, progressive illness. The goal of palliative care is to help them achieve the best possible quality of life through minimizing suffering, controlling symptoms, and restoring functional capacity, while remaining sensitive to personal, cultural, and religious values, beliefs, and practices."

Nursing Skills in Caring for the Dying

Regardless of the setting, nurses take on a primary role in the delivery of palliative care at a time in which aggressive, curative medical care is no longer feasible or appropriate. According to the Hospice and Palliative Nurses Association (HPNA) position statement on the *Value of Professional Nurse in End-of-Life Care* "Achieving quality of life, especially at the end of life, is contingent upon competent, 'state of the art' professional nursing care" (HPNA, 2003, p. 1). Nursing pioneers in palliative care Florence Wald, Cicely Saunders (also a physician), and Jeanne Quint Benoliel emphasized that those in need of care at the end of life deserve "the most competent, expert, evidence-based care provided in a way that embodies compassion, respect for dignity, and an appreciation for the whole person and the family" (Ferrell, 2001, p. xii). Further specialized nursing skills required to deliver effective care are defined as follows:

> *Competency-based nursing practice at the end of life includes expert assessment skills, critical thinking, comprehensive pain and symptom management, and the acquisition of knowledge, attitudes, and skills in areas related to the phases of wellness and illness at the end of life. End-stage illness usually presents with not only one, but multiple and often complex symptoms that affect the body, mind, and spirit. This requires the professional nurse to use specialized skills and provide holistic care that is consistent with the goals of the patient and family. Individualized professional nursing care at this time of life has never been so critical to maximize autonomy, dignity, healing, and comfort, which are generally accepted quality-of-life indicators (HPNA, 2003, p. 1).*

CULTURAL AND HISTORICAL PERSPECTIVES ON DEATH AND DYING

During the last hundred years, society has witnessed significant change in the perception and management of death. Before the 20th century, death was more readily accepted as an inevitable and normal part of life. Illness and death were family centered, with care provided by family members in their homes. As health care has became more sophisticated, a shift has occurred. Hospital-based care provided by physicians, nurses, and other professionals has replaced the family caregiving model. This **medicalization** of end-of-life care has had a major impact on the dying experience in the last 3 to 4 decades: end-of-life experiences in formal health care facilities are often technologically driven and dehumanized (Saunderson & Brener, 2007).

Nursing is a leading force in the palliative care movement—a natural fit given the holistic tradition of the profession. In the past 2 to 3 decades, as hospice has grown, so has a realization that the end of life can be positively affected by returning to basics. Goals are slowly refocusing on comfort, companionship, and caring, with nurses in a pivotal role. This **rehumanizing** of death and dying recognizes and respects the process as an important and meaningful stage of the continuum of human life. Box 29-1 presents strategies for rehumanizing death.

Demographics of Death and Dying

Changing demographics in the United States during the last century have inspired the recent interest in and emphasis on end-of-life care. For example, dramatic increases in life expectancy and changes in the causes of death (as discussed in Chapter 1) have led to a larger population that is spending

Box 29-1
Strategies for Rehumanizing Death

- Reintroduce a peaceful sense of harmony between dying people and the process of dying.
- Provide the support of community participation in dying rituals.
- Support the harmonious acceptance of death as ordinary and natural, not a social evil.
- Emphasize the comforting roles of fellowship, ritual, and ceremony.
- Facilitate, even mandate, the notion that dying should be a culturally shared community experience.
- Culturally legitimize the pain and suffering that often accompanies dying.
- Provide a common base of participation and sense of belonging; attach the dying person to the community of living.

From Saunderson, C. A., & Brener, T. H. (Eds.). (2007). *End of life: A nurse's guide to compassionate care* (p. 281). Philadelphia: Lippincott Williams & Wilkins.

longer periods of time in poor health. This fact has implications for the end-of-life and palliative care needs of society (Wilke & TNEEL Investigators, 2003). In older adults, death is usually associated with the cumulative effects of chronic illness and many interacting conditions, rather than a single cause. The need for palliative care to improve comfort and quality of life for this population is significant and growing rapidly (see Chapter 27 for a discussion of this topic).

Sites of Death and Dying

Since the beginning of the 20th century, when most people died in their homes, the place of death has gradually shifted, so that by the 1990s only 20% of people died at home or in noninstitutional settings. However, that trend is reversing, and in 1999 25% of deaths occurred in private homes (Wilke & TNEEL Investigators, 2003). According to the report by the Robert Wood Johnson Foundation Last Acts Task Force (2002), a national coalition to improve care and caring near the end of life, 50% of Americans 65 years of age and older die in hospitals, although more than 70% state their desire to die at home. The deaths are often preceded by multiple physician visits and expensive life-prolonging treatments. A growing percentage of people, 20% to 25%, die in nursing homes.

Death is a subject that not only is often avoided, but is influenced by many misperceptions. Nurses need to examine their own attitudes towards death, in addition to the perspectives of society, older adults, and other health care professionals.

Views of Death and Dying in Western Culture

As a result of many interacting factors, Western culture has tended to deny or ignore the universality of death. During the last several decades, responsibility for the dying experience has been informally and more exclusively delegated to clinicians, with a majority of deaths occurring in hospitals. In health care settings, physicians are usually the major decision makers because of their medical expertise. Many older adults revere physician suggestions and recommendations for treatment, even though they do not always fully understand the issues, options, or potential consequences. Older adults are often reluctant to question physicians, and they may set aside their personal values, ideas, and wishes to follow the advice of their doctor. Consequently, they may not explore their options of dying in places other than hospitals or institutional settings.

In studies of social gerontology, Markson (2003) identified four contemporary societal values or beliefs that shape the general outlook on aging and death. First, because work and activity are intertwined with personal self-worth, chronic illness or disability is often associated with the end of productivity and loss of purpose. As a result of these associations, people may avoid acknowledging illness and aging because they are viewed as predecessors to death.

In addition, Markson (2003) cites a mythologic belief that many Americans share, which is that through self-determination and individual responsibility, anyone can do anything if he or she tries hard enough. Because human life has inherent limitations, this false mentality is a major underpinning to the denial of aging and death in the 21st century.

The belief that modern technology gives us the ability to control or modify the environment has expanded with the medical advances of the last several decades. The implication is that aging, illness, and even death can be manipulated, managed, and controlled (Markson, 2003).

Finally, over time the authority over and responsibility for death has subtly transferred from religious leaders to physicians. The ability to cure illness and prolong life has imbued life and death with qualities that are more humanistic and less spiritual (Markson, 2003).

In some ways, society is more accepting of an older adult's death compared with that of a younger person. The rationale for this attitude is that older people have had an opportunity to "live their lives." As the aging process works on the body, sometimes death is viewed as a blessing, taking an older adult out of a situation of suffering and reduced capacity. Caregivers often express relief when death occurs, stating that "he wouldn't have wanted to live like this."

In spite of these prevalent attitudes and beliefs, in the past 20 to 30 years society in general has begun to culturally acknowledge and integrate an increasing acceptance of life's end. This change has been largely provoked by the baby boom generation facing its own aging process, while simultaneously dealing with their parents' aging and health issues. Ethical questions and challenges have surfaced as a result of problems in care and rising associated costs. For example, in the midst of the assisted suicide debate, society has begun asking a second layer of questions: "What value is there in the last phase of life? Can there be any meaning and value in the process of dying? Can there be value in grieving? Can there be value in caring for people as they die?" (Byock, 2006). The changing demographics and sheer increase in the numbers of older adults dying will be an impetus for continued discussion and changes in social policies.

Older Adults' Perspective on Death and Dying

How do older adults view death when mortality becomes imminent? Common stereotypes about old age contribute to the myth that older adults are ready to die because their lives have lost their value. These beliefs have been proven to be ageist. On the contrary, although studies have suggested that death anxiety decreases with advancing age, older adults' feelings about death vary according to individual social circumstances and life experiences (Markson, 2003). In spite of their chronologic years, many older adults have life goals they expect to fulfill and consequently are not ready to die.

Whereas younger generations may feel a sense of entitlement to a long life, many older adults hold the opposite view. They may be more accepting of the possibility of imminent death, viewing long life as a privilege. Young people tend to place life and death on opposite ends of the spectrum, and feel threatened and cheated by death because of the opportunity for living that is lost. From their vantage point, older adults more frequently view death as a natural part of life's continuum, and the process of dying as a period of self-actualization. Even though physical decline is a main theme of aging and dying, for many older adults this time of life is one of growth and fulfillment. From this holistic perspective on death and dying, old age can be turned into an opportunity for development, and death into an ultimate accomplishment.

Health Care Professionals' Perspective on Death and Dying

Health care facilities have been institutionally designed to be centers for disease care and disease cure. Given this orientation, practitioners and health care professionals often view death as something to be avoided because it symbolizes professional and personal incompetence or failure. Prolonging life, even at the expense of quality, was thought to be the ultimate accomplishment: a symbol of success for patients, families, and the health care teams involved.

In recent decades, palliative and end-of-life care have become part of the medical mainstream, and health care professionals realize they can find meaning and satisfaction in caring for people who are dying and their loved ones. As experts, professionals in the disciplines of hospice and palliative care play a key role in promoting awareness and understanding in this process of social, cultural, and professional maturation. Standards of care define and guide health professionals' practice to include clear communication, ethical decision making, technical competence, and intensive management of symptoms, respecting the dying individual's autonomy. The issue of quality of life versus quantity of life at all costs has redefined the professional perspective.

To provide effective end-of-life care, nurses need to examine their own feelings and attitudes, which may affect the care they provide. Personal beliefs about death are shaped by experiences from the time of birth, with the family as the primary influence. Religious affiliations, popular media and culture, and ethnic background contribute to one's reactions to death and dying. Whether death is discussed as part of normal life, or whether it is seen as "the enemy," influences care. Nurses need to not only learn about clinical aspects of end-of-life care, but they must take time to process their own feelings and concerns. Some questions to ponder for self-awareness and insight include the following (Ohio State University Health Sciences Center, 2003):

- When you hear the word "death," what comes to mind? What do you personally fear the most? What are you most curious about?
- How old were you the first time someone close to you died? How was grief handled in your family? What do you believe happens to you when you die?
- Have you ever seen anyone die? What was that like for you?
- How do your own attitudes and previous experiences affect the way you work with dying patients now?

Because of the nature of their work as care providers, nurses are in an ideal position to serve primary roles in achieving quality end-of-life experiences for older adults.

> **A Student's Perspective**
>
> *This week, I learned that it is okay to accept that an elderly patient is ready to die and that is his wish. I had a patient who requested that we not perform any measures—just give him his beer with lunch, wine with dinner, and some pain medicine to make him comfortable. He stated that he has led a good life and is ready to go see God. That is really hard for me because it's my job to help people and save lives. The other aspect of that is helping people die a dignified death—it's just a really TOUGH aspect!!!*
>
> *Sarah E.*

Culturally Diverse Perspectives on Death and Dying

Nurses providing holistic care to older adults at the end of life need to acknowledge the effects of culture on the dying experience. Attitudes, beliefs, reactions, and decisions are influenced by an individual's cultural heritage. Culture is multidimensional. Its commonly identified components include race, ethnicity, age, differing abilities, sexual orientation, religion and spirituality, and socioeconomic factors. In addition, nurses must consider two additional perspectives. One is the culture of the health care system, which may be defined by the type, location, and mission of the facility; skill level and size of staff; and characteristics of the patient base. Another is the generational difference in opinions, values, and lifestyle, all of which are influenced by life experiences. Nurses need to recognize and address these differences in relation to end-of-life care. Cultural Considerations 29-1 summarizes some beliefs and attitudes about death that are associated with cultural groups. The experience of death and dying is very individualized, but nurses should incorporate these considerations into individualized assessments and be aware of diverse beliefs and attitudes associated with the experience of death and dying.

QUALITY OF CARE AT THE END OF LIFE

Preferences for end-of-life care are strongly influenced by the availability of resources in the community (Robert Wood Johnson Foundation Last Acts Task Force, 2002). Several large-scale studies have identified serious problems with end-of-life care in the United States. The 1997 Institute of

Cultural Considerations 29-1

Perspectives on Death and Dying

- Cultural factors may determine a "line of communication" about pending death; for example, a male relative or the head of a family (e.g., eldest son) may be the one who summons other family members, or close friends may be told before the family so they can provide emotional support.
- Even when death is accepted as expected and inevitable, dying patients or their families may also believe that it should be prevented or delayed by biomedical interventions; this may affect decisions about resuscitation.
- Some families may prefer that death occur in a hospital so they do not feel responsible.
- Cultural groups may have rituals for the time immediately after death (e.g., summoning a religious leader, burning candles, saying prayers, have the body face a certain direction, calling all family to the bedside).
- Some cultural groups have special rituals for care of the body after death; nurses need to ask families if the institutional protocol needs to be adapted for cultural considerations.
- Families may prefer to care for the body after death, or they may need to arrange for a designated person (e.g., a religious leader) to prepare the body.
- In some cultural groups, it is taboo to talk about death before it occurs; in these situations, the concept of hospice is usually unacceptable.
- Muslims and many of other religious groups may believe that when their time comes, they must go to the other world where God is calling them; this belief may make it easier for families to "let go."
- Cultural or religious factors may prohibit autopsy or organ donation.

Medicine (IOM) report, which examined the dying experience in various settings, concluded that many people experienced discomfort and suffering from end-of-life symptoms (Field & Cassell, 1997). This report also found that health care professionals did not possess the skills and knowledge required to meet the needs of a dying person. Additional problems identified were poor symptom control, patient and family stress, lack of coordination among health care professionals, inadequate preparation for the dying process, and drained financial and emotional resources.

The Study to Understand Prognoses and Preferences for Outcomes and Risks of Treatments (SUPPORT), which was conducted in the mid-1990s, also found deficiencies in end-of-life care (SUPPORT Principal Investigators, 1995). A more recent study, "Family Perspectives on End-of-Life Care at the Last Place of Care," concluded that in spite of increasing awareness and educational opportunities, people dying in this country continue to have their needs poorly met (Teno et al., 2004).

To address some of the problems, the Nathan Cummings Foundation and the Robert Wood Johnson Foundation developed a toolkit to help assess the quality of the end-of-life experience. TIME (the Toolkit of Instruments for Measuring End-of-life Care) provides measurement tools that can be used to identify opportunities for improving care, examining the impact of interventions, and holding facilities accountable for the quality of care provided (see the Educational Resources section at the end of this chapter).

The Role of Nursing

For many older adults, a "good death" is part of the process of "good aging," but both processes are very individualized and strongly influenced by cultural and spiritual factors. In the continuum of life, the experiences of aging, the end of life, and death are opportunities for self-actualization. Defining a "good death" for older adults is extremely personal and often dependent on the effects of aging and illness on the person's level of function and independence. The goal of nursing is to support this stage of life and help patients maintain optimal personal dignity. Studies of patient and family satisfaction have confirmed "death with dignity" as perhaps the most critically important characteristic of a good death. A **death with dignity** is specifically characterized by a dying experience in which (Wilke & TNEEL Investigators, 2003):

- The patient's and family's wishes are respected.
- The patient and family feel a sense of control over the situation.
- The patient is physically comfortable.
- The patient is psychologically comfortable.
- The patient has spiritual support available according to her or his wishes.

These characteristics are in accordance with the "Dying Patient's Bill of Rights," a document created at a workshop on "The Terminally Ill Patient and the Helping Person" by Linda Austin (1975) to identify concretely the dignified care that dying people deserve (Box 29-2). This document continues to be helpful as a fundamental guide for defining goals and interventions for individualized end-of-life care.

Patient comfort, which has always been a core nursing responsibility, is an essential component of death with dignity. The word "patient" is derived from the Latin word *patiens*, which means "one who endures" or "one who suffers." The word "comfort" comes from the Latin *confortare*, which means "to strengthen." Literally, then, nurses who provide comfort to patients are strengthening those who suffer. This definition is particularly appropriate for nurses who provide care for patients at the end of life that is built on the following beliefs (Wilke & TNEEL Investigators, 2003):

- The dying are not people for whom "nothing can be done."
- Patients deserve to be assured that *everything* will be done to prevent them from dying in pain, without dignity.
- Patients will not die alone, isolated from those they love and who love them.

Box 29-2
The Dying Person's Bill of Rights

I have the right to be treated as a living human being until I die.
I have the right to maintain a sense of hopefulness, however changing its focus may be.
I have the right to express my feelings and emotions about my approaching death in my own way.
I have the right to participate in decisions concerning my care.
I have the right to expect continuing medical and nursing attention even though cure goals must be changed to comfort goals.
I have the right not to die alone.
I have the right to be free from pain.
I have the right to have my questions answered honestly.
I have the right not to be deceived.
I have the right to have help from and for my family in accepting my death.
I have the right to die in peace and with dignity.
I have the right to retain my individuality and not be judged for my decisions which may be contrary to the beliefs of others.
I have the right to be cared for by caring, sensitive, knowledgeable people who will attempt to understand my needs and will be able to gain some satisfaction in helping me face my death.
I have the right to be cared for by those who can maintain a sense of hopefulness, however changing this might be.
I have the right to expect that the sanctity of the human body will be respected after death.
I have the right to discuss and enlarge my religious and/or spiritual experiences, whatever these may mean to others.

From Austin, L. (1975).

Hospice Care

Hospice refers to a philosophy of care that seeks to support dignified dying or a good death experience for those with terminal illnesses. Hospice care involves a core interdisciplinary team of professionals and volunteers who provide medical, psychological, and spiritual support, as well as support for the patient's family. These services are provided by public and private agencies in home- or facility-based care settings, or in free-standing, short-term residential facilities.

The term *hospice* (from the same linguistic root as "hospitality") was first applied to specialized care for dying patients in the 1960s by physician and nurse Dame Cicely Saunders, who founded the first modern hospice—St. Christopher's—in a residential suburb of London. During a guest lecture for medical students, nurses, social workers, and chaplains at Yale University, Saunders introduced the idea of hospice care and emphasized holistic services and symptom control. This lecture sparked interest, which led to the development of hospice care as it is known today.

In 1969, psychiatrist Elisabeth Kübler-Ross published "On Death and Dying." This book, based on interviews with dying patients, identified five stages through which many terminally ill patients progress: denial, anger, bargaining, depression, and acceptance (Kübler-Ross, 1969). The book was well received by all disciplines and drew attention to the needs of dying people. In 1972, Kübler-Ross testified at the first national hearings conducted by the U.S. Senate Special Committee on Aging, on the subject of death with dignity. In her testimony she stated,

> *We live in a very particular death-denying society. We isolate both the dying and the old, and it serves a purpose. They are reminders of our own mortality. We should not institutionalize people. We can give families more help with home care and visiting nurses, giving the families and the patients the spiritual, emotional, and financial help in order to facilitate the final care at home (National Hospice and Palliative Care Organization [NHPCO], n.d.).*

In 1982, Congress created a Medicare hospice benefit, which provided federal financial support to people dying of a terminal illness. Hospice benefits have become increasingly available and are now supported by many health insurance plans. Advantages of these services include:

- Hospice treats the person, not the disease; focuses on the family, not the individual; and emphasizes the quality of life, not the duration.
- Hospice care relies on the combined knowledge and skill of an interdisciplinary team of professionals, including physicians, nurses, home care aides, social workers, counselors, and volunteers.
- Hospice care is a cost-effective alternative to the high costs associated with hospitals and traditional institutional care.

Hospice eligibility criteria, which are defined by Medicare, require a physician referral, including a statement that a patient is terminally ill and has a life expectancy of 6 months or less. This requirement is problematic because it is difficult to predict a time period. As a result, many patients have missed opportunities for services and had their benefits delayed until the last few weeks of life. An important role of nurses in this regard is to advocate for referrals to engage hospice support earlier for the benefit of older adult patients and their families. Hospice programs offer the following services:

- Physician and nursing care
- Home health aide
- Therapies such as music, art, and other supportive services
- Social work and counseling services
- Spiritual care
- Volunteer support
- Bereavement counseling, including support programs for 1 year after death
- Medical equipment and supplies
- Drugs related to the disease
- Inpatient care for symptom management, caregiver respite, or both

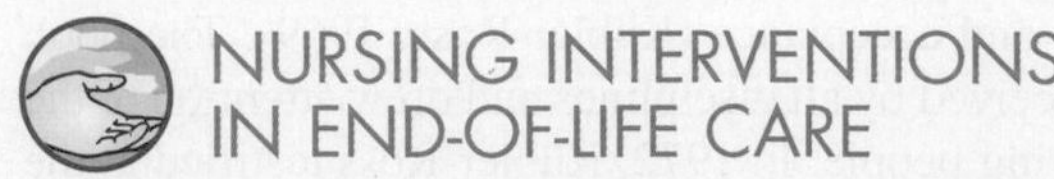

NURSING INTERVENTIONS IN END-OF-LIFE CARE

To assist patients and their families in attaining death with dignity in a caring manner, the nurse must possess the following skills: interpersonal communication abilities; expertise in the assessment and treatment of the physical, psychosocial, and spiritual dimensions of dying; the ability to relate prognoses to patients and families; and knowledge of resources. Nurses assist patients and families with end-of-life tasks, such as identifying sources of support (e.g., hospice), managing symptoms, supporting life-closure processes, and planning for rites and rituals at the time of death and after. Nurses have primary roles not only in assisting with these tasks, but in teaching families about the signs of imminent death and management of the dying processes.

McSteen and Peden-McAlpine (2006) discuss the primary role of nurses as advocates serving as guides, liaisons, and supporters during the dying experience. Guiding activities include providing and clarifying information and options in a manner that supports the decision making of the dying individual and his or her family. In addition, the nurse advocate serves as a liaison between the family and members of the health care team. Including family members in their loved ones' dying process ultimately has a positive impact on the experience. Finally, the nurse advocate acts to support the choices and decision making of patients and families, setting aside his or her own perspective as a health care professional.

Nurses will gain personal and professional satisfaction from serving as care providers, coordinators, and advocates for older adults at the end of life. Fulfillment can be obtained from knowing that patients die in comfort, with their dignity intact and their wishes and values respected.

Promoting Communication

The National Institutes of Health consensus statement on improving end-of-life care (National Institutes of Health Consensus Development Program, 2004) identified numerous transitions that people face at the end of life, including physical, emotional, spiritual, and financial. Nurses have many opportunities to intervene in each of these realms by using communication strategies and interpersonal skills. These interventions include presence, compassion, touch, recognition of an individual's autonomy, and honesty (Box 29-3).

Communication is the cornerstone of interpersonal relationship building. When caring for people who are dying, communication is critically important to all involved, and its importance is magnified by the unpredictability of the situation. Nurses can help dying patients express their needs by using open, honest, direct, and empathetic communication, even when they may be uncertain about what to say. (See Box 29-4 for examples of what to say as well as not to say.) Dying patients value the ability to express themselves; in particular, older adults value the opportunity to achieve closure and say good-bye.

In addition to sensory challenges that can interfere with communication (as discussed in Chapters 16 and 17), some barriers that affect communication at the end of life include the overall stress of the situation, physical symptoms (e.g., pain, fatigue), difficulty expressing thoughts and feelings, difficulty assimilating what is going on in the immediate surroundings, and hierarchical role definitions (e.g., older adults

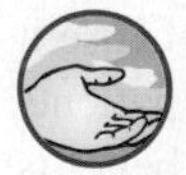

Box 29-3 Supportive Interventions for Relationship Building

Presence	A core nursing intervention, presence can be described as a "gift of self" in which the nurse is available and open to the situation. Presence can be demonstrated through verbal communication, valuing what the patient says, accepting the patient's meaning for things, and remembering or reflecting.
Compassion	The nurse strives to be totally and compassionately *with* the patient and family, allowing the most positive experience.
Touch	A powerful therapeutic intervention, touch communicates an offer of unconditional acceptance. It can be both healing and life affirming, a means of communicating genuine care and compassion.
Recognition of autonomy	The nurse realizes and respects the individual's right to make all end-of-life decisions.
Honesty	The nurse is often in a front-line position to communicate/explain what can be expected. Compassionate honesty builds trust with the older adult facing death and his or her family.
Expert communication	At any given moment, nurses need to be able to assess the patient and family, implement a plan to comfort them, and communicate clearly and supportively throughout.
Assisting in transcendence	At the highest level of care, nurses provide emotional support that facilitates the experience of self-transcendence and a sense of triumph over death.

Adapted from Saunderson, C. A., & Brener, T. H. (Eds.). (2007). *End of life: A nurse's guide to compassionate care* (p. 6). Philadelphia: Lippincott Williams & Wilkins.

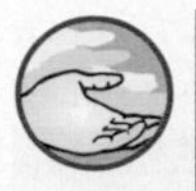

Box 29-4
Communicating With Dying Patients and Their Families

What to Say

- What do you need me to do for you?
- Is there anyone I can call for you?
- I'm here to listen.
- No need to rush. Take your time.
- It's okay to cry. Let me get you a tissue.
- Would you like to be left alone?
- Would you like to share some memories?

What Not to Say

- She's in a better place now.
- He lived a full life.
- She's out of her pain.
- It'll be all right.
- Don't cry.
- Be strong.
- He'd want you to get on with your life.

From Saunderson, C. A., & Brener, T. H. (Eds.). (2007). *End of life: A nurse's guide to compassionate care* (p. 18). Philadelphia: Lippincott Williams & Wilkins.

or family members may feel overwhelmed or intimidated by health care professionals or the setting) (Mauk, 2003).

Nurses can use the following guidelines to address potential barriers (Mauk, 2003):

- Understand yourself and speak honestly.
- Consider the timing and communicate according to the patient's readiness.
- Establish a comfortable environment (e.g., limit noise and distraction; sit at eye level).
- Use good verbal and nonverbal communication skills (use body language purposefully, focus on one point or issue to facilitate concentration).
- Do not make assumptions about what the patient/family know.
- Ask and listen, listen and ask.
- Listen attentively.
- Use understandable terminology.
- Use silence liberally.
- Tell people what to expect.
- Assume that the patient can hear during the entire dying process.

Offering Spiritual Support

The spiritual support provided by nurses is an important component of end-of-life care because it contributes to the dying person's quality of life (Norris et al., 2004). **Spiritual well-being** at the end of life includes meaningful existence, the ability to find meaning in daily experience, and the ability to transcend physical discomfort and prepare for death (Ferrell & Coyle, 2006). Nurses assess spiritual needs both initially and on an ongoing basis because these needs are likely to change during the end-of-life process. Nurses can apply information from Chapter 13 to assess spirituality in older adults. In addition, nurses can use formal spiritual assessment tools, as suggested by Gaskamp and colleagues (2004).

Three nursing diagnoses pertinent to spiritual care during the end of life are Risk for Spiritual Distress, Spiritual Distress, and Readiness for Enhanced Spiritual Well-being (Ackley & Ladwig, 2004). Interventions relevant to the care of the older adult are facilitating forgiveness, instilling hope, and praying (Table 29-1). Nurses also make referrals for pastoral care, hospital chaplains, parish nurses, or other spiritual support resources when appropriate. Outcomes of addressing spirituality for older adults at the end of life include decreased depression, finding or clarifying meaning in life, use of spiritual resources, and improved quality of life (Gaskamp et al., 2004).

Managing Symptoms

Although the end-of-life period and dying are very individualized and unpredictable processes, some symptoms occur commonly and require expert and timely nursing care, particularly for older adults who may experience more symptoms (Ogle & Hopper, 2005). Symptoms, which can occur at any time, include fatigue and weakness, constipation, dyspnea, nausea and vomiting, dehydration, decreased appetite, and pain. Because these symptoms usually occur in combination, management is challenging and it is not always possible to control every symptom completely. Although not every patient will have a peaceful passing, nurses and other health care professionals must make every effort to manage symptoms and alleviate distress to the extent possible.

Nurses can use information in Table 29-2 and the following sections as a guide to nursing assessment and interven-

TABLE 29-1 The Nursing Process: Providing Spiritual Support

Interventions	Specific Actions
Facilitating forgiveness	• Be available. • Listen when the person expresses self-doubt or guilt. • Provide guidance in the forgiveness of others and oneself (e.g., offer to pray with those who are seeking forgiveness).
Instilling hope	• Acknowledge older adult's spirituality, which facilitates hope. • Assist an older adult in coping with grief from personal loss. • Refer the patient to support groups (cultural, religious, or community affiliated).
Prayer	• Participate in prayer with the older adult. • Support/facilitate spiritual expressions such as art, writing, reflection, guided imagery, religious or spiritual readings, rituals, or connection to others and God. • Respect a person's time for quiet and prayer.

From Ackley, B., & Ladwig, G. (2004). *Nursing diagnosis handbook* (6th ed.). St. Louis: Mosby.

TABLE 29-2 Guide to Nursing Assessment and Interventions for Common Symptoms at the End of Life

Symptom	Nursing Assessment	Nursing Interventions	Pharmacologic Interventions
Fatigue (asthenia)	Assess for associated conditions, including infection, fever, pain, depression, insomnia, anxiety, dehydration, hypoxia, medication effects.	Inform older adult and family of the normality of fatigue at end of life. Pace activities and care according to tolerance. Exercise if tolerated. Promote optimal sleep, with regular times of rest, sleep, and waking.	Corticosteroids, although generally contraindicated in older adults, may decrease fatigue in patients with cancer. Treat associated conditions (e.g., with antibiotics, antidepressants).
Constipation	Identify risks (e.g., chronic laxative users, medications). Perform abdominal assessment, including palpation for distention, tenderness, or masses; and auscultation of bowel sounds and pitch. Assess patients taking pain medications daily. Monitor the character of the bowel movements. Check the rectum if the older adult has not had a bowel movement in more than 3 days or is leaking liquid stool (which can occur with an impaction).	Anticipate and prevent constipation with emphasis on fiber, fluid intake, and activity, but recognize that patients may have difficulty tolerating the optimal interventions. Promote regular routine. Strongest propulsive contractions occur after breakfast; provide patient privacy at this time.	Individualize laxative regimen based on the cause(s) of constipation, history, and preferences. Use bulk-forming and stool-softening agents for patients with normal peristalsis. A laxative regimen (with stimulant laxative) may be ordered for patients taking a pain medication known to cause constipation. Stimulant laxatives are the most appropriate for opioid-induced constipation.
Dyspnea	*Respiratory:* Assess vital signs, including oxygen saturation, breathing pattern, and use of accessory muscles. Auscultate breath sounds. Assess cough (type, if present). Check for tachypnea and cyanosis. *General:* Assess for restlessness, anxiety, and activity tolerance.	Pace activities and rest. Provide oxygen, usually at 2–4 L per cannula (avoid using face mask because of discomfort and sensation of smothering). Provide calm reassurance. Use a fan to circulate air and help reduce the feeling of breathlessness. Position for optimal respiratory function (e.g., leaning forward over a table with a pillow on top is helpful for COPD; on the side with head slightly elevated for unresponsive patient). Teach patient to use pursed lip breathing, and encourage relaxation techniques to reduce muscle tightness and associated sensation of breathlessness.	Treat causes. Treat symptoms with morphine or hydromorphone, which relieves the breathless sensation in almost all cases. Use anti-anxiety agents or antidepressants if appropriate (and if perception of breathlessness is exaggerated because of anxiety or depression). Corticosteroids can be used for their anti-inflammatory effects in certain conditions (e.g., COPD, radiation pneumonitis).
Nausea and vomiting	Assess for potential cause (e.g., constipation, bowel obstruction). Palpate abdomen and check for distention. Assess vomitus for fecal odor. Assess heartburn and nausea, which may occur after meals in squashed stomach syndrome. Assess pain (e.g., pain on swallowing may indicate oral thrush; pain on standing may be caused by mesenteric traction). Hiccups occur with uremia.	Offer frequent, small meals; serve foods cold or at room temperature. Apply damp, cool cloth to face when nauseated. Provide oral care after vomiting.	Medications need to be specific to the cause: • Squashed stomach syndrome, gastritis, and functional bowel obstruction: metoclopramide (contraindicated in full bowel obstruction) • Chemical causes such as morphine, hypercalcemia, or renal failure: haloperidol • If caused by dysfunction of vomiting center (e.g., associated with mechanical bowel obstruction, increased intracranial pressure, motion sickness): meclizine or diphenhydramine

continued on following page

TABLE 29-2 Guide to Nursing Assessment and Interventions for Common Symptoms at the End of Life (continued)

Symptom	Nursing Assessment	Nursing Interventions	Pharmacologic Interventions
Dehydration	Assess for clinical signs of hydration (e.g., skin turgor over the upper chest or forehead). Assess buccal membranes for moistness. Assess vital signs: pulse, orthostatic blood pressure.	Encourage fluids as tolerated; offer ice chips and popsicles if swallowing. Provide frequent oral care; use swabs or moistened toothettes.	Give intravenous fluids or administer clysis per advance directives. Discuss continued diuretic use with physician.
Anorexia and cachexia	Assess for weight loss. Assess for levels of weakness and fatigue. Conduct physical examination for decreased fat, muscle wasting, decreased strength. Assess mental status, including depression.	Remove unpleasant odors. Provide frequent oral care. Treat pain optimally. Provide frequent, small meals. Provide companionship. Serve meals in a place that is separate from the bed area. Involve patient with meal planning. Collaborate with dietician for nutritional analysis and meal planning. Encourage culturally appropriate foods. Consider using an alcoholic beverage before meals.	Medications that are used to stimulate appetite, promote weight gain, and provide a sense of well-being: megestrol acetate, corticosteroids, and mirtazapine. Metoclopramide is used to improve gastric motility and appetite.

COPD, chronic obstructive pulmonary disease.

tions for some of the commonly occurring symptoms. In addition, nurses can use information in Chapter 28 to address pain, which is a symptom that occurs frequently at the end of life and is one of the most feared symptoms associated with death. This chapter addresses the symptoms only in relation to the end of life; other pertinent topics are discussed more comprehensively in other chapters: confusion (Chapter 14), depression (Chapter 15), constipation (Chapter 18), and sleep problems (Chapter 24).

Fatigue (Asthenia)

Fatigue is one of the most commonly reported symptoms at the end of life. Fatigue is often described as tiredness, or lack of physical strength and endurance, or decreased mental concentration. Older adults may have reduced energy or activity tolerance caused by usual aging changes, so it is important for the nurse to establish a baseline for comparison and meaningful interpretation. Fatigue is generally a symptom with underlying causes related to disease processes or conditions, such as anemia, malnutrition, infection, drug therapy, or depression. Other concurrent end-of-life symptoms, such as pain and dyspnea, may exacerbate fatigue.

Constipation

Constipation, a reduced frequency of bowel movements, can include passing hard stools, straining to pass a stool, or impaction (hard stool that is blocked). Constipation may be accompanied by pain, abdominal fullness, and reduced bowel sounds. In general, older adults are at increased risk for constipation because of medications, dietary patterns, and decreased physical activity. Factors that increase the risk for constipation at the end of life include pain medications (discussed in Chapter 28), dehydration, kidney failure, elevated calcium levels, and disease effects (e.g., ascites, spinal cord damage, colon or pelvic cancers).

Dyspnea

Dyspnea is a sensation of shortness of breath or breathlessness. It has been described as a sensation of suffocation or being smothered that can generate fear that death is occurring. Dyspnea may result from abnormalities or imbalanced states in the pulmonary, cardiac, neuromuscular, or metabolic systems, as well as arising from psychological causes.

Nausea and Vomiting

Nausea and vomiting are common symptoms associated with terminal illness. Causes of nausea and vomiting at the end of life include the following:

- Irritation/obstruction of gastrointestinal tract (bowel obstruction, constipation, cancer tumor, delayed emptying of stomach from ascites, tumor pressure [often called *squashed stomach syndrome*])
- Medication side effect (especially opioids like morphine)
- Ear infection or labyrinthitis
- Electrolyte imbalance, sepsis
- Kidney failure, liver failure
- Increased intracranial pressure (brain tumor, cerebral edema, intracranial bleeding, metastasis)
- Foul odors
- Anxiety, fear

Dehydration

Because older adults normally have an age-related decrease in body water, they become dehydrated more easily. Causes of dehydration at the end of life include reduced or inadequate oral intake, medications such as diuretics, vomiting, diarrhea, and fever. Symptoms of dehydration can interfere with comfort by causing dry mouth, constipation, confusion, and skin impairment.

Anorexia and Cachexia

Additional symptoms include anorexia, a lack of appetite that progresses to the inability to eat, and cachexia, which is a general state of malnutrition in which there is loss of fat, muscle, and bone mineral content. People with cachexia usually do not respond to increased intake or nutritional supplements (Ferrell & Coyle, 2006). Even before the terminal illness, older adults often have less lean tissue, so there is less reserve and malnutrition can progress quickly. Factors that contribute to anorexia and cachexia include nausea and vomiting, constipation, dehydration, weakness, depression, pain, oral candidiasis or dry mouth, gastritis, and medication side effects.

Symptoms During the Active Dying Process

When it becomes apparent that a dying person has only a few days to live, it is especially important that the nurse work closely with the individual and his or her family to help them understand the dying process and anticipate changes. Guidance about what to expect helps reduce fear and anxiety (Ogle & Hopper, 2005). Characteristic physical signs indicate the "active dying" process. In most situations, the individual has become totally dependent on others for all aspects of care, with less wakeful or alert time. Levels of consciousness may change or fluctuate. The person has little or no interest in the oral intake of food or fluids. Physiologic changes occur in breathing patterns, circulation slows, sensory awareness decreases, and muscle weakness occurs as a result of decreased tone. Table 29-3 summarizes some signs and symptoms that occur within days of death. Nurses should describe plans for care to give reassurance that comfort needs will be met. The overall focus of nursing care at this point is to continue to promote physiologic and psychological comfort, while assisting the older adult in achieving a peaceful, dignified death. The Dying Person's Bill of Rights (see Box 29-2) continues to provide guidance for care in the final hours of life.

When death does not occur suddenly, the older adult may have opportunities for final closure. Reminiscence and life review can promote self-actualization during this time. Participation in decisions concerning the person's death, as well as those concerning the continuation of life for loved ones, can assist in bringing inner peace. Older adults often reach a point of readiness and anticipation of death, and they may communicate that they are ready to make the transition from life to death. Nurses can use therapeutic communication techniques to acknowledge their expressions in a genuine and supportive manner. Final good-byes to family members and friends are also difficult for those being left behind. Nurses can offer and coordinate grief support through the hospice or palliative care team, or through chaplains or other meaningful religious and spiritual resources.

TABLE 29-3 Signs and Symptoms of Death Within Days

Physiologic Change	Signs and Symptoms
Altered breathing patterns	• Breathing initially becomes more shallow. • Cheyne-Stokes respirations • Noisy breathing (death rattle)
Changing circulation	• Limbs, ears, and nose become cold to touch or mottled in appearance. • Decreased blood pressure • Pulse may weaken and become irregular. • Diaphoresis • Possible increase in dependent edema • No urine output or small amount of very dark urine (anuria or oliguria)
Decreased muscle tone	• Relaxed facial muscles, lower jaw drops, mouth open • Decreased/loss of gag reflex • Difficulty swallowing • Abdominal distention due to decreased gastrointestinal activity • Possible urinary and fecal incontinence due to relaxation of sphincter muscles
Decreased senses	• Reduced level of consciousness • Blurred or distorted vision • Decreased taste and smell (probable continued sense of hearing)

From Saunderson, C. A., & Brener, T. H. (Eds.). (2007). *End of life: A nurse's guide to compassionate care.* Philadelphia: Lippincott Williams & Wilkins.

Part I: Mr. Bauer is a 91-year-old man with medical diagnoses including hypertension, type 2 diabetes mellitus, history of cerebrovascular accident, and benign prostatic hyperplasia. He was taking the following medications, lisinopril, 20 mg daily; aspirin, 81 mg daily; furosemide, 40 mg daily; potassium, 20 mEq daily; and acetaminophen p.r.n. for arthritis pain. He has lived at home by himself for the last 15 years since the death of his wife. He has three adult children, all living out of state, who visit on average on a monthly basis. He is very well known in his neighborhood as the older man who helps everyone. He loves his home and spends his days "keeping house." His favorite chores include mowing the grass in the sum-

(case study continues on page 603)

mer and blowing the snow in the winter. He owns and drives a car to the local supermarket and barber and to the cemetery to visit his wife's grave. In late summer he had an accident with his lawn mower that drew his family's attention to the fact that he was losing his strength. While mowing his grass, he had fallen over the lawn mower, scraping his face on the cement. He required emergency department (ED) evaluation and treatment, including stitches for facial lacerations. He later admitted that, before his fall, he had been experiencing dizziness, especially when getting up out of his easy chair.

Three weeks after his ED evaluation, Mr. Bauer's daughter came to visit. She was shocked to see her father looking so "thin and gaunt." Mr. Bauer admitted that he had lost a few pounds over the summer and still didn't have much energy. He stated that he wasn't sleeping well at night, with his sleep disrupted every 30 to 45 minutes because of the need to urinate. To control his urination, he had decided to limit his drinking fluids to less than 8 oz per day. Mr. Bauer's daughter noticed that in spite of his weight loss, his abdomen was very large and distended. "Do you have any aches?" she asked her father. He nodded yes and grabbed his lower abdomen.

THINKING POINTS

- Based on symptoms and history, what points would you address in your nursing assessment?
- What nursing problems would you address in Mr. Bauer's nursing care plan?
- What are some probable causes of Mr. Bauer's abdominal discomfort?
- What would the appropriate nursing interventions be?
- What health teaching would you provide?

Part II: Mr. Bauer and his daughter have a follow-up office visit with his primary care physician. On arrival, his vital signs are as follows: temperature, 98 PO; apical pulse, 82 beats per minute and irregularly irregular; respirations, 24 per minute; and blood pressure sitting, 98/50. When standing to walk to the scale for his weight measurement, he swayed a bit, grabbed the wall, and then steadied himself. "I just got a little dizzy," he admitted. As the office nurse, you immediately grabbed the blood pressure cuff and took his blood pressure in the standing position. It was 70/40. Mr. Bauer's pulse at that time was 90 and irregular. Noting the vital sign changes, the physician ordered some laboratory tests, which were drawn in the office. With results pending, no changes were made in his medical care at that time.

THINKING POINTS

- What are your immediate nursing concerns for Mr. Bauer based on information about his decline during the past 6 months?
- What risk factors are likely to be contributing to Mr. Bauer's dizziness?
- What patient teaching is indicated at this time?

Part III: Mr. Bauer's laboratory results come back the next day, confirming dehydration and malnutrition:

- Sodium: 150
- Potassium: 3.7
- Serum albumin: 3.0
- Prealbumin: 14
- Blood urea nitrogen: 35
- Serum creatinine: 1.7

The physician discontinued Mr. Bauer's Lasix and lisinopril and suggested a follow-up visit in 2 weeks. Two days before his next appointment, his daughter called the office to relay that her father had fallen and was taken to the hospital for evaluation. A workup revealed that he had a transient ischemic attack and was now too weak to eat and experiencing difficulty swallowing. The family declined a feeding tube and a hospice referral was made.

THINKING POINTS

- Identify two priority nursing diagnoses appropriate for Mr. Bauer at this time.
- For each diagnosis, list two to three nursing interventions.

Mr. Bauer died in the hospital 1 week after his fall, on the day he was scheduled for discharge.

CHAPTER HIGHLIGHTS

End-of-Life Transitions

- The end of life is the period in which there is little likelihood of cure, and comfort is the primary goal.

Cultural and Historical Perspectives on Death and Dying

- There is a gradual trend toward dying at home, which is where most people say they want to die, and where most people did die during the early part of the 20th century.
- American society is moving beyond the culture of denial of death and finding ways to address death as an integral part of life (Box 29-1).
- Cultural factors significantly affect attitudes toward death and dying (Cultural Considerations 29-1).

Quality of Care at the End of Life

- Nurses and other health care professionals have strong roles in supporting death with dignity (Box 29-2).
- Hospice is a philosophy of care whose goal is to support dignified dying and a good death experience for people who are terminally ill.

Nursing Interventions in End-of-Life Care

- Nurses use many interventions, including verbal and nonverbal communication (Boxes 29-3 and 29-4 and Table 29-1), to address the complex needs of patients who are dying and their families.
- Nurses assess and address common symptoms that occur during the end of life, including fatigue, constipation, dyspnea, nausea and vomiting, dehydration, and anorexia (Table 29-2).
- Nurses holistically address needs of patients and families during the immediate end-of-life process (Table 29-3).

Critical Thinking Exercises

1. Review the section on Health Care Professionals' Perspective on Death and Dying and spend a few minutes answering the questions for self-reflection.
2. Review Cultural Considerations 29-1 and think about how each of the points listed applies to your personal perspectives on death and dying.
3. From a nursing perspective, identify the ways in which caring for patients at the end of life differs from caring for patients with acute care needs.
4. From a nursing perspective, identify the ways in which caring for patients at the end of life differs from caring for patients who have chronic illnesses.

Educational Resources

American Association of Colleges of Nursing, End-of-Life Care
www.aacn.nche.edu/elnec

Hospice and Palliative Nurses Association
www.hpna.org

National Association for Home Care & Hospice
www.nahc.org

TIME: Toolkit of Instruments for Measuring End-of-life Care
www.chcr.brown.edu/pcoc/toolkit.htm

References

Ackley, B., & Ladwig, G. (2004). *Nursing diagnosis handbook* (6th ed.). St. Louis: Mosby.

American Geriatrics Society (AGS). (2002, November). *Position statement: The care of dying patients.* Available at www.americangeriatrics.org/products/positionpapers/careofd.shtml. Accessed January 19, 2007.

Austin, L. (1975). *Dying patient's bill of rights.* Created at The Terminally Ill Patient and the Helping Person Workshops. Sponsored by the Southwest Michigan Inservice Education Council in Lansing, MI.

Byock, I. (2006). Where do we go from here? A palliative care perspective. *Critical Care Medicine, 34,* S416–S420.

Ferrell, B. R., & Coyle, N. (2006). *Textbook of palliative nursing* (2nd ed.). New York: Oxford University Press.

Ferrell, B. R. (2001). Forward. In M. Matzo & D. Sherman (Eds.). *Palliative care nursing: Quality care to the end of life* (pp. xii–xv). New York: Springer.

Field, M., & Cassell, C. (Eds.). (1997). *Approaching death; Improving care at the end of life (Report of the Institute of Medicine Task Force).* Washington, DC: National Academy Press.

Gaskamp, C. D., Sutter, R., & Meraviglia, M. (2004). *Promoting spirituality in the older adult.* Iowa City, IA: University of Iowa Gerontological Nursing Interventions Research Center, Research Dissemination Core. Available at www.guideline.gov.

Hospice and Palliative Nurses Association (HPNA). (2003, October). *Position statement: Value of professional nurse in end-of life care.* Available at www.hpna.org. Accessed February 6, 2007.

Kübler-Ross, E. (1969). *On death and dying.* New York: Macmillan.

Markson, E. (2003). *Social gerontology today.* Los Angeles: Roxbury.

Mauk, J. (2003). Communication at the end of life. In D. C. Sheehan & W. B. Forman (Eds.), *Hospice and palliative care concepts and practice* (pp. 67–85). Sudbury, MA: Jones and Bartlett.

McSteen, K., & Peden-McAlpine, C. (2006). The role of the nurse as advocate in ethically difficult care situations with dying patients. *Journal of Hospice and Palliative Nursing, 8,* 259–269.

Meier, D. E. (2004, May 15). Variability in end of life care [editorial]. *British Medical Journal, 328,* E296–E297. Available at www.bmj.com/cgi/content/full/328/7449/E296. Accessed January 3, 2007.

National Hospice and Palliative Care Organization (NHPCO). (n.d.). *The history of hospice care.* Available at http://www.nhpco.org. Accessed January 18, 2007.

National Institutes of Health Consensus Development Program. (2004, December 6–8). *National Institutes of Health state-of-the-science conference statement on improving end-of-life care.* Available at http://consensus.nih.gov/2004/2004EndOfLifeCareSOS024html.htm. Accessed December 28, 2006.

Norris, K., Strohmaier, G., Asp, C. & Byock, I. (2004, July-August). Spiritual care at the end of life. *Health Progress.* Available at www.lifes-end.org/pdf/press/spcare.pdf. Accessed January 3, 2007.

Ogle, K., & Hopper, K. (2005). End of life care for older adults. *Primary Care: Clinics in Office Practice, 32,* 811–828.

Ohio State University Health Sciences Center, Office of Geriatrics & Gerontology. (2003). Series to understand, nurture and support end-of-life transitions (SUNSET). Available at http://sunset.osu.edu. Accessed December 18, 2006.

Robert Wood Johnson Foundation Last Acts Task Force. (2002, November). *Means to a better end: A report on dying in America today.* Available at www.rwjf.org/files/publications/other/meansbetterend.pdf. Accessed December 28, 2006.

Saunderson, C. A., & Brener, T. H. (Eds.). (2007). *End of life: A nurse's guide to compassionate care.* Philadelphia: Lippincott Williams & Wilkins.

SUPPORT Principal Investigators. (1995). A controlled trial to improve care for seriously ill hospitalized patients: The Study to Understand Prognoses and Preferences for Outcomes and Risks of Treatments (SUPPORT). *Journal of the American Medical Association, 274,* 1591–1598.

Teno, J. M., Clarridge, B. R., Casey, V., Welch, L. C., Wetle, T., Shield, R., et al. (2004). Family perspectives on end-of-life care at the last place of care. *Journal of the American Medical Association, 291,* 88–93.

Wilke, D., & TNEEL Investigators. (2003). *Toolkit for nurturing excellence at end-of-life transition (TNEEL).* University of Washington School of Nursing. Available at www.tneel.uic.edu/tneel.asp. Accessed December 15, 2006.

APPENDIX

Age-Related Variations in Laboratory Values

Nurses incorporate information about normal age-related changes in their assessments of older adults so they can better identify the factors that are likely to respond to interventions. Parts 3 through 5 of this book discuss age-related changes affecting specific aspects of functioning. In addition to understanding this information, nurses need to be aware of age-related variations in laboratory values that are pertinent in assessing the health status of older adults. Nurses can use the following table as a guide to these variations.

Test Values Ages 20 to 40 Years	Age-Related Changes	Considerations
Serum		
Albumin 3.5 to 5 g/dL	Younger than age 65: Higher in men Older than age 65: Equal levels that then decrease at same rate	Increased dietary protein intake needed in older patients if liver function is normal; edema: a sign of low albumin level
Alkaline phosphatase 13 to 39 IU/L	Increases 8 to 10 IU/L	May reflect liver function decline or vitamin D malabsorption and bone demineralization
Beta globulin 2.3 to 3.5 g/dL	Increases slightly	Increases in response to decrease in albumin if liver function is normal; increased dietary protein intake needed
Blood urea nitrogen Men: 10 to 25 mg/dL Women: 8 to 20 mg/dL	Increases, possibly to 69 mg/dL	Slight increase acceptable in absence of stressors, such as infection or surgery
Cholesterol 120 to 220 mg/dL	Men: Increases to age 50, then decreases Women: Lower than men until age 50, increases to age 70, then decreases	Rise in cholesterol level (and increased cardiovascular risk) in women as a result of postmenopausal estrogen decline; dietary changes, weight loss, and exercise needed
Creatine kinase 17 to 148 U/L	Increases slightly	May reflect decreasing muscle mass and liver function
Creatinine 0.6 to 1.5 mg/dL	Increases, possibly to 1.9 mg/dL in men	Important factor to prevent toxicity when giving drugs excreted in urine
Creatinine clearance 104 to 125 mL/min	Men: Decreases; formula: (140 − age) × kg body weight/72 × serum creatinine Women: 85% of men's rate	Reflects reduced glomerular filtration rate; important factor to prevent toxicity when giving drugs excreted in urine
Glucose tolerance (fasting plasma glucose) 1 hr: 160 to 170 mg/dL 2 hr: 115 to 125 mg/dL 3 hr: 70 to 110 mg/dL	Rises faster in first 2 hours, then drops to baseline more slowly	Reflects declining pancreatic insulin supply and release and diminishing body mass for glucose uptake (Rapid rise can quickly trigger hyperosmolar hyperglycemic nonketotic syndrome. Rapid decline can result from certain drugs, such as alcohol, beta-adrenergic blockers, and monoamine oxidase inhibitors.)
Hematocrit Men: 45% to 52% Women: 37% to 48%	May decrease slightly (unproven)	Reflects decreased bone marrow and hematopoiesis, increased risk of infection (because of fewer and weaker lymphocytes and immune system changes that diminish antigen–antibody response)
Hemoglobin Men: 13 to 18 g/dL Women: 12 to 16 g/dL	Men: Decreases by 1 to 2 g/dL Women: Unknown	Reflects decreased bone marrow, hematopoiesis, and (for men) androgen levels
High-density lipoprotein 80 to 310 mg/dL	Levels higher in women than in men but equalize with age	Compliance with dietary restrictions required for accurate interpretation of test results

continued on following page 606

Test Values Ages 20 to 40 Years	Age-Related Changes	Considerations
Lactate dehydrogenase 45 to 90 U/L	Increases slightly	May reflect declining muscle mass and liver function
Leukocyte count 4300 to 10,800/mcL	Decreases to 3100 to 9000/mcL	Decrease proportionate to lymphocyte count
Lymphocyte count T cells: 500 to 2400/mcL B cells: 50 to 200/mcL	Decreases	Decrease proportionate to leukocyte count
Platelet count 150,000 to 350,000/mm^3	Change in characteristics: decreased granular constituents, increased platelet-release factors	May reflect diminished bone marrow and increased fibrinogen levels
Potassium 3.5 to 5.5 mEq/L	Increases slightly	Requires avoidance of salt substitutes composed of potassium, vigilance in reading food labels, and knowledge of hyperkalemia's signs and symptoms
Thyroid-stimulating hormone 0.3 to 5 mcIU/mL	Increases slightly	Suggests primary hypothyroidism or endemic goiter at much higher levels
Thyroxine 4.5 to 13.5 mcg/dL	Decreases 25%	Reflects declining thyroid function
Triglycerides 40 to 150 mg/dL	Range widens: 20 to 200 mg/dL	Suggests abnormalities at any other levels, requiring additional tests such as serum cholesterol
Triiodothyronine 90 to 220 ng/dL	Decreases 25%	Reflects declining thyroid function
Urine		
Glucose 0 to 15 mg/dL	Decreases slightly	May reflect renal disease or urinary tract infection (UTI); unreliable check for older diabetic people because glucosuria may not occur until plasma glucose level exceeds 300 mg/dL
Protein 0 to 5 mg/dL	Increases slightly	May reflect renal disease or UTI
Specific gravity 1.032	Decreases to 1.024 by age 80	Reflects 30% to 50% decrease in number of nephrons available to concentrate urine

From *Handbook of geriatric nursing care* (2nd ed., Appendix B, pp. 627–629). (2003). Philadelphia: Lippincott Williams & Wilkins.

Nurses also need to know which laboratory values for older adults remain within the normal range so they can avoid falsely attributing abnormal laboratory values to aging. The following laboratory values are *not* affected by increased age*:

- Prothrombin time
- Partial thromboplastin time
- Serum chloride
- Serum carbon dioxide
- Serum acid phosphatase
- Aspartate aminotransferase
- Total serum protein

Data from *Handbook of geriatric nursing care* (2nd ed.). Philadelphia: Lippincott Williams & Wilkins.

Index

Page numbers followed by the letter *b* denote boxes, those followed by *f* denote figures, and those followed by *t* denote tables.

O

Q

R

T